ESSENTIALS OF PHYSIOLOGY
for Dental Students

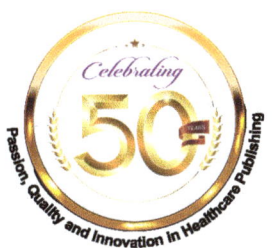

ESSENTIALS OF PHYSIOLOGY
for Dental Students

Third Edition

K Sembulingam PhD

Formerly at

MR Medical College, Kalaburagi, Karnataka, India
Sri Ramachandra Medical College and Research Institute, Chennai, Tamil Nadu, India
School of Health Sciences, Universiti Sains Malaysia, Kelantan, Malaysia
Sri Lakshmi Narayana Institute of Medical Sciences, Puducherry, India
Sri Manakula Vinayagar Medical College and Hospital, Puducherry, India
Shri Sathya Sai Medical College and Research Institute, Nellikuppam, Tamil Nadu, India
Madha Medical College and Research Institute, Chennai, Tamil Nadu, India

Prema Sembulingam PhD

Formerly at

MR Medical College, Kalaburagi, Karnataka, India
Sri Ramachandra Medical College and Research Institute, Chennai, Tamil Nadu, India
School of Health Sciences, Universiti Sains Malaysia, Kelantan, Malaysia
Sri Lakshmi Narayana Institute of Medical Sciences, Puducherry, India
Sathyabama University Dental College and Hospital, Chennai, Tamil Nadu, India
Sri Manakula Vinayagar Medical College and Hospital, Puducherry, India
Shri Sathya Sai Medical College and Research Institute, Nellikuppam, Tamil Nadu, India
Madha Medical College and Research Institute, Chennai, Tamil Nadu, India

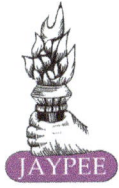

JAYPEE BROTHERS MEDICAL PUBLISHERS

The Health Sciences Publisher

New Delhi | London

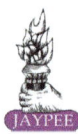
Jaypee Brothers Medical Publishers (P) Ltd

Headquarters

Jaypee Brothers Medical Publishers (P) Ltd
EMCA House, 23/23-B
Ansari Road, Daryaganj
New Delhi - 110 002, INDIA
Landline: +91-11-23272143,+91-11-23272703, +91-11-23282021,+91-11-23245672
Head Office : 011-43574357
Email: jaypee@jaypeebrothers.com

Corporate Office

Jaypee Brothers Medical Publishers (P) Ltd
4838/24, Ansari Road, Daryaganj
New Delhi 110 002, India
Phone: +91-11-43574357
Fax: +91-11-43574314
Email: jaypee@jaypeebrothers.com

Overseas Office

J.P. Medical Ltd
83 Victoria Street, London
SW1H 0HW (UK)
Phone: +44 20 3170 8910
Fax: +44 (0)20 3008 6180
Email: info@jpmedpub.com

Website: www.jaypeebrothers.com
Website: www.jaypeedigital.com

© 2021, Jaypee Brothers Medical Publishers

The views and opinions expressed in this book are solely those of the original contributor (s)/author (s) and do not necessarily represent those of editor (s) of the book.

All rights reserved. No part of this publication may be reproduced, stored or transmitted in any form or by any means, electronic, mechanical, photocopying, recording or otherwise, without the prior permission in writing of the publishers/editors.

All brand names and product names used in this book are trade names, service marks, trademarks or registered trademarks of their respective owners. The publisher is not associated with any product or vendor mentioned in this book.

Medical knowledge and practice change constantly. This book is designed to provide accurate, authoritative information about the subject matter in question. However, readers are advised to check the most current information available on procedures included and check information from the manufacturer of each product to be administered, to verify the recommended dose, formula, method and duration of administration, adverse effects and contraindications. It is the responsibility of the practitioner to take all appropriate safety precautions. Neither the publisher nor the author (s)/editor (s) assume any liability for any injury and/or damage to persons or property arising from or related to use of material in this book.

This book is sold on the understanding that the publisher is not engaged in providing professional medical services. If such advice or services are required, the services of a competent medical professional should be sought.

Every effort has been made where necessary to contact holders of copyright to obtain permission to reproduce copyright material. If any have been inadvertently overlooked, the publisher will be pleased to make the necessary arrangements at the first opportunity. The **CD/DVD-ROM** (if any) provided in the sealed envelope with this book is complimentary and free of cost. **Not meant for sale.**

Inquiries for bulk sales may be solicited at: jaypee@jaypeebrothers.com

Essentials of Physiology for Dental Students

First Edition: 2011

Second Edition: 2016

Third Edition: **2021**

ISBN: 978-93-86150-57-8

In Loving Memory of

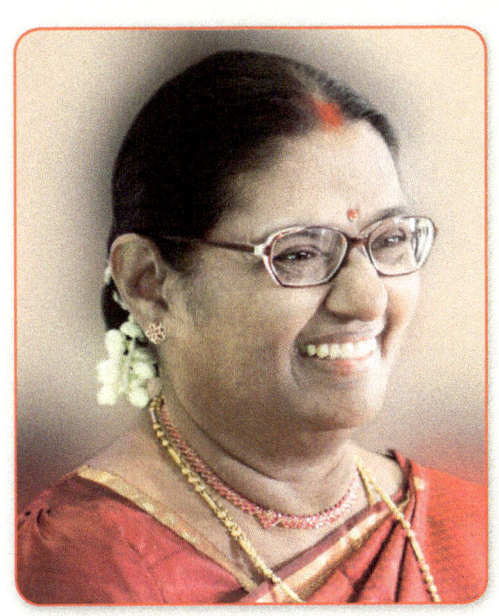

Dr Prema Sembulingam

Dedicated to

Our beloved students

Preface *to the third edition*

A Journey from Good to Better!

In 1999 we took the venture to publish our first textbook *Essentials of Medical Physiology*. The book started as a 'National book' has become an 'International book'. Thanks for the whole hearted support from faculty and students of medical institutes, in and out of country, and the publishers.

Slowly, this book gained its due recognition among the students of other medical and allied courses, such as homeopathy, Indian medicine, dental, nursing, physiotherapy and other paramedical courses.

However, revelation started by the feeling that *Essentials of Medical Physiology* was too voluminous for the dental and paramedical courses. So, requests and suggestions started pouring in to reduce the volume without compromising on the essence of the subject. That is how the first edition of the textbook *Essentials of Physiology for Dental Students* emerged in 2011. Now is the time to venture into the task of upgrading the book into its Third edition in the same format followed in our textbook *Essentials of Medical Physiology*.

Long back, we planned to update and bring out Third Edition of the book. But it was possible to execute it now only due to various reasons.

It could not have been possible to bring out this book without efforts and hard work by my life partner and the co-author of all our books Dr Prema Sembulingam. Her encouragement and emotional support in upgrading book will be evergreen in memory.

Though we miss her now, the efforts and work rendered by her for this book also could not be forgotten. That made me to mention "We" in this preface.

We wish to continue our services to the students' community through this book. We are confident that the opinions, comments and valuable suggestions from one and all coming across for this book will help us improve it further to meet the need of students.

We are grateful to **Shri Jitendar P Vij** (Group Chairman), **Mr Ankit Vij** (Managing Director), **Mr MS Mani** (Group President) and **Ms Chetna Malhotra Vohra** (Associate Director–Content Strategy) of M/s Jaypee Brothers Medical Publishers (P) Ltd, New Delhi, India for publishing the book in the same format as we wanted.

We are also grateful to **Dr Madhu Choudhary** (Publishing Head–Education), **Ms Pooja Bhandari** (Production Head) and **Ms Sunita Katla** (Executive Assistant to Group Chairman and Publishing Manager) for coordinating the processing of this edition. We thank **Dr Sneha Kashyap** (Development Editor), **Mr Rajesh Sharma** (Production Coordinator), **Ms Seema Dogra** (Cover Visualizer), **Ms Geeta Srivastava** (Proofreader), **Ms Neelam Kakriya** (Proofreader), **Mr Deepak Saxena** (Typesetter), **Mr Varun Rajoria** (Graphic Designer) and all other staff of M/s Jaypee Brothers Medical Publishers (P) Ltd, New Delhi, India for their wholehearted contribution while formatting the book.

K Sembulingam
DrSembu@gmail.com

Preface to the first edition

We, the authors of *Essentials of Medical Physiology* are proud to bring out another textbook in Physiology, titled *Essentials of Physiology for Dental Students*. This is the outcome of requests, wishes and friendly orders from different category of people including the dental and paramedical students and faculties.

Physiology is different from other biomedical sciences as it deals with the functional aspects of various systems in the living body along with the emphasis on the regulatory mechanism that maintain the normalcy of the functions within narrow limits. It forms the strong foundation on which other medical fields are constructed.

The primary aim of this book is to meet the needs of the dental, paramedical and health science students precisely in the examination point of view, in getting knowledge of recent developments in the field of Physiology and in knowing the important applied aspects of various topics.

The descriptive diagrams are given in such a way that the students can easily understand and reproduce them wherever necessary. The explanation of the topics is supported with the flowcharts and tables which makes the reading a pleasure and stress-free.

In the starting of each chapter, we have included the topics that are to be learnt in that particular chapter which will help the reader to remember the contents while revising the topic. At the end of each section, the long questions and short questions are given for the follow-up of the topics.

This venture is possible only because of blessings of professors, best wishes and cooperation of our friends and co-teachers and the students who know what they want and where to get them. We are grateful and thankful to one and all for being the well-wishers of us.

We wish to continue our services to the students' community through this book. We are confident that the opinions, comments and valuable suggestions from one and all coming across for this book will help us to improve it further to meet the needs of everyone who has Physiology as subject in their career.

K Sembulingam
ksembu@yahoo.com

Prema Sembulingam
premsem@yahoo.com

Contents

Section 1 – General Physiology

1. Cell 1
2. Cell Junctions 12
3. Transport through Cell Membrane 15
4. Homeostasis 22

Section 2 – Blood and Body Fluids

5. Body Fluids 27
6. Blood 33
7. Plasma Proteins 37
8. Red Blood Cells 40
9. Erythropoiesis 44
10. Hemoglobin and Iron Metabolism 48
11. Erythrocyte Sedimentation Rate, Packed Cell Volume and Blood Indices 52
12. Anemia 55
13. Hemolysis and Fragility of Red Blood Cells 58
14. White Blood Cells 60
15. Immunity 65
16. Platelets 73
17. Hemostasis 76
18. Coagulation of Blood 78
19. Blood Groups 85
20. Blood Transfusion 91
21. Reticuloendothelial System, Tissue Macrophage and Spleen 93
22. Lymphatic System and Lymph 96
23. Tissue Fluid and Edema 99

Section 3 – Muscle Physiology

24. Classification of Muscles 103
25. Structure of Skeletal Muscle 105
26. Properties of Skeletal Muscle 110
27. Changes During Muscular Contraction 116
28. Neuromuscular Junction 122
29. Smooth Muscle 126

Section 4 – Digestive System

30. Overview of Digestive System 133
31. Mouth and Salivary Secretion 137
32. Stomach and Gastric Secretion 144
33. Pancreas and Pancreatic Secretion 152
34. Liver and Biliary System 157

35. Small Intestine and its Secretion 166
36. Large Intestine and its Secretion 170
37. Movements of Gastrointestinal Tract 172

Section 5 – Renal Physiology and Skin

38. Overview of Renal System 181
39. Nephron 183
40. Juxtaglomerular Apparatus 187
41. Renal Circulation 190
42. Urine Formation 193
43. Concentration of Urine 200
44. Acidification of Urine and Role of Kidney in Acid-base Balance 205
45. Renal Function Tests, Renal Failure, Dialysis and Diuretics 209
46. Micturition 213
47. Skin 218
48. Body Temperature 222

Section 6 – Endocrinology

49. Overview of Endocrine System 227
50. Pituitary Gland 233
51. Thyroid Gland 243
52. Parathyroid Glands and Physiology of Bone 251
53. Endocrine Functions of Pancreas 260
54. Adrenal Cortex 266
55. Adrenal Medulla 274
56. Endocrine Functions of Other Organs 278
57. Local Hormones 281

Section 7 – Reproductive System

58. Male Reproductive System 285
59. Female Reproductive System 295
60. Menstrual Cycle 301
61. Pregnancy and Parturition 310
62. Mammary Glands and Lactation 315
63. Fertility Control 318

Section 8 – Cardiovascular System

64. Overview of Cardiovascular System 325
65. Properties of Cardiac Muscle 331
66. Cardiac Cycle 335
67. Heart Sounds and Cardiac Murmur 340
68. Electrocardiogram and Arrhythmia 344
69. Cardiac Output 351
70. Heart Rate 356
71. Arterial Blood Pressure 362
72. Venous Blood Pressure and Capillary Blood Pressure 371
73. Arterial Pulse and Venous Pulse 374

74. Regional Circulation..378
75. Fetal Circulation and Respiration...384
76. Hemorrhage, Circulatory Shock and Heart Failure..387
77. Cardiovascular Adjustments During Exercise..391

Section 9 – Respiratory System and Environmental Physiology

78. Respiratory Tract and Pulmonary Circulation..395
79. Mechanics of Respiration..400
80. Pulmonary Function Tests..405
81. Ventilation and Dead Space..411
82. Exchange and Transport of Respiratory Gases..414
83. Regulation of Respiration...421
84. Diseases and Disorders of Respiration..427
85. High Altitude and Deep Sea Physiology...434
86. Effects of Exposure to Cold and Heat..438
87. Artificial Respiration..440
88. Effects of Exercise on Respiration..443

Section 10 – Nervous System

89. Overview of Nervous System..445
90. Neuron and Neuroglia...447
91. Receptors..456
92. Synapse and Neurotransmitters...461
93. Reflex Activity..468
94. Spinal Cord..473
95. Somatosensory System and Somatomotor System...489
96. Physiology of Pain...496
97. Thalamus...500
98. Hypothalamus...503
99. Cerebellum..509
100. Basal Ganglia..513
101. Cerebral Cortex and Limbic System...516
102. Reticular Formation...525
103. Proprioceptors, Posture and Equilibrium..527
104. Vestibular Apparatus...533
105. Electroencephalogram (EEG) and Epilepsy...539
106. Physiology of Sleep..542
107. Higher Intellectual Functions..546
108. Cerebrospinal Fluid...550
109. Autonomic Nervous System...553

Section 11 – Special Senses

110. Eye..559
111. Visual Process and Field of Vision...567
112. Visual Pathway..572
113. Pupillary Reflexes...576
114. Color Vision...580

115. Refractive Errors 582
116. Ear 585
117. Auditory Pathway 589
118. Mechanism of Hearing and Auditory Defects 591
119. Sensation of Taste 595
120. Sensation of Smell 598

Index 603

SECTION 1: GENERAL PHYSIOLOGY

CHAPTER 1: Cell

CHAPTER OUTLINE

- CELL, TISSUE, ORGAN AND SYSTEM
- STRUCTURE OF THE CELL
- CELL MEMBRANE
- CYTOPLASM
- ORGANELLES IN CYTOPLASM
- ORGANELLES WITH LIMITING MEMBRANE
- ORGANELLES WITHOUT LIMITING MEMBRANE
- NUCLEUS
- DEOXYRIBONUCLEIC ACID: DNA
- GENE
- RIBONUCLEIC ACID: RNA
- GENE EXPRESSION
- CELL DEATH

CELL, TISSUE, ORGAN AND SYSTEM

CELL

Cell is defined as the structural and functional unit of the living body. All living organisms are composed of many blocks of cells. Each single has all the characteristics of life.

TISSUE

Tissue is the group of cells having similar function. Tissues are classified into four primary tissues.

Primary tissues are:

1. *Muscle tissue:* Skeletal muscle, smooth muscle and cardiac muscle.
2. *Nervous tissue:* Neurons and supporting cells.
3. *Epithelial tissue:* Squamous, columnar and cuboidal epithelial cells.
4. *Connective tissue:* Connective tissue proper, cartilage, bone and blood.

ORGAN

An organ is defined as the structure that is formed by two or more primary types of tissues. Some organs are composed of all the four types of primary tissues. Organs may be tubular like intestine or hollow like stomach.

SYSTEM

Organ system is defined as group of organs that work together to carry out specific functions of the body. Each system performs a specific function.

Digestive system is concerned with digestion of food particles. Excretory system eliminates unwanted substances. Cardiovascular system is responsible for transport of substances between the organs. Respiratory system is concerned with the supply of oxygen and removal of carbon dioxide. Reproductive system is involved in the reproduction of species. Endocrine system is concerned with growth of the body and regulation and maintenance of normal life. Musculoskeletal system is responsible for stability and movements of the body. Nervous system controls the locomotion and other activities including the intellectual functions.

STRUCTURE OF THE CELL

Each cell is formed by a cell body and a cell membrane or plasma membrane that covers the cell body. The important parts of the cell are (Fig. 1.1):

I. Cell membrane.
II. Nucleus.
III. Cytoplasm with organelles.

CELL MEMBRANE

Cell membrane is a protective sheath that envelops the cell body. It separates the fluid outside the cell called extracellular fluid (ECF) and the fluid inside the cell called intracellular fluid (ICF). It is a **semipermeable membrane** and allows free exchange of certain substances between ECF and ICF (Fig. 1.2). Thickness of the cell membrane varies from 75 to 111Å.

Section 1: General Physiology

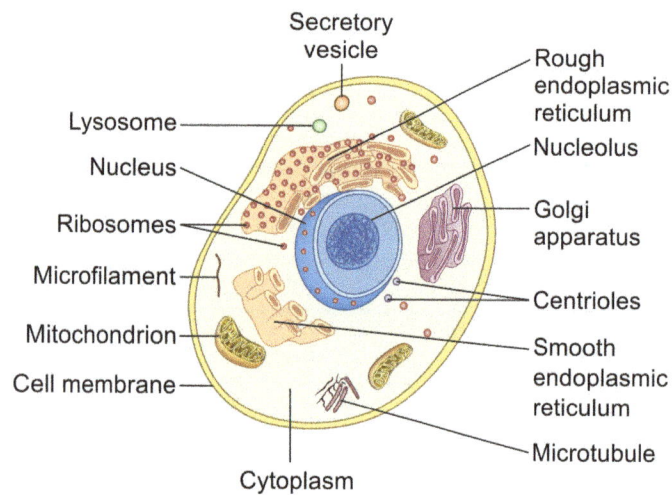

FIGURE 1.1: Structure of the cell.

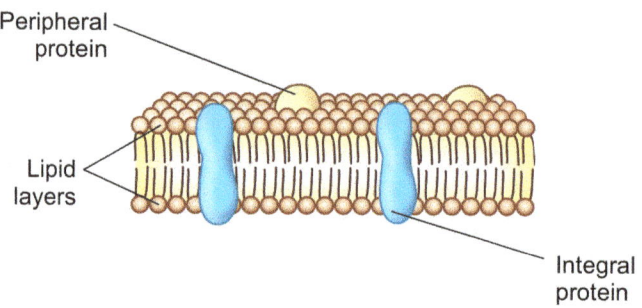

FIGURE 1.2: Diagram of the cell membrane.

■ COMPOSITION OF CELL MEMBRANE

Cell membrane is composed of three substances:

1. Proteins (55%).
2. Lipids (40%).
3. Carbohydrates (5%).

■ STRUCTURE OF CELL MEMBRANE

On the basis of structure, cell membrane is called a **unit membrane** or a three-layered membrane.

Electron microscopic study reveals three layers in the cell membrane namely, **one electron-lucent lipid layer** in the center and two **electron-dense layers**. The two electron-dense protein layers are placed on either side of the central layer. Carbohydrate molecules are found on the surface of the cell membrane.

Lipid Layer of Cell Membrane

It is a bilayered structure formed by a thin film of lipids (Fig. 1.2). It is fluid in nature and the portions of the membrane along with the dissolved substances move to all areas of the cell membrane.

Major lipids are:

1. Phospholipids.
2. Cholesterol.

1. Phospholipids

The phospholipid molecules are formed by phosphorus and fatty acids. Each phospholipid molecule resembles

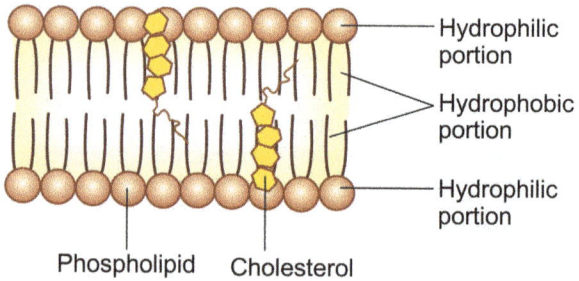

FIGURE 1.3: Lipids of the cell membrane.

a headed pin in shape (Fig. 1.3). The outer part of the phospholipid molecule is the head portion which is water soluble (hydrophilic) and the inner part is the tail portion that is not soluble in water (hydrophobic). The hydrophobic tail portions meet in the center of the membrane. The hydrophilic head portions of outer layer face the ECF and those of the inner layer face the cytoplasm.

Two layers of phospholipids are arranged in such a way that the hydrophobic tail portions meet in the center of the membrane. Hydrophilic head portions of outer layer face the ECF and those of the inner layer face ICF (cytoplasm).

2. Cholesterol

Cholesterol molecules are arranged in between the phospholipid molecules. As phospholipids are soft and oily in nature, cholesterol helps to 'pack' the phospholipids in the membrane and maintain the structural integrity of cell membrane.

Functions of lipid layer

The lipid layer is semipermeable in nature and allows only the fat-soluble substances such as oxygen, carbon dioxide and alcohol to pass through it. It does not allow the water-soluble materials like glucose, urea and electrolytes to pass through it.

Protein Layers of the Cell Membrane

Protein layers of the cell membrane are electron-dense layers situated on either side of the central lipid layer. The protein molecules present in these layers are mostly glycoproteins.

Protein molecules are classified into two categories:

1. Integral proteins.
2. Peripheral proteins.

1. Integral proteins

Integral proteins, also known as **transmembrane proteins** or intrinsic proteins, are tightly bound with the cell membrane. These protein molecules pass through the entire thickness of the cell membrane from one side to the other side.

2. Peripheral proteins

Peripheral proteins or **peripheral membrane proteins** do not penetrate the cell membrane but are embedded partially in the outer and inner surfaces of the cell membrane. These protein molecules are loosely bound with the cell membrane and so dissociate readily from the cell membrane.

Functions of protein layers

1. Integral proteins provide the structural integrity of the cell membrane.
2. Channel proteins help in the diffusion of water-soluble substances such as glucose and electrolytes (Chapter 3).
3. Carrier or transport proteins help in the transport of substances across the cell membrane by means of active or passive transport (Chapter 3).
4. Some carrier proteins act as pumps, by which ions are transported actively across the cell membrane.
5. Receptor proteins serve as the receptor sites for hormones and neurotransmitters.
6. Some of the protein molecules form the enzymes and control chemical (metabolic) reactions within the cell membrane.
7. Some proteins act as antigens and induce the process of antibody formation.
8. Some proteins called cell adhesion molecules are responsible for attachment of cells to their neighbors or to basal lamina.

Carbohydrates of the Cell Membrane

Carbohydrate molecules form a thin loose covering over the entire surface of the cell membrane called **glycocalyx**. Some carbohydrate molecules are attached with proteins and form **glycoproteins** and some are attached with lipids and form **glycolipids**.

Functions of carbohydrates

1. Carbohydrate molecules are negatively charged and do not permit the negatively charged substances to move in and out of the cell.
2. The glycocalyx from the neighboring cells helps in the tight fixation of cells with one another.
3. Some of the carbohydrate molecules form the receptors for some hormones.

■ FUNCTIONS OF CELL MEMBRANE

Functions of proteins in cell membrane are listed in **Box 1.1**.

■ CYTOPLASM

Cytoplasm of the cell present inside the cell contains a clear liquid portion called **cytosol** which contains various substances like proteins, carbohydrates, lipids and electrolytes. Apart from these substances, many organelles are also present in cytoplasm. The cytoplasm is distributed as peripheral **ectoplasm** just beneath the cell membrane and inner **endoplasm** between the ectoplasm and the nucleus.

■ ORGANELLES IN CYTOPLASM

All the cells in the body contain some common structures called organelles in the cytoplasm. Some organelles are bound by limiting membrane and others do not have

BOX 1.1: Functions of cell membrane.

1. Protective function
Cell membrane protects the cytoplasm and the organelles present in the cytoplasm
2. Selective permeability
Cell membrane acts as a semipermeable membrane, which allows only some substances to pass through it and acts as a barrier for other substances
3. Absorptive function
Nutrients are absorbed into the cell through the cell membrane
4. Excretory function
Metabolites and other waste products from the cell are excreted out through the cell membrane
5. Exchange of gases
Oxygen enters the cell from blood and carbon dioxide leaves the cell and enters blood through the cell membrane
6. Maintenance of shape and size of cell
Cell membrane is responsible for the maintenance of shape and size of the cell

BOX 1.2: Cytoplasmic organelles.

Organelles with limiting membrane
1. Endoplasmic reticulum 2. Golgi apparatus 3. Lysosome 4. Peroxisome 5. Secretory vesicles 6. Mitochondria 7. Nucleus
Organelles without limiting membrane
1. Ribosomes 2. Centrosome 3. Cytoskeleton

limiting membrane **(Box 1.2)**. The organelles carry out the various functions of the cell **(Table 1.1)**.

■ ORGANELLES WITH LIMITING MEMBRANE

■ 1. ENDOPLASMIC RETICULUM

Endoplasmic reticulum is made up of tubules and microsomal vesicles. These structures form an interconnected network which forms the link between the organelles and cell membrane.

Types of Endoplasmic Reticulum

Endoplasmic reticulum is of two types namely, rough endoplasmic reticulum and smooth endoplasmic reticulum.

Rough Endoplasmic Reticulum

It is the endoplasmic reticulum with rough, bumpy or bead-like appearance. Rough appearance is due to the attachment of granular ribosomes to its outer surface. Hence, it is also called the **granular endoplasmic**

TABLE 1.1: Functions of cytoplasmic organelles.

Organelles	Functions
Rough endoplasmic reticulum	1. Synthesis of proteins 2. Degradation of worn-out organelles
Smooth endoplasmic reticulum	1. Synthesis of lipids and steroids 2. Role in cellular metabolism 3. Storage and metabolism of calcium 4. Catabolism and detoxification of toxic substances
Golgi apparatus	1. Processing, packaging, labelling and delivery of proteins and lipids
Lysosomes	1. Degradation of macromolecules 2. Degradation of worn-out organelles in cytoplasm 3. Removal of excess of secretory products 4. Secretion of perforin, granzymes, melanin and serotonin 5. Degradation of own cell
Peroxisomes	1. Breakdown of excess fatty acids 2. Detoxification of hydrogen peroxide and other metabolic products 3. Oxygen utilization 4. Acceleration of gluconeogenesis 5. Degradation of purine to uric acid 6. Role in the formation of myelin 7. Role in the formation of bile acids
Mitochondria	1. Production of energy 2. Synthesis of ATP 3. Initiation of apoptosis
Ribosomes	1. Synthesis of proteins
Centrosome	1. Movement of chromosomes during cell division
Cytoskeleton	1. Determination of shape of the cell 2. Provide support and stability of the cell 3. Movement of substances within the cell 4. Role in mitosis
Nucleus	1. Control of all activities of the cell 2. Synthesis of RNA 3. Sending genetic instruction to cytoplasm for protein synthesis 4. Formation of subunits of ribosomes 5. Control of cell division 6. Storage of hereditary information in genes (DNA)

reticulum (Fig. 1.4). Rough endoplasmic reticulum is vesicular or tubular in structure.

Functions of rough endoplasmic reticulum

I. Rough endoplasmic reticulum is concerned with the **synthesis of proteins** in the cell. Examples are synthesis of insulin from β-cells of islets of Langerhans in pancreas and antibodies from B lymphocytes.
II. It also plays an important role in degradation of worn-out cytoplasmic organelles. It wraps itself around the worn-out organelles and forms a vacuole which is called the **autophagosome**. It is digested by lysosomal enzymes.

Smooth Endoplasmic Reticulum

Smooth endoplasmic reticulum is also called as agranular endoplasmic reticulum because of its smooth appearance without the attachment of ribosome. It is formed by many interconnected tubules. So, it is also called tubular endoplasmic reticulum.

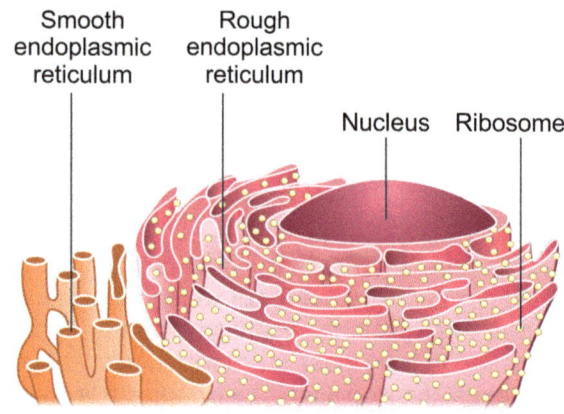

FIGURE 1.4: Endoplasmic reticulum.

Functions of smooth endoplasmic reticulum

i. It is responsible for synthesis of cholesterol and steroid.
ii. It is concerned with various metabolic processes of the cell because of the presence of many enzymes on the outer surface.

iii. It is concerned with the storage and metabolism of calcium.
iv. It is also concerned with catabolism and **detoxification** of toxic substances like some drugs and **carcinogens** (cancer producing substances) in liver.

Rough endoplasmic reticulum and smooth endoplasmic reticulum are interconnected and continuous with one another. Depending upon the activities of the cells, the rough endoplasmic reticulum changes to smooth endoplasmic reticulum and *vice versa*.

■ 2. GOLGI APPARATUS

Golgi apparatus (Golgi body or Golgi complex) is present in all the cells except red blood cells. It consists of 5 to 8 flattened membranous sacs called **cisternae** (Fig. 1.5).

Golgi apparatus is situated near the nucleus. It has two ends or faces namely, **cis face** and **trans face**. The cis face is positioned near the endoplasmic reticulum.

Reticular vesicles from endoplasmic reticulum enter the Golgi apparatus through cis face. The trans face is situated near the cell membrane. The processed substances make their exit from Golgi apparatus through trans face.

Functions of Golgi Apparatus

i. Golgi apparatus is concerned with the processing and delivery of substances like proteins and lipids to different parts of the cell.
ii. It functions like a **post office** because, it packs the processed materials into the secretory granules, secretory vesicles, and lysosomes and dispatch them either out of the cell or to another part of the cell.
iii. Golgi apparatus also functions like a **shipping department** of the cell because it sorts out and labels the materials for distribution to their proper destinations (Fig. 1.6).

■ 3. LYSOSOMES

Lysosomes are small vesicular structures filled with enzymes lysosomal enzymes. Lysosomal enzymes are synthesized in rough endoplasmic reticulum and transported to the Golgi apparatus. Here, these enzymes

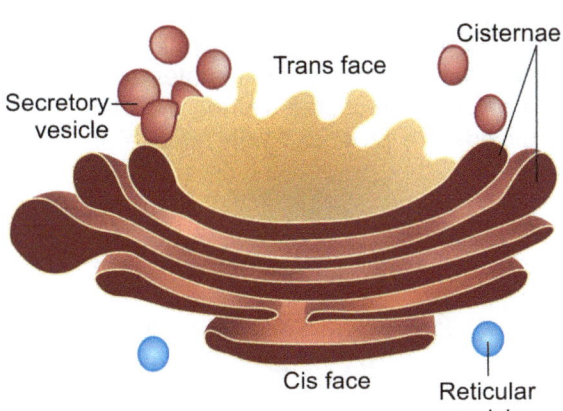

FIGURE 1.5: Golgi apparatus.

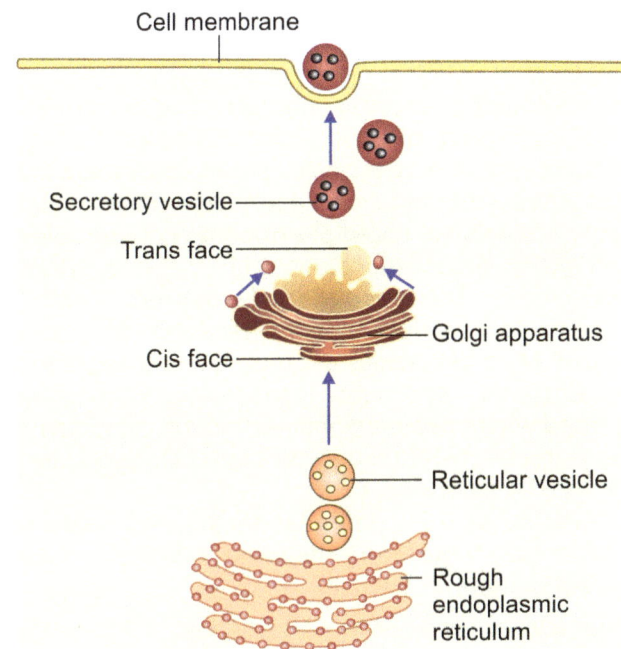

FIGURE 1.6: Integrated function of endoplasmic reticulum and Golgi apparatus.

are processed and packed in the form of small vesicles. Then, the vesicles are pinched off from Golgi apparatus and become the lysosomes.

Types of Lysosomes

Lysosomes are of two types:
i. Primary lysosome which is pinched off from Golgi apparatus. It is inactive in spite of having the hydrolytic enzymes.
ii. Secondary lysosome which is active lysosome formed by the fusion of a primary lysosome with phagosome or endosome.

Functions of Lysosomes

Lysosomes contain about 50 different hydrolytic enzymes. Functions of lysosomes are executed through these enzymes.

Important lysosomal enzymes

i. Proteases, which hydrolyze the proteins into amino acids.
ii. Lipases, which hydrolyze the lipids into fatty acids and glycerides.
iii. Amylases, which hydrolyze the polysaccharides into glucose.
iv. Nucleases, which hydrolyze the nucleic acids into mononucleotides.

Mechanism of lysosomal function

Lysosomal functions involve two mechanisms:

i. Heterophagy: Digestion of extracellular materials engulfed by the cell via endocytosis.
ii. Autophagy: Digestion and degradation of intracellular materials such as worn-out cytoplasmic organelles.

Specific Functions of Lysosomes

i. Degradation of macromolecules

Macromolecules such as bacteria are engulfed by the cell by means of endocytosis (Chapter 3). Macromolecules engulfed by the cell via endocytosis are called **endosomes**. Other macromolecules engulfed by the cell via phagocytosis are called **phagosomes** or **vacuoles.**

Primary lysosome fuses with the endosome or phagosome to form **secondary lysosome.** Secondary lysosome becomes acidic and the lysosomal enzymes are activated. Macromolecules are digested and degraded by these enzymes. Secondary lysosome containing these **degraded waste products** moves through cytoplasm and fuses with cell membrane. Now the waste products are eliminated by **exocytosis**.

Because of their degradation activity, lysosomes are often called **'garbage disposal system'** or **'waste disposal system'** of the cell.

ii. Degradation of worn-out organelles

The rough endoplasmic reticulum wraps itself around the worn-out organelles and form **autophagosomes**. One **primary lysosome** fuses with one autophagosome and form the **secondary lysosome**. Enzymes in the secondary lysosome are activated. Now, these enzymes digest the contents of autophagosome.

iii. Removal of excess secretory products in the cells

Lysosomes in the cells of the secretory glands remove the excess secretory products by degrading the secretory granules.

iv. Secretory function: Secretory lysosomes

Lysosomes having secretory function called secretory lysosomes are found in some of the cells, particularly in cells of immune system. The conventional lysosomes are modified into secretory lysosomes by combining with secretory granules (which contain the particular secretory product of the cell).

Examples of secretory lysosomes:

  a. Lysosomes in the cytotoxic T lymphocytes and natural killer (NK) cells secrete perforin and **granzymes,** which destroy both viral-infected cells and tumor cells.
  b. Secretory lysosomes of melanocytes secrete melanin.
  c. Secretory lysosomes of mast cells secrete serotonin, which is a vasoconstrictor substance and inflammatory mediator.

v. Degradation of own cells

When a cell is damaged and about to die, lysosomes are burst and release the enzymes. These enzymes digest and degrade their own cell. Hence, the lysosomes are also called "**suicidal bags**" of the cell.

4. PEROXISOMES

Peroxisomes or **microbodies** are pinched off from endoplasmic reticulum. Peroxisomes contain some **oxidative enzymes** such as catalase, urate oxidase and D-amino acid oxidase.

Functions of Peroxisomes

Peroxisomes:
  i. Degrade the toxic substances like hydrogen peroxide and other metabolic products by means of detoxification.
  ii. Form the major site of oxygen utilization in the cells.
  iii. Breakdown the excess fatty acids.
  iv. Accelerate gluconeogenesis from fats.
  v. Degrade purine to uric acid.
  vi. Participate in the formation of myelin.
  vii. Are involved in the formation of bile acids.

5. SECRETORY VESICLES

Secretory vesicles are globular structures, formed in the endoplasmic reticulum, and processed and packed in Golgi apparatus. When necessary, the secretory vesicles rupture and release the secretory substances into the cytoplasm.

6. MITOCHONDRION

Mitochondrion (plural 'mitochondria') is a rod or oval-shaped structure with a diameter of 0.5 to 1 μ. It is covered by a double layered membrane **(Fig. 1.7)**. The outer membrane is smooth and encloses the contents of mitochondrion. It contains many enzymes such as acetyl-CoA synthetase and glycerophosphate acetyltransferase.

Inner membrane forms many folds called **cristae** and covers the **inner matrix space**. The cristae also contain many enzymes and other protein molecules which are involved in respiration and ATP synthesis. Because of these functions, the enzymes and other protein molecules in cristae are collectively known as **respiratory chain** or electron transport system.

Mitochondria move freely in the cytoplasm of the cell and are capable of reproducing themselves. The mitochondria contain their own DNA which is responsible for many enzymatic actions.

Functions of Mitochondrion

i. Production of energy

Mitochondrion is called the '**power house of the cell**' because it produces the energy required for the cellular activities. The energy is produced by oxidation of the food substances like proteins, carbohydrates and lipids by the oxidative enzymes in cristae. During oxidation, water and carbon dioxide are produced with release of energy. The

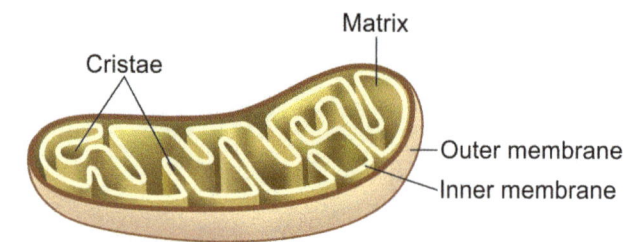

FIGURE 1.7: Structure of mitochondrion.

released energy is stored in mitochondria and used later for synthesis of ATP.

ii. Synthesis of ATP

Components of respiratory chain in the mitochondrion are responsible for the synthesis of ATP by utilizing the energy through oxidative phosphorylation. The ATP molecules defuse throughout the cell from mitochondrion. Whenever energy is needed for cellular activity, the ATP molecules are broken down.

iii. Apoptosis

Mitochondria are involved in apoptosis (see below) also.

■ ORGANELLES WITHOUT LIMITING MEMBRANE

■ 1. RIBOSOMES

Ribosomes are small granular structures with a diameter of 15 nm. Some ribosomes are attached to rough endoplasmic reticulum while others are present as free ribosomes in the cytoplasm. The ribosomes are made up of proteins (35%) and ribonucleic acid (RNA) (65%). The RNA present in ribosomes is called **ribosomal RNA** (rRNA).

Functions of Ribosomes

Ribosomes are called **protein factories** because of their role in the synthesis of proteins. Messenger RNA passes the genetic code for protein synthesis from nucleus to the ribosomes. Ribosomes, in turn arrange the amino acids into small units of proteins. The ribosomes attached with endoplasmic reticulum are involved in the synthesis of proteins like the enzymatic proteins, hormonal proteins, lysosomal proteins and the proteins of the cell membrane.

Free ribosomes are responsible for the synthesis of proteins in hemoglobin, peroxisome and mitochondria.

■ 2. CENTROSOME

Centrosome is situated near the center of the cell close to the nucleus. It consists of two cylindrical structures called centrioles which are responsible for the movement of chromosomes during cell division.

■ 3. CYTOSKELETON

Cytoskeleton of the cell is a complex network that gives shape, support and stability to the cell. It is also essential for the cellular movements and the response of the cell to external stimuli.

Cytoskeleton consists of three major protein components, viz.:

a. Microtubules.
b. Intermediate filaments.
c. Microfilaments.

Microtubules

Microtubules are straight and hollow tubular structures formed by bundles of globular protein called α- and β-tubulin **(Fig. 1.8)**.

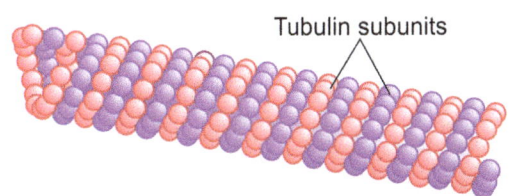

FIGURE 1.8: Microtubule.

Functions of microtubules

Microtubules:
  i. Determine the shape of the cell.
  ii. Give structural strength to the cell.
  iii. Act like **conveyor belts** which allow the movement of granules, vesicles, protein molecules and some organelles like mitochondria to different parts of the cell.
  iv. Form the spindle fibers, which separate the chromosomes during mitosis.

Intermediate Filaments

Intermediate filaments form a network around the nucleus and extend to the periphery of the cell. These are formed by fibrous proteins **(Fig. 1.9)**.

Functions or intermediate filaments

Intermediate filaments help to maintain the shape of the cell. These filaments also connect the adjacent cells through desmosomes.

Microfilaments

Microfilaments are long and fine thread-like structures, which are made up of nontubular contractile proteins called actin and myosin **(Fig. 1.10)**. Actin is more abundant than myosin.

Functions or microfilaments

Microfilaments:
  i. Give structural strength to the cell.

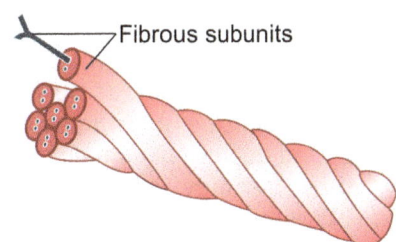

FIGURE 1.9: Intermediate filament.

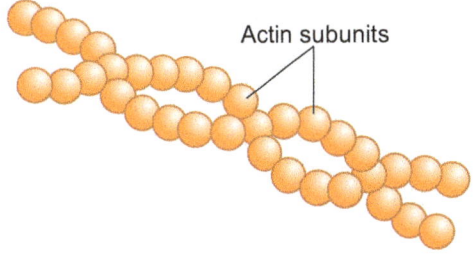

FIGURE 1.10: Microfilament of ectoplasm.

ii. Provide resistance to the cell against the pulling forces.
iii. Responsible for cellular movements like contraction, gliding and cytokinesis (partition of cytoplasm during cell division).

■ NUCLEUS

Nucleus is present in all the cells in the body except the red blood cells. The cells with nucleus are called **eukaryotes** and those without nucleus are known as **prokaryotes**. Presence of nucleus is necessary for cell division.

Most of the cells have only one nucleus (**uninucleated**). Few types of cells like skeletal muscle cells have many nuclei (**multinucleated**). Generally, the nucleus is located near the center of the cell. It is mostly spherical in shape. However, the shape and situation of nucleus vary in different cells.

■ STRUCTURE OF NUCLEUS

Nuclear Membrane

Nucleus is covered by a double layered membrane called nuclear membrane. It encloses the fluid called nucleoplasm. Nuclear membrane is porous and permeable in nature and it allows nucleoplasm to communicate with the cytoplasm.

Nucleoplasm

Nucleoplasm is a highly viscous fluid that forms the ground substance of nucleus. It is similar to cytoplasm present outside the nucleus. It surrounds chromatin and nucleolus.

Chromatin

Chromatin is a thread-like material made up of large molecules of **deoxyribonucleic acid (DNA)**. The DNA molecules are compactly packed with the help of a specialized basic protein called **histone**. It forms the major bulk of nuclear material. Just before cell division, the chromatin condenses to form chromosome.

Chromosomes

Chromosome is the rod-shaped nuclear structure that carries a complete blueprint of all the hereditary characteristics of that species. A chromosome is formed from a single DNA and each DNA contains many genes.

Normally, chromosomes are not visible in the nucleus under microscope. Only during cell division, the chromosomes are visible under microscope. This is because DNA becomes more tightly packed just before cell division, which makes the chromosome visible during cell division.

Diploid cells and haploid cells

All the dividing cells of the body except reproductive cells contain 23 pairs of chromosomes. Each pair consists of one chromosome inherited from mother and one from father. The cells with 23 pairs of chromosomes are called diploid cells. Reproductive cells called gametes or sex cells contain only 23 single chromosomes. These cells are called haploid cells.

Sex chromosomes and autosomes

Among the 23 pairs of chromosomes, one pair is concerned with determination of sex of the person. These chromosomes are called sex chromosomes. Remaining 22 pair of chromosomes that are not concerned with sex determination are named as autosomes.

Among the sex chromosomes, one is called X chromosome and another one is called Y chromosomes. The cells of females have two X chromosomes and cells of males have one X chromosome and one Y chromosome.

Nucleolus

Nucleolus is a small, round granular structure of the nucleus. Each nucleus contains one or more nucleoli. The nucleolus contains **ribonucleic acid** (RNA) and some proteins, which are similar to those found in ribosomes. The RNA is synthesized by five different pairs of chromosomes and stored in the nucleolus. Later, it is condensed to form the subunits of ribosomes. All the subunits formed in the nucleolus are transported to cytoplasm through the pores of nuclear membrane. In the cytoplasm, these subunits fuse to form ribosomes, which play an essential role in the formation of proteins.

■ FUNCTIONS OF NUCLEUS

Nucleus is considered as brain of the cells. Major functions of nucleus are the control of cellular activities and storage of hereditary material. So, it is also called control center. Functions of nucleus are listed in **Box 1.3**.

■ DEOXYRIBONUCLEIC ACID: DNA

Deoxyribonucleic acid (DNA) is a nucleic acid that carries the genetic information to the offspring of an organism. DNA forms the chemical basis of hereditary characters. It contains the instruction for the synthesis of proteins in the ribosomes. Gene is a part of a DNA molecule.

DNA is present in mitochondria and the nucleus (chromosome) of the cell. DNA in mitochondria is called **non-chromosomal DNA**. DNA present in the nucleus forms the component of chromosomes, which carries the hereditary information. The hereditary information that is

BOX 1.3: Functions of nucleus.

Functions of nucleus
1. Control of all the cellular activities that include metabolism, protein synthesis, growth and reproduction (cell division)
2. Synthesis of ribonucleic acid (RNA)
3. Formation of subunits of ribosomes
4. Sending genetic instruction to the cytoplasm for protein synthesis through messenger RNA (mRNA)
5. Control of the cell division through genes
6. Storage of hereditary information (in genes) and transformation of this information from one generation of the species to the next.

Chapter 1: Cell

encoded in DNA is called **genome.** Each DNA molecule is divided into discrete units called **genes**.

STRUCTURE OF DNA

DNA is a double-stranded complex nucleic acid. It is formed by deoxyribose, phosphoric acid and four types of bases. Each DNA molecule consists of two polynucleotide chains, which are twisted around one another in the form of a double helix. The two chains are formed by the sugar deoxyribose and phosphate. These two substances form the backbone of DNA molecule. Both chains of DNA are connected with each other by some organic bases **(Fig. 1.11)**.

Each chain of DNA molecule consists of many nucleotides.

Each nucleotide is formed by:

1. Deoxyribose: Sugar.
2. Phosphate.
3. One of the following organic (nitrogenous) bases:

    Purines:
      i. Adenine (A)
      ii. Guanine (G
    Pyrimidines:
      i. Thymine (T)
      ii. Cytosine (C).

Strands of DNA are arranged in such a way that both are bound by specific pairs of bases. The adenine of one strand binds specifically with thymine of opposite strand. Similarly, the cytosine of one strand binds with guanine of the other strand.

GENE

Gene is the basic **hereditary unit** of the cell. It is a portion of DNA molecule that contains the message or code for the synthesis of a specific protein from amino acids. It is like a book that contains the information necessary for protein synthesis.

GENETIC DISORDERS

Genetic disorder is a disease or condition that occurs due to absence of a gene or a defective gene or by a chromosomal abnormality. Refer **Table 1.2** for different types of genetic disorders.

Causes of Genetic Disorders

Genetic disorders occur due to two causes.

1. Genetic variation

Genetic variation means the presence of a gene that differs from normal gene.

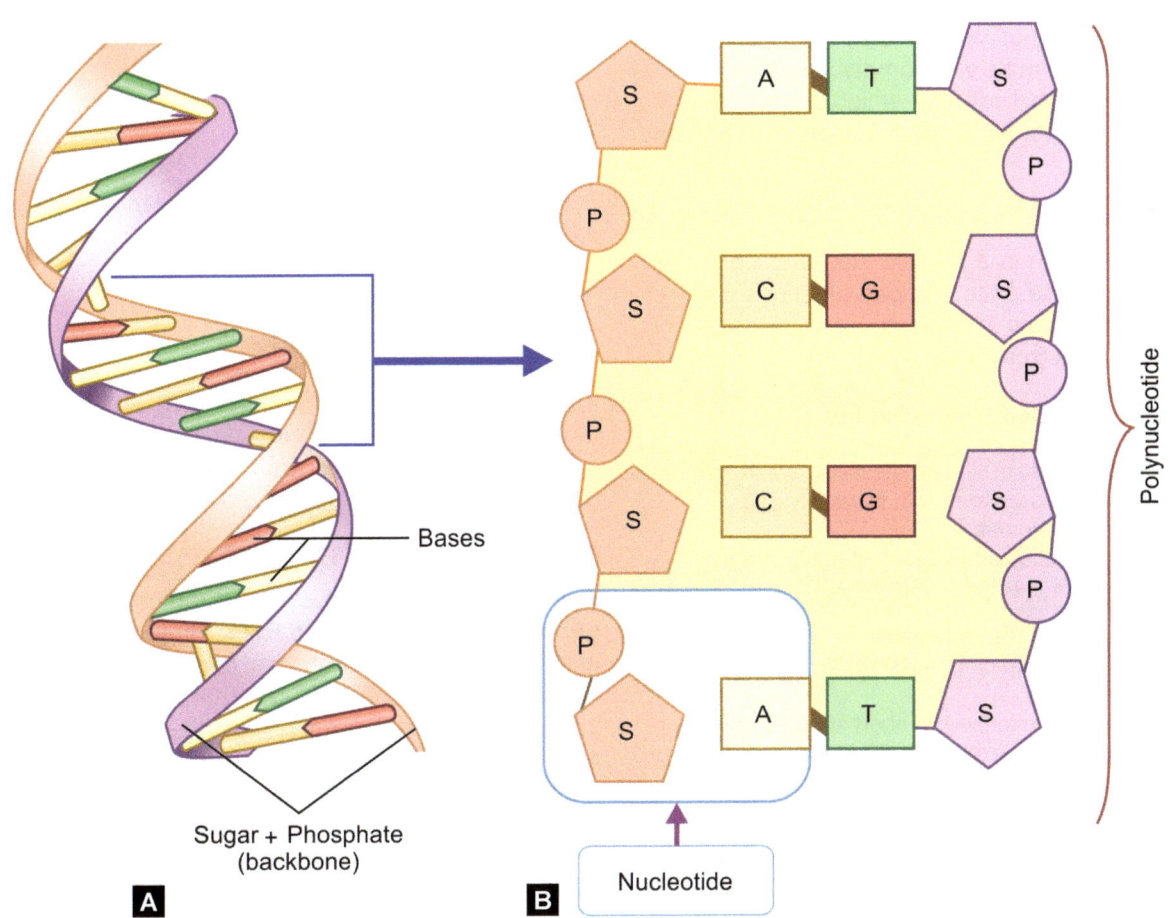

FIGURE 1.11: Structure of DNA. **A.** Double helical structure of DNA. **B.** Magnified view of the components of DNA.
A = Adenine, C = Cytosine, G = Guanine, P = Phosphate, S = Sugar, T = Thymine.

TABLE 1.2: Genetic disorders.

Type	Examples
1. Single gene or mendelian or monogenic disorders	a. Sickle cell anemia b. Huntington's disease
2. Multifactorial genetic or polygenic disorders	a. Coronary heart disease b. Alzheimer's disease c. Arthritis d. Diabetes
3. Chromosomal disorders	a. Chromosome instability syndromes b. Turner's syndrome c. Down syndrome
4. Mitochondrial DNA disorders	a. Kearns-Sayre syndrome b. Leber's hereditary optic neuropathy

2. Genetic mutation

Generally, mutation means an alteration or a change in nature, form, or quality. Genetic mutation refers to change of the DNA sequence within a gene or chromosome of an organism, which results in the creation of a new character.

CHROMOSOMAL DISORDERS

Chromosomal disorder is a genetic disorder caused by abnormalities in chromosome. It may be due to any change in structure (structural abnormality) or number (numerical abnormality) of chromosomes. It is also called **chromosomal abnormality,** anomaly or aberration. It often results in genetic disorders, which involve physical or mental abnormalities. Refer **Box 1.4** for chromosomal disorders.

RIBONUCLEIC ACID: RNA

Ribonucleic acid (RNA) is a nucleic acid that contains a long chain of nucleotide units. Various functions coded in the genes are carried out in the cytoplasm of the cell by RNA. RNAs is formed from DNA.

BOX 1.4: Chromosomal disorders.

1. Chromosome instability syndromes
- Inherited diseases associated with instability and breakage of chromosomes
- These diseases cause certain types of malignancies

2. Turner's syndrome
- Genetic disorder that affects females
- It is due to partial or complete missing of one of the two sex (X) chromosomes
- This disorder is characterized by short stature, infertility, heart abnormalities, renal problems and learning difficulties

3. Down syndrome
- Genetic disorder that occurs due to the presence of an extra copy of chromosome 21
- The person has 47 chromosomes instead of usual 46
- It is characterized by physical disabilities and mental retardation

TYPES OF RNA

RNA is of three types. Each type of RNA plays a specific role in protein synthesis. Three types of RNA are given below.

1. *Messenger RNA (mRNA)*

Messenger RNA carries the **genetic code** of the amino acid sequence for synthesis of protein from the DNA to the cytoplasm.

2. *Transfer RNA (tRNA)*

Transfer RNA is responsible for decoding the genetic message present in mRNA.

3. *Ribosomal RNA (rRNA)*

Ribosomal RNA is present within the ribosome and forms a part of the structure of ribosome. It is responsible for the assembly of protein from amino acids in the ribosome.

STRUCTURE OF RNA

Each RNA molecule consists of a single strand of poly nucleotide unlike the double-stranded DNA.

Each nucleotide in RNA is formed by:

1. Ribose: Sugar.
2. Phosphate.
3. One of the following organic bases:
   Purines:
   i. Adenine (A)
   ii. Guanine (G).
   Pyrimidines:
   i. Uracil (U)
   ii. Cytosine (C).

Uracil replaces the thymine of DNA and it has similar structure of thymine.

GENE EXPRESSION

Gene expression is the process by which the information (code word) encoded in the gene is converted into functional gene product or document of instruction (RNA) that is used for protein synthesis.

Gene expression involves two steps namely, transcription and translation.

TRANSCRIPTION OF GENETIC CODE

Transcription means copying. It indicates the copying of genetic code from DNA to RNA. Proteins are synthesized in the ribosomes which are present in the cytoplasm. However, the synthesis of different proteins depends upon information (**sequence of codon**) encoded in the genes of the DNA which is present in the nucleus. Since DNA is a macromolecule, it cannot pass through the pores of the nuclear membrane and enter the cytoplasm. But, the information from DNA must be sent to ribosome. So, the gene has to be transcribed (copied) into mRNA which is developed from DNA.

Thus, the first stage in the protein synthesis is transcription of genetic code. It involves the formation of mRNA and simultaneous copying or transfer of information from DNA to mRNA. The mRNA enters the cytoplasm from the nucleus and activates the ribosome resulting in protein synthesis.

■ TRANSLATION OF GENETIC CODE

Translation is the process by which protein synthesis occurs in the ribosome of the cell under the direction of genetic instruction carried by mRNA from DNA. Or, it is the process by which the mRNA is read by ribosome to produce a protein. This involves the role of other two types of RNA, namely tRNA and rRNA.

The mRNA moves out of nucleus into the cytoplasm. Now, a group of ribosomes called **polysome** gets attached to mRNA. The sequence of **codons** in mRNA are exposed and recognized by the complementary sequence of base in tRNA. The complementary sequence of base is called **anticodon.** According to the sequence of bases in anticodon, different amino acids are transported from the cytoplasm into the ribosome by tRNA that acts as a carrier. With the help of rRNA, the protein molecules are assembled from amino acids. The protein synthesis occurs in the ribosomes which are attached to rough endoplasmic reticulum.

■ CELL DEATH

Cell death occurs by two distinct processes:

1. Apoptosis.
2. Necrosis.

■ APOPTOSIS

Apoptosis is defined as the **programmed cell death** under genetic control. Originally apoptosis (means 'falling leaves' in Greek) refers to the process by which the leaves fall from trees in autumn. It is also called 'cell suicide' since the genes of the cell play a major role in the death.

This type of programmed cell death is a normal phenomenon and it is essential for normal development of the body.

Functional Significance of Apoptosis

Main function of apoptosis is to remove unwanted cells without causing any stress or damage to the neighboring cells.

Functional significance of apoptosis are:

1. Apoptosis plays a vital role in cellular homeostasis. About 10 million cells are produced every day in human body by mitosis. An equal number of cells die by apoptosis. This helps in cellular homeostasis.
2. It is useful for removal of a cell that is damaged by a virus or a toxin beyond repair.
3. It is an essential event during the development and in adult stage. For example, a large number of neurons are produced during the development of central nervous system. But up to 50% of the neurons are removed by apoptosis during the formation of synapses between neurons.

■ NECROSIS

Necrosis (means 'dead' in Greek) is the uncontrolled and **unprogrammed cell death** due to unexpected and accidental damage. It is also called '**cell murder**' because the cell is killed by extracellular or external events. After necrosis, the harmful chemical substances released from the dead cells cause damage and inflammation of neighboring tissues.

Causes for Necrosis

Common causes of necrosis are injury, infection, inflammation, infarction and cancer. Necrosis is induced by both physical and chemical events such as heat, radiation, trauma, hypoxia due to lack of blood flow, and exposure to toxins.

CHAPTER 2

Cell Junctions

CHAPTER OUTLINE

- **DEFINITION AND CLASSIFICATION**
- **OCCLUDING JUNCTIONS**
  - TIGHT JUNCTION
- **COMMUNICATING JUNCTIONS**
  - GAP JUNCTION
  - CHEMICAL SYNAPSE
- **ANCHORING JUNCTIONS**
  - ADHERENS JUNCTIONS
  - FOCAL ADHESIONS
  - DESMOSOME
  - HEMIDESMOSOME

■ DEFINITION AND CLASSIFICATION

Cell junction is defined as the connection between neighboring cells or the contact between the cell and extracellular matrix. It is also called **membrane junction**.

Connection between two cells is called **intercellular junctions**. Tight junction, gap junction, adherence junction and desmosome are intercellular junctions. Contact between the cell and extracellular matrix are focal adherence and hemidesmosome. Cells junctions are mostly formed by cell junction proteins.

Cell junctions are classified into three types:
  I. Occluding junction.
  II. Communicating junction.
  III. Anchoring junction.

■ OCCLUDING JUNCTIONS

Cell junctions which prevent the movement of ions and molecules from one cell to another cell are called the occluding junctions. Tight junctions belong to this category.

■ TIGHT JUNCTION

Tight Junction is formed by the tight fusion of the cell membranes from the adjacent cells. The area of the fusion is very tight and forms a ridge. This type of junction is present in the apical margins of epithelial cells in intestinal mucosa, wall of renal tubule, capillary wall and choroid plexus **(Fig. 2.1)**.

Proteins involved in tight junction are listed in **Table 2.1**.

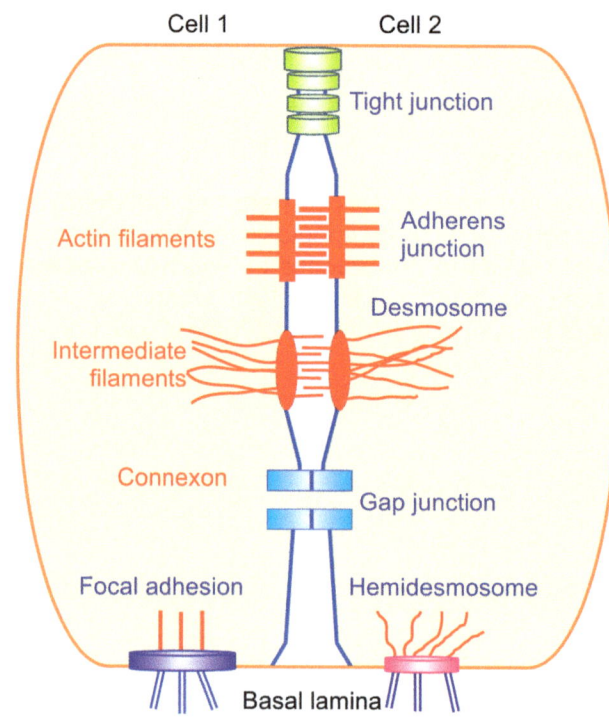

FIGURE 2.1: Different types of cell junctions.

Functions of Tight Junction

1. The tight junction holds the neighboring cells of the tissues firmly and thus provide strength and stability to the tissues.
2. It provides the barrier or **gate function** by which the interchange of ions, water and macromolecules between the cells is regulated.

TABLE 2.1: Cell junctions.

Junction types	Proteins involved	Functions	Examples
Tight junction	1. Occludin 2. Claudin 3. JAMs 4. Cingulin 5. Symplekin 6. ZO -1, 2, 3	1. Strength and stability to tissues 2. Selective permeability 3. Fencing function 4. Maintenance of cell polarity 5. Formation of blood-brain barrier	1. Epithelial lining of intestinal mucosa and renal tubule 2. Endothelium in capillary wall and choroid plexus
Gap junction	1. Connexins	1. Allows passage of small molecules, ions and chemical messengers 2. Propagation of action potential	1. Epithelial lining 2. Syncytium of heart 3. Epithelium in intestine
Adherens junction	1. Cadherins	1. Cell to cell attachment	1. Epithelial lining 2. Intercalated disks in cardiac muscle 3. Epidermis
Focal adhesions	1. Integrins	Cell attachment to: 1. Basal lamina 2. Extracellular matrix	1. Epithelial lining
Desmosome	1. Cadherins	1. Cell to cell attachment	1. Epithelial lining 2. Skin
Hemidesmosome	1. Integrins	Cell attachment to: 1. Basal lamina 2. Extracellular matrix	1. Epithelial lining

JAMs = Junctional adhesion molecules.

3. It acts like a fence by preventing the lateral movement of integral membrane proteins and lipids from cell membrane.
4. By the **fencing function**, the tight junctions maintain the cell polarity by keeping the proteins in the apical region of the cell membrane.
5. Tight junctions in the brain capillaries form the **blood-brain barrier** (BBB) which prevents the entrance of many harmful substances from the blood into the brain tissues.

COMMUNICATING JUNCTIONS

Cell junctions, which permit the movement of ions and molecules from one cell to another cell, are called communicating junctions.

Communication junctions are of two types:

1. Gap junction or Nexus.
2. Chemical synapse.

GAP JUNCTION OR NEXUS

Gap junction is also called **nexus**. It is present in heart, basal part of epithelial cells of intestinal mucosa, etc.

Structure of Gap Junction

Membranes of the two adjacent cells lie very close to each other and the **intercellular space** becomes a narrow channel. Cytoplasm of both the cells is interconnected and molecules move from one cell to another cell through these channels without having contact with extracellular fluid (ECF). The channel is surrounded by 6 subunits of proteins which are called **connexins** or **connexons**.

Functions of Gap Junction

1. Diameter of the channel in the gap junction is about 1.5 to 3 nm. So, the substances having molecular weight less than 1,000 such as glucose can pass through this junction easily.
2. It helps in the exchange of chemical messengers between the cells.
3. It helps in rapid propagation of action potential from one cell to another cell.

CHEMICAL SYNAPSE

Chemical synapse is the junction between a nerve fiber and a muscle fiber or between two nerve fibers, through which the signals are transmitted by the release of chemical transmitter. Refer Chapter 28 for details.

ANCHORING JUNCTIONS

Anchoring junctions are the junctions, which provide firm structural attachment between two cells or between a cell and the extracellular matrix.

Anchoring junctions are divided into four types:

1. Adherens junctions (cell to cell).
2. Focal adhesions (cell to matrix).

3. Desmosomes (cell to cell).
4. Hemidesmosomes (cell to matrix).

ADHERENS JUNCTIONS

Adherens junction is a **cell to cell junction** that is the junction found between the cells. The connection occurs through the **actin filaments**. Adherens junctions are present in the intercalated disk of cardiac muscles (Chapter 64) and epidermis of the skin.

FOCAL ADHESIONS

Focal adhesion is a **cell to matrix junction** that is junction between the cell and the extracellular matrix. The connection occurs through the **actin filaments**. This type of junction is seen in epithelia of various organs.

DESMOSOME

Desmosome is also **cell to cell junction**, but here the membranes of the cells are thickened and connected by **intermediate filaments**. So, desmosome functions like tight junction. This type of junction is found in areas subjected for stretching such as the skin.

HEMIDESMOSOME

Hemidesmosome is also **cell to matrix junction** and the connection is through **intermediate filaments**. It is like half desmosome because here, the membrane of only one cell thickens. So, this is known as hemidesmosome or half desmosome. Mostly, the hemidesmosome connects the cells with their basal lamina.

Chapter 3: Transport through Cell Membrane

CHAPTER OUTLINE

- **IMPORTANCE OF TRANSPORT MECHANISM**
- **BASIC MECHANISM OF TRANSPORT**
- **PASSIVE TRANSPORT**
  - **SIMPLE DIFFUSION**
  - **FACILITATED OR CARRIER MEDIATED DIFFUSION**
  - **FACTORS AFFECTING RATE OF DIFFUSION**
  - **SPECIAL TYPES OF PASSIVE TRANSPORT**
- **ACTIVE TRANSPORT**
  - **MECHANISM OF ACTIVE TRANSPORT**
- **CARRIER PROTEINS**
- **SUBSTANCES TRANSPORTED BY ACTIVE TANSPORT**
- **TYPES OF ACTIVE TRANSPORT**
- **PRIMARY ACTIVE TRANSPORT**
- **SECONDARY ACTIVE TRANSPORT**
- **SPECIAL CATEGORIES OF ACTIVE TRANSPORT**

■ IMPORTANCE OF TRANSPORT MECHANISM

Transport mechanism in the body is necessary for the supply of essential substances such as nutrients, water, oxygen, electrolytes, etc. and to remove the unwanted substances like waste materials, carbon dioxide, etc. from the tissues.

■ BASIC MECHANISM OF TRANSPORT

Mechanism of transport of substances across the cell membrane is of two types:

I. Passive transport.
II. Active transport.

■ PASSIVE TRANSPORT

Passive transport is the transport of substances along the concentration gradient or electrical gradient or both (electrochemical gradient). During this, the substances move from the region of higher concentration to the region of lower concentration. It is also known as **diffusion** or **downhill movement**. It does not need energy.

Passive transport of diffusion is of two types:

A. Simple diffusion.
B. Facilitated diffusion.

■ SIMPLE DIFFUSION

Simple diffusion is of two types:

1. Simple diffusion through lipid layer.
2. Simple diffusion through protein layer.

Simple Diffusion through Lipid Layer

Lipid soluble substances such as oxygen, carbon dioxide and alcohol are transported by simple diffusion trough the lipid layer of the cell membrane **(Fig. 3.1A)**.

Simple Diffusion through Protein Layer

There are specific protein channels that extend from cell membrane through which the simple diffusion takes place. Water-soluble substances like electrolytes are transported through these channels. The protein channels are selectively permeable to only one type of ion. Accordingly, the channels are named after the ions diffusing through these channels such as sodium channels, potassium channels, etc.

Protein Channels

Protein channels are of two types:

1. Ungated channels which are opened continuously.
2. Gated channels which are closed all the time and are opened only when required **(Fig. 3.1B)**.

Gated channels

Gated channels are divided into three categories **(Fig. 3.1C)**:

1. **Voltage-gated channels** which opens by change in the electrical potential.
   Examples: Calcium channels present in neuromuscular junction (Chapter 28).

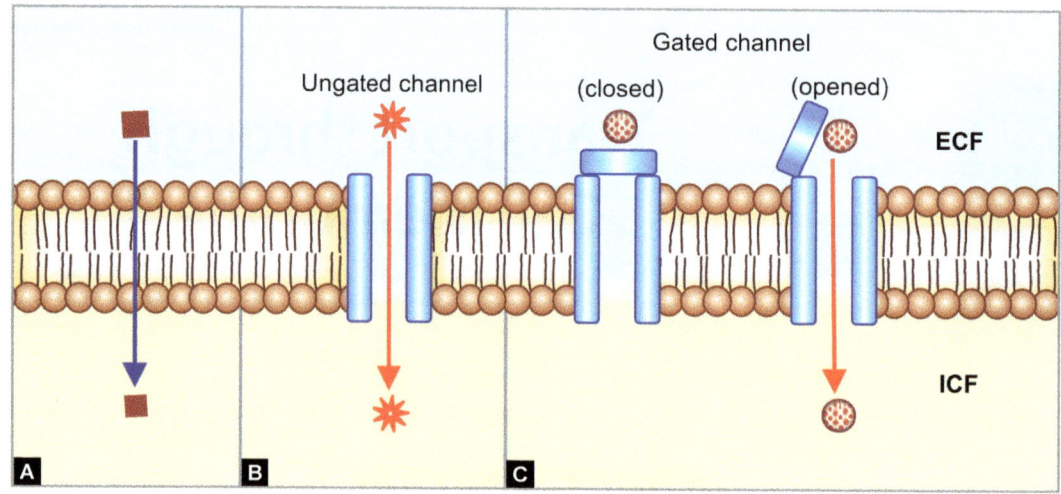

FIGURE 3.1: Hypothetical diagram of simple diffusion through the cell membrane. **A.** Diffusion through lipid layer. **B.** Diffusion through ungated channel. **C.** Diffusion through gated channel.

2. **Ligand-gated channels** that opens in the presence of hormonal substances (ligand).
   Examples: Sodium channels which are opened by acetylcholine in neuromuscular junction.
3. **Mechanically gated channels** which are opened by some mechanical factors such as pressure and force.
   Examples: Sodium channels in pressure receptors called Pacinian corpuscles (Chapter 91).

■ FACILITATED OR CARRIER MEDIATED DIFFUSION

In this type of diffusion, some carrier proteins help the transport of substances. The water-soluble substances with larger molecules cannot pass through the protein channels by simple diffusion. Such substances are transported with the help of carrier proteins. This type of diffusion is faster than the simple diffusion. Glucose and amino acids are transported by this method **(Fig. 3.2)**.

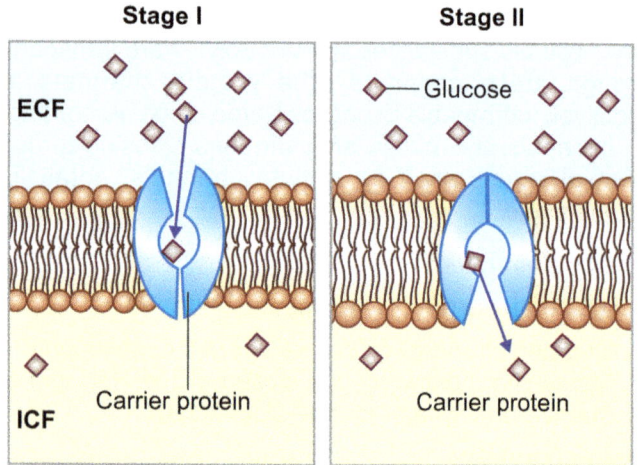

FIGURE 3.2: Hypothetical diagram of facilitated diffusion from higher concentration to lower concentration. **Stage I**: Glucose binds with carrier protein. **Stage II**: Conformational change occurs in the carrier protein and glucose is released into ICF. ECF = Extracellular fluid, ICF = Intracellular fluid.

■ FACTORS AFFECTING RATE OF DIFFUSION

Rate of diffusion of substances through the cell membrane is **directly proportional** to the following factors:

1. Permeability of the cell membrane.
2. Body temperature.
3. Concentration gradient or electrical gradient of the substance across the cell membrane.
4. Solubility of the substance.

Rate of diffusion of substances through the cell membrane is **inversely proportional** to the following factors:

1. Thickness of the cell membrane.
2. Charge of the ions.
3. Size of the molecules.

■ SPECIAL TYPES OF PASSIVE TRANSPORT

In additions to diffusion, there are some special types of passive transport, viz.:

1. Bulk flow.
2. Filtration.
3. Osmosis.

1. Bulk Flow

Bulk flow is the movement of large quantity of substances from a region of high pressure to the region of low pressure. Bulk flow is due to the pressure gradient of the substance across the cell membrane. The best example for this is the exchange of gases across the respiratory membrane in lungs (Chapter 82).

2. Filtration

Filtration is the process by which water and solutes move from an area of high hydrostatic pressure to an area of low hydrostatic pressure. The hydrostatic pressure is developed by weight of the fluid. Filtration process is seen at the arterial end of the capillaries where movement of fluid occurs along with dissolved substances from blood into the

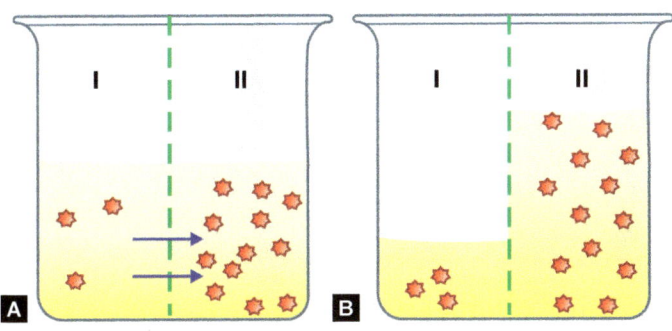

FIGURE 3.3: Osmosis. Red objects = Solute. Yellow shade = Water. Green dotted line = Semipermeable membrane. **A.** Concentration of solute is high in compartment II and low in compartment I. So, water moves from I to II through semipermeable membrane. **B.** Entrance of water into II exerts osmotic pressure.

interstitial fluid (Chapter 23). It also occurs in glomeruli of kidneys (Chapter 42).

3. Osmosis

Osmosis is defined as movement of water or any other solvent from an area of lower concentration to an area of higher concentration through a semipermeable membrane **(Fig. 3.3)**.

Osmosis is of two types:
  i. **Endosmosis** by which water moves into the cell.
  ii. **Exosmosis** by which water moves out of the cell.

Osmotic Pressure

Osmotic pressure is the pressure created by the solutes in a fluid. During osmosis, when water or any other solvent moves from the area of lower concentration to the area of higher concentration, the solutes in the area of higher concentration, get dissolved in the solvent. This creates a pressure which is known as osmotic pressure.

Colloidal Osmotic Pressure and Oncotic Pressure

Colloidal osmotic pressure is the osmotic pressure exerted by **colloidal substances** in the body.

Oncotic pressure is the osmotic pressure exerted by the colloidal substances (proteins) of the plasma. It is about 25 mm Hg.

■ ACTIVE TRANSPORT

Active transport is the transport of substances against the chemical or electrical or electrochemical gradient. It is also called **uphill transport (Table 3.1)**. Active transport requires energy, which is obtained mainly by breakdown of ATP. It also needs a carrier protein.

Active Transport vs Facilitated Diffusion

Active transport mechanism is different from facilitated diffusion by two ways **(Table 3.2)**.

■ MECHANISM OF ACTIVE TRANSPORT

When a substance that has to be transported across the cell membrane comes near the cell, it combines with the

TABLE 3.1: Passive transport vs active transport.

Description	Passive transport	Active transport
Definition	Transport along concentration or electrical or electrochemical gradient	Transport against concentration or electrical or electrochemical gradient
Another name	Downhill movement	Uphill movement
Energy	Does not require energy	Requires energy
Substances transported	Oxygen Carbon dioxide Alcohol Water Electrolytes	Ionic substances: Sodium Potassium Calcium Hydrogen Chloride Iodide Non-ionic substances: Glucose Amino acids Urea Macromolecules

TABLE 3.2: Active transport vs facilitated diffusion.

Description	Active transport	Facilitated diffusion
Definition	Transport against concentration or electrical or electrochemical gradient	Transport along concentration or electrical or electrochemical gradient
Energy	Requires energy	Does not require energy

carrier protein of the cell membrane and forms substance-protein complex. This complex moves towards the inner surface of the cell membrane. Now, the substance is released from the carrier proteins. The same carrier protein moves back to the outer surface of the cell membrane to transport another molecule of the substance.

■ CARRIER PROTEINS

Carrier proteins involved in active transport are of two types:
  1. Uniport.
  2. Symport or antiport.

Uniport

Uniport is the carrier protein that can carry only one substance in a single direction. It is also known as uniport pump.

Symport or Antiport

Symport is the carrier protein that transports two different substances in the same direction. Antiport is the carrier

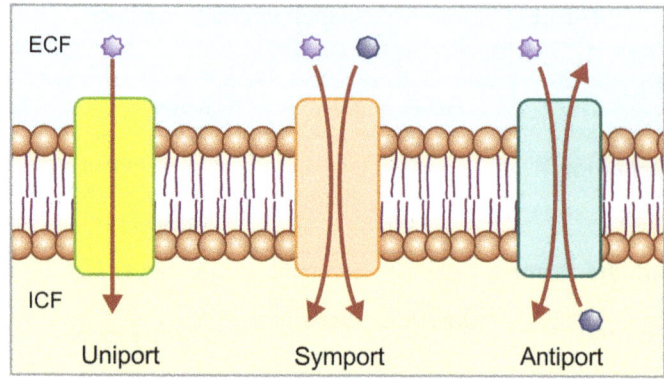

FIGURE 3.4: Carrier proteins of active transport. ECF = Extracellular fluid, ICF = Intracellular fluid.

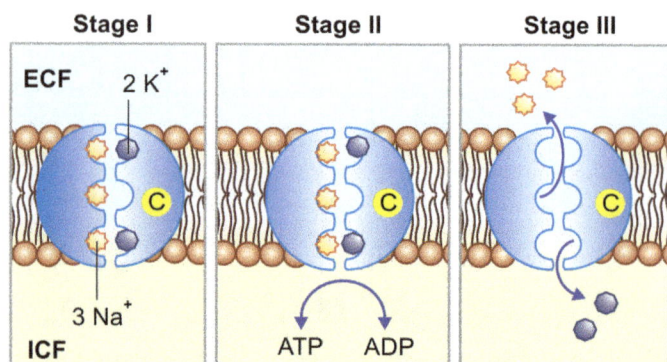

FIGURE 3.5: Hypothetical diagram of sodium-potassium (Na^+-K^+) pump. C = Carrier protein. **Stage I:** Three Na^+ from intracellular fluid (ICF) and two K^+ from extracellular fluid (ECF) bind with 'C'. **Stage II:** Binding of Na^+ and K^+ to 'C' activates the enzyme ATPase. ATPase causes breakdown of ATP into adenosine diphosphate (ADP) with the release of one high-energy phosphate. **Stage III:** Conformational change occurs in 'C' followed by release of Na^+ into ECF and K^+ into ICF.

protein that transports two different substances in opposite directions (Fig. 3.4).

■ SUBSTANCES TRANSPORTED BY ACTIVE TRANSPORT

Substances transported by active transport are in ionic form and non-ionic form. The substances in ionic form are sodium, potassium, calcium, hydrogen, chloride and iodide. The substances in non-ionic form are glucose, amino acids and urea.

■ TYPES OF ACTIVE TRANSPORT

Active transport is of two types:

A. Primary active transport.
B. Secondary active transport.

■ PRIMARY ACTIVE TRANSPORT

Primary active transport is the type of transport mechanism in which the energy is liberated directly from breakdown of ATP. By this method, the substances such as sodium, potassium, calcium, hydrogen and chloride are transported across the cell membrane.

Primary Active Transport of Sodium and Potassium: Sodium-potassium Pump

Sodium (Na^+) and potassium (K^+) ions are transported across the cell membrane by sodium-potassium (Na^+-K^+) pump which is also called Na^+-K^+ ATPase pump. This pump is formed by a carrier protein and it is present in all cells of the body.

Mechanism of action of Na^+-K^+ pump

Three sodium ions from the cell get attached to the receptor sites of sodium ions on the inner surface of the carrier protein. Two potassium ions outside the cell bind to the receptor sites of potassium ions located on the outer surface of the carrier protein **(Fig. 3.5, Stage I)**.

Binding of sodium and potassium ions to carrier protein activates the enzyme ATPase. The ATPase causes breakdown of ATP into adenosine diphosphate (ADP) with the release of one high-energy phosphate **(Fig. 3.5, Stage II)**. Now, the energy liberated causes some sort of conformational change in the molecule of the carrier protein. Because of this, the outer surface of the molecule (with potassium ions) now faces the inner side of the cell. And, the inner surface of the protein molecule (with sodium ions) faces the outer side of the cell **(Fig. 3.5, Stage III)**. Now, dissociation and release of the ions take place, so that the sodium ions are released outside the cell (ECF) and the potassium ions are released inside the cell (ICF). Exact mechanisms involved in the dissociation and release of ions are not yet known.

Electrogenic activity of Na^+-K^+ pump

The Na^+-K^+ pump moves three sodium ions outside the cell and two potassium ions inside cell. Thus, when the pump works once, there is a net loss of one positively charged ion from the cell. Continuous activity of the Na^+-K^+ pumps causes reduction in the number of positively charged ions inside the cell, leading to increase in the negativity inside the cell. This activity is called the electrogenic activity of Na^+-K^+ pump.

Transport of Calcium Ions

Calcium ions are actively transported from inside to outside the cell by **calcium pump** with the help of a separate carrier protein. The energy is obtained from ATP.

Transport of Hydrogen Ions

Hydrogen ions are actively transported across the cell membrane by **hydrogen pump** with the help of another carrier protein. It also obtains energy from ATP.

■ SECONDARY ACTIVE TRANSPORT

Secondary active transport is the transport of a substance along with sodium ions by a common carrier protein.

Secondary active transports if of two types:

1. ***Cotransport***: Transport of the substance in the same direction along with sodium.
2. ***Countertransport***: Transport of the substance in the opposite direction to that of sodium.

Sodium Cotransport

In this, along with sodium, another substance is carried with the help of a carrier protein called symport (the protein that transports two different molecules in the same direction across the cell membrane).

Examples: Transport of glucose, amino acids, chloride, iodine, iron and urate ions **(Fig. 3.6)**.

Sodium Countertransport

In this process, the substances are transported across the cell membrane in exchange for sodium ions by the carrier protein called antiport (the carrier protein that transports two different ions or molecules in opposite direction across the cell membrane).

Examples: Sodium-calcium countertransport and sodium-hydrogen counter transport in the tubular cells **(Figs. 3.7 and 3.8)**.

■ SPECIAL CATEGORIES OF ACTIVE TRANSPORT

In addition to primary and secondary active transport systems, some special categories of active transport systems also exist in the body.

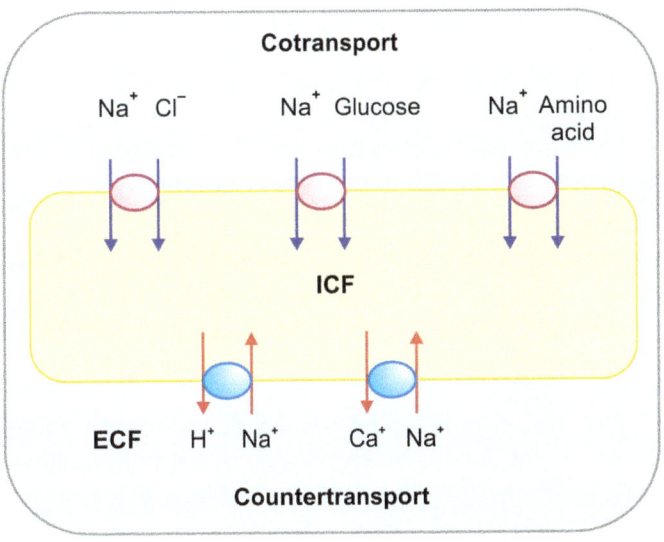

FIGURE 3.8: Sodium cotransport and countertransport by carrier proteins.

Special categories of active transport are:
1. Endocytosis.
2. Exocytosis.
3. Transcytosis.

1. Endocytosis

Endocytosis is the transport mechanism by which the **macromolecules** enter the cell. The substances with larger molecules are called macromolecules and these substances cannot pass through the cell membrane either by active or by passive transport mechanism. Such substances are transported into the cell by endocytosis.

Endocytosis is of three types:
a. Pinocytosis.
b. Phagocytosis.
c. Receptor-mediated endocytosis.

a. Pinocytosis

Pinocytosis is the process by which macromolecules such as bacteria and antigens are taken into the cells. It is otherwise called **cell drinking**.

Mechanism of pinocytosis
i. Macromolecules (in the form of droplets of fluid) bind to the outer surface of the cell membrane.
ii. Now, the cell membrane evaginates and engulfs the droplets.
iii. Engulfed droplets are converted into vesicles and vacuoles, which are called **endosomes (Fig. 3.9)**.

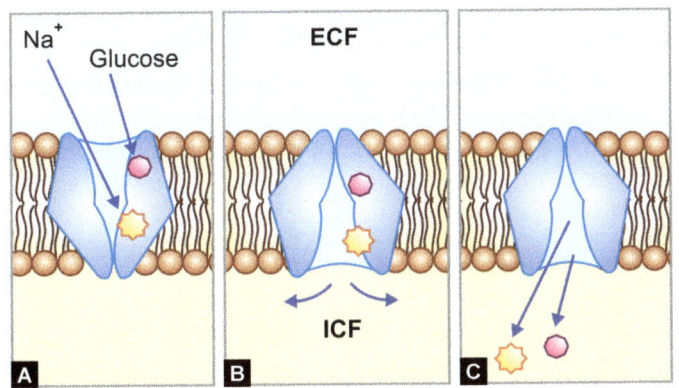

FIGURE 3.6: Sodium (Na+) cotransport. A. Na+ and glucose from extracellular fluid (ECF) bind with carrier protein. B. Conformational change occurs in the carrier protein. C. Na+ and glucose are released into intracellular fluid (ICF).

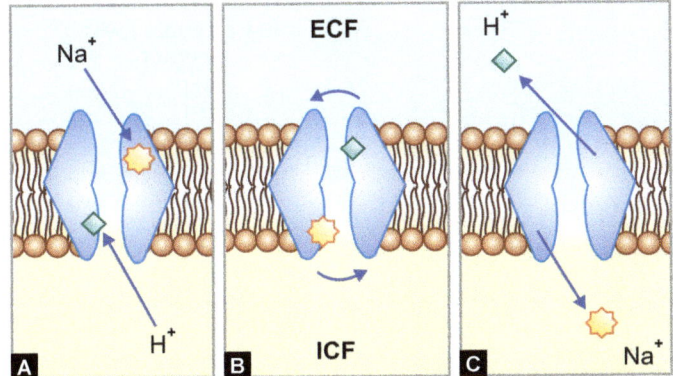

FIGURE 3.7: Sodium (Na+) countertransport. A. Na+ from extracellular fluid (ECF) and hydrogen (H+) from intracellular fluid (ICF) bind with carrier protein. B. Conformational change occurs in the carrier protein. C. Na+ enters ICF and H+ enters ECF.

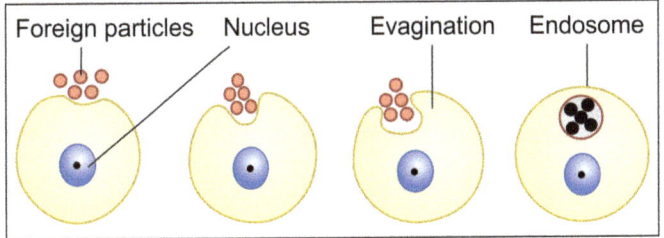

FIGURE 3.9: Process of pinocytosis.

iv. Endosome travels into the interior of the cell.
v. **Primary lysosome** in the cytoplasm fuses with the endosome and forms the **secondary lysosome**.
vi. Now, hydrolytic enzymes present in the secondary lysosome are activated resulting in digestion and degradation of the **endosomal contents**.

b. Phagocytosis

Phagocytosis is the process by which particles larger than macromolecules are engulfed into the cells. It is also called **cell eating**. Larger bacteria, larger antigens and other larger foreign bodies are taken inside the cell by means of phagocytosis.

Only few cells in the body such as neutrophils, monocytes and the tissue macrophages show phagocytosis. Among these cells, the **macrophages** are the largest phagocytic cells.

Mechanism of phagocytosis

i. When the bacteria or the foreign body enters the body, first the phagocytic cell sends pseudopodium (cytoplasmic extension) around the bacteria or the foreign substance.
ii. Then, these particles are engulfed and are converted into endosome-like vacuole. The vacuole is very large and it is usually called the **phagosome**.
iii. Phagosome travels into the interior of the cell.
iv. **Primary lysosome** fuses with this phagosome and forms **secondary lysosome**.
v. Hydrolytic enzymes present in the secondary lysosome are activated resulting in digestion and degradation of the **phagosomal contents (Fig. 3.10)**.

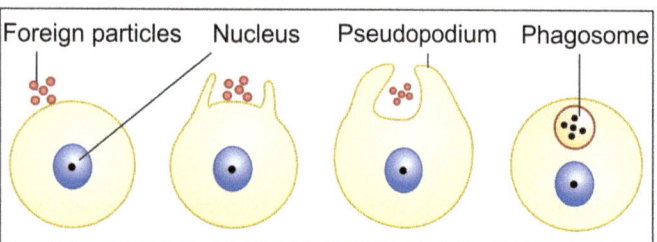

FIGURE 3.10: Process of phagocytosis.

c. Receptor-mediated endocytosis

Receptor-mediated endocytosis is the transport of macromolecules with the help of a receptor protein. The surface of cell membrane has some pits which contain a receptor protein called **clathrin**. Together with a receptor protein, each pit is called **receptor coated pit**. The coated pits are involved in the receptor-mediated endocytosis.

Mechanism of receptor-mediated endocytosis

i. Receptor-mediated endocytosis is induced by substances like ligands **(Fig. 3.11-I)**.
ii. Ligand molecules approach the cell and bind to receptors in the coated pits and form ligand-receptor complex **(Fig. 3.11-II)**.
iii. Ligand-receptor complex gets aggregated in the coated pits. Then, the pit is detached from cell membrane and becomes the coated vesicle. This coated vesicle forms the endosome **(Fig. 3.11-III)**.
iv. Endosome travels into the interior of the cell. Primary lysosome in the cytoplasm fuses with endosome and forms secondary lysosome **(Fig. 3.11-IV)**.
v. Now, the hydrolytic enzymes present in secondary lysosome are activated resulting in release of ligands into the cytoplasm **(Fig. 3.11-V)**.
vi. Receptor may move to a new pit of the cell membrane **(Fig. 3.11-VI)**.

Receptor-mediated endocytosis plays an important role in the transport of various types of macromolecules such as hormones, antibodies, lipids, growth factors, toxins, bacteria and viruses.

2. Exocytosis

Exocytosis is the process by which the substances are expelled from the cell. In this process, the substances are extruded from the cell without passing through the cell membrane **(Fig. 3.12)**. This is the reverse of endocytosis.

Mechanism of exocytosis

Secretory substances from the cells are released by exocytosis. The secretory substances of the cell are stored

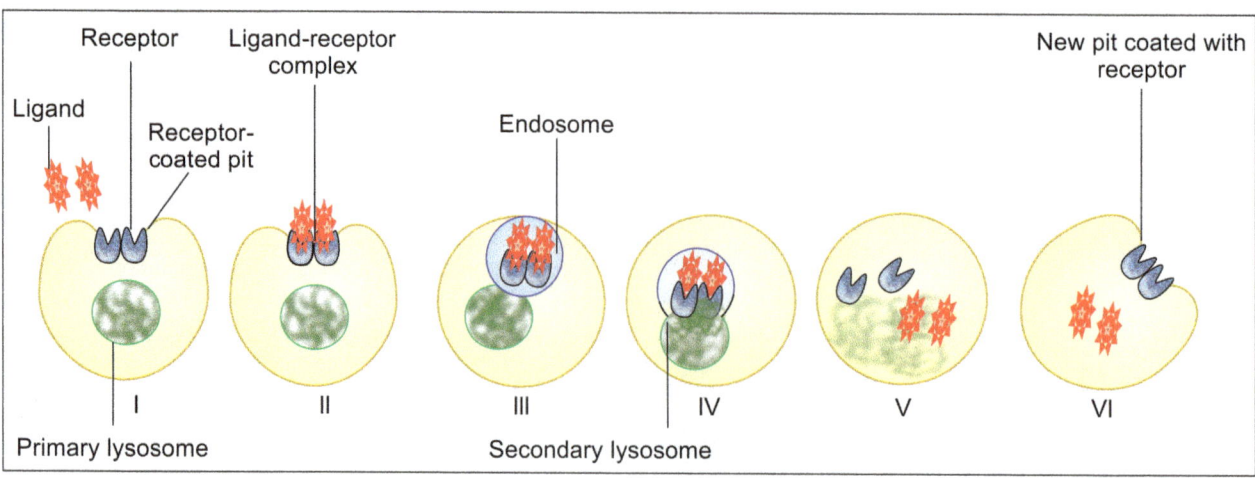

FIGURE 3.11: Mechanism of receptor-mediated endocytosis.

in the form of secretory vesicles in the cytoplasm. When required, the vesicles move towards the cell membrane and get fused with it. Later, the contents of the vesicles are released out of the cell **(Fig. 3.13)**.

3. Transcytosis

Transcytosis is a transport mechanism in which an extracellular macromolecule enters through one side of a cell, migrates across cytoplasm of the cell and exits through the other side by means of exocytosis.

Examples are movement of proteins and pathogens like HIV from capillary blood into interstitial fluid through endothelial cells of the capillary.

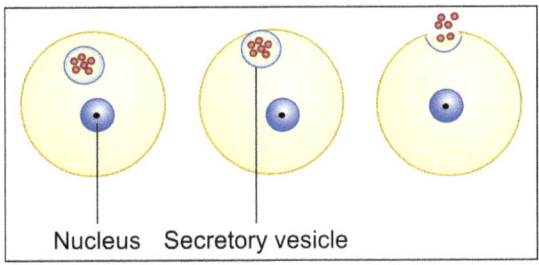

FIGURE 3.12: Process of exocytosis.

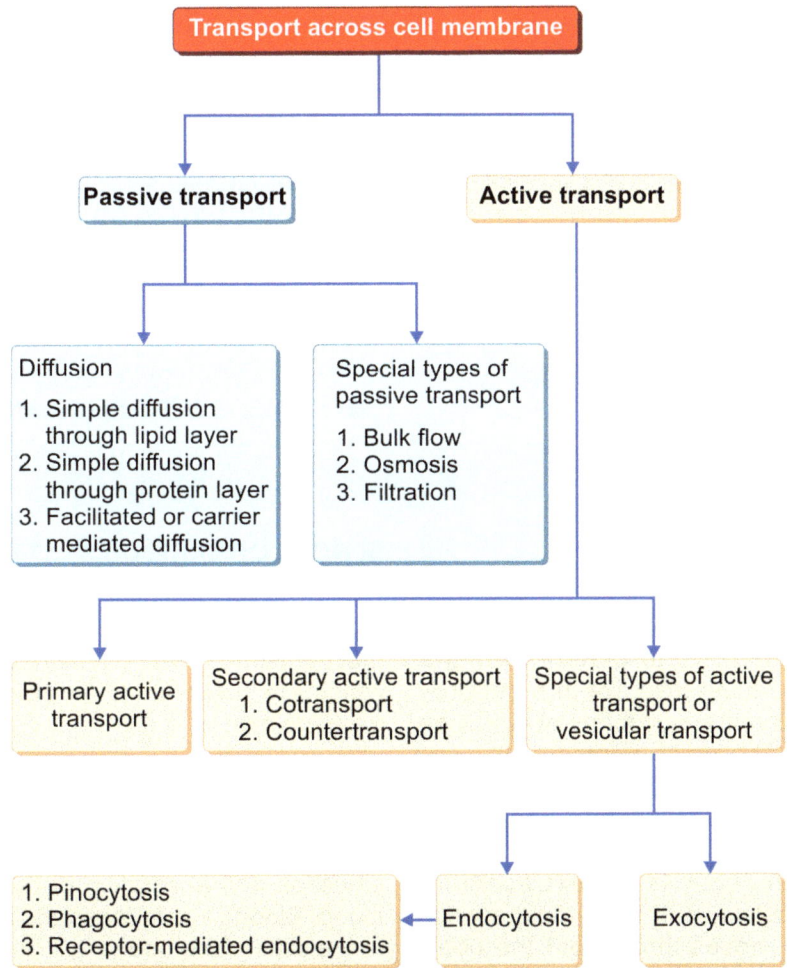

FIGURE 3.13: Types of transport mechanisms across cell membrane.

Chapter 4: Homeostasis

CHAPTER OUTLINE

- **DEFINITION**
- **INTERNAL ENVIRONMENT**
- **ROLE OF VARIOUS SYSTEMS OF THE BODY IN HOMEOSTASIS**
  - DIGESTIVE SYSTEM
  - RESPIRATORY SYSTEM
  - EXCRETORY SYSTEM
  - SKIN
  - BLOOD AND CIRCULATORY SYSTEM
  - LYMPHATIC SYSTEM
- ENDOCRINE SYSTEM
- SKELETAL MUSCLES
- NERVOUS SYSTEM
- **COMPONENTS OF HOMEOSTATIC SYSTEM**
- **MECHANISM OF ACTION OF HOMEOSTATIC SYSTEM**
  - NEGATIVE FEEDBACK
  - POSITIVE FEEDBACK
  - FEED-FORWARD CONTROL
- **HOMEOSTATIC IMBALANCE**

■ DEFINITION

'**Homeostasis**' means the maintenance of constant **internal environment** of the body (**homeo** means same; stasis means standing). According to **Claude Bernard**, multicellular organisms including man live in a perfectly organized and controlled internal environment which he called '**Milieu interieur**'. The word 'homeostasis' was introduced by **Walter B Cannon** in 1930.

■ INTERNAL ENVIRONMENT

Internal environment in the body is the **extracellular fluid (ECF)** in which the cells live. It is the fluid outside the cell and it constantly moves throughout the body. ECF includes blood, which circulates in the vascular system and **interstitial fluid** which is present in between the cells. ECF contains nutrients, ions and all other substances necessary for the survival of the cells.

Normal healthy living of large organisms including human beings depends upon constant maintenance of internal environment within the physiological limits. If the internal environment deviates beyond the **set limits,** body suffers from malfunction or dysfunction. Therefore, the ultimate goal of an organism is to have a normal healthy living, which is achieved by the maintenance of internal environment within set limits.

■ ROLE OF VARIOUS SYSTEMS OF THE BODY IN HOMEOSTASIS

Many systems of the body are involved in homeostatic mechanism of each function. Functions of each system which are responsible for homeostatic mechanism are given below:

■ 1. DIGESTIVE SYSTEM

Nutrients are essential for various activities of the cell and growth of the tissues. Digestive system is responsible for digestion and absorption of nutritive substances into the blood. Blood in turn transports supplies these substances to the cells of the body.

■ 2. RESPIRATORY SYSTEM

Respiratory system is responsible supply of oxygen to the cells for metabolism of the nutrients. Simultaneously, carbon dioxide is removed from the cells and expelled out of body via lungs.

Respiratory system is also responsible for maintenance of water balance, acid balance and temperature of the body.

■ 3. EXCRETORY SYSTEM

Kidneys and other excretory organs are involved in the excretion of waste products. Kidneys are also responsible for maintenance of water balance, electrolyte balance, acid-base balance and osmolality of body fluids.

4. SKIN

Skin covers and protects all organs of the body from mechanical blow, bacteria, toxic substances and ultraviolet rays. By secreting sweat skin plays an important role in regulation of body temperature and water balance. Skin also forms the largest sense organ. It has many receptors which convey many sensations to brain via afferent nerves.

5. BLOOD AND CIRCULATORY SYSTEM

Circulatory system includes heart and blood vessels. Heart is responsible for flow of blood in blood vessels throughout the body. Blood transports nutritive substances, oxygen and other important substances such as hormones to all cells of the body. Simultaneously, from cells it removes carbon dioxide, metabolic and other waste products which are to be excreted.

White blood cells are responsible for protection of the body from invading organisms and development immunity against pathogenic agents.

6. LYMPHATIC SYSTEM

Lymphatic system includes closed system of lymphatic vessels and lymph nodes through which lymph flows. Major function of lymph is to return proteins from tissue space into blood. It is also responsible for redistribution of fluid in body.

Lymph nodes form defense barriers of the body by destructing bacteria and other toxic agents.

7. ENDOCRINE SYSTEM

Many hormones secreted by endocrine glands and other structures are essential for the metabolism of nutrients and other substances necessary for the cells. Hormones also are necessary for growth and functions of various tissues of the body.

8. SKELETAL MUSCLES

Skeletal muscles help the organism to move around in search of food. It also helps to protect the organism from adverse surroundings, thus preventing damage or destruction.

9. NERVOUS SYSTEM

Central nervous system, which includes brain and spinal cord plays an important role in homeostasis. Sensory system detects the state of the body or surroundings. Brain integrates and interprets the pros and cons of these information and commands the body to act accordingly through motor system so that, the body can avoid the damage.

Autonomic nervous system regulates all vegetative functions of the body essential for homeostasis.

COMPONENTS OF HOMEOSTATIC SYSTEM

Homeostatic system in the body includes three components:

1. *Sensors or Detectors or Receptors*

Sensors recognize the deviation in any activity in internal environment and transmit the message to control center (Fig. 4.1).

2. *Control Center or Integrator Center*

Control center receives the message from receptors and immediately sends commands to concerned effectors.

3. *Effectors*

Effectors receive the commands from the center and either accelerate or inhibit the activity so that normalcy is restored.

MECHANISM OF ACTION OF HOMEOSTATIC SYSTEM

Homeostatic mechanism in the body maintains the normalcy of various systems. Whenever there is any change in behavioral pattern of any system, the effectors bring back the normalcy either by inhibiting and reversing the change or by supporting and accelerating the change.

Homeostatic mechanism functions by two types of feedback control systems:

1. Negative feedback.
2. Positive feedback.

NEGATIVE FEEDBACK

Negative feedback mechanism is the one by which a particular system reacts in such a way as to stop the change or reverse the direction of change. After receiving a message, the effectors send the inhibitory signals back to the system. Now, the system stabilizes its own function either by stopping the signals or by reversing the signals.

For example, thyroid-stimulating hormone (TSH) released from pituitary gland stimulates thyroid gland, which in turn secretes thyroxin. When thyroxin level increases in blood, it inhibits the secretion of TSH from

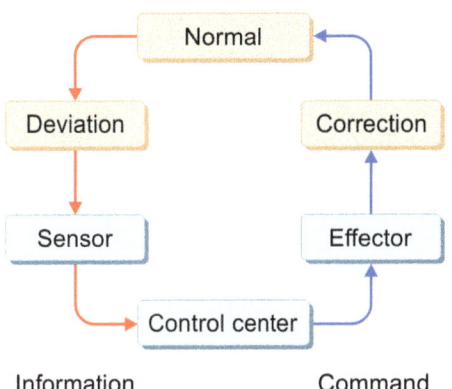

FIGURE 4.1: Components of homeostatic system.

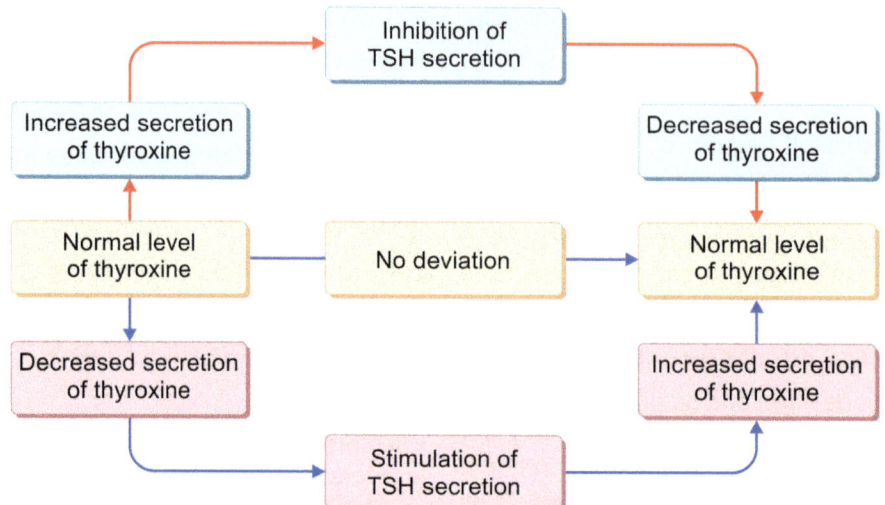

FIGURE 4.2: Negative feedback mechanism: Secretion of thyroxine.
TSH = Thyroid-stimulating hormone.

pituitary so that, the secretion of thyroxine from thyroid gland decreases **(Fig. 4.2)**. On the other hand, if thyroxin secretion is less, it induces pituitary gland to release TSH. Now, TSH stimulates thyroid gland to secrete thyroxin. Refer Chapter 51 for details. Another example for negative feedback mechanism is maintenance of water balance in the body **(Fig. 4.3)**.

■ POSITIVE FEEDBACK

Positive feedback mechanism is the one in which the system reacts in such a way as to amplify (increase the intensity of) the change in the same direction. Positive feedback is less common than the negative feedback. However, it has its own significance, particularly during emergency conditions.

One of the positive feedbacks occurs during the blood clotting. Blood clotting is necessary to arrest bleeding during injury and it occurs in three stages:

1. Formation of prothrombin activator.
2. Conversion of prothrombin into thrombin.
3. Conversion of fibrinogen into fibrin by thrombin.

Thrombin formed in the second stage stimulates the formation of more prothrombin activator in addition to converting fibrinogen into fibrin **(Fig. 4.4)**. It causes formation of more and more amount of prothrombin activator so that the blood clotting process is accelerated and blood loss is prevented quickly (Chapter 18). Other processes where positive feedback occurs are milk ejection reflex (Chapter 50) and parturition **(Fig. 4.5)** and both the processes involve oxytocin secretion.

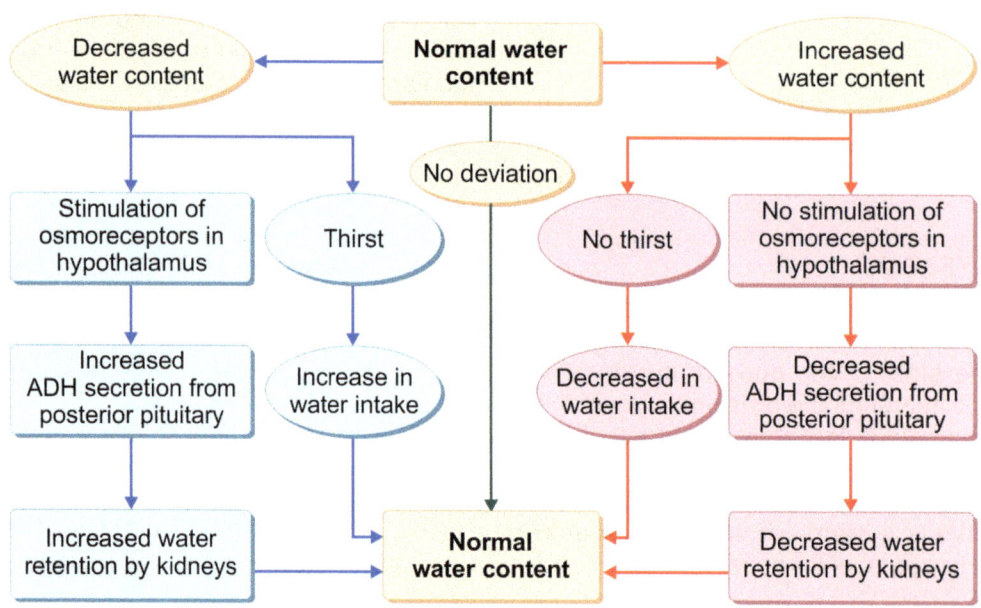

FIGURE 4.3: Negative feedback mechanism: Maintenance of water balance.
ADH = Antidiuretic hormone.

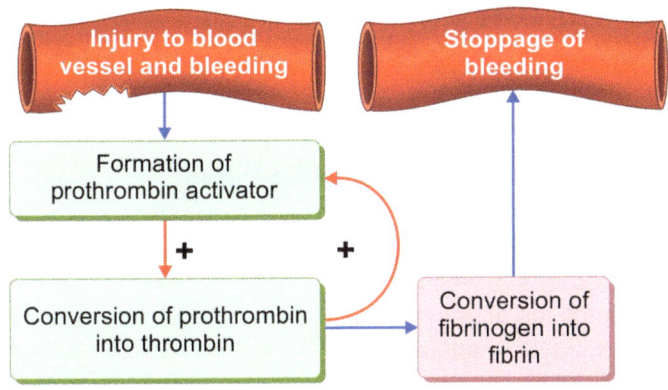

FIGURE 4.4: Positive feedback mechanism: Coagulation of blood. Once formed, thrombin induces the formation of more prothrombin activator.

■ FEED-FORWARD CONTROL

In addition to positive and negative feedback, homeostasis mechanism has feed-forward control system also.

Feed-forward control system is the control system in homeostasis that anticipates the change or deviation that may occur in a later stage and takes appropriate control action to avoid the disturbance. Whereas the feedback control systems detect the deviation only when it happens.

Examples of Feed-forward Control

1. Preadaptation before onset of exercise such as changes in cardiovascular system in order to prepare the body for exercise.
2. Secretion of gastric juice (along with salivary secretion) even before entrance of food in mouth.
3. Increase in secretion of luteinizing hormone prior to ovulation.

■ HOMEOSTATIC IMBALANCE

Homeostatic imbalance is the failure of the body to maintain constant internal environment. It is the starting point of

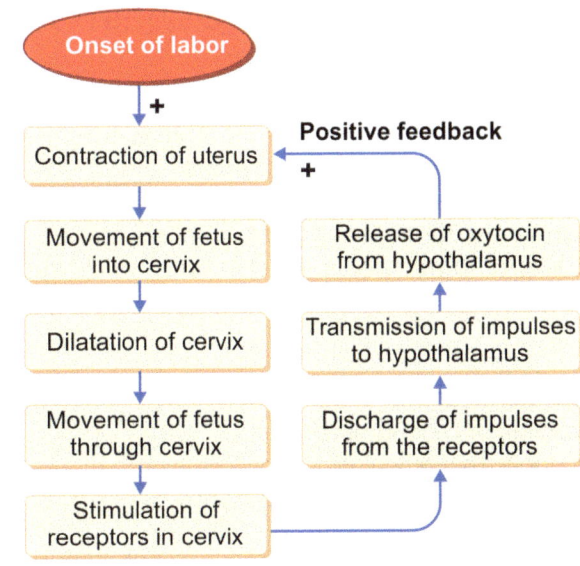

FIGURE 4.5: Positive feedback mechanism: Parturition.

BOX 4.1: Homeostatic imbalance.

Common causes	
1. Stress	6. Lack of water intake
2. Altered eating habits	7. Hypoxia
3. Alcohol consumption	8. Long-term illness
4. Sleeplessness	9. Genetic mutation
5. Over-exercise	10. Aging
Common consequences	
1. Acidosis	6. Hypertension
2. Diabetes mellitus	7. Heart failure
3. Hypoglycemia	8. Gout
4. Hyperglycemia	9. Infections
5. Dehydration	10. Disease caused by toxins

disorders and diseases in the body. Details of homeostatic imbalance are given in **Box 4.1**.

MODEL QUESTIONS IN GENERAL PHYSIOLOGY

■ LONG QUESTIONS

1. Describe the mechanism of active transport of substances through cell membrane.
2. Describe the mechanism of passive transport of substances through cell membrane.
3. Explain homeostasis in the body with suitable examples.

■ SHORT QUESTIONS

1. Cell membrane.
2. Proteins of cell membrane.
3. Endoplasmic reticulum.
4. Ribosomes.
5. Mitochondria.
6. Golgi apparatus.
7. Cytoskeleton.
8. Tight junctions.
9. Gap junctions.
10. Sodium-potassium pump.
11. Factors affecting rate of diffusion.
12. Endocytosis.
13. Negative feedback.
14. Positive feedback.

■ VERY SHORT ANSWER QUESTIONS

1. Integral proteins.
2. List the organelles present in cytoplasm.
3. Functions of lysosomes.
4. Functions of peroxisomes.
5. Functions of nucleus.
6. Apoptosis.
7. Cellular necrosis.
8. Proteins of tight junctions.
9. Adherence junction.
10. Focal adhesion.
11. Desmosome.
12. Hemidesmosome.
13. Protein channels.
14. Facilitated diffusion.
15. Active transport vs facilitated diffusion.
16. Phagocytosis.
17. Exocytosis.
18. Transcytosis.

SECTION 2: BLOOD AND BODY FLUIDS

Chapter 5: Body Fluids

CHAPTER OUTLINE

- **TOTAL BODY WATER**
- **COMPARTMENTS OF BODY FLUIDS**
- **COMPOSITION OF BODY FLUIDS**
  - ORGANIC SUBSTANCES
  - INORGANIC SUBSTANCES
- **MEASUREMENT OF BODY FLUID VOLUME**
  - INDICATOR DILUTION METHOD
  - MEASUREMENT OF TOTAL BODY WATER
  - MEASUREMENT OF EXTRACELLULAR FLUID VOLUME
  - MEASUREMENT OF PLASMA VOLUME
  - MEASUREMENT OF BLOOD VOLUME
- **MEASUREMENT OF INTRACELLULAR FLUID VOLUME**
- **MEASUREMENT OF INTERSTITIAL FLUID VOLUME**
- **CONCENTRATION OF BODY FLUIDS**
  - OSMOLALITY
  - OSMOLARITY
  - TONICITY
- **MAINTENANCE OF WATER BALANCE**
- **APPLIED PHYSIOLOGY**
  - DEHYDRATION
  - OVERHYDRATION OR WATER INTOXICATION

TOTAL BODY WATER

Body is formed by solids and fluids. Fluid part is more than two third of the whole body. Water forms most of the fluid part of the body.

In human beings, the total body water varies from 45 to 75% of body weight. In a normal young adult male, body contains 60 to 65% of water and 35 to 40% of solids. In a normal young adult female, the water is 50 to 55% and solids are 45 to 50%.

Total quantity of body water in an average human being weighing about 70 kg is about 40 L.

COMPARTMENTS OF BODY FLUIDS: DISTRIBUTION OF BODY FLUIDS

Compartments and distribution of body fluids with the quantity is given in **Table 5.1**. Water moves between different compartments **(Fig. 5.1)**. Total body water (40 L) is distributed into two major fluid compartments:

1. **Intracellular fluid** (ICF) forming 55% of the total body water (22 L).
2. **Extracellular fluid** (ECF) forming 45% of the total body water (18 L). ECF is divided into five subunits. Refer **Table 5.1** for details.

TABLE 5.1: Subunits of extracellular fluid.

Subunit of ECF	%	L
I. Interstitial fluid and lymph	20.0	12.0
II. Plasma	7.5	2.75
III. Fluids in bones	7.5	
IV. Fluid in dense connective tissues such as cartilage	7.5	
V. Transcellular fluid 　1. Cerebrospinal fluid 　2. Intraocular fluid 　3. Digestive juices 　4. Serous fluid 　　a. Intrapleural fluid 　　b. Pericardial fluid 　　c. Peritoneal fluid 　5. Synovial fluid in joints 　6. Fluid in urinary tract	2.5	3.25

ECF 45% of body fluid. Total quantity of ECF is 18 L.

COMPOSITION OF BODY FLUIDS

Body fluids contain water and solids. Solids are organic and inorganic substances.

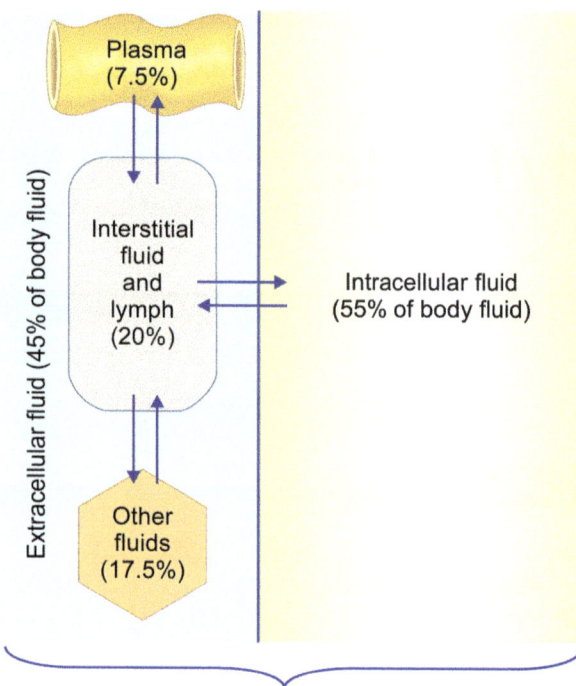

FIGURE 5.1: Body fluid compartments and movement of fluid between different compartments. Other fluids = Transcellular fluid, fluid in bones and fluid in connective tissue.

■ ORGANIC SUBSTANCES

Organic substances present in body fluids are glucose, amino acids and other proteins, fatty acids and other lipids, hormones and enzymes.

■ INORGANIC SUBSTANCES

Inorganic substances present in body fluids are sodium, potassium, calcium, magnesium, chloride, bicarbonate, phosphate and sulfate. Differences between ECF and ICF are given in the **Table 5.2**.

■ MEASUREMENT OF BODY FLUID VOLUME

Volume of different compartments of the body fluid is measured by indicator dilution method or dye dilution method.

■ INDICATOR DILUTION METHOD

Principle

A known quantity of a substance such as a dye is administered into a specific body fluid compartment. This substance is called the **marker substance** or **indicator** **(Table 5.3)**. After administration into the fluid, the marker substance is allowed to mix thoroughly with the fluid compartment. Then, a sample of fluid is drawn and the concentration of the marker substance is determined. The substances whose concentration can be determined by using colorimeter or radioactive substances are generally used as marker substances.

TABLE 5.2: Differences between extracellular fluid (ECF) and intracellular fluid (ICF).

Substance	ECF	ICF
Sodium	142 mEq/L	10 mEq/L
Calcium	5 mEq/L	1 mEq/L
Potassium	4 mEq/L	140 mEq/L
Magnesium	3 mEq/L	28 mEq/L
Chloride	103 mEq/L	4 mEq/L
Bicarbonate	28 mEq/L	10 mEq/L
Phosphate	4 mEq/L	75 mEq/L
Sulfate	1 mEq/L	2 mEq/L
Proteins	2 g/dL	16 g/dL
Amino acids	30 mg/dL	200 mg/dL
Glucose	90 mg/dL	0 to 20 mg/dL
Lipids	0.5 g/dL	2 to 95 g/dL
Partial pressure of oxygen	35 mm Hg	20 mm Hg
Partial pressure of carbon dioxide	46 mm Hg	50 mm Hg
Water	15 to 20 L (18)	20 to 25 L (22)
pH	7.4	7.0

TABLE 5.3: Marker substances used to measure body fluid compartments.

Fluid compartment	Marker substances
Total body water	1. Deuterium oxide (D_2O) 2. Tritium oxide (T_2O) 3. Antipyrine
Extracellular fluid	1. Radioactive sodium, chloride, bromide, sulfate and thiosulfate 2. Non-metabolizable saccharides such as inulin, mannitol, raffinose and sucrose
Plasma	1. Radioactive iodine ($_{131}I$) 2. Evans blue (T-1824)

Formula to Measure the Body Fluid Volume by Indicator Dilution Method

Quantity of fluid in the compartment is measured by using the formula:

$$V = \frac{M}{C}$$

Where,
- V = The volume of fluid in the compartment
- M = Mass or total quantity of marker substance injected
- C = Concentration of the marker substance in the sample fluid

Correction factor

Some amount of marker substance is lost through urine during distribution. So, the formula is corrected as follows:

$$\text{Volume} = \frac{M - \text{Amount of substance excreted}}{C}$$

Uses of Indicator Dilution Method

Indicator dilution or dye dilution method is used to measure ECF volume, plasma volume and the volume of total body water.

Characteristics of Marker Substances

Dye or any substance used as a marker substance should have some qualities which are listed in **Box 5.1**.

■ MEASUREMENT OF TOTAL BODY WATER

Marker substance for measuring TBW should be distributed through all the compartments of body fluid.

Such marker substances are:

1. Deuterium oxide.
2. Tritium oxide.
3. Antipyrine.

Deuterium oxide and tritium oxide mix with fluids of all the compartments within few hours after injection. Since plasma is part of total body fluid, the concentration of marker substances can be obtained from sample of plasma. And, the formula for indicator dilution method is applied to calculate total body water.

■ MEASUREMENT OF EXTRACELLULAR FLUID VOLUME

ECF volume is measured by using the substances, which can pass through the capillary membrane freely and remain only in the ECF but not enter into the cell.

Such marker substances are:

1. Radioactive sodium, chloride, bromide, sulfate and thiosulfate.
2. Non-metabolizable saccharides like inulin, mannitol, raffinose and sucrose.

When any of the above substances is injected into blood, it mixes with the fluid of all sub-compartments of ECF

BOX 5.1: Characteristics of marker substance.

Marker substance
1. Must be nontoxic
2. Must mix with the fluid compartment thoroughly within reasonable time
3. Should not be excreted rapidly
4. Should be excreted from the body completely within reasonable time
5. Should not change the color of the body fluid
6. Should not alter the volume of the body fluid

within 30 minutes to 1 hour. The indicator dilution method is applied to calculate ECF volume. Since ECF includes plasma, the concentration of the marker substance can be obtained in the sample of plasma.

Some marker substances such as sodium, chloride, inulin and sucrose diffuse more widely throughout all sub-compartments of ECF. So, the measured volume of ECF by using these substances is called **sodium space**, **chloride space**, **inulin space** and **sucrose space**.

Example for Measurement of ECF Volume

Quantity of sucrose injected (M)   : 150 mg
Urinary excretion of sucrose   : 10 mg
Concentration of sucrose in plasma (C)   : 0.01 mg/mL

$$\text{Sucrose space} = \frac{\text{Mass} - \text{Amount lost in urine}}{\text{Concentration of sucrose in plasma}}$$

$$= \frac{150 - 10 \text{ mg}}{0.01 \text{ mg/mL}}$$

$$= 14{,}000 \text{ ML}$$

Therefore, the ECF volume = 14 L.
Sucrose space = 14,000 mL
Therefore, the ECF volume = 14 L

■ MEASUREMENT OF PLASMA VOLUME

The substance, which binds with plasma proteins strongly and diffuses into interstitium only in small quantities or does not diffuse at all, is used to as marker substance to measure plasma volume.

Measurement of plasma volume by indicator or dye dilution technique

Principles and other details of this technique are same as that of ECF volume. The dye which is used to measure plasma volume is Evans blue or T-1824.

Procedure

A small quantity of blood (3 to 4 mL) is drawn from the subject and a known quantity of the dye is added. This is used as control sample in the procedure. Then, a known volume of dye is injected intravenously. After 10 minutes, a sample of blood is drawn. Then, another 4 samples of blood are collected at the interval of 10 minutes. All the 5 samples are centrifuged and plasma is separated from the samples. In each sample of plasma, the concentration of the dye is measured by colorimetric method and the average concentration is found. The subject's urine is collected and the amount of dye excreted in the urine is measured.

Calculation

Plasma volume is determined by using the formula:

$$\text{Volume} = \frac{\text{Amount of dye injected} - \text{Amount excreted}}{\text{Average concentration of dye in plasma}}$$

MEASUREMENT OF BLOOD VOLUME

Measurement of total blood volume involves two steps:
1. Determination of plasma volume.
2. Determination of blood cell volume.

Plasma volume is determined by indicator dilution technique as mentioned above. Blood cell volume is determined by hematocrit value.

It is usually done by centrifuging the blood and measuring the packed cell volume (Chapter 11). PCV is expressed in percentage. If this is deducted from 100, the percentage of plasma is known. From this, and from the volume of plasma, the amount of total blood is calculated by using the formula:

$$\text{Blood volume} = \frac{100 \times \text{Amount of plasma}}{100 - \text{PCV}}$$

MEASUREMENT OF INTRACELLULAR FLUID VOLUME

Intracellular fluid volume cannot be measured directly. It is calculated from the values of volume of total body water and ECF volume:

ICF volume = Total fluid volume − ECF volume

MEASUREMENT OF INTERSTITIAL FLUID VOLUME

Interstitial fluid volume also cannot be measured directly. It is calculated from the values of ICF volume and plasma volume as given below:

Interstitial fluid volume = ICF volume − Plasma volume

CONCENTRATION OF BODY FLUIDS

Concentration of body fluids is expressed in three ways:
1. Osmolality.
2. Osmolarity.
3. Tonicity.

OSMOLALITY

Osmolality is the concentration of osmotically active substance in a solution. It is expressed as the number of particles (osmoles) per kilogram of solvent (osmoles/kg H_2O).

OSMOLARITY

Osmolarity is another term to express the osmotic concentration. It is the number of particles (osmoles) per liter of solution (osmoles/L).

Osmotic pressure in solutions depends upon osmolality. However, in practice, the osmolarity and not osmolality is considered to determine the osmotic pressure.

Often, these two terms are used interchangeably. Change in osmolality of ECF affects the volume of both ECF and ICF. When osmolality of ECF increases, water moves from ICF to ECF. When the osmolality decreases in ECF, water moves from ECF to ICF. Water movement continues until the osmolality of these two fluid compartments becomes equal.

Mole and Osmole

A mole (mol) is the molecular weight of a substance in gram. Millimole (mMol) is 1/1,000 of a mole. One osmole (Osm) is the expression of amount of osmotically active particles. It is the molecular weight of a substance in grams divided by number of freely moving particles liberated in solution of each molecule. One milliosmole (mOsm) is 1/1,000 of an osmole.

TONICITY

Tonicity is the measure of effective osmolality. In terms of tonicity, the solutions are classified into three categories:
1. Isotonic fluid.
2. Hypertonic fluid.
3. Hypotonic fluid.

1. Isotonic Fluid

Fluid which has the same effective osmolality (tonicity) as body fluids is called isotonic fluid. Examples are 0.9% sodium chloride solution (normal saline) and 5% glucose solution.

Red blood cells or other cells placed in isotonic fluid (normal saline) neither gain nor lose water by osmosis **(Fig. 5.2)**. This is because of **osmotic equilibrium** between inside and outside the cell across the cell membrane.

2. Hypertonic Fluid

Fluid which has greater effective osmolality than the body fluids is called hypertonic fluid. Example is 2% sodium chloride solution.

When red blood cells or other cells are placed in hypertonic fluid, **exosmosis** occurs resulting in shrinkage of the cells (crenation) **(Fig. 5.2)**.

3. Hypotonic Fluid

Fluid which has less effective osmolality than the body fluids is called hypotonic fluid. Example is 0.3% sodium chloride solution.

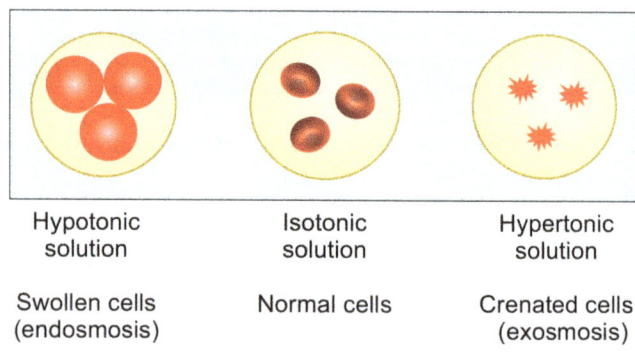

FIGURE 5.2: Effect of isotonic, hypertonic and hypotonic solutions on red blood cells.

When red blood cells or other cells are placed in hypotonic fluid, **endosmosis** occurs resulting in swelling of the cells **(Fig. 5.2)**. Now the red blood cells become globular and get ruptured (hemolysis).

■ MAINTENANCE OF WATER BALANCE

Body has several mechanisms which work together to maintain the water balance. The important mechanisms involve hypothalamus (Chapters 4, 98) and kidneys (Chapter 43).

■ APPLIED PHYSIOLOGY

Fluid balance exists in the body because of equal intake and removal of fluid. Abnormal level of fluids in the body is called fluid imbalance **(Box 5.2)**.

Fluid imbalance results in:

1. Dehydration or
2. Water intoxication.

■ DEHYDRATION

Definition

Dehydration is defined as excessive loss of water from the body. Body requires certain amount of fluid intake daily for normal functions. Minimum daily requirement of water intake is about 1 L. This varies with the age and activity of the individual. The most active individuals need 2 to 3 L of water intake daily. Dehydration occurs when fluid loss is more than what is consumed.

Classification of Dehydration

Basically, dehydration is of three types:

1. Mild dehydration

It occurs when fluid loss is about 5% of total body fluids. Dehydration is not very serious and can be treated easily by rehydration.

2. Moderate dehydration

Moderate dehydration occurs when fluid loss is about 10%. Dehydration becomes little serious and immediate treatment should be given by rehydration.

3. Severe dehydration

It occurs when fluid loss is about 15%. Dehydration becomes severe and requires hospitalization and emergency treatment. When fluid loss is more than 15%, dehydration becomes very severe and life threatening.

BOX 5.2: Fluid imbalance.

- Abnormal level of fluids in the body is referred as fluid imbalance
- Body is losing fluid constantly through breathing, sweating and urination
- It should be replaced by intake of equal quantity of fluid; otherwise, it will cause dehydration (refer text)
- If the body cannot excrete the fluid, it accumulates in the body causing fluid (water) intoxication (refer text)

Causes of Dehydration

1. Severe diarrhea and vomiting due to gastrointestinal disorders.
2. Excess urinary output due to renal disorders.
3. Excess loss of water through urine due to endocrine disorders such as diabetes mellitus, diabetes insipidus and adrenal insufficiency.
4. Insufficient intake of water.
5. Prolonged physical activity without consuming adequate amount of water in hot environment.
6. Prolonged exposure to heat: Severe sweating and dehydration occur while spending longer periods on regular basis in the saunas. Excess sweating leads to **heat frustration** (extreme loss of water, heat and energy).
7. Use of laxatives or diuretics in order to lose weight quickly. This is common in athletes.

Signs and Symptoms of Dehydration

Mild and moderate dehydration

1. Dryness of the mouth.
2. Excess thirst.
3. Decrease in sweating.
4. Decrease in urine formation.
5. Headache.
6. Dizziness.
7. Weakness.
8. Cramps in legs and arms.

Severe dehydration

1. Decrease in blood volume.
2. Decrease in cardiac output.
3. Low blood pressure.
4. Hypovolemic cardiac shock.
5. Fainting.

Very severe dehydration

1. Damage of organs like brain, liver and kidneys.
2. Mental depression and confusion.
3. Renal failure.
4. Convulsions.
5. Coma.

Dehydration in Infants

Infants suffering from severe diarrhea and vomiting caused by bacterial or viral infection, develop dehydration. It becomes life threatening if the lost body fluids are not replaced. This happens when parents are unable to recognize the signs.

Already volume of ECF is decreased during first 6 months after birth. And, dehydration affects the infants severely. So, immediate treatment must be given to save the infant.

Aging Effects on Dehydration

Elders are at higher risk for dehydration even if they are healthy. It is because of increased fluid loss and decreased fluid intake. In some cases, severe dehydration in old age may be fatal.

Treatment of Dehydration

Treatment depends upon the severity of dehydration. In mild dehydration, the best treatment is drinking of water and stopping fluid loss. However, in severe dehydration drinking water alone is ineffective because it cannot compensate the salt loss. So, the effective treatment for severe dehydration is oral rehydration therapy.

Oral Rehydration Therapy

Oral rehydration therapy (ORT) is the treatment for dehydration in which an **oral rehydration solution (ORS)** is administered orally. ORS was formulated by World Health Organization (WHO). This solution contains anhydrous glucose, sodium chloride, potassium chloride and trisodium citrate.

In case of very severe dehydration, proper treatment is intravenous administration of necessary fluid and electrolytes.

■ OVERHYDRATION OR WATER INTOXICATION

Definition

Overhydration, hyperhydration, water excess or water intoxication is defined as the condition in which body has too much water.

Causes for Water Intoxication

Overhydration occurs when more fluid is taken than that can be excreted. It also develops in some conditions such as heart failure, renal disorders and hypersecretion of antidiuretic hormone.

Common Features of Water Intoxication

1. Since the brain is more vulnerable to the effects of water intoxication, behavioral changes appear first.
2. Person becomes drowsy and inattentive.
3. Nausea and vomiting occur.
4. There is sudden loss of weight, followed by weakness and blurred vision.
5. Anemia, acidosis, cyanosis, hemorrhage and shock are also common.
6. Muscular symptoms such as weakness, cramps, twitching, poor coordination and paralysis develop.
7. Severe conditions of water intoxication result in:
    i. **Delirium** (extreme mental condition characterized by confused state and illusion).
    ii. **Seizures** (sudden uncontrolled involuntary muscular contractions).
    iii. **Coma** (profound state of unconsciousness, in which the person fails to respond to external stimuli and cannot perform voluntary actions).

Treatment of Water Intoxication

Mild water intoxication requires only fluid restriction. In very severe cases, the treatment includes:

1. Administration of diuretics to increase water loss through urine.
2. Administration of antidiuretic hormone (**ADH**) **receptor antagonists** to prevent ADH-induced reabsorption of water from renal tubules.
3. Intravenous administration of saline to restore sodium.

Chapter 6

Blood

CHAPTER OUTLINE

- **DEFINITION**
- **PROPERTIES OF BLOOD**
- **COMPOSITION OF BLOOD**
  - BLOOD CELLS
  - PLASMA
- **BLOOD VOLUME**
  - NORMAL BLOOD VOLUME
  - VARIATION OF BLOOD VOLUME
  - REGULATION OF BLOOD VOLUME
  - MEASUREMENT OF BLOOD VOLUME
- **FUNCTIONS OF BLOOD**
  - NUTRITIVE FUNCTION
  - RESPIRATORY FUNCTION
  - EXCRETORY FUNCTION
  - TRANSPORT OF HORMONES AND ENZYMES
  - REGULATION OF WATER BALANCE
  - REGULATION OF ACID-BASE BALANCE
  - REGULATION OF BODY TEMPERATURE
  - STORAGE FUNCTION
  - DEFENSIVE FUNCTION

DEFINITION

Blood is defined as a red color fluid that circulates through vascular system in humans and other vertebrates, carrying nutrients and oxygen to all parts of the body and waste products including carbon dioxide from all parts of the body.

Blood is a connective tissue in fluid form. It is considered as the **fluid of life**, because it carries oxygen from lungs to all parts of the body and carbon dioxide from all parts of the body to the lungs.

PROPERTIES OF BLOOD

1. Color

Blood is red in color. Arterial blood is scarlet red because of more O_2 and venous blood is purple red because of more CO_2.

2. Volume

See below for details of blood volume.

3. Reaction and pH

Blood is slightly alkaline and its pH in normal conditions is 7.4.

4. Specific Gravity

Specific gravity of total blood : 1.052 to 1.061
Specific gravity of blood cells : 1.092 to 1.101
Specific gravity of plasma : 1.022 to 1.026

5. Viscosity

Blood is five times more viscous than water. It is mainly due to red blood cells and plasma proteins.

COMPOSITION OF BLOOD

Blood contains the blood cells which are called formed elements and the liquid portion known as plasma.

BLOOD CELLS

Three types of cells are present in the blood:

1. Red blood cells (RBCs) or erythrocytes.
2. White blood cells (WBCs) or leukocytes.
3. Platelets or thrombocytes.

Hematocrit Value

Hematocrit is the volume of RBCs in blood expressed in percentage. It is also called **packed cell volume** (PCV). Its normal value is 45%.

If blood is collected in a hematocrit tube along with a suitable anticoagulant and centrifuged for 30 minutes at a speed of 3,000 revolutions per minute (rpm), the red blood cells settle down at the bottom leaving clear plasma at the top. Plasma forms 55% and red blood cells form 45% of the total blood. In between the plasma and the red blood cells, there is a thin layer of white buffy coat **(Fig. 11.2)**. This white buffy coat is formed by the aggregation of white blood cells and platelets.

PLASMA

Plasma is a straw-colored clear liquid part of blood. It contains 91% to 92% of water and 8% to 9% of solids (**Fig. 6.1**). The solids are the organic substances (**Box 6.1**) and inorganic substances (**Box 6.2**). Plasma also has some gases (**Box 6.2**).

Table 6.1 gives the normal values of some important substances in blood.

Serum

Serum is the clear fluid that oozes out from blood clot. When the blood is shed or collected in a container, it clots because of the conversion of fibrinogen into fibrin. After about 45 minutes, serum oozes out of the clot. For clinical investigations, serum is separated from blood cells by centrifuging. Volume of the serum is almost the same as that of plasma (55%). It is different from plasma only by the absence of fibrinogen, i.e. serum contains all the other constituents of plasma except fibrinogen. Fibrinogen is absent in serum because it is converted into fibrin during blood clotting. Thus,

Serum = Plasma – Fibrinogen

BLOOD VOLUME

NORMAL BLOOD VOLUME

Average volume of blood in a normal adult is 5 L. Total amount of blood present in the circulatory system, blood reservoirs, organs and tissues together constitute blood volume.

In newborn baby it is 450 mL. It increases during growth and reaches 5 L at the time of puberty. Blood volume is about 8% of the body weight in a normal young healthy adult male weighing about 70 kg. In females it is slightly less and is about 4.5 L.

VARIATIONS OF BLOOD VOLUME

Physiological Variations

1. *Age*: Blood volume is less at birth and it increases as the age advances. At birth and at 24 hours after birth, the blood volume is about 80 mL/kg body weight. At the age of 15 years, the blood volume is about 70 mL/kg body weight, which is almost the adult volume.
2. *Sex*: In males, blood volume is slightly more than in females because of increase in erythropoietic activity, body weight and surface area of the body. In females, it is slightly less because of loss of blood through menstruation, more fats and less body surface area.

BOX 6.1: Organic substances present in plasma.

I. Plasma proteins
1. Albumin
2. Globulin
3. Fibrinogen

II. Amino acids
1. Essential amino acids
2. Non-essential amino acids

III. Carbohydrates
1. Glucose

IV. Fats
1. Triglycerides
2. Cholesterol
3. Phospholipids

V. Internal secretions
1. Hormones

VI. Enzymes
1. Amylase
2. Carbonic anhydrase
3. Acid phosphatase
4. Alkaline phosphatase
5. Lipase
6. Esterase
7. Protease
8. Transaminase

VII. Non-protein nitrogenous substances
1. Ammonia
2. Creatine
3. Creatinine
4. Xanthi
5. Hypoxanthine
6. Urea
7. Uric acid

VIII. Antibodies

BOX 6.2: Inorganic substances and gases present in plasma.

Inorganic substances	
1. Sodium	6. Chloride
2. Calcium	7. Phosphate
3. Potassium	8. Iodide
4. Magnesium	9. Iron
5. Bicarbonate	10. Copper

Gases
1. Oxygen
2. Carbon dioxide
3. Nitrogen

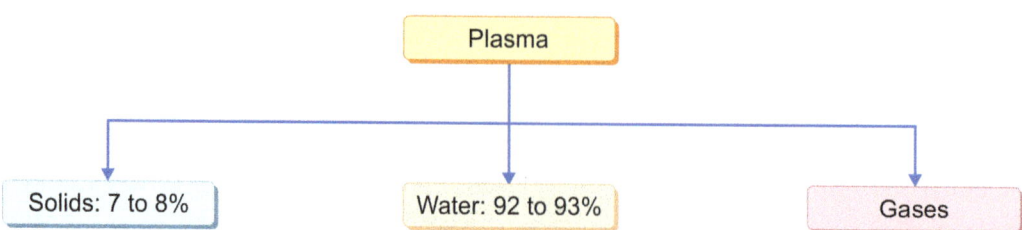

FIGURE 6.1: Composition of plasma.

TABLE 6.1: Normal values of some important substances in blood.

Substance	Normal value
1. Fasting glucose	70 to 100 mg/dL
2. Creatinine	0.5 to 1.5 mg/dL
3. Urea	15 to 40 mg/dL
4. Cholesterol	Up to 200 mg/dL
5. Plasma proteins	6.4 to 8.3 g/dL
6. Bilirubin	0.5 to 1.5 mg/dL
7. Iron	50 to 150 µg/dL
8. Copper	100 to 200 mg/dL
9. Calcium	9 to 11 mg/dL 4.5 to 5.5 mEq/L
10. Sodium	135 to 145 mEq/L
11. Potassium	3.5 to 5.0 mEq/L
12. Magnesium	1.5 to 2.0 mEq/L
13. Chloride	100 to 110 mEq/L
14. Bicarbonate	22 to 26 mEq/L

3. *Surface area of the body:* Blood volume is directly proportional to the surface area of the body.
4. *Body weight*: Blood volume is directly proportional to body weight.
5. *Atmospheric temperature:* Exposure to cold environment reduces the blood volume and exposure to warm environment increases the blood volume.
6. *Pregnancy*: During early stage of pregnancy, blood volume increases by 20 to 30%.
7. *Exercise:* Exercise increases the blood volume by increasing the release of erythropoietin and production of more RBCs.
8. *Posture:* Standing (erect posture) for long time reduces the blood volume by about 15%.
9. *High altitude:* Blood volume increases in high altitude.
10. *Emotion:* Excitement increases blood volume.

Pathological Variations

Hypervolemia

Increase in blood volume is called hypervolemia. It occurs in the following pathological conditions.

1. Hyperthyroidism.
2. Hyperaldosteronism.
3. Cirrhosis of the liver.
4. Congestive cardiac failure.

Hypovolemia

Decrease in blood volume is called hypovolemia. It occurs in the following pathological conditions.

1. Hemorrhage or blood loss.
2. Fluid loss.
3. Hemolysis.
4. Anemia.
5. Hypothyroidism.

REGULATION OF BLOOD VOLUME

Various mechanisms are involved in the regulation of blood volume. Important ones are the renal and hormonal mechanisms. Hypothalamus plays a vital role in the activation of these two mechanisms during the regulation of blood volume.

When blood volume increases, hypothalamus causes loss of fluid from the body. When the blood volume reduces, hypothalamus induces retention of water. Hypothalamus regulates the extracellular fluid (ECF) volume and blood volume by acting mainly through kidneys and sweat glands and by inducing thirst. This function of hypothalamus is described in Chapter 98.

Hormones also are involved in the regulation of blood volume through the regulation of ECF volume.

Hormones regulating blood volume through ECF volume are:

1. Antidiuretic hormone (Chapter 50).
2. Aldosterone (Chapter 54).
3. Cortisol (Chapter 54).
4. Atrial natriuretic peptide (Chapter 56).

MEASUREMENT OF BLOOD VOLUME

Refer Chapter 5 for measurement blood volume.

FUNCTIONS OF BLOOD

1. NUTRITIVE FUNCTION

Nutritive substances such as glucose, amino acids, lipids and vitamins derived from digested food are absorbed from gastrointestinal tract and carried by blood to different parts of the body for growth and production of energy.

2. RESPIRATORY FUNCTION

Transport of respiratory gases is done by the blood. It carries oxygen from alveoli of lungs to different tissues and carbon dioxide from tissues to alveoli.

3. EXCRETORY FUNCTION

Waste products formed in the tissues during various metabolic activities are removed by blood and carried to the excretory organs like kidney, skin, liver, etc. for excretion.

4. TRANSPORT OF HORMONES AND ENZYMES

Hormones which are secreted by ductless (endocrine) glands are released directly into the blood. The blood transports these hormones to their target organs/ tissues. Blood also transports enzymes.

5. REGULATION OF WATER BALANCE

This helps in the regulation of water content of the body.

6. REGULATION OF ACID-BASE BALANCE

Plasma proteins and hemoglobin act as buffers and help in the regulation of acid-base balance.

7. REGULATION OF BODY TEMPERATURE

Because of the high specific heat of blood. It is responsible for maintaining the thermoregulatory mechanism in the body, i.e. the balance between heat loss and heat gain in the body.

8. STORAGE FUNCTION

Water and some important substances like proteins, glucose, sodium and potassium are constantly required by the tissues. Blood serves as a readymade source for these substances. And, these substances are taken from blood during the conditions like starvation, fluid loss, electrolyte loss, etc.

9. DEFENSIVE FUNCTION

Blood plays an important role in the defense of the body. The white blood cells are responsible for this function. Neutrophils and monocytes engulf the bacteria by phagocytosis. Lymphocytes are involved in development of immunity. Eosinophils are responsible for detoxification; disintegration and removal of foreign proteins (Chapters 14 and 15).

Chapter 7: Plasma Proteins

CHAPTER OUTLINE

- DIFFERENT PLASMA PROTEINS
- NORMAL VALUES
- ORIGIN
- PROPERTIES
- FUNCTIONS
- PLASMAPHERESIS AND THERAPEUTIC PLASMA EXCHANGE
- APPLIED PHYSIOLOGY

DIFFERENT PLASMA PROTEINS

Plasma proteins are:

1. Serum albumin.
2. Serum globulin.
3. Fibrinogen.

Serum (Chapter 6) contains only albumin and globulin. Fibrinogen is absent in serum because, it is converted into fibrin during blood clotting. Because of this, the albumin and globulin are usually called **serum albumin** and **serum globulin**.

Globulin is of three types namely, α-globulin, β-globulin and γ-globulin.

NORMAL VALUES OF PLASMA PROTEINS

Normal values of the plasma proteins are given in **Table 7.1**.

Albumin/Globulin Ratio

The ratio between plasma level of albumin and globulin is called albumin/globulin (A/G) ratio. It is an important indicator of some liver and kidney diseases. Normal A/G ratio is 2:1.

TABLE 7.1: Normal value and molecular weight of plasma proteins.

Plasma protein	Normal value	Molecular weight
Serum albumin	4.7 g/dL	69,000
Serum globulin	2.3 g/dL	1,56,000
Fibrinogen	0.3 g/dL	4,00,000
Total proteins	7.3 g/dL (6.4 to 8.3 g/dL)	---

ORIGIN OF PLASMA PROTEINS

IN EMBRYO

In embryonic stage, plasma proteins are synthesized by the **mesenchyme cells**.

IN ADULTS

In adults, the plasma proteins are synthesized mainly from reticuloendothelial cells of liver and also from spleen, bone marrow, disintegrating blood cells and general tissue cells. Gamma globulin is synthesized from B lymphocytes.

PROPERTIES OF PLASMA PROTEINS

1. MOLECULAR WEIGHT

Molecular weight of plasma proteins is given in **Table 7.1**. Molecular weight of fibrinogen is greater than that of other two proteins.

2. ONCOTIC PRESSURE

Plasma proteins exert oncotic or osmotic pressure in the blood (Chapter 3). Normally, it is about 25 mm Hg. Albumin plays a major role in exerting oncotic pressure (see below).

3. SPECIFIC GRAVITY

Specific gravity of the plasma proteins is 1.026.

4. BUFFER ACTION

Acceptance of hydrogen ions is called buffer action. Plasma proteins have 1/6 of total buffering action of the blood.

FUNCTIONS OF PLASMA PROTEINS

1. ROLE IN COAGULATION OF BLOOD

Fibrinogen is essential for the coagulation of blood (Chapter 18).

2. ROLE IN DEFENSE MECHANISM OF BODY

Gamma globulins play an important role in the defense mechanism of the body by acting as antibodies. Gamma globulins are also called **immunoglobulins** (Chapter 15).

3. ROLE IN TRANSPORT MECHANISM

Plasma proteins are essential for transport of various substances in the blood. Albumin, alpha globulin and beta globulin are responsible for the transport of the hormones, enzymes, etc. The alpha and beta globulins transport metals in the blood.

4. ROLE IN MAINTENANCE OF ONCOTIC PRESSURE IN BLOOD

At the capillary level, most of the substances are exchanged between blood and tissues. However, because of their large size, the plasma proteins cannot pass through the capillary membrane easily and remain in the blood. In the blood, the proteins exert oncotic pressure or colloidal osmotic pressure. Albumin generates about 70% of oncotic pressure. Oncotic pressure exerted by the plasma proteins is about 25 mm Hg. Refer Chapter 3 for definition of osmotic pressure and oncotic pressure.

Since the concentration of albumin is more than the other plasma proteins, it exerts maximum pressure. It contributes about 70 to 80% of osmotic pressure. Globulin is the next and fibrinogen exerts least pressure.

5. ROLE IN REGULATION OF ACID-BASE BALANCE

Plasma proteins, particularly the albumin, play an important role in regulating the acid-base balance in the blood. This is because of the virtue of their buffering action.

6. ROLE IN VISCOSITY OF BLOOD

Plasma proteins provide viscosity to the blood, which is important to maintain the blood pressure. Albumin provides maximum viscosity than the other plasma proteins.

7. ROLE IN ERYTHROCYTE SEDIMENTATION RATE (ESR)

Globulin and fibrinogen accelerate the tendency of **rouleaux formation** by the red blood cells. Rouleaux formation is responsible for ESR, which is an important diagnostic and prognostic tool (Chapter 8).

8. ROLE IN SUSPENSION STABILITY OF RED BLOOD CELLS

During circulation, red blood cells remain suspended uniformly in the blood. This property of the red blood cells is called the suspension stability. Globulin and fibrinogen help in the suspension stability of the red blood cells.

9. ROLE IN PRODUCTION OF TREPHONE SUBSTANCES

Trephone substances are necessary for nourishment of tissue cells in culture. These substances are produced by leukocytes from the plasma proteins.

10. ROLE AS RESERVE PROTEINS

During fasting, inadequate food intake or inadequate protein intake, the plasma proteins are utilized by the body tissues as the last source of energy. The plasma proteins are split into amino acids by the tissue macrophages. The amino acids are taken back by blood and distributed throughout the body to form cellular protein molecules. Because of this, the plasma proteins are called the **reserve proteins**.

PLASMAPHERESIS AND THERAPEUTIC PLASMA EXCHANGE

PLASMAPHERESIS

Plasmapheresis is an experimental procedure done in animals to demonstrate the importance of plasma proteins.

Procedure

Plasmapheresis is demonstrated in dogs. Blood is removed completely from the body of the dog. Red blood cells are separated from plasma and are washed in saline and reinfused into the body of the same dog along with a physiological solution called **Locke's solution.**

Due to sudden lack of proteins, the animal undergoes a state of shock. If the animal is fed with diet containing sufficiently high quantity of proteins, the normal level of plasma proteins is restored within 7 days and the animal survives. The new plasma proteins are also synthesized by the liver of the dog.

If the experiment is done in animals after removal of liver, even if the diet contains adequate quantity of proteins, the plasma proteins are not produced. The shock persists in the animal and leads to death.

Thus, this experiment 'plasmapheresis' is used to demonstrate:

1. Importance of plasma proteins for survival.
2. Synthesis of plasma proteins by the liver.

THERAPEUTIC PLASMA EXCHANGE

Therapeutic plasma exchange is a blood purification procedure by which plasma is replaced by blood substitutes. Patient's blood is passed through a machine which removes the plasma and returns the blood cells to patient's blood stream along with blood substitutes. This procedure is used for an effective temporary treatment of many autoimmune diseases.

In an **autoimmune disease**, the immune system attacks body's own tissues through antibodies (Chapter 15). The antibodies that are proteins in nature circulate in the bloodstream before attacking the target tissues. This procedure is used to remove these antibodies from the blood.

Though purification producer is used to remove antibodies from the blood, it cannot prevent the production of antibodies by the immune system of the body. So, it can provide only a temporary benefit of protecting the tissues from the antibodies. The patients must go for repeated sessions of this treatment.

APPLIED PHYSIOLOGY: VARIATIONS IN PLASMA PROTEIN LEVEL

Level of plasma proteins vary independently of one another. However, in several conditions, the quantity of albumin and globulin change in opposite direction. Elevation of all fractions of plasma proteins is called **hyperproteinemia** and decrease in all fractions of plasma proteins is called **hypoproteinemia**.

Chapter 8: Red Blood Cells

CHAPTER OUTLINE

- **DEFINITION**
- **NORMAL COUNT**
- **MORPHOLOGY**
- **PROPERTIES**
- **LIFESPAN**
- **FATE**
- **FUNCTIONS**
- **VARIATIONS IN NUMBER**
- **VARIATIONS IN SIZE**
- **VARIATIONS IN SHAPE**

■ DEFINITION

Red blood cells (RBCs) or **erythrocytes** are the **non-nucleated** formed elements in the blood. Red color of the RBC is due to the presence of hemoglobin.

■ NORMAL RBC COUNT

RBC count ranges between 4 and 5.5 million/cu mm of blood. In adult males, it is 5 million/cu mm and in adult females it is 4.5 million/cu mm.

■ MORPHOLOGY OF RED BLOOD CELLS

■ NORMAL SHAPE

Normally, RBCs are disk shaped and biconcave (**dumbbell shaped**). The central portion is thinner and periphery is thicker. The biconcave contour of RBCs has some mechanical and functional advantages.

Advantages of Biconcave Shape of RBCs

Biconcave shape of RBCs has some functional advantages which are given in **Box 8.1**.

■ NORMAL SIZE

Diameter : 7.2 μ (6.9 μ to 7.4 μ)
Thickness : At the periphery it is thicker with 2.2 μ and at the center it is thinner with 1 μ (**Fig. 8.1**). This difference in thickness is because of the biconcave shape
Surface area : 120 sq μ
Volume : 85 cu μ to 90 cu μ

■ NORMAL STRUCTURE

RBC is a non-nucleated cell. Because of the absence of nucleus, the DNA is also absent. Other organelles such as

BOX 8.1: Advantages of biconcave shape of RBCs.

1. Biconcave shape helps in equal and rapid diffusion of oxygen and other substances into the interior of the cell.
2. Large surface area is provided for absorption or removal of different substances from the cell
3. Minimal tension is offered on the membrane when the volume of cell alters.
4. Because of biconcave shape, while passing through minute capillaries, RBCs squeeze through the capillaries very easily without getting damaged.

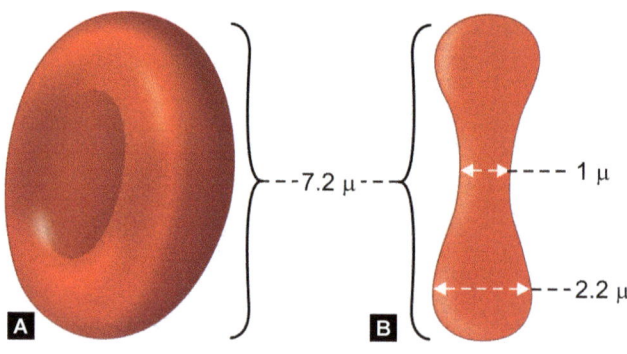

FIGURE 8.1: Dimensions of RBC. **A.** Surface view; **B.** Sectioned view.

mitochondria and Golgi apparatus also are absent in RBC. Since, mitochondria are absent, the energy is produced from glycolytic process.

■ PROPERTIES OF RED BLOOD CELLS

■ 1. ROULEAUX FORMATION

When blood is taken out of the blood vessel, the RBCs pile up one above another like the pile of coins. This property of

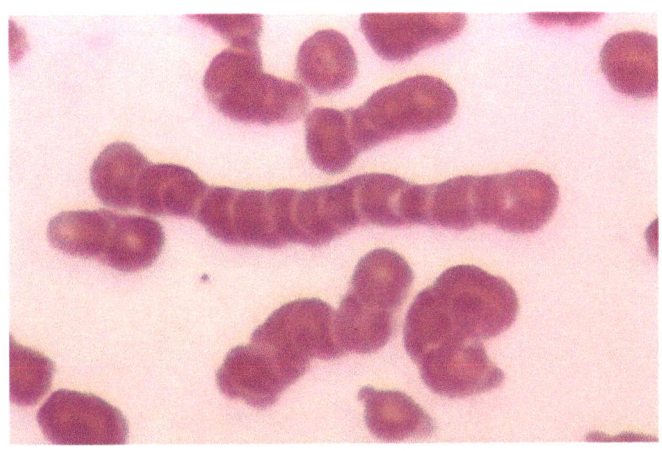

FIGURE 8.2: Rouleaux formation
(*Courtesy:* Dr Nivaldo Medeiros).

the RBCs is called rouleaux (pleural = rouleau) formation **(Fig. 8.2)**. It is accelerated by plasma proteins namely globulin and fibrinogen.

■ 2. SPECIFIC GRAVITY

Specific gravity of RBC is 1.092 to 1.101.

■ 3. PACKED CELL VOLUME

Packed cell volume (PCV) is the volume of the RBCs expressed in percentage. It is also called **hematocrit** value. It is 45% of the blood and the plasma volume is 55% (Chapter 11).

■ 4. SUSPENSION STABILITY

During circulation, the RBCs remain suspended or dispersed uniformly in the blood. This property of the RBCs is called the suspension stability (Chapter 11).

■ LIFESPAN OF RED BLOOD CELLS

Average lifespan of RBC is about 120 days. After the lifetime, the senile (old) RBCs are destroyed in reticuloendothelial system.

■ FATE OF RED BLOOD CELLS

When the RBCs become older (120 days), the cell membrane becomes very fragile. So, these cells are destroyed while trying to squeeze through the capillaries which have lesser or equal diameter as that of RBC. The destruction occurs mainly in the capillaries of spleen because these capillaries are very much narrow. Hence, the spleen is called **graveyard of RBCs**.

Destroyed RBCs are fragmented and hemoglobin is released from the fragmented parts.

Hemoglobin is degraded into iron, **globin** and **porphyrin**. Iron combines with the protein called **apoferritin** to form **ferritin** which is stored in the body and reused later. Globin enters the protein depot for later use **(Fig. 8.3)**. The porphyrin is degraded into **bilirubin**, which is excreted by liver through bile (Chapter 34).

Daily 10% of senile RBCs are destroyed in normal young healthy adults. It causes release of about 0.6 g/dL

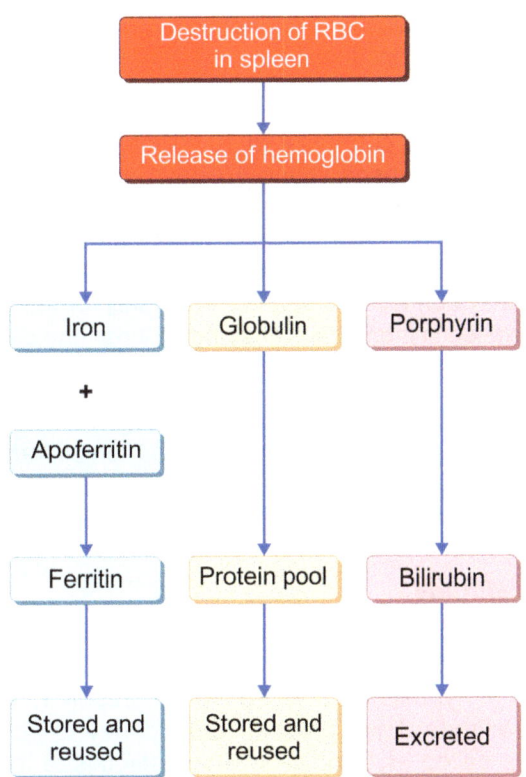

FIGURE 8.3: Fate of RBC.

of hemoglobin into the plasma. From this 0.9 mg/dL to 1.5 mg/dL bilirubin is formed.

■ FUNCTIONS OF RED BLOOD CELLS

1. *Transport of O_2 from the Lungs to the Tissues*

Hemoglobin combines with oxygen to form **oxyhemoglobin** which is transported in blood. About 97% of oxygen is transported in blood as oxyhemoglobin (Chapter 82).

2. *Transport CO_2 from the Tissues to the Lungs*

Hemoglobin combines with carbon dioxide and form **carbhemoglobin**.

3. *Buffering Action in Blood*

Hemoglobin functions as a good buffer. By this action, it regulates the hydrogen ion concentration and thereby plays a role in the maintenance of acid-base balance.

4. *In Blood Group Determination*

RBCs carry the blood group antigens like A antigen, B antigen and Rh factor. This helps in determination of blood group and enables to prevent the reactions due to incompatible blood transfusion (Chapter 19).

■ VARIATIONS IN NUMBER OF RED BLOOD CELLS
■ PHYSIOLOGICAL VARIATIONS

A. *Increase in RBC Count: Polycythemia*

Increase in the RBC count is known as polycythemia. It occurs in both physiological and pathological conditions. When it occurs in physiological conditions it is called **physiological polycythemia**. The increase in number during this condition is marginal and temporary. It occurs in the following conditions.

1. Age

At birth, the RBC count is 8 to 10 million/cu mm of blood. The count decreases within 10 days after birth due to destruction of RBCs. Because of excess destruction of RBCs and liberation of bilirubin, **physiological jaundice** develops in some newborn babies between 2 to 3 days after birth. Such type of jaundice lasts only for few days.

However, in infants and growing children, the cell count is more than that in adults.

2. Sex

Before puberty and after menopause, in females the RBC count is similar to that in males. During reproductive period of females, the count is less than in males (4.5 million/cu mm).

3. High altitude

In people living in mountains (above 10,000 feet from mean sea level), the RBC count is more than 7 million/cu mm. It is due to hypoxia (decreased oxygen supply to tissues) in high altitude. Hypoxia stimulates kidney to secrete a hormone called erythropoietin which stimulates the bone marrow to produce more RBCs **(Fig. 8.4)**.

4. Muscular exercise

RBC count increases after muscular exercise. It is because of mild hypoxia which increases the sympathetic activity secretion of adrenaline from adrenal medulla. Adrenaline contracts spleen and RBCs are released into blood. Hypoxia also causes secretion of erythropoietin which stimulates the bone marrow to produce more RBCs.

5. Emotional conditions

The RBC count increases during the emotional conditions such as anxiety. It is because of increase in the sympathetic activity and contraction of spleen **(Fig. 8.5)**.

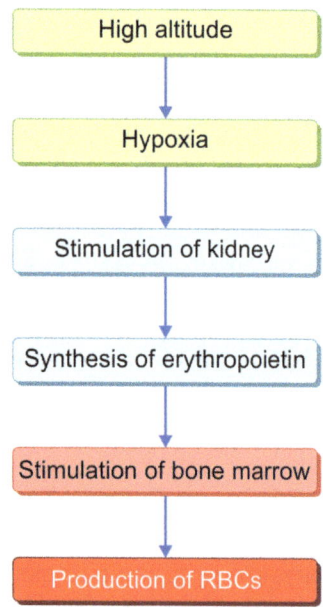

FIGURE 8.4: Physiological polycythemia in high altitude.

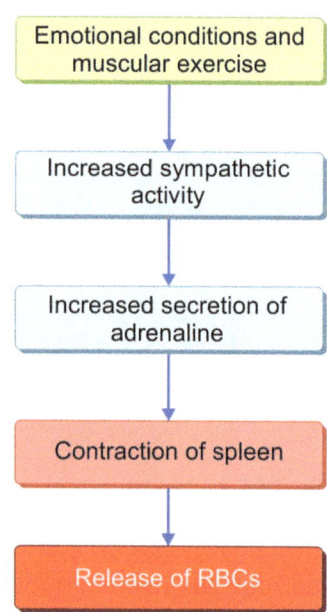

FIGURE 8.5: Physiological polycythemia in emotional conditions and exercise.

6. Increased environmental temperature

Generally increased temperature increases all the activities in the body including production of RBCs.

7. After meals

There is a slight increase in the RBC count after taking meals. It is because of need for more oxygen for metabolic activities.

B. Decrease in RBC Count

Decrease in RBC count occurs in the following physiological conditions.

1. High barometric pressures

At high barometric pressures as in deep sea, where the oxygen tension of blood is higher, the RBC count decreases.

2. During sleep

Generally, all the activities of the body are decreased during sleep including production of RBCs.

3. Pregnancy

In pregnancy, the RBC count decreases. It is because of increase in ECF volume. Increase in ECF volume, increases the plasma volume also resulting in **hemodilution**. So, there is a relative reduction in the RBC count.

■ PATHOLOGICAL VARIATIONS

Pathological Polycythemia

Pathological polycythemia is the abnormal increase in the RBC count. The count increases above 7 million/cu mm of the blood. Polycythemia is of two types, the primary polycythemia and secondary polycythemia.

Primary polycythemia: Polycythemia vera

Primary polycythemia is otherwise known as polycythemia vera. It is a disease characterized by persistent increase in

RBC count above 14 million/cu mm of blood. This is always associated with increased WBC count above 24,000/cu mm of blood. Polycythemia vera occurs due to malignancy of red bone marrow.

Secondary polycythemia

It is the pathological condition in which polycythemia occurs because of diseases in some other system such as:

1. Respiratory disorders like emphysema.
2. Congenital heart disease.
3. **Ayerza's disease**, a condition associated with hypertrophy of right ventricle and obstruction of blood flow to lungs.
4. Chronic carbon monoxide poisoning.
5. Poisoning by chemicals such as phosphorus and arsenic.
6. Repeated mild hemorrhages.

All these conditions lead to hypoxia which stimulates release of erythropoietin. Erythropoietin stimulates the bone marrow resulting in increased RBC count.

Anemia

Anemia is the abnormal decrease in RBC count. It is described in Chapter 12.

VARIATIONS IN SIZE OF RED BLOOD CELLS

Under physiological conditions, the size of RBCs in venous blood is slightly larger than those in arterial blood. In pathological conditions, the variations in size of RBCs are:

1. Microcytes   : Smaller cells.
2. Macrocytes   : Larger cells.
3. Anisocytosis : Cells without uniform size.

1. Microcytes

Microcytes are present in:

a. Iron deficiency anemia.
b. Prolonged forced breathing.
c. Increased osmotic pressure in blood.

2. Macrocytes

Macrocytes are present in:

a. Megaloblastic anemia.
b. Muscular exercise.
c. Decreased osmotic pressure in blood.

3. Anisocytes

Anisocytes occurs in pernicious anemia.

VARIATIONS IN SHAPE OF RED BLOOD CELLS

Shape of RBCs is altered in many conditions including different types of anemia:

1. **Crenation**: Shrinkage as in hypertonic conditions.
2. **Spherocytosis**: Globular form as in hypotonic conditions.
3. **Elliptocytosis**: Elliptical shape as in certain types of anemia.
4. **Sickle cell**: Crescentic shape as in sickle cell anemia.
5. **Poikilocytosis**: Unusual variations in shape due to deformed cell membrane. The shape will be of flask, hammer or any other unusual shape.

Chapter 9

Erythropoiesis

CHAPTER OUTLINE

- DEFINITION
- SITE OF ERYTHROPOIESIS
  - IN FETAL LIFE
  - IN NEWBORN BABIES, CHILDREN AND ADULTS
- PROCESS OF ERYTHROPOIESIS
  - STEM CELLS
- CHANGES DURING ERYTHROPOIESIS
- STAGES OF ERYTHROPOIESIS
- FACTORS NECESSARY FOR ERYTHROPOIESIS
  - STIMULATING FACTORS
  - MATURATION FACTORS
  - FACTORS NECESSARY FOR HEMOGLOBIN FORMATION

DEFINITION

Erythropoiesis is the process of origin, development and maturation of erythrocytes. **Hemopoiesis** is the process of origin, development and maturation of all the blood cells.

SITE OF ERYTHROPOIESIS

IN FETAL LIFE

In fetal life, the erythropoiesis occurs in different sites in different periods.

1. Mesoblastic Stage

During the first 2 or 3 months (first trimester) of intrauterine life, the RBCs are produced from mesenchymal cells of **yolk sac**.

2. Hepatic Stage

During the next 3 months (second trimester) of intrauterine life, RBCs are produced mainly from the liver. Some cells are produced from the spleen and lymphoid organs are also.

3. Myeloid Stage

During the last 3 months (third trimester) of intrauterine life, the RBCs are produced from red bone marrow and liver.

IN NEWBORN BABIES, CHILDREN AND ADULTS

1. Up to the age of 20 years: RBCs are produced from red bone marrow of all bones.
2. After the age of 20 years: RBCs are produced from all the membranous bones and ends of long bones.

PROCESS OF ERYTHROPOIESIS

STEM CELLS

In bone marrow, RBCs develop from **hematopoietic stem cells (Fig. 9.1)** which are called uncommitted **pluripotent hematopoietic stem cells** (PHSC). PHSC are not designed to form a particular type of blood cell; hence the name **uncommitted PHSC**. When the cells are designed to form a particular type of blood cell, the uncommitted PHSCs are called **committed PHSC**.

Committed PHSCs are of two types:

1. **Lymphoid stem cells** (LSC) which give rise to lymphocytes and natural killer (NK) cells.
2. **Colony-forming blastocytes**, which give rise to blood cells other than lymphocytes. When grown in cultures, these cells form colonies hence, name colony-forming blastocytes. Different units of colony-forming cells are:
   i. Colony-forming unit-erythrocytes (CFU-E) from which RBCs develop.
   ii. Colony-forming unit-granulocytes/monocytes (CFU-GM) from which granulocytes (neutrophils, basophils and eosinophils) and monocytes develop.
   iii. Colony-forming unit-megakaryocytes (CFU-M) from which platelets develop.

CHANGES DURING ERYTHROPOIESIS

When the cells of CFU-E pass through different stages and finally become the matured RBCs, four important changes are noticed:

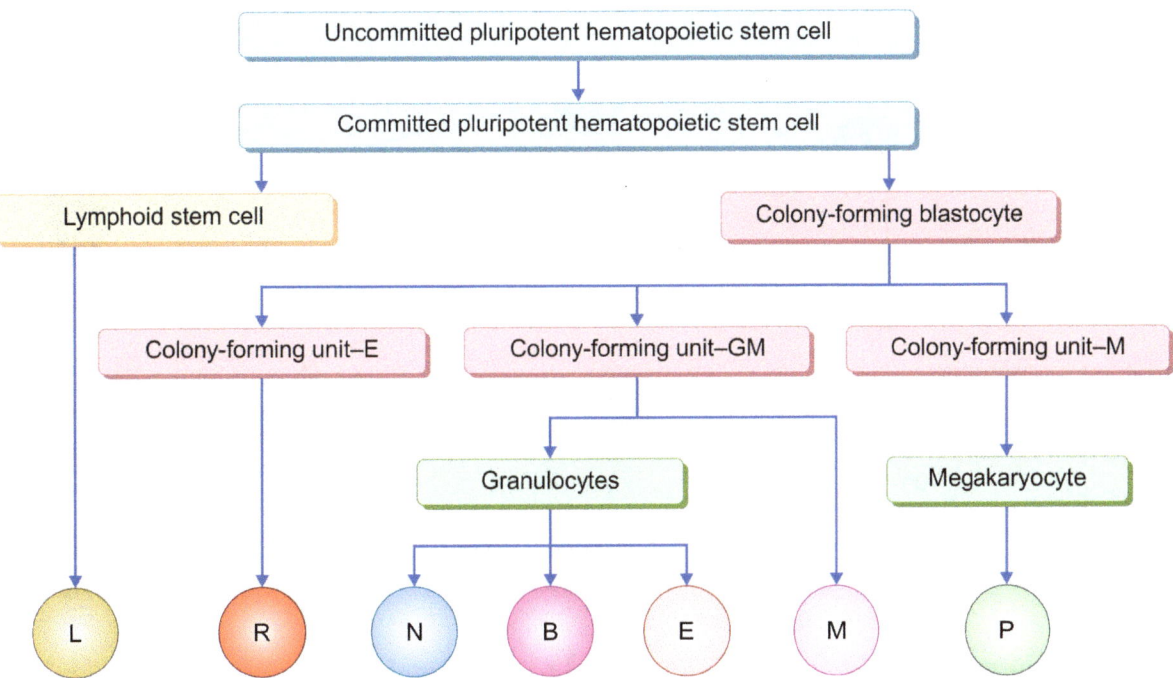

FIGURE 9.1: Stem cells. L = Lymphocyte, R = Red blood cell, N = Neutrophil, B = Basophil, E = Eosinophil, M = Monocyte. P = Platelet.

1. Diameter of the cell is reduced to 7.2 μ from 25 μ.
2. Disappearance of nucleoli and nucleus.
3. Appearance of hemoglobin.
4. Change in the staining properties of the cytoplasm.

■ STAGES OF ERYTHROPOIESIS

Various stages between CFU-E cells and matured RBC are:

1. Proerythroblast.
2. Early normoblast.
3. Intermediate normoblast.
4. Late normoblast.
5. Reticulocyte.
6. Matured erythrocyte.

1. Proerythroblast (Megaloblast)

Proerythroblast or megaloblast is very large in size with a diameter of about 20 μ. A large nucleus with two or more nucleoli and a **chromatin network** is present. Hemoglobin is absent. The cytoplasm is **basophilic** in nature. The proerythroblast multiplies several times and finally forms the cell of next stage called early normoblast **(Fig. 9.2)**.

2. Early Normoblast

It is smaller than proerythroblast with a diameter of about 15 μ. The nucleoli disappear from the nucleus and condensation of chromatin network occurs. The condensed network becomes dense. The cytoplasm is **basophilic** in nature. So, this cell is also called **basophilic erythroblast**. This cell develops into the next stage called intermediate normoblast.

3. Intermediate Normoblast

It is smaller than the early normoblast with a diameter of 10 to 12 μ. The nucleus is still present. But the chromatin network shows further condensation. This stage is marked by the appearance of hemoglobin. Because of the presence of small quantity of acidic hemoglobin, the cytoplasm which is basophilic becomes **polychromatic**, i.e. both acidic and basic in nature. So, this cell is called polychromophilic or **polychromatic erythroblast**. This cell develops into the next stage called late normoblast.

4. Late Normoblast

Diameter of the cell decreases further to about 8 to 10 μ. Nucleus becomes very small with very much condensed chromatin network and is called **ink spot nucleus**. Quantity of hemoglobin increases making the cytoplasm almost **acidophilic**. So, the cell is now called **orthochromatic erythroblast**. At the end of late normoblastic stage, just before it passes to the next stage, the nucleus disintegrates and disappears by the process called **pyknosis**. The final remnant is extruded from the cell. Late normoblast develops into the next stage called reticulocyte.

5. Reticulocyte

It is slightly larger than matured RBC and it is otherwise known as **immature RBC**. It is called reticulocyte because, the **reticular network** or reticulum that is formed from the disintegrated organelles are present in the cytoplasm.

In newborn babies, the reticulocyte count is 2 to 6% of RBCs, i.e. 2 to 6 reticulocytes are present for every 100 RBCs. The number of reticulocytes decreases during the 1st week after birth. Later, the reticulocyte count remains constant at or below 1%. The number increases whenever the erythropoietic activity increases. Reticulocytes can enter the capillaries through the capillary membrane from the site of production by diapedesis.

Important events during erythropoiesis are given in **Table 9.1**.

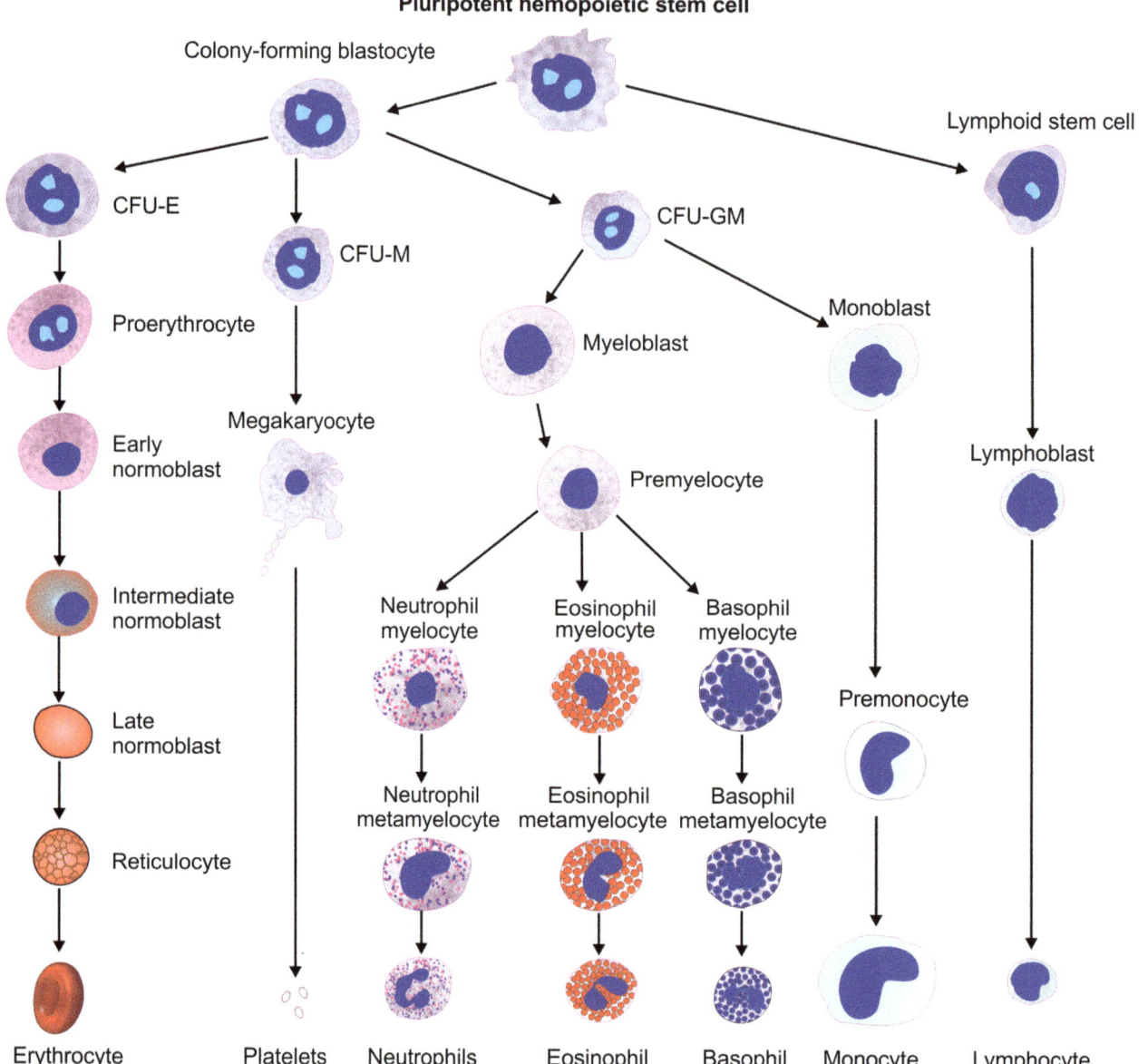

FIGURE 9.2: Stages of hemopoiesis. CFU-E = Colony-forming unit-erythrocyte, CFU-M = Colony-forming unit-megakaryocyte, CFU-GM = Colony-forming unit-granulocyte/monocyte.

TABLE 9.1: Changes during erythropoiesis.

Stage of erythropoiesis	Diameter (μ)	Nucleus	Staining property	Important event
1. Proerythroblast	20	Has two or more nucleoli and chromatin network	Basophilic	Synthesis of hemoglobin starts
2. Early normoblast	15	No nucleoli Dense chromatin network	Basophilic	Nucleoli disappear
3. Intermediate normoblast	10 to 12	Further condensation of chromatin network	Polychromophilic or polychromatic	Hemoglobin starts appearing
4. Late normoblast	8 to 10	Small with very much condensed chromatin Ink-spot nucleus	Acidophilic	Nucleus disappears by pyknosis
5. Reticulocyte	7 to 7.5	Absent	Basophilic	Reticulum is formed Cell enters capillary from site of production
6. Matured RBC	7.2	Absent	Acidophilic	Reticulum disappears Cell attains biconcavity

6. Matured Erythrocyte

Cell decreases in size with the diameter of 7.2 µ. The reticular network disappears and the cell becomes matured RBC with biconcave shape and hemoglobin but without nucleus. It requires 7 days for the proerythroblast to become fully developed and matured of RBC.

■ FACTORS NECESSARY FOR ERYTHROPOIESIS

Development and maturation of erythrocytes require many factors which are classified into three categories:

I. Stimulating factors.
II. Maturation factors.
III. Factors necessary for hemoglobin formation.

■ STIMULATING FACTORS

1. Hypoxia

Hypoxia is the decreased availability of oxygen to the tissues. It is the most important stimulating factor for erythropoiesis. It stimulates erythropoiesis by inducing secretion of erythropoietin from kidney.

2. Erythropoietin

Erythropoietin is a hormone secreted by peritubular capillaries in the kidney. And a small quantity is also secreted from liver and brain. Hypoxia is the stimulant for the secretion of erythropoietin.

Erythropoietin promotes the following processes:

i. Production of proerythroblasts from CFU-E of the bone marrow.
ii. Development of proerythroblasts into matured RBCs through the several stages.
iii. Release of matured erythrocytes into blood. Some reticulocytes are also released along with matured RBCs.

3. Thyroxine

Being a general metabolic hormone, thyroxine accelerates the process of erythropoiesis at many levels.

4. Role of Sex Hormones

Testosterone has mild erythropoietic action after puberty. Action of estrogen on erythropoiesis in not clearly understood. In animals, estrogen suppresses erythropoiesis.

5. Hematopoietic Growth Factors

Hematopoietic growth factors or **growth inducers** are the interleukins 3, 6 and 11 and **stem cell factor** (steel factor). Generally, these factors induce the proliferation of PHSCs.

6. Vitamins

Vitamins B_3, B_6, C, D and E are necessary for erythropoiesis **(Table 9.2)**. Deficiency of these vitamins causes anemia.

■ MATURATION FACTORS

Vitamin B_{12}, intrinsic factor and folic acid are necessary for the maturation of RBCs.

1. Vitamin B_{12} (Cyanocobalamin)

Vitamin B_{12} is essential for synthesis of DNA, cell division and maturation in RBCs. It is also called **extrinsic factor** because it is obtained mostly from diet. It is also produced in the large intestine by the intestinal flora. It is absorbed from the small intestine in the presence of intrinsic factor of Castle. Vitamin B_{12} is stored mostly in liver and in small quantity in muscle. Deficiency of vitamin B_{12} causes **pernicious anemia** (macrocytic anemia) in which the cells remain larger with fragile and weak cell membrane.

2. Intrinsic Factor of Castle

Intrinsic factor is produced in gastric mucosa by the parietal cells of the gastric glands. It is essential for the absorption of vitamin B_{12} from intestine. Absence of intrinsic factor also leads to pernicious anemia because of failure of vitamin B_{12} absorption. The deficiency of intrinsic factor occurs in conditions like severe gastritis, ulcer and gastrectomy.

3. Folic Acid

Folic acid is also essential for the synthesis of DNA. Deficiency of folic acid decreases the DNA synthesis causing maturation failure. Here the cells are larger and remain in megaloblastic (proerythroblastic) stage which leads to **megaloblastic anemia**.

■ FACTORS NECESSARY FOR HEMOGLOBIN FORMATION

Various materials are essential for the formation of hemoglobin in the RBCs such as:

1. First class proteins and amino acids of high biological value are required for formation of globin.
2. Iron is necessary for formation of heme part of the hemoglobin.
3. Copper helps absorption of iron from GI tract.
4. Cobalt and nickel help utilization of iron during hemoglobin synthesis.
5. Vitamins C, B_2, B_3, and B_6 are essential for hemoglobin synthesis.

TABLE 9.2: Factors necessary for erythropoiesis.

Stimulating factors	Maturation factors	Factors necessary for hemoglobin formation
1. Hypoxia 2. Erythropoietin 3. Thyroxine 4. Hematopoietic growth factors 5. Vitamins: B_3, B_6, C, D and E	1. Vitamin B_{12} 2. Intrinsic factor 3. Folic acid	1. First class proteins and amino acids 2. Iron 3. Copper 4. Cobalt and nickel 5. Vitamins: C, B_2, B_3 and B_6

Chapter 10: Hemoglobin and Iron Metabolism

CHAPTER OUTLINE

- DEFINITION
- NORMAL HEMOGLOBIN CONTENT
- FUNCTIONS
- STRUCTURE
- TYPES OF NORMAL HEMOGLOBIN
- ABNORMAL HEMOGLOBIN
- ABNORMAL HEMOGLOBIN DERIVATIVES
- SYNTHESIS
- DESTRUCTION
- IRON METABOLISM

DEFINITION

Hemoglobin (Hb) is the iron-containing coloring pigment of red blood cell. It forms 95% of dry weight of RBC and 30 to 34% of wet weight. Molecular weight of hemoglobin is 68,000.

NORMAL HEMOGLOBIN CONTENT

Average hemoglobin content in blood is 14 to 16 g/dL. However, it varies depending upon age and sex of the individual and the number of RBCs.

Age

At birth	: 25 g/dL
After 3rd month	: 20 g/dL
After 1 year	: 17 g/dL
From puberty onwards	: 14 to 16 g/dL

At the time of birth, infants and growing children, hemoglobin content is high because of increased number of RBCs (Chapter 8).

Sex

In adult males	: 15 g/dL
In adult females	: 14.5 g/dL

FUNCTIONS OF HEMOGLOBIN

TRANSPORT OF RESPIRATORY GASES

Major function of hemoglobin is the transport of respiratory gases. It transports:

1. Oxygen from the lungs to tissues.
2. Carbon dioxide from tissues to lungs (Chapter 82).

BUFFER ACTION

Hemoglobin acts as a buffer and plays an important role in acid-base balance.

STRUCTURE OF HEMOGLOBIN

Hemoglobin is a conjugated protein. It consists of a protein called **globin** and an iron-containing pigment called **heme**.

Globin is made up of four polypeptide chains. Among the four polypeptide chains, two are α-chains and two are β-chains **(Table 10.1)**.

Iron is present in an unstable ferrous (Fe^{2+}) form. Heme part is called **porphyrin**. It is formed by four **pyrrole rings** (tetrapyrrole). The iron is attached to each pyrrole ring and globin molecule.

TYPES OF NORMAL HEMOGLOBIN

Hemoglobin is of two types:

1. **Adult hemoglobin** (HbA).
2. **Fetal hemoglobin** (HbF).

Both the types of hemoglobin differ from each other structurally and functionally.

TABLE 10.1: Molecular weight and number of amino acids of polypeptide chains of globin.

Polypeptide chain	Molecular weight	Amino acids
α-chain	15,126	141
β-chain	15,866	146

Structural Difference

In adult hemoglobin, the globin contains two α-chains and two β-chains. In fetal hemoglobin, there are two α-chains and two γ-chains instead of β-chains **(Table 10.2)**.

Functional Difference

Functionally, fetal hemoglobin has more affinity for oxygen than adult hemoglobin. And, the oxygen-hemoglobin dissociation curve of fetal blood is shifted to left (Chapter 82).

■ ABNORMAL HEMOGLOBIN

Abnormal types of hemoglobin are produced because of structural changes in the polypeptide chains caused by mutation in the genes of the globin chains.

Abnormal hemoglobin is of two categories:

1. Abnormal hemoglobin in hemoglobinopathies.
2. Abnormal hemoglobin in thalassemia and related disorders.

1. Abnormal Hemoglobin in Hemoglobinopathies

Hemoglobinopathy is a genetic disorder caused by abnormal polypeptide chains of hemoglobin. Some of the hemoglobinopathies are HbS, HbC, HbE, HbH and HbM.

2. Abnormal Hemoglobin in Thalassemia and Related Disorders

In thalassemia, different types of abnormal hemoglobin are present. The polypeptide chains are decreased, absent or abnormal (Chapter 12).

■ ABNORMAL HEMOGLOBIN DERIVATIVES

Abnormal hemoglobin formed by the combination of hemoglobin with substances other than oxygen and carbon dioxide is called **hemoglobin derivative**. Abnormal hemoglobin derivatives are formed by carbon monoxide poisoning or due to the combination of some drugs like nitrites, nitrates and sulfonamides with hemoglobin.

High levels of hemoglobin derivatives in blood produce serious effects by preventing the transport of oxygen. It results in oxygen lack in tissues, which may be fatal.

Abnormal hemoglobin derivatives are:

1. Carboxyhemoglobin
2. Methemoglobin
3. Sulfhemoglobin

TABLE 10.2: Types of normal hemoglobin.

Type	Polypeptide chains in globin
HbA: Adult hemoglobin	Two α-chains and Two β-chains
HbF: Fetal hemoglobin	Two α-chains and Two γ-chains

■ CARBOXYHEMOGLOBIN

Carboxyhemoglobin or **carbon monoxyhemoglobin** is the abnormal hemoglobin derivative formed by the combination of carbon monoxide with hemoglobin **(Table 10.3)**. Carbon monoxide is a colorless and odorless gas. Since hemoglobin has 200 times more affinity for **carbon monoxide** than oxygen, it hinders the transport of oxygen resulting in tissue hypoxia (Chapter 82).

Sources of Carbon Monoxide

Some of the sources of carbon monoxide are charcoal burning, coal mines, deep wells, underground drainage system, exhaust of gasoline engines, gases from guns and other weapons, heating system with poor or improper ventilation, smoke from fire and tobacco smoking.

Signs and Symptoms of Carbon Monoxide Poisoning

1. While breathing air with less than 1% of carbon monoxide, the hemoglobin saturation is 15 to 20% and mild symptoms such as headache and nausea appear.
2. While breathing air with more than 1% carbon monoxide, the hemoglobin saturation is 30 to 40%. It causes severe symptoms like convulsions, cardiorespiratory arrest, unconsciousness and coma.
3. When hemoglobin saturation increases above 50%, death occurs.

■ METHEMOGLOBIN

Methemoglobin is the abnormal hemoglobin derivative formed when iron molecule of hemoglobin is oxidized from normal ferrous state to ferric state. Methemoglobin is also called **ferrihemoglobin**. Normal methemoglobin level is less than 3% of total hemoglobin.

Some of the sources of methemoglobin are contaminated well waters with nitrates and nitrites, matchsticks, explosives, naphthalene balls and irritant gases like nitrous oxide.

■ SULFHEMOGLOBIN

Sulfhemoglobin is the abnormal hemoglobin derivative formed by the combination of hemoglobin with hydrogen sulfide. It is caused by drugs such as sulfonamides. Normal sulfhemoglobin level is less than 1% of total hemoglobin.

TABLE 10.3: Formation of abnormal hemoglobin derivatives.

Derivative	Formation
Carboxyhemoglobin	By combination of hemoglobin with carbon monoxide
Methemoglobin	By oxidation of hemoglobin from ferrous state to ferric state
Sulfhemoglobin	By combination of hemoglobin with hydrogen sulfide

SYNTHESIS OF HEMOGLOBIN

Synthesis of hemoglobin actually starts in proerythroblastic stage. However, hemoglobin appears only in the intermediate normoblastic stage. Synthesis of the hemoglobin is continued until the stage of reticulocyte. The heme portion of hemoglobin is synthesized in mitochondria. And the protein part (globin) is synthesized in ribosomes.

SYNTHESIS OF HEME

Heme is synthesized from **succinyl-CoA** and glycine in the mitochondria.

FORMATION OF GLOBIN

The polypeptide chains of globin are produced in the ribosomes. There are four types of polypeptide chains namely, alpha, beta, gamma and delta chains. Each globin molecule is formed by the combination of 2 pairs of chains. Adult hemoglobin contains two alpha chains and two beta chains. Fetal hemoglobin contains two alpha chains and two gamma chains.

CONFIGURATION

Each polypeptide chain combines with one heme molecule. Thus, after the complete configuration, each hemoglobin molecule contains 4 polypeptide chains and 4 heme molecules.

SUBSTANCES NECESSARY FOR HEMOGLOBIN SYNTHESIS

Various factors are essential for the formation of hemoglobin in the RBC. Refer Chapter 9 for details.

DESTRUCTION OF HEMOGLOBIN

After the lifespan of 120 days, the RBC is destroyed in the reticuloendothelial system, particularly in spleen and the hemoglobin is released into plasma. Soon, the hemoglobin is degraded in the reticuloendothelial cells and split into globin, iron and porphyrin **(Fig. 8.3)**.

Globin is utilized for the resynthesis of hemoglobin. Iron is stored in the body. Porphyrin is converted into **biliverdin**. Most of the biliverdin is converted into **bilirubin**. Bilirubin and biliverdin are together called the bile pigments (Chapter 34).

IRON METABOLISM

IMPORTANCE OF IRON

Iron is an essential mineral and an important component of proteins, involved in oxygen transport. Iron is important for the formation of hemoglobin and myoglobin. Iron is also necessary for the formation of other substances such as cytochrome, cytochrome oxidase, peroxidase and catalase.

NORMAL VALUES AND DISTRIBUTION OF IRON IN THE BODY

Total quantity of iron in the body is about 4 g.

Approximate distribution of iron in the body:

1. In blood : 50 to 150 µg/dL
2. In the hemoglobin : 65 to 68%
3. In the muscle as myoglobin : 4%
4. As intracellular oxidative heme compound : 1%
5. In the plasma as transferrin : 0.1%
6. Stored in reticuloendothelial system : 25 to 30%

DIETARY IRON

Dietary iron is available in two forms called heme and nonheme.

Heme Iron

Heme iron is present in fish, meat and chicken. Heme iron is absorbed easily from intestine.

Nonheme Iron

Iron in the form of nonheme is available in vegetables, grains and cereals. Nonheme iron is not absorbed easily as heme iron. Cereals, flours and products of grains which are enriched or fortified (strengthened) with iron, become good dietary sources of nonheme iron, particularly for children and women.

ABSORPTION OF IRON

Iron is absorbed mainly from the small intestine. It is absorbed through the intestinal cells (enterocytes) by pinocytosis and transported into the blood. Bile is essential for the absorption of iron.

Iron is present mostly in ferric (Fe^{3+}) form. It is converted into ferrous form (Fe^{2+}) which is absorbed into the blood.

TRANSPORT OF IRON

Immediately after absorption into blood, iron combines with a **β-globulin** called **apotransferrin** (secreted by liver) resulting in the formation of **transferrin.** And iron is transported in blood in the form of transferrin. Iron combines loosely with globin and can be released easily at any region of the body.

STORAGE OF IRON

Iron is stored in large quantities in reticuloendothelial cells and hepatocytes in liver. It is stored in other cells also but in small quantities. In the cytoplasm of the cell, iron is stored as ferritin in large amount. Small quantity of iron is also stored as **hemosiderin**.

DAILY LOSS OF IRON

In males, about 1 mg of iron is excreted everyday through feces. In females, the amount of iron loss is very much high. This is because of the menstruation. During every menstrual cycle, about 50 mL of blood is lost by which 25 mg of iron is lost. This is why the iron content is always less in females than in males.

Iron is lost during hemorrhage and blood donation also. If 450 mL of blood is donated, about 225 mg of iron is lost.

■ REGULATION OF TOTAL IRON IN THE BODY

Absorption and excretion of iron are maintained almost equally under normal physiological conditions. When the iron storage is saturated in the body, it automatically reduces further absorption of iron from the gastrointestinal tract by feedback mechanism.

■ APPLIED PHYSIOLOGY: IRON DEFICIENCY ANEMIA

Deficiency of iron causes decrease in hemoglobin synthesis resulting in iron deficiency anemia. Refer Chapter 12 for details.

CHAPTER 11

Erythrocyte Sedimentation Rate, Packed Cell Volume and Blood Indices

CHAPTER OUTLINE

- **ERYTHROCYTE SEDIMENTATION RATE**
  - DEFINITION
  - DETERMINATION
  - NORMAL VALUES
  - SIGNIFICANCE OF DETERMINING ESR
  - APPLIED PHYSIOLOGY: VARIATIONS
  - FACTORS AFFECTING ESR
- **PACKED CELL VOLUME**
  - DEFINITION
  - METHOD OF DETERMINATION
  - SIGNIFICANCE OF DETERMINING PCV
  - NORMAL VALUES
  - APPLIED PHYSIOLOGY: VARIATIONS
- **BLOOD INDICES**
  - IMPORTANCE OF BLOOD INDICES
  - DIFFERENT BLOOD INDICES

ERYTHROCYTE SEDIMENTATION RATE

DEFINITION

Erythrocyte sedimentation rate (ESR) is the rate at which the erythrocytes settle down. Normally, when the blood is in circulation, the red blood cells (RBCs) remain suspended uniformly. This property of RBCs is called **suspension stability** of RBCs. If blood is mixed with an anticoagulant and allowed to stand undisturbed on a vertical tube, the red cells settle down due to gravity with a supernatant layer of clear plasma.

DETERMINATION OF ESR

ESR is determined by two methods:

1. Westergren method.
2. Wintrobe method.

1. Westergren Method

In this method, **Westergren tube** is used to determine ESR. This tube is 300 mm long and opened on both ends **(Fig. 11.1A)**. It is marked 0 to 200 mm from above downwards. 1.6 mL of blood is mixed with 0.4 mL of 3.8% **sodium citrate** (anticoagulant). The ratio of blood and anticoagulant is 4:1. This blood is loaded in the Westergren tube up to '0' mark above. Tube is placed vertically in the **Westergren stand** and left undisturbed and reading is taken after 1 hour.

2. Wintrobe Method

In this method, **Wintrobe tube** is used to determine ESR. This tube is a short and opened on one end and closed on the other end **(Fig. 11.1B)**. It is 110 mm long with 3 mm bore. It is used for determining ESR and PCV. It is marked on both sides. On one side, the marking is 0 to 100 (for ESR) and on other side, 100 to 0 (for PCV) from above downwards.

About 1 mL of blood is mixed with an anticoagulant called **ethylenediaminetetra-acetic acid** (**EDTA**). Blood is loaded in the tube up to '0' mark above. Tube is placed on the **Wintrobe stand** and left undisturbed and reading is taken after 1 hour.

NORMAL VALUES OF ESR

Normal values of ESR in both Westergren method and Wintrobe method are given in **Table 11.1**.

SIGNIFICANCE OF DETERMINING ESR

ESR is an easy, inexpensive test which helps in diagnosis as well as prognosis. **Prognosis** means monitoring the course of disease and response of the patient to therapy. Determination of ESR is especially helpful in assessing the progress of patients treated for certain chronic disorders such as pulmonary tuberculosis and rheumatoid arthritis.

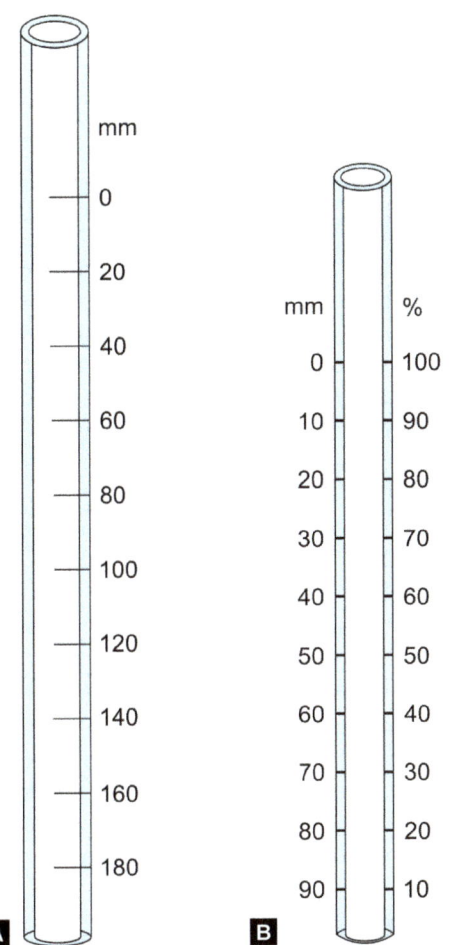

FIGURE 11.1: ESR tubes. **A.** Westergren tube: Used to determine ESR; **B.** Wintrobe tube: Used to determine ESR and PCV.

TABLE 11.1: Normal values of erythrocyte sedimentation rate (ESR).

ESR	Westergren method (mm in 1 hour)	Wintrobe method (mm in 1 hour)
Males	3 to 7	0 to 9
Females	5 to 9	0 to 15
Infants	0 to 2	0 to 5

■ APPLIED PHYSIOLOGY: VARIATIONS OF ESR

Physiological Variation

1. *Age*: ESR is less in children and infants because of large number of RBCs.
2. *Sex*: ESR is more in females than in males because of decreased number of RBCs.
3. *Menstruation*: ESR increases during menstruation because of loss of blood and RBCs.
4. *Pregnancy*: From 3rd month to parturition, ESR increases up to 35 mm in 1 hour because of hemodilution.

Pathological Variation

ESR increases in the following diseases:

1. Tuberculosis.
2. All types of anemia, except sickle cell anemia.
3. Malignant tumors.
4. Rheumatoid arthritis.
5. Rheumatic fever.
6. Liver diseases.

ESR decreases in the following diseases:

1. Allergic conditions.
2. Sickle cell anemia.
3. Peptone shock.
4. Polycythemia.
5. Severe leukocytosis.

■ FACTORS AFFECTING ESR

Following factors increase the ESR:

1. Specific gravity of RBC.
2. Rouleaux formation.
3. Increase in size of RBC.
4. Decrease in RBC count.

Following factors decrease the ESR:

1. Viscosity of blood.
2. Increase in RBC count.

■ PACKED CELL VOLUME
■ DEFINITION

Packed cell volume (PCV) is the volume of the RBCs in the blood that is expressed in percentage. It is also called hematocrit value.

■ METHOD OF DETERMINATION

Blood is mixed with the anticoagulant EDTA or **heparin** and filled in Wintrobe tube up to the 100 or 0 mark above. The tube with the blood is centrifuged at a speed of 3,000 revolutions per minute (rpm) for 30 minutes.

At the end of 30 minutes, the tube is taken out and the reading is taken. RBCs are packed at the bottom and this is the backed cell volume. The plasma remains above this. In between the RBCs and the plasma, there is a **white buffy coat**, which is formed by white blood cells (WBCs) and the platelets **(Fig. 11.2)**.

■ SIGNIFICANCE OF DETERMINING PCV

Determination of PCV helps in:

1. Diagnosis and treatment of anemia.
2. Diagnosis and treatment of polycythemia.
3. Determination of severity of dehydration and recovery from dehydration after treatment.
4. Decision of blood transfusion.

■ NORMAL VALUES OF PCV

Normal PCV:
    In males   : 40 to 45%
    In females   : 38 to 42%

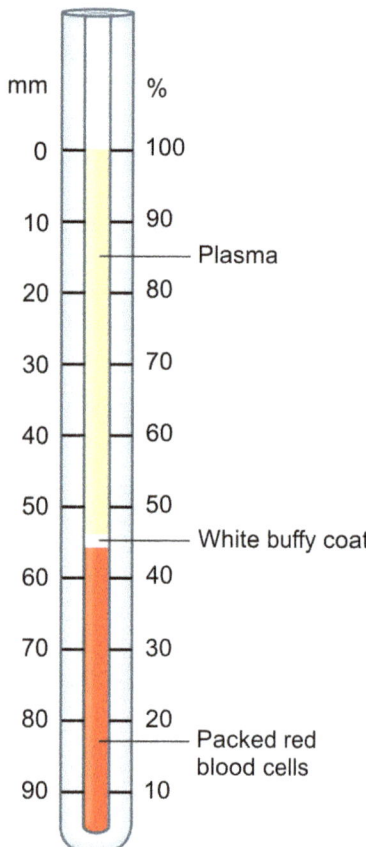

FIGURE 11.2: Packed cell volume.

APPLIED PHYSIOLOGY: VARIATIONS IN PCV

PCV increases in:

1. Polycythemia.
2. Dehydration.
3. **Dengue shock syndrome** (dengue fever of grade III or IV severity). **Dengue fever** is a tropical disease caused by flavivirus, transmitted by mosquito *Aedes aegypti*.

PCV decreases in:

1. Anemia.
2. Cirrhosis of liver.
3. Pregnancy.

BLOOD INDICES

Blood indices are the calculations derived from RBC count, hemoglobin content of blood and PCV.

IMPORTANCE OF BLOOD INDICES

Blood indices help in diagnosis of the type of anemia.

DIFFERENT BLOOD INDICES

Blood indices are:

1. Mean corpuscular volume (MCV).
2. Mean corpuscular hemoglobin (MCH).
3. Mean corpuscular hemoglobin concentration (MCHC).
4. Color index (CI).

1. Mean Corpuscular Volume

Mean corpuscular volume (MCV) is the average volume of a single RBC and it is expressed in cubic micron (cu μ).

Normal MCV: 90 cu μ (78 cu μ to 90 cu μ).

When MCV is normal, the RBC is called **normocyte**. When MCV increases, the cell is known as a **macrocyte** and when it decreases, the cell is called **microcyte**.

In pernicious anemia and megaloblastic anemia, the RBCs are macrocytic in nature. In iron deficiency anemia, the RBCs are microcytic.

2. Mean Corpuscular Hemoglobin

Mean corpuscular hemoglobin (MCH) is the quantity or amount of hemoglobin present in one RBC. It is expressed in picogram (pg).

Normal MCH: 30 pg (27 pg to 32 pg).

3. Mean Corpuscular Hemoglobin Concentration

Mean corpuscular hemoglobin concentration (MCHC) is the concentration of hemoglobin in one RBC. It is the amount of hemoglobin expressed in relation to the volume of one RBC. So, the unit of expression is percentage. This is the most important absolute value in the diagnosis of anemia.

Normal value MCHC: 30% (30 to 38%).

When MCHC is normal, the RBC is **normochromic**. When MCHC decreases, the RBC is known as **hypochromic**. In pernicious anemia and megaloblastic anemia, RBCs are macrocytic and normochromic or hypochromic. In iron deficiency anemia, RBCs are microcytic and hypochromic. A single RBC cannot be hyperchromic because, the amount of hemoglobin cannot increase beyond normal level.

4. Color Index

Color index (CI) is the ratio between the percentage of hemoglobin and the percentage of RBCs in the blood. Actually, it is the average hemoglobin content in one cell of a patient compared to the average hemoglobin content in one cell of a normal person.

Normal color index: 1.0 (0.8 to 1.2).

It is useful in determining the type of anemia. It increases in macrocytic (pernicious) anemia and megaloblastic anemia. It is reduced in iron deficiency anemia. And it is normal in normocytic normochromic anemia.

Chapter 12: Anemia

CHAPTER OUTLINE

- DEFINITION
- CLASSIFICATION
  - MORPHOLOGICAL CLASSIFICATION
  - ETIOLOGICAL CLASSIFICATION
- SIGNS AND SYMPTOMS
  - SKIN
  - HAIR AND NAILS
- CARDIOVASCULAR SYSTEM
- RESPIRATORY SYSTEM
- DIGESTIVE SYSTEM AND METABOLISM
- KIDNEY
- REPRODUCTIVE SYSTEM
- NEUROMUSCULAR SYSTEM

DEFINITION

Anemia is a blood disorder characterized by the reduction in red blood cell count, hemoglobin content and packed cell volume.

CLASSIFICATION OF ANEMIA

Anemia is classified by two methods:

A. Morphological classification.
B. Etiological classification.

MORPHOLOGICAL CLASSIFICATION

By this method, anemia is classified by the morphology (size and color) of RBC. Size of RBC is expressed as mean corpuscular volume (MCV). Color of RBC depends upon hemoglobin concentration in RBC and it is expressed as mean corpuscular hemoglobin concentration (MCHC).

By this method, anemia is classified into four types:

1. Normocytic normochromic anemia.
2. Macrocytic normochromic anemia.
3. Macrocytic hypochromic anemia.
4. Microcytic hypochromic anemia (Table 12.1).

ETIOLOGICAL CLASSIFICATION

In this method, anemia is classified by the cause. Etiology means the study of cause or origin of any disease.

By method, anemia is classified into five types.

1. Hemorrhagic anemia.
2. Hemolytic anemia.
3. Nutrition deficiency anemia.
4. Aplastic anemia.
5. Anemia due to chronic diseases.

1. Hemorrhagic Anemia

Hemorrhage means excessive loss of blood (Chapter 76). Anemia due to hemorrhage is known as hemorrhagic anemia or **blood loss anemia**. It occurs both in acute and chronic hemorrhagic conditions.

TABLE 12.1: Morphological classification of anemia.

Type of anemia	Size of RBC	MCV (cu μ)	Color of RBC	MCHC (%)
Normocytic normochromic	Normal	90	Normal	30
Macrocytic normochromic	Large	More than 90	Normal	30
Macrocytic hypochromic	Large	More than 90	Less	Less than 30
Microcytic hypochromic	Small	Less than 78	Less	Less than 30

Acute hemorrhage

Acute hemorrhage means sudden loss of large quantity of blood as in case of accidents. RBCs are **normocytic** and **normochromic (Table 12.2)**.

Chronic hemorrhage

Chronic hemorrhage refers to loss of blood over a long period of time. Blood loss occurs by internal or external bleeding as in conditions such as peptic ulcer, purpura, hemophilia and menorrhagia. RBCs are **microcytic** and **hypochromic**.

2. Hemolytic Anemia

Hemolysis means destruction of RBCs. Anemia due to excess destruction of RBCs is called hemolytic anemia.

It is classified into two types:

A. Extrinsic hemolytic anemia.
B. Intrinsic hemolytic anemia.

A. Extrinsic hemolytic anemia

This type of anemia caused by destruction of RBCs by external factors. Healthy RBCs are hemolyzed by factors outside the blood cells such as antibodies, chemicals and drugs.

Common causes of extrinsic hemolytic anemia:

i. Liver failure.
ii. Renal disorder.
iii. Hypersplenism.
iv. Burns.
v. Infections like hepatitis, malaria and septicemia.
vi. Drugs such as penicillin, antimalarial drugs and sulfa drugs.
vii. Poisoning by chemical substances such as lead, coal and tar.
viii. Presence of isoagglutinins like anti-Rh.
ix. Autoimmune diseases such as rheumatoid arthritis and ulcerative colitis.

B. Intrinsic hemolytic anemia

This type of anemia is caused by destruction of RBCs due to defective RBCs. There is production of unhealthy RBCs, which are short lived and are destroyed soon. Intrinsic hemolytic anemia is often inherited and it includes sickle cell anemia and thalassemia.

Because of the abnormal shape in sickle cell anemia and thalassemia, the RBCs become more fragile and susceptible for hemolysis.

Sickle cell anemia

Sickle cell anemia is an inherited blood disorder characterized by sickle-shaped RBCs. It occurs when a person inherits two abnormal genes (one from each parent). It is also called **hemoglobin SS disease** or **sickle cell disease**. It is common in people of African origin.

In sickle cell anemia, hemoglobin becomes abnormal with normal α-chains and abnormal β-chains. Because

TABLE 12.2: Etiological classification of anemia.

Type of anemia	Causes		Morphology of RBC
Hemorrhagic anemia	Excess loss of blood by internal or external bleeding		Acute loss: Normocytic and normochromic
			Chronic loss: Microcytic and hypochromic

Hemolytic anemia	Extrinsic hemolytic anemia:
	  i. Liver failure
	  ii. Renal disorder
	  iii. Hypersplenism
	  iv. Burns
	  v. Infections: Hepatitis, malaria and septicemia
	  vi. Drugs: Penicillin, antimalarial drugs and sulfa drugs
	  vii. Poisoning by lead, coal and tar
	  viii. Presence of isoagglutinins like anti-Rh
	  ix. Autoimmune diseases: Rheumatoid arthritis and ulcerative colitis
			Normocytic, normochromic

	Intrinsic hemolytic anemia Hereditary disorders	Sickle cell anemia	Sickle shape
		Thalassemia	Irregular, microcytic and hypochromic
Nutrition deficiency anemia	Iron deficiency		Microcytic, hypochromic
	Protein deficiency		Macrocytic, hypochromic
	Vitamin B_{12} deficiency		Macrocytic, normochromic/hypochromic
	Folic acid deficiency		Megaloblastic, hypochromic
Aplastic anemia	Bone marrow disorder		Normocytic, normochromic
Anemia due to chronic diseases	i. Non-infectious inflammatory diseases: Rheumatoid arthritis ii. Chronic infections: Tuberculosis iii. Chronic renal failure iv. Neoplastic disorders: Hodgkin's disease		Normocytic, normochromic

of this, RBCs attain sickle (crescent) shape and become more fragile leading to hemolysis.

Thalassemia

Thalassemia is an inherited disorder characterized by abnormal hemoglobin. In normal hemoglobin, the number of α- and β-polypeptide chains is equal. In thalassemia, the number of these chains is not equal. This causes the precipitation of the polypeptide chains leading to defective formation of RBCs or hemolysis of the matured RBCs.

It is also known as **Cooley's anemia** or **Mediterranean anemia**. It is more common in Thailand and to some extent in Mediterranean countries.

Thalassemia is of two types:
 i. α-thalassemia.
 ii. β-thalassemia.

The β-thalassemia is more common among these two types.

3. Nutrition Deficiency Anemia

Anemia that occurs due to deficiency of a nutritive substance necessary for erythropoiesis is called nutrition deficiency anemia. Such substances are iron, proteins and vitamins like C, B_{12} and folic acid. The types of nutrition deficiency anemia are detailed below.

Iron deficiency anemia

Iron deficiency anemia is the most common type of anemia. It develops due to inadequate availability of iron for hemoglobin synthesis. RBCs are **microcytic and hypochromic**.

Protein deficiency anemia

Protein deficiency decreases the hemoglobin synthesis. RBCs are **macrocytic and hypochromic**.

Vitamin B_{12} deficiency: Pernicious anemia

Vitamin B_{12} is a maturation factor for RBC and deficiency of this causes pernicious anemia, which is also called **Addison's anemia**. It occurs because of less intake of vitamin B_{12} or poor absorption of vitamin B_{12}. Vitamin B_{12} is absorbed from the stomach with the help of intrinsic factor of Castle, which is secreted in the gastric mucosa. Decrease in the production of intrinsic factor causes poor absorption of vitamin B_{12}. RBCs are **macrocytic and normochromic/hypochromic**.

Folic acid deficiency: Megaloblastic anemia

Folic acid is necessary for the maturation of RBC. Deficiency of this leads to defective DNA synthesis making the nucleus to remain immature. RBCs are **megaloblastic and hypochromic**.

4. Aplastic Anemia

Aplastic anemia is due to the bone marrow disorder. The red bone marrow is reduced and replaced by fatty tissues. It occurs in conditions such as repeated exposure to X-ray or γ-ray radiation, tuberculosis and viral infections like hepatitis and HIV infections. RBCs are **normocytic and normochromic**.

5. Anemia due to Chronic Diseases

Anemia occurs due to some chronic diseases such as rheumatoid arthritis, tuberculosis and chronic renal failure. RBCs are **normocytic and normochromic (Table 12.2)**.

■ SIGNS AND SYMPTOMS OF ANEMIA

■ 1. SKIN

In anemic patients, the color of the skin becomes pale which is observed prominently in buccal cavity, pharyngeal mucous membrane, conjunctivae, lips, ear lobes, palm and nail bed. Skin also loses the elasticity and becomes thin and dry.

■ 2. HAIR AND NAILS

Loss of hair is common with thinning and early graying. The nails become brittle and easily breakable.

■ 3. CARDIOVASCULAR SYSTEM

There is increase in heart rate and cardiac output. Heart is dilated and cardiac murmurs are produced. The velocity of blood flow is increased.

■ 4. RESPIRATORY SYSTEM

Rate and force of respiration increases. Sometimes, it leads to breathlessness and **dyspnea** (difficulty in breathing). Oxygen-hemoglobin dissociation curve is shifted to right.

■ 5. DIGESTIVE SYSTEM AND METABOLISM

Anorexia (loss of appetite), nausea, vomiting, abdominal discomfort and constipation are common. In pernicious anemia, there is atrophy of papillae in tongue. In aplastic anemia, necrotic lesions appear in mouth and pharynx. Basal metabolic rate increases in severe anemia.

■ 6. KIDNEY

Kidney function is disturbed. Albuminuria is common.

■ 7. REPRODUCTIVE SYSTEM

In females, the menstrual cycle is disturbed. There may be menorrhagia, oligomenorrhea or amenorrhea (Chapter 60).

■ 8. NEUROMUSCULAR SYSTEM

Common neuromuscular symptoms are headache, lack of concentration, restlessness, irritability, drowsiness, dizziness or vertigo, especially when standing, increased sensitivity to cold and fainting. Muscles become weak and the patient feels lack of energy and fatigued quite often and quite easily.

Chapter 13: Hemolysis and Fragility of Red Blood Cells

CHAPTER OUTLINE

- DEFINITION
- HEMOLYSIS IN NORMAL CONDITIONS
- HEMOLYSIS IN ABNORMAL CONDITIONS
  - HEMOLYSINS
  - ABNORMAL SHAPE OF RBC
  - DISEASES
- MECHANICAL FACTORS
- FRAGILITY
- DEFINITION
- TYPES
- FRAGILITY TEST

DEFINITION

Hemolysis is the rupture of the blood cells, particularly erythrocytes with the release of hemoglobin into the blood. Hemolysis occurs both in normal and abnormal conditions.

HEMOLYSIS IN NORMAL CONDITIONS

Normally, rupture of red blood cells occurs after the life span of 120 days. The cell membrane of the **senile RBC** becomes fragile and it cannot withstand the stress of squeezing through the thin capillaries. So, the cell ruptures and releases hemoglobin. This process occurs mostly in spleen.

In this way, only 10% of the total RBCs are hemolyzed and so it does not cause any adverse effect in the body.

HEMOLYSIS IN ABNORMAL CONDITIONS

Hemolysis occurs during some abnormal conditions due to the presence of some external factors. In this process, even younger RBCs are broken down in large number and a large quantity of hemoglobin is released into the blood. This may lead to the clinical conditions such as **hemolytic jaundice** and **hemolytic anemia**.

Abnormal hemolysis occurs because of:

1. Hemolysins.
2. Abnormal shape of RBCs.
3. Diseases.
4. Mechanical factors.

1. HEMOLYSINS

Hemolysins or **hemolytic agents** are the substances which cause destruction of RBCs.

Hemolysins are of three types:

i. Hemolysins of bacterial origin.
ii. Hemolysins of animal origin.
iii. Hemolysins in the form of chemical substances.

i. Hemolysins of Bacterial Origin

During bacterial infection, many bacteria produce some toxic substances which become the hemolysins and destroy RBCs. Bacteria which produce hemolysins are gram-positive bacteria like *Streptococcus* species, *Staphylococcus aureus*, *Listeria* species, *Bacillus cereus* and *Clostridium tetani* and gram-negative bacteria like *E. coli*, *Serratia* species, *Proteus* spp and *Pseudomonas aeruginosa*.

ii. Hemolysins of Animal Origin

Venom of poisonous snakes such as cobra and viper contain hemolysins.

iii. Hemolysins in the Form of Chemical Substances

Some of the chemical substances act as hemolysins and cause the death of RBCs. Examples are alcohol, ether, benzene, chloroform, either, acids, alkalis, bile salts and saponin. Some chemical poisons such as arsenic preparations, carbolic acid, nitrobenzene and resin also act like hemolysins.

2. ABNORMAL SHAPE OF RBC

Normal biconcave shape of RBC is essential to prevent hemolysis. But in some hereditary disorders such as sickle cell anemia and thalassemia, RBCs attain abnormal shape like sickle shape, oval shape, elliptical shape, round

TABLE 13.1: Results of fragility test.

Type of observations	Observations	Result
Direct observation	1. Fluid in the tube appears turbid	No hemolysis
	2. Turbidity is reduced	Onset of hemolysis
	3. Fluid becomes clear	Completion of hemolysis
Observations after centrifugation	1. Cells sediment at the bottom with clear colorless fluid above	No hemolysis
	2. Cell sedimentation is less and fluid becomes slightly reddish because of the release of small amount of hemoglobin from few hemolyzed RBCs	Onset of hemolysis
	3. Fluid becomes more reddish without any sedimentation due to release of hemoglobin from all hemolyzed cells	Completion of hemolysis

shape, etc. Membranes of these cells become more fragile resulting in hemolysis.

3. DISEASES

Diseases which cause hemolysis are autoimmune diseases, infections and severe renal failure that needs hemodialysis. Some medications such as cephalosporins, levodopa, non-steroidal anti-inflammatory drugs, penicillin can cause hemolysis by producing antibodies against red blood cells.

4. MECHANICAL FACTORS

Some mechanical factors like physical stress and compression of muscles during severe exercise also can induce hemolysis. This occurs in cases of repeated mechanical movements like prolonged marching, marathon running, and bongo drumming. Freezing the blood at near to 0° temperature is one of the most important mechanical factors in causing destruction of RBCs.

Rarely hemolysis occurs in conditions that involve using artificial kidney for hemodialysis or heart lung bypass machine during cardiac surgery. In such conditions, hemolysis might be induced either mechanically or chemically.

FRAGILITY

DEFINITION

Fragility refers to tendency of RBC to break easily or susceptibility (to be affected) of RBC to hemolysis (Fragile = easily broken).

TYPES OF FRAGILITY

Fragility is of two types:

1. **Osmotic fragility**, which occurs due to exposure to hypotonic saline.

2. **Mechanical fragility**, which occurs due to **mechanical trauma** (wound or injury).

Normally, plasma and RBCs are in osmotic equilibrium. When the osmotic equilibrium is disturbed, the cells are affected. For example, when the RBCs are immersed in hypotonic saline the cells swell and rupture by bursting because of endosmosis. Hemoglobin is released from the ruptured RBCs.

FRAGILITY TEST

Fragility test is a test that measures the resistance of erythrocytes in hypotonic saline solution. It is done by using sodium chloride solution at different concentrations from 1.2% to 0.2%. The solutions at different concentrations are taken in series of **Cohn's tubes**. Then one drop of blood to be tested is added to each tube. The sodium chloride solution and the blood in each tube are mixed well and left undisturbed for some time.

Results can be analyzed by observing the tubes directly or by centrifuging the tubes after 15 minutes **(Table 13.1)**.

Index for Fragility

After 20 minutes:
- No hemolysis : Up to 0.6%
- Onset of hemolysis : Around 0.45%
- Completion of hemolysis : Around 0.35%

At 0.45%, only the older cells are destroyed because, their membrane is fragile. So, these cells cannot withstand this hypotonicity. But younger cells are not affected. At 0.35%, even the younger cells are destroyed.

Chapter 14: White Blood Cells

CHAPTER OUTLINE

- WBC VS RBC
- CLASSIFICATION
- MORPHOLOGY
- NORMAL COUNT
- APPLIED PHYSIOLOGY: VARIATIONS
- LIFESPAN
- PROPERTIES
- FUNCTIONS
- LEUKOPOIESIS

■ WBC VS RBC

White blood cells (WBCs) or **leukocytes** are the colorless and nucleated formed elements of blood (leuko means white or colorless).

Compared to red blood cells (RBCs), the WBC is larger in size and lesser in number. Yet functionally, WBC is as important as RBC. WBCs play important role in defense mechanism of body by acting like soldiers and protecting the body from invading organisms.

WBCs differ from RBCs in many aspects. Differences between these two types of blood cells are given in **Table 14.1**.

■ CLASSIFICATION OF WHITE BLOOD CELLS

White blood cells are classified into two groups depending upon the presence or absence of granules in the cytoplasm:

I. Granulocytes with granules.
II. Agranulocytes without granules.

Granulocytes

Depending upon the staining property of granules, the granulocytes are classified into three types:

1. Neutrophils : Granules take both acidic and basic stains.
2. Eosinophils : Granules take acidic stain.
3. Basophils : Granules take basic stain.

Agranulocytes

Agranulocytes have plain cytoplasm without granules. Agranulocytes are of two types:

1. Monocytes.
2. Lymphocytes.

TABLE 14.1: Differences between white blood cell and red blood cell.

Feature	WBC	RBC
1. Color	Colorless	Red
2. Number	Less: 4,000 to 11,000/cu mm	More: 4.5 to 5.5 million/cu mm
3. Size	Larger with maximum diameter of 18 μ	Smaller with maximum diameter of 7.4 μ
4. Shape	Irregular	Disk shaped and biconcave
5. Hemoglobin	Absent	Present
6. Nucleus	Present	Absent
7. Granules	Present in some types	Absent
8. Types	Many types	Only one type
9. Lifespan	Shorter Ranges from ½ to 15 days	Longer 120 days
10. Functions	Defense and immunity	Transport of oxygen and carbon dioxide Buffering action

■ MORPHOLOGY

Morphology of each white blood cell is different from others.

NEUTROPHILS

Neutrophils are also known as **polymorphonuclear leukocytes** because the nucleus is multilobed. Number of lobes in the nuclei varies from 1 to 6 **(Fig. 14.1)**. Granules are fine or small in size. When stained with **Leishman's stain** which contains acidic eosin and basic methylene blue, the granules take both the stains equally. So, the granules appear violet in color. Diameter of cell is 10 to 12 μ. Neutrophils are ameboid and phagocytic in nature.

EOSINOPHILS

Eosinophils have coarse (larger) granules in the cytoplasm, which stain pink or reddish orange with eosin. Normally, the nucleus is bilobed and spectacle shaped. Rarely trilobed nucleus may be present. Diameter of this cell varies between 10 μ and 14 μ.

BASOPHILS

Basophils also have coarse granules in the cytoplasm and the granules stain purple blue with methylene blue. Nucleus is bilobed. Diameter of this cell is 8 μ to 10 μ.

MONOCYTES

Monocytes are the largest leukocytes with diameter of 14 μ to 18 μ. The cytoplasm is clear without granules. The nucleus is round, oval, horseshoe shaped, bean shaped or kidney shaped. Nucleus is placed either in the center of the cell or pushed to one side and a large amount of cytoplasm is seen.

LYMPHOCYTES

Lymphocytes also do not have granules in cytoplasm. Nucleus is oval, bean shaped or kidney shaped and occupies the whole of the cytoplasm. A rim of cytoplasm may or may not be seen.

Depending upon the size, the lymphocytes are divided into two types:

1. *Large lymphocytes*: Younger cells with a diameter of 10 μ to 12 μ.
2. *Small lymphocytes*: Older cells with a diameter of 7 μ to 10 μ.

NORMAL LEUKOCYTE COUNT

1. *Total leukocyte count (TC)*: 4,000 to 11,000/cu mm of blood.
2. *Differential WBC count (DC)*: Given in **Table 14.2**.

APPLIED PHYSIOLOGY: VARIATIONS IN LEUKOCYTE COUNT

Leukocytosis

Leukocytosis is the increase in total WBC count. Leukocytosis occurs in both physiological and pathological conditions.

Leukopenia

Leukopenia is the decrease in total WBC count. Generally, the term leukopenia is used for pathological conditions only.

PHYSIOLOGICAL VARIATIONS

1. *Age:* In infants and children, total WBC count is more; it is about 20,000/cu mm in infants and about 10,000 to 15,000/ cu mm of blood in children.
2. *Sex:* WBC count is slightly more in males than in females.
3. *Diurnal variation:* WBC count is minimum in early morning and maximum in the afternoon.
4. *Exercise:* Count increases slightly.
5. *Sleep:* Count decreases slightly.
6. *Emotional conditions like anxiety:* WBC count increases slightly.
7. *Pregnancy:* WBC count increases.
8. *Menstruation:* Count increases.
9. *Parturition:* Count increases.

PATHOLOGICAL VARIATIONS

Leukocytosis

It occurs in the following pathological conditions:

1. Infections.
2. Allergy.

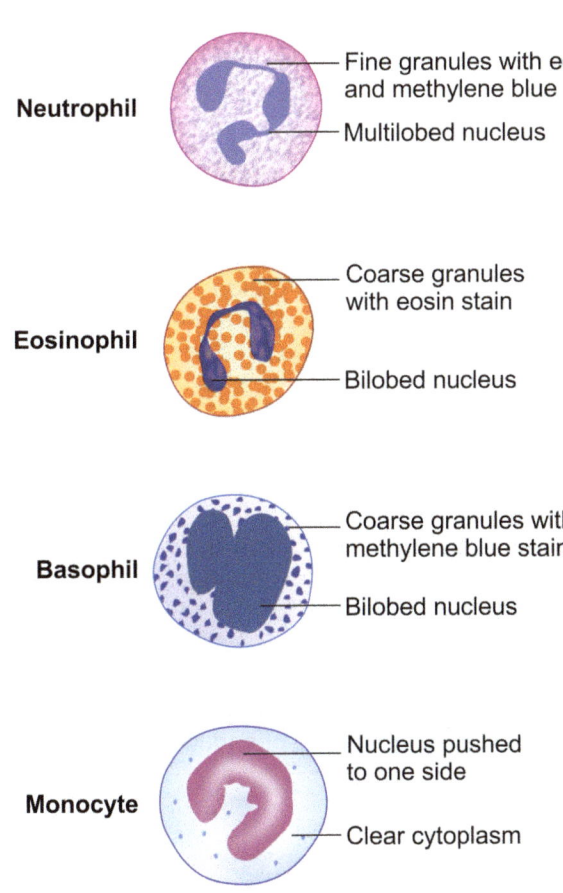

FIGURE 14.1: Different white blood cells.

3. Common cold.
4. Tuberculosis.
5. Glandular fever.

Leukopenia

Leukopenia occurs in the following pathological conditions:

1. Anaphylactic shock.
2. Cirrhosis of liver.
3. Disorders of spleen.
4. Pernicious anemia.
5. Typhoid and paratyphoid.
6. Viral infections.

Leukemia

Leukemia is a type of **blood cancer** characterized by production of large number of leukocytes including immature and abnormal leukocytes. Leukocyte count increases more than 10,00,000/ cu mm.

Leukemia is caused by genetic mutation in DNA of bone marrow cells.

LIFESPAN OF WHITE BLOOD CELLS

Lifespan of WBCs is not constant. It depends upon the demand in the body and their function. Lifespan of different WBCs is given in **Table 14.2**.

PROPERTIES OF WHITE BLOOD CELLS

1. Diapedesis

Diapedesis is the process by which the leukocytes squeeze through the narrow blood vessels.

2. Ameboid Movement

Neutrophils, monocytes and lymphocytes show amebic movement characterized by protrusion of the cytoplasm and change in the shape.

3. Chemotaxis

Chemotaxis is the attraction of WBCs towards injured tissues by the chemical substances released at the site of injury.

4. Phagocytosis

Neutrophils and monocytes engulf the foreign bodies by means of phagocytosis. Refer Chapter 3 for phagocytosis.

FUNCTIONS OF WHITE BLOOD CELLS

WBCs play an important role in defense mechanism. These cells protect the body from invading organisms or foreign bodies either by destroying or inactivating them. However, in defense mechanism, each type of WBCs acts in a different way.

FUNCTIONS OF NEUTROPHILS

Along with monocytes, the neutrophils provide the **first line of defense** against the invading microorganisms. Neutrophils wander freely all over the body through the tissue.

Neutrophils move by diapedesis towards the site of infection by means of **chemotaxis**. Chemotaxis occurs due to the attraction by some chemical substances called **chemoattractants**, which are released from the infected area. After reaching the area, the neutrophils engulf the bacteria and then destroy them by means of **phagocytosis** (Chapter 3).

Pus and Pus Cells

Pus cells are the dead WBCs killed by toxins released from bacteria during the battle between WBCs and bacteria.

Pus is the whitish yellow fluid formed in the area of infected tissue. It consists of dead WBCs, bacteria or foreign bodies, serum and cellular debris.

FUNCTIONS OF EOSINOPHILS

Eosinophils provide defense to the body by acting against the parasitic infections and during allergic conditions such as asthma. Eosinophils are responsible for detoxification, disintegration and removal of foreign proteins.

Eosinophils attack the invading organisms by secreting some of **cytotoxic substances** which destroy the invading organisms such as parasites.

FUNCTIONS OF BASOPHILS

Basophils are involved in **healing processes** and acute **hypersensitivity reactions** (allergy).

Basophils execute the functions by releasing some important substances from their granules such as heparin and histamine.

FUNCTIONS OF MONOCYTES

Monocytes are the largest leukocytes. Like neutrophils, monocytes also are motile and phagocytic in nature. These

TABLE 14.2: Normal count, diameter and lifespan of white blood cells.

WBC	Percentage	Absolute value (per cu mm)	Diameter (μ)	Lifespan (days)
1. Neutrophils	50 to 70	3,000 to 6,000	10 to 2	2 to 5
2. Eosinophils	2 to 4	150 to 300	10 to 14	7 to 12
3. Basophils	0 to 1	0 to 100	8 to 10	12 to 15
4. Monocytes	2 to 6	200 to 600	14 to 15	2 to 5
5. Lymphocytes	20 to 30	1,500 to 3,000	7 to 12	½ to 1

cells wander freely through all tissues of the body and provide the **first line of defense** along with neutrophils.

Monocytes are the precursors of the **tissue macrophages**. The matured monocytes stay in the blood only for few hours. Afterwards these cells enter the tissues from the blood and become tissue macrophages.

Examples of tissue macrophages are **Kupffer cells** in liver, **alveolar macrophages** in lungs and macrophages in spleen. Functions of macrophages are discussed in Chapter 21.

FUNCTIONS OF LYMPHOCYTES

Lymphocytes are responsible in development of immunity. Depending upon the function, the lymphocytes are divided into two types:

1. T lymphocytes which are concerned with cellular immunity.
2. B lymphocytes which are concerned with humoral immunity.

Functions of these two types of lymphocytes are explained in detail in Chapter 15.

LEUKOPOIESIS

Leukopoiesis is the development and maturation of leukocytes **(Fig. 14.2)**.

STEM CELLS

Committed pluripotent stem cell gives rise to leukocytes through various stages. Details of stem cells are given in Chapter 9.

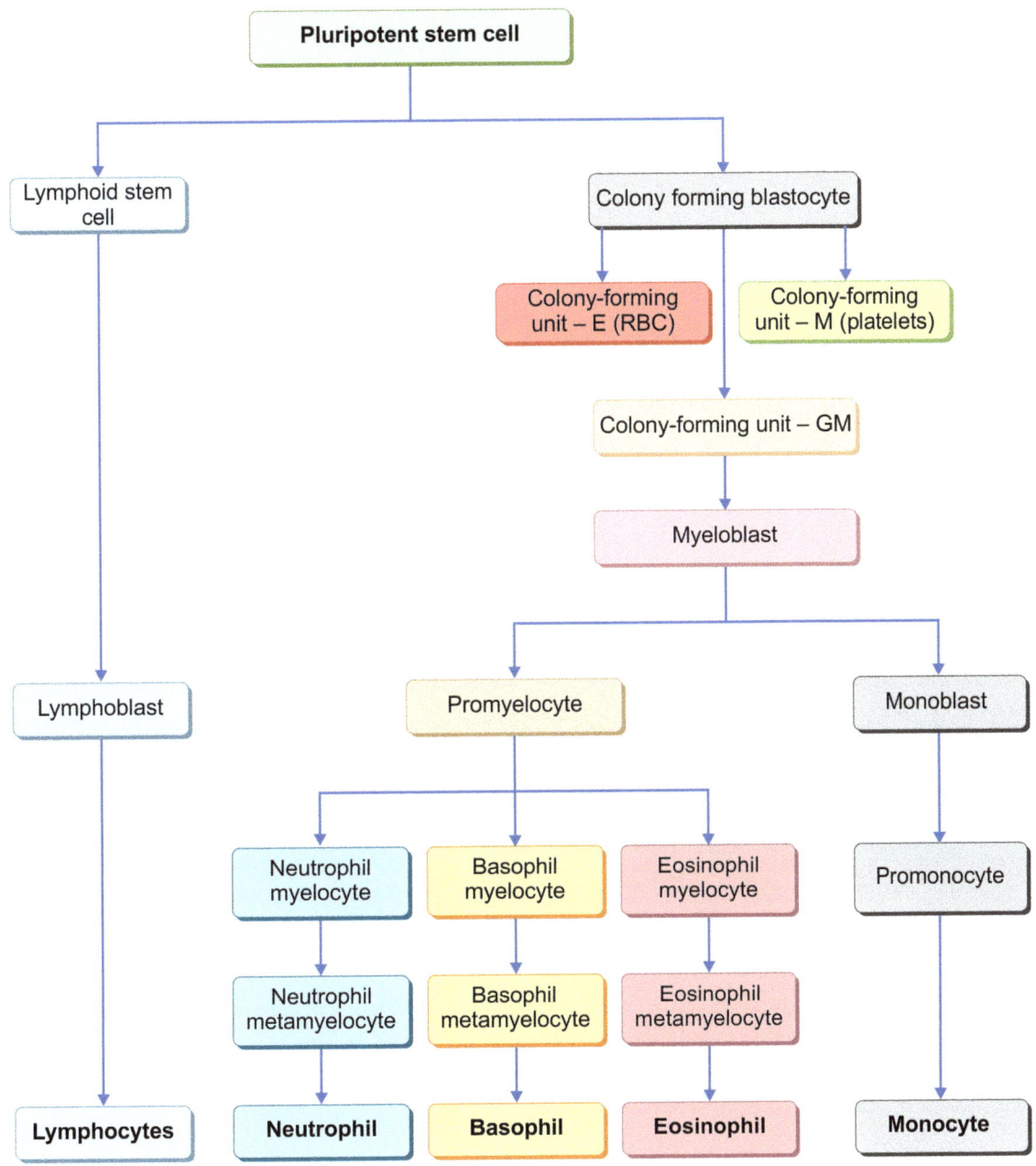

FIGURE 14.2: Leucopoiesis. E = Erythrocytes, M = Magakaryocyte, GM = Granulocyte/Monocyte, RBC = Red blood cell.

■ FACTORS NECESSARY FOR LEUKOPOIESIS

Leukopoiesis is influenced by **hematopoietic growth factors** and colony-stimulating factors (CSFs). Hematopoietic growth factors are discussed in Chapter 9.

Colony-stimulating Factors

Colony-stimulating factors are proteins which cause the formation of **colony-forming blastocytes**.

Colony-stimulating factors are of three types:

1. **Granulocyte-CSF** (G-CSF) secreted by monocytes and endothelial cells.
2. **Granulocyte-monocyte-CSF** (GM-CSF) secreted by monocytes, endothelial cells and T lymphocytes.
3. **Monocyte-CSF** (M-CSF) secreted by monocytes and endothelial cells.

Chapter 15: Immunity

CHAPTER OUTLINE

- DEFINITION AND TYPES OF IMMUNITY
- DEVELOPMENT AND PROCESSING OF LYMPHOCYTES
- ANTIGENS
- DEVELOPMENT OF CELL-MEDIATED IMMUNITY
- DEVELOPMENT OF HUMORAL IMMUNITY
- NATURAL KILLER CELL
- CYTOKINES
- IMMUNIZATION
- IMMUNE DEFICIENCY DISEASES
- AUTOIMMUNE DISEASES

■ DEFINITION AND TYPES OF IMMUNITY

Immunity is defined as the capacity of the body to resist the **pathogenic agents**. It is the ability of the body to resist the entry of different types of foreign bodies such as bacteria, virus, toxic substances, etc.

Immunity is of two types:
I. Innate immunity.
II. Acquired immunity.

■ INNATE IMMUNITY OR NON-SPECIFIC IMMUNITY

Innate immunity is the inborn capacity of the body to resist the pathogens. By chance, if any organism enters the body, innate immunity eliminates it before the development of any disease.

This type of immunity represents the first line of defense against any type of pathogens. Therefore, it is also called **non-specific immunity**.

Examples of Innate Immunity

1. Destruction of toxic substances or organisms entering digestive tract through food by enzymes in digestive juices.
2. Destruction of bacteria by salivary lysozyme.
3. Destruction of bacteria by acidity in urine and vaginal fluid.

■ ACQUIRED IMMUNITY OR SPECIFIC IMMUNITY

Acquired immunity is the resistance developed in the body against any specific foreign body like bacteria, viruses, toxins, vaccines or transplanted tissues. So, this type of immunity is also known as **specific immunity**.

It is the most powerful immune mechanism that protects the body from invading organisms or toxic substances. Lymphocytes are responsible for acquired immunity **(Fig. 15.1)**.

Types of Acquired Immunity

Two types of acquired immunity develop in the body:
I. Cell-mediated immunity or cellular immunity.
II. Humoral immunity.

■ DEVELOPMENT AND PROCESSING OF LYMPHOCYTES

In fetus, lymphocytes develop from bone marrow. All the lymphocytes are released in the circulation and are differentiated into two categories:

A. T lymphocytes.
B. B lymphocytes.

■ T LYMPHOCYTES

T lymphocytes are processed in **thymus**. The processing occurs during the period between just before birth and few months after birth.

Thymus secretes **thymosin**, which accelerates the proliferation and activation of lymphocytes in thymus. It also increases the activity of lymphocytes in lymphoid tissues.

Types of T Lymphocytes

During the processing, T lymphocytes are transformed into four types:

1. Helper T cells or inducer T cells.

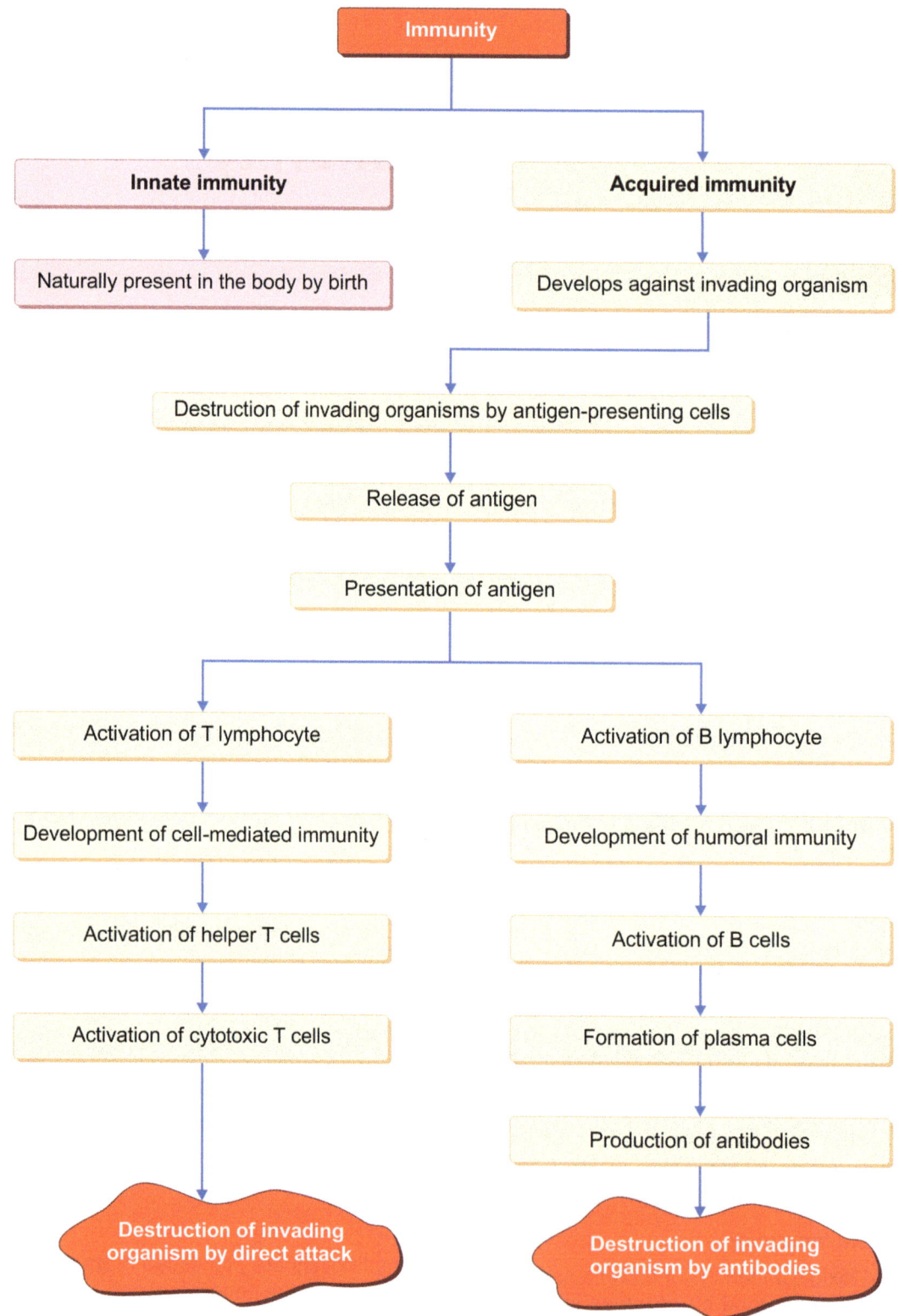

FIGURE 15.1: Schematic diagram showing development of immunity.

2. Cytotoxic T cells or killer T cells.
3. Suppressor T cells.
4. Memory T cells.

Storage of T Lymphocytes

After the transformation, all the types of T lymphocytes leave the thymus and are stored in lymphoid tissues of lymph nodes, spleen, bone marrow and the gastrointestinal (GI) tract.

■ B LYMPHOCYTES

B lymphocytes were first discovered in the **bursa of Fabricius** in birds, hence the name B lymphocytes. The bursa of Fabricius is a lymphoid organ situated near the cloaca of birds. The bursa is absent in mammals, and the processing of B lymphocytes takes place in bone marrow and liver.

Types of B Lymphocytes

After processing, the B lymphocytes are transformed into two types:

1. Plasma cells.
2. Memory cells.

Storage of B Lymphocytes

After the transformation, B lymphocytes are stored in the lymphoid tissues of lymph nodes, spleen, bone marrow and the GI tract.

ANTIGENS

DEFINITION AND TYPES

Antigens are the substances, which induce specific immune reactions in the body. The antigens are mostly the conjugated proteins such as lipoproteins, glycoproteins and nucleoproteins.

Antigens are of two types:

1. **Autoantigens** or **self-antigens** which are present on the body's own cells like 'A' antigen and 'B' antigen on the RBCs.
2. **Foreign antigens** or **non-self-antigens** which enter the body from outside.

DEVELOPMENT OF CELL-MEDIATED IMMUNITY

Cell-mediated immunity is offered by T lymphocytes. It involves several types of cells such as macrophages, T lymphocytes and natural killer cells and hence the name cell-mediated immunity. It is also called **cellular immunity** or **T cell immunity**. It does not involve antibodies.

Cellular immunity is the major defense mechanism against infections by viruses, fungi and few bacteria. It is also responsible for **delayed allergic reactions** and **rejection of transplanted tissues**.

Cell-mediated immunity starts developing when T cells come in contact with the antigens. Usually, the invading microbial or non-microbial organisms carry the **antigenic materials**. These antigenic materials are released from invading organisms and are presented to the helper T cells by antigen-presenting cells.

ANTIGEN-PRESENTING CELLS

Antigen-presenting cells are the special type of cells in the body which induce the release of antigenic materials from invading organisms and later present these materials to the helper T cells. Major antigen-presenting cells are **macrophages**. **Dendritic cells** in spleen, lymph nodes and skin also function like antigen-presenting cells.

Role of Antigen-presenting Cells

Invading foreign organisms are either engulfed by macrophages through phagocytosis or trapped by dendritic cells. Later, the antigen from these organisms is digested into small peptides. The antigenic peptide products are moved towards the surface of the antigen-presenting cells and loaded on a genetic matter of the antigen-presenting cells called **human leukocyte antigen** (HLA). The HLA is present in the molecule of class II **major histocompatibility complex** (MHC) which is situated on the surface of the antigen-presenting cells.

Presentation of Antigen

Antigen-presenting cells present their class II MHC molecules together with antigen bound HLA to the helper T cells. This activates the helper T cells through series of events **(Fig. 15.2)**.

Sequence of Events during Activation of Helper T Cells

1. Helper T cell recognizes the antigen bound to class II MHC molecule which is displayed on the surface of the antigen-presenting cell. It recognizes the antigen with the help of its own surface receptor protein called **T cell receptor**.
2. Recognition of the antigen by the helper T cell initiates a complex interaction between the helper T cell receptor and the antigen. This reaction activates helper T cells.
3. At the same time, macrophages (the antigen presenting cells) release interleukin-1 which facilitates the activation and proliferation of helper T cells.
4. Activated helper T cells proliferate and the proliferated helper T cells enter the circulation for further actions.
5. Simultaneously the antigen bound to class II MHC molecules activate the B cells also resulting in development of humoral immunity (see below).

ROLE OF HELPER T CELLS

Helper T cells which enter the circulation, activate all the other T cells and B cells.

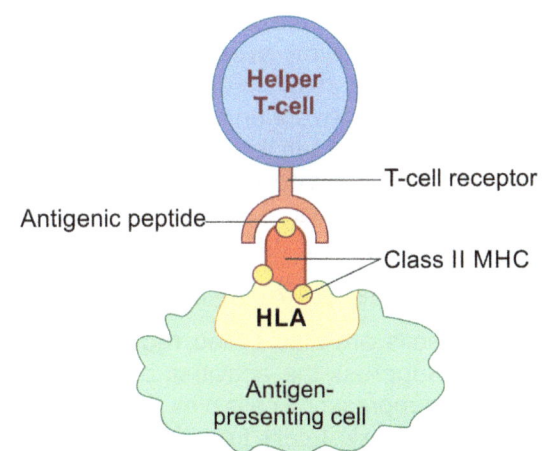

FIGURE 15.2: Antigen presentation. Antigen-presenting cells present their class II MHC molecules together with antigen-bound HLA to the helper T cells.

MHC = Major histocompatibility complex, HLA = Human leukocyte antigen.

Helper T cells are of two types:
1. Helper-1 (TH1) cells.
2. Helper-2 (TH2) cells.

Role of TH1 Cells

TH1 cells are concerned with cellular immunity and secrete two substances:

   i. **Interleukin-2** which activates the other T cells.
  ii. **Gamma interferon** which stimulates the phagocytic activity of cytotoxic cells, macrophages and natural killer (NK) cells.

Role of TH2 Cells

TH2 cells are concerned with humoral immunity and secrete interleukin-4 and interleukin-5 which are concerned with:

   i. Activation of B cells.
  ii. Proliferation of plasma cells.
 iii. Production of antibodies by plasma cell.

ROLE OF CYTOTOXIC T CELLS

Cytotoxic T cells that are activated by helper T cells circulate through blood, lymph and lymphatic tissues and destroy the invading organisms by attacking them directly.

Mechanism of Action of Cytotoxic T Cells

1. Receptors situated on the outer membrane of cytotoxic T cells bind the antigens or organisms tightly with cytotoxic T cells.
2. Then, the cytotoxic T cells enlarge and release cytotoxic substances such as lysosomal enzymes.
3. These substances destroy the invading organisms.
4. Like this, each cytotoxic T cell can destroy a large number of microorganisms one after another.

Other Actions of Cytotoxic T Cells

1. Cytotoxic T cells also destroy cancer cells, transplanted cells such as those of transplanted heart or kidney or any other cells, which are foreign bodies.
2. Cytotoxic T cells destroy even the body's own tissues which are affected by the foreign bodies, particularly the viruses. Many viruses are entrapped in the membrane of affected cells. The antigen of the viruses attracts the T cells. And the cytotoxic T cells kill the affected cells also along with viruses. Because of this, cytotoxic T cell is called **killer cell**.

ROLE OF SUPPRESSOR T CELLS

Suppressor T cells are also called **regulatory T cells**. These T cells suppress the activities of the cytotoxic T cells. Thus, the suppressor T cells play an important role in preventing the cytotoxic T cells from destroying the body's own tissues along with invaded organisms. Suppressor cells suppress the activities of helper T cells also.

ROLE OF MEMORY T CELLS

Some of the T cells activated by an antigen do not enter the circulation, but remain in lymphoid tissue. These T cells are called memory T cells.

In later periods, the memory cells migrate to various lymphoid tissues throughout the body. When the body is exposed to the same organism for the second time, the memory cells identify the organism and immediately activate the other T cells. So, the invading organism is destroyed very quickly. The response of the T cells is also more powerful this time.

SPECIFICITY OF T CELLS

Each T cell is designed to be activated only by one type of antigen. It is capable of developing immunity against that antigen only. This property is called the specificity of T cells.

DEVELOPMENT OF HUMORAL IMMUNITY

Humoral immunity is the immunity mediated by antibodies. **Antibodies** are secreted by B lymphocytes and released into the blood and lymph. The blood and lymph are the body fluids (humours or humors in Latin). Since the B lymphocytes provide immunity through humors, this type of immunity is called humoral immunity or **B cell immunity**.

The antibodies are the gamma globulins produced by B lymphocytes. These anti-bodies fight against the invading organisms. The humoral immunity is the major defense mechanism against the bacterial infection.

As in the case of cell-mediated immunity, the macrophages and other antigen-presenting cells play an important role in the development of humoral immunity also.

ROLE OF ANTIGEN-PRESENTING CELLS

Ingestion of foreign organisms and digestion of their antigen by the antigen-presenting cells are already explained.

Presentation of Antigen

The antigen-presenting cells present their class II MHC molecules together with antigen bound HLA to B lymphocytes. This activates the B lymphocytes through series of events.

Sequence of Events during Activation of B Cells

1. B cell recognizes the antigen bound to class II MHC molecule which is displayed on the surface of the antigen-presenting cell. It recognizes the antigen with the help of its own surface receptor protein called **B-cell receptor**.
2. Recognition of the antigen by the B cell initiates a complex interaction between the B-cell receptor and the antigen. This reaction activates B cells.
3. At the same time, macrophages (the antigen-presenting cells) release interleukin-1 which facilitates the activation and proliferation of B cells.
4. Activated B cells proliferate and the proliferated B cells carry out the further actions.
5. Simultaneously the antigen bound to class II MHC molecules activates the helper T cells also resulting in development of cell-mediated immunity (already explained).

Transformation B Cells

Proliferated B cells are transformed into two types of cells:
1. Plasma cells.
2. Memory cells.

ROLE OF PLASMA CELLS

Plasma cells destroy the foreign organisms by producing the antibodies. Antibodies are globulin in nature. The rate of the antibody production is very high, i.e. each plasma cell produces about 2,000 molecules of antibodies per second. Antibodies are released into lymph and then transported into the circulation. Antibodies are produced until the end of lifespan of each plasma cell which may be from several days to several weeks.

ROLE OF MEMORY B CELLS

Memory B cells occupy the lymphoid tissues throughout the body. Memory cells are in inactive condition until the body is exposed to the same organism for the second time.

During the second exposure, the memory cells are activated by the antigen and produce more quantity of antibodies at a faster rate, than in the first exposure. The antibodies produced during the second exposure to the foreign antigen are also more potent than those produced during first exposure. This phenomenon forms the basic principle of vaccination against the infections.

ROLE OF HELPER T CELLS

Helper T cells are simultaneously activated by antigen. Activated helper T cells secrete two substances called interleukin-2 and B cell growth factor, which promote:

1. Activation of a greater number of B lymphocytes.
2. Proliferation of plasma cells.
3. Production of antibodies.

ANTIBODIES OR IMMUNOGLOBULINS

An antibody is defined as a protein that is produced by B lymphocytes in response to the presence of an antigen. Antibody is γ-globulin in nature and so it is also called **immunoglobulin** (Ig). Immunoglobulins form 20% of the total plasma proteins. The antibodies enter almost all the tissues of the body.

Structure of Antibodies

Antibodies are formed by two pairs of chains, namely one pair of heavy or long chains and one pair of light or short chains. Each heavy chain consists of about 400 amino acids and each light chain consists of about 200 amino acids.

Actually, each antibody has two halves, which are identical. The two halves are held together by **disulfide bonds** (S–S). Each half of the antibody consists of one heavy chain (H) and one light chain (L). The two chains in each half are also joined by disulfide bonds (S–S). The disulfide bonds allow the movement of amino acid chains. In each antibody, the light chain is parallel to one end of the heavy chain. The light chain and the part of heavy chain parallel to it form one arm. The remaining part of the heavy chain forms another arm. A hinge joins both the arms **(Fig. 15.3)**.

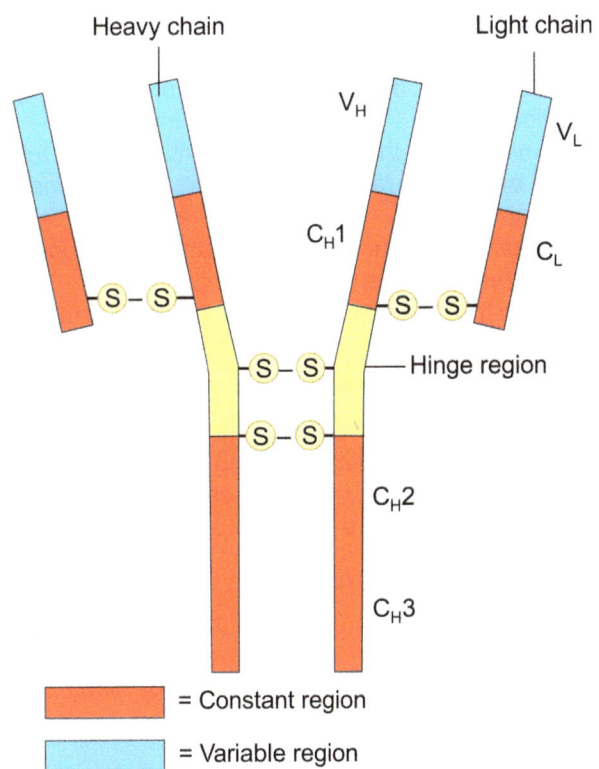

FIGURE 15.3: Structure of antibody (IgG) molecule. V_L = Variable region of light chain, V_H = Variable region of heavy chain, C_L = Constant region of light chain, C_H1, C_H2 and C_H3 = Constant regions of heavy chains.

Each chain of the antibody includes two regions:
1. Constant region.
2. Variable region.

Types and Functions of Antibodies

Antibodies are of five types:

1. **IgA (Ig alpha):** This antibody plays a role in localized defense mechanism in external secretions like tear.
2. **IgD (Ig delta):** It is involved in recognition of antigen by B lymphocytes.
3. **IgE (Ig epsilon):** IgE is involved in allergic reactions
4. **IgG (Ig gamma):** This is responsible for complement fixation.
5. **IgM (Ig mu):** This antibody is also responsible for complement fixation.

Among these antibodies, IgG forms 75% of the antibodies in the body.

Mechanism of Actions of Antibodies

Antibodies protect the body from the invading organisms in two ways:

1. By direct actions.
2. Through complement system.

1. Direct actions of antibodies

Antibodies directly inactivate the invading organism by any one of the following methods:

i. *Agglutination:* In this, the foreign bodies such as RBCs (from a donor) or bacteria, with antigens on their surfaces, are held together in a clump by the antibodies.
ii. *Precipitation:* In this, the soluble antigens like tetanus toxin are converted into insoluble forms and then precipitated.
iii. *Neutralization:* During this, the antibodies cover the toxic sites of antigenic products.
iv. *Lysis:* In this, the antibodies rupture the cell membrane of organisms and then destroy them.

2. Actions of antibodies through complement system

Complement system is the one that enhances or accelerates various activities during the fight against the invading organisms. It contains plasma enzymes, which are identified by numbers from C1 to C9.

Specificity of B Lymphocytes

Each B lymphocyte is designed to be activated only by one type of antigen. It is also capable of producing antibodies against that antigen only. This property is called **B lymphocyte specificity**.

NATURAL KILLER CELL

Natural killer (NK) cell is a large granular cell with indented nucleus. It is considered as the third type of lymphocyte. It is not a phagocytic cell, but its granules contain hydrolytic enzymes which causes lysis of cells of invading organisms.

Functions of NK Cell

Natural killer cell:

1. Destroys the viruses.
2. Destroys the viral infected or damaged cells, which might form tumors.
3. Destroys the malignant cells and prevents development of cancerous tumors.
4. Secretes cytokines such as interleukin-2, interferons, colony-stimulating factor (GM-CSF) and tumor necrosis factor-α.

CYTOKINES

Cytokines are the hormone-like small proteins acting as intercellular messengers (cell signaling molecules) by binding to specific receptors of target cells. These **non-antibody proteins** are secreted by WBCs and some other types of cells. Their major function is the activation and regulation of general immune system of the body.

Cytokines are distinct from the other cell signaling molecules such as growth factors and hormones.

Cytokines are classified into several types:

1. Interleukins.
2. Interferons.
3. Tumor necrosis factors.
4. Chemokines.
5. Defensins.
6. Cathelicidins.
7. Platelet-activating factor.

Refer **Table 15.1** for source of secretion and actions of all these types of cytokines.

IMMUNIZATION

Immunization is a procedure by which the body is prepared to fight against a specific disease. It is used to induce immune resistance of the body to a specific disease.

Immunization is of two types:

I. Passive immunization.
II. Active immunization.

PASSIVE IMMUNIZATION

Passive immunization or immunity is produced without challenging the immune system of the body. It is done by administration of serum or gamma globulins from a person who is already immunized (affected by the disease) to a non-immune person. Passive immunization is acquired either naturally or artificially.

1. Passive Natural Immunization

Passive natural immunization is acquired from the mother before and after birth. Before birth, maternal antibodies (mainly IgG) are transported to fetus through placenta. After birth, the antibodies (IgA) are transported through breast milk.

2. Passive Artificial Immunization

Passive artificial immunization is developed by injecting previously prepared antibodies using serum from humans or animals.

ACTIVE IMMUNIZATION

Active immunization or immunity is acquired by activating the immune system of body. Body develops resistance against disease by producing antibodies following the exposure to antigens.

Active immunity is acquired either naturally or artificially.

1. Active Natural Immunization

Naturally acquired active immunity involves activation of immune system in the body to produce antibodies. It is achieved during infections.

2. Active Artificial Immunization

Active artificial immunization is a type of immunization achieved by the administration of vaccines or toxoids.

Vaccines

Vaccine is a substance that is administered into the body in order to develop or increase immunity against a particular disease. Vaccine is prepared from dead pathogens or live but attenuated (artificially weakened) organisms. Vaccine induces immunity against the pathogen, either by production of antibodies or by activation of T lymphocytes.

Vaccines are used to prevent many diseases such as smallpox, measles, mumps, poliomyelitis, tuberculosis, smallpox, rubella, yellow fever, rabies, typhoid, influenza, hepatitis B, etc.

TABLE 15.1: Cytokines.

Cytokines	Sources of secretion	Actions
Interleukins	1. T cells 2. B cells 3. Eosinophils 4. Basophils 5. Monocytes 6. Mast cells 7. Macrophages 8. NK cells	1. Activation of T cells, macrophages and natural killer (NK) cells 2. Promotion of growth of hematopoietic cells and B cells 3. Acceleration of inflammatory response by activating eosinophils 4. Chemotaxis of neutrophils, eosinophils, basophils and T cells 5. Destruction of invading organisms
Interferons	1. WBCs 2. NK cells 3. Fibroblasts	1. Fighting against viral infection by suppressing virus multiplication in target cells 2. Inhibition of multiplication of parasites and cancer cells 3. Promotion of phagocytosis by monocytes and macrophages 4. Activation of NK cells
Tumor necrosis factors	1. T cells 2. B cells 3. Mast cells 4. Macrophages 5. NK cells 6. Platelets	1. Causing necrosis of tumor 2. Activation of general immune system 3. Production of vascular effects 4. Promotion of inflammation
Chemokines	1. T cells 2. B cells 3. Monocytes 4. Macrophages	1. Attraction of WBCs by chemotaxis
Defensins	1. Neutrophils 2. Macrophages 3. Paneth cells in small intestine 4. Airway epithelial cells 5. Salivary glands 6. Cutaneous cells	1. Role in innate immunity in airway surface and lungs 2. Killing the phagocytosed bacteria 3. Anti-inflammatory actions 4. Promotion of wound healing 5. Attraction of monocytes and T cells by chemotaxis
Cathelicidins	1. Neutrophils 2. Macrophages 3. Airway epithelial cells	1. Antimicrobial activity in air passage and lungs
Platelet-activating factor	1. Neutrophils 2. Monocytes	1. Acceleration of agglutination and aggregation of platelets

Toxoids

Toxoid is a substance which is processed to destroy its toxicity, but retains its capacity to induce antibody production by immune system. Toxoid consists of weakened components or toxins secreted by the pathogens. Toxoids are used to develop immunity against diseases like diphtheria, tetanus, cholera, etc.

Active artificial immunity may be effective life-long or for short period. It is effective lifelong against the diseases such as mumps, measles, smallpox, tuberculosis and yellow fever. It is effective only for short period against some diseases such as cholera (about 6 months) and tetanus (about 1 year).

IMMUNE DEFICIENCY DISEASES

Immune deficiency diseases are group of diseases in which some components of immune system are missing or defective. Normally, defense mechanism protects the body from invading pathogenic organism. When the defense mechanism fails or becomes faulty (defective), the organisms of even low virulence produce severe disease. Such organisms, which take advantage of defective defense mechanism, are called **opportunists**.

Immune deficiency diseases caused by opportunists are of two types:

1. Congenital immune deficiency diseases.
2. Acquired immune deficiency diseases.

CONGENITAL IMMUNE DEFICIENCY DISEASES

Congenital diseases are inherited and occur due to the defects in B cell or T cell, or both. The common examples are **Di George's syndrome** (due to absence of thymus) and severe combined immune deficiency (due to lymphopenia or the absence of lymphoid tissue).

ACQUIRED IMMUNE DEFICIENCY DISEASES

Acquired immune deficiency diseases occur due to infection by some organisms. The most common disease of this type is acquired immune deficiency syndrome (AIDS).

Acquired Immune Deficiency Syndrome

AIDS is an infectious disease caused by **human immune deficiency virus** (HIV). AIDS is the most common problem throughout the world because of rapid increase in the number of victims. Infection occurs when a glycoprotein from HIV binds to surface receptors of T lymphocytes, monocytes, macrophages and dendritic cells leading to destruction of these cells. It causes slow progressive decrease in immune function resulting in opportunistic infections of various types. The common **opportunistic infections** which kill the AIDS patient are pneumonia and skin cancer.

■ AUTOIMMUNE DISEASES

Autoimmune disease is defined as condition in which the immune system mistakenly attacks body's own cells and tissues. Normally, an antigen induces the immune response in the body. The condition in which the immune system fails to give response to an antigen is called tolerance. This is true with respect to body's own antigens that are called **self-antigens** or **autoantigens**.

Normally, body has the tolerance against self-antigen. However, in some occasions, the tolerance fails or becomes incomplete against self-antigen. This state is called **autoimmunity** and it leads to the activation of T lymphocytes or production of **autoantibodies** from B lymphocytes. T lymphocytes (cytotoxic T cells) or autoantibodies attack the body's normal cells whose surface contains the self-antigen or autoantigen.

Common Autoimmune Diseases

1. Diabetes mellitus.
2. Myasthenia gravis.
3. Hashimoto's thyroiditis.
4. Graves' disease.
5. Rheumatoid arthritis.

Chapter 16: Platelets

CHAPTER OUTLINE

- MORPHOLOGY
- STRUCTURE AND COMPOSITION
- NORMAL COUNT AND VARIATIONS
- PROPERTIES
- FUNCTIONS
- DEVELOPMENT
- LIFESPAN AND FATE
- APPLIED PHYSIOLOGY: PLATELET DISORDERS

MORPHOLOGY OF PLATELETS

Platelets or **thrombocytes** are the formed elements of blood. Platelets are small, colorless, nonnucleated and moderately refractive bodies, which are considered to be the fragments of cytoplasm.

Size of Platelets

Diameter : 2.5 μ (2 μ to 4 μ)
Volume : 7.5 cu μ (7 cu μ to 8 cu μ)

Shape of Platelets

Normally, platelets are of several shapes, viz. spherical or rod shaped and become oval or disc shaped when inactivated. Sometimes, the platelets have dumbbell shape, comma shape, cigar shape or any other unusual shape.

STRUCTURE AND COMPOSITION OF PLATELETS

Platelets are constituted by cell membrane or surface membrane, microtubules and cytoplasm.

CELL MEMBRANE

Cell membrane is 6 nm thick and contains lipids in the form of phospholipids, cholesterol and glycolipids, carbohydrates as glycocalyx, and glycoproteins and proteins.

MICROTUBULES

Microtubules form a ring around cytoplasm below cell membrane. These tubules are made up of proteins called **tubulin**. Microtubules provide structural support for inactivated platelets to maintain the disk-like shape (**Fig. 16.1**).

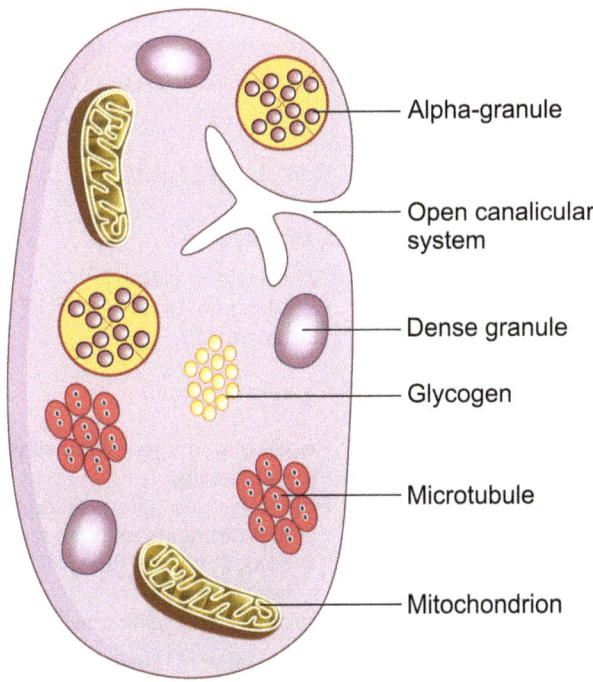

FIGURE 16.1: Platelet under electron microscope.

CYTOPLASM

Cytoplasm of the platelets contains the cellular organelles, Golgi apparatus, endoplasmic reticulum, mitochondria, microtubule, microvessels, filaments and granules. Platelet granules are of two types namely alpha-granules and dense granules. Granules of each type contain different substances. Cytoplasm also contains some chemical substances as given below.

I. Proteins

Details of proteins present in cytoplasm of platelets are given in **Table 16.1**.

II. Enzymes

1. ATPase.
2. Enzymes necessary for synthesis of prostaglandins.

III. Hormonal Substances

1. Adrenaline.
2. 5-HT (serotonin).
3. Histamine.

IV. Other Chemical Substances

1. Glycogen.
2. Substances like blood group antigens.
3. Inorganic substances such as calcium, copper, magnesium and iron.

V. Platelet Granules

1. Alpha-granules
2. Beta-granules.

TABLE 16.1: Proteins present in cytoplasm of platelets and their actions.

Proteins	Actions
1. Contractile proteins	
i. Actin	Contraction of platelets
ii. Myosin	
iii. Thrombosthenin	Clot retraction
2. von Willebrand factor	Adherence of platelets Regulation of plasma level of factor VIII
3. Fibrin-stabilizing factor	Clotting factor XIII
4. Platelet-derived growth factor (PDGF)	Repair of damaged blood vessels Wound healing Potent mitogen (chemical agent that promotes mitosis) for smooth muscle fibers of blood vessels Proliferation of connective tissue
5. Platelet-activating factor (PAF)	Aggregation of platelets during injury of blood vessels, resulting in prevention of excess loss of blood
6. Vitronectin (serum-spreading factor)	Adhesion of platelets Spreading of tissue cells in culture
7. Thrombospondin	Inhibition of angiogenesis: (formation of new blood vessels from pre-existing vessels)

TABLE 16.2: Substances present in platelet granules.

Alpha-granules	Dense granules
1. Clotting factors: Fibrinogen, V and XIII 2. Platelet-derived growth factor 3. Vascular endothelial growth factor 4. Basic fibroblast growth factor 5. Endostatin 6. Thrombospondin	1. Nucleotides 2. Serotonin 3. Phospholipid 4. Calcium 5. Lysosomes

Substances present in platelet granules are listed in **Table 16.2**.

NORMAL COUNT AND VARIATIONS OF PLATELETS

Normal platelet count is 2,50,000. It ranges between 2,00,000/cu mm and 4,00,000/cu mm of blood.

PHYSIOLOGICAL VARIATIONS

1. *Age:* Platelets are less in infants (1,50,000/cu mm to 2,00,000/cu mm) and reaches normal level at 3rd month after birth.
2. *Sex:* There is no difference in the platelet count between males and females. In females, it is reduced during menstruation.
3. *High altitude:* Platelet count increases.
4. *After meals:* After taking food, the platelet count increases.

PATHOLOGICAL VARIATIONS

Refer applied physiology of this chapter.

PROPERTIES OF PLATELETS

1. ADHESIVENESS

Adhesiveness is the property of sticking to a rough surface. While coming in contact with any rough surface the platelets are activated and stick to the surface.

2. AGGREGATION

Aggregation is the grouping of platelets. Activated platelets group together and become sticky.

3. AGGLUTINATION

Agglutination is the clumping together of platelets.

FUNCTIONS OF PLATELETS

1. ROLE IN BLOOD CLOTTING

Platelets are responsible for the formation of intrinsic **prothrombin activator**. This substance is responsible for the onset of blood clotting (Chapter 18).

2. ROLE IN CLOT RETRACTION

In the blood clot, the blood cells including platelets are entrapped in between the fibrin threads. The cytoplasm of platelets contains the contractile proteins namely actin, myosin and thrombosthenin which are responsible for clot retraction (Chapter 18).

3. ROLE IN PREVENTION OF BLOOD LOSS (HEMOSTASIS)

Platelets accelerate hemostasis by three ways:
i. Platelets secrete 5-HT, which causes the constriction of blood vessels.
ii. Due to the adhesive property, the platelets seal the damage in blood vessels like capillaries.
iii. By formation of temporary plug also platelets seal the damage in blood vessels (Chapter 17).

4. ROLE IN REPAIR OF RUPTURED BLOOD VESSEL

Platelet-derived growth factor (PDGF) formed in cytoplasm of platelets is useful for the repair of the endothelium and other structures of the ruptured blood vessels.

5. ROLE IN DEFENSE MECHANISM

By the property of agglutination, platelets encircle the foreign bodies and destroy them by phagocytosis.

DEVELOPMENT OF PLATELETS

Platelets are formed from bone marrow. The pluripotent stem cell gives rise to the CFU-M. This develops into **megakaryocyte**. The cytoplasm of megakaryocyte form pseudopodium. A portion of pseudopodium is detached to form platelet, which enters the circulation **(Fig. 9.2)**.

Production of platelets is influenced by **thrombopoietin**. Thrombopoietin is a glycoprotein like erythropoietin, which is secreted by liver and kidneys.

LIFESPAN AND FATE OF PLATELETS

Average lifespan of platelets is about 10 days. Older platelets are destroyed by tissue macrophage system in spleen.

APPLIED PHYSIOLOGY: PLATELET DISORDERS

Platelet disorders occur because of pathological variation in platelet count and dysfunction of platelets. Platelet disorders are given in **Box. 16.1**.

BOX 16.1: Platelet disorders.

Thrombocytopenia

Decrease in platelet count

Occurs in:
1. Acute infections
2. Acute leukemia
3. Aplastic and pernicious anemia
4. Chickenpox
5. Smallpox
6. Splenomegaly
7. Scarlet fever
8. Typhoid
9. Tuberculosis
10. Purpura
11. Gaucher's disease

Leads to thrombocytopenic purpura (Chapter 18)

Thrombocytosis

Increase in platelet count

Occurs in:
1. Allergic conditions
2. Asphyxia
3. Hemorrhage
4. Bone fractures
5. Surgical operations
6. Splenectomy
7. Rheumatic fever
8. Trauma (wound or injury or damage caused by external force)

Thrombocythemia

Persistent and abnormal increase in platelet count

Occurs in:
1. Carcinoma
2. Chronic leukemia
3. Hodgkin's disease

Glanzmann's thrombasthenia

Inherited hemorrhagic disorder, caused by structural or functional abnormality of platelets

Platelet count is normal

Characterized by:
  Normal clotting time
  Normal or prolonged bleeding time
  But defective clot retraction.

Leads to thrombasthenic purpura (Chapter 18).

Chapter 17: Hemostasis

CHAPTER OUTLINE

- DEFINITION
- STAGES OF HEMOSTASIS
  - VASOCONSTRICTION
- FORMATION OF PLATELET PLUG
- COAGULATION OF BLOOD

DEFINITION

Hemostasis is defined as arrest or stoppage of bleeding.

STAGES OF HEMOSTASIS

When a blood vessel is injured, the injury initiates a series of reactions resulting in hemostasis.

Hemostasis occurs in three stages:

1. Vasoconstriction.
2. Formation of platelet plug.
3. Coagulation of blood.

1. VASOCONSTRICTION

Immediately after injury, the blood vessel constricts and decreases the loss of blood from damaged portion. Usually, arterioles and small arteries constrict. The vasoconstriction is purely a local phenomenon. When the blood vessels are cut, the endothelium is damaged and the collagen is exposed. The platelets adhere to this collagen, and get activated. The activated platelets secrete **serotonin** and other vasoconstrictor substances which cause constriction of the blood vessels **(Fig. 17.1)**. The adherence of platelets to the collagen is accelerated by **von Willebrand factor**. This factor acts as a bridge between a specific glycoprotein present on the surface of platelet and collagen fibrils.

2. FORMATION OF PLATELET PLUG

The platelets get adhered to the collagen of ruptured blood vessel and secrete **ADP** and **thromboxane A$_2$**. These two substances attract more and more platelets and activate them. All these platelets aggregate together and form a loose temporary platelet plug or temporary hemostatic plug, which closes the vessel and prevents further blood loss. The platelet aggregation is accelerated by **platelet-activating factor** (PAF).

3. COAGULATION OF BLOOD

During this process, the fibrinogen is converted into fibrin. The fibrin threads get attached to the loose platelet plug, which blocks the ruptured part of blood vessels and prevents further blood loss completely. The mechanism of blood coagulation is explained in the next chapter.

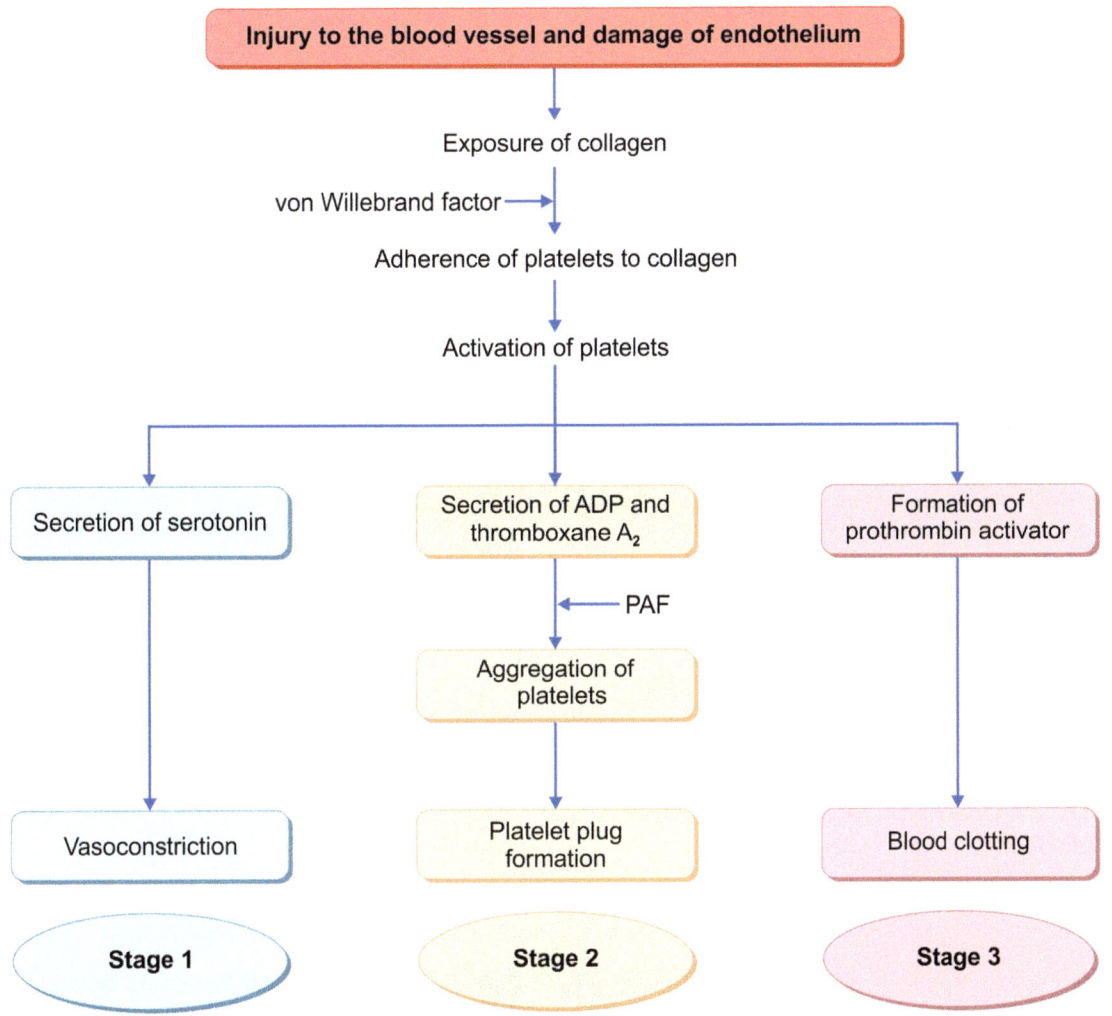

FIGURE 17.1: Stages of hemostasis.
ADP = Adenosine diphosphate, PAF = Platelet-activating factor.

Chapter 18: Coagulation of Blood

CHAPTER OUTLINE

- DEFINITION
- FACTORS INVOLVED IN BLOOD CLOTTING
- SEQUENCE OF CLOTTING MECHANISM
  - ENZYME CASCADE THEORY
  - STAGE 1: FORMATION OF PROTHROMBIN ACTIVATOR
  - STAGE 2: CONVERSION OF PROTHROMBIN INTO THROMBIN
  - STAGE 3: CONVERSION OF FIBRINOGEN INTO FIBRIN
- BLOOD CLOT
- ANTICLOTTING MECHANISM IN THE BODY
- ANTICOAGULANTS
- PHYSICAL METHODS TO PREVENT BLOOD CLOTTING
- PROCOAGULANTS
- TESTS FOR CLOTTING
- APPLIED PHYSIOLOGY

DEFINITION

Blood coagulation or **blood clotting** is defined as the process in which blood loses its fluidity and becomes a jelly-like mass few minutes after it is shed out or collected in a container.

FACTORS INVOLVED IN BLOOD CLOTTING

Coagulation of blood occurs through a series of reactions due to the activation of a group of substances. The substances necessary for clotting are called **clotting factors**. Thirteen clotting factors are identified and listed in **Table 18.1**.

The clotting factors were named after the scientists who discovered them or as per the activity except factor IX. Christmas factor (factor IX) was named after the patient in whom it was discovered.

SEQUENCE OF CLOTTING MECHANISM

ENZYME CASCADE THEORY

Most of the clotting factors are proteins in the form of enzymes. Normally, all the factors are present in the form of inactive proenzymes. These proenzymes must be activated into enzymes to enforce blood clotting. It is carried out by series of proenzyme – enzyme conversion reactions. The first one of the series is converted into an active enzyme that activates the second one, which activates the third one; this continues till the final active enzyme thrombin is formed.

Enzyme cascade theory explains how various reactions involved in the conversion of proenzymes to active enzymes take place in the form of a cascade. **Cascade** refers to a process that occurs through a series of steps, each step initiating the next, until the final step is reached.

TABLE 18.1: Clotting factors.

Factors	Name
I	Fibrinogen
II	Prothrombin
III	Thromboplastin (tissue factor)
IV	Calcium
V	Labile factor (proaccelerin or accelerator globulin)
VI	Presence has not been proved
VII	Stable factor
VIII	Antihemophilic factor (antihemophilic globulin)
IX	Christmas factor
X	Stuart-Prower factor
XI	Plasma thromboplastin antecedent
XII	Hageman factor (contact factor)
XIII	Fibrin-stabilizing factor (fibrinase)

Chapter 18: Coagulation of Blood

Stages of Blood Clotting

In general, blood clotting occurs in three stages:
1. Formation of prothrombin activator.
2. Conversion of prothrombin into thrombin.
3. Conversion of fibrinogen into fibrin.

■ STAGE 1: FORMATION OF PROTHROMBIN ACTIVATOR

Blood clotting commences with the formation of a substance called prothrombin activator. This process is initiated by substances produced either within the blood itself or outside the blood.

Thus, formation of prothrombin activator occurs through two pathways:

A. Intrinsic pathway.
B. Extrinsic pathway.

Intrinsic Pathway for the Formation of Prothrombin Activator

In this, the formation of prothrombin activator is initiated by platelets, which are within the blood itself **(Fig. 18.1)**.

Sequence of events in intrinsic pathway

i. During injury, the blood vessel is ruptured. Endothelium is damaged and collagen beneath the endothelium is exposed.
ii. When factor XII (**Hageman factor**) comes in contact with collagen, it is converted into activated factor XII in the presence of **kallikrein** and **HMW kininogen** (high molecular weight kininogen).

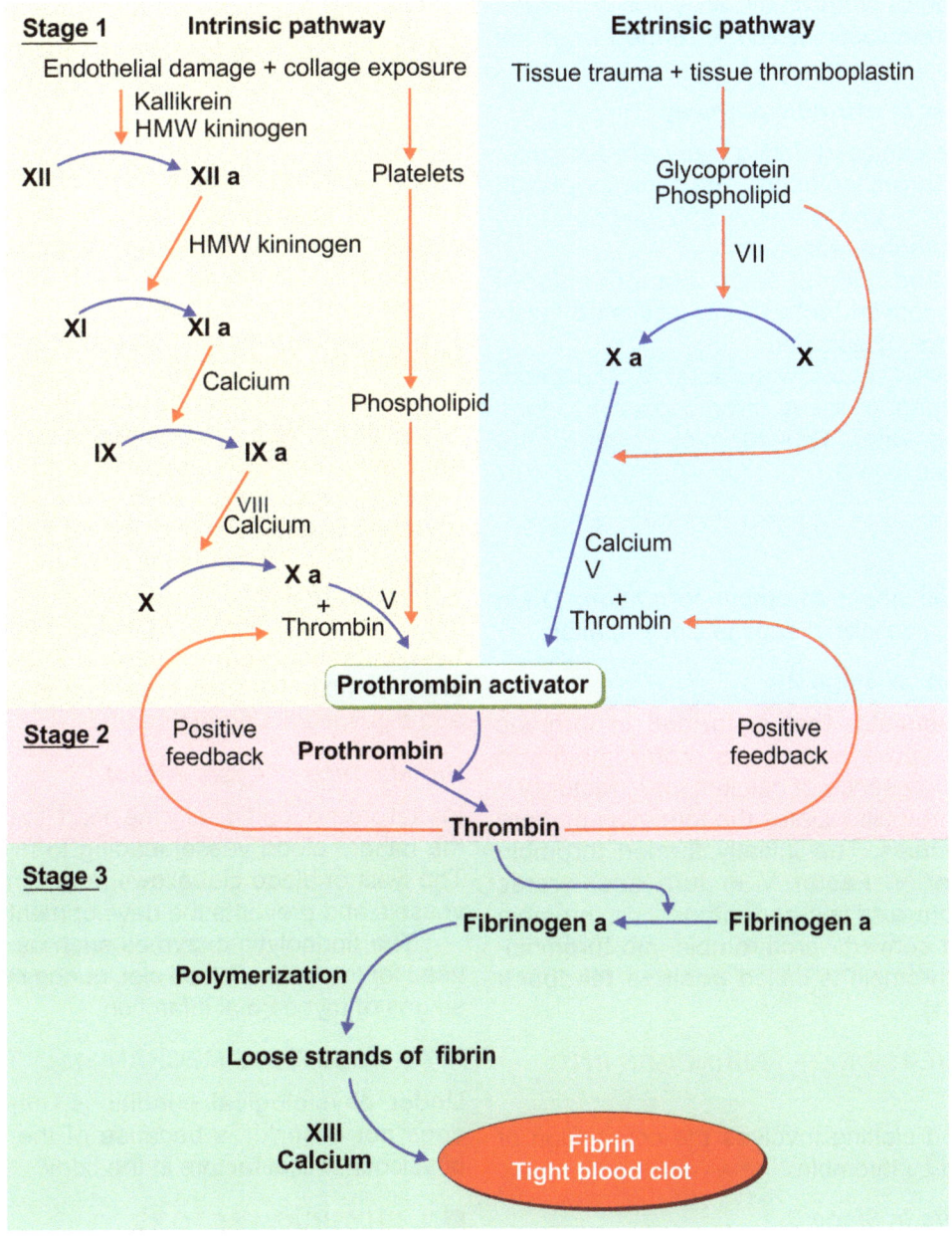

FIGURE 18.1: Stages of blood coagulation.
+ = Thrombin induces formation of more thrombin (positive feedback), a = Activated, HMW = High molecular weight.

iii. Activated factor XII converts factor XI into activated factor XI in the presence of HMW kininogen.
iv. Activated factor XI activates factor IX in the presence of factor IV (calcium).
v. Activated factor IX activates factor X in the presence of factor VIII and calcium.
vi. When platelet comes in contact with collagen of damaged blood vessel, it gets activated and releases phospholipids.
vii. Now, the activated factor X reacts with platelet phospholipid and factor V to form prothrombin activator. This needs presence of calcium ions.
viii. Factor V is also activated by positive feedback effect of thrombin (see below).

Extrinsic Pathway for the Formation of Prothrombin Activator

In this, the formation of prothrombin activator is initiated by the tissue thromboplastin which is formed from the injured tissues.

Sequence of events in extrinsic pathway

i. Tissues that are damaged during injury release factor III, i.e. tissue thromboplastin. The thromboplastin contains proteins, phospholipid and glycoprotein, which act as proteolytic enzymes.
ii. Glycoprotein and phospholipid components of thromboplastin convert factor X into activated factor X, in the presence of factor VII.
iii. Activated factor X reacts with factor V and phospholipid component of tissue thromboplastin to form prothrombin activator. This reaction requires the presence of calcium ions.

STAGE 2: CONVERSION OF PROTHROMBIN INTO THROMBIN

Blood clotting is all about thrombin formation. Once thrombin is formed, it definitely leads to clot formation.

Sequence of Events in Stage 2

i. Prothrombin activator that is formed in intrinsic and extrinsic pathways converts prothrombin into thrombin in the presence of calcium ions (factor IV).
ii. Once formed thrombin initiates the formation of more thrombin molecules. The initially formed thrombin activates factor V. Factor V in turn accelerates formation of both extrinsic and intrinsic prothrombin activator which converts prothrombin into thrombin. This effect of thrombin is called **positive feedback effect (Fig. 18.1)**.

STAGE 3: CONVERSION OF FIBRINOGEN INTO FIBRIN

Final stage of blood clotting involves the conversion of fibrinogen into fibrin by thrombin.

Sequence of Events in Stage 3

i. Thrombin converts fibrinogen into **activated fibrinogen** which is called **fibrin monomer**.
ii. Fibrin monomer polymerizes with other monomer molecules and form loosely arranged strands of fibrin.
iii. Later these loose strands are modified into dense and tight fibrin threads by fibrin-stabilizing factor (factor XIII) in the presence of calcium ions **(Fig. 18.1)**. All the tight fibrin threads are aggregated to form a meshwork of stable clot.

BLOOD CLOT

DEFINITION AND COMPOSITION OF BLOOD CLOT

Blood clot is defined as the mass of coagulated blood which contains RBCs, WBCs and platelets entrapped in fibrin meshwork.

The RBCs and WBCs are not necessary for clotting process. However, when clot is formed, these cells are trapped in it along with platelets. The trapped RBCs are responsible for the red color of the clot.

External blood clot is also called **scab**. It adheres to the opening of damaged blood vessel and prevents blood loss.

CLOT RETRACTION

Clot retraction is the process which involves contraction of blood clot 30 to 45 minutes after formation and oozing of **serum** out of clot. The contractile proteins namely, actin, myosin and **thrombosthenin** in the cytoplasm of platelets are responsible for clot retraction.

FIBRINOLYSIS

Fibrinolysis is the process that involves breakdown and dissolution of blood clot inside the blood vessel. It helps to remove the clot from lumen of the blood vessel.

Fibrinolysis requires a substance called **plasmin** or **fibrinolysin**. Plasmin is derived from inactivated glycoprotein called **plasminogen**. Plasminogen is synthesized in liver and it is incorporated with other proteins in the blood clot. Plasminogen is converted into plasmin by **tissue plasminogen activator** (t-PA), lysosomal enzymes and thrombin. Plasmin causes lysis of clot by dissolving and digesting the fibrin threads.

Significance of Lysis of Clot

In vital organs, particularly the heart, the blood clot obstructs the minute blood vessel leading to myocardial infarction. The lysis of blood clot allows reopening of affected blood vessels and prevents the development of infarction.

The fibrinolytic enzymes such as **streptokinase** are used for the lysis of blood clot, during the treatment in early stages of myocardial infarction.

ANTICLOTTING MECHANISM IN THE BODY

Under physiological conditions, intravascular clotting does not occur. It is because of the presence of some physicochemical factors in the body.

1. PHYSICAL FACTORS

i. Continuous circulation of blood.
ii. Smooth endothelial lining of the blood vessels.

2. CHEMICAL FACTORS

i. Presence of natural anticoagulant called heparin that is produced by the liver.
ii. Production of **thrombomodulin** by endothelium of the blood vessels (except in brain capillaries). Thrombomodulin is a **thrombin binding protein**. It binds with thrombin and forms a thrombomodulin–thrombin complex. This complex activates **protein-C**. Activated protein-C along with its cofactor **protein-S** inactivates factor V and factor VIII. Inactivation of these two clotting factors prevents clot formation.
iii. All the clotting factors are in inactive state.

ANTICOAGULANTS

Anticoagulants are the substances, which prevent or postpone coagulation of blood.

Anticoagulants are of three types:

I. Anticoagulants used to prevent blood clotting inside the body, i.e. in vivo.
II. Anticoagulants used to prevent clotting of blood that is collected from the body, i.e. in vitro.
III. Anticoagulants used to prevent blood clotting both in vivo and in vitro.

1. HEPARIN

Heparin is a naturally produced anticoagulant in the body. It is produced by **mast cells**, which are the wandering cells situated immediately outside the capillaries in many tissues or organs that contain more connective tissue. These cells are abundant in liver and lungs. Basophils also secrete heparin.

Heparin is a conjugated polysaccharide. The commercial heparin is prepared from the liver and other organs of animals. The commercial preparation is available in liquid form or dry form as sodium, calcium, ammonium or lithium salts.

Mechanism of Action of Heparin

Heparin:

i. Prevents blood clotting by its anti-thrombin activity. It directly suppresses the activity of thrombin.
ii. Combines with antithrombin III present in circulation and removes thrombin from circulation.
iii. Activates antithrombin III.
iv. Inactivates the active form of other clotting factors like IX, X, XI and XII **(Fig. 18.2)**.

Uses of Heparin

Heparin is used as an anticoagulant both in vivo and in vitro.

Clinical use

Intravenous injection of heparin (0.5 to 1 mg/kg body weight) postpones clotting for 3 to 4 hours (until it is destroyed by the enzyme heparinase). So, it is widely used as an anticoagulant in clinical practice for many purposes such as:

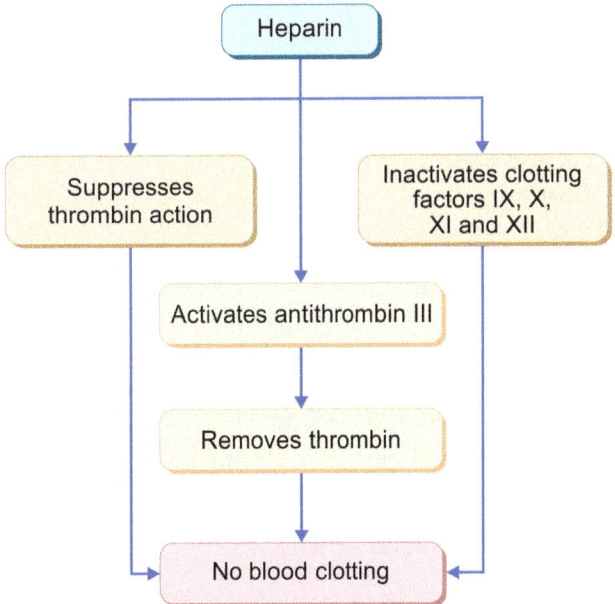

FIGURE 18.2: Mechanism of action of heparin.

i. To prevent intravascular blood clotting during surgery.
ii. During dialysis when blood is passed through artificial kidney.
iii. During cardiac surgery, that involves passing the blood through heart lung machine.
iv. To preserve the blood before transfusion.

Use in the laboratory

Heparin is also used as anticoagulant in vitro while collecting blood for various investigations. Heparin is the most expensive anticoagulant.

2. COUMARIN DERIVATIVES

Dicoumoral and warfarin are the derivatives of coumarin.

Mechanism of Action

The coumarin derivatives prevent blood clotting by inhibiting the action of vitamin K. Vitamin K is essential for the formation of various clotting factors namely, II, VII, IX and X.

Uses

Dicoumoral and warfarin are the commonly used **oral anticoagulants** (in vivo).

3. EDTA

Ethylenediaminetetra acetic acid (EDTA) is a strong anticoagulant.

It is available in two forms:

i. Disodium salt (Na_2 EDTA).
ii. Tripotassium salt (K_3 EDTA).

Mechanism of Action of EDTA

These substances prevent blood clotting by removing calcium from blood.

Uses of EDTA

EDTA is used as an anticoagulant both in vivo and in vitro:

i. It is administered intravenously in cases of lead poisoning (in vivo).
ii. It is also used as an anticoagulant in the laboratory (in vitro).

4. OXALATE COMPOUNDS

Oxalate compounds prevent coagulation by forming calcium oxalate, which is precipitated later. Thus, these compounds reduce the blood calcium level.

A mixture of ammonium oxalate and potassium oxalate in the ratio of 3:2 is used. Each salt is an anticoagulant by itself. But, potassium oxalate alone causes shrinkage of RBCs. Ammonium oxalate alone causes swelling of RBCs. But together, these substances do not alter the cellular activity.

Mechanism of Action of Oxalate Compounds

Oxalate combines with calcium and forms insoluble calcium oxalate. Thus, oxalate removes calcium from blood and lack of calcium prevents coagulation.

Uses of Oxalate Compounds

Oxalate compounds are used as in vitro anticoagulants. Oxalate is poisonous so it cannot be used in vivo.

5. CITRATES

Sodium, ammonium and potassium citrates are used as anticoagulants.

Mechanism of Action of Citrates

Citrate combines with calcium in blood to form insoluble calcium citrate. Like oxalate, citrate also removes calcium from blood and prevents coagulation.

Uses of Citrates

Citrates are used as an anticoagulant both in vivo and in vitro:

i. Used to store blood in the **blood bank**. It is available in two forms:
   a. Acid citrate dextrose (ACD).
   b. Citrate phosphate dextrose (CPD).
ii. Used in laboratory in vitro for RBC and platelet counts.

6. OTHER SUBSTANCES, WHICH PREVENT BLOOD CLOTTING

Peptone, proteins from venom of copper-head snake and hirudin (from leech) are the known anticoagulants.

PHYSICAL METHODS TO PREVENT BLOOD CLOTTING

Coagulation of blood is postponed or prevented by the following physical methods.

1. COLD

Reducing the temperature to about 5°C postpones coagulation of blood.

2. COLLECTING BLOOD IN A CONTAINER WITH SMOOTH SURFACE

Collecting the blood in a container with smooth surface like a **silicon-coated container** prevents clotting. The smooth surface inhibits the activation of factor XII and platelets. So, the formation of prothrombin activator is prevented.

PROCOAGULANTS

Procoagulants or **hemostatic agents** are the substances, which accelerate the process of blood coagulation.

Procoagulants are:

1. Thrombin.
2. Snake venom.
3. Extracts of lungs and thymus.
4. Sodium or calcium alginate.
5. Oxidized cellulose.

TESTS FOR CLOTTING

1. BLEEDING TIME

Bleeding time is the time interval from oozing of blood after a cut or injury till arrest of bleeding. Usually, it is determined by **Duke method** using blotting paper or filter paper method. Its normal duration is 3 to 6 minutes. It is prolonged in **purpura**.

2. CLOTTING TIME

Clotting time is the time interval from oozing of blood after a cut or injury till the formation of clot. It is usually determined by capillary tube method. Its normal duration is 3 to 8 minutes. And it is prolonged in **hemophilia**.

3. PROTHROMBIN TIME

It is the time taken by blood to clot after adding tissue thromboplastin to it. Blood is collected and oxalated so that, the calcium is precipitated and prothrombin is not converted into thrombin. Thus, the blood clotting is prevented. Then a large quantity of tissue thromboplastin with calcium is added to this blood. Calcium nullifies the effect of oxalate. The tissue thromboplastin activates prothrombin and blood clotting occurs.

During this procedure, the time taken by blood to clot after adding tissue thromboplastin is determined. Prothrombin time indicates the total quantity of prothrombin present in the blood.

Normal duration of prothrombin time is about 12 seconds. It is prolonged in deficiency of prothrombin and other factors such as factors I, V, VII and X. However, it is normal in hemophilia.

APPLIED PHYSIOLOGY
BLEEDING DISORDERS

Bleeding disorders are the diseases characterized by prolonged bleeding time or clotting time. The bleeding disorders are of three types.

1. Hemophilia

Hemophilia is a group of sex-linked inherited blood disorders characterized by prolonged clotting time. However, bleeding time is normal in hemophilia. In this disorder males are affected and the females are the carriers. Because of prolonged clotting time, even a mild trauma causes excess bleeding which can lead to death. Damage of skin while falling or extraction of a tooth may cause excess bleeding for few weeks. Easy bruising and hemorrhage in muscles and joints are also common in this disease.

Cause for hemophilia

Lack of prothrombin activator is the cause for hemophilia. The formation of prothrombin activator is affected due to the deficiency of factor VIII, IX or XI.

Types of hemophilia

Depending upon the deficiency of the factor involved, hemophilia is classified into three types:

  i. Hemophilia A or classic hemophilia that is due to the deficiency of factor VIII. 85% of people with hemophilia are affected by hemophilia A.
  ii. Hemophilia B or **Christmas disease** which is due to the deficiency of factor IX. 15% of people with hemophilia are affected by hemophilia B.
  iii. Hemophilia C which is due to the deficiency of factor XI. It is a very rare blood disorder.

2. Purpura

It is a disorder characterized by prolonged bleeding time. However, the clotting time is normal. The characteristic feature of this disease is spontaneous bleeding under the skin from ruptured capillaries. It causes small tiny hemorrhagic spots under the skin which are called **purpuric spots** (purple colored patch-like appearance). That is why this disease is called purpura.

Types and causes of purpura

Purpura is classified into different types depending upon the causes.

i. Thrombocytopenic purpura

Thrombocytopenic purpura is due to the deficiency of platelets (thrombocytopenia). In bone marrow disease, platelet production is affected leading to deficiency of platelets.

ii. Idiopathic thrombocytopenic purpura

Purpura due to some unknown cause is called idiopathic thrombocytopenic purpura. It is believed that platelet count decreases due to the development of antibodies against platelets, which occurs after blood transfusion.

iii. Thrombasthenic purpura

This type of purpura is due to structural or functional abnormality of platelets. However, the platelet count is normal. It is characterized by normal clotting time, normal or prolonged bleeding time, but defective clot retraction.

3. von Willebrand Disease

von Willebrand disease is a bleeding disorder characterized by excess bleeding even with a mild injury. It is due to inherited deficiency of **von Willebrand factor** which is a protein secreted by endothelium of damaged blood vessels and platelets. This protein is responsible for adherence of platelets to endothelium of blood vessels during hemostasis after an injury. It is also responsible for the survival and maintenance of factor VIII in plasma.

The deficiency of von Willebrand factor suppresses platelet adhesion. It also causes deficiency of factor VIII. This results in excess bleeding which resembles the bleeding that occurs during platelet dysfunction or hemophilia.

THROMBOSIS

Thrombosis or **intravascular blood clotting** refers to coagulation of blood inside the blood vessels. Normally, blood does not clot in the blood vessel because of some factors which are already explained. But some abnormal conditions can cause thrombosis.

Causes of Thrombosis

1. Injury to blood vessels.
2. Roughened endothelial lining.
3. Sluggishness of blood flow.
4. Agglutination of RBCs.
5. Poisons like snake venom, mercury, and arsenic compounds.
6. Congenital absence of protein C.

Complications of Thrombosis

1. Thrombus

During thrombosis, lumen of blood vessels is occluded. The solid mass of platelets, red cells and/or clot, which obstructs the blood vessel, is called thrombus. The thrombus formed due to agglutination of RBC is called **agglutinative thrombus**.

2. Embolism and embolus

Embolism is the process in which the thrombus or part of it is detached and carried in bloodstream and occludes the small blood vessels resulting in arrests of blood flow to any organ or region of the body. Embolus is the thrombus or part of it, which arrests the blood flow. The obstruction of blood flow by embolism is common in lungs (**pulmonary embolism**), brain (**cerebral embolism**) and heart (**coronary embolism**).

3. Ischemia

Insufficient blood supply to an organ or area of body by the obstruction of blood vessels is called ischemia. Ischemia results in tissue damage because of hypoxia (lack of oxygen). Ischemia also causes discomfort, pain and tissue death. Death of body tissue is called necrosis.

4. Necrosis and infarction

Necrosis is a general term that refers to tissue death caused by loss of blood supply, injury, infection, inflammation, physical agents or chemical substances.

Infarction means the tissue death due to loss of blood supply. Loss blood supply is usually caused by occlusion of an artery by thrombus or embolus and sometimes by atherosclerosis (Chapter 51). The area of tissue that undergoes infarction is called infarct. Infarction commonly occurs in heart, brain, lungs, kidneys and spleen.

Chapter 19: Blood Groups

CHAPTER OUTLINE

- **BLOOD GROUP SYSTEMS**
- **ABO BLOOD GROUPS**
  - LANDSTEINER'S LAW
  - ABO SYSTEM
  - DETERMINATION OF THE ABO GROUP
  - IMPORTANCE OF ABO GROUPS IN BLOOD TRANSFUSION
  - MATCHING AND CROSSMATCHING
  - INHERITANCE OF ABO AGGLUTINOGENS AND AGGLUTININS
- **Rh FACTOR**
  - INHERITANCE OF Rh ANTIGEN
- **APPLIED PHYSIOLOGY**
  - TRANSFUSION REACTIONS DUE TO ABO INCOMPATIBILITY
  - TRANSFUSION REACTIONS DUE TO Rh INCOMPATIBILITY
- **OTHER BLOOD GROUPS**
  - LEWIS BLOOD GROUP
  - BOMBAY GROUP: H ANTIGEN
  - OTHER MINOR BLOOD GROUPS
- **IMPORTANCE OF KNOWING BLOOD GROUP**

BLOOD GROUP SYSTEMS

Blood groups were discovered by Austrian Scientist **Karl Landsteiner** in 1901. He was honored with Nobel Prize in 1930 for this discovery.

More than 20 genetically determined blood group systems are known today. But, Landsteiner discovered two blood group systems called ABO system and Rh system. These two blood group systems are the most important ones that are determined before blood transfusions.

ABO BLOOD GROUPS

Determination of ABO blood groups depends upon the immunological reaction between **antigen** and **antibody**. Landsteiner found two antigens on the surface of RBCs and named them as A antigen and B antigen. These antigens are also called **agglutinogens** because of their capacity to cause agglutination of RBCs. He noticed the **corresponding antibodies** or **agglutinins** in the plasma and named them anti-A or α antibody and anti-B or β antibody. However, a particular agglutinogen and the corresponding agglutinin cannot be present together. If present, it causes clumping of the blood. Based on this, Landsteiner classified the blood groups. Later it has become the 'Landsteiner's Law' for grouping the blood.

LANDSTEINER'S LAW

Landsteiner's law states that:

1. If a particular antigen (agglutinogen) is present in the RBCs, corresponding antibody (agglutinin) must be absent in the serum.
2. If a particular antigen is absent in the RBCs, the corresponding antibody must be present in the serum.

Though the second part of Landsteiner's law is a fact, it is not applicable to Rh factor.

ABO SYSTEM

Based on the presence or absence of antigen A and antigen B, blood is divided into four groups:

1. 'A' group.
2. 'B' group.
3. 'AB' group.
4. 'O' group.

Blood having antigen A is called A group. This group has β antibody in the serum. The blood with antigen B and α antibody is called B group. If both the antigens are present, the blood group is called AB group and serum of this group does not contain any antibody. If both antigens are absent, the blood group is called O group and both α

TABLE 19.1: Antigen and antibody present in ABO blood groups.

Group	Antigen in RBC	Antibody in serum
A	A	Anti-B (β)
B	B	Anti-A (α)
AB	A and B	No antibody
O	No antigen	Anti-A and anti-B

TABLE 19.2: Percentage of people having different blood groups.

Population	A	B	AB	O
Indians	23	33	7	37
Asians	25	25	5	45
Europeans	42	9	3	46

All Indians in Peru (South American country) have only "O" blood group.

and β antibodies are present in the serum. The antigens and antibodies present in different groups of ABO system are given in **Table 19.1**. Percentage of people among Asian and European population belonging to different blood groups is given in **Table 19.2**.

'A' group has two subgroups namely 'A_1' and 'A_2'. Similarly, 'AB' group has two subgroups namely 'A_1B' and 'A_2B'.

■ DETERMINATION OF THE ABO GROUP

Determination of the ABO group is also called blood grouping, blood typing or blood matching.

Principle of Blood Typing: Agglutination

The blood typing is done on the basis of agglutination. **Agglutination** means the collection of separate particles like RBCs into clumps or masses. Agglutination occurs if an antigen is mixed with its corresponding antibody which is called **isoagglutinin**. Agglutination occurs when A antigen is mixed with anti-A or when B antigen is mixed with anti-B.

Requisites for Blood Typing

To determine the blood group of a person, a suspension of his RBC and testing antisera are required. Suspension of RBC is prepared by mixing blood drops with isotonic saline (0.9%).

Test sera are:
1. Antiserum A, containing anti-A.
2. Antiserum B, containing anti-B.

Procedure

1. One drop of antiserum A is placed on one end of a tile or glass slide. And, one drop of antiserum B is placed on the other end of tile or slide.
2. One drop of RBC suspension is mixed with each antiserum. The tile is slightly rocked for 2 minutes. The presence or absence of agglutination is observed by

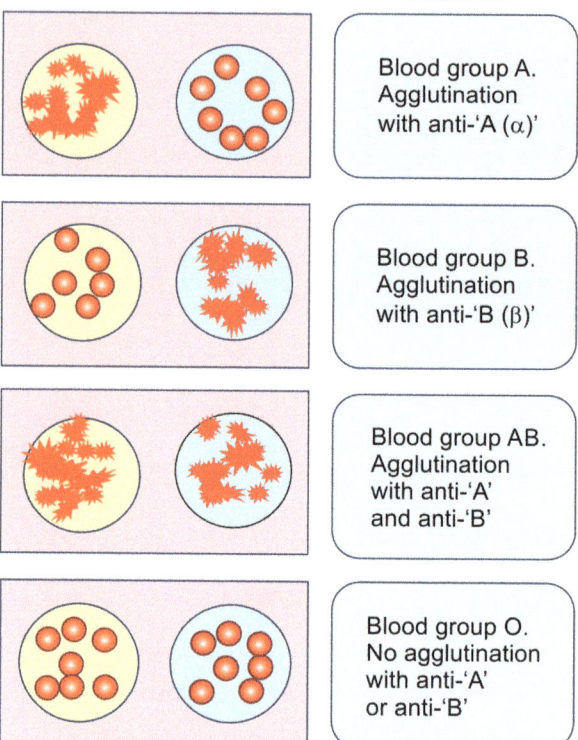

FIGURE 19.1: Determination of blood group.

naked eyes and if necessary, it is confirmed by using microscope.
3. Presence of agglutination is confirmed by the presence of clumping of RBCs.
4. Absence of agglutination is confirmed by clear mixture with dispersed RBCs.

Results

1. *If agglutination occurs with antiserum A:*
   The antiserum A contains anti-A or α antibody. The agglutination occurs if the RBC contains A antigen. So, the blood group is A **(Fig. 19.1)**.
2. *If agglutination occurs with antiserum B:*
   The antiserum B contains anti-B or β antibody. The agglutination occurs if the RBC contains B antigen. So, the blood group is B.
3. *If agglutination occurs with both antisera A and B:*
   The RBC contains both A and B antigens to cause agglutination. And, the blood group is AB.
4. *If agglutination does not occur either with antiserum A or antiserum B:*
   The agglutination does not occur if the RBC does not contain any antigen. The blood group is O.

■ IMPORTANCE OF ABO GROUPS IN BLOOD TRANSFUSION

During blood transfusion, only compatible blood must be used. The one who gives blood is called the donor and the one who receives the blood is called recipient.

While transfusing the blood, antigen of the donor and the antibody of the recipient are considered. The antibody of the donor and antigen of the recipient are ignored mostly.

Thus, RBC of 'O' group has no antigen and so agglutination does not occur with any other group of blood. So, 'O' group blood can be given to any blood group persons and the people of this group blood are called **universal donors**.

The plasma of AB group blood has no antibody. This does not cause agglutination of RBC from any other group of blood. The people of AB group can receive blood from any blood group persons. So, people with this group blood are called **universal recipients**.

MATCHING AND CROSSMATCHING

Blood matching or **blood typing** is a laboratory test done to determine the blood group of a person. When the person needs blood transfusion, another test called crossmatching is done after the blood is typed. It is done to find out whether the person's body will accept the donor's blood or not.

For blood matching, RBC of the individual (recipient) and test sera are used. Crossmatching is done by mixing the serum of the recipient and the RBCs of donor. Crossmatching is always done before blood transfusion. If agglutination of RBCs from a donor occurs during crossmatching, the blood from that person is not used for transfusion.

Matching = Recipient's RBC + Test sera
Crossmatching = Recipient's serum + Donor's RBC

INHERITANCE OF ABO AGGLUTINOGENS AND AGGLUTININS

Blood group of a person depends upon the two genes inherited from each parent. Gene A and gene B are dominant by themselves and gene O is recessive. The inheritance of blood group is represented schematically as given in **Table 19.3**.

Rh FACTOR

Rh factor is an antigen present in RBC. This antigen was discovered by Landsteiner and Wiener. It was first discovered in **rhesus monkey** and hence the name Rh factor. There are many Rh antigens but only the D is more antigenic in human.

The persons having **D antigen** are called Rh positive and those without D antigen are called Rh negative. Among Asian population, 85% of people are Rh positive and 15% are Rh negative.

Rh group system is different from ABO group system because, the antigen D does not have corresponding natural antibody (anti-D). However, if Rh positive blood is transfused to a Rh negative person for the first time, then anti-D is formed in that person. On the other hand, there is no risk of complications if Rh positive person receives Rh negative blood.

INHERITANCE OF Rh ANTIGEN

Rhesus factor is an inherited dominant factor. It may be homozygous Rhesus positive with DD or heterozygous Rhesus positive with Dd **(Fig. 19.2)**. Rhesus

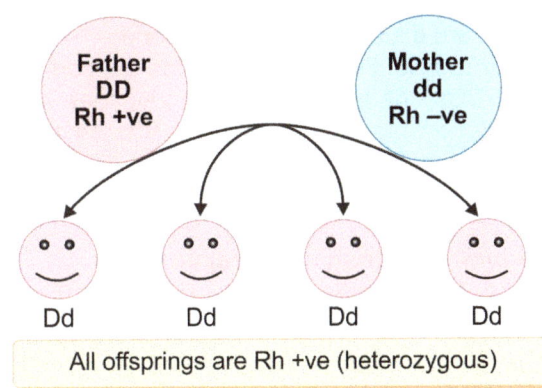

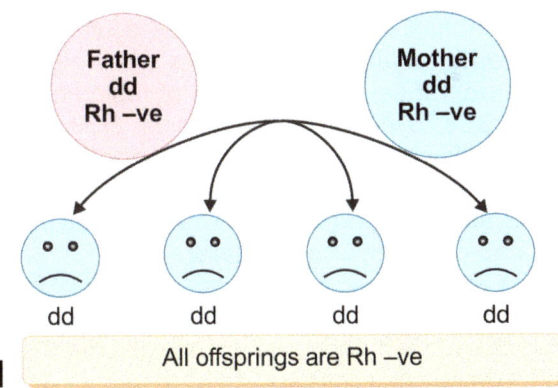

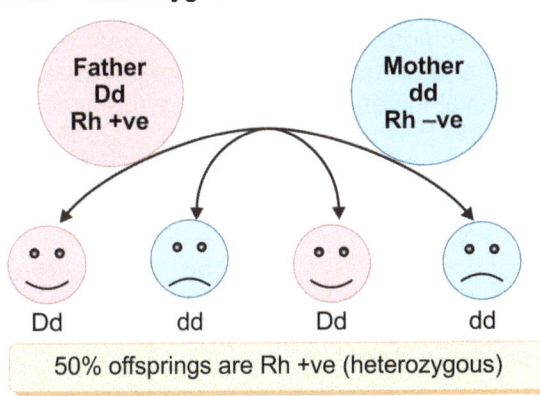

FIGURE 19.2: Inheritance of Rh antigen. **A.** If father is homozygous with DD; **B.** If father is homozygous with dd; **C.** If father is heterozygous with Dd.

TABLE 19.3: Inheritance of ABO group.

Gene from parents	Group of offspring	Genotype
A + A A + O	A	AA or AO
B + B B + O	B	BB or BO
A + B	AB	AB
O + O	O	OO

negative occurs only with complete absence of D (i.e. with homozygous dd).

■ APPLIED PHYSIOLOGY

■ TRANSFUSION REACTIONS DUE TO ABO INCOMPATIBILITY

Transfusion reactions are the adverse reactions in the body which occur due to transfusion of incompatible (mismatched) blood. The reactions may vary from fever and **hives** (skin disorder characterized by itching) to renal failure, shock and death.

In mismatched transfusion, the transfusion reactions occur between donor's RBC and recipient's plasma. So, if the donor's plasma contains antibody against recipient's RBC, agglutination does not occur because these antibodies are diluted in recipient's blood.

But, if recipient's plasma contains antibodies against donor's RBCs, the immune system launches a response against the new blood cells. Donor RBCs are agglutinated and hemolyzed.

Signs and Symptoms of Transfusion Reactions

Non-hemolytic transfusion reaction

Non-hemolytic transfusion reaction develops within a few minutes to hours after the commencement of blood transfusion. Common symptoms are fever, difficulty in breathing and itching.

Hemolytic transfusion reaction

Hemolytic transfusion reaction may be acute or delayed. The acute hemolytic reaction occurs within few minutes of transfusion. It develops because of rapid hemolysis of donor's RBCs. Symptoms include fever, chills, increased heart rate, low blood pressure, shortness of breath, bronchospasm, nausea, vomiting, red urine, chest pain, back pain and rigor. Some patients may develop pulmonary edema and congestive cardiac failure.

Delayed hemolytic reaction occurs from 1 to 5 days after transfusion. The hemolysis of RBCs results in release of large amount of hemoglobin into the plasma. This leads to the following complications.

1. Jaundice

Normally, hemoglobin released from destroyed RBC is degraded and bilirubin is formed from it. When the serum bilirubin level increases above 2 mg/dL, jaundice occurs (Chapter 34).

2. Cardiac Shock

Simultaneously, the hemoglobin released into the plasma increases the viscosity of blood. This increases the workload on the heart leading to cardiac shock.

3. Renal Shutdown

Dysfunction of kidneys is called renal shutdown. The toxic substances from hemolyzed cells cause constriction of blood vessels in kidney. In addition, the toxic substances along with free hemoglobin are filtered through glomerular

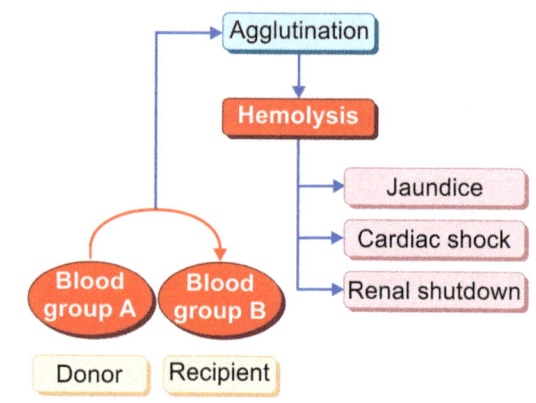

FIGURE 19.3: Complications of mismatched blood transfusion.

membrane and enter renal tubules. Because of poor rate of reabsorption from renal tubules, all these substances precipitate and obstruct the renal tubule. This suddenly stops formation of urine (anuria).

If not treated with artificial kidney, the person dies within 10 to 12 days because of jaundice, circulatory shock and more specifically due to renal shutdown and anuria **(Fig. 19.3)**.

■ TRANSFUSION REACTIONS DUE TO Rh INCOMPATIBILITY

When a person with Rh negative blood receives Rh positive blood for the first time, he is not affected much, since the reactions do not occur immediately. But the Rh antibodies develop within one month. The transfused RBCs, which are still present in recipient's blood are agglutinated. These agglutinated cells are lysed by macrophages. So, a delayed transfusion reaction occurs. But, it is usually mild and does not affect the recipient. However, antibodies developed in the recipient remain in the body for ever. So, when this person receives Rh positive blood for the second time, the donor RBCs are agglutinated and severe transfusion reactions occur immediately **(Fig. 19.4)**. These reactions

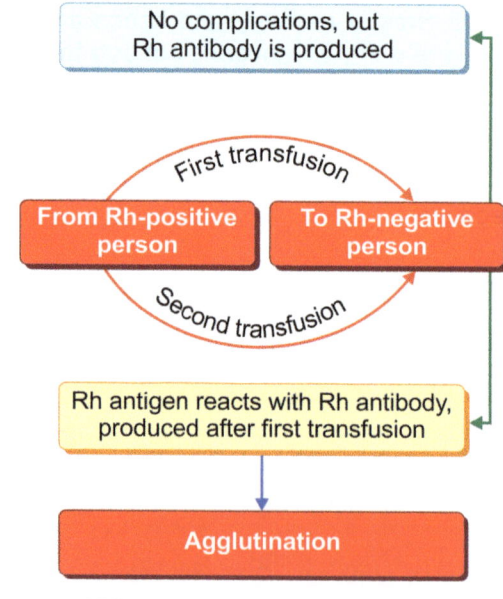

FIGURE 19.4: Rh incompatibility.

are similar to the reactions of ABO incompatibility (see above).

Hemolytic Disease of Fetus and Newborn: Erythroblastosis Fetalis

Hemolytic disease is the disease in fetus and newborn characterized by abnormal hemolysis of RBCs. It is due to Rh incompatibility. Hemolytic disease leads to erythroblastosis fetalis.

Erythroblastosis fetalis is a disorder in fetus characterized by the presence of **erythroblasts** in blood. When a mother is Rh negative and fetus is Rh positive (Rh factor being inherited from the father), first child of the lady escapes the complications of Rh incompatibility. This is because the Rh antigen cannot pass from fetal blood into the mother's blood through the placental barrier.

However, at the time of parturition (delivery of the child) the Rh antigen from fetal blood may leak into mother's blood because of placental detachment. During postpartum period, i.e. within a month after delivery, the mother develops Rh antibody in her blood.

When the mother conceives for the second time and if the fetus happens to be Rh positive again, the Rh antibody from mother's blood crosses placental barrier and enters the fetal blood. Thus, the Rh antigen cannot cross the placental barrier whereas Rh antibody can cross it.

The Rh agglutinins which enter the fetus cause agglutination of fetal RBCs resulting in hemolysis.

Severe hemolysis in the fetus causes jaundice. To compensate the hemolysis of greater number of RBCs, there is rapid production of RBCs, not only from bone marrow, but also from spleen and liver. Now, many large and immature cells in **proerythroblastic** stage are released into circulation. Because of this, the disease is called erythroblastosis fetalis.

Complications of Erythroblastosis Fetalis

Ultimately due to excessive hemolysis severe complications develop, viz.:

1. Severe anemia.
2. Hydrops fetalis.
3. Kernicterus.

1. Severe Anemia

Excess hemolysis results in anemia. And the infant dies when anemia becomes severe.

2. Hydrops Fetalis

It is a serious condition in fetus characterized by edema. Severe hemolysis results in the development of edema, enlargement of liver and spleen and cardiac failure. When this condition becomes more severe it may lead to intrauterine death of fetus.

3. Bilirubin Encephalopathy: Kernicterus

Bilirubin encephalopathy is a neurological disorder characterized by brain damage in infants caused by severe jaundice. If the baby survives anemia in erythroblastosis fetalis (see above), encephalopathy develops because of high bilirubin content.

Bilirubin encephalopathy is often called as kernicterus. The term kernicterus refers to yellow staining of brain tissues caused by bilirubin.

Prevention or Treatment for Erythroblastosis Fetalis

i. If mother is found to be Rh negative and fetus is Rh positive, **anti-D** (antibody against D antigen) should be administered to the mother at 28th and 34th weeks of gestation as **prophylactic measure**. If Rh negative mother delivers Rh positive baby, then anti D should be administered to the mother within 48 hours of delivery. This develops passive immunity and prevents the formation of Rh antibodies in mother's blood. So, the hemolytic disease of newborn does not occur in a subsequent pregnancy.

ii. If the baby is born with erythroblastosis fetalis, the treatment is given by means of **exchange transfusion** (Chapter 20). Rh negative blood is transfused into the infant replacing infant's own Rh positive blood. It will now take at least 6 months for the infant's new Rh positive blood to replace the transfused Rh negative blood. By this time all the molecules of Rh antibody derived from the mother get destroyed.

■ OTHER BLOOD GROUPS

■ LEWIS BLOOD GROUP

Lewis blood group was first found in a subject named Lewis. The antibody that was found in this lady reacted with the antigens found on RBCs and in body fluids such as saliva, gastric juice, etc. The antigens, which are named Lewis antigens are formed in the tissues, released in the body secretions and then absorbed by the RBC membrane. Because of secretion along with body secretions, these antigens are also known as **secretor antigens**. Presence of Lewis antigens in children leads to some complications such as retarded growth. Sometimes, it causes transfusion reactions also.

■ BOMBAY GROUP: H ANTIGEN

H antigen is the precursor of ABO group antigens, i.e. antigen A and antigen B. H antigen is present in RBCs of all individuals. If a person has the gene for A antigen or B antigen or both, these antigens are formed from H antigen. If there is no gene for A and B antigens, the person will not have A or B antigen in spite of having H antigen. The blood of this person belongs to O group.

Rarely, in some persons A, B and H antigens are absent in red blood cells. This group is called Bombay group, since it was first discovered in Bombay in the year 1952.

Serum of this Bombay group contains anti-A, anti-B and anti-H antibodies. Sera of these persons will agglutinate the RBCs of all other groups except Bombay group as the red cells of Bombay group do not contain H antigen. While typing the blood group these persons are seen as

O group as antigens are absent in RBCs. So, RBCs are agglutinated while typing. However, during crossmatching sera of this group will agglutinate the RBCs of all other groups.

OTHER MINOR BLOOD GROUPS

In addition, many more blood group systems were found. However, these systems of blood groups do not have much clinical importance.

Other blood groups include:

1. MNS group.
2. Auberger groups.
3. Diego group.
4. Duffy group.
5. Lutheran group.
6. P group.
7. Kell group.
8. I group.
9. Kidd group.
10. Sutter group.
11. Xg group.

IMPORTANCE OF KNOWING BLOOD GROUP

Nowadays, knowledge of blood group is very essential medically and socially.

Importance of knowing blood group is:

1. Medically, it is important during blood transfusions and in tissue transplants to save life.
2. Socially, one should know his/her own blood group and become a member of the Blood Donor's Club so that he/she can be approached for blood donation during emergency conditions.
3. Among the couple, knowledge of blood groups helps to prevent the complications due to Rh incompatibility and save the child from the disorders like erythroblastosis fetalis.

Chapter 20: Blood Transfusion

CHAPTER OUTLINE

- DEFINITION AND TYPES
- INDICATIONS OF BLOOD TRANSFUSION
- PRECAUTIONS
  - PRECAUTIONS TO BE TAKEN BEFORE TRANSFUSION OF BLOOD
  - PRECAUTIONS TO BE TAKEN WHILE TRANSFUSING BLOOD
- HAZARDS OF BLOOD TRANSFUSION
- BLOOD SUBSTITUTES
- EXCHANGE TRANSFUSION
  - PROCEDURE
  - INDICATIONS OF EXCHANGE TRANSFUSION
- AUTOLOGOUS BLOOD TRANSFUSION

DEFINITION AND TYPES

Blood transfusion is a process by which blood or blood components are transfused from one person (donor) into the bloodstream of another person (recipient). Transfusion may be done as a **lifesaving procedure** to replace blood cells or blood products lost through bleeding.

Blood transfusion is of four types:

1. *Whole blood transfusion*: Used in hemorrhage.
2. *Red cell transfusion*: Used in anemia.
3. *Platelet transfusion*: Used in bleeding disorders.
4. *Plasma transfusion*: Used during burns, liver diseases and surgical procedures particularly heart surgery.

INDICATIONS OF BLOOD TRANSFUSION

Indications means the symptoms or condition of a disease that indicate or suggest the necessity of medical treatment. Following are the indications of exchange transfusion:

1. Anemia.
2. Hemorrhage.
3. Trauma.
4. Burns.
5. Surgery.

PRECAUTIONS

PRECAUTIONS TO BE TAKEN BEFORE TRANSFUSION OF BLOOD

1. Donor must be healthy, without any diseases like
    i. Sexually transmitted diseases such as syphilis.
    ii. Diseases caused by virus like hepatitis, AIDS, etc.
2. Only compatible blood must be transfused. Rh compatibility also must be confirmed.
3. Both matching and crossmatching must be done.

PRECAUTIONS TO BE TAKEN WHILE TRANSFUSING BLOOD

1. Apparatus for transfusion must be sterile.
2. Temperature of blood to be transfused must be same as body temperature.
3. Transfusion of blood must be slow. Sudden rapid infusion of blood into the body increases the load on the heart resulting in many complications.

HAZARDS OF BLOOD TRANSFUSION

Hazards of blood transfusion are of four types:

1. Reactions due to mismatched (incompatible) blood transfusion (transfusion reactions).
2. Reactions due to massive blood transfusion.
3. Reactions due to faulty techniques during blood transfusion.
4. Transmission of infections.

BLOOD SUBSTITUTES

Blood substitutes are the substances infused as a replacement for blood or to expand blood volume.

Commonly used Blood Substitutes

1. Human plasma.
2. 0.9% sodium chloride solution (saline)
3. 5% glucose.

4. Colloids like gum acacia, isinglass, albumin and animal gelatin.

EXCHANGE TRANSFUSION

Exchange transfusion is the procedure which involves removal of patient's blood completely and replacement with fresh blood or plasma of the donor. It is otherwise known as **replacement transfusion.** It is an important lifesaving procedure carried out in conditions such as severe jaundice, sickle cell anemia, erythroblastosis fetalis, etc.

PROCEDURE FOR EXCHANGE TRANSFUSION

Procedure involves both removal and replacement of affected blood in stages. Exchange transfusion is carried out in short cycles of few minutes duration as given below:

1. Affected person's blood is slowly drawn out in small quantities of 5 to 20 mL, depending upon the age and size of the person and the severity of the condition.
2. Equal quantity of fresh, pre-warmed blood or plasma is infused through intravenous catheter. This is carried out for few minutes.
3. Catheter is left in place and the transfusion is repeated within few hours.
4. This procedure is continued till the whole or predetermined volume of blood is exchanged.

INDICATIONS OF EXCHANGE TRANSFUSION

Following are the indications of exchange transfusion:

1. Hemolytic disease of the newborn (erythroblastosis fetalis).
2. Severe sickle cell anemia.
3. Severe polycythemia (replacement with saline, plasma or albumin).
4. Toxicity of certain drugs.
5. Severe jaundice in newborn babies.

AUTOLOGOUS BLOOD TRANSFUSION

Autologous blood transfusion is the collection and reinfusion of patient's own blood. It is also called self blood donation. The conventional transfusion of blood that is collected from persons other than the patient is called allogeneic or **heterologous blood transfusion**.

Autologous blood transfusion is used for planned surgical procedures. Patient's blood is withdrawn in advance and stored. Later, it is infused during surgery if necessary.

This type of blood transfusion prevents the transmission of viruses such as HIV or hepatitis B. It also eliminates transfusion reactions.

Chapter 21: Reticuloendothelial System, Tissue Macrophage and Spleen

CHAPTER OUTLINE

- **DEFINITION AND DISTRIBUTION**
  - RETICULOENDOTHELIAL SYSTEM OR TISSUE MACROPHAGE SYSTEM
  - TISSUE MACROPHAGE
- **CLASSIFICATION OF RETICULOENDOTHELIAL CELLS**
  - FIXED RETICULOENDOTHELIAL CELLS: TISSUE MACROPHAGE
- **WANDERING RETICULOENDOTHELIAL CELLS**
- **FUNCTIONS OF RETICULOENDOTHELIAL SYSTEM**
- **SPLEEN**
  - FUNCTIONAL ANATOMY
  - FUNCTIONS
  - APPLIED PHYSIOLOGY

DEFINITION AND DISTRIBUTION

RETICULOENDOTHELIAL SYSTEM OR TISSUE MACROPHAGE SYSTEM

Reticuloendothelial system or tissue macrophage system is the system of primitive phagocytic cells which play important role in defense mechanism of the body.

Structures having Reticuloendothelial Cells

1. Endothelial lining of vascular and lymph channels.
2. Connective tissue and some organs such as spleen, liver, lungs, lymph nodes and bone marrow, etc.

Reticular cells in these tissues form the tissue macrophage system.

TISSUE MACROPHAGE

Macrophage is a large phagocytic cell, derived from monocyte (Chapter 14). Monocytes leave the blood and enter tissues and transform into larger macrophages. Tissue macrophages have long lifespan ranging from months to years.

CLASSIFICATION OF RETICULOENDOTHELIAL CELLS

Reticuloendothelial cells are classified into two types:

I. Fixed reticuloendothelial cells or tissue macrophages.
II. Wandering reticuloendothelial cells.

FIXED RETICULOENDOTHELIAL CELLS: TISSUE MACROPHAGES

Fixed reticuloendothelial cells are also called tissue macrophages or **fixed histiocytes**, because these cells are usually located in the tissues.

Tissue macrophages are:

1. Reticuloendothelial cells in connective tissues and in serous membranes like pleura, omentum and mesentery.
2. Endothelial cells of blood sinusoid in bone marrow, liver, spleen, lymph nodes, adrenal glands and pituitary glands. **Kupffer cells** in liver belong to this category.
3. Cells in the reticulum of spleen, lymph node and bone marrow.
4. **Meningocytes** of meninges and **microglia** in brain.
5. Alveolar cells in lungs.
6. Subcutaneous tissue cells.

WANDERING RETICULOENDOTHELIAL CELLS

Wandering reticuloendothelial cells are also called **free histiocytes**.

Wandering reticuloendothelial cells are of two types:

1. Free histiocytes of blood:
   i. Neutrophils.
   ii. Monocytes, which become macrophages and migrate to the site of injury or infection.
2. Free histiocytes of solid tissue.

During emergency, the fixed histiocytes from connective tissue and other organs become wandering cells and enter the circulation.

FUNCTIONS OF RETICULOENDOTHELIAL SYSTEM

Reticuloendothelial system plays an important role in the defense mechanism of the body. Most of the functions of the reticuloendothelial system are carried out by the tissue macrophages which are detailed below.

1. PHAGOCYTIC FUNCTION

Macrophages play an important role in defense of the body by phagocytosis. When any foreign body invades, macrophages ingest them by phagocytosis and liberate the antigen from the organism. Antigens activate the helper T lymphocytes and B lymphocytes. Refer Chapter 15 for details.

Lysosomes of macrophages contain proteolytic enzymes and lipases which digest the bacteria and other foreign bodies.

2. ANTIGEN PRESENTATION

Macrophages play an important role in development of immunity by presenting the antigenic substances to helper T cells (Chapter 15).

3. SECRETION OF BACTERICIDAL AGENTS

In addition to proteolytic enzymes. tissue macrophages secrete many bactericidal agents, which kill the bacteria. Important bactericidal agents secreted by macrophages are the **free radicals**. Free radicals are also called **reactive oxygen species** (ROS).

Free Radicals Secreted by Macrophages

  i. Superoxide (O_2^-)
  ii. Hydrogen peroxide (H_2O_2).
  iii. Hydroxyl ions (OH^-).

These **radicals** are the most potent bactericidal agents. So, even the bacteria which cannot be digested by lysosomal enzymes are degraded by these oxidants.

4. SECRETION OF INTERLEUKINS

Tissue macrophages secrete interleukin-1, 6 and 12 which help in immunity.

5. SECRETION OF TUMOR NECROSIS FACTORS

Tissue macrophages secrete tumor necrosis factor-α and tumor necrosis factor-β which cause necrosis of tumor.

6. SECRETION OF TRANSFORMING GROWTH FACTOR

Tissue macrophages secrete transforming growth factor, which prevents rejection of transplanted tissues or organs by immunosuppression.

7. SECRETION OF COLONY-STIMULATING FACTOR

Macrophages secrete the colony-stimulating factor (M-CSF) which accelerates growth of granulocytes, monocytes and macrophages.

8. SECRETION OF PLATELET-DERIVED GROWTH FACTOR

Tissue macrophages secrete the platelet-derived growth factor (PDGF), which accelerates repair of damaged blood vessel and wound healing.

9. REMOVAL OF CARBON PARTICLES AND SILICON

Macrophages ingest the substances like carbon dust particles and silicon which enter the body.

10. DESTRUCTION OF SENILE RBC

Reticuloendothelial cells, particularly those in spleen destroy the senile RBCs and release hemoglobin (Chapter 8).

11. DESTRUCTION OF HEMOGLOBIN

Hemoglobin released from broken senile RBCs is degraded by the reticuloendothelial cells (Chapter 10).

SPLEEN
FUNCTIONAL ANATOMY

Spleen is the largest lymphoid organ in the body and it is highly vascular. It also contains reticuloendothelial cells. Spleen is covered by an outer serous coat and an inner fibromuscular capsule. From the capsule, the trabeculae and trabecular network arise. All the three structures, viz. capsule, trabeculae and trabecular network contain collagen fibers, elastic fibers, smooth muscle fibers and reticular cells. The parenchyma of spleen is divided into red and white pulp.

Red Pulp

Red pulp consists of venous sinus and cords of structures such as blood cells, macrophages and mesenchymal cells.

White Pulp

Structure of white pulp is similar to that of lymphoid tissue. It has a central artery, which is surrounded by **splenic corpuscles** or **Malpighian corpuscles**. These corpuscles contain lymphocytes and macrophages.

FUNCTIONS OF SPLEEN

1. *Formation of Blood Cells*

Spleen has the hemopoietic function in embryo. During the hepatic stage, spleen produces blood cells along with liver. In myeloid stage, it produces the blood cells along with liver and bone marrow.

2. Destruction of Blood Cells

Older RBCs, lymphocytes and thrombocytes are destroyed in the spleen. When the RBCs become old (120 days), the cell membrane becomes more fragile. Diameter of most of the capillaries is less or equal to that of RBC. Fragile old cells are destroyed while trying to squeeze through the capillaries because these cells cannot withstand the stress of squeezing.

Destruction occurs mainly in the capillaries of spleen because the splenic capillaries have a thin lumen. So, the spleen is known as **graveyard of RBCs**.

3. Blood Reservoir Function

In animals, spleen stores large amount of blood. However, this function is not significant in humans. But, a large number of RBCs are stored in spleen. RBCs are released from spleen into circulation during the emergency conditions like hypoxia and hemorrhage.

4. Role in Defense of Body

Spleen filters the blood by removing the microorganisms. Macrophages in splenic pulp destroy the microorganisms and other foreign bodies by phagocytosis. Spleen contains about 25% of T lymphocytes and 15% of B lymphocytes and forms the site of antibody production.

■ APPLIED PHYSIOLOGY

Splenomegaly and Hypersplenism

Splenomegaly refers to enlargement of spleen. Increase in the activities of spleen is called hypersplenism.

Diseases such as malaria, typhoid, tuberculosis and rheumatoid arthritis cause splenomegaly resulting in hypersplenism.

Hyposplenism and Asplenia

Hyposplenism or **hyposplenia** means to diminished functioning of spleen. It occurs after partial removal of spleen due to trauma or cyst. Asplenia means absence of spleen. Functional asplenia means absence of splenic functions.

Chapter 22: Lymphatic System and Lymph

CHAPTER OUTLINE

- **LYMPHATIC SYSTEM**
  - ORGANIZATION
  - DRAINAGE
- **LYMPH NODES**
  - STRUCTURE
  - FUNCTION
  - APPLIED PHYSIOLOGY
- **LYMPH**
  - DEFINITION
  - FORMATION
  - RATE OF FLOW
  - COMPOSITION
  - FUNCTIONS

◼ LYMPHATIC SYSTEM

Lymphatic system is a closed system of **lymph channels** or **lymph vessels** through which lymph flows. It is a one-way system and allows the lymph flow from tissue spaces towards the blood.

◼ ORGANIZATION OF LYMPHATIC SYSTEM

Lymphatic system arises from tissue spaces as a meshwork of delicate vessels. These vessels are called **lymph capillaries**.

Lymph capillaries start from tissue spaces as enlarged blind-ended terminals called **capillary bulbs**. These bulbs contain valves, which allow flow of lymph in only one direction. There are some muscle fibers around the capillary bulbs. These muscle fibers cause contraction of bulbs, so that lymph is pushed through the vessels.

Lymph capillaries are lined by endothelial cells. Capillaries unite to form large lymphatic vessels. Lymphatic vessels become larger and larger because of the joining of many tributaries along their course.

Structure of lymph capillaries is slightly different from that of the blood capillaries. Lymph capillaries are more porous and the cells lie overlapping on one another. This allows the fluid to move into lymph capillaries and not in the opposite direction.

◼ DRAINAGE OF LYMPHATIC SYSTEM

Larger lymph vessels ultimately form the **right lymphatic duct** and **thoracic duct**. Right lymphatic duct opens into right subclavian vein and the thoracic duct opens into left subclavian vein. Thoracic duct drains the lymph from more than two-third of the tissue spaces in the body **(Fig. 22.1)**.

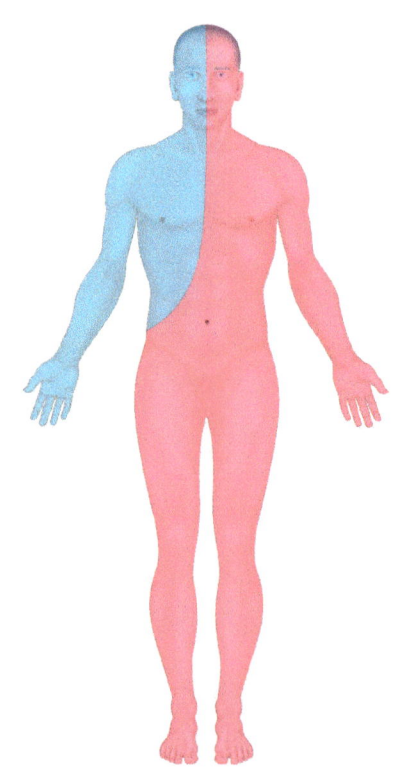

FIGURE 22.1: Lymph drainage.
Blue area = Drained by right lymphatic duct.
Pink area = Drained by thoracic duct.

LYMPH NODES

Lymph nodes are small glandular structures located in the course of lymph vessels. Lymph nodes are also called **lymph glands** or lymphatic nodes.

STRUCTURE OF LYMPH NODES

Each lymph node constitutes masses of lymphatic tissue, covered by a dense connective tissue capsule. The structures are arranged in three layers namely cortex, paracortex and medulla **(Fig. 22.2)**.

Cortex

Cortex of lymph node consists of primary and secondary **lymphoid follicles.** Primary follicle develops first. When some antigens enter the body and reach the lymph nodes, the cells of primary follicle proliferate. The active proliferation of the cells occurs in a particular area of the follicle called the **germinal center**. After proliferation of cells, the primary follicles become the secondary follicles. Cortex also contains some B lymphocytes, which are usually aggregated into the primary follicles. Macrophages are also found in the cortex.

Paracortex

Paracortex is in between the cortex and medulla. Paracortex contains T lymphocytes.

Medulla

Medulla contains B and T lymphocytes and macrophages. Blood vessels of lymph node pass through medulla.

Lymphatic Vessels to Lymph Node

Lymph node receives lymph through one or two lymphatic vessels called afferent vessels. Afferent vessels divide into small channels. Lymph passes through afferent vessels and small channels and reaches the cortex. It circulates through cortex, paracortex and medulla of the lymph node. From medulla, the lymph leaves the node via one or two efferent vessels.

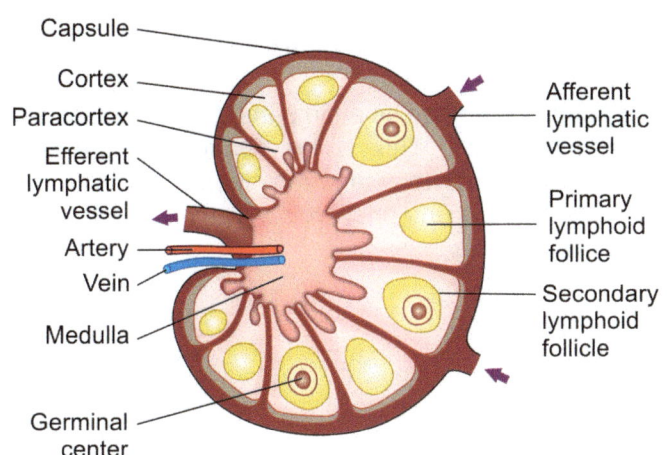

FIGURE 22.2: Structure of a lymph node.

Distribution of Lymph Nodes

Lymph nodes are present along the course of lymphatic vessels in elbow, axilla, knee and groin. Lymph nodes are also present in certain points in abdomen, thorax and neck, where many lymph vessels join.

FUNCTIONS OF LYMPH NODES

Lymph nodes serve as filters which filter bacteria and toxic substances from the lymph.

Functions of the lymph nodes:

1. When lymph passes through lymph nodes, it is filtered, i.e. the water and electrolytes are removed. But proteins and lipids are retained in the lymph.
2. Bacteria and other toxic substances are destroyed by macrophages of lymph nodes. Because of this, lymph nodes are called defense barriers.

APPLIED PHYSIOLOGY: SWELLING OF LYMPH NODES

During infection or any other processes in a particular region of the body, activities of the lymph nodes in that region increase. This causes swelling of the lymph nodes. Sometimes, the swollen lymph nodes cause pain.

Most common cause of swollen lymph nodes is infection. Lymph nodes situated near an infected area swell immediately. When the body recovers from infection, the lymph nodes restore their original size gradually, in 1 or 2 weeks.

LYMPH

DEFINITION

Lymph is an alkaline clear fluid that is derived from interstitial fluid and flowing to bloodstream through lymphatic vessels.

FORMATION OF LYMPH

Lymph is formed from interstitial fluid, due to the permeability of lymph capillaries. When blood passes via blood capillaries in the tissues, 9/10th of fluid passes into venous end of capillaries from arterial end. And, the remaining 1/10th of the fluid passes into lymph capillaries, which have more permeability than blood capillaries.

So, when lymph passes through lymph capillaries, the composition of lymph is more or less similar to that of interstitial fluid including protein content. Proteins present in the interstitial fluid cannot enter the blood capillaries because of their larger size. So, these proteins enter lymph vessels, which are permeable to large particles also.

Addition of Proteins and Fats

Tissue fluid in liver and gastrointestinal tract (GIT) contains more protein and lipid substances. So, proteins and lipids enter the lymph vessels of liver and GIT in

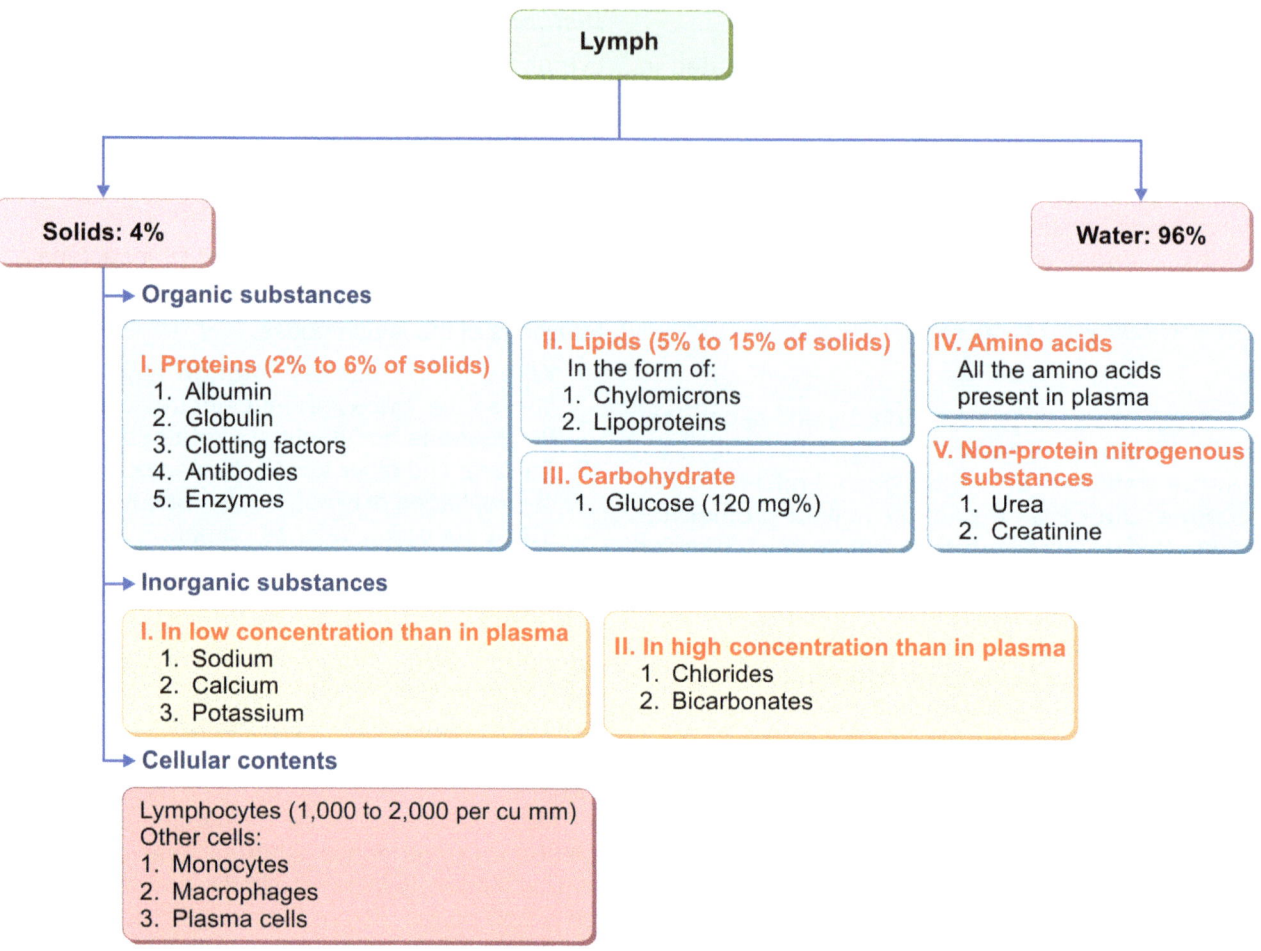

FIGURE 22.3: Composition of lymph.

large quantities. Thus, lymph in larger vessels has more proteins and lipids.

Concentration of Lymph

When the lymph passes through the lymph nodes, it is concentrated because of absorption of water and the electrolytes. However, the proteins and lipids are not absorbed.

■ RATE OF LYMPH FLOW

About 120 mL of lymph flows into blood per hour. Out of this, about 100 mL/h flows through thoracic duct and 20 mL/h flows through the right lymphatic duct.

■ COMPOSITION OF LYMPH

Usually, lymph is a clear and colorless fluid. It is formed by 96% water and 4% solids. Some blood cells are also present in lymph **(Fig. 22.3)**.

■ FUNCTIONS OF LYMPH

1. Important function of lymph is to return proteins from tissue spaces into the blood.
2. Lymph flow plays an important role in redistribution of fluid in the body.
3. Through lymph, bacteria, toxins and other foreign bodies are removed from tissues.
4. Lymph flow is responsible for the maintenance of structural and functional integrity of tissue. Obstruction to lymph flow affects various types of tissues, particularly myocardium, nephrons and the hepatic cells.
5. Lymph flow serves as an important route for intestinal fat absorption. This is the reason for the milky appearance of lymph after fatty meal.
6. Lymph plays an important role in immunity by transport of lymphocytes.

Chapter 23: Tissue Fluid and Edema

CHAPTER OUTLINE

- **DEFINITION**
- **FUNCTIONS**
- **FORMATION**
  - FILTRATION
  - REABSORPTION
- **APPLIED PHYSIOLOGY: EDEMA**
  - DEFINITION
  - TYPES
  - PITTING AND NON-PITTING EDEMA

DEFINITION

Tissue fluid is the medium in which cells are bathed. It is otherwise known as **interstitial fluid**. It forms about 20% of ECF.

FUNCTIONS OF TISSUE FLUID

Because of the capillary membrane, there is no direct contact between blood and cells. And the tissue fluid acts as a medium for exchange of various substances between the cells and the blood in the capillary loop. Oxygen and nutritive substances diffuse from the arterial end of capillary through the tissue fluid and reach the cells. Carbon dioxide and waste materials diffuse from the cells into the venous end of capillary through this fluid.

FORMATION OF TISSUE FLUID

Formation of tissue fluid involves two processes:

1. Filtration.
2. Reabsorption.

FILTRATION

Tissue fluid is formed by the process of filtration. Normally, blood pressure (also called hydrostatic pressure) in arterial end of the capillary is about 30 mm Hg. This hydrostatic pressure is the driving force for filtration of water and other substances from blood into tissue spaces **(Fig. 23.1)**.

REABSORPTION

Fluid filtered at the arterial end of capillaries is reabsorbed back into the blood at the venous end of capillaries. Here also, the pressure gradient plays an important role. At the venous end of capillaries, the hydrostatic pressure is less (15 mm Hg) and the **oncotic pressure** is more (25 mm Hg). Due to the pressure gradient of 10 mm Hg, the fluid is reabsorbed along with waste materials from the tissue fluid into the capillaries. About 10% of filtered fluid enters the lymphatic vessels.

Reabsorption at the venous end helps to maintain the volume of tissue fluid.

APPLIED PHYSIOLOGY: EDEMA

DEFINITION

Edema is defined as the swelling caused by excess accumulation of fluid in tissues. It may be generalized or local. Edema that involves the entire body is called **generalized edema**. **Local edema** is the one that occurs is specific areas of the body such as abdomen, lungs and extremities like feet, ankles and legs. Accumulation of fluid may be inside or outside the cell.

TYPES OF EDEMA

Edema is classified into two types depending upon the body fluid compartment where accumulation of excess fluid occurs:

A. Intracellular edema.
B. Extracellular edema.

Intracellular Edema

Intracellular edema is the accumulation of fluid inside the cell. It occurs because of three reasons **(Box 23.1)**.

Extracellular Edema

Extracellular edema is defined as the accumulation of fluid outside the cell. It occurs because of abnormal leakage of

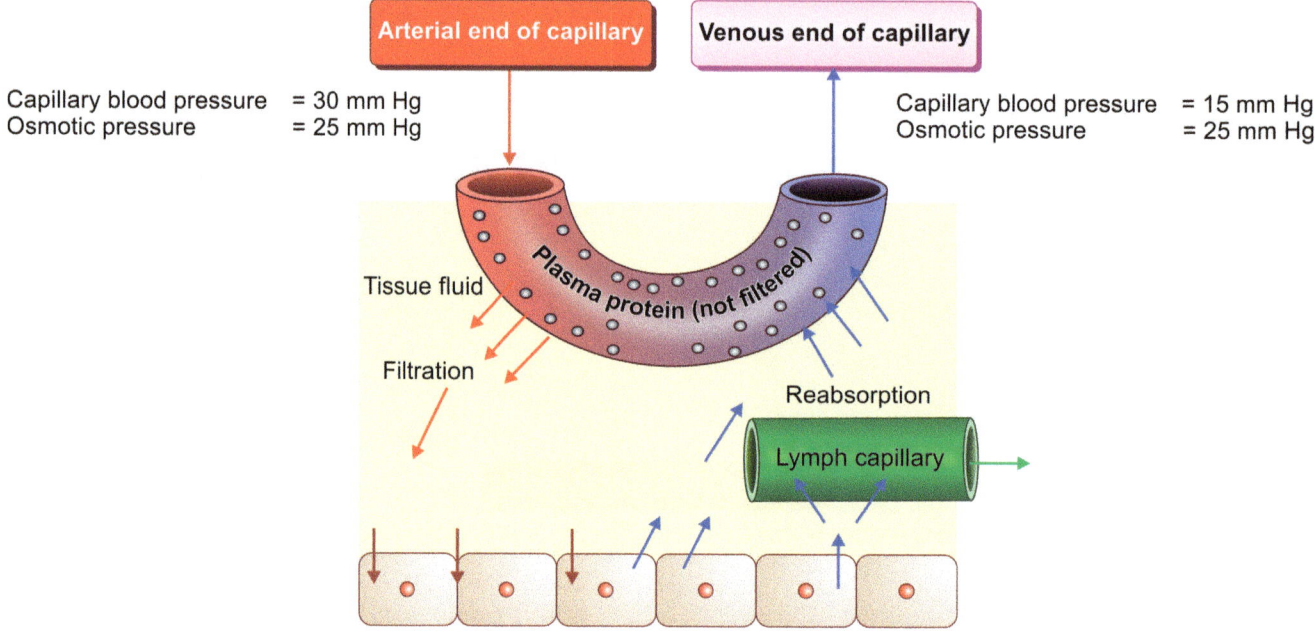

FIGURE 23.1: Formation of tissue fluid. Plasma proteins remain inside the blood capillary, as the capillary membrane is not permeable to plasma proteins.

fluid from capillaries into interstitial space and obstruction of lymphatic vessels that prevents return of fluid from interstitial fluid back into blood. Common conditions which leads to extracellular edema are given in **Box 23.1**.

■ PITTING AND NON-PITTING EDEMA

Interstitial fluid is present in the form of a gel that is almost like a semisolid substance. It is because the interstitial fluid is not present in fluid form, but is bound in a **proteoglycan meshwork**. It does not allow any free space for the movement of fluid.

When interstitial fluid volume increases, most of the fluid becomes free fluid that is not bound to proteoglycan meshwork. It flows freely through tissue spaces, producing a swelling called edema. This type of edema is known as pitting edema, because when this area is pressed with the finger, displacement of fluid occurs producing a depression or pit. When the finger is removed, the pit remains for few seconds, sometimes as long as 1 minute, till the fluid flows back into that area.

BOX 23.1: Intracellular and extracellular edema.

Intracellular edema
1. Edema due to malnutrition
2. Edema due to poor metabolism
3. Edema due to inflammation of the tissues
Extracellular edema
1. Edema due to right-sided heart failure: Peripheral edema
2. Edema due to left-sided heart failure: Pulmonary edema
3. Edema due to renal disease: Generalized edema
4. Edema due to decreased amount of plasma proteins: Peripheral edema
5. Lymphatic obstruction: Lymphedema
6. Increased endothelial permeability: Peripheral edema

Edema also develops due to swelling of the cells or clotting of interstitial fluid in the presence of fibrinogen. This is called non-pitting edema, because it is hard and a pit is not formed while pressing.

MODEL QUESTIONS IN BLOOD AND BODY FLUIDS

LONG QUESTIONS

1. What are the compartments of body fluid? Enumerate the differences between ECF and ICF and explain the measurement of ECF volume.
2. What is indicator dilution technique? How is it applied in the measurement of total body water? Describe dehydration briefly.
3. Give a detailed account of erythropoiesis.
4. Define erythropoiesis. List the different stages of erythropoiesis. Describe the changes, which take place in each stage and the factors necessary for erythropoiesis.
5. Describe the morphology, development and functions of leukocytes.
6. Describe the development of cell-mediated immunity.
7. Describe the development of humoral immunity.
8. Define blood coagulation. Describe the mechanisms involved in coagulation. Add a note on anticoagulants.
9. Enumerate the factors involved in blood coagulation and describe the intrinsic mechanism of coagulation.
10. Give an account of extrinsic mechanism of coagulation of blood. Give a brief description of bleeding disorders.

SHORT QUESTIONS

1. Dye or indicator dilution technique.
2. Measurement of total body water.
3. Measurement of ECF volume.
4. Measurement of ICF volume.
5. Measurement of blood volume.
6. Dehydration.
7. Water intoxication.
8. Functions of blood.
9. Plasma proteins.
10. Polycythemia.
11. Factors necessary for erythropoiesis.
12. Abnormal hemoglobin derivatives.
13. Pernicious anemia.
14. Erythrocyte sedimentation rate.
15. Packed cell volume or hematocrit.
16. Anemia.
17. Hemolysins.
18. Types and morphology of WBCs.
19. Functions of WBCs.
20. T lymphocytes.
21. B lymphocytes.
22. Role of macrophages in immunity.
23. Immunoglobulins or antibodies.
24. Immune deficiency diseases.
25. Autoimmune diseases.
26. Cytokines.
27. Platelets.
28. Hemostasis.
29. Fibrinolysis.
30. Tests for coagulation.
31. Anticoagulants.
32. Hemophilia.
33. Purpura.
34. ABO blood groups.
35. Rh factor.
36. Transfusion reactions.
37. Exchange transfusion.
38. Erythroblastosis fetalis.
39. Tissue macrophage.
40. Lymph.
41. Tissue fluid.
42. Edema.

VERY SHORT ANSWER QUESTIONS

1. Characteristics of marker substances.
2. Marker substances used to measure body fluid compartments.
3. Measurement of total body water.
4. Formula for indicator dilution method.
5. Measurement of volume of interstitial fluid and intracellular fluid.
6. Hematocrit value.
7. Albumin/globulin ratio.
8. Therapeutic plasma exchange.
9. Advantages of biconcave shape of RBCs.
10. Functions of RBCs.
11. Fate of RBCs.
12. Life span of RBCs.
13. Physiological variations of RBC count.
14. Important changes taking place during erythropoiesis.
15. Reticulocytes.
16. Erythropoietin.
17. Functions of hemoglobin.
18. Types of normal hemoglobin.
19. Types of abnormal hemoglobin.
20. Destruction of hemoglobin.
21. Sickle cell anemia.
22. Thalassemia.
23. Iron deficiency anemia.
24. Pernicious anemia.
25. Granulocytes.
26. Monocytes.
27. Lymphocytes.
28. Types of T lymphocytes and B lymphocytes.
29. Macrophage.
30. Antigen presentation.
31. NK cell.
32. AIDS.
33. Vaccines/Toxoids.
34. Properties of platelets.
35. von Willebrand factor.
36. Blood clot.

37. Heparin.
38. Procoagulants.
39. Hemophilia.
40. Purpura.
41. von Willebrand disease.
42. Landsteiner's law.
43. Crossmatching.
44. Bilirubin encephalopathy/Kernicterus.
45. H antigen.
46. Exchange transfusion/Autologous transfusion.
47. Functions of spleen.
48. Functions of lymph.
49. Formation of tissue fluid.
50. Pitting and non-pitting edema.

SECTION 3: MUSCLE PHYSIOLOGY

Chapter 24: Classification of Muscles

CHAPTER OUTLINE

- CLASSIFICATION OF MUSCLES
- CLASSIFICATION DEPENDING UPON STRIATIONS
- CLASSIFICATION DEPENDING UPON CONTROL
- CLASSIFICATION DEPENDING UPON SITUATION

CLASSIFICATION OF MUSCLES

Muscles perform many useful functions and help us in doing everything in day to day life. Human body has got more than 600 muscles.

Muscles are classified by three different methods based on different factors:

I. Depending upon presence or absence of striations.
II. Depending upon control.
III. Depending upon function.

CLASSIFICATION OF MUSCLES DEPENDING UPON STRIATIONS

Depending upon presence or absence of cross striations, the muscles are divided into two groups:

1. Striated muscle.
2. Non-striated muscle.

1. STRIATED MUSCLE

Striated muscle is the muscle which has a large number of cross striations (transverse lines). **Skeletal muscle** and **cardiac muscle** belong to this category.

2. NON-STRIATED MUSCLE

Muscle which does not have cross striations is called non-striated muscle. It is also called **plain muscle** or **smooth muscle**. It is found in the wall of the visceral organs.

CLASSIFICATION OF MUSCLES DEPENDING UPON CONTROL

Depending upon control, the muscles are classified into two types:

1. Voluntary muscle.
2. Involuntary muscle.

1. VOLUNTARY MUSCLE

Voluntary muscle is the muscle that is controlled by the will. Skeletal muscles are the voluntary muscles. Voluntary muscles are innervated by somatic nerves.

2. INVOLUNTARY MUSCLE

Muscle that cannot be controlled by the will is called involuntary muscle. Cardiac muscle and smooth muscle are involuntary muscles. Involuntary muscles are innervated by autonomic nerves.

CLASSIFICATION OF MUSCLES DEPENDING UPON SITUATION

Depending upon situation, the muscles are classified into three types:

1. Skeletal muscle.
2. Cardiac muscle.
3. Smooth muscle.

1. SKELETAL MUSCLE

Skeletal muscles are situated in association with bones forming the skeletal system. Skeletal muscles from 40 to 50% of body mass. These muscles are **striated** and **voluntary**. Skeletal muscles are supplied by somatic nerves.

Fibers of the skeletal muscles are arranged in parallel. In most of the skeletal muscles, the muscle fibers are attached to tendons on either end. Skeletal muscles are anchored to the bones by the tendons.

2. CARDIAC MUSCLE

Cardiac muscle forms the musculature of the heart. These muscles are **striated** and **involuntary**. Cardiac muscles are supplied by autonomic nerve fibers.

3. SMOOTH MUSCLE

Smooth muscle is situated in association with viscera. It is also called visceral muscle. Smooth muscle is **non-striated and involuntary**. It is different from skeletal and cardiac muscles because of the absence of cross striations, hence the name smooth muscle. Smooth muscles are supplied by autonomic nerve fibers. Smooth muscles form the main contractile units of wall of the various visceral organs.

Features of skeletal, cardiac and smooth muscles are given in **Table 24.1**.

TABLE 24.1: Features of skeletal, cardiac and smooth muscle fibers.

Features	Skeletal muscle	Cardiac muscle	Smooth muscle
Location	In association with bones	In the heart	In the visceral organs
Shape	Cylindrical and unbranched	Branched	Spindle shaped, unbranched
Length	1 to 4 cm	80 to 100 μ	50 to 200 μ
Diameter	10 to 100 μ	15 to 20 μ	2 to 5 μ
Number of nucleus	> 1	1	1
Cross-striations	Present	Present	Absent
Myofibrils	Present	Present	Absent
Sarcomere	Present	Present	Absent
Troponin	Present	Present	Absent
Sarcotubular system	Well developed	Well developed	Poorly developed
T-tubules	Long and thin	Short and broad	Absent
Depolarization	Upon stimulation	Spontaneous	Spontaneous
Fatigue	Possible	Not possible	Not possible
Summation	Possible	Not possible	Possible
Tetanus	Possible	Not possible	Possible
Resting membrane potential	Stable	Stable	Unstable
To trigger contraction, calcium binds with	Troponin	Troponin	Calmodulin
Source of calcium	Sarcoplasmic reticulum	Sarcoplasmic reticulum	Extracellular fluid
Speed of contraction	Quick	Intermediate	Slow
Neuromuscular junction	Well defined	Ill defined	Ill defined
Action	Voluntary action	Involuntary action	Involuntary action
Control of action	Neurogenic	Myogenic	Neurogenic and myogenic
Nerve supply	Somatic nerves	Autonomic nerves	Autonomic nerves

Chapter 25: Structure of Skeletal Muscle

CHAPTER OUTLINE

- **MUSCLE MASS**
- **MUSCLE FIBER**
- **MYOFIBRIL**
  - DEFINITION
  - MORPHOLOGY
  - MICROSCOPIC STRUCTURE
- **SARCOMERE**
  - DEFINITION
  - EXTENT
  - COMPONENTS
  - ELECTRON MICROSCOPIC STUDY
- **CONTRACTILE ELEMENTS (PROTEINS) OF MUSCLE**
  - MYOSIN MOLECULE
  - ACTIN MOLECULE
  - TROPOMYOSIN
  - TROPONIN
- **OTHER PROTEINS OF THE MUSCLE**
- **SARCOTUBULAR SYSTEM**
  - T-TUBULES
  - L-TUBULES OR SARCOPLASMIC RETICULUM
- **COMPOSITION OF MUSCLE**

MUSCLE MASS

Muscle mass (or tissue) is made up of many individual muscle cells or **myocytes**. **Muscle cells** are commonly called **muscle fibers** because of their long and slender in appearance. **Skeletal muscle** fibers are multinucleated and arranged parallel to one another with some connective tissue in between.

Muscle mass is separated from neighboring tissues by a thick fibrous tissue layer known as **fascia**. Beneath this fascia, the muscle is covered by a connective tissue sheath called **epimysium**. In each muscle, the muscle fibers are arranged in different groups called the bundles or **fasciculi**. Connective tissue sheath that covers each fasciculus is called **perimysium**. Each muscle fiber is covered by the connective tissue layer called the **endomysium (Figs. 25.1 and 25.2)**.

MUSCLE FIBER

Each muscle fiber or muscle cell is cylindrical in shape. Length of the muscle fiber is between 1 cm and 4 cm depending upon length of the muscle. Diameter of the muscle fiber varies from 10 μ to 100 μ. Muscle fibers are attached to bone by a tough cord of connective tissue called tendon.

Each muscle fiber is enclosed by a cell membrane called plasma membrane or **sarcolemma** that lies beneath the endomysium **(Fig. 25.3)**. Cytoplasm of muscle fiber is known as **sarcoplasm**. Many structures are embedded within the sarcoplasm:

Structures embedded within sarcoplasm are:

1. Nuclei.
2. Myofibril.
3. Golgi apparatus.
4. Mitochondria.
5. Sarcoplasmic reticulum.
6. Ribosomes.
7. Glycogen droplets.
8. Occasional lipid droplets.

Each muscle fiber has got one or more nuclei. In long muscle fibers, many nuclei are seen. Nuclei are oval or elongated and situated just beneath the sarcolemma. Usually in other cells, nucleus is in the interior of cell.

MYOFIBRIL

DEFINITION

Myofibrils or **myofibrillae** are very fine filaments arranged parallelly in cytoplasm of muscle fibers.

MORPHOLOGY

Myofibrils run through entire length of the muscle fiber. **Diameter** of the myofibril is 0.2 μ to 2 μ. **Length** of a myofibril varies between 1 cm and 4 cm, depending upon the length of the muscle fiber **(Table 25.1)**.

Section 3: Muscle Physiology

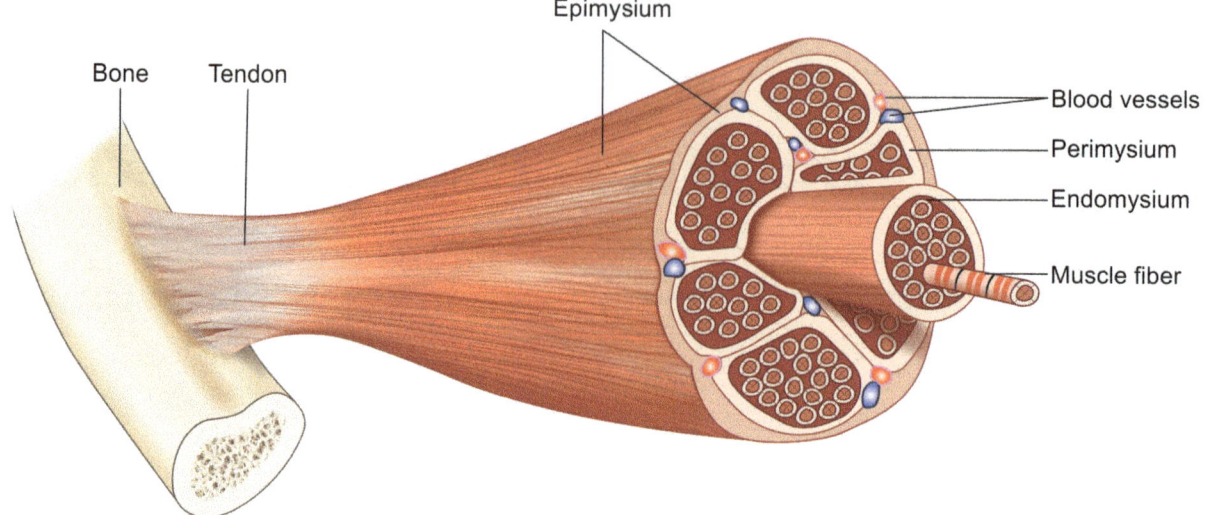

FIGURE 25.1: Structure of a skeletal muscle.

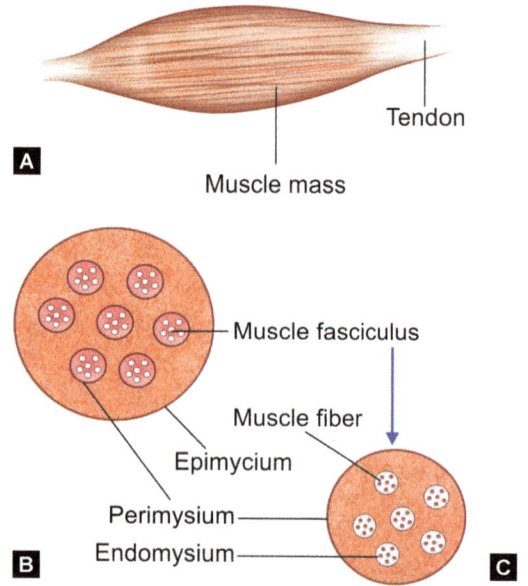

FIGURE 25.2: Diagram showing. **A.** Skeletal muscle mass. **B.** Cross-section of muscle. **C.** One muscle fasciculus.

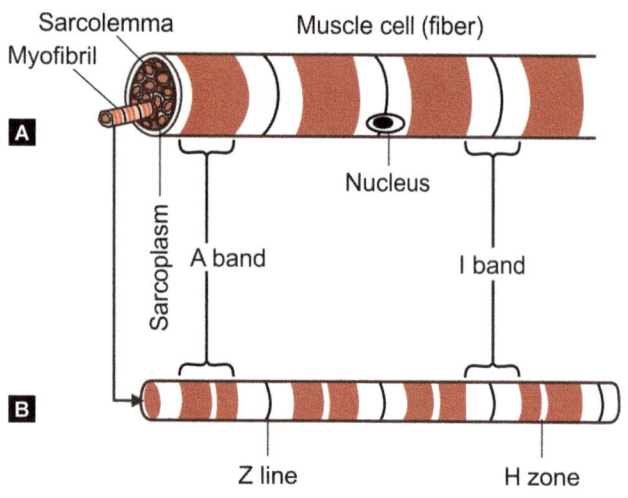

FIGURE 25.3: Diagram showing: **A.** One muscle cell. **B.** One myofibril.

TABLE 25.1: Dimensions of structures in skeletal muscle.

Structure	Length	Diameter
Muscle fiber	1 cm to 4 cm	10 µ to 100 µ
Myofibril	1 cm to 4 cm	0.2 µ to 2 µ
Actin filament	1 µ	20 Å
Myosin filament	1.5 µ	115 Å

■ MICROSCOPIC STRUCTURE OF A MYOFIBRIL

Light microscopic studies show that, each myofibril consists of a number of two alternating bands.

Bands in myofibril:

1. Light band or 'I' band.
2. Dark band or 'A' band.

Light Band or 'I' Band

Light band in myofibril is called 'I' band because it is isotropic to **polarized light**. When a polarized light is passed through the muscle fiber at this area, all the light rays are refracted at the same angle.

Dark Band or 'A' Band

Dark band is called 'A' band because it is anisotropic to polarized light. When a polarized light is passed through the muscle fiber at this area, the light rays are refracted at different directions (an = not, iso = it, trops = turning).

In an intact muscle fiber, 'I' band and 'A' band of adjacent myofibrils are placed side by side. It gives the appearance of characteristic cross striations in muscle fiber.

'I' band is divided into two portions by a narrow dark line called '**Z' line** or 'Z' disk (in German zwischenscheibe = between disks). The 'Z' line is formed by a protein disk which does not permit passage of light. The portion of myofibril in between two 'Z' lines is called sarcomere.

SARCOMERE

Definition

Sarcomere is the structural and functional unit of the skeletal muscle.

EXTENT OF SARCOMERE

Each sarcomere extends between two 'Z' lines of myofibril **(Fig. 25.4)**. Thus, each myofibril contains many sarcomeres arranged in series throughout its length. When the muscle is in relaxed state, average length of each sarcomere is 2 microns to 3 microns.

COMPONENTS OF SARCOMERE

Each sarcomere consists of:

1. One half of light 'I' band.
2. One dark 'A' band.
3. One half of light 'I' band.

In the middle of 'A' band, there is a light area called 'H' zone (H = hell = light—in German, H = Henson, the discoverer). In the middle of 'H' zone lies the middle part of myosin filament. This is called 'M' line (in German mittel = middle). 'M' line is formed by myosin binding proteins.

ELECTRON MICROSCOPIC STUDY OF SARCOMERE

Electron microscopic studies reveal that the sarcomere consists of many thread-like structures called myofilaments.

Myofilaments are of two types:

1. Actin filaments.
2. Myosin filaments.

Actin Filaments

Actin filaments are the thin filaments that extend from either side of the 'Z' lines, run through 'I' band and enter into 'A' band up to 'H' zone. Each actin filament has a diameter of 20 Å and a length of 1 μ.

Myosin Filaments

Myosin filaments are thick filaments and are situated in 'A' band. Each myosin filament has a diameter of 115 Å and a length of 1.5 μ **(Table 25.1.)**

Some lateral processes (projections) or **cross bridges** arise from myosin filaments. These bridges have enlarged structures called myosin heads at their tips. Myosin heads attach themselves to actin filaments. These heads pull the actin filaments during contraction of the muscle by means of a mechanism called sliding mechanism or ratchet mechanism (Chapter 27).

CONTRACTILE ELEMENTS (PROTEINS) OF MUSCLE

Myosin filaments are formed by one type of protein namely myosin molecules. However, actin filaments are formed by three types of proteins called actin, tropomyosin and troponin. These four proteins together constitute the muscle proteins or the contractile elements of the muscle.

In addition to the contractile proteins, the sarcomere contains some more proteins.

MYOSIN MOLECULE

Each myosin filament consists of about 200 myosin molecules. Myosin is a globulin which is made up of 6 polypeptide chains. Out of these, two are heavy chains and four are light chains. Both the heavy chains twist around each other to form a double helix **(Fig. 25.5)**. At one end, the two chains remain twisted around one another and form the tail portion. At the other end, both the chains turn away in opposite directions and form the globular head portion. To each part of this head, are attached two light chains.

Each **myosin head** has two attachment sites. One site is for actin filament and the other one is for one ATP molecule **(Fig. 25.6)**. In the central part of the myosin filament, i.e. in the 'H' zone, the myosin head is absent.

ACTIN MOLECULE

Actin molecules are the major constituents of the thin actin filaments. Each actin molecule is called **F-actin** and it is derived from **G-actin**. There are about 300 to 400 actin

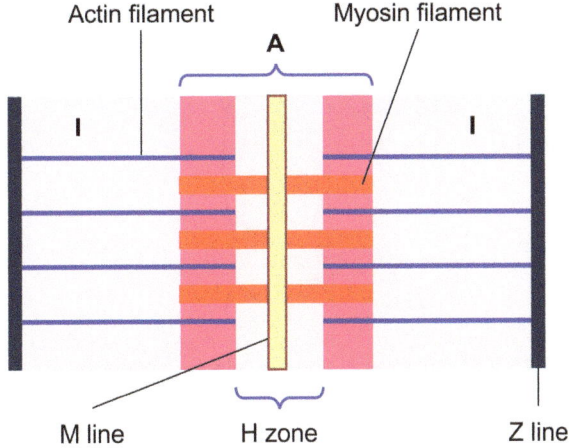

FIGURE 25.4: One sarcomere. A = A band. I = I band.

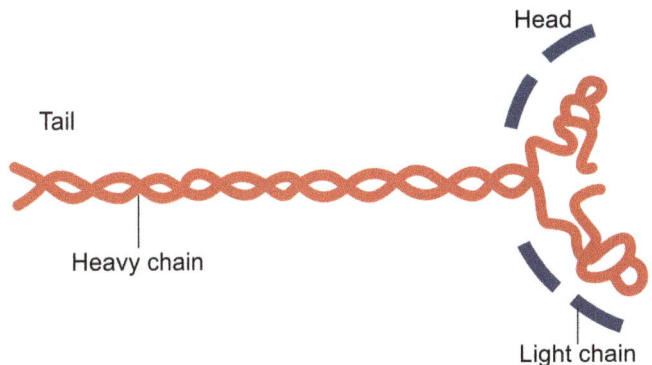

FIGURE 25.5: Myosin molecule formed by two heavy chains and four light chains of polypeptides.

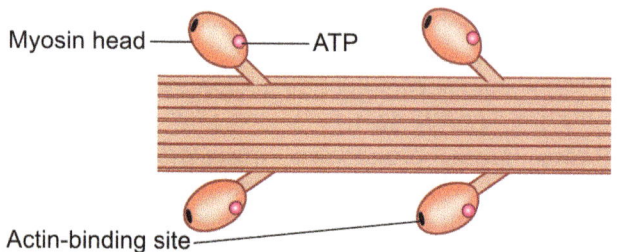

FIGURE 25.6: Diagram showing myosin filament. ATP = Adenosine triphosphate.

molecules in each actin filament. Actin molecules in the actin filament are also arranged in the form of a double helix. Each F-actin molecule has an active site to which the myosin head is attached.

TROPOMYOSIN

There are about 40 to 60 tropomyosin molecules situated along the double helix strand of actin filament. In relaxed condition of the muscle, the tropomyosin molecules cover all active sites of F actin molecules **(Fig. 25.7)**.

TROPONIN

Troponin is formed by three subunits:

1. Troponin I which is attached to F-actin.
2. Troponin T which is attached to tropomyosin.
3. Troponin C which is attached to calcium ions.

SARCOTUBULAR SYSTEM

Sarcotubular system is a system of membranous structures in the form of vesicles and tubules in sarcoplasm of the muscle fiber. It surrounds the myofibrils embedded in the sarcoplasm.

Structures of Sarcotubular System

Sarcotubular system is formed mainly by two types of structures:

1. T-tubules.
2. L-tubules or sarcoplasmic reticulum.

T-TUBULES

T-tubules or **transverse tubules** are narrow tubules formed by invagination of the sarcolemma. T-tubules penetrate all the way from one side of the muscle fiber to other side. Because of their origin from sarcolemma, T-tubules open to the exterior of the muscle cell. Therefore, the ECF runs through their lumen.

Functions of T-Tubules

T-tubules are responsible for rapid transmission of impulse in the form of action potential from sarcolemma to the myofibrils.

L-TUBULES OR SARCOPLASMIC RETICULUM

L-tubules or **longitudinal tubules** are the closed tubules that run in long axis of muscle fiber forming sarcoplasmic reticulum. These tubules form a closed tubular system around each myofibril and do not open to exterior like T-tubules.

L-tubules correspond to the endoplasmic reticulum of other cells. At regular intervals, throughout the length of the myofibrils, the L-tubules dilate to form a pair of lateral sacs called **terminal cisternae**.

Each pair of terminal cisternae is in close contact with T-tubule. T-tubule along with the cisternae on either side is called the **triad of skeletal muscle**. Calcium ions are stored in L-tubule and the amount of calcium ions is more in cisternae **(Fig. 25.8)**.

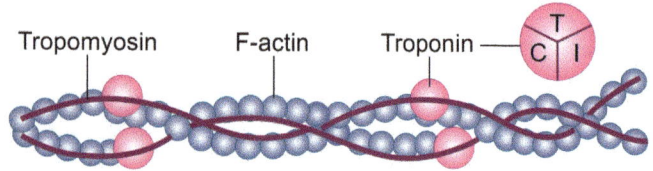

FIGURE 25.7: Part of actin filament. Troponin has three subunits T, C and I.

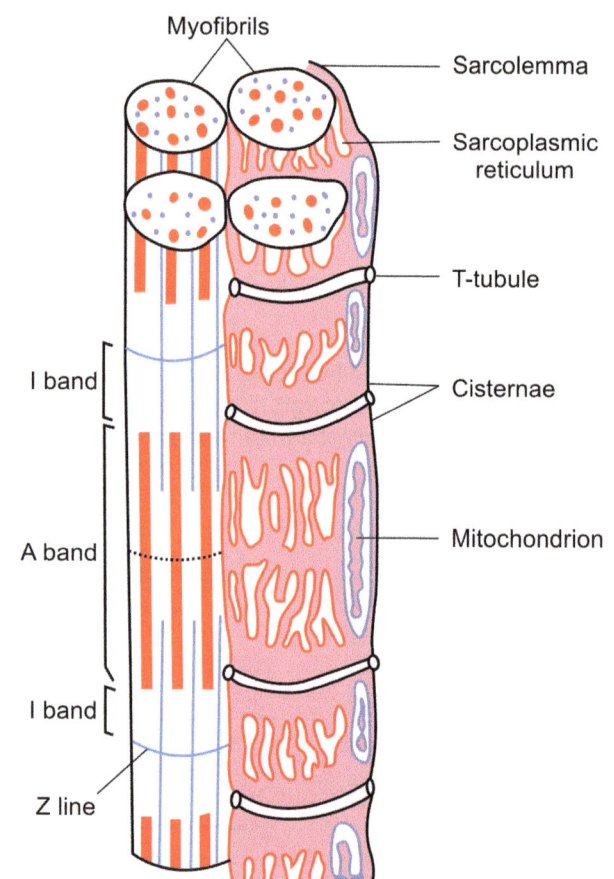

FIGURE 25.8: Diagram showing the relation between sarcotubular system and parts of sarcomere. Only few myofilaments are shown in the myofibril drawn on the right side of the diagram.

Functions of L-tubules

L-tubules store a large quantity of calcium ions. When action potential reaches the cisternae of L-tubule, calcium ions are released into the sarcoplasm. These calcium ions trigger the processes involved in contraction of the muscle. The process by which the calcium ions cause contraction of muscle is called excitation contraction coupling (Chapter 27).

COMPOSITION OF MUSCLE

Skeletal muscle is formed by 75% of water and 25% of solids. Solids are 20% of proteins and 5% of organic substances other than proteins and inorganic substances (Fig. 25.9).

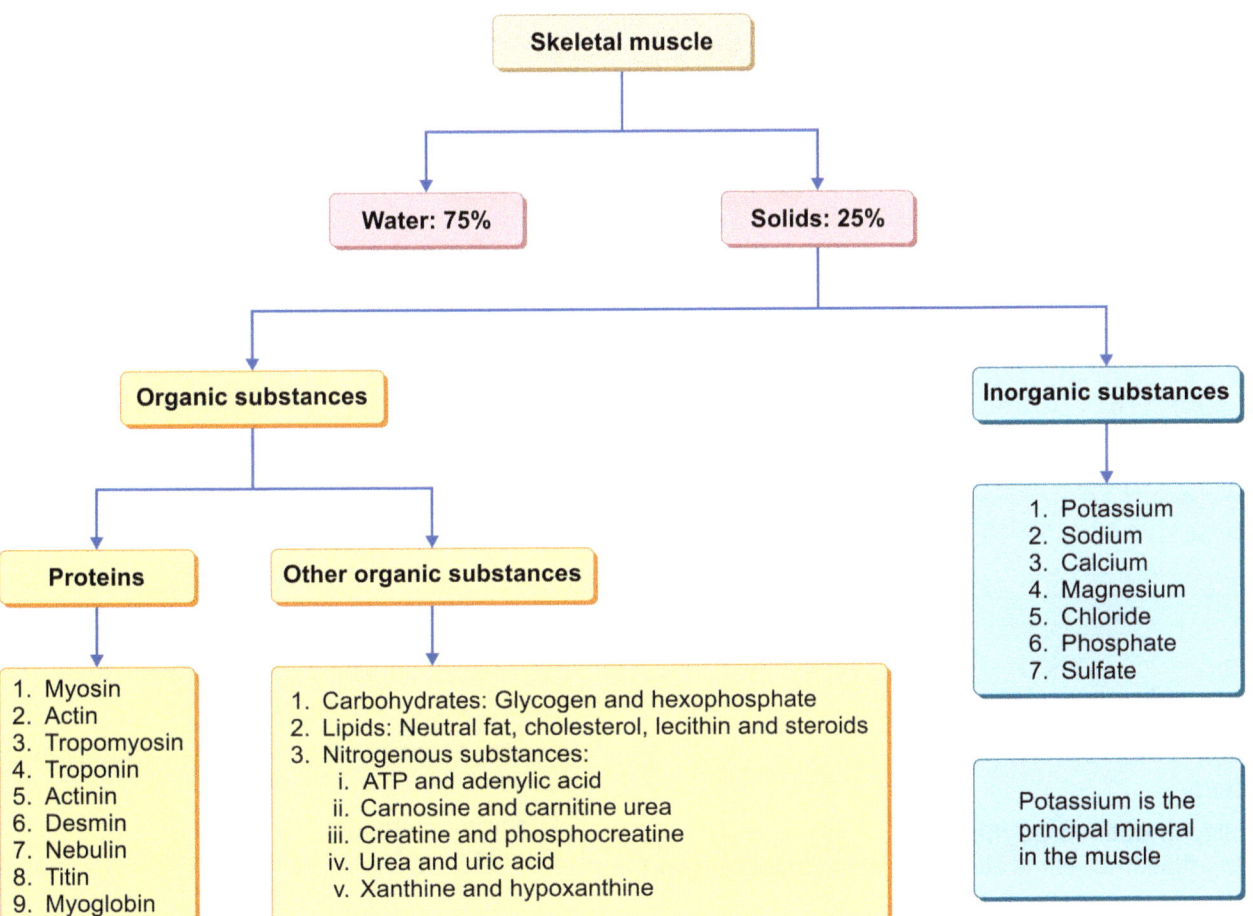

FIGURE 25.9: Composition of skeletal muscle.

Chapter 26: Properties of Skeletal Muscle

CHAPTER OUTLINE

- **EXCITABILITY**
  - **DEFINITIONS**
  - **TYPES OF STIMULUS**
  - **QUALITIES OF STIMULUS**
  - **EXCITABILITY CURVE OR STRENGTH-DURATION CURVE**
- **CONTRACTILITY**
  - **TYPES OF CONTRACTION**
  - **SIMPLE MUSCLE CONTRACTION**
  - **CONTRACTION TIME: RED MUSCLE AND PALE MUSCLE**
- **FACTORS AFFECTING FORCE OF CONTRACTION**
- **REFRACTORY PERIOD**
- **MUSCLE TONE**
  - **DEFINITION**
  - **MAINTENANCE OF MUSCLE TONE**
  - **APPLIED PHYSIOLOGY: DISEASES INVOLVING MUSCLE TONE**

EXCITABILITY

DEFINITIONS

Excitability

Excitability is defined as the reaction or response of a tissue to irritation or stimulation. It is a **physicochemical** change.

Stimulus

Stimulus is the change in environment. It is defined as an agent or influence or act which causes the response in an excitable tissue.

TYPES OF STIMULUS

Stimulus, which can excite a living tissue is of four types:

1. Mechanical stimulus (pinching).
2. Electrical stimulus (electric shock).
3. Thermal stimulus (by applying heated glass rod or ice piece).
4. Chemical stimulus (by applying chemical substances such as acids).

Electrical stimulus is commonly used for experimental purposes.

QUALITIES OF STIMULUS

To excite a tissue, the stimulus must possess two characters:

I. Intensity or strength
II. Duration.

1. Intensity of Stimulus

Intensity or strength of a stimulus is of five types:

1. Subminimal stimulus.
2. Minimal stimulus.
3. Submaximal stimulus.
4. Maximal stimulus.
5. Supramaximal stimulus.

The stimulus whose strength (or voltage) is sufficient to excite the tissue is called **threshold** or liminal or minimal stimulus.

2. Duration of Stimulus

Whatever may be the strength, the stimulus, must be applied for a minimum duration to excite the tissue. However, the duration of a stimulus depends upon the strength of the stimulus. For a weak stimulus, duration is longer and for a stronger stimulus, the duration is shorter. The relationship between the strength and duration of stimulus is demonstrated by means of **excitability curve** or **strength-duration curve**.

EXCITABILITY CURVE OR STRENGTH-DURATION CURVE

Excitability curve is the graph that demonstrates the exact relationship between the strength and the duration of a stimulus. So, it is also called the strength-duration curve **(Fig. 26.1)**.

In this curve, the strength of the stimulus is plotted (in volts) vertically on Y axis and the duration (in milliseconds) horizontally on X axis.

Characteristic Features of the Curve

Following are the important features to be observed in excitability curve:

1. Rheobase.
2. Utilization time.
3. Chronaxie.

1. Rheobase

Rheobase is the **minimum strength** (voltage) of stimulus which can excite the tissue. The voltage below this cannot excite the tissue, whatever may be the duration of the stimulus. Rheobasic strength is also called **threshold strength**.

2. Utilization Time

Utilization time is the **minimum time** required for rheobasic strength of stimulus (threshold strength) to excite the tissue.

3. Chronaxie

Chronaxie is the **minimum time** required for a stimulus with double the rheobasic strength (voltage) to excite the tissue.

Importance of chronaxie

Measurement of chronaxie determines the **excitability** of the tissues. It is used to compare the excitability in different tissues. Longer the chronaxie, lesser is the excitability.

CONTRACTILITY

Contractility is the response of the skeletal muscle to a stimulus by change in either length or tension of muscle fibers.

TYPES OF CONTRACTION

Muscular contraction is classified into two types based on change in length of muscle fibers or tension of muscle:

1. Isotonic contraction.
2. Isometric contraction.

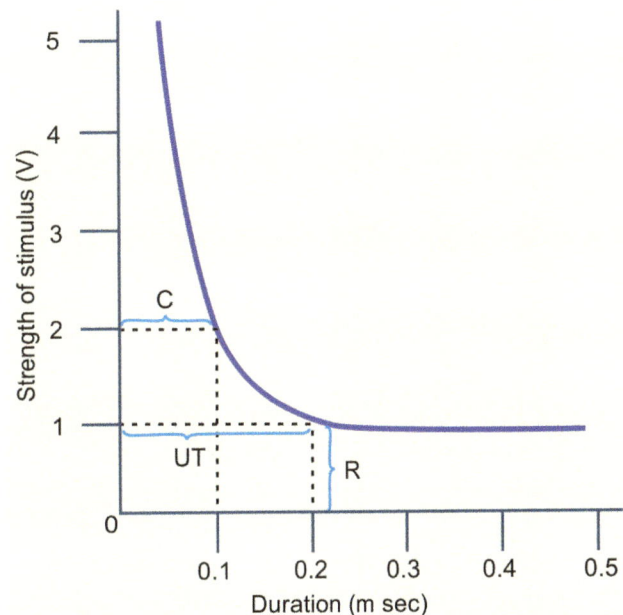

FIGURE 26.1: Strength-duration curve.
R = Rheobase. UT = Utilization time. C = Chronaxie.

1. Isotonic Contraction

Isotonic contraction is the type of muscular contraction in which tension remains the same and length of the muscle fiber is altered (Iso = same, Tonic = tension). For example, during simple flexion of arm, shortening of muscle fibers occurs but the tension does not change.

2. Isometric Contraction

Isometric contraction is the type of muscular contraction in which length of muscle fibers remains the same and tension is increased. Example is pulling any heavy object when muscles become stiff and strained with increased tension but the length does not change.

SIMPLE MUSCLE CONTRACTION

Contractile property of the muscle is studied by using **gastrocnemius-sciatic preparation** from frog. It is also called muscle-nerve preparation.

When a **threshold stimulus** is applied, the muscle contracts and then relaxes. These activities are recorded graphically by using suitable instruments.

Contraction is recorded as upward deflection from the base line. And, relaxation is recorded as downward deflection back to the base line **(Fig. 26.2)**.

Simple contraction of the muscle is called **simple muscle twitch** and the graphical recording of this is called **simple muscle curve**.

Important Points in Simple Muscle Curve

Four points are to be observed in simple muscle curve:

1. *Point of stimulus (PS):* Time when the stimulus is applied

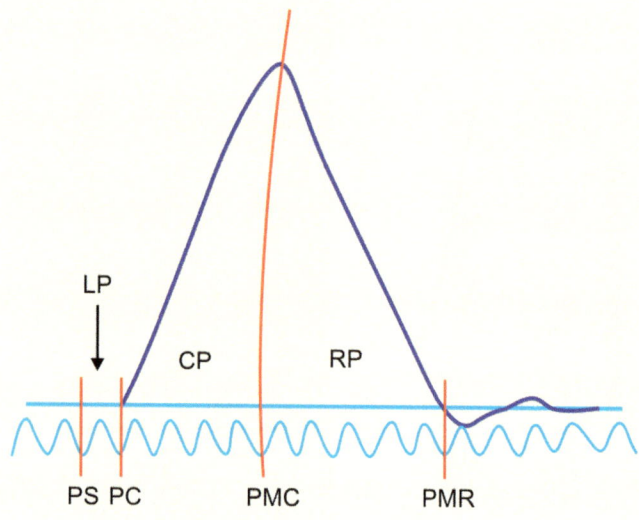

FIGURE 26.2: Isotonic simple muscle curve.
PS: Point of stimulus. PC: Point of contraction. PMC: Point of maximum contraction. PMR: Point of maximum relaxation. LP: Latent period (0.01 sec). CP: Contraction period (0.04 sec). RP: Relaxation period (0.05 sec).

2. *Point of contraction (PC):* Time when the muscle begins to contract
3. *Point of maximum contraction (PMC):* Point up to which the muscle contracts. It also indicates the beginning of relaxation of the muscle
4. *Point of maximum relaxation (PMR):* Point when muscle relaxes completely.

Periods of Simple Muscle Curve

All the four points mentioned above divide the entire simple muscle curve into three periods:

1. Latent period (LP)
2. Contraction period (CP)
3. Relaxation period (RP).

1. Latent period

Latent period is the time interval between the point of stimulus and point of contraction. Muscle does not show any mechanical activity during this period.

2. Contraction period

Contraction period is the interval between point of contraction and point of maximum contraction. Muscle contracts during this period.

3. Relaxation period

Relaxation period is the interval between point of maximum contraction and point of maximum relaxation. Muscle relaxes during this period.

Duration of different periods in a typical simple muscle curve:

Latent period	: 0.01 sec
Contraction period	: 0.04 sec
Relaxation period	: <u>0.05 sec</u>
Total twitch period	: **0.10 sec**

Contraction period is always shorter than relaxation period. It is because the contraction is an active process and relaxation is a passive process.

Causes of Latent Period

1. Latent period is the time taken by the impulse to travel along the nerve from place of stimulation to muscle
2. It is the time taken for the onset of initial chemical changes in the muscle
3. It is due to the delay in the conduction of impulse at the neuromuscular junction
4. It is due to the resistance offered by viscosity of the muscle
5. It is also due to the inertia of the recording instrument.

■ CONTRACTION TIME: RED MUSCLE AND PALE MUSCLE

Contraction time or total twitch period varies from species to species. It is less in homeothermic animals than in poikilothermic animals (Chapter 48). In the same animal, it varies in different groups of muscles.

Based on contraction time, the **skeletal muscles** are classified into two types:

1. Red muscles
2. Pale muscles.

1. Red Muscles

Red muscles are the muscles which contain large quantity of myoglobin. These muscles have large number of **type I fibers**. Red muscles are also called **slow muscles** or slow twitch muscles. Contraction time is longer in this type of muscles.

Examples are back muscles and gastrocnemius muscles.

2. Pale Muscles

Pale or **white muscles** are the muscles which contain less quantity of myoglobin. Pale muscles have large number of **type II fibers**. These muscles are also called **fast muscles** or fast twitch muscles. Contraction time is shorter in this type of muscles.

Examples are hand muscles and ocular muscles.

Characteristic features of red and pale muscles are given in **Table 26.1**.

■ FACTORS AFFECTING FORCE OF CONTRACTION

Force of contraction of the skeletal muscle is affected by the following factors:

A. Strength of stimulus.
B. Number of stimulus.
C. Temperature.
D. Load.

A. Effect of Strength of Stimulus

Force of contraction is directly proportional to strength of stimulus.

TABLE 26.1: Features of red and pale muscles.

No.	Red (slow) muscle	Pale (fast) muscle
1.	Type I fibers are more	Type II fibers are more
2.	Myoglobin content is high. So, it is red	Myoglobin content is less. So, it is pale
3.	Sarcoplasmic reticulum is less extensive	Sarcoplasmic reticulum is more extensive
4.	Blood vessels are more extensive	Blood vessels are less extensive
5.	Mitochondria are more in number	Mitochondria are less in number
6.	Response is slow with long-latent period	Response is rapid with short-latent period
7.	Contraction is less Powerful	Contraction is more Powerful
8.	Undergoes sustained contraction by prolonged and continued activity	Relaxes immediately and does not show prolonged and continued activity
9.	Fatigue occurs slowly	Fatigue occurs quickly
10.	Depends on cellular respiration for ATP production	Depends on glycolysis for ATP production

B. Effect of Number of Stimulus

Contractility of the muscle varies, depending upon the number of stimuli. If a single stimulus is applied, muscle contracts once (simple muscle twitch). Two or more than two (multiple) stimuli produce two different effects.

When a muscle is stimulated by multiple stimuli, two types of effects are obtained depending upon the frequency of stimuli:

1. Fatigue.
2. Tetanus.

1. Fatigue

Definition

Fatigue is defined as the decrease in muscular activity due to repeated stimuli. When the stimuli are applied continuously, after some time, the muscle does not show any response to the stimulus. This condition is called fatigue.

Causes for fatigue

  i. Exhaustion of acetylcholine in motor endplate.
 ii. Accumulation of metabolites such as lactic acid and phosphoric acid.
iii. Lack of nutrients like glycogen.
 iv. Lack of oxygen.

Site (seat) of fatigue

In the intact body, the sites of fatigue are in the following order:

  i. **Betz cells** (pyramidal cells) in cerebral cortex.
 ii. Anterior gray horn cells (motor neurons) of spinal cord.
iii. Neuromuscular junction.
 iv. Muscle.

Recovery of the muscle after fatigue

Fatigue is a reversible phenomenon. The fatigued muscle recovers if given rest and nutrition.

Causes of recovery

  i. Removal of metabolites.
 ii. Formation of acetylcholine at the neuromuscular junction.
iii. Re-establishment of normal polarized state of the muscle.
 iv. Availability of nutrients.
  v. Availability of oxygen.
 vi. In the intact body, all the processes involved in recovery are achieved by circulation itself.

2. Tetanus

Definition

Tetanus is defined as the **sustained contraction** of muscle due to repeated stimuli with high frequency. When the multiple stimuli are applied at a higher frequency in such a way that the successive stimuli fall during contraction period of previous twitch, the muscle remains in state of tetanus, i.e. all the contractions are fused. Muscle relaxes only after stoppage of stimulus or when the muscle is fatigued.

If the frequency of stimuli is less, partial fusion of contractions takes place leading to **incomplete tetanus** or **clonus**.

Frequency of stimuli necessary to cause tetanus and clonus

In gastrocnemius muscle of human being, the frequency required to cause tetanus is 60/second. And for clonus, the frequency of stimuli necessary is 55/second.

C. Effect of Variations in Temperature

If the temperature of muscle is altered, the force of contraction is also affected.

Warm temperature

At warm temperature of about 40°C, force of contraction increases because of the following reasons:

1. Excitability of muscle increases.
2. Chemical processes involved in muscular contraction are accelerated.
3. Viscosity of muscle decreases.

Cold temperature

At cold temperature of about 10°C, force of contraction decreases because of the following reasons:

1. Excitability of muscle decreases.
2. Chemical processes are slowed or delayed.
3. Viscosity of the muscle increases.

High or hot temperature: Heat rigor

At high temperatures, heat rigor occurs in the muscle. **Rigor** refers to shortening and stiffening of muscle fibers. Heat rigor is the rigor that occurs due to increased temperature above 60°C. Cause of heat rigor is the coagulation of muscle proteins actin and myosin. It is an irreversible phenomenon.

Other types of rigors are:

1. **Cold rigor** that occurs due to the exposure to severe cold. It is a reversible phenomenon.
2. **Calcium rigor** which is due to increased calcium content. It is also reversible.
3. Rigor mortis which develops after death.

Rigor mortis

Rigor mortis is the after-death condition of the body which is characterized by stiffness of muscles and joints (Latin word, rigor = stiff). It occurs due to stoppage of aerobic respiration, which causes changes in the muscles.

Soon after death, the cell membrane becomes highly permeable to calcium. So, a large number of calcium ions enters the muscle fibers and promotes formation of actomyosin complex resulting in contraction of the muscles.

Few hours after death, all the muscles of body undergo severe contraction and become rigid. Joints also become stiff and locked.

Normally for relaxation, muscle needs to drive out the calcium which requires ATP. But during continuous muscular contraction and other cellular processes after death, the ATP molecules are completely exhausted. New ATP molecules cannot be produced because of lack of oxygen. So, in the absence of ATP, muscles remain in contracted state until the onset of decomposition.

Medicolegal importance of rigor mortis

Rigor mortis is useful in determining the time of death. Onset of stiffness starts between 10 minutes and 3 hours after death depending upon the condition of the body and environmental temperature at the time of death. If the body is active or the environmental temperature is high at the time of death, the stiffness sets in quickly.

Stiffness develops first in facial muscles and then spreads to other muscles. Maximum stiffness occurs around 12 to 24 hours after death. Stiffness of muscles and joints continues for 1 to 3 days.

Afterwards, the decomposition of general tissues starts. Now the lysosomal intracellular hydrolytic enzymes like cathepsins and calpains are released. These enzymes hydrolyze the muscle proteins, actin and myosin resulting in breakdown of actomyosin complex. It relieves the stiffness of the muscles. This process is known as **resolution of rigor**.

D. *Effect of Load*

Load acting on muscle is of two types:

1. After load.
2. Free load.

After load

After load is the load, that acts on the muscle after the beginning of muscular contraction. Example of after load is lifting any object from the ground. Load acts on muscles of arm only after lifting the object off the ground, i.e. only after beginning of the muscular contraction.

Free load

Free load is the load, which acts on muscle freely, even before onset of contraction of the muscle. It is otherwise called **fore load**. Example of free load is filling water from a tap by holding the bucket in hand.

Muscle in free loaded condition works better than the muscle in after loaded condition. It is because, in free loaded condition, the muscle fibers are stretched and initial length of muscle fibers is increased. So, force of contraction and work done by the muscles are increased. It is in accordance with Frank-Starling law.

Frank-Starling law

Frank-Starling law states that the force of contraction is directly proportional to initial length of muscle fibers within physiological limits.

■ REFRACTORY PERIOD

Refractory period is the period at which the muscle does not show any response to a stimulus. It is because already one action potential is in progress and the muscle is in depolarized state during this period. Muscle is unexcitable to further stimulation until it is repolarized.

Refractory period is of two types:

1. Absolute refractory period.
2. Relative refractory period.

1. *Absolute Refractory Period*

Absolute refractory period is the period during which the muscle does not show any response at all, whatever may be the strength of stimulus.

2. *Relative Refractory Period*

Relative refractory period is the period during which the muscle shows some response if the strength of stimulus is increased to maximum.

■ MUSCLE TONE

■ DEFINITION

Muscle tone is defined as continuous and partial contraction of the muscles with certain degree of vigor and tension. More details on muscle tone are given in Chapter 103.

■ MAINTENANCE OF MUSCLE TONE

In Skeletal Muscle

Maintenance of tone in skeletal muscle is neurogenic. It is due to continuous discharge of impulses from **gamma motor neurons** in anterior gray horn of spinal cord. Gamma motor neurons in spinal cord are controlled by higher centers in brain.

In Cardiac Muscle

In cardiac muscle, maintenance of tone is purely myogenic, i.e. the muscles themselves control the tone. The tone is not under nervous control in cardiac muscle.

In Smooth Muscle

In smooth muscle, tone is myogenic. It depends upon calcium level and number of cross bridges.

■ APPLIED PHYSIOLOGY: DISEASES INVOLVING MUSCLE TONE

Abnormalities of muscle tone leads to:

1. Hypertonia.
2. Hypotonia.
3. Myotonia.

Hypertonia

Hypertonia or hypertonicity is a muscular disease characterized by increased muscle tone and inability of the muscle to stretch.

Causes for hypertonia

Hypertonia occurs in upper motor neuron lesion (Chapter 95). During the lesion of upper motor neuron, inhibition of lower motor neurons (gamma motor neurons in the spinal cord) is lost. It causes exaggeration of lower motor neuron activity, resulting in hypertonia.

In children, hypertonia is associated with **cerebral palsy**. Cerebral palsy is a permanent disorder characterized by muscular impairment. It is caused by damage of cerebral cortex, which occurs at or before birth. Here also, the motor pathway is affected. Such children usually have speech and language delays, with lack of communication skills.

Hypertonia and spasticity

Hypertonia may be related to spasticity, but it is present with or without spasticity. **Spasticity** is a motor disorder characterized by stiffness of certain muscles due to continuous contraction. Hypertonicity is one of the major symptoms of spasticity. **Paralysis** (complete loss of function) of the muscle due to hypertonicity is called **spastic paralysis**.

2. Hypotonia

Hypotonia is the muscular disease characterized by decreased muscle tone. Tone of the muscle is decreased or lost. Muscle offers very little resistance to stretch. Muscle becomes flaccid (lack of firmness) and the condition is called **flaccidity**.

Causes for hypotonia

Major cause for hypotonia is lower motor neuron lesion (Chapter 95). Paralysis of muscle with hypotonicity is called **flaccid paralysis** and it results in **muscle wastage**.

Hypotonia may also occur because of central nervous system dysfunction, genetic disorders or muscular disorders.

Important clinical conditions associated with hypotonia

i. **Down syndrome**: Chromosomal disorder, characterized by physical disabilities and mental retardation.
ii. **Myasthenia gravis**: Autoimmune disease of neuromuscular junction caused by antibodies to cholinergic receptors (Chapter 28).
iii. **Kernicterus**: Brain damage caused by jaundice in infants (Chapters 19 and 100).
iv. **Cerebellar ataxia**: Lack of coordination of movements.
v. **Muscular dystrophy**: Muscular disease characterized by progressive degeneration of muscle fibers.

3. Myotonia

Myotonia is a congenital disease characterized by continuous contraction of muscle and slow relaxation even after the cessation of voluntary act. Main feature of this disease is the muscle stiffness, which is sometimes referred as **cramps**. Muscle relaxation is delayed.

This type of muscular stiffness with delayed relaxation causes discomfort during simple actions like walking, grasping and chewing. Muscles are enlarged (hypertrophy) because of continuous contraction.

Cause for Myotonia

Myotonia is caused by mutation in the genes of channel proteins in sarcolemma. Such disorders are called **channelopathies**.

Chapter 27: Changes During Muscular Contraction

CHAPTER OUTLINE

- **CHANGES TAKING PLACE DURING MUSCULAR CONTRACTION**
- **ELECTRICAL CHANGES**
  - RESTING MEMBRANE POTENTIAL
  - IONIC BASIS OF RESTING MEMBRANE POTENTIAL
  - ACTION POTENTIAL
  - ACTION POTENTIAL CURVE
  - IONIC BASIS OF ACTION POTENTIAL
- **TYPES OF ACTION POTENTIAL**
- **GRADED POTENTIAL**
- **PHYSICAL CHANGES**
- **HISTOLOGICAL OR MOLECULAR CHANGES**
  - ACTOMYOSIN COMPLEX
  - MOLECULAR BASIS OF MUSCULAR CONTRACTION
- **CHEMICAL CHANGES**
- **THERMAL CHANGES**

CHANGES TAKING PLACE DURING MUSCULAR CONTRACTION

Muscle contracts when it is stimulated. Contraction of the muscle is a **physical or mechanical** event. In addition, several other changes occur in the muscle when it is stimulated.

Changes taking place during muscular contraction:

1. Electrical changes.
2. Physical changes.
3. Histological or molecular changes.
4. Chemical changes.
5. Thermal changes.

ELECTRICAL CHANGES DURING MUSCULAR CONTRACTION

When the muscle is in resting condition, the electrical potential is called resting membrane potential (RMP). When the muscle is stimulated, electrical changes occur which are collectively called action potential.

RESTING MEMBRANE POTENTIAL

Resting membrane potential is the electrical potential difference (voltage) across the cell membrane (between inside and outside of the cell) under resting condition. It is also called **membrane potential** or **transmembrane potential**.

Resting muscle shows negativity inside and positivity outside. This condition of the muscle during resting membrane potential is called **polarized state**. In human skeletal muscle, the resting membrane potential is – 90 mV.

IONIC BASIS OF RESTING MEMBRANE POTENTIAL

In a muscle fiber or a neuron, resting membrane potential is developed and maintained by movement of ions, which produces ionic imbalance across the cell membrane. This results in the development of more positivity outside and more negativity inside the cell.

Ionic imbalance is produced by two factors:

1. Sodium-potassium pump.
2. Selective permeability of cell membrane.

1. Sodium-Potassium Pump

Sodium and potassium ions are actively transported in opposite directions across the cell membrane by means of an electrogenic pump called sodium-potassium pump. It moves three sodium ions out of the cell and two potassium ions inside the cell by using energy from ATP. Since more positive ions (cations) are pumped outside, a net deficit of positive ions occurs inside the cell. It leads to negativity inside and positivity outside the cell. More details of this pump are given in Chapter 3.

2. Selective Permeability of Cell Membrane

Permeability of cell membrane depends largely on the transport channels. Transport channels are selective for movement of some specific ions. Most of the channels are gated channels and the specific ions can move across the membrane only when these gated channels are opened.

Channels for major anions (negatively charged substances)

Channels for some of the negatively charged large substances such as proteins, organic phosphate and sulfate compounds are absent or closed. So, such substances remain inside the cell and cause development and maintenance of negativity inside the cell (resting membrane potential).

Channels for ions

In addition, the channels for three important ions, i.e. sodium, chloride and potassium also play an important role in maintaining the resting membrane potential.

ACTION POTENTIAL

Action potential is defined as a series of electrical changes that occur when the muscle or nerve is stimulated.

Action potential occurs in two phases:

1. Depolarization.
2. Repolarization.

Depolarization

Depolarization is the initial phase of action potential in which the inside of the muscle becomes positive and outside becomes negative. That is, the **polarized state** (resting membrane potential) is **abolished** resulting in depolarization.

Repolarization

Repolarization is the phase of action potential when the potential inside the muscle reverses back to the resting membrane potential. That is, within a short time after depolarization, the interior of muscle becomes negative and outside becomes positive. So, the **polarized state** of the muscle is **re-established**.

Properties of Action Potential

Properties of action potential are listed in **Table 27.1**.

TABLE 27.1: Properties of action potential and graded potential.

Action potential	Graded potential
Propagative	Non-propagative
Long-distance signal	Short-distance signal
Consists of both depolarization and repolarization	Consists of either depolarization or hyperpolarization
Obeys all-or-none law	Does not obey all-or-none law
Summation is not possible	Summation is possible
Has refractory period	Has no refractory period

ACTION POTENTIAL CURVE

Action potential curve is the graphical registration of electrical activity that occurs in an excitable tissue after stimulation.

Action potential curve has three major segments:

1. Latent period.
2. Depolarization.
3. Repolarization.

Resting membrane potential in skeletal muscle is – 90 mV and it is recorded as a straight baseline **(Fig. 27.1)**.

1. Latent Period

Latent period is the period during which no change occurs in the electrical potential immediately after applying the

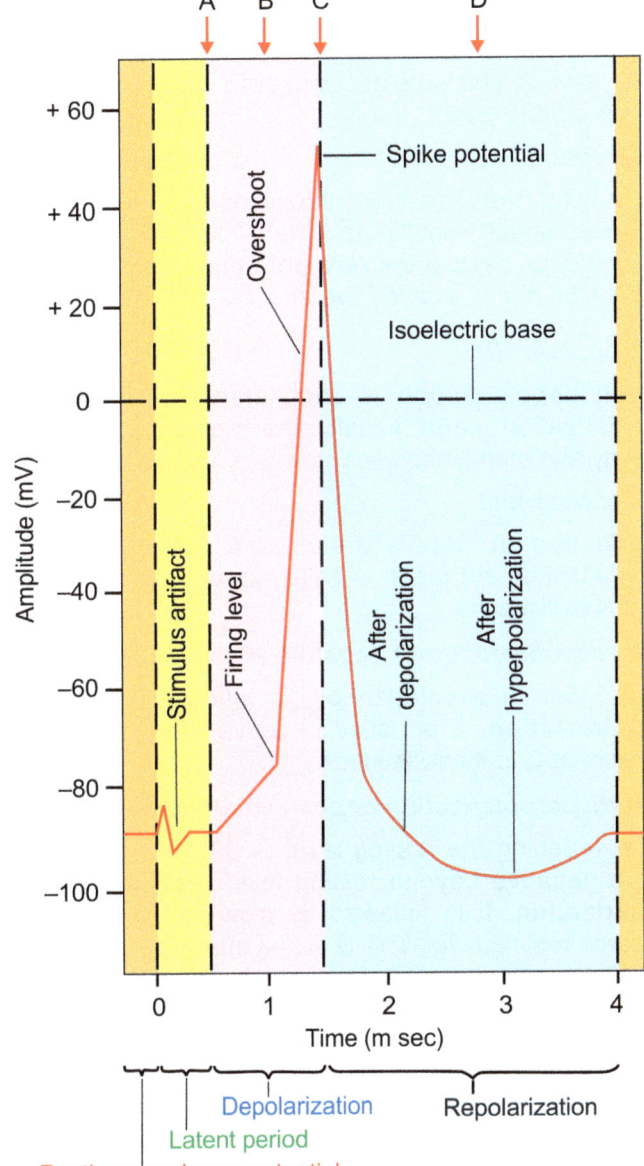

FIGURE 27.1: Action potential in a skeletal muscle.
A = Opening of few Na$^+$ channels.
B = Opening of many Na$^+$ channels.
C = Closure of Na$^+$ channels and opening of K$^+$ channels.
D = Closure of K$^+$ channels.

stimulus. It is a very short period with duration of 0.5 to 1 millisecond.

Stimulus artifact

Resting membrane potential is recorded as a straight baseline at – 90 mV **(Fig. 27.1)**. When a stimulus is applied, there is a slight irregular deflection of baseline for a very short period. This is called stimulus artifact. This artifact is due to leakage of current from stimulating electrode to the recording electrode. The stimulus artifact is followed by latent period.

2. Depolarization

Depolarization starts after the latent period. Initially, it is very slow and the muscle is depolarized for about 15 mV.

Firing level

After the initial slow depolarization for about 15 mV (up to – 75 mV), the rate of depolarization increases suddenly. This point, at which the depolarization increases suddenly is called firing level.

Overshoot

From firing level, the curve reaches **isoelectric potential** (zero potential) rapidly. And then, the curve shoots up (overshoots) beyond the **zero potential** (isoelectric base) up to + 55 mV. It is called overshoot.

3. Repolarization

When depolarization is completed (+ 55 mV), the repolarization starts. Initially, the repolarization occurs rapidly and then it becomes slow.

Spike potential

Rapid rise in depolarization and the rapid fall in repolarization are together called spike potential. It lasts for 0.4 millisecond.

Afterdepolarization or negative afterpotential

Rapid fall in repolarization is followed by a **slow repolarization**. It is called negative afterpotential. Its duration is 2 to 4 milliseconds.

Afterhyperpolarization or positive afterpotential

After reaching the resting level (– 90 mV), it becomes more negative beyond resting level leading to **hyperpolarization**. It is followed by slow rise in the curve towards resting level. This is called afterhyperpolarization or positive afterpotential. This lasts for more than 50 milliseconds. After this, the normal RMP is restored slowly.

■ IONIC BASIS OF ACTION POTENTIAL

Voltage-gated Na^+ channels and voltage-gated K^+ channels play important role in the development of action potential.

Depolarization

During the onset of depolarization, voltage-gated Na^+ channels open and there is slow influx of Na^+. When depolarization reaches 7 to 10 mV, the voltage-gated Na^+ channels start opening at a faster rate. It is called **Na^+ channel activation**. When the firing level is reached, the influx of Na^+ is very great and it leads to overshoot.

Repolarization

The Na^+ transport is short lived. It is because of rapid inactivation of Na^+ channels. Thus, the Na^+ channels open and close quickly. At the same time, K^+ channels start opening. This leads to efflux of K^+ out of the cell, causing repolarization.

Unlike Na+ channels, the K^+ channels remain open for longer duration. These channels remain opened for few more milliseconds after completion of repolarization. It causes efflux of greater number of K^+ producing more negativity inside, i.e. **hyperpolarization**.

■ TYPES OF ACTION POTENTIAL

Action potential is of three types:
1. Monophasic action potential.
2. Biphasic action potential.
3. Compound action potential.

1. Monophasic Action Potential

Monophasic action potential is the series of electrical changes occurring in a single phase when a muscle or a nerve is stimulated. It is characterized by either positive deflection or negative deflection.

Monophasic action potential is recorded by placing one electrode on its surface and the other inside. Action potential in the muscle discussed above belongs to this category.

2. Biphasic Action Potential

Biphasic or diphasic action potential is the series of electrical changes occurring in two phases when a muscle or a nerve is stimulated. It is characterized by both positive and negative deflections.

It is recorded by placing both the recording electrodes on the surface of muscle or nerve fiber.

3. Compound Action Potential

Compound action potential is the algebraic summation of all action potentials produced by all nerve fibers. Each nerve is made up of thousands of nerve fibers (axons). While stimulating the whole nerve, all nerve fibers are activated and produce action potential.

Compound action potential is obtained by recording all the action potentials simultaneously.

■ GRADED POTENTIAL

Graded potential is a mild local change in the membrane potential that develops in receptors, synapse or neuromuscular junction when stimulated. It is also called **graded membrane potential** or **graded depolarization**. The graded potential is distinct from the action potential and the properties of these two potentials are given in **Table 27.1**. In most of the cases, the graded potential is responsible for the generation of action potential. However, in some cases the graded potential hyperpolarizes the membrane potential (more negativity than resting membrane potential).

Examples of graded potentials are:

1. Endplate potential in neuromuscular junction (Chapter 28).
2. Receptor potential (Chapter 91).
3. Excitatory postsynaptic potential (Chapter 92).
4. Inhibitory postsynaptic potential (Chapter 92).

■ PHYSICAL CHANGES DURING MUSCULAR CONTRACTION

Physical change, which takes place during muscular contraction, is the change in length of muscle fibers or change in tension developed in the muscle. Depending upon this, the muscular contraction is classified into two types, namely **isotonic contraction** and **isometric contraction**. Refer Chapter 26 for details.

■ HISTOLOGICAL OR MOLECULAR CHANGES DURING MUSCULAR CONTRACTION

■ ACTOMYOSIN COMPLEX

Actomyosin complex is defined as a complex protein in skeletal muscle formed by actin and myosin.

During relaxed state of the muscle, thin actin filaments from opposite ends of the sarcomere are away from each other leaving a broad 'H' zone.

During contraction of the muscle, actin (thin) filaments glide over the myosin (thick) filaments and form actomyosin complex.

■ MOLECULAR BASIS OF MUSCULAR CONTRACTION

Molecular mechanism is responsible for formation of actomyosin complex that results in muscular contraction.

It includes three stages:

1. Excitation-contraction coupling.
2. Role of troponin and tropomyosin.
3. Sliding mechanism.

1. Excitation-Contraction Coupling

Excitation-contraction coupling is the process that occurs in between the excitation and contraction of the muscle. This process involves series of activities which are responsible for the contraction of the excited muscle.

Sequence of excitation-contraction coupling

When the impulse passes through a motor neuron and reaches the neuromuscular junction, **acetylcholine** is released from motor endplate of neuromuscular junction. Acetylcholine causes opening of ligand-gated sodium channels. So, sodium ions enter the neuromuscular junction. It leads to the development of **endplate potential**. Endplate potential causes generation of action potential in the muscle fiber.

Action potential spreads over sarcolemma and also into the muscle fiber through T-tubules. T-tubules are responsible for rapid spread of action potential into the muscle fiber. When action potential reaches the cisternae of L-tubules, these cisternae are excited. Now, calcium ions stored in cisternae are released into the sarcoplasm. Calcium ions from the sarcoplasm move towards actin filaments to produce the muscular contraction.

Role of calcium ion

Thus, calcium ion forms the link or coupling material between excitation and contraction of muscle. Hence, the calcium ions are said to form the basis of excitation contraction coupling.

2. Role of Troponin and Tropomyosin

Normally, head of myosin molecules has a strong tendency to get attached with active site of F-actin. However, in relaxed condition, the active site of F-actin is covered by the tropomyosin. Therefore, the myosin head cannot combine with actin molecule.

Large number of calcium ions, which are released from L-tubules during excitation of the muscle, bind with troponin 'C'. Loading of troponin 'C' with calcium ions produces some changes in the position of troponin molecule. It in turn, pulls tropomyosin molecule away from F-actin. Due to the movement of tropomyosin, active site of F-actin is uncovered and immediately the head of myosin gets attached to actin **(Fig. 27.2)**.

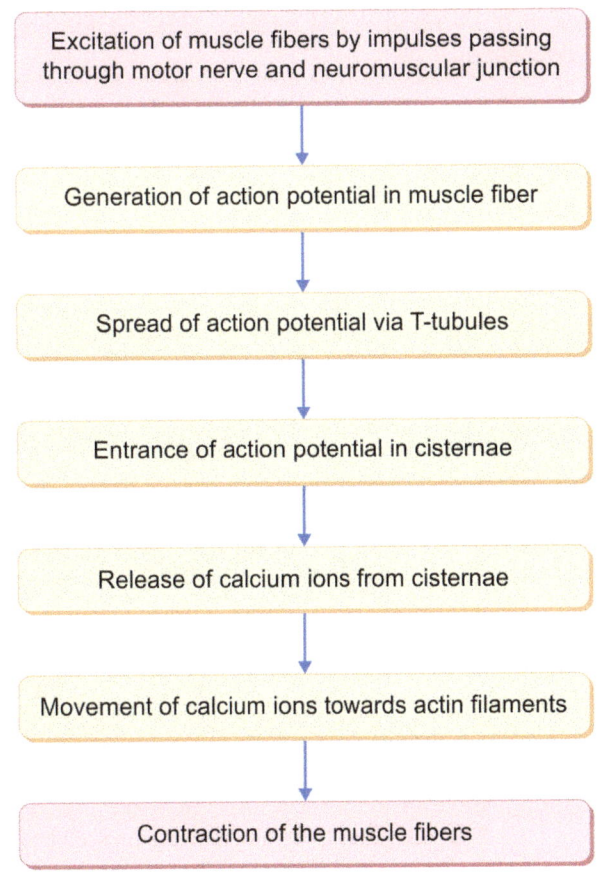

FIGURE 27.2: Excitation-contraction coupling.

3. Sliding Mechanism and Formation of Actomyosin Complex: Sliding Theory

Sliding theory explains how actin filaments slide over myosin filaments and form the actomyosin complex during muscular contraction. It is also called **ratchet theory** or **walk along theory**.

Each **cross bridge** from the myosin filaments has got three components namely, a hinge, an arm and a head.

Power stroke

After binding with active site of F-actin, myosin head is tilted towards the arm, so that the actin filament is dragged along with it **(Fig. 27.3)**. This tilting of head is called power stroke.

Formation of actomyosin complex

After tilting, the head immediately breaks away from the active site and returns to the original position. Now, it combines with a new active site on the actin molecule. And tilting movement occurs again. Thus, the head of cross bridge bends back and forth, and pulls the actin filament towards center of sarcomere.

In this way, all the actin filaments of both ends of sarcomere are pulled. So, the actin filaments of opposite sides overlap and form actomyosin complex. Formation of actomyosin complex results in contraction of the muscle.

When the muscle shortens further, actin filaments from opposite ends of the sarcomere approach each other. So, the 'H' zone becomes narrow. And, the two 'Z' lines come closer with reduction in length of the sarcomere. However, the length of 'A' band is not altered. But, the length of 'I' band decreases.

Changes in sarcomere during muscular contraction

When the muscular contraction becomes severe, the actin filaments from opposite ends overlap and, the 'H' zone disappears.

Following changes occur in sarcomere during muscular contraction:

1. Length of all the sarcomeres decreases, as 'Z' lines come close to each other.
2. Length of 'I' band decreases, since the actin filaments from opposite side overlap.
3. 'H' zone either decreases or disappears.
4. Length of 'A' band remains the same.

Summary of sequence of events during muscular contraction by sliding mechanism is given in **Figure 27.4**.

Energy for Muscular Contraction

Energy for movement of myosin head (power stroke) is obtained by breakdown of **adenosine triphosphate** (ATP) into **adenosine diphosphate** (ADP) and inorganic phosphate (Pi).

Head of myosin has a site for ATP. Actually, head itself can act as the enzyme ATPase and catalyze the breakdown of ATP. Even before the onset of contraction, an ATP molecule binds with myosin head.

When tropomyosin moves to expose the active sites, head is attached to the active site. Now ATPase cleaves ATP into ADP and Pi, which remains in head itself. Energy released during this process is utilized for contraction.

When head is tilted, the ADP and Pi are released and a new ATP molecule binds with head. This process is repeated until the muscular contraction is completed.

Relaxation of the Muscle

Relaxation of the muscle occurs when calcium ions are pumped back into the L-tubules. When calcium ions enter the L-tubules, calcium content in sarcoplasm decreases leading to the release of calcium ions from the troponin. It causes detachment of myosin from actin followed by relaxation of the muscle **(Fig. 27.5)**. Detachment of myosin from actin obtains energy from breakdown of ATP. Thus, the chemical process of muscular relaxation is an active process, although the physical process is said to be passive.

■ CHEMICAL CHANGES DURING MUSCULAR CONTRACTION

■ LIBERATION OF ENERGY

Energy necessary for muscular contraction is liberated during process of breakdown and resynthesis of ATP.

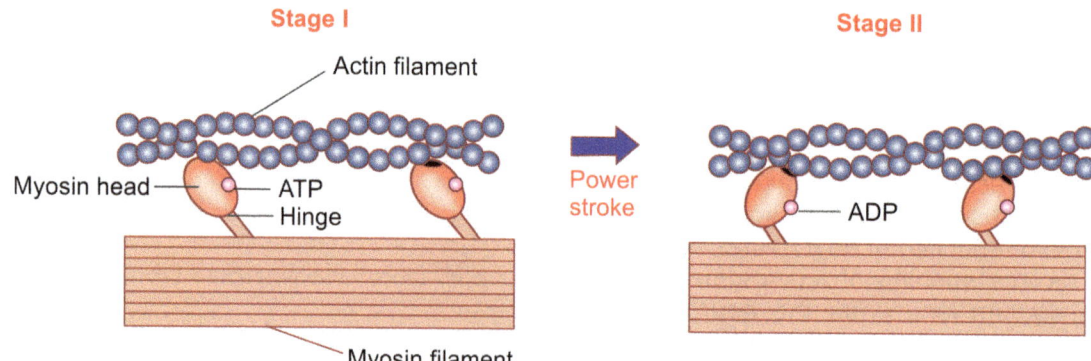

FIGURE 27.3: Diagram showing power stroke by myosin head. Stage I: Myosin head binds with actin. Stage II: Tilting of myosin head (power stroke) drags the actin filament.
ATP = Adenosine triphosphate. ADP = Adenosine diphosphate.

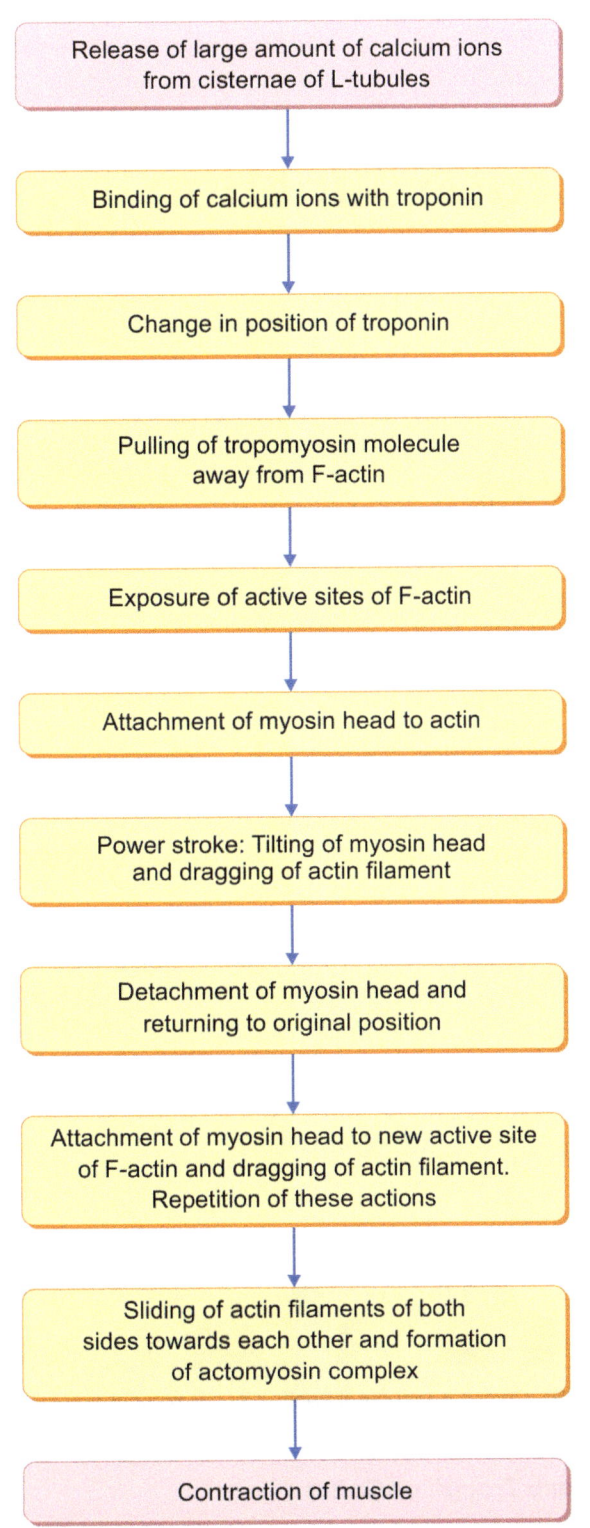

FIGURE 27.4: Muscle contraction by sliding mechanism.

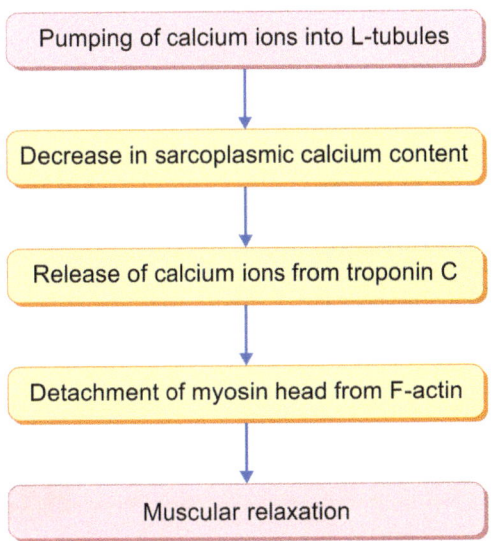

FIGURE 27.5: Sequence of events during muscular relaxation.

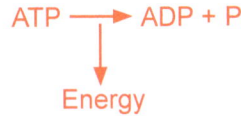

Energy liberated by breakdown of ATP is responsible for the following activities during muscular contraction:

1. Spread of action potential into the muscle.
2. Liberation of calcium ions from cisternae of L-tubules into the sarcoplasm.
3. Movements of myosin head.
4. Sliding mechanism.

Resynthesis of ATP

Adenosine diphosphate, which is formed during ATP breakdown, is immediately utilized for the resynthesis of ATP. But, for resynthesis of ATP, the ADP cannot combine with Pi. It should combine with a **high-energy phosphate** radical. There are two sources from which the high-energy phosphate is obtained namely, **creatine phosphate** and carbohydrate metabolism.

■ THERMAL CHANGES DURING MUSCULAR CONTRACTION

During muscular contraction, heat is produced. Not all the heat is liberated at a time.

Heat is released in three stages:

1. *Resting heat*: Heat produced in the muscle during resting condition. It is due to basal metabolic process in the muscle.
2. *Initial heat*: Heat produced during initiation of muscular contraction and during muscular contraction.
3. *Recovery heat*: Heat produced after muscular contraction.

Breakdown of ATP

During muscular contraction, the energy is supplied from breakdown of ATP. ATP is broken into ADP and Pi and energy is liberated:

Chapter 28: Neuromuscular Junction

CHAPTER OUTLINE

- **DEFINITION AND STRUCTURE**
  - DEFINITION
  - STRUCTURE
- **NEUROMUSCULAR TRANSMISSION**
  - RELEASE OF ACETYLCHOLINE
  - ACTION OF ACETYLCHOLINE
  - DEVELOPMENT ENDPLATE POTENTIAL
  - DEVELOPMENT MINIATURE ENDPLATE POTENTIAL
  - DESTRUCTION OF ACETYLCHOLINE
- **NEUROMUSCULAR BLOCKERS**
- **DRUGS STIMULATING NEUROMUSCULAR JUNCTION**
- **MOTOR UNIT**
  - DEFINITION
  - NUMBER OF MUSCLE FIBERS IN MOTOR UNIT
- **APPLIED PHYSIOLOGY: DISORDERS OF NEUROMUSCULAR JUNCTION**
  - MYASTHENIA GRAVIS
  - EATON-LAMBERT MYASTHENIC SYNDROME

DEFINITION AND STRUCTURE

DEFINITION

Neuromuscular junction is the junction between the terminal branch of nerve fiber and muscle fiber.

STRUCTURE

Skeletal muscle fibers are innervated by the motor nerve fibers. Each nerve fiber (axon) divides into many terminal branches. Each terminal branch innervates one muscle fiber through the neuromuscular junction **(Fig. 28.1)**.

Axon Terminal and Motor Endplate

Terminal branch of nerve fiber is called axon terminal. When the axon comes close to the muscle fiber, it loses the myelin sheath. So, the axis cylinder is exposed. This portion of the axis cylinder is expanded like a bulb which is called **motor endplate**.

Axon terminal contains **mitochondria** and **synaptic vesicles**. Synaptic vesicles contain the neurotransmitter substance, **acetylcholine**. Acetylcholine is synthesized by mitochondria present in the axon terminal and stored in the vesicles.

Mitochondria contain ATP which is the source of energy for the synthesis of acetylcholine.

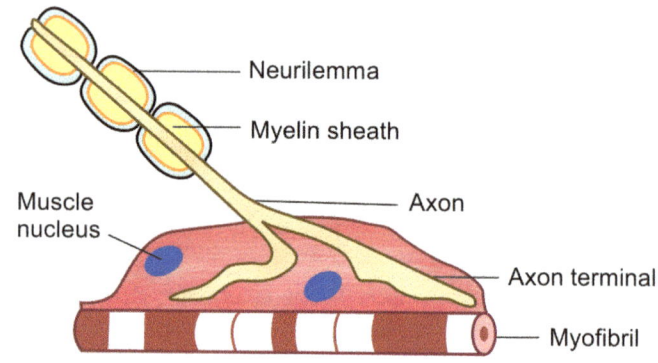

FIGURE 28.1: Longitudinal section of neuromuscular junction.

Synaptic Trough or Gutter

Motor endplate invaginates inside the muscle fiber and forms a depression which is known as synaptic trough or synaptic gutter. Membrane of the muscle fiber below the motor endplate is thickened.

Synaptic Cleft

Membrane of the nerve ending is called the **presynaptic membrane**. Membrane of the muscle fiber is called **postsynaptic membrane**. Space between these two is called synaptic cleft. Synaptic cleft contains **basal lamina**.

It is a thin layer of spongy reticular matrix through which the extracellular fluid diffuses. Large quantity of an enzyme called **acetylcholinesterase** is attached to the matrix of basal lamina.

Subneural Clefts

Postsynaptic membrane is the membrane of the muscle fiber. It is thrown into numerous folds called subneural clefts. Postsynaptic membrane contains the receptors called nicotinic **acetylcholine receptors (Fig. 28.2)**.

■ NEUROMUSCULAR TRANSMISSION

Neuromuscular transmission is defined as the transfer of information from motor nerve ending to the muscle fiber through neuromuscular junction. It is the mechanism by which the motor nerve impulses initiate muscle contraction.

Series of events take place in the neuromuscular junction during this process **(Fig. 28.3)**:

Events of Neuromuscular Transmission

1. Release of acetylcholine.
2. Action of acetylcholine.
3. Development of endplate potential.
4. Development of miniature endplate potential.
5. Destruction of acetylcholine.

■ 1. RELEASE OF ACETYLCHOLINE

When action potential reaches axon terminal, it opens the **voltage-gated calcium channels** in membrane of the axon terminal. Calcium ions enter the axon terminal from extracellular fluid and cause bursting of synaptic vesicles. Now, acetylcholine is released from the vesicles and diffuses through presynaptic membrane and enters the synaptic cleft by **exocytosis**.

Each vesicle contains about 10,000 acetylcholine molecules. And, at a time, about 300 vesicles open and release acetylcholine.

■ 2. ACTION OF ACETYLCHOLINE

After entering synaptic cleft, the acetylcholine molecules bind with **nicotinic receptors** present in postsynaptic membrane and form **acetylcholine-receptor complex**. This complex opens the ligand-gated channels for sodium in the postsynaptic membrane. Now, sodium ions from extracellular fluid enter the neuromuscular junction through these channels. And there, the sodium ions produce an electrical potential called endplate potential.

■ 3. DEVELOPMENT OF ENDPLATE POTENTIAL

Endplate potential is the change in the resting membrane potential when an impulse reaches the neuromuscular junction. Resting membrane potential at the neuromuscular junction is – 90 mV. When sodium ions enter inside, slight depolarization occurs up to – 60 mV which is called endplate potential.

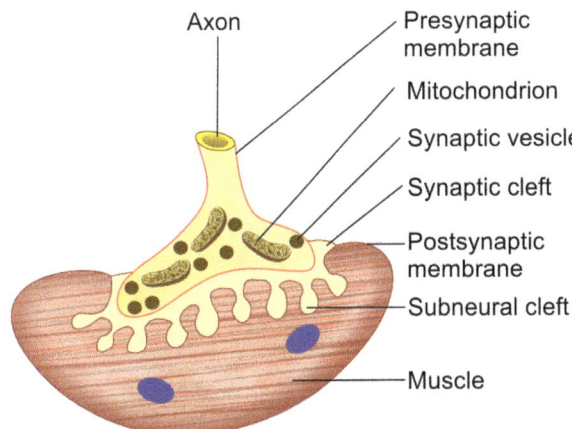

FIGURE 28.2: Structure of neuromuscular junction.

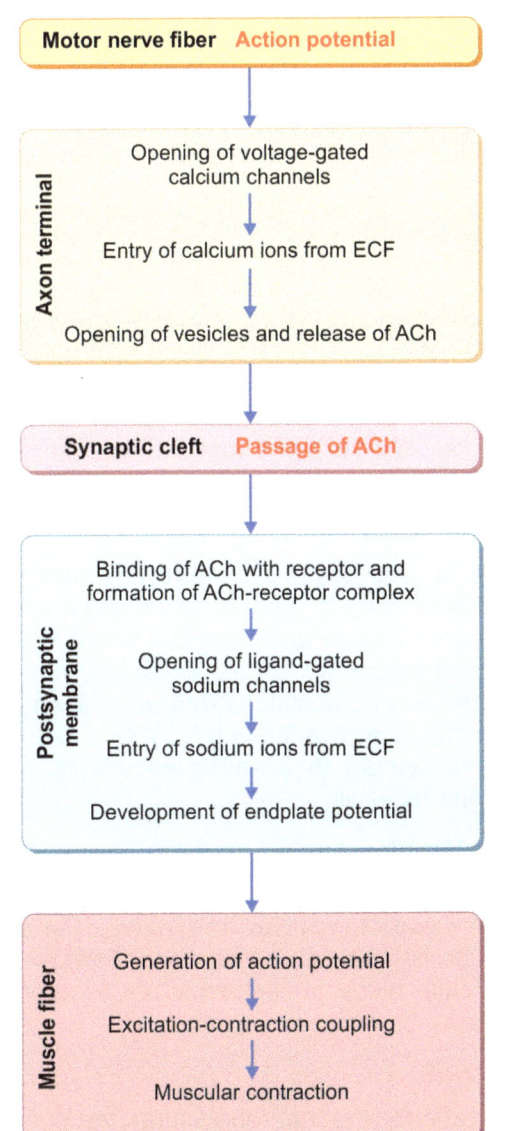

FIGURE 28.3: Sequence of events during neuromuscular transmission.
Ach: Acetylcholine. ECF: Extracellular fluid.

Properties of Endplate Potential

Endplate potential is a **graded potential** (Chapter 27) and it is not action potential. Refer **Table 27.1** for properties of graded potential.

Significance of Endplate Potential

Endplate potential is non-propagative. But it causes the development of action potential in the muscle fiber.

4. DEVELOPMENT MINIATURE ENDPLATE POTENTIAL

Miniature endplate potential is a weak endplate potential in neuromuscular junction that is developed by the release of a small quantity of acetylcholine from axon terminal. And, each quantum of this neurotransmitter produces a weak miniature endplate potential. Amplitude of this potential is only up to 0.5 mV.

Miniature endplate potential cannot produce action potential in the muscle. When more and more quanta of acetylcholine are released continuously, the miniature endplate potentials are added together and finally produce endplate potential resulting in action potential in the muscle.

5. DESTRUCTION OF ACETYLCHOLINE

Acetylcholine released into the synaptic cleft is destroyed very quickly within 1 millisecond by the enzyme, **acetylcholinesterase**. However, the acetylcholine is so potent, that even this short duration of 1 millisecond is sufficient to excite the muscle fiber. Rapid destruction of acetylcholine is functionally significant because it prevents repeated excitation of the muscle fiber and allows the muscle to relax.

Reuptake Process

Reuptake is a process in neuromuscular junction, by which a degraded product of neurotransmitter re-enters the presynaptic axon terminal where it is reused. Acetylcholinesterase splits (degrades) acetylcholine into inactive choline and acetate. **Choline** is taken back into axon terminal from synaptic cleft by reuptake process. There, it is reused in synaptic vesicle to form new acetylcholine molecule.

NEUROMUSCULAR BLOCKERS

Neuromuscular blockers are the drugs, which can prevent the transmission of impulses from nerve fiber to muscle fiber through neuromuscular junctions. Following are the neuromuscular blockers commonly used in surgery and in research.

1. CURARE

Curare prevents the neuromuscular transmission by combining with acetylcholine receptors. So, acetylcholine cannot combine with the receptors. And, the endplate potential cannot develop. Since curare blocks the neuromuscular transmission by acting on acetylcholine receptors hence it is called **receptor blocker**.

2. BUNGAROTOXIN

It is a toxin from the venom of deadly snakes. It affects neuromuscular transmission by blocking the acetylcholine receptors.

3. SUCCINYLCHOLINE AND CARBAMYLCHOLINE

These drugs block the neuromuscular transmission by acting like acetylcholine and keeping the muscle in a depolarized state. But these drugs are not destroyed by cholinesterase. So, the muscle remains in a depolarized state for a long time.

4. BOTULINUM TOXIN

It is derived from the bacteria **Clostridium botulinum**. It prevents release of acetylcholine from axon terminal into the neuromuscular junction.

DRUGS STIMULATING NEUROMUSCULAR JUNCTION

Neuromuscular junction can be stimulated by some drugs like **neostigmine**, **physostigmine** and diisopropyl fluorophosphate. These drugs inactivate the enzyme, acetylcholinesterase. So, acetylcholine is not hydrolyzed. It leads to repeated stimulation and continuous contraction of the muscle.

These drugs are also called **cholinesterase inhibitors**.

MOTOR UNIT
DEFINITION

One single motor neuron, its axon terminals and the muscle fibers innervated by it are together called motor unit. Each motor neuron activates a group of muscle fibers through the axon terminals. Stimulation of a motor neuron causes contraction of all the muscle fibers innervated by that neuron.

NUMBER OF MUSCLE FIBERS IN MOTOR UNIT

Number of muscle fiber in each motor unit varies depending upon the functions of the muscles.

In Muscles Concerned with Fine Movements

Number of muscle fiber is small in the motor units of muscles concerned with fine, graded and precise movements.

Examples are:

1. Laryngeal muscles : 2 to 3 muscle fibers per motor unit
2. Pharyngeal muscles : 2 to 6 muscle fibers per motor unit
3. Ocular muscles   : 3 to 6 muscle fibers per motor unit

In Muscles Concerned with Crude Movements

Muscles concerned with crude or coarse movements have motor units with large number of muscle fibers. There are about 120 to 165 muscle fibers in each motor unit in these muscles. Examples of muscles concerned with crude movements are leg muscles and back muscles.

APPLIED PHYSIOLOGY: DISORDERS OF NEUROMUSCULAR JUNCTION

Disorders of neuromuscular junction include:

1. Myasthenia gravis.
2. Eaton-Lambert myasthenic syndrome.

1. MYASTHENIA GRAVIS

Myasthenia gravis is an autoimmune disorder of neuromuscular junction caused by antibodies to cholinergic receptors. It is characterized by grave weakness of the muscle due to the inability of neuromuscular junction to transmit impulses from nerve to the muscle.

2. EATON-LAMBERT MYASTHENIC SYNDROME

Eaton-Lambert myasthenic syndrome is also an autoimmune disorder of neuromuscular junction. It is caused by antibodies to calcium channels in axon terminal. This disease is characterized by features of myasthenia gravis. In addition, the patients have blurred vision and dry mouth.

Chapter 29: Smooth Muscle

CHAPTER OUTLINE

- DISTRIBUTION
- FUNCTIONS
- STRUCTURE
- TYPES
- ELECTRICAL ACTIVITY IN SINGLE-UNIT SMOOTH MUSCLE
- ELECTRICAL ACTIVITY IN MULTIUNIT SMOOTH MUSCLE
- CONTRACTILE PROCESS
- NEUROMUSCULAR JUNCTION
- CONTROL OF SMOOTH MUSCLE ACTIVITIES

■ DISTRIBUTION SMOOTH MUSCLE

Smooth muscles are **nonstriated** (plain) and **involuntary muscles** present in almost all the organs in the form of sheets, bundles or sheaths around other tissues. These muscles form major contractile tissues of various organs.

■ STRUCTURES HAVING SMOOTH MUSCLE FIBERS

1. Wall of organs such as esophagus, stomach and intestine in gastrointestinal tract.
2. Ducts of digestive glands.
3. Trachea, bronchial tube and alveolar ducts of respiratory tract.
4. Ureter, urinary bladder and urethra in excretory system.
5. Wall of the blood vessels in circulatory system.
6. Arrector pilorum of skin.
7. Mammary glands, uterus, genital ducts, prostate gland and scrotum in reproductive system.
8. Iris and ciliary body of the eye.

■ FUNCTIONS OF SMOOTH MUSCLE

Smooth muscles are concerned with very important functions in different parts of the body such as:

■ 1. IN CARDIOVASCULAR SYSTEM

Smooth muscle fibers around the blood vessels regulate blood pressure and blood flow through different organs and regions of the body.

■ 2. IN RESPIRATORY SYSTEM

Contraction and relaxation of smooth muscle fibers of the air passage alter the diameter of air passage and regulate the inflow and outflow of air.

■ 3. IN DIGESTIVE SYSTEM

Smooth muscle fibers in digestive tract help in:
  i. Movement of food substances.
  ii. Mixing of food substance with digestive juices.
  iii. Absorption of digested material.
  iv. Elimination of unwanted substances.

Sphincters along the digestive tract regulate the flow of materials.

■ 4. IN RENAL SYSTEM

Smooth muscle fibers in renal blood vessels regulate renal blood flow and glomerular filtration. Smooth muscles in the ureters propel urine from kidneys to urinary bladder through ureters. Smooth muscles present in urinary bladder help in voiding urine to the exterior.

■ 5. IN REPRODUCTIVE SYSTEM

In males, smooth muscle fibers facilitate the movement of sperms and secretions from accessory glands along the reproductive tract. In females, these muscles accelerate the movement of sperms through genital tract after sexual act, movement of ovum into uterus through fallopian tube, expulsion of menstrual fluid and delivery of the baby.

■ STRUCTURE OF SMOOTH MUSCLE

Smooth muscle fibers are fusiform or elongated cells. Nucleus is single and elongated and it is centrally placed. Normally, two or more nucleoli are present in the nucleus **(Fig. 29.1)**. Smooth muscle fibers are generally very small, measuring 2 to 5 microns in diameter and 50 to 200 microns

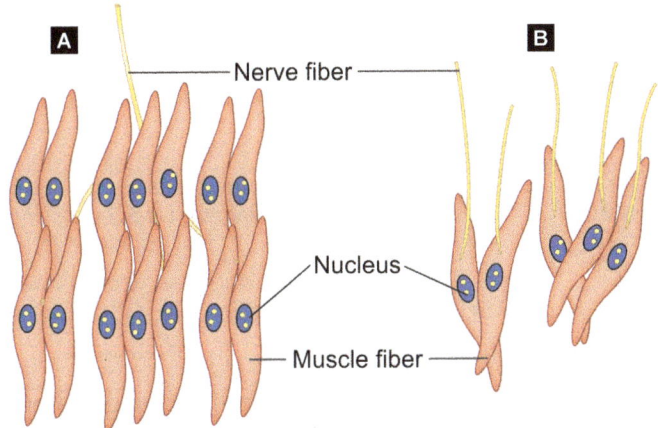

FIGURE 29.1: Smooth muscle fibers. **A.** Single-unit smooth muscle fibers. **B.** Multiunit smooth muscle fibers.

in length. Smooth muscle fibers are covered by connective tissue, but tendons are absent.

Myofibrils and Sarcomere

Well-defined myofibrils and sarcomere are absent in smooth muscles. So, the alternate dark and light bands are absent.

Absence of dark and light bands gives the non-striated appearance to the smooth muscle.

Myofilaments and Contractile Proteins

Contractile proteins in smooth muscle fiber are actin, myosin and tropomyosin. But troponin or troponin-like substance is absent.

Thick and thin filaments are present in smooth muscle. However, these filaments are not arranged in orderly fashion as in skeletal muscle. Thick filaments are formed by myosin molecules and have many numbers of cross bridges than in skeletal muscle. Thin filaments are formed by actin and tropomyosin molecules.

Dense Bodies

Dense bodies are the special structures of smooth muscle fibers to which the actin and tropomyosin molecules of thin filaments are attached.

Sarcotubular System

Sarcotubular system in smooth muscle fibers is in the form of network. T-tubules are absent and L-tubules are poorly developed **(Table 24.1)**.

■ TYPES OF SMOOTH MUSCLE FIBERS

Smooth muscle fibers are of two types:

1. Single-unit or visceral smooth muscle fibers.
2. Multiunit smooth muscle fibers.

■ SINGLE-UNIT OR VISCERAL SMOOTH MUSCLE FIBERS

Single-unit smooth muscle fibers are the fibers with interconnecting **gap junctions**. Gap junctions allow rapid spread of action potential throughout the tissue so that all the muscle fibers show synchronous contraction as a single unit. Single-unit smooth muscle fibers are also called **visceral smooth muscle fibers**.

Features of Single-unit Smooth Muscle Fibers

i. Muscle fibers are arranged in sheets or bundles.
ii. Cell membrane of adjacent fibers fuses at many points to form **gap junctions**. Through the gap junctions, ions move freely from one cell to the other. Thus, a functional **syncytium** is developed. Syncytium contracts as a single unit. In this way, the visceral smooth muscle resembles cardiac muscle more than the skeletal muscle.

Single-unit smooth muscle fibers are in the walls of the organs such as gastrointestinal organs, uterus, ureters, respiratory tract, etc.

■ MULTIUNIT SMOOTH MUSCLE FIBERS

Multiunit smooth muscle fibers are the muscle fibers without interconnecting gap junctions. These smooth muscle fibers resemble the skeletal muscle fibers in many ways.

Features of Multiunit Smooth Muscle Fibers

i. Muscle fibers are individual fibers.
ii. Each muscle fiber is innervated by a single nerve ending.
iii. Each muscle fiber has got an outer membrane made up of glycoprotein, which helps to insulate and separate the muscle fibers from one another.
iv. Control of the muscle fibers is mainly by nerve signals.
v. Smooth muscle fibers do not exhibit spontaneous contractions.

Multiunit muscle fibers are in ciliary muscles of the eye, iris of the eye, nictitating membrane (in cat), arrector pili and smooth muscles of the blood vessels and urinary bladder. Differences between single-unit smooth muscle and multiunit smooth muscle are listed in **Table 29.1**.

■ ELECTRICAL ACTIVITY IN SINGLE-UNIT SMOOTH MUSCLE

Usually 30 to 40 smooth muscle fibers are simultaneously depolarized which leads to development of self-propagating action potential. It is possible because of gap junctions and syncytial arrangements of single-unit smooth muscles.

■ RESTING MEMBRANE POTENTIAL

Resting membrane potential in single-unit smooth muscle fiber is very much unstable and ranges between – 50 mV and – 75 mV. Sometimes, it reaches low level of – 25 mV.

■ CAUSE FOR UNSTABLE RESTING MEMBRANE POTENTIAL: SLOW-WAVE RHYTHM

Unstable resting membrane potential in single-unit smooth muscle fiber is caused by appearance of some wave-like fluctuations called **slow waves**. These slow waves occur in a rhythmic fashion at a frequency of 4 to 10 per minute with the amplitude of 10 to 15 mV **(Fig. 29.2)**. **Slow-wave rhythm** may be due to the rhythmic modulations in the

Section 3: Muscle Physiology

TABLE 29.1: Differences between single-unit smooth muscle and multiunit smooth muscle.

Features	Single-unit smooth muscle	Multiunit smooth muscle
Presence	More common	Less common
Appearance	Arranged like sheets or bundles of tissue	Discrete individual muscle fibers
Situation	In small blood vessels and walls of hollow organs such as of gastrointestinal tract, urinary system, reproductive system, respiratory tract, etc.	Ciliary muscles of the eye, iris of the eye, nictitating membrane (in cat), arrector pili and larger blood vessels
Interconnection	Has gap junctions, which allow rapid passage of action potential	No gap junctions, each muscle fiber is innervated by single nerve ending
Pacemaker cells	Self-excitable pacemaker cells are present; so, spontaneous rhythmical contractions occur	No pacemaker cells and so no spontaneous contractions
Control of action	Myogenic	Neurogenic
Resting membrane potential	Unstable resting membrane potential with slow spike potentials due to rhythmic modulations in sodium-potassium pump	Stable resting membrane potential
Action potential	Can be generated spontaneously Can be elicited by electrical or hormonal stimulation Spreads rapidly throughout the sheet of cells and make the cells to contract as a single unit Occurs with a plateau due to long depolarization and slow repolarization	Cannot be generated spontaneously Can be elicited by neural and hormonal stimulation Selective activation of each muscle fiber that can contract independently of each other No plateau

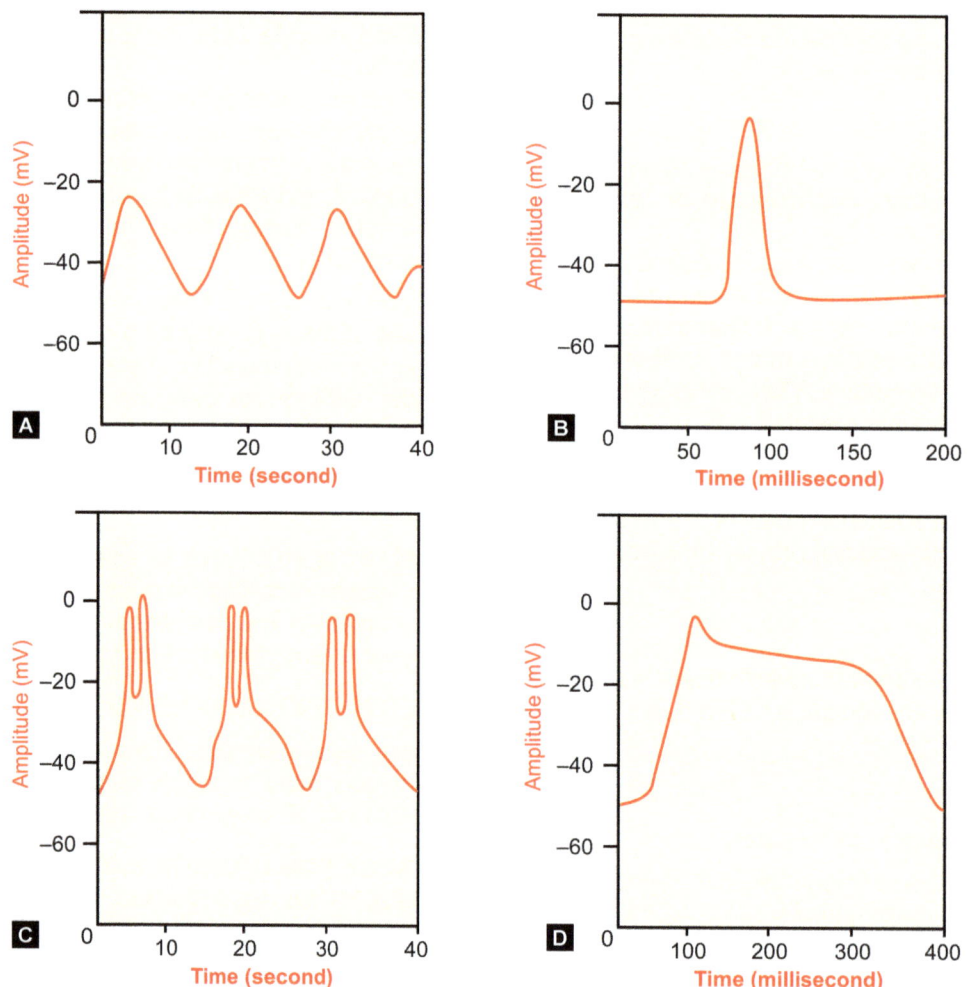

FIGURE 29.2: Electrical activities in smooth muscle. **A.** Slow-wave rhythm of resting membrane potential. **B.** Spike potential. **C.** Spike potential initiated by slow-wave rhythm. **D.** Action potential with plateau.

activities of sodium-potassium pump. Slow wave is not action potential and it cannot cause contraction of the muscle. But it initiates the action potential (see below).

ACTION POTENTIAL

Three types of action potential occur in single-unit smooth muscle fibers:

1. Spike potential.
2. Spike potential initiated by slow-wave rhythm.
3. Action potential with plateau.

1. Spike Potential

Spike potential in single-unit smooth muscle is different from that in skeletal muscles. In smooth muscle, the average duration of spike potential varies between 30 milliseconds and 50 milliseconds. Its amplitude is very low and it does not reach the isoelectric base. It is due to nervous and other stimuli and it leads to contraction of the muscle.

2. Spike Potential Initiated by Slow-wave Rhythm

Sometimes the slow-wave rhythm of resting membrane potential initiates the spike potentials, which lead to contraction of the muscle. Spike potentials appear rhythmically at a rate of about one or two spikes at the peak of each slow wave. These potentials initiated by the slow-wave rhythm cause rhythmic contractions of smooth muscles. This type of potentials appears mostly in smooth muscles, which are self-excitatory and contract themselves without any external stimuli. So, the spike potentials initiated by slow-wave rhythm are otherwise called **pacemaker waves**. Smooth muscles showing rhythmic contractions are present in some of the visceral organs such as intestine.

3. Action Potential with Plateau

This type of action potential starts with rapid depolarization as in the case of skeletal muscle. But repolarization does not occur immediately. Muscle remains depolarized for long periods of about 100 to 1,000 milliseconds. This forms the plateau (stable period) in action potential. This type of action potential is responsible for sustained contraction of smooth muscle fibers. After long depolarized state, slow repolarization occurs.

TONIC CONTRACTION OF SMOOTH MUSCLE WITHOUT ACTION POTENTIAL

Smooth muscles of some visceral organs maintain a state of partial contraction called **tonus** or **tone**. It is due to the tonic contraction of the muscle that occurs without any action potential or any stimulus. Sometimes, the tonic contraction occurs due to the action of some hormones.

IONIC BASIS OF ACTION POTENTIAL

Important difference between the action potential in skeletal muscle and single-unit smooth muscle lies in the ionic basis of depolarization. In skeletal muscle, the depolarization occurs due to opening of sodium channels and entry of sodium ions from extracellular fluid into the muscle fiber. But in single-unit smooth muscle, the depolarization is due to entry of calcium ions rather than sodium ions. Unlike the fast sodium channels, the calcium channels open and close slowly. It is responsible for the prolonged action potential with plateau in smooth muscles. Calcium ions play an important role during the contraction of the smooth muscle.

ELECTRICAL ACTIVITY IN MULTIUNIT SMOOTH MUSCLE

Electrical activity in multiunit smooth muscle is different from that in the single-unit smooth muscle. Electrical changes leading to contraction of multiunit smooth muscle are triggered by nervous stimuli. Nerve endings secrete neurotransmitters such as acetylcholine and noradrenaline. These neurotransmitters depolarize the membrane of smooth muscle fiber slightly leading to contraction. Action potential does not develop. This type of depolarization is called **local depolarization** of **junctional potential**. Local depolarization travels throughout the entire smooth muscle fiber and causes contraction. Local depolarization is developed because the multiunit smooth muscle fibers are too small to develop action potential.

CONTRACTILE PROCESS IN SMOOTH MUSCLE

Compared to skeletal muscles, in smooth muscles, the contraction and relaxation processes are slow.

MOLECULAR BASIS OF SMOOTH MUSCLE CONTRACTION

Process of excitation and contraction is very slow in smooth muscles because of poor development of L-tubules (sarcoplasmic reticulum). So, the calcium ions, which are responsible for **excitation-contraction coupling**, must be obtained from the extracellular fluid. It makes the process of excitation-contraction coupling slow.

Calcium-Calmodulin Complex

Stimulation of ATPase activity of myosin in smooth muscle is different from that in the skeletal muscle. In smooth muscle, the myosin has to be phosphorylated for the activation of **myosin ATPase**. **Phosphorylation** of myosin occurs in the following manner.

1. Calcium, which enters the sarcoplasm from the extracellular fluid combines with a protein called **calmodulin** and forms calcium-calmodulin complex **(Fig. 29.3)**.
2. It activates an enzyme called calmodulin-dependent **myosin light chain kinase**.
3. This enzyme in turn causes phosphorylation of myosin followed by activation of myosin ATPase.
4. Now, the sliding of actin filaments starts.

The phosphorylated myosin gets attached to the actin molecule for longer period. It is called **latch-bridge**

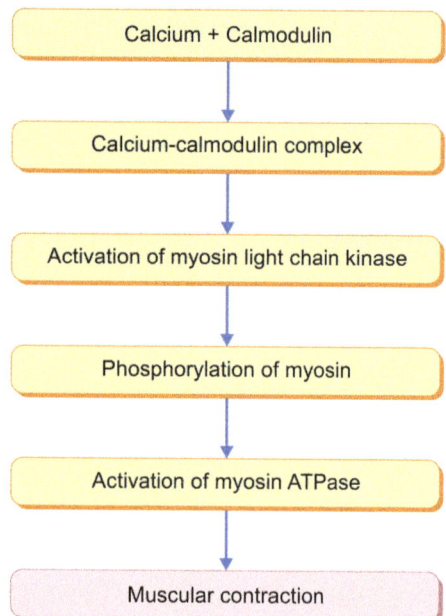

FIGURE 29.3: Molecular basis of smooth muscle contraction.

mechanism and it is responsible for the sustained contraction of the muscle with expenditure of little energy.

Relaxation of the muscle occurs due to the dissociation of calcium-calmodulin complex.

Length-Tension Relationship: Plasticity

Smooth muscle fibers have the property of plasticity. Plasticity is the adaptability of smooth muscle fibers to a wide range of lengths. If the smooth muscle fiber is stretched, it adapts to this new length and contracts when stimulated. This adaptability exists to a wide range of lengths. Because of this property, tension produced in the muscle fiber is not directly proportional to resting length of the muscle fiber. In other words, **Starling's law** is not applicable to smooth muscle. In skeletal and cardiac muscles Starling's law is applicable and the tension or force of contraction is directly proportional to initial length of the muscle fibers.

■ NEUROMUSCULAR JUNCTION IN SMOOTH MUSCLE

Well-defined neuromuscular junctions are absent in smooth muscle. Nerve fibers (axons) do not end in the form of endplate. Instead, these nerve fibers end on smooth muscle fibers in three different ways:

1. In some smooth muscles, nerve fibers diffuse on the sheet of smooth muscle fibers without making any direct contact with the muscle. These **diffused nerve fibers** form **diffused junctions** which contain neurotransmitters.
2. In some smooth muscle fibers, axon terminal ends in the form of many **varicosities** which contain the neurotransmitter.
3. In some of the multiunit smooth muscle fibers, a gap is present between varicosities and the membrane of smooth muscle fibers which resembles the synaptic cleft in skeletal muscle. This gap is called **contact junction** and it functions as neuromuscular junction of skeletal muscle.

■ CONTROL OF SMOOTH MUSCLE ACTIVITIES

Smooth muscle fibers are controlled by:
1. Nervous factors.
2. Humoral factors.

■ NERVOUS FACTORS

Single-unit smooth muscle and multiunit smooth muscle are innervated by nerves of both the divisions of autonomic nervous system. All these nerves initiate the contraction of multiunit smooth muscles only. Nerves supplying single-unit smooth muscles do not initiate contraction. But these nerves can modify or regulate the rate and force of contraction.

■ HUMORAL FACTORS

Activity of smooth muscle is also controlled by humoral factors which include hormones, neurotransmitters and other humoral factors.

Action of the hormones and neurotransmitters depends upon the type of receptors present in membrane of smooth muscle fibers in particular area. The receptors are of two types, excitatory and inhibitory receptors.

If excitatory receptors are present, the hormones or the neurotransmitters contract the muscle by producing depolarization. If inhibitory receptors are present, the hormones or the neurotransmitters relax the muscles by producing hyperpolarization.

Humoral Factors which Cause Contraction of Smooth Muscles

Humoral factors which cause contraction of smooth muscles are:
1. Acetylcholine.
2. Antidiuretic hormone (ADH).
3. Adrenaline.
4. Angiotensin II, III and IV.
5. Endothelin.
6. Histamine.
7. Noradrenaline.
8. Oxytocin.
9. Serotonin.

Humoral Factors which Cause Relaxation of Smooth Muscles

Humoral factors which relax the smooth muscles are:
1. Lack of oxygen.
2. Excess of carbon dioxide.
3. Increase in hydrogen ion concentration.
4. Adenosine.
5. Lactic acid.
6. Excess of potassium ion.
7. Decrease in calcium ion.
8. Nitric oxide (NO), the endothelium-derived relaxing factor (EDRF).

MODEL QUESTIONS IN MUSCLE PHYSIOLOGY

LONG QUESTIONS

1. Enumerate the properties of muscles and give an account of contractile property of the skeletal muscle.
2. Explain the molecular basis of contraction.
3. Describe the electrical changes during muscular contraction.
4. Explain the ionic basis of electrical events during contraction of skeletal muscle.
5. Describe the neuromuscular junction with a suitable diagram. Add a note on neuromuscular transmission.

SHORT QUESTIONS

1. Classify muscles by different methods.
2. Sarcomere.
3. Muscle proteins.
4. Sarcotubular system.
5. Composition of muscle.
6. Differences between pale and red muscles.
7. Rigor.
8. Effects of repeated stimuli on skeletal muscle.
9. Fatigue.
10. Tetanus.
11. Refractory period.
12. Resting membrane potential.
13. Action potential in skeletal muscle.
14. Actomyosin complex.
15. Excitation-contraction coupling.
16. Sliding theory of muscular contraction.
17. Electrical activity in smooth muscle.
18. Molecular basis of smooth muscular contraction.
19. Neuromuscular junction.
20. Neuromuscular transmission.

VERY SHORT ANSWER QUESTIONS

1. Compare skeletal muscle and cardiac muscle.
2. Compare skeletal muscle and smooth muscle.
3. Microscopic structure of myofibril.
4. Contractile elements of the muscle.
5. Composition of skeletal muscle.
6. Sarcoplasmic reticulum.
7. Define excitability and stimulus.
8. Types of muscular contraction.
9. Latent period and its causes.
10. Types of skeletal muscle. Give examples for each type.
11. Medicolegal importance of rigor mortis.
12. Free load and afterload. Which is beneficial? Why?
13. Starlings law of muscle.
14. Define muscle tone. How it is maintained in different types of muscles?
15. Name the changes taking place during muscular contraction.
16. Resting membrane potential.
17. Graded potentials.
18. Actomyosin complex.
19. Endplate potential.
20. Motor units.
21. Neuromuscular blockers.
22. Motor unit.
23. Disorders of neuromuscular junction.
24. Types of smooth muscle.
25. Myasthenia gravis.
26. Hypotonia.
27. Hypertonia.
28. Myotonia.

SECTION 4: DIGESTIVE SYSTEM

Chapter 30: Overview of Digestive System

CHAPTER OUTLINE

- DIGESTION AND DIGESTIVE PROCESS
- FUNCTIONAL ANATOMY
  - GASTROINTESTINAL TRACT
  - ACCESSORY DIGESTIVE ORGANS
- WALL OF GASTROINTESTINAL TRACT
  - MUCUS LAYER
  - SUBMUCUS LAYER
- MUSCULAR LAYER
- SEROUS OR FIBROUS LAYER
- NERVE SUPPLY TO GASTROINTESTINAL TRACT
  - INTRINSIC NERVE SUPPLY
  - EXTRINSIC NERVE SUPPLY

DIGESTION AND DIGESTIVE PROCESS

Digestion is defined as the process by which food is broken down into simple chemical substances that can be absorbed and used as nutrients by the body. Most of the substances in diet cannot be utilized as such. These substances must be broken into smaller particles. Then only these substances can be absorbed into blood and distributed to various parts of the body for utilization. Digestive system is responsible for these functions.

Digestive process is accomplished by mechanical and enzymatic breakdown of food particles into simpler chemical compounds. A normal young healthy adult consumes about 1 kg of solid diet and about 1 to 2 L of liquid diet every day. All these food materials are subjected to digestive process, before being absorbed into blood and distributed to the tissues of the body. Digestive system plays the major role in the digestion and absorption of food substances.

FUNCTIONS OF DIGESTIVE SYSTEM

Functions of digestive system include:

1. Ingestion or consumption of food substances.
2. Breaking them into small particles.
3. Secretion of necessary enzymes and other substances for digestion.
4. Digestion of food particles.
5. Absorption of digested products (nutrients).
6. Removal of unwanted substances from body.

FUNCTIONAL ANATOMY OF DIGESTIVE SYSTEM

Digestive system is made up of **gastrointestinal tract** (GI tract) or **alimentary canal** and **accessory digestive organs** (Fig. 30.1).

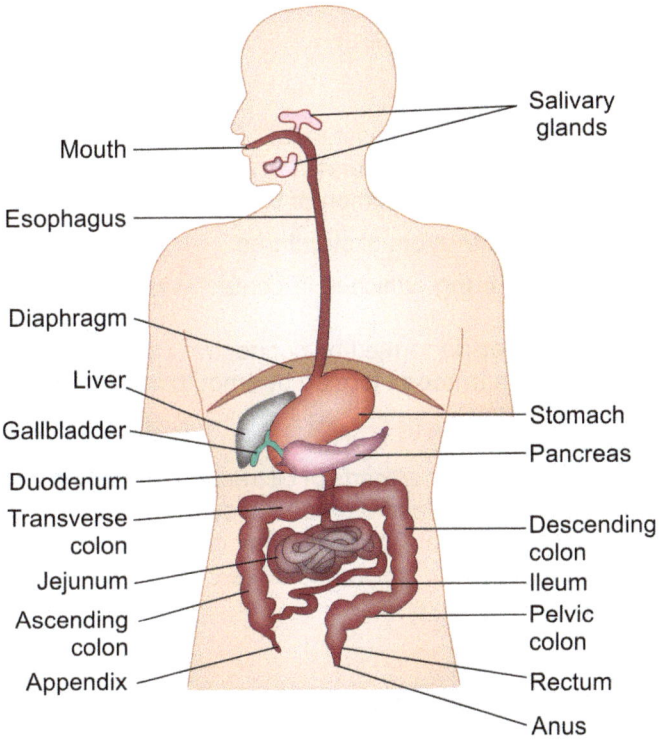

FIGURE 30.1: Gastrointestinal tract.

GASTROINTESTINAL TRACT

GI tract is a tubular structure extending from the mouth up to anus with a length of about 30 feet. It opens to external environment at both the ends. Gastrointestinal tract includes the **primary digestive organs** where actual digestion takes place.

Primary digestive organs are:

1. Mouth.
2. Pharynx.
3. Esophagus.
4. Stomach.
5. Small intestine.
6. Large intestine.

ACCESSORY DIGESTIVE ORGANS

Accessory digestive organs are the organs which help the primary digestive organs in the process of digestion.

Accessory digestive organs are:

1. Teeth.
2. Tongue.
3. Salivary glands.
4. Exocrine part of pancreas.
5. Liver.
6. Gallbladder.

WALL OF GASTROINTESTINAL TRACT

In general, wall of the GI tract is formed by four layers, which are from inside out:

1. Mucus layer.
2. Submucus layer.
3. Muscular layer.
4. Serous or fibrous layer.

1. MUCUS LAYER

Mucus layer is the innermost layer of the wall of GI tract. It is also called **gastrointestinal mucosa** or **mucous membrane**. It faces the lumen of GI tract.

Mucosa has three layers of structures:

  i. **Epithelial lining**, which is in contact with contents of GI tract.
 ii. **Lamina propria** formed by connective tissue.
iii. **Muscularis mucosa** formed by smooth muscle fibers.

2. SUBMUCUS LAYER

This layer is present in all parts of GI tract except mouth and pharynx. Submucus layer contains loose collagen fibers, elastic fibers, reticular fibers and few cells of connective tissue. Blood vessels, lymphatic vessels and nerve plexus are present in this layer.

3. MUSCULAR LAYER

Muscular layer in lips, cheeks and wall of pharynx consists of **skeletal muscle** fibers. Esophagus has both skeletal and smooth muscle fibers. Wall of the stomach and intestine is formed by **smooth muscle** fibers only.

In Stomach

Smooth muscle fibers in stomach are arranged in three layers:

  i. Inner oblique layer.
 ii. Middle circular layer.
iii. Outer longitudinal layer.

In Intestine

Smooth muscle fibers in the intestine are arranged in two layers:

  i. Inner circular layer.
 ii. Outer longitudinal layer.

Smooth muscle fibers present in inner circular layer of anal canal constitute **internal anal sphincter**. **External anal sphincter** is formed by skeletal muscle fibers.

4. SEROUS OR FIBROUS LAYER

Outermost layer of the wall of GI tract is either serous or fibrous in nature. Serous layer is formed by connective tissue and **mesoepithelial cells**. It is also called **serosa**, **serous membrane**.

NERVE SUPPLY TO GASTROINTESTINAL TRACT

GI tract has two types of nerve supply:

A. Intrinsic nerve supply.
B. Extrinsic nerve supply.

INTRINSIC NERVE SUPPLY: ENTERIC NERVOUS SYSTEM

Enteric nervous system is present within the wall of GI tract from esophagus to anus. Nerve fibers of this system are interconnected and form two major networks called:

1. Auerbach's plexus.
2. Meissner's plexus.

These two nerve plexuses contain nerve cell bodies, processes of nerve cells and the receptors. Receptors in the GI tract are **stretch receptors** and **chemoreceptors**. Enteric nervous system is controlled by extrinsic nerves.

1. *Auerbach's Plexus*

It is also known as **myenteric nerve plexus**. It is present in between the inner circular muscle layer and the outer longitudinal muscle layer **(Fig. 30.2)**.

Functions of Auerbach's plexus

Major function of this plexus is to regulate the movements of GI tract. Some nerve fibers of this plexus accelerate the movements by secreting the excitatory neurotransmitter substances such as acetylcholine, serotonin and substance P. Other fibers of this plexus inhibit the GI motility by secreting the inhibitory neurotransmitters such as vasoactive intestinal polypeptide (VIP), neurotensin and enkephalin.

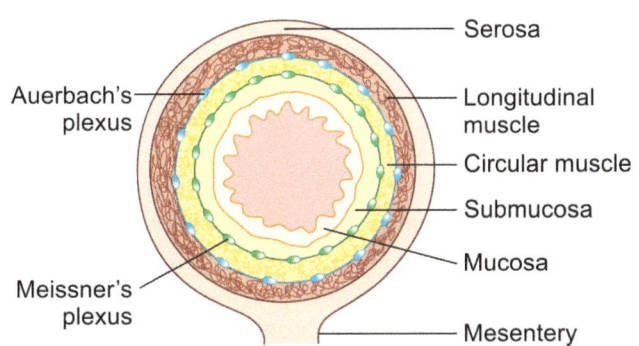

FIGURE 30.2: Structure of intestinal wall with intrinsic nerve plexus.

2. Meissner's Nerve Plexus

Meissner's plexus is otherwise called **submucus nerve plexus**. It is situated in between the muscular layer and submucosal layer of GI tract.

Functions of Meissner's plexus

Meissner's plexus regulates secretory functions of GI tract. It also causes constriction of blood vessels of GI tract.

EXTRINSIC NERVE SUPPLY

Extrinsic nerves that control the enteric nervous system are from autonomic nervous system. Both sympathetic and parasympathetic divisions of the autonomic nervous system innervate GI tract **(Fig. 30.3)**.

Sympathetic Nerve Fibers

Preganglionic sympathetic nerve fibers to GI tract arise from lateral horns of spinal cord between fifth thoracic and second lumbar segments (T5 to L2). From here, the fibers leave the spinal cord, pass through the ganglia of sympathetic chain without having any synapse and then terminate in the **celiac ganglion** and **mesenteric ganglia**. The postganglionic fibers from these ganglia are distributed throughout the GI tract.

Functions of sympathetic nerve fibers

Sympathetic nerve fibers inhibit the movements and decrease the secretions of GI tract by secreting the neurotransmitter noradrenaline.

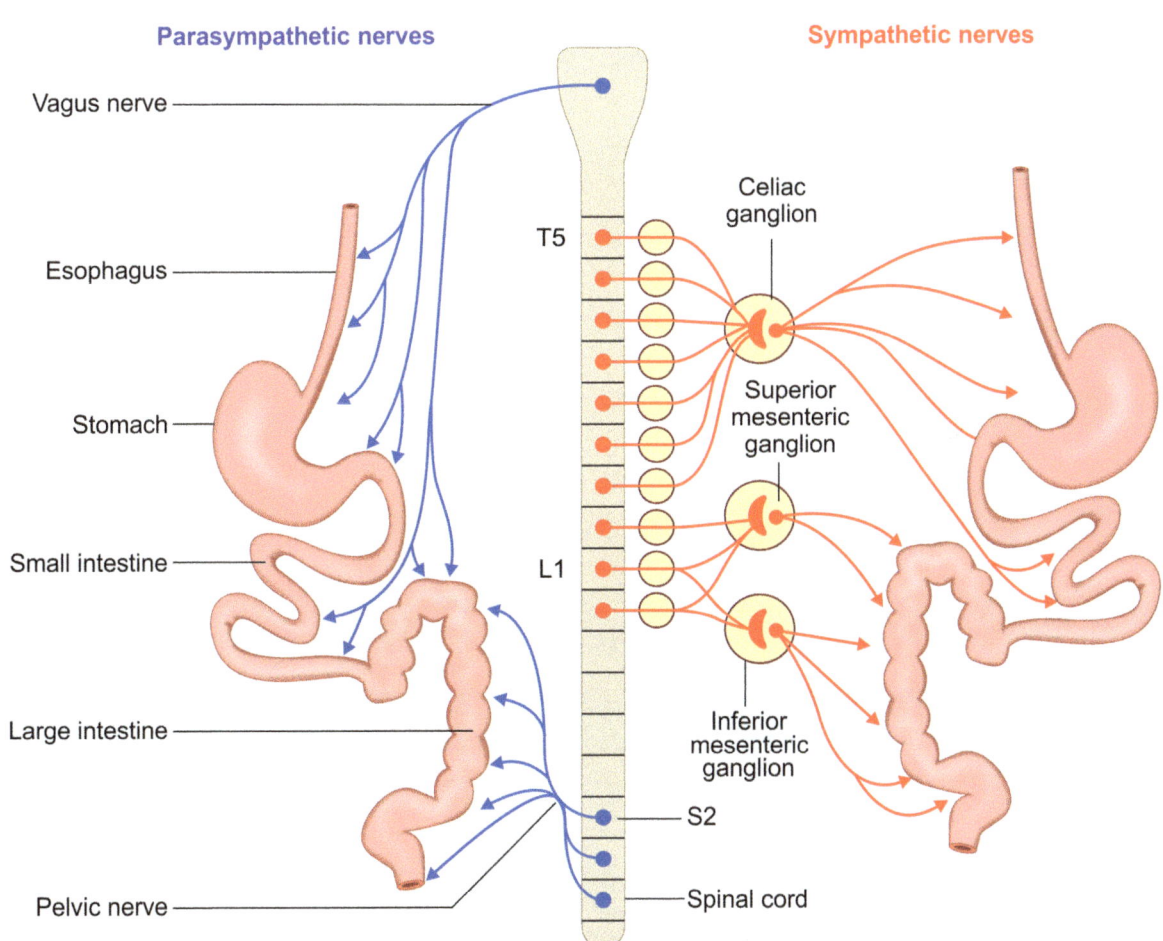

FIGURE 30.3: Extrinsic nerve supply to GI tract.
T5: 5th thoracic segment of spinal cord.
L1: 1st lumbar segment of spinal cord.
S2: 2nd sacral segment of spinal cord.

Parasympathetic Nerve Fibers

Parasympathetic nerve fibers to GI tract pass through some of the cranial nerves and sacral nerves. Preganglionic and postganglionic parasympathetic nerve fibers to mouth and salivary glands pass through **facial nerve** and **glossopharyngeal nerve**.

Preganglionic parasympathetic nerve fibers to esophagus, stomach, small intestine and upper part of large intestine pass through **vagus nerve**. Preganglionic nerve fibers to lower part of large intestine arise from second, third and fourth sacral segments (S2, S3 and S4) of spinal cord and pass through **pelvic nerve**. All these preganglionic parasympathetic nerve fibers synapse with the postganglionic nerve cells in the myenteric and submucus plexus.

Functions of parasympathetic nerve fibers

Parasympathetic nerve fibers accelerate movements and increase the secretions of GI tract. Neurotransmitter secreted by the parasympathetic nerve fibers is acetylcholine.

Chapter 31: Mouth and Salivary Secretion

CHAPTER OUTLINE

- FUNCTIONAL ANATOMY OF MOUTH
- FUNCTIONS OF MOUTH
- SALIVARY GLANDS
- PROPERTIES AND COMPOSITION OF SALIVA
- FUNCTIONS OF SALIVA
- REGULATION OF SALIVARY SECRETION
- EFFECTS OF DRUGS AND CHEMICALS ON SALIVARY SECRETION
- APPLIED PHYSIOLOGY: DISORDERS OF SALIVARY SECRETION

FUNCTIONAL ANATOMY OF MOUTH

Mouth is otherwise known as **oral cavity** or **buccal cavity**. It is formed by cheeks, lips and palate. It encloses the teeth, tongue and salivary glands. It opens anteriorly to the exterior through lips and posteriorly through fauces into the pharynx.

Digestive juice present in the mouth is saliva which is secreted by the salivary glands.

FUNCTIONS OF MOUTH

Primary function of mouth is eating. It has few other important functions also. Refer **Table 31.1** for details.

SALIVARY GLANDS

In humans, saliva is secreted by three pairs of major (larger) salivary glands and some minor (small) salivary glands in the oral and pharyngeal mucous membrane.

TABLE 31.1: Functions of mouth.

Function	Process
1. Mastication	Teeth cut and grind the food Lips and cheeks hold food in the mouth with the help of tongue Muscles of the mouth along with jaw movements help in chewing the food properly and mixing the food with saliva Saliva lubricates and softens the food to facilitate chewing and swallowing
2. Taste	Taste buds present on tongue and other structures of mouth help to appreciate and differentiate the taste of food Saliva helps in appreciation of taste by dissolving the foodstuffs
3. Speech	Mouth coordinates with larynx, pharynx, lips and tongue during speech Saliva helps in speech by moistening and lubricating soft parts of mouth and lips
4. Appearance	Shape of the mouth along with jaws, lips and teeth together contribute to the appearance of face
5. Expression	Facial expressions such as smiling and laughing are mostly centered on mouth along with movements of lips and cheeks
6. Breathing	Occasionally, when nose breathing is inadequate, as in case of running or nasal block, mouth is used for breathing

Major salivary glands are:

1. Parotid glands.
2. Submaxillary or submandibular glands.
3. Sublingual glands.

1. PAROTID GLANDS

Parotid glands are the largest of all salivary glands situated at the side of face just below and in front of ear. Secretions from these glands are emptied into the oral cavity by **Stensen's duct** that opens inside the cheek against the upper second molar tooth **(Fig. 31.1)**.

2. SUBMAXILLARY GLANDS

Submaxillary glands or **submandibular glands** are located in submaxillary triangle medial to mandible. Saliva from these glands is emptied into the oral cavity by **Wharton's duct**. This duct opens at the side of frenulum of tongue by means of a small opening on the summit of papilla called **caruncula sublingualis**.

3. SUBLINGUAL GLANDS

Sublingual glands are the smallest salivary glands situated in the mucosa at the floor of mouth. Saliva from these glands is poured into 5 to 15 small ducts called **ducts of Rivinus**. These ducts open on small papillae beneath the tongue. One of the ducts is larger and it is called **Bartholin's duct (Table 31.2)**. It drains the anterior part of the gland and opens on caruncula sublingualis near the opening of **Wharton's duct**.

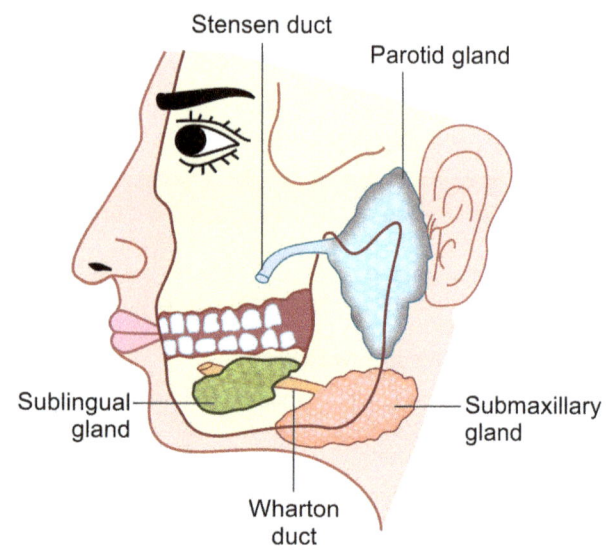

FIGURE 31.1: Major salivary glands.

TABLE 31.2: Ducts of major salivary glands.

Gland	Duct
Parotid gland	Stensen's duct
Submaxillary gland	Wharton's duct
Sublingual gland	Ducts of Rivinus/Bartholin's duct

MINOR SALIVARY GLANDS

1. **Lingual mucus glands** situated in posterior 1/3 of the tongue, behind circumvallate papillae and at the tip and margins of tongue.
2. **Lingual serous glands** located near circumvallate papillae and filiform papillae.
3. **Buccal glands** present between the mucus membrane and buccinator muscle. Four to five of these are larger and situated outside buccinator around terminal part of parotid duct. These glands are called **molar glands**.
4. **Labial glands** situated beneath the mucous membrane around the orifice of mouth.
5. **Palatal glands** found beneath the mucous membrane of the soft palate.

CLASSIFICATION OF SALIVARY GLANDS

Salivary glands are classified into three types based on the type of secretion.

1. Serous Glands

Serous glands are predominately made up of **serous cells**. Serous glands secrete thin and **watery saliva**. Parotid glands and lingual (serous) glands are the serous glands.

2. Mucus Glands

Mucus glands are made up of mainly the **mucus cells**. These glands secrete thick, **viscus saliva** with high mucin content. Lingual mucus glands, buccal glands and palatal glands belong to this type.

3. Mixed Glands

Mixed glands are made up of both **serous** and **mucus cells**. Submandibular, sublingual and labial glands are the mixed glands.

STRUCTURE AND DUCT SYSTEM OF SALIVARY GLANDS

Salivary glands are made up of **acini** or **alveoli**. Each acinus is formed by a small group of cells which surround a central cavity. Central cavity of each acinus is continuous with the lumen of the duct. Fine duct draining each acinus is called **intercalated duct**. Many intercalated ducts join together to form **intralobular duct**. Few intralobular ducts join to form **interlobular ducts**, which unite to form the main duct of the gland **(Fig. 31.2)**. Gland with this type of structure and duct system is called **racemose type** (racemose = bunch of grapes).

PROPERTIES AND COMPOSITION OF SALIVA

PROPERTIES OF SALIVA

1. *Volume:* 1,000 to 1,500 mL of saliva is secreted per day and it is approximately about 1 mL/min.

    Contribution by each major salivary gland is:
    i. Parotid glands : 25%
    ii. Submaxillary glands : 70%
    iii. Sublingual glands : 5%

2. *Reaction:* Mixed saliva from all the glands is slightly acidic with pH of 6.35 to 6.85.
3. *Specific gravity:* It ranges between 1.002 and 1.012.
4. *Tonicity:* Saliva is hypotonic to plasma.

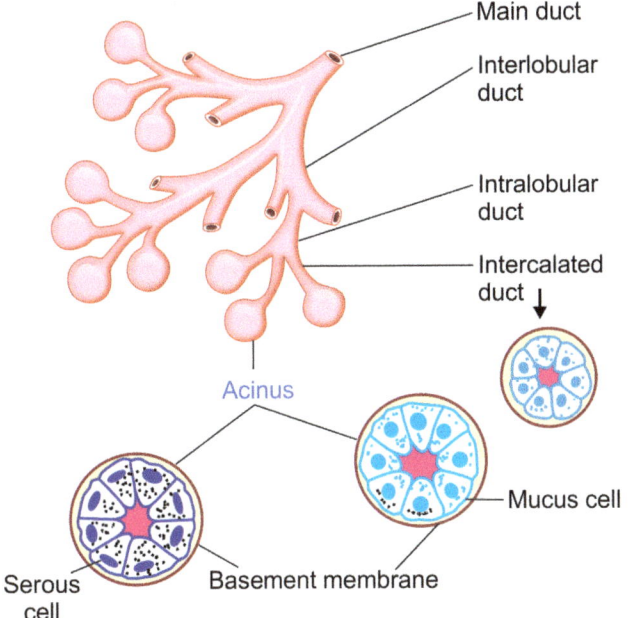

FIGURE 31.2: Diagram showing acini and duct system in salivary glands.

COMPOSITION OF SALIVA

Mixed saliva contains 99.5% water and 0.5% solids. Composition of saliva is given in **Figure 31.3**.

FUNCTIONS OF SALIVA

Saliva is an essential digestive juice. Since it has many functions, its absence leads to many inconveniences.

1. PREPARATION OF FOOD FOR SWALLOWING

When food is taken into the mouth, it is moistened and dissolved by saliva. Mucous membrane of mouth is also moistened by saliva. It facilitates **chewing**. By the movement of tongue, moistened and masticated food is rolled into a **bolus**. **Mucin** of saliva lubricates the bolus and facilitates swallowing.

2. APPRECIATION OF TASTE

Taste is a chemical sensation. Saliva, by its solvent action, dissolves the solid food substances, so that dissolved substances can stimulate the taste buds. The stimulated taste buds recognize the taste.

3. DIGESTIVE FUNCTION

Saliva has three digestive enzymes namely, salivary amylase, maltase and lingual lipase **(Table 31.3)**.

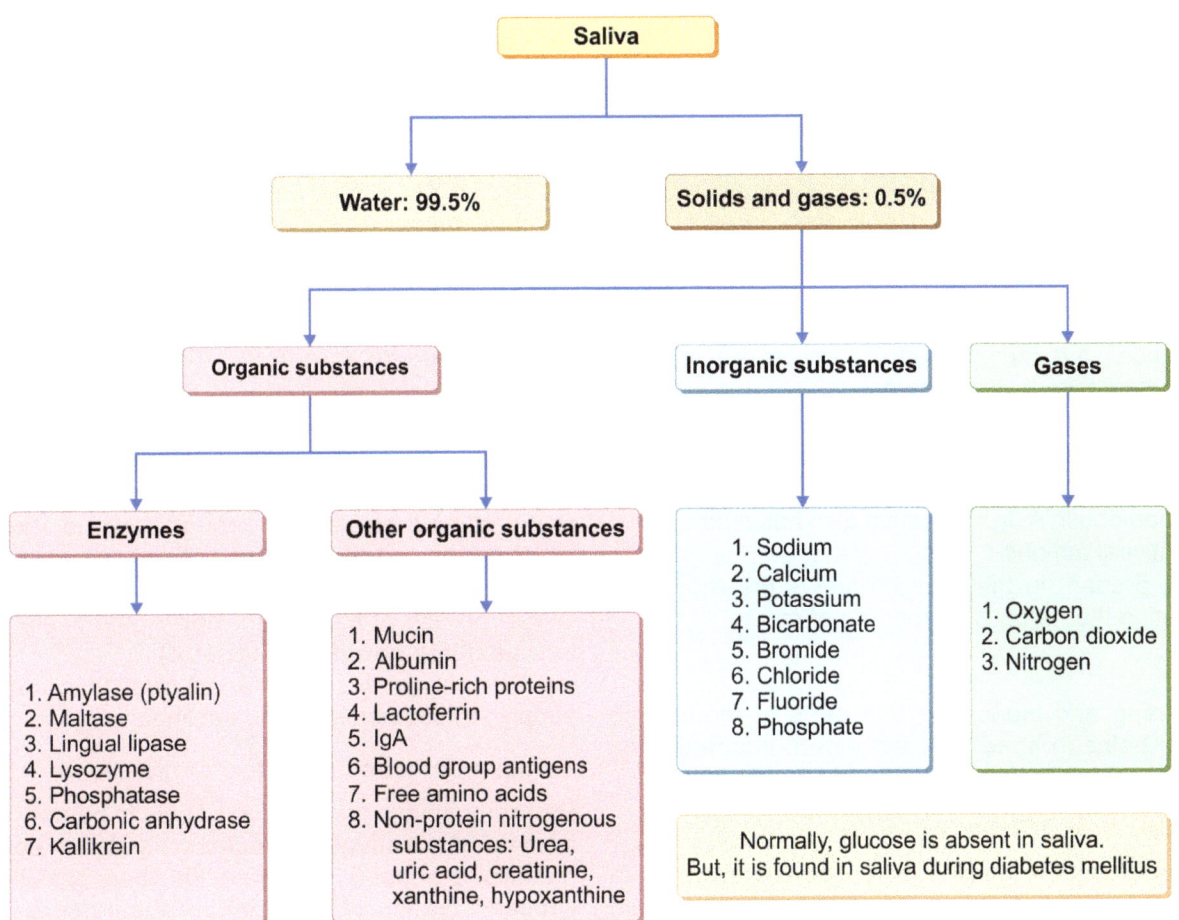

FIGURE 31.3: Composition of saliva.

TABLE 31.3: Digestive enzymes of saliva.

Enzyme	Source of secretion	Activation	Action
Salivary amylase	All salivary glands	Acid medium	Converts starch into maltose
Maltase	Major salivary glands	Acid medium	Converts maltose into glucose
Lingual lipase	Lingual glands	Acid medium	Converts triglycerides of milk fat into fatty acids and diacylglycerol

Salivary Amylase

Salivary amylase is an **amylolytic enzyme** (carbohydrate digesting enzyme). It acts on cooked or **boiled starch** and converts it into dextrin and maltose. Though starch digestion starts in the mouth, major part of it occurs in the stomach, because food stays only for a short time in the mouth.

Optimum pH necessary for the activation of salivary amylase is 6. Salivary amylase cannot act on **cellulose**.

Maltase

Maltase is present only in traces in human saliva. It converts maltose into glucose.

Lingual Lipase

Lingual lipase is a **lipolytic enzyme** (lipid digesting enzyme). It digests **milk fats** which are the **pre-emulsified fats**. It hydrolyzes triglycerides into fatty acids and diacylglycerol **(Table 31.3)**.

■ 4. CLEANSING AND PROTECTIVE FUNCTIONS

i. Due to the constant secretion of saliva, the mouth and teeth are rinsed and kept free of food debris, shed epithelial cells and foreign particles. In this way, saliva prevents bacterial growth by removing materials, which may serve as culture media for the bacterial growth.
ii. Enzyme **lysozyme** of saliva kills some bacteria such as *Staphylococcus, Streptococcus* and *Brucella*.
iii. **Proline-rich proteins** present in saliva have antimicrobial property and neutralize the toxic substances, e.g. tannins. Tannins are present in many food substances including fruits.
iv. **Lactoferrin** of saliva also has antimicrobial property.
v. Proline-rich proteins and lactoferrin protect the teeth by stimulating enamel formation.
vi. Immunoglobulin A (IgA) in saliva also has antibacterial and antiviral actions.
vii. **Mucin** present in the saliva protects the mouth by lubricating the mucous membrane of mouth.

■ 5. ROLE IN SPEECH

By moistening and lubricating soft parts of mouth and lips, saliva helps in speech. If the mouth becomes dry, articulation and pronunciation become difficult.

■ 6. EXCRETORY FUNCTION

Many organic and inorganic substances are excreted in saliva. It excretes substances such as mercury, potassium iodide, lead and thiocyanate. Saliva also excretes some viruses such as those causing rabies and mumps.

In some pathological conditions, saliva excretes certain substances, which are not found in saliva under normal conditions such as glucose in diabetes mellitus. In certain conditions, some of the normal constituents of saliva are excreted in large quantities. For example, excess urea is excreted in saliva during nephritis and excess calcium is excreted during hyperparathyroidism.

■ 7. REGULATION OF BODY TEMPERATURE

In dogs and cattle, excessive dripping of saliva during **panting** helps in loss of heat and regulation of body temperature. However, in human being, saliva does not play any role in this function.

■ 8. REGULATION OF WATER BALANCE

When the body water content decreases, salivary secretion also decreases. This causes dryness of the mouth and induces thirst. When the water is taken, it quenches the thirst and restores the body water content.

■ REGULATION OF SALIVARY SECRETION

Salivary secretion is regulated only by nervous mechanism. Autonomic nervous system is involved in the regulatory function.

■ NERVE SUPPLY TO SALIVARY GLANDS

Salivary glands are supplied by parasympathetic and sympathetic divisions of autonomic nervous system.

■ PARASYMPATHETIC FIBERS

Parasympathetic Fibers to Submandibular and Sublingual Glands

Parasympathetic preganglionic fibers to submandibular and sublingual glands arise from **superior salivatory nucleus** situated in pons. After taking origin from this nucleus, the preganglionic fibers run through **nervus intermedius of Wrisberg**, **geniculate ganglion**, the motor fibers of facial nerve, **chorda tympani** branch of **facial nerve** and lingual branch of **trigeminal nerve** and finally reach the **submaxillary ganglion (Fig. 31.4)**.

Postganglionic fibers arise from this ganglion and supply the submaxillary and sublingual glands.

Parasympathetic Fibers to Parotid Gland

Parasympathetic preganglionic fibers to parotid gland arise from **inferior salivatory nucleus** situated in upper part of medulla oblongata. From here, the fibers pass through the tympanic branch of **glossopharyngeal nerve**, **tympanic plexus** and **lesser petrosal nerve**, and end in **otic ganglion (Fig. 31.5)**.

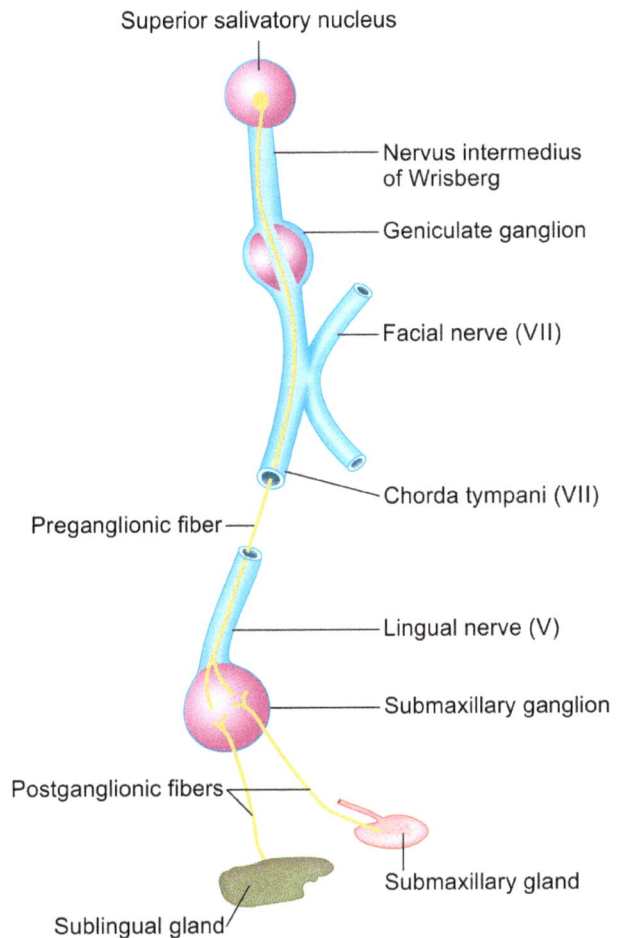

FIGURE 31.4: Parasympathetic nerve supply to submaxillary and sublingual glands.

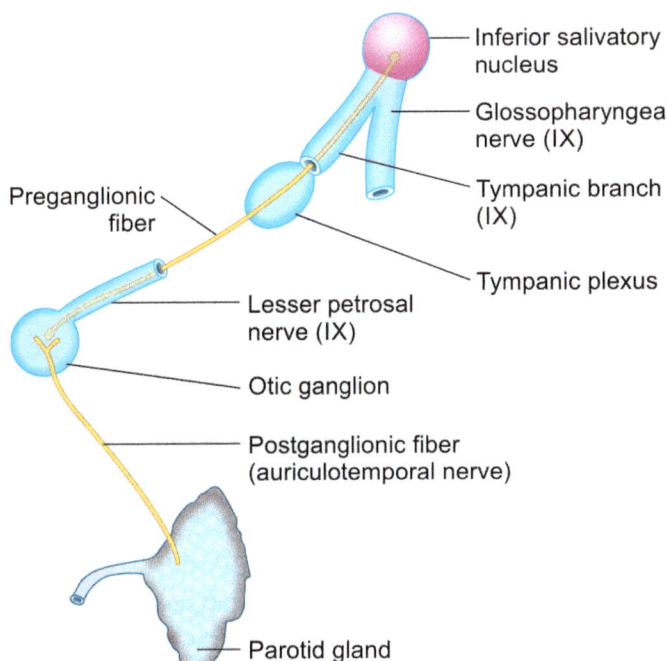

FIGURE 31.5: Parasympathetic nerve supply to parotid gland.

Postganglionic fibers arise from otic ganglion and reach the parotid gland by passing through auriculotemporal branch in mandibular division of **trigeminal nerve**.

Functions of Parasympathetic Fibers

When the parasympathetic fibers of salivary glands are stimulated, a large quantity of watery saliva is secreted with less quantity of organic constituents. It is because, parasympathetic fibers activate acinar cells and cause vasodilatation in salivary glands. The neurotransmitter is **acetylcholine**.

■ SYMPATHETIC FIBERS

Sympathetic preganglionic fibers to salivary glands arise from lateral horns of first and second thoracic segments of spinal cord. These fibers leave the cord through anterior nerve roots and end in **superior cervical ganglion** of sympathetic chain.

Postganglionic fibers from this ganglion are distributed to salivary glands along the nerve plexus around arteries supplying the glands.

Functions of Sympathetic Fibers

Stimulation of sympathetic fibers causes less secretion of saliva, which is thick and rich in mucus. It is because these fibers activate the acinar cells and cause vasoconstriction in salivary glands by secreting **noradrenaline**.

■ REFLEX REGULATION OF SALIVARY SECRETION

Salivary secretion is regulated by nervous mechanism through reflex action.

Salivary reflexes are of two types:

1. Unconditioned reflex.
2. Conditioned reflex.

1. Unconditioned Reflex

Unconditioned reflex is the inborn reflex that is present since birth. It does not need any previous experience. This reflex induces salivary secretion when any substance is placed in the mouth. It is due to the stimulation of nerve endings in mucous membrane of the oral cavity.

Examples include:

i. When food is taken.
ii. When any unpleasant or unpalatable substance enters the mouth.
iii. When the oral cavity is handled with instruments by dentists.

2. Conditioned Reflex

Conditioned reflex is acquired by experience and it needs previous experience (Chapter 107). Presence of food in the mouth is not necessary to elicit this reflex. Stimulus for this reflex is the sight, smell, hearing or thought of food. It is due to the impulses arising from eyes, nose, ears, etc.

■ EFFECTS OF DRUGS AND CHEMICALS ON SALIVARY SECRETION

Substances which Increase the Salivary Secretion

1. Sympathomimetic drugs like adrenaline and ephedrine.
2. Parasympathomimetic drugs like acetylcholine, pilocarpine, muscarine and physostigmine.
3. Histamine.

Substances which Decrease the Salivary Secretion

1. Sympathetic depressants like ergotamine and dibenamine.
2. Parasympathetic depressants like atropine and scopolamine.
3. Anesthetics such as chloroform and ether stimulate the secretion of saliva. However, deep anesthesia decreases the secretion due to central inhibition.

APPLIED PHYSIOLOGY: DISORDERS OF SALIVARY SECRETION

HYPOSALIVATION

Hyposalivation is the reduction in secretion of saliva. It is of two types, namely, the temporary hyposalivation and the permanent hyposalivation:

Temporary Hyposalivation

Temporary hyposalivation occurs in:

1. Emotional conditions such as fear.
2. Fever.
3. Dehydration.

Permanent Hyposalivation

Permanent hyposalivation occurs in:

1. **Sialolithiasis**: Obstruction of salivary duct by the formation of salivary calculus (stone).
2. Congenital absence or hypoplasia of salivary glands.
3. **Bell's palsy**: Paralysis of facial nerve.

Dental caries is the common consequence of hyposalivation.

HYPERSALIVATION

Hypersalivation is the excess secretion of saliva. Physiological condition when hypersalivation occurs is pregnancy. Hypersalivation in pathological conditions is called **ptyalism** or **sialorrhea**.

Hypersalivation occurs in the following conditions:

1. **Decay of tooth** or **neoplasm** (abnormal new growth or tumor) in mouth or tongue: Due to continuous irritation of nerve endings in the mouth.
2. Disease of esophagus, stomach and intestine.
3. Neurological disorders such as mental retardation, cerebral stroke and parkinsonism.
4. Some psychological and psychiatric conditions.
5. Nausea and vomiting.

OTHER DISORDERS

In addition to hyposalivation and hypersalivation, salivary secretion is affected by some other disorders also which include the following.

1. Xerostomia

Xerostomia means dry mouth. It is also called **pasties** or **cottonmouth**. It is due to hyposalivation or absence of salivary secretion (**aptyalism**).

Causes of xerostomia

i. Dehydration or renal failure.
ii. Sjögren's syndrome (see below).
iii. Radiotherapy.
iv. Trauma to salivary gland or their ducts.
v. Side effect of drugs like antihistamines, antidepressants and antiparkinsonian drugs.
vi. Shock.
vii. After smoking **marijuana** (psychoactive compound from the plant cannabis).

Xerostomia causes difficulties in mastication, swallowing and speech. It also causes **halitosis** (bad breath).

2. Drooling

Uncontrolled flow of saliva outside the mouth is called drooling. Drooling occurs because of excess production of saliva in association with inability to retain saliva within the mouth.

Drooling occurs in the following conditions:

i. During teeth eruption in children.
ii. Upper respiratory tract infection or nasal allergies in children.
iii. Difficulty in swallowing.
iv. Tonsillitis.
v. Peritonsillar abscess.

3. Chorda Tympani Syndrome

Chorda tympani syndrome is the condition characterized by sweating while eating. During trauma or surgical procedure, some of the parasympathetic nerve fibers to salivary glands may be severed. And during regeneration, some of these nerve fibers, which run along with chorda tympani branch of facial nerve, may deviate and join with the nerve fibers supplying sweat glands. So, when the food is placed in the mouth, salivary secretion is associated with sweat secretion.

4. Paralytic Secretion of Saliva

When the parasympathetic nerve to salivary gland is cut in experimental animals, salivary secretion increases for first 3 weeks and later diminishes. Finally, the secretion stops at about 6th week. The increased secretion of saliva after cutting the parasympathetic nerve fibers is called paralytic secretion. It is because of hyperactivity of sympathetic nerve fibers to salivary glands when parasympathetic fibers are cut.

5. Augmented Secretion of Saliva

If the nerves supplying salivary glands are stimulated twice, the amount of saliva secreted by the second stimulus is more than the amount secreted by the first stimulus. It is because the first stimulus increases excitability of acinar cells, so that when the second stimulus is applied, the salivary secretion is augmented.

6. Mumps

Mumps is the acute viral infection affecting parotid glands. The virus causing this disease is **paramyxovirus**. It is common in children who are not immunized. It occurs in adults also. Features of mumps are puffiness of cheeks (due to swelling of parotid glands), fever, sore throat and weakness. Mumps affects meninges, gonads and pancreas also.

7. Sjögren's Syndrome

It is an autoimmune disorder in which the immune cells destroy exocrine glands such as salivary glands and lacrimal glands. Common symptoms of this syndrome are dryness of the mouth due to lack of saliva (xerostomia), persistent cough and dryness of eyes. In severe conditions, organs like kidneys, lungs, liver, pancreas, thyroid, blood vessels and brain are affected.

Chapter 32: Stomach and Gastric Secretion

CHAPTER OUTLINE

- FUNCTIONAL ANATOMY OF STOMACH
- GLANDS OF STOMACH
- NERVE SUPPLY TO STOMACH
- FUNCTIONS OF STOMACH
- PROPERTIES AND COMPOSITION OF GASTRIC JUICE
- FUNCTIONS OF GASTRIC JUICE
- SECRETION OF GASTRIC JUICE
- REGULATION OF GASTRIC SECRETION
- COLLECTION OF GASTRIC JUICE
- GASTRIC FUNCTION TESTS: GASTRIC ANALYSIS
- APPLIED PHYSIOLOGY: GASTRIC DISORDERS

■ FUNCTIONAL ANATOMY OF STOMACH

Stomach is a hollow organ situated just below diaphragm on the left side in abdominal cavity. Volume of empty stomach is 50 mL. Under normal conditions, it can expand to accommodate 1 to L of solids and liquids. However, it is capable of expanding still further up to 4 liters.

■ PARTS OF STOMACH

In humans, stomach has four parts:

1. Cardiac region.
2. Fundus.
3. Body or corpus.
4. Pyloric region.

1. Cardiac Region

Cardiac region or **cardiac end** of stomach is the upper part of stomach where esophagus opens. This opening is guarded by a sphincter called **cardiac sphincter** which opens only towards stomach. **Sphincter** is a circular muscle that surrounds and closes a tube or an opening in the body.

2. Fundus

Fundus is a small dome-shaped structure. It is elevated above the level of esophageal opening.

3. Body or Corpus

Body or corpus of the stomach is the largest part of stomach forming about 75 to 80% of the whole stomach. It extends from just below the fundus up to the pyloric region **(Fig. 32.1)**.

4. Pyloric Region

Pyloric region has two parts, antrum and pyloric canal. Body of the stomach ends in antrum. The junction between body and antrum is marked by an angular notch called incisura angularis. Antrum is continued as the narrow canal which is called pyloric canal or pyloric end or **pylorus**. Pyloric canal opens into first part of small intestine called duodenum. The opening of pyloric canal is guarded by a sphincter called **pyloric sphincter**. It opens towards duodenum.

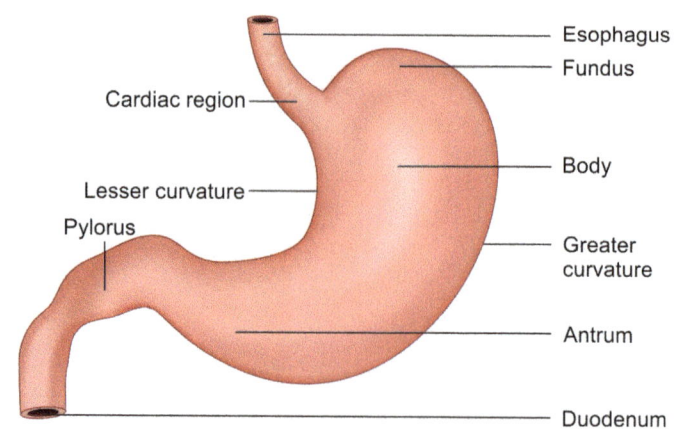

FIGURE 32.1: Parts of stomach.

Stomach has two curvatures. One on the right side is lesser curvature and other one on the left side is greater curvature.

STRUCTURE OF STOMACH WALL

Wall of the stomach is formed by four layers of structures:

1. Outer serous layer formed by **peritoneum**.
2. Muscular layer made up of three layers of smooth muscle fibers namely, inner oblique, middle circular and outer longitudinal layers.
3. Submucus layer formed by areolar tissue, blood vessels and lymph vessels.
4. Inner mucus layer lined by mucus-secreting columnar epithelial cells. Gastric glands are situated in this layer. Inner surface of mucus layer is covered by 2 mm thick **mucus**.

GLANDS OF STOMACH

Glands of the stomach or **gastric glands** are tubular structures made up of different types of cells. Gastric glands open into the stomach cavity through **gastric pits**.

CLASSIFICATION OF GLANDS OF THE STOMACH

Gastric glands are classified into three types depending upon their situation:

A. Fundic glands situated in body and fundus of stomach.
B. Pyloric glands present in pyloric part of the stomach.
C. Cardiac glands located in cardiac region of the stomach.

STRUCTURE OF GASTRIC GLANDS

Fundic Glands

Fundic glands or **oxyntic glands** of the stomach are considered as typical gastric glands **(Fig. 32.2)**. These glands are long and tubular glands. Each fundic gland has three parts, viz. body, neck and isthmus.

Cells present in fundic glands

Fundic gland is formed by the following types of cell:

1. **Chief cells** or **pepsinogen cells**
2. Parietal cells or **oxyntic cells**
3. **Mucus neck cells**
4. **Enteroendocrine cells**
5. **Enterochromaffin cells** (EC cells) or **Kulchitsky cells**
6. **Enterochromaffin-like cells** (ECL cells)
7. Stem cells.

Stem cells divide and replace other cells in gastric glands. Secretory functions of other cells mentioned above are given in **Table 32.1**.

Parietal cells are different from other cells of the gland because of the presence of **canaliculi** (singular = canaliculus). Parietal cells empty their secretions into the lumen of the gland through the canaliculi. But other cells empty their secretions directly into lumen of the gland.

Pyloric Glands

Pyloric glands of stomach are short and tortuous in nature. Pyloric glands are formed by **G cells**, mucus cells, EC cells and ECL cells.

Cardiac Glands

Cardiac glands of the stomach are also short and tortuous in structure with many mucus cells. EC cells, ECL cells and chief cells are also present in the cardiac glands.

Enteroendocrine cells, enterochromaffin cells and enterochromaffin like cells

Enteroendocrine cells, enterochromaffin cells and enterochromaffin like cells are the hormone-secreting cells present in glands or mucosa of gastrointestinal tract

TABLE 32.1: Secretory functions of cells in gastric glands.

Cells	Secretory products
Chief cells or pepsinogen cells	Pepsinogen Rennin Lipase Gelatinase Urase
Parietal cells or oxyntic cells	Hydrochloric acid Intrinsic factor of Castle
Mucus neck cells	Mucin
Enterochromaffin (EC) cells	Serotonin
Enterochromaffin-like (ECL) cells	Histamine
Enteroendocrine cells	
G cells	Gastrin
D cells	Somatostatin
A cells	Glucagon
Ghrelin producing cells	Ghrelin
Unnamed cells	Vasoactive intestinal polypeptide

Vasoactive intestinal polypeptide is also secreted by nerve endings in stomach.

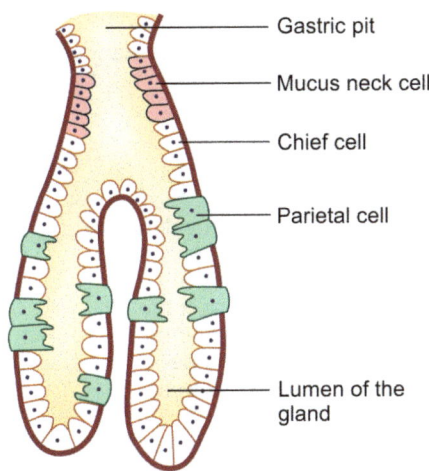

FIGURE 32.2: Gastric glands.

particularly stomach and intestine. Secretory functions of these types of cells in glands of the stomach are given in **Table 32.1**.

■ NERVE SUPPLY TO STOMACH

Stomach receives sympathetic fibers through **splanchnic nerve**. Parasympathetic fibers to stomach pass through branches of anterior and posterior **vagal trunks**.

■ FUNCTIONS OF STOMACH

■ 1. MECHANICAL FUNCTION

i. Storage Function

Food is stored in the stomach for a long period, i.e. for 3 to 4 hours and emptied into the intestine slowly. The maximum capacity of stomach is up to 1.5 L. Slow emptying of stomach provides enough time for proper digestion and absorption of food substances in the small intestine.

ii. Formation of Chyme

Peristaltic movements of stomach mix the bolus with gastric juice and convert it into the semisolid material known as chyme.

■ 2. DIGESTIVE FUNCTION

Refer functions of gastric juice.

■ 3. PROTECTIVE FUNCTION

Refer functions of gastric juice.

■ 4. HEMOPOIETIC FUNCTION

Refer functions of gastric juice.

■ 5. EXCRETORY FUNCTION

Many substances like toxins, alkaloids and metals are excreted through gastric juice.

■ PROPERTIES AND COMPOSITION OF GASTRIC JUICE

Gastric juice is the mixture of secretions from different gastric glands.

■ PROPERTIES OF GASTRIC JUICE

Volume : 1,200 to 1,500 mL/day
Specific gravity : 1.002 to 1.004
Reaction : Gastric juice is highly acidic with pH of 0.9 to 1.2 due to hydrochloric acid

■ COMPOSITION OF GASTRIC JUICE

Gastric juice contains 99.5% of water and 0.5% solids. The solids are organic and inorganic substances. Refer **Figure 32.3** for composition of gastric juice.

■ FUNCTIONS OF GASTRIC JUICE

■ 1. DIGESTIVE FUNCTION

Gastric juice acts mainly on proteins. **Proteolytic enzymes** of the gastric juice are pepsin and **rennin (Table 32.2)**. Gastric juice also contains some other enzymes like gastric lipase, gelatinase, urase and gastric amylase.

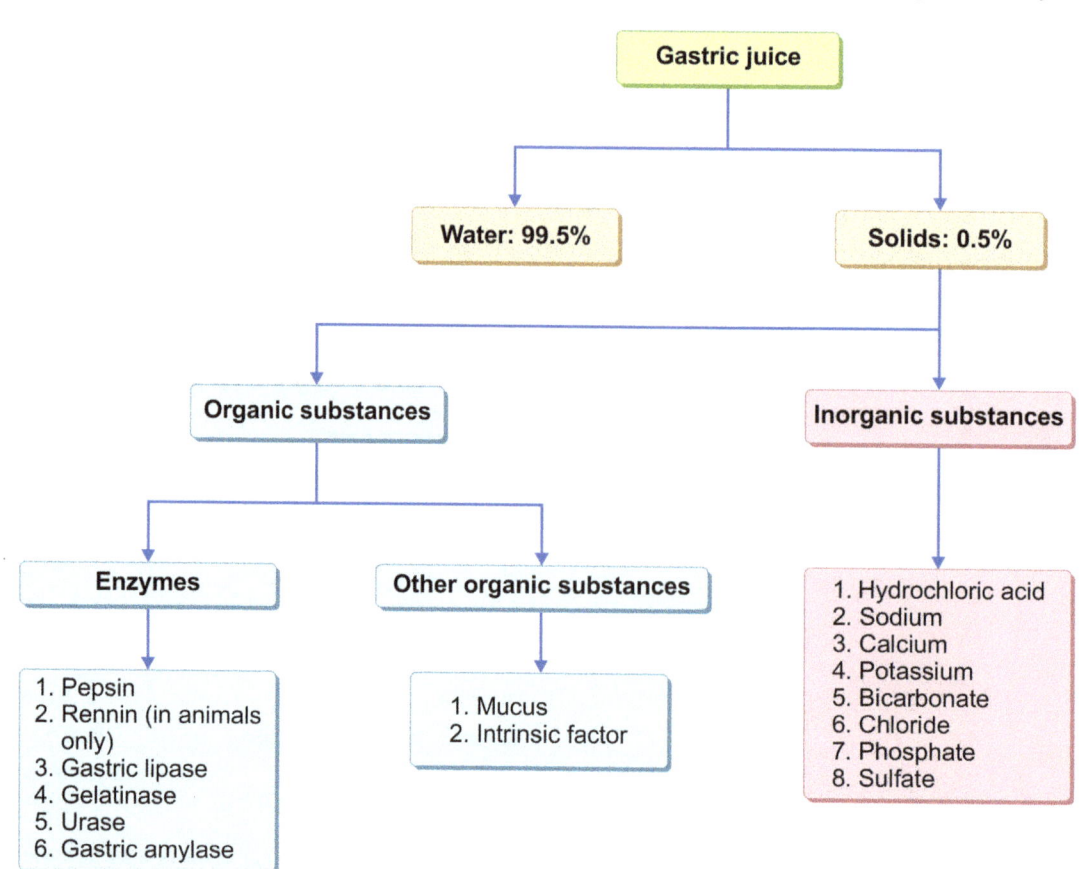

FIGURE 32.3: Composition of gastric juice.

TABLE 32.2: Digestive enzymes of gastric juice.

Enzyme	Activator	Substrate	End products
Pepsin	Hydrochloric acid	Proteins	Proteoses, peptones and polypeptides
Gastric lipase	Acid medium	Triglycerides of butter	Fatty acids and glycerols
Gastric amylase	Acid medium	Starch	Dextrin and maltose (negligible action)
Gelatinase	Acid medium	Gelatin and collagen of meat	Peptides
Urase	Acid medium	Urea	Ammonia

Pepsin

Pepsin is secreted as inactive **pepsinogen**. Pepsinogen is converted into pepsin by hydrochloric acid which is secreted by parietal cells. Optimum pH for activation of pepsinogen is below 6.

Action of pepsin

Pepsin converts proteins into proteoses, peptones and polypeptides. Pepsin also causes curdling and digestion of milk (**casein**).

Gastric Lipase

Gastric lipase is a weak **lipolytic enzyme**. It needs acidic medium with pH is between 4 and 5 for its action. But, it becomes inactive when the pH falls below 2.5. Gastric lipase acts on **tributyrin** (**butter fat**) and hydrolyzes it into fatty acids and glycerols.

Other Enzymes of Gastric Juice

i. Gelatinase: Degrades gelatin and collagen into peptides.
ii. Urase: Acts on urea and produces ammonia.
iii. Gastric amylase: Degrades starch (but its action is insignificant).
iv. Rennin: Curdles milk (present in animals only).

2. HEMOPOIETIC FUNCTION

Intrinsic factor of Castle secreted by parietal cells of gastric glands plays an important role in erythropoiesis. It is necessary for absorption of vitamin B_{12} (which is called **extrinsic factor**) from GI tract into the blood. Vitamin B_{12} is an important maturation factor during erythropoiesis. Absence of intrinsic factor in gastric juice causes deficiency of vitamin B_{12} leading **to pernicious anemia** (Chapter 12).

3. PROTECTIVE FUNCTION: FUNCTION OF MUCUS

Mucus present in gastric juice protects gastric wall by the following functions:

i. It protects wall of the stomach from irritation or mechanical injury by virtue of its high viscosity.
ii. It prevents the digestive action of pepsin on gastric mucosa.
iii. It protects the gastric mucosa from hydrochloric acid of gastric juice because of its alkaline nature and its acid-combining power.

4. FUNCTIONS OF HYDROCHLORIC ACID

Hydrochloric acid present in gastric juice has following functions:

i. Bactericidal action: HCl kills some bacteria that enter the stomach along with food substances.
ii. It activates pepsinogen into pepsin.
iii. HCl provides acid medium necessary for the action of hormones.

SECRETION OF GASTRIC JUICE

SECRETION OF PEPSINOGEN

Pepsinogen is synthesized from amino acids in the ribosomes attached to endoplasmic reticulum in chief cells. Pepsinogen molecules are packed into **zymogen granules** by Golgi apparatus.

When zymogen granule is secreted into stomach from chief cells, the granule is dissolved and pepsinogen is released into gastric juice. Pepsinogen is activated into pepsin by hydrochloric acid.

SECRETION OF HYDROCHLORIC ACID

Hydrochloric acid secretion is an active process that takes place in the canaliculi of parietal cells in gastric glands. Energy for this is derived from oxidation of glucose.

In parietal cells, the carbon dioxide is formed from metabolic activity. It is also derived from blood. Carbon dioxide combines with water to form **carbonic acid** in the presence of **carbonic anhydrase**. This enzyme is present in high concentration in **parietal cells**. Carbonic acid is the most unstable compound and, immediately it splits into hydrogen ion and bicarbonate ion. Hydrogen ion is actively pumped into the canaliculus of parietal cell.

Simultaneously, the chloride ion is also pumped into canaliculus actively. Chloride is derived from sodium chloride in the blood. Now, the hydrogen ion combines with chloride ion to form hydrochloric acid. To compensate the loss of chloride ion, bicarbonate ion from parietal cell enters the blood and combines with sodium to form sodium bicarbonate. Thus, the entire process is summarized as (**Fig. 32.4**):

$$CO_2 + H_2O + NaCl \longrightarrow HCl + NaHCO_3$$

REGULATION OF GASTRIC SECRETION

Regulation of gastric secretion and intestinal secretion is studied by some experimental procedures.

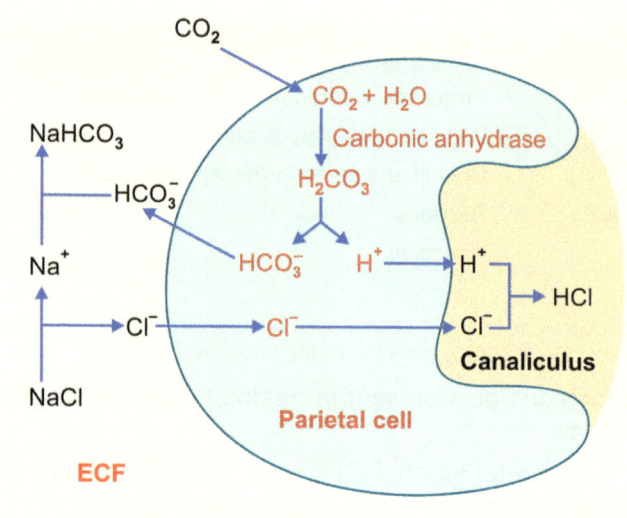

FIGURE 32.4: Secretion of hydrochloric acid in parietal cell of gastric gland.

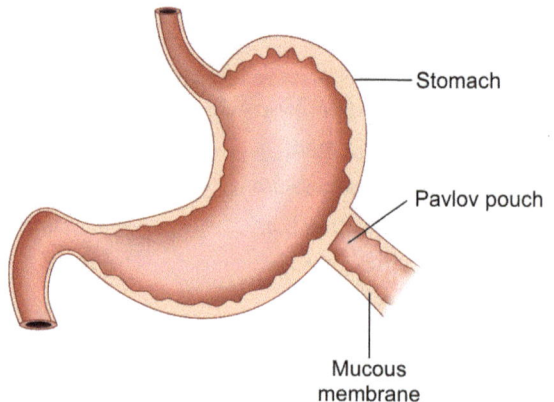

FIGURE 32.5: Pavlov pouch.

■ METHODS OF STUDY

Russian scientist **Pavlov** has designed some methods in dogs during his studies on conditioned reflexes. Important methods followed by Pavlov are given here.

1. Pavlov Pouch

Pavlov pouch is a small part of the stomach that is incompletely separated from the main portion and made into a small bag-like pouch **(Fig. 32.5)**. A small part of muscular coat called isthmus is retained. Isthmus connects the two parts.

Nerve supply of Pavlov pouch

Pavlov pouch receives parasympathetic (vagus) nerve fibers through isthmus and sympathetic fibers through blood vessels.

Use of Pavlov pouch

Pavlov pouch is used to demonstrate the different phases of gastric secretion particularly the cephalic phase and used to demonstrate the role of vagus in cephalic phase.

2. Farrell and Ivy Pouch

Farrell and Ivy pouch is prepared by removing the part of Pavlov pouch from the stomach and transplanting it in the subcutaneous tissue of abdominal wall or thoracic wall in the same animal. It is used for experimental purpose, when the new blood vessels are developed.

Uses of Farrell and Ivy pouch

This pouch is useful to study the role of hormones during gastric and intestinal phases of gastric secretion.

3. Sham Feeding

Sham feeding means the false feeding. It is another experimental procedure devised by Pavlov to demonstrate the regulation of gastric secretion.

Procedure for sham feeding

i. A hole is made in the neck of an anesthetized dog.
ii. Esophagus is transversely cut. The cut ends are drawn out through the hole in the neck.
iii. When the dog eats food, it comes out through the cut end of the esophagus. But the dog has the satisfaction of eating the food. It is called sham feeding.

This experimental procedure is supported by the preparation of Pavlov pouch with a fistula from the stomach. The fistula opens to the exterior and it is used to observe the gastric secretion. The animal is used for experimental purpose after a week time when healing is completed.

Uses of sham feeding

Sham feeding is useful to demonstrate the secretion of gastric juice during cephalic phase. In the same animal after vagotomy, sham feeding does not induce gastric secretion. It proves the role of vagus nerve during cephalic phase.

■ PHASES OF GASTRIC SECRETION

Gastric juice is secreted in three different phases:
  I. Cephalic phase.
 II. Gastric phase.
III. Intestinal phase.

In human beings, a fourth phase called interdigestive phase exists. All the phases are regulated by neural mechanism or hormonal mechanism or both.

■ CEPHALIC PHASE

Secretion of gastric juice by the stimuli arising from head region (**cephalus**) is called cephalic phase **(Fig. 32.6)**. This phase is regulated by nervous mechanism. During this phase 30% of total amount of gastric juice is secreted.

During this phase, gastric secretion occurs even without the presence of food in the stomach. Quantity of the juice is less but it is rich in enzymes and hydrochloric acid. The nervous mechanism that regulates cephalic phase operates through reflex action.

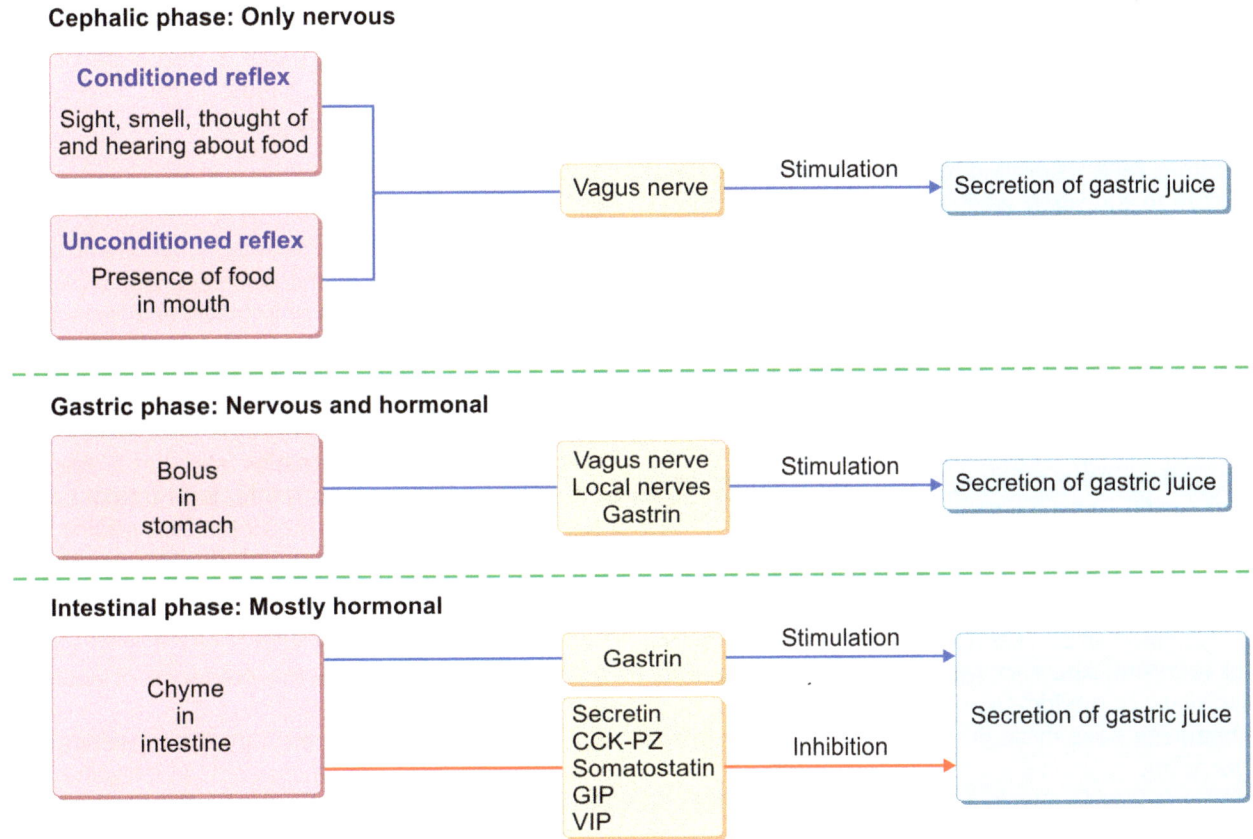

FIGURE 32.6: Schematic diagram showing the regulation of gastric secretion.
CCK-PZ = Cholecystokinin-pancreozymin, GIP = Gastric inhibitory peptide, VIP = Vasoactive intestinal peptide.

Two types of reflexes occur:
a. Unconditioned reflex.
b. Conditioned reflex.

Unconditioned Reflex

Unconditioned reflex is the inborn reflex. When food is placed in the mouth, it induces salivary secretion (Chapter 31). Simultaneously, gastric secretion also occurs.

Stages of the reflex action

1. Presence of food in mouth stimulates the taste buds and other receptors in the mouth.
2. Sensory (afferent) impulses from mouth pass via afferent nerve fibers of glossopharyngeal and facial nerves to appetite center present in amygdala and hypothalamus.
3. From here, efferent impulses pass through dorsal nucleus of vagus and vagal efferent nerve fibers to the wall of the stomach.
4. Acetylcholine is secreted at the vagal efferent nerve endings stimulates gastric glands to increase the secretion.

This is experimentally proved by Pavlov pouch and sham feeding.

Conditioned Reflex

Conditioned reflex is the reflex acquired by previous experience (Chapter 107). Presence of food in the mouth is not necessary to elicit this reflex. Sight, smell, hearing or thought of food which induce salivary secretion also induce gastric secretion.

Stages of reflex action

1. Impulses from the special sensory organs (eye, ear and nose) pass through afferent fibers of neural circuits to the cerebral cortex. Thinking of food stimulates the cerebral cortex directly.
2. From cerebral cortex the impulses pass through dorsal nucleus of vagus and vagal efferents and reach stomach wall.
3. Vagal nerve endings secrete acetylcholine. It stimulates the gastric glands to increase its secretion.

Conditioned reflex of gastric secretion is proved by Pavlov pouch and bell dog experiment (Chapter 107).

■ GASTRIC PHASE

Secretion of gastric juice when food enters the stomach is called gastric phase. This phase is regulated by both nervous and hormonal mechanisms. Gastric juice secreted during this phase is rich in pepsinogen and hydrochloric acid. During gastric phase 60% of total amount of gastric juice is secreted.

Mechanisms involved in this phase are:

1. Nervous mechanism.
2. Hormonal mechanism.

1. Nervous Mechanism

Nervous mechanism controls the secretion during gastric phase through local myenteric reflex and vagovagal reflex.

Local myenteric reflex

Local myenteric reflex is elicited by stimulation of myenteric nerve plexus in stomach wall. After entering stomach, food particles stimulate the local nerve plexus (Chapter 30) present in the wall of the stomach. These nerve fibers release acetylcholine, which stimulates the gastric glands to secrete a large quantity of gastric juice. Simultaneously, acetylcholine stimulates **G cells** to secrete gastrin (see below).

Vagovagal reflex

Vagovagal reflex is the reflex in which both afferent and efferent vagal fibers are involved. Presence of food in stomach stimulates the sensory (afferent) nerve endings of vagus which generate sensory impulses. These sensory impulses are transmitted to the brainstem via sensory fibers of vagus. Brainstem in turn sends efferent impulses through the motor (efferent) fibers of vagus back to stomach and cause secretion of gastric juice. Since, both afferent and efferent impulses pass through vagus, this reflex is called vagovagal reflex.

2. Hormonal Mechanism: Gastrin

Hormonal mechanism involves a gastrointestinal hormone called gastrin. It is secreted by the G cells which are present in pyloric glands of stomach. Small amount of gastrin is also secreted in mucosa of upper small intestine. Gastrin is a polypeptide containing G14, G17 or G34 amino acids.

Gastrin is released when food enters stomach. The mechanism involved in the release of gastrin may be the local nervous reflex or vagovagal reflex. Nerve endings release the neurotransmitter called **gastrin-releasing peptide** which stimulates the G cells to secrete gastrin.

Actions of gastrin on gastric secretion

Gastrin stimulates the secretion of pepsinogen and hydrochloric acid by the gastric glands.

Experimental evidences of gastric phase

Nervous mechanism of gastric secretion during gastric phase is proved by Pavlov pouch. Hormonal mechanism of gastric secretion is proved by Farrell and Ivy pouch.

■ INTESTINAL PHASE

Intestinal phase is the secretion of gastric juice when chyme enters the intestine. When chyme enters the intestine initially gastric secretion increases and later it stops. Intestinal phase of gastric secretion is under both nervous and hormonal control.

Initial Stage of Intestinal Phase

Chyme entering intestine stimulates the duodenal mucosa to release gastrin which is transported to stomach through blood. Gastrin increases gastric secretion. During this phase 10% of total amount of gastric juice is secreted.

Later Stage of Intestinal Phase

After the initial increase, there is decrease or complete stoppage of secretion of gastric juice. Two factors are responsible for the inhibition:

1. Enterogastric reflex.
2. GI hormones.

1. Enterogastric reflex

It is a reflex that inhibits the secretion and movements of stomach due to distention or irritation of intestinal mucosa. It is mediated by myenteric nerve (Auerbach's) plexus and vagus.

2. GI hormones

Presence of chyme in intestine stimulates the secretion of many GI hormones from intestinal mucosa and other structures. All these hormones inhibit the gastric secretion. Some of these hormones inhibit the gastric motility also.

GI hormones which inhibit gastric secretion:

1. Secretin: Secreted by the presence of acid chyme in the intestine.
2. Cholecystokinin: Secreted by the presence of chyme containing fats and amino acids in intestine.
3. Gastric inhibitory peptide (GIP): Secreted by the presence of chyme containing glucose and fats in the intestine.
4. Vasoactive intestinal polypeptide (VIP): Secreted by the presence of acidic chyme in intestine.
5. Peptide YY: Secreted by the presence of fatty chyme in intestine.

In addition to these hormones, pancreas also secretes a hormone called **somatostatin** during intestinal phase. It also inhibits gastric secretion.

Intestinal phase of gastric secretion is demonstrated by Farrell and Ivy pouch.

■ INTERDIGESTIVE PHASE

Secretion of small amount of gastric juice in between meals (or during period of fasting) is called interdigestive phase. Gastric secretion during this phase is mainly due to the hormones like gastrin. This phase of gastric secretion is demonstrated by Farrell and Ivy pouch.

■ COLLECTION OF GASTRIC JUICE

In human beings, gastric juice is collected by using **Ryle tube.** This tube is made out of rubber or plastic. It is passed through nostril or mouth and through esophagus into the stomach. A line is marked in the tube. Entrance of the tip of the tube into stomach is indicated when this line comes near the mouth. Then, the contents of stomach are collected by means of aspiration.

■ GASTRIC FUNCTION TESTS: GASTRIC ANALYSIS

For analysis, gastric juice is collected from patient only in the morning. Analysis of the gastric juice is done for the diagnosis of ulcer and other disorders of stomach.

Gastric juice is analyzed for the following:

1. Measurement of **peptic activity**
2. Measurement of **gastric acidity**: Total acid, free acid (hydrochloric acid) and combined acid.

Fractional Test Meal (FTM): Fractional Gastric Analysis

Fractional gastric analysis is the common method of gastric analysis. It is carried out with fractional test meal.

After overnight fasting, gastric juice is collected. Then, the patient takes a small test meal called fractional test meal. After the ingestion of a test meal, gastric juice is collected at every 15th minute for a period of 2½ hours. All these samples are analyzed for peptic activity and acidity.

APPLIED PHYSIOLOGY: GASTRIC DISORDERS

1. GASTRITIS

Inflammation of gastric mucosa is called gastritis. It may be acute or chronic.

Causes of Gastritis

i. Infection with bacterium **Helicobacter pylori**.
ii. Excess consumption of alcohol.
iii. Excess or long-term administration **non-steroidal anti-inflammatory drugs** (NSAIDs).
iv. Trauma by nasogastric tubes.
v. Autoimmune disease.

Features of Gastritis

i. Abdominal upset or pain.
ii. Nausea.
iii. Vomiting.
iv. **Anorexia** (loss of appetite).
v. Indigestion.
vi. Discomfort or feeling of fullness in the epigastric region.
vii. **Belching** (process to relieve swallowed air that is accumulated in stomach).

2. GASTRIC ATROPHY

Gastric atrophy is the condition in which muscles of the stomach shrink and become weak. Gastric glands also shrink resulting in the deficiency of gastric juice.

Causes of Gastric Atrophy

Gastric atrophy is caused by chronic gastritis and autoimmune disease.

Features of Gastric Atrophy

Gastric atrophy causes **achlorhydria** (absence of hydrochloric acid in gastric juice) and pernicious anemia. Some patients develop **gastric cancer**.

3. PEPTIC ULCER

Ulcer means erosion of the surface of any organ due to shedding or sloughing of inflamed necrotic tissue that lines the organ. Peptic ulcer means an ulcer in the wall of stomach or duodenum caused by digestive action of gastric juice. Peptic ulcer found in stomach is called **gastric ulcer** and that found in duodenum it is called **duodenal ulcer**.

Common Causes of Peptic Ulcer

i. Increased peptic activity.
ii. Hyperacidity of gastric juice.
iii. Reduced alkalinity of duodenal content.
iv. Decreased mucin content in gastric juice.
v. Constant physical and emotional stress.
vi. Food with excess spices or smoking.
vii. Long-term use of NSAIDs (see above).
viii. Chronic inflammation due to *Helicobacter pylori*.

Features of Peptic Ulcer

Most common feature of peptic ulcer is severe burning pain in epigastric region. In gastric ulcer, pain occurs while eating or drinking. In duodenal ulcer, pain is felt 1 or 2 hours after food intake and during night.

Other symptoms of peptic ulcer accompanying pain sensation are:

i. Nausea.
ii. Vomiting.
iii. **Hematemesis** (vomiting blood).
iv. **Heartburn** (burning pain in chest due to regurgitation of acid from stomach into esophagus).
v. Anorexia (loss of appetite).
vi. Loss of weight.

4. ZOLLINGER-ELLISON SYNDROME

Zollinger-Ellison syndrome is a gastric disorder characterized by secretion of excess hydrochloric acid in the stomach.

Cause of Zollinger-Ellison Syndrome

This disorder is caused by **pancreatic tumor** which produces a large quantity of gastrin. Gastrin increases the hydrochloric acid secretion in stomach by stimulating the parietal cells.

Features of Zollinger-Ellison Syndrome

i. Abdominal pain.
ii. Diarrhea (frequent and watery, loose bowel movements).
iii. Difficulty in eating.
iv. Occasional hematemesis (see above).

Chapter 33: Pancreas and Pancreatic Secretion

CHAPTER OUTLINE

- DUAL FUNCTIONS OF PANCREAS
- FUNCTIONAL ANATOMY OF EXOCRINE PART OF PANCREAS
- NERVE SUPPLY TO PANCREAS
- PROPERTIES AND COMPOSITION OF PANCREATIC JUICE
- FUNCTIONS OF PANCREATIC JUICE
- REGULATION OF PANCREATIC SECRETION
- COLLECTION OF PANCREATIC JUICE
- PANCREATIC EXOCRINE FUNCTIONS TESTS
- APPLIED PHYSIOLOGY: DISORDERS OF PANCREAS

DUAL FUNCTIONS OF PANCREAS

Pancreas is a dual organ having two functions, endocrine function and exocrine function. **Endocrine function** is concerned with production of the hormones. Refer Chapter 53 for details. **Exocrine function** is concerned with secretion of digestive juice called pancreatic juice and it is explained in this chapter.

FUNCTIONAL ANATOMY OF EXOCRINE PART OF PANCREAS

Exocrine part of pancreas is made up of **acini** or **alveoli** like salivary glands. Each acinus has a single layer of acinar cells with a lumen in the center. **Acinar cells** contain **zymogen granules**, which possess digestive enzymes.

Duct System in Pancreas

A small duct arises from lumen of each alveolus. Some of these ducts from neighboring alveoli unite to form **intralobular duct**. All the intralobular ducts unite to form the main **pancreatic duct** or **Wirsung's duct**. Pancreatic duct joins **common bile duct** to form **ampulla of Vater**, which opens into duodenum **(Fig. 34.3)**.

NERVE SUPPLY TO PANCREAS

Pancreas is supplied by both sympathetic and parasympathetic nerve fibers. Sympathetic nerve fibers are supplied through **splanchnic nerve** and parasympathetic nerve fibers are supplied through **vagus nerve**.

PROPERTIES AND COMPOSITION OF PANCREATIC JUICE

PROPERTIES OF PANCREATIC JUICE

Volume : 500 to 800 mL/day
Reaction : Highly alkaline with pH of 8 to 8.3
Specific gravity : 1.010 to 1.018

COMPOSITION OF PANCREATIC JUICE

Pancreatic juice contains 99.5% of water and 0.5% of solids. Solids are the organic and inorganic substances. Composition of pancreatic juice is given in **Figure 33.1**.

Bicarbonate content is very high in pancreatic juice. It is about 110 to 150 mEq/L against the concentration of 24 mEq/L in plasma. This high concentration of **bicarbonate** is responsible for the **alkalinity** of pancreatic juice.

FUNCTIONS OF PANCREATIC JUICE

Pancreatic juice has digestive functions and the neutralizing action.

DIGESTIVE FUNCTIONS OF PANCREATIC JUICE

Pancreatic juice plays an important role in the digestion of proteins and lipids. It also has mild action on carbohydrate digestion.

DIGESTION OF PROTEINS

Proteolytic enzymes of pancreatic juice are trypsin and chymotrypsin; and other proteolytic enzymes are carboxypeptidases, nuclease, elastase and collagenase.

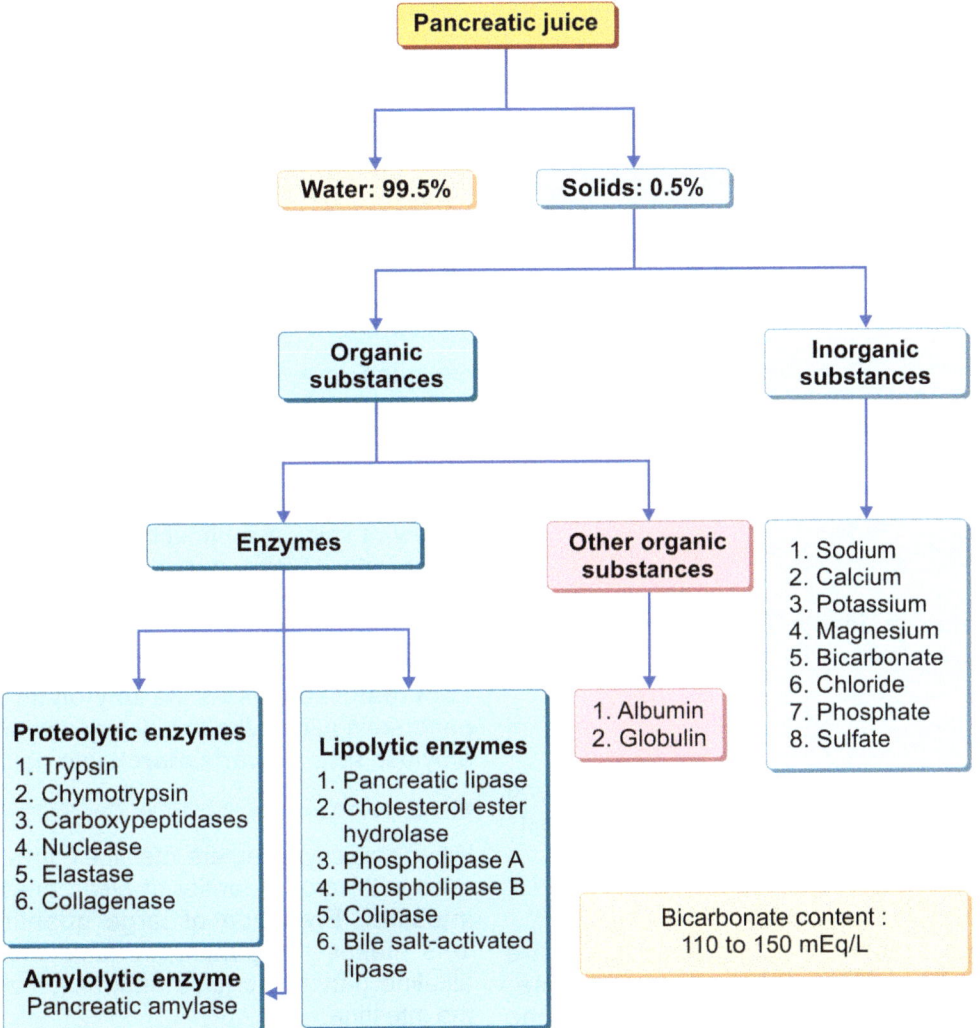

FIGURE 33.1: Composition of pancreatic juice.

1. Trypsin

Trypsin is a single polypeptide with a molecular weight of 25,000. It contains 229 amino acids.

It is secreted as inactive **trypsinogen** which is converted into active trypsin by **enterokinase**. Enterokinase is also called **enteropeptidase** and it is secreted by the **brush bordered cells** of duodenal mucus membrane.

Actions of trypsin

i. Digestion of proteins: Trypsin is the most powerful **proteolytic enzyme**. It is an **endopeptidase** and breaks the interior bonds of protein molecules. And it converts proteins into proteoses and polypeptides.
ii. Curdling of milk: It converts **caseinogens** in the milk into casein.
iii. It accelerates blood clotting.
iv. It activates other enzymes of pancreatic juice:
   a. Chymotrypsinogen into chymotrypsin.
   b. Procarboxypeptidases into carboxypeptidases.
   c. Proelastase into elastase.
   d. Procolipase into colipase.

Trypsin also activates collagenase, phospholipase A and phospholipase B.

Autocatalytic action of trypsin

Once formed trypsin itself converts trypsinogen into trypsin. This action is called autocatalytic or **autoactive action**.

2. Chymotrypsin

Chymotrypsin is a polypeptide with a molecular weight of 25,700 and 246 amino acids. It is secreted as inactive **chymotrypsinogen** and activated into chymotrypsin by trypsin.

Actions of chymotrypsin

i. *Digestion of proteins:* Chymotrypsin is also an **endopeptidase** and it breaks the proteins into polypeptides.
ii. *Digestion of milk:* Chymotrypsin digests casein faster than trypsin. The combination of both enzymes causes more rapid digestion of milk.
iii. *On blood clotting:* No action.

3. Carboxypeptidases

Carboxypeptidases are carboxypeptidase A and carboxypeptidase B. These two enzymes are secreted as procarboxypeptidase A and procarboxypeptidase B. Inactive **procarboxypeptidases** are activated into carboxypeptidases by trypsin.

Actions of carboxypeptidases

Carboxypeptidases are **exopeptidases** and split the polypeptides and other proteins into amino acids.

4. Nucleases

Nucleases of pancreatic juice are ribonuclease and deoxyribonuclease, which are responsible for the digestion of nucleic acids. These enzymes convert the ribonucleic acid (RNA) and deoxyribonucleic acid (DNA) into mononucleotides.

5. Elastase

Elastase is secreted as inactive **proelastase** and is activated into active elastase by trypsin. It digests the elastic fibers.

6. Collagenase

Collagenase is secreted as inactive **procollagenase** and is activated into active collagenase by trypsin. It digests collagen.

■ DIGESTION OF LIPIDS

Lipolytic enzymes present in pancreatic juice are pancreatic lipase, cholesterol ester hydrolase, phospholipase A, phospholipase B and a coenzyme called colipase.

1. Pancreatic Lipase

Pancreatic lipase is a powerful **lipolytic enzyme**. It digests the triglycerides into monoglycerides and fatty acids. Activity of pancreatic lipase is accelerated in the presence of bile. Optimum pH required for activity of this enzyme is 7 to 9.

Digestion of fat by pancreatic lipase requires two more factors:

i. Bile salts which are responsible for the emulsification of fat prior to their digestion.
ii. Colipase which is a coenzyme necessary for the pancreatic lipase to hydrolyze the dietary lipids. Colipase is secreted as an inactive procolipase which activated into colipase by trypsin.

About 80% of fat is digested by pancreatic lipase. Deficiency or absence of this enzyme leads to **steatorrhea** (see below).

2. Cholesterol Ester Hydrolase

Cholesterol ester hydrolase or cholesterol esterase converts cholesterol ester into free cholesterol and fatty acid by hydrolysis.

3. Phospholipase A

It is activated by trypsin. Phospholipase A digests phospholipids namely **lecithin** and **cephalin** and converts them into **lysolecithin** and **lysocephalin** respectively.

4. Phospholipase B

Phospholipase B is also activated by trypsin. This enzyme converts lysolecithin and lysocephalin into **phosphoryl choline** and free fatty acids.

5. Colipase

Colipase is a small **coenzyme**, which facilitates the hydrolysis of fats by pancreatic lipase.

6. Bile Salt-activated Lipase

This enzyme has a weak lipolytic action. It digests a variety of lipids like phospholipids, cholesterol esters and triglycerides. Since, it is activated bile salt it is known as bile salt-activated lipase **(Table 33.1)**.

■ DIGESTION OF CARBOHYDRATES

Pancreatic amylase is the **amylolytic enzyme** present in pancreatic juice. Like to salivary amylase, the pancreatic amylase also converts **starch** into dextrin and maltose.

■ NEUTRALIZING ACTION OF PANCREATIC JUICE

When acid chyme enters intestine from stomach, pancreatic juice with large quantity of bicarbonate is released into intestine. Presence of large quantity of bicarbonate ions makes the pancreatic juice highly alkaline. This alkaline pancreatic juice neutralizes acidity of chyme in the intestine.

Neutralizing action is an important function of pancreatic juice, because it protects the intestine from the destructive action of acid in the chyme.

■ REGULATION OF PANCREATIC SECRETION

Pancreatic secretion occurs in three stages:

I. Cephalic phase.
II. Gastric phase.
III. Intestinal phase.

Each phase is regulated by nervous mechanism or hormonal mechanism or both.

■ CEPHALIC PHASE

As in case of gastric secretion, cephalic phase of pancreatic secretion is regulated by nervous mechanism through reflex action. During this phase, 20% of total amount pancreatic juice is secreted.

Two types of reflexes occur:

1. Unconditioned reflex.
2. Conditioned reflex.

1. Unconditioned Reflex

Unconditioned reflex is the inborn reflex. When food is placed in the mouth, it induces salivary secretion

Chapter 33: Pancreas and Pancreatic Secretion

TABLE 33.1: Digestive enzymes of pancreatic juice.

Enzyme	Activator	Acts on (substrate)	End products
Trypsin	Enterokinase Trypsin	Proteins	Proteoses Polypeptides
Chymotrypsin	Trypsin	Proteins	Polypeptides
Carboxypeptidases	Trypsin	Polypeptides	Amino acids
Nucleases	Trypsin	RNA and DNA	Mononucleotides
Elastase	Trypsin	Elastin	Amino acids
Collagenase	Trypsin	Collagen	Amino acids
Pancreatic lipase	Alkaline medium	Triglycerides	Monoglycerides Fatty acids
Cholesterol ester hydrolase	Alkaline medium	Cholesterol ester	Cholesterol Fatty acids
Phospholipase A	Trypsin	Phospholipids	Lysophospholipids
Phospholipase B	Trypsin	Lysophospholipids	Phosphoryl choline Free fatty acids
Colipase	Trypsin	Facilitates action of pancreatic lipase	-
Bile salt-activated lipase	Bile salt	Phospholipids	Lysophospholipids
		Cholesterol esters	Cholesterol Fatty acids
		Triglycerides	Monoglycerides Fatty acids
Pancreatic amylase	Acid medium	Starch	Dextrin Maltose

(Chapter 31), gastric secretion (Chapter 32). Simultaneously it induces pancreatic secretion also.

2. Conditioned Reflex

Conditioned reflex is the reflex response acquired by previous experience (Chapter 107). Presence of food in the mouth is not necessary to elicit this reflex. Sight, smell, hearing or thought of food which induce salivary secretion and gastric secretion also induces pancreatic secretion **(Fig. 33.2)**.

Impulses from mouth (during unconditioned reflex) or from cerebral cortex (during conditioned reflex) reach the dorsal nucleus of vagus. From the dorsal nucleus of vagus, efferent impulses reach the pancreas via efferent fibers of vagus nerve. Vagal nerve endings release acetylcholine which stimulates the acinar cells to release the enzymes.

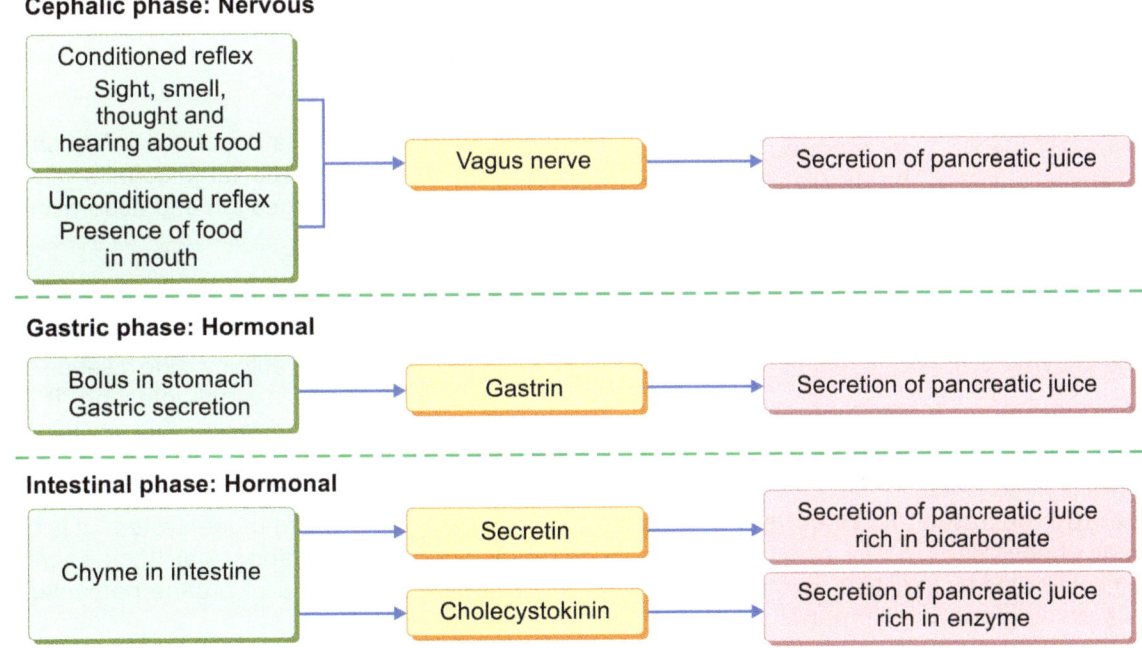

FIGURE 33.2: Schematic diagram showing the regulation of pancreatic secretion.

GASTRIC PHASE

Secretion of pancreatic juice when food enters the stomach is known as gastric phase. This phase of pancreatic secretion is under **hormonal control**. Hormone involved is **gastrin**.

When food enters stomach, gastrin is secreted from stomach (Chapter 32). When gastrin is transported to pancreas through blood, it stimulates the pancreatic secretion. Pancreatic juice secreted during gastric phase is rich in enzymes. During gastric phase, only 10% of pancreatic juice is secreted.

INTESTINAL PHASE

Intestinal phase is the secretion of pancreatic juice when the chyme enters the intestine. This phase is also under **hormonal control**. In this phase, 70% of total amount of pancreatic juice is secreted.

When **chyme** enters the intestine, many hormones are released. Some hormones stimulate the pancreatic secretion and some hormones inhibit the pancreatic secretion.

Hormones Stimulating Pancreatic Secretion

1. Secretin.
2. Cholecystokinin.

1. Secretin

Secretin is produced by **S cells** of mucous membrane in duodenum and jejunum. It is produced in an inactive **prosecretin** which is activated into secretin by acid chyme.

Stimulant for the release and activation of prosecretin is the acid chyme entering intestine. The products of protein digestion also stimulate the hormonal secretion.

Action of secretin

Secretin stimulates the secretion of watery pancreatic juice which contains high concentration of bicarbonate ion.

2. Cholecystokinin

Cholecystokinin (CCK) is also called **cholecystokinin-pancreozymin** (CCK-PZ). It is secreted by **I cells** in duodenal and jejunal mucosa. The stimulant for the release of this hormone is the chyme containing digestive products such as fatty acids, peptides and amino acids.

Action of cholecystokinin

Cholecystokinin stimulates the secretion of pancreatic juice which is rich in enzyme and less in volume.

Hormones Inhibiting Pancreatic Secretion

1. **Pancreatic polypeptide** secreted by **PP cells** in islets of Langerhans of pancreas.
2. **Somatostatin** secreted by **D cells** in islets of Langerhans of pancreas.
3. **Peptide YY** secreted by intestinal mucosa.
4. Peptides such as **ghrelin** and **leptin**.

COLLECTION OF PANCREATIC JUICE

Pancreatic juice is collected by a **multilumen tube**. This tube is inserted through nose or mouth, till tip of the tube reaches intestine near the **ampulla of Vater**. The tube has a marking. Entrance of the tip of tube into the intestine near the ampulla is indicated when this line comes near mouth.

This tube has three lumens. Small balloons are attached to the two outer lumens. When balloons are inflated by air, the intestine near the ampulla is enlarged. Now, the pancreatic juice is collected through the middle lumen by means of aspiration.

PANCREATIC EXOCRINE FUNCTIONS TESTS

1. Blood tests:
   i. Amylase test.
   ii. Serum lipase test.
2. Lundh test: After giving a test meal, duodenal content is aspirated and tested for trypsin activity.
3. Stool tests.

APPLIED PHYSIOLOGY: DISORDERS OF PANCREAS

PANCREATITIS

Pancreatitis is the inflammation of pancreatic acini resulting in absence of pancreatic enzymes. Common causes of pancreatitis are long-time consumption of alcohol, congenital abnormalities of pancreatic duct and **malnutrition** (poor nutrition; mal = bad).

Features of Pancreatitis

1. Steatorrhea.
2. Severe abdominal pain.
3. Nausea and vomiting.
4. Loss of appetite and weight.
5. Fever.
6. Shock.

STEATORRHEA

Steatorrhea is the formation of bulky, foul smelling, frothy and clay colored stools with large quantity of undigested fat because of impaired digestion and absorption of fat.

Causes of Steatorrhea

1. Lack of pancreatic lipase.
2. Liver disease affecting secretion of bile.
3. **Celiac disease**: An autoimmune disease characterized by damage of villi in small intestine. It is caused by gluten intake.
4. **Cystic fibrosis**: A genetic disorder affecting the functions of many organs such as lungs, pancreas and biliary system and immune system. It is characterized by production of abnormal thick secretions which impair the functions of organs particularly lungs and pancreas.

Chapter 34

Liver and Biliary System

CHAPTER OUTLINE

- DUAL FUNCTIONS OF LIVER
- FUNCTIONAL ANATOMY OF LIVER AND BILIARY SYSTEM
- BLOOD SUPPLY TO LIVER
- NERVE SUPPLY TO LIVER
- PROPERTIES AND COMPOSITION OF BILE
- SECRETION OF BILE
- STORAGE OF BILE
- BILE SALTS
- BILE PIGMENTS
- FUNCTIONS OF BILE
- FUNCTIONS OF LIVER
- GALLBLADDER
- REGULATION OF BILE SECRETION
- LIVER FUNCTION TESTS
- APPLIED PHYSIOLOGY: DISORDERS OF LIVER AND GALLBLADDER

■ DUAL FUNCTIONS OF LIVER

Liver is a dual organ having dual functions. It has both secretory and excretory functions.

■ FUNCTIONAL ANATOMY OF LIVER AND BILIARY SYSTEM

Liver is the largest gland in the body weighing about 1.5 kg in man. It is situated in the upper and right side of the abdominal cavity immediately beneath diaphragm.

Liver is made up of many lobes called **hepatic lobes** (Fig. 34.1). Each lobe consists of many lobules called **hepatic lobules**.

Hepatic lobule is the structural and functional unit of liver. It is a honeycomb-like structure and it is made up of liver cells called **hepatocytes**. Hepatocytes are arranged in **hepatic plates**. Each plate is made up of two columns of cells. In between the two columns of each plate lies a **bile canaliculus** (Fig. 34.2).

In between the neighboring plates, a blood space called **sinusoid** is present. Sinusoid is lined by the endothelial cells. In between the endothelial cells, macrophages called **Kupffer cells** are present.

Portal Triads

Each lobule is surrounded by many portal triads.

Each portal triad consists of three vessels:

1. A branch of hepatic artery.

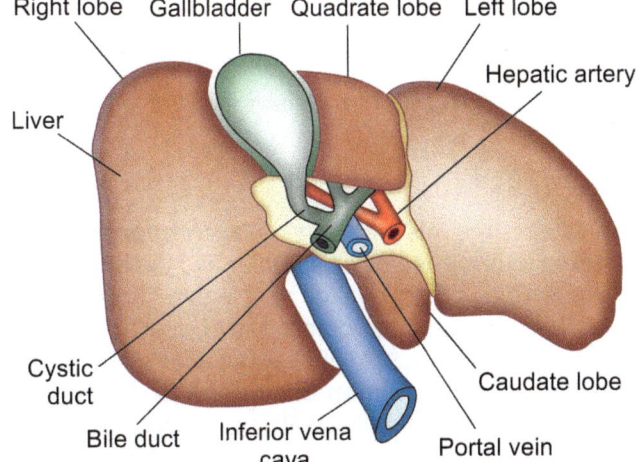

FIGURE 34.1: Posterior surface of liver.

2. A branch of portal vein.
3. A tributary of bile duct.

Branches of hepatic artery and portal vein open into the sinusoid. Sinusoid opens into the central vein. Central vein empties into hepatic vein. Bile is secreted by hepatic cells and emptied into **bile canaliculus**. From canaliculus, the bile enters the tributary of bile duct. Tributaries of bile duct from canaliculi of neighboring lobules unite to form small **bile ducts**. These small bile ducts join together and finally form left and right **hepatic ducts** which emerge out of liver.

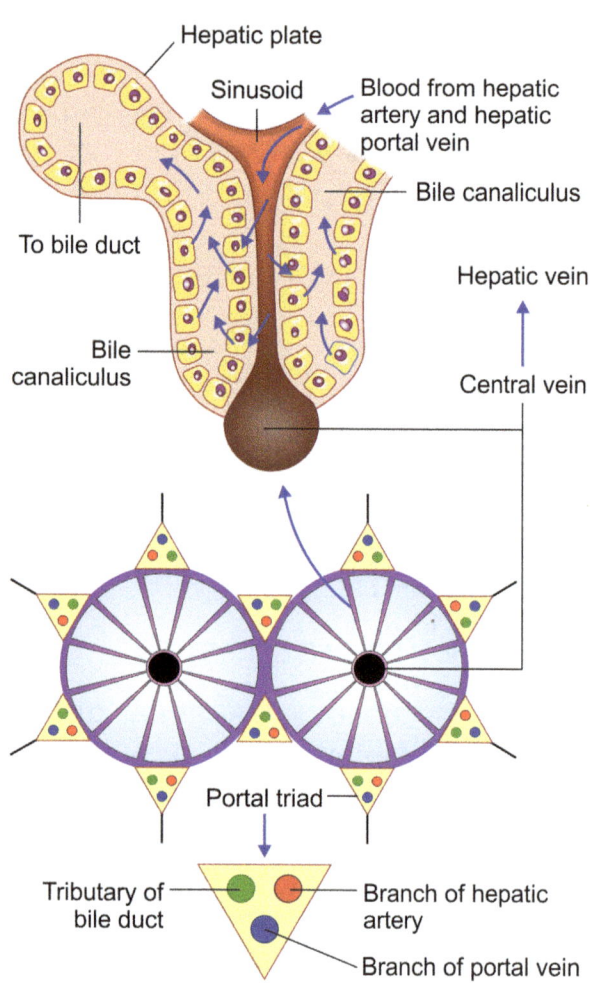

FIGURE 34.2: Hepatic lobule.

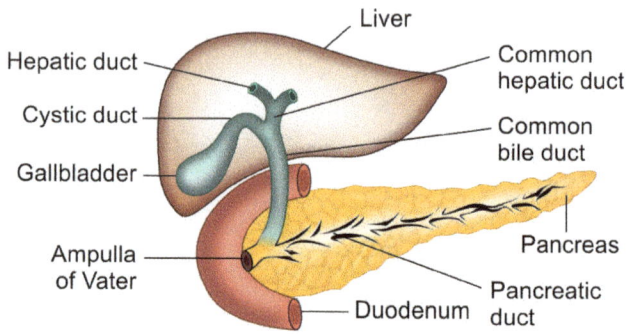

FIGURE 34.3: Biliary system.

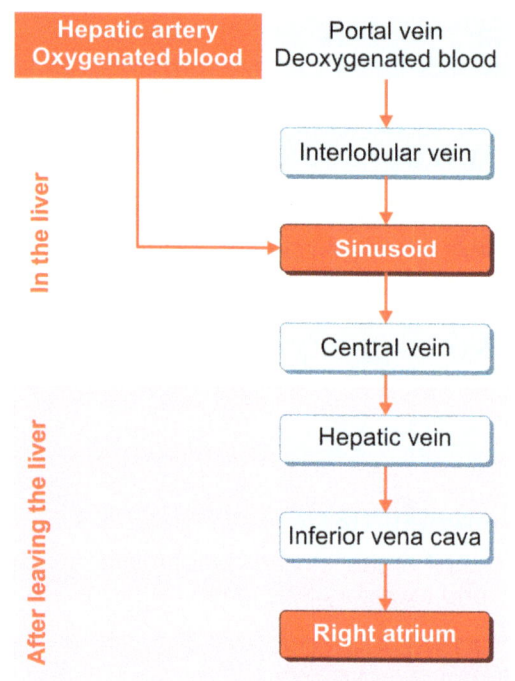

FIGURE 34.4: Schematic diagram of blood flow through liver.

■ BILIARY SYSTEM

Biliary system is also known as **extrahepatic biliary apparatus**. It is formed by gallbladder and the extrahepatic bile ducts (bile ducts outside the liver). Right and left hepatic bile ducts which come out of liver join to form **common hepatic duct**. It unites with the **cystic duct** from gallbladder to form **common bile duct (Fig. 34.3)**.

Common bile duct unites with pancreatic duct to form the common hepatopancreatic duct or **ampulla of Vater** which opens into the duodenum.

There is a sphincter called **sphincter of Oddi** at the lower part of common bile duct, before it joins the pancreatic duct. It is formed by smooth muscle fibers of common bile duct. Sphincter of Oddi is normally kept closed, so that bile secreted from liver enters gallbladder where it is stored. Upon appropriate stimulation the sphincter opens and allows flow of bile from gallbladder into the intestine.

■ BLOOD SUPPLY TO LIVER

Liver receives the maximum blood supply of about 1,500 mL/min. It receives blood from two sources, namely the hepatic artery and portal vein **(Fig. 34.4)**.

■ HEPATIC ARTERY

Hepatic artery arises directly from aorta and supplies **oxygenated blood** to liver. After entering the liver, hepatic artery divides into many branches. Each branch enters a portal triad.

■ HEPATIC PORTAL VEIN

Hepatic portal vein is formed by superior mesenteric vein and splenic vein. It brings **deoxygenated blood** from stomach, intestine, spleen and pancreas to liver. Blood from hepatic artery mixes with the blood from portal vein in the hepatic sinusoids. Hepatic cells obtain oxygen and nutrients from the sinusoid.

■ HEPATIC VEIN

Substances synthesized by hepatic cells, waste products and carbon dioxide are discharged into sinusoids. Sinusoids drain them into central vein of the lobule. **Central**

veins from many lobules unite to form bigger veins, which ultimately form hepatic veins (right and left) which open into inferior vena cava.

ENTEROHEPATIC CIRCULATION

Enterohepatic circulation is the circulation of substances such as bile salts and bilirubin that are absorbed from intestine and transported to liver through hepatic portal vein. These substances are excreted or secreted in bile and enter intestine again **(Fig. 34.5)**.

Significance of Enterohepatic Circulation

Enterohepatic circulation is responsible for recycling of both metabolized and nonmetabolized substances. Many important substances that are secreted or excreted by liver into small intestine through bile are brought back to liver via enterohepatic circulation.

NERVE SUPPLY TO LIVER

Parenchyma of liver is supplied by sympathetic fibers from **celiac plexus** and parasympathetic fibers from anterior and posterior trunks of **vagus**. All these nerve fibers reach the hepatic tissues by passing through hepatic nerve plexus which runs along hepatic artery and hepatic portal vein.

PROPERTIES AND COMPOSITION OF BILE

Bile is a golden yellow or greenish fluid. It enters the digestive tract along with pancreatic juice through ampulla of Vater.

PROPERTIES OF BILE

Volume : 800 to 1,200 mL/day
Reaction : Alkaline
pH : 8 to 8.6
Specific gravity : 1.010 to 1.011

COMPOSITION OF BILE

Bile contains 97.6% of water and 2.4% of solids. Solids include organic and inorganic substances. Refer **Figure 34.6** for details.

SECRETION OF BILE

Bile is secreted by **hepatocytes**. Initial bile secreted by hepatocytes contains large quantity of bile acids, bile pigments, cholesterol, lecithin and fatty acids. From hepatocytes, bile passes through canaliculi and hepatic ducts to reach common hepatic duct. From here it may enter the intestine or gallbladder **(Fig. 34.7)**.

Sodium, bicarbonate and water are added to bile when it passes through the ducts. These substances are secreted by the epithelial cells of the ducts. The addition of sodium, bicarbonate and water increases the total quantity of bile **(Fig. 34.8)**.

STORAGE OF BILE

Most of the bile from liver enters the gallbladder where it is stored. It is released from gallbladder into the intestine whenever it is required.

Changes Taking Place in Bile during Storage at Gallbladder

When bile is stored in gallbladder, it undergoes many changes both in quality and quantity such as:

1. Volume is reduced because of absorption of large amount of water and electrolytes (except calcium and potassium).
2. Concentration of bile salts, bile pigments, cholesterol, fatty acids and lecithin is increased because of absorption of water.
3. The pH is slightly decreased.

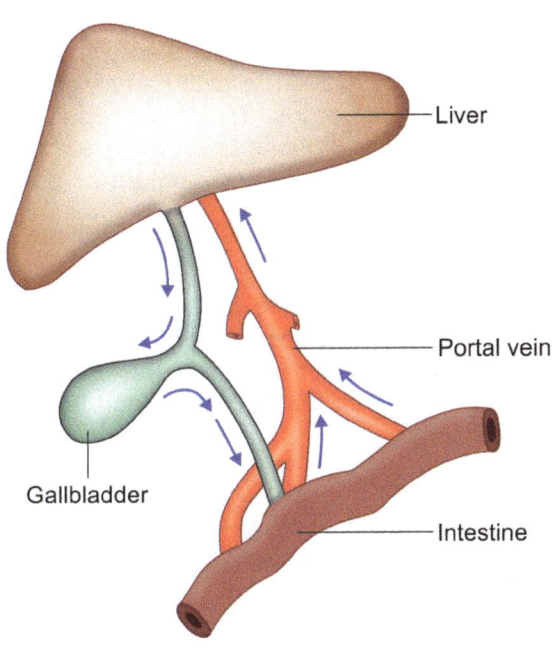

FIGURE 34.5: Enterohepatic circulation.

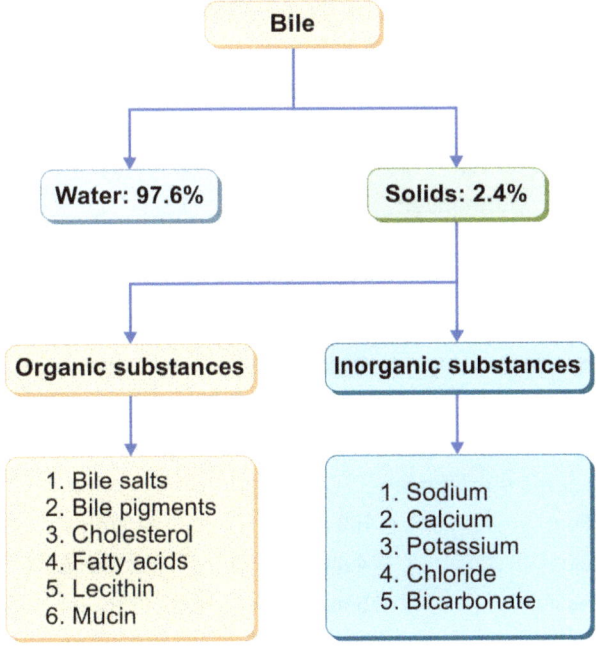

FIGURE 34.6: Composition of bile.

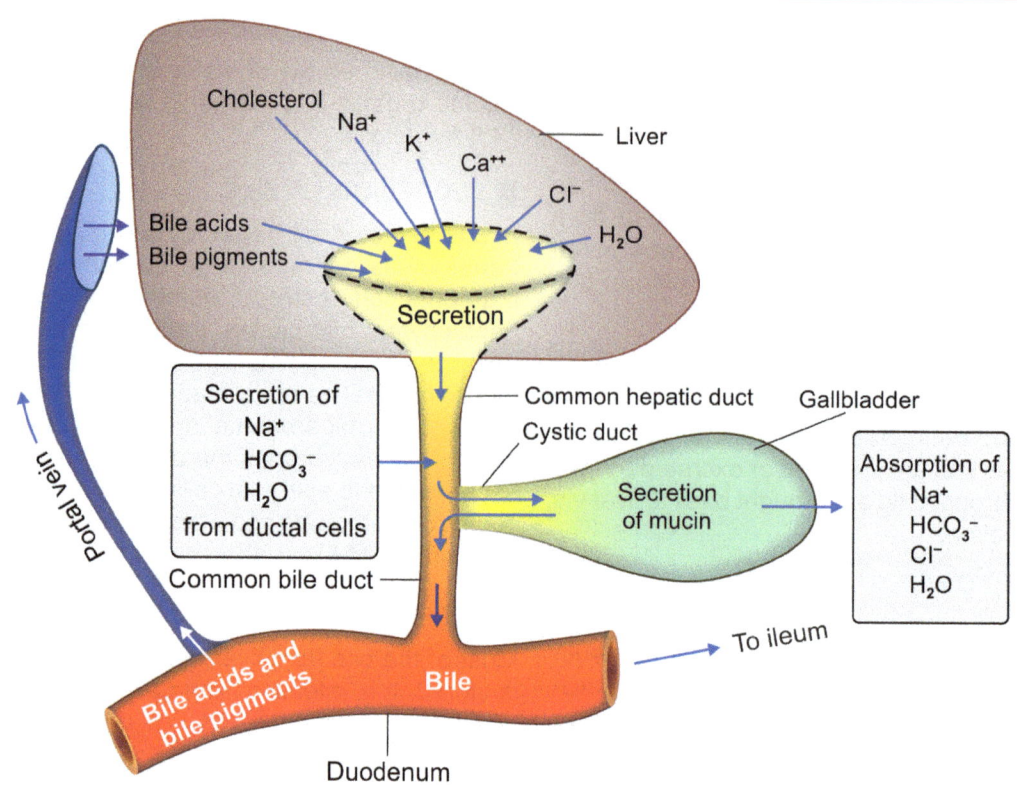

FIGURE 34.7: Diagram showing the formation of bile from liver and changes taking place in the composition of gallbladder bile.

4. Specific gravity is increased.
5. Mucin is added **(Table 34.1)**.

■ BILE SALTS

Bile salts are the sodium and potassium salts of bile acids, which are conjugated with glycine or taurine. Bile salts are formed in liver.

TABLE 34.1: Differences between liver bile and gallbladder bile.

Entities	Liver bile	Gallbladder bile
pH	8 to 8.6	7 to 7.6
Specific gravity	1,010 to 1,011	1,026 to 1,032
Water content	97.6%	89%
Solids	2.4%	11%
Organic substances		
Bile salts	0.5 g/dL	6.0 g/dL
Bile pigments	0.05 g/dL	0.3 g/dL
Cholesterol	1 g/dL	0.5 g/dL
Fatty acids	2 g/dL	1.2 g/dL
Lecithin	0.05 g/dL	0.4 g/dL
Mucin	Absent	Present
Inorganic substances		
Sodium	150 mEq/L	135 mEq/L
Calcium	4 mEq/L	22 mEq/L
Potassium	5 mEq/L	12 mEq/L
Chloride	100 mEq/L	10 mEq/L
Bicarbonate	30 mEq/L	10 mEq/L

■ FORMATION OF BILE SALTS

Bile salts are formed from the **primary bile acids**, namely **cholic acid** and **chenodeoxycholic** acid which are formed in liver and enter the intestine through bile. Due to the bacterial action in the intestine, these primary bile acids are converted into **secondary bile acids**:

Cholic acid ⟶ Deoxycholic acid

Chenodeoxycholic acid ⟶ Lithocholic acid

Secondary bile acids from intestine are transported back to liver through enterohepatic circulation. In the liver the secondary bile acids are conjugated with **glycine** or **taurine** and form conjugated bile acids namely **glycocholic acid** and **taurocholic acids**. These bile acids combine with sodium or potassium ions to form the salts, sodium or potassium **glycocholate** and sodium or potassium **taurocholate**.

■ ENTEROHEPATIC CIRCULATION OF BILE SALTS

About 90 to 95% of bile salts from intestine are transported to liver through enterohepatic circulation. Remaining 5 to 10% of the bile salts enter large intestine. Here, the bile salts are converted into **deoxycholate** and **lithocholate** and excreted in feces.

■ FUNCTIONS OF BILE SALTS

Bile salts are required for digestion and absorption of fats in the intestine. Functions of bile salts are:

1. *Emulsification of Fats: Detergent Action*

Emulsification is the process by which fat globules are broken down into minute droplets and made in the form of a milky fluid called **emulsion**. Emulsification of fats occurs in small intestine by the action of bile salts.

Fats cannot be digested directly by lipolytic enzymes of GI tract, because the fats are insoluble in water due to the surface tension. Bile salts reduce the **surface tension of fats** due to their **detergent action**. Because of this, the lipid granules are broken into minute particles which can be easily digested by lipolytic enzymes. Emulsification of fats by bile salts needs the presence of lecithin from bile.

2. Absorption of Fats

Bile salts help in the absorption of digested fats from intestine into blood. Bile salts combine with fats and make complexes of fats called **micelles**. Fats in the form of micelles can be absorbed easily.

3. Choleretic Action

Bile salts stimulate the secretion of bile from liver. This action is called choleretic action.

4. Cholagogue Action

Cholagogue is an agent, which causes contraction of gallbladder and release of bile into the intestine. Bile salts act as cholagogues indirectly by stimulating the secretion of hormone cholecystokinin. This hormone causes contraction of gallbladder resulting in release of bile.

5. Laxative Action

Laxative is an agent which induces **defecation**. Bile salts act as laxatives by stimulating peristaltic movements of the intestine.

6. Prevention of Gallstone Formation

Bile salts prevent formation of gallstone by keeping the cholesterol and lecithin in solution. In the absence of bile salts, cholesterol precipitates along with lecithin and forms gallstone.

■ BILE PIGMENTS

Bile pigments are the **excretory products** in bile. Bile pigments are bilirubin and biliverdin. And, bilirubin is the major bile pigment in human being.

Bile pigments are formed during the breakdown of hemoglobin, which is released from the destroyed RBCs in the reticuloendothelial system **(Fig. 34.8)**.

■ FORMATION AND EXCRETION OF BILE PIGMENTS

Stages of Formation and Circulation of Bile Pigments

1. Senile erythrocytes are destroyed in reticuloendothelial system and hemoglobin is released from them.
2. Hemoglobin is broken into globin and heme.
3. Heme is split into iron and the pigment biliverdin.
4. Iron goes to iron pool and is reused.
5. First formed pigment **biliverdin** is reduced to **bilirubin**.
6. Bilirubin is released into blood from reticuloendothelial cells.
7. Bilirubin circulating in the blood is called **free bilirubin** or **unconjugated bilirubin**.

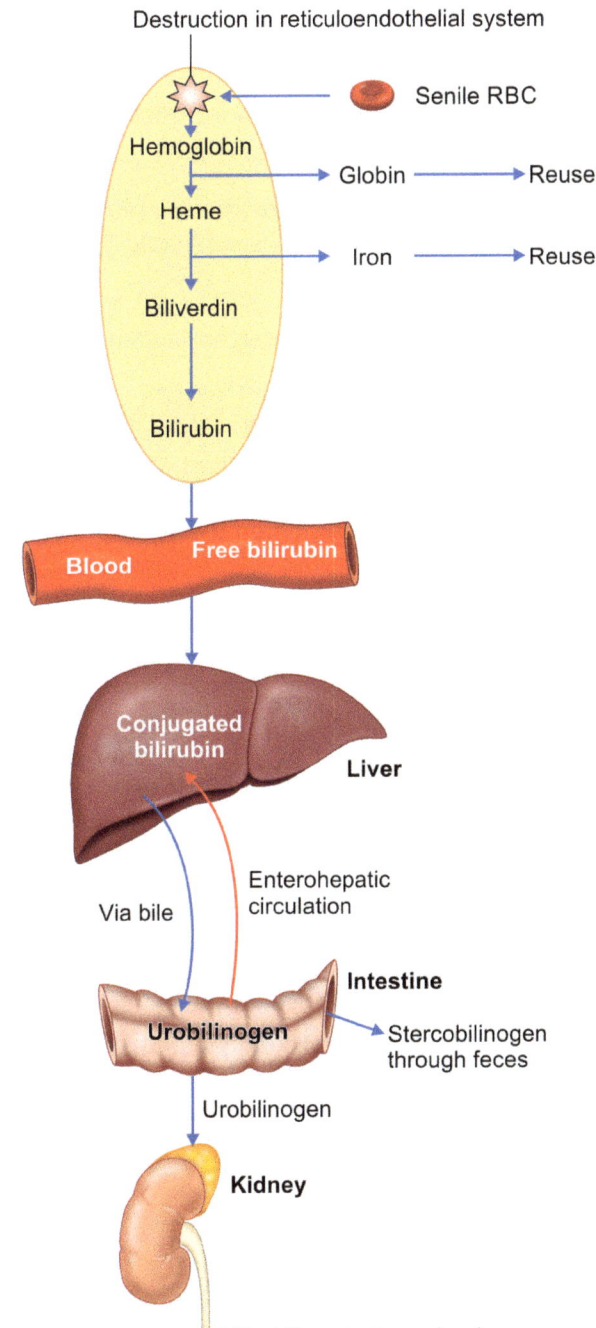

FIGURE 34.8: Formation and circulation of bile pigments.

8. Within few hours the free bilirubin is taken up by the liver cells.
9. In the liver, it is conjugated with glucuronic acid to form **conjugated bilirubin** or **direct bilirubin**.
10. Conjugated bilirubin is then excreted into intestine through bile.

■ FATE OF CONJUGATED BILIRUBIN

Stages of Excretion of Conjugated Bilirubin

1. In the intestine, 50% of conjugated bilirubin is converted into **urobilinogen** by intestinal bacteria. First the conjugated bilirubin is deconjugated into free bilirubin which is later reduced into urobilinogen.

2. Remaining 50% of conjugated bilirubin from intestine enters the liver through enterohepatic circulation. From liver, it is re-excreted in bile.
3. Most of the urobilinogen from intestine enters liver via enterohepatic circulation. Later, it is re-excreted through bile.
4. About 5% of urobilinogen is excreted by kidney through urine. In urine, urobilinogen is converted into urobilin by oxidation due to the exposure to air.
5. Some of the urobilinogen is excreted in feces as **stercobilinogen**. In feces, stercobilinogen is oxidized to stercobilin.

NORMAL PLASMA LEVELS OF BILIRUBIN

Normal bilirubin (total bilirubin) content in plasma is 0.5 to 1.5 mg/dL. When it exceeds 1 mg/dL, the condition is called **hyperbilirubinemia**. When it exceeds 2 mg/dL, **jaundice** occurs.

FUNCTIONS OF BILE

Most of the functions of bile are due to the bile salts.

1. DIGESTIVE FUNCTION

Bile salts are responsible for digestion of fats by lipolytic enzymes of GI tract. Refer functions of bile salts for details.

2. ABSORPTIVE FUNCTIONS

Bile salts are responsible for absorption of digested fats from intestine into blood. Refer functions of bile salts for details.

3. EXCRETORY FUNCTIONS

Bile pigments are the major excretory products of the bile.

Other substances excreted in bile are:
 i. Heavy metals such as copper and iron.
 ii. Some bacteria such as typhoid bacteria.
 iii. Some toxins.
 iv. Cholesterol.
 v. Lecithin.
 vi. Alkaline phosphatase.

4. LAXATIVE ACTION

Bile salts act as laxatives (see above).

5. ANTISEPTIC ACTION

Bile inhibits the growth of certain bacteria in the lumen of intestine by its natural detergent action.

6. CHOLERETIC ACTION

Bile salts have the choleretic action (see above).

7. MAINTENANCE OF pH IN GASTROINTESTINAL TRACT

As the bile is highly alkaline, it neutralizes acid chyme which enters the intestine from stomach. Thus, an optimum pH is maintained for the action of digestive enzymes.

8. PREVENTION OF GALLSTONE FORMATION

Refer function of bile salts.

9. LUBRICATION FUNCTION

Mucin in bile acts as a lubricant for the chyme in intestine.

10. CHOLAGOGUE ACTION

Bile salts act as cholagogues (see above).

FUNCTIONS OF LIVER

Liver is the largest gland and one of the vital organs of the body. It performs many vital metabolic and homeostatic functions, which are summarized below.

1. METABOLIC FUNCTION

Liver is the organ where maximum metabolic reactions are carried out such as metabolism of carbohydrates, proteins, fats, vitamins and many hormones.

2. STORAGE FUNCTION

Many substances like glycogen, amino acids, iron, folic acid and vitamins A, B_{12}, and D are stored in liver.

3. SYNTHETIC FUNCTION

Liver produces glucose by gluconeogenesis. It synthesizes all the plasma proteins and other proteins (except immunoglobulins) such as clotting factors, complement factors and hormone-binding proteins. It also synthesizes steroids, somatomedin and heparin.

4. SECRETION OF BILE

Liver secretes bile, which contains bile salts, bile pigments, cholesterol, fatty acids and lecithin. Functions of bile are mainly due to the bile salts. Bile salts are required for digestion and absorption of fats in the intestine. Bile helps to carry away waste products and breakdown fats, which are excreted through feces or urine.

5. EXCRETORY FUNCTION

Liver excretes cholesterol, bile pigments, heavy metals (like lead, arsenic and bismuth), toxins, bacteria and virus through bile.

6. HEAT PRODUCTION

Liver is the organ where maximum heat is produced because of the metabolic reactions.

7. HEMOPOIETIC FUNCTION

In fetus (hepatic stage), liver produces the blood cells (Chapter 9). It stores vitamin B_{12} necessary for erythropoiesis and iron necessary for synthesis of hemoglobin. Liver produces **thrombopoietin** that promotes production of thrombocytes.

8. HEMOLYTIC FUNCTION

The senile RBCs after the lifespan of 120 days are destroyed by reticuloendothelial cells (Kupffer cells) of liver.

9. INACTIVATION OF HORMONES AND DRUGS

Liver catabolizes the hormones such as growth hormone, parathormone, cortisol, insulin, glucagon and estrogen. It also inactivates the drugs particularly fat-soluble drugs. Fat-soluble drugs are converted into water-soluble substances, which are excreted through bile or urine.

10. DEFENSIVE AND DETOXIFICATION FUNCTIONS

Kupffer cells (reticuloendothelial cells) of the liver play an important role in the defense of the body. Liver is also involved in the detoxification of foreign bodies:

i. Foreign bodies such as bacteria or antigens are swallowed and digested by reticuloendothelial cells of liver by means of phagocytosis.
ii. Reticuloendothelial cells of liver are also involved in production of some substances like interleukins and tumor necrosis factors, which activate the immune system of the body (Chapter 15).
iii. Liver cells are involved in removal of toxic property of various harmful substances. Removal of toxic property of the harmful agent is known as detoxification.

GALLBLADDER

Bile secreted from liver is stored in gallbladder. Capacity of gallbladder is approximately 50 mL. Gallbladder is not essential for life. **Cholecystectomy** (removal of gallbladder) is often done in patients suffering from gallbladder dysfunction. After cholecystectomy, patients do not suffer from any major disadvantage. In some species, gallbladder is absent.

FUNCTIONS OF GALLBLADDER

Major functions of gallbladder are the storage and concentration of bile.

1. Storage of Bile

Bile is continuously secreted from liver. But it is released into intestine only intermittently and most of the bile is stored in gallbladder till it is required.

2. Concentration of Bile

Bile is concentrated while it is stored in gallbladder. Mucosa of gallbladder rapidly reabsorbs water and electrolytes except calcium and potassium. But the bile salts, bile pigments, cholesterol and lecithin are not reabsorbed. So, the concentration of these substances in bile increases 5 to 10 times **(Fig. 34.7)**.

3. Alteration of pH of Bile

The pH of bile decreases from 8–8.6 to 7–7.6 and it becomes less alkaline when it is stored in gallbladder.

4. Secretion of Mucin

Gallbladder secretes mucin into the bile. Mucin acts as a lubricant for movement of chyme in the intestine.

5. Maintenance of Pressure in Biliary System

Due to the concentrating capacity, gallbladder maintains a pressure of about 7 cm H_2O in biliary system. This pressure in the biliary system is essential for the release of bile into the intestine.

REGULATION OF BILE SECRETION

Bile secretion is a continuous process though the amount secreted may be less during fasting. It starts increasing 3 hours after the meals. Secretion of bile from the liver and release of bile from the gallbladder are influenced by some chemical factors which are categorized into three groups:

1. Choleretics.
2. Cholagogues.
3. Hydrocholeretic agents.

1. Choleretics

Choleretic is the substance, which increases secretion of bile from liver.

Effective choleretic agents are:

i. Acetylcholine.
ii. Secretin.
iii. Cholecystokinin.
iv. Acid chyme in intestine.
v. Bile salts.

2. Cholagogues

Cholagogue is an agent, which increases the release of bile from gallbladder into intestine by contracting the gallbladder.

Common cholagogues are:

i. Bile salts.
ii. Calcium.
iii. Fatty acids.
iv. Amino acids.
v. Inorganic acids.

All these substances stimulate the secretion of cholecystokinin, which in turn causes contraction of gallbladder and flow of bile into intestine.

3. Hydrocholeretic Agents

Hydrocholeretic agent is a substance, which causes secretion of bile from liver with large amount of water and less quantity of solids. Hydrochloric acid is a hydrocholeretic agent.

LIVER FUNCTION TESTS

Liver function tests or hepatic function tests are the group of blood tests to assess the health and normal functioning of liver.

Following are the liver functions tests:

1. Total bilirubin.
2. Total protein.
3. Total albumin.

4. Albumin/Globulin ratio.
5. Alkaline phosphatase (ALP).
6. Alanine transaminase (ALT).
7. Aspartate aminotransferase (ALP).
8. Gamma glutamyl transferase (GGT).

APPLIED PHYSIOLOGY: DISORDERS OF LIVER AND GALLBLADDER

JAUNDICE OR ICTERUS

Jaundice or icterus is the condition characterized by yellow coloration of the skin, mucous membrane and deeper tissues due to increased bilirubin level in blood. The word jaundice is derived from the French word 'jaune' meaning yellow.

Normal serum bilirubin level is 0.5 to 1.5 mg/dL. Jaundice occurs when bilirubin level exceeds 2 mg/dL.

Types of Jaundice

Jaundice is classified into three types:

1. Prehepatic or hemolytic jaundice.
2. Hepatic or hepatocellular jaundice.
3. Posthepatic or obstructive jaundice.

1. Prehepatic or Hemolytic Jaundice

Hemolytic jaundice is the type of jaundice that occurs because of excess destruction of RBCs resulting in increased blood level of free (unconjugated) bilirubin. Function of liver is normal. Since the quantity of bilirubin increases enormously, liver cells cannot excrete that much bilirubin rapidly. So, bilirubin accumulates in the blood resulting in jaundice.

Causes of prehepatic or hemolytic jaundice

Any condition that causes hemolytic anemia can lead to hemolytic jaundice.

Common causes of hemolytic jaundice are:

i. Renal disorder.
ii. Hypersplenism.
iii. Burns.
iv. Infections such as malaria.
v. Hemoglobin abnormalities such as sickle cell anemia or thalassemia.
vi. Drugs or chemical substances causing red cell damage.
vii. Autoimmune diseases.

2. Hepatic or Hepatocellular or Cholestatic Jaundice

This is the type of jaundice that occurs due to damage of hepatic cells. Because of the damage, conjugated bilirubin from liver cannot be excreted and it returns to blood.

Causes of hepatic or hepatocellular or cholestatic jaundice

i. Viral hepatitis.
ii. Alcoholic hepatitis.
iii. Cirrhosis of liver.
iv. Exposure to toxic materials.

3. Posthepatic or Obstructive or Extrahepatic Jaundice

This type of jaundice occurs because of the obstruction of bile flow at any level of the biliary system. The bile cannot be excreted into small intestine **(Fig. 34.9)**. So, bile salts and bile pigments enter the circulation. The blood contains more amount of conjugated bilirubin **(Table 34.2)**.

Causes of posthepatic or obstructive or extrahepatic jaundice

i. Gallstones.
ii. Cancer of biliary system or pancreas.

Jaundice in Newborn Babies

In newborn babies, because of high count, RBCs are destroyed in large numbers. This increases blood level of bilirubin. And, they develop jaundice because their liver is not fully developed to excrete that much of bilirubin. Refer **Box 34.1** for details of jaundice in newborn babies.

HEPATITIS

Hepatitis is the liver damage characterized by swelling and inadequate functioning of liver. It is caused by several factors such as viral infection, bacterial infection and excess alcohol.

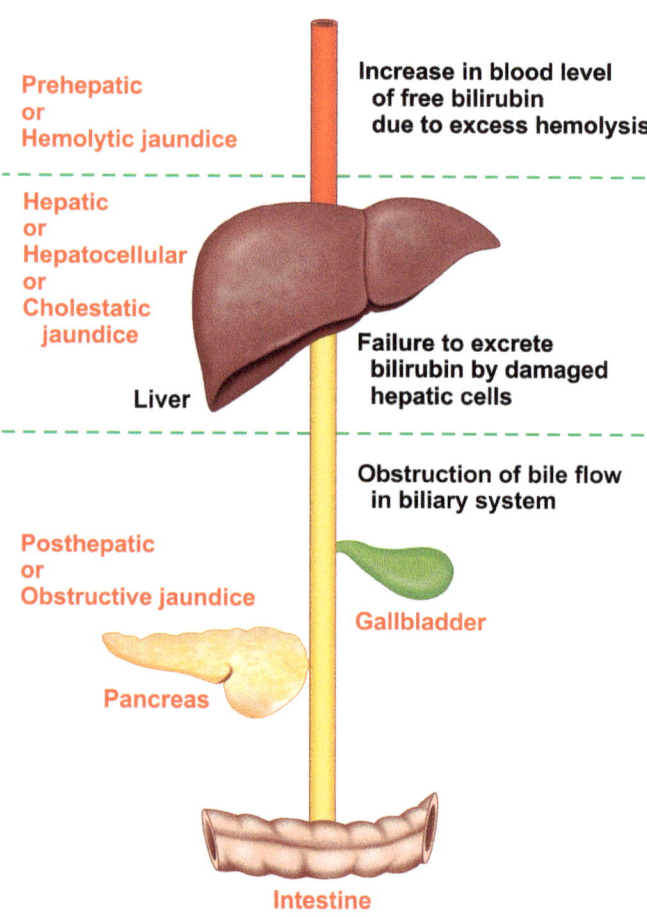

FIGURE 34.9: Types of jaundice.

TABLE 34.2: Features of different types of jaundice.

Feature	Prehepatic jaundice (hemolytic)	Hepatic jaundice (hepatocellular)	Posthepatic jaundice (obstructive)
Cause	Excess breakdown of RBCs	Liver damage	Obstruction of bile ducts
Type of bilirubin in blood	Unconjugated	Conjugated and unconjugated	Conjugated
Urinary excretion of urobilinogen	Increases	Decreases	Decreases Absent in severe obstruction
Fecal excretion of stercobilinogen	Increases	Decreases (pale feces)	Absent (clay-colored feces)
van den Bergh reaction	Indirect – positive	Biphasic	Direct – positive
Liver functions	Normal	Abnormal	Exaggerated
Blood picture	Anemia Reticulocytosis Abnormal RBC	Normal	Normal
Plasma albumin and globulin	Normal	Albumin : Increases Globulin : Increases A:G ratio: Decreases	Normal
Hemorrhagic tendency	Absent	Present due to lack of vitamin K	Present due to lack of vitamin K

BOX 34.1: Jaundice in newborn babies.

Physiological jaundice

Physiological jaundice develops if bilirubin level increases between 6 to 8 mg/L within 48 to 72 hours after birth (Chapter 8)

Physiological jaundice lasts only for few days

Pathological jaundice

High bilirubin level results in pathological jaundice

When bilirubin level increases above 15 mg/dL, immediate treatment is required

Pathological jaundice in infants may lead to bilirubin encephalopathy and kernicterus (Chapter 19).

Common features of hepatitis are fever, nausea, vomiting, diarrhea, loss of appetite, jaundice. Liver failure and death occur in severe conditions.

■ CIRRHOSIS OF LIVER

Cirrhosis of liver refers to inflammation and damage of parenchyma of liver resulting in degeneration of hepatic cells and dysfunction of liver. It is caused by infection, obstruction of biliary system and liver enlargement due to intoxication.

Features of cirrhosis of liver are fever, nausea and vomiting, jaundice, portal hypertension, muscular weakness and wasting of muscles. Coma occurs in advanced stages.

■ GALLSTONES

Definition

Gallstone is a solid crystal deposit that is formed by cholesterol, calcium ions and bile pigments in the gallbladder or bile duct. **Cholelithiasis** is the presence of gallstones in gallbladder.

Formation of Gallstones

Normally, cholesterol is water soluble. Under some abnormal conditions, it precipitates resulting in the formation of crystals in the mucosa of gallbladder. Bile pigments and calcium are attached to these crystals resulting in formation of gallstones.

Causes for Gallstone Formation

1. Reduction in bile salts.
2. Excess of cholesterol or disturbed cholesterol metabolism.
3. Excess of calcium ions due to increased concentration of bile.
4. Damage or infection of gallbladder epithelium.
5. Obstruction of bile flow from the gallbladder.

Features of Gallstone

Common feature of gallstone is the pain in stomach area or in upper right part of the belly under the ribs. Other features include nausea, vomiting, abdominal bloating and indigestion.

Chapter 35: Small Intestine and its Secretion

CHAPTER OUTLINE

- FUNCTIONAL ANATOMY
- INTESTINAL VILLI AND GLANDS
- PROPERTIES AND COMPOSITION OF SUCCUS ENTERICUS
- FUNCTIONS OF SUCCUS ENTERICUS
- FUNCTIONS OF SMALL INTESTINE
- REGULATION OF SECRETION OF SUCCUS ENTERICUS
- APPLIED PHYSIOLOGY: DISORDERS OF SMALL INTESTINE

■ FUNCTIONAL ANATOMY OF SMALL INTESTINE

Small intestine is the part of GI tract extending between **pyloric sphincter** of stomach and **ileocecal valve**, which opens into large intestine. It is called small intestine because its diameter is smaller than that of large intestine. But it is longer than large intestine. Its length is about 6 meters.

Functional importance of small intestine is absorption. Maximum absorption of digested food products takes place in small intestine.

■ PARTS OF SMALL INTESTINE

Small intestine consists of three portions:

1. Proximal part known as **duodenum**.
2. Middle part known as **jejunum**.
3. Distal part known as **ileum**.

Ileum of small intestine opens into cecum of large intestine through ileocecal valve. Ileocecal valve is a sphincter like structure present in **ileocecal junction**. Wall of the small intestine has all the four layers as in stomach (Chapter 30).

■ INTESTINAL VILLI AND GLANDS OF SMALL INTESTINE

■ INTESTINAL VILLI

Mucous membrane of small intestine is covered by minute projections called **villi**.

Villi in small intestine are lined by columnar cells, which are called **enterocytes**. Each enterocyte gives rise to hair-like projections called **microvilli**. Within each villus, there is a central channel called **lacteal**. The lacteal opens into lymphatic vessels. It contains blood vessels also.

■ CRYPTS OF LIEBERKÜHN OR INTESTINAL GLANDS

Crypts of Lieberkühn or intestinal glands are simple tubular glands of intestine. These glands open into lumen of intestine between the villi. Intestinal glands are lined by columnar cells. Lining of each gland is continuous with epithelial lining of the villi **(Fig. 35.1)**.

Epithelial cells lining the intestinal glands undergo division by mitosis at a faster rate. Newly formed cells push

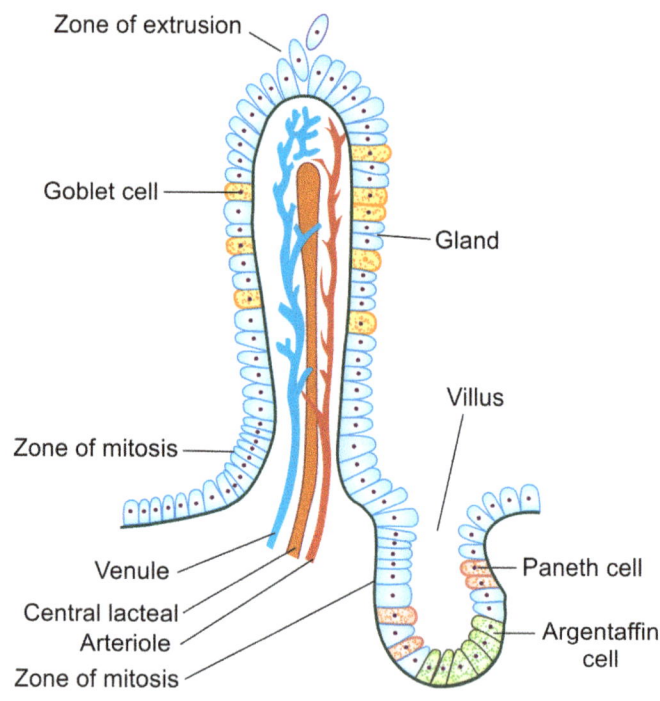

FIGURE 35.1: Intestinal gland and villus.

the older cells upward over the lining of villi. The cells which move to villi are called **enterocytes**.

Enterocytes secrete the enzymes. Old enterocytes are continuously shed into lumen along with enzymes.

Types of Cells in Intestinal Glands

Different types of cells are interposed between columnar cells of intestinal glands. Types of cells present in intestinal glands and their secretory functions are given in **Table 35.1**.

Three types of cells are interposed between columnar cells of the glands:

1. **Argentaffin cells** which are otherwise known as **enterochromaffin cells**. These cells secrete intrinsic factor that is essential for the absorption of vitamin B_{12}.
2. **Goblet cells** which secrete mucus.
3. **Paneth cells** which secrete the cytokines called defensins.

■ BRUNNER'S GLANDS

In addition to intestinal glands, the first part of duodenum contains some mucus glands, called Brunner's glands. Brunner's glands secrete mucus and traces of enzymes.

TABLE 35.1: Secretory function of cells in intestinal glands.

Cells	Secretory products
Enterocytes (columnar cells)	Pepsinogen Rennin Lipase Gelatinase Urase
Argentaffin cells	Intrinsic factor of Castle
Goblet cells	Mucus
Paneth cells	Cytokines: Defensins Lysosomal enzymes
Enterochromaffin (EC) cells	Serotonin
Enterochromaffin-like (ECL) cells	Histamine
Enteroendocrine cells	
G cells	Gastrin
S cells	Secretin
I cells	Cholecystokinin
K cells	Glucose-dependent insulinotropic hormone or gastric inhibitory peptide
M cells	Motilin
L cells	Glucagon-like polypeptide-1 Glucagon-like polypeptide-2 Peptide YY
Unnamed cells	Vasoactive intestinal polypeptide

Nerve endings in small intestine secrete vasoactive intestinal polypeptide and substance P.

■ PROPERTIES AND COMPOSITION OF SUCCUS ENTERICUS

Secretion from small intestine is called succus entericus.

■ PROPERTIES OF SUCCUS ENTERICUS

Volume : 1,800 mL/day
Reaction : Alkaline
pH : 8.3

■ COMPOSITION OF SUCCUS ENTERICUS

Succus entericus contains water (99.5%) and solids (0.5%). Solids include organic and inorganic substances. Refer **Figure 35.2** for details. Bicarbonate concentration is slightly high in succus entericus.

■ FUNCTIONS OF SUCCUS ENTERICUS

■ 1. DIGESTIVE FUNCTION

Enzymes of succus entericus act on the partially digested food and convert them into final digestive products.

Proteolytic Enzymes

Proteolytic enzymes in succus entericus are the **peptidases** which convert peptides into amino acids **(Fig. 35.2)**.

Amylolytic Enzymes

Amylolytic enzymes of succus entericus are listed in **Figure 35.2**. **Lactase**, **sucrase** and **maltase** convert the disaccharides (lactose, sucrose and maltose) into two molecules of monosaccharides **(Table 35.2)**.

Dextrinase converts dextrin, maltose and maltotriose into glucose. **Trehalase** or **trehalose glucohydrolase** causes hydrolysis of trehalose (carbohydrate present in mushrooms and yeast) and converts it into glucose.

Lipolytic Enzyme

Lipolytic enzyme in small intestine is called **intestinal lipase**. It acts on triglycerides and converts them into fatty acids.

■ 2. PROTECTIVE FUNCTION

i. Mucus present in the succus entericus protects intestinal wall from the acid chyme, which enters the intestine from stomach; thereby it prevents the intestinal ulcer.
ii. Paneth cells of intestinal glands secrete **defensins** which are the antimicrobial peptides.

■ 3. ACTIVATOR FUNCTION

Enterokinase present in intestinal juice activates trypsinogen into trypsin. Trypsin which in turn activates other enzymes (Chapter 33).

■ 4. HEMOPOIETIC FUNCTION

The **intrinsic factor of Castle**, which is present in the intestine, plays an important role in erythropoiesis (Chapter 9).

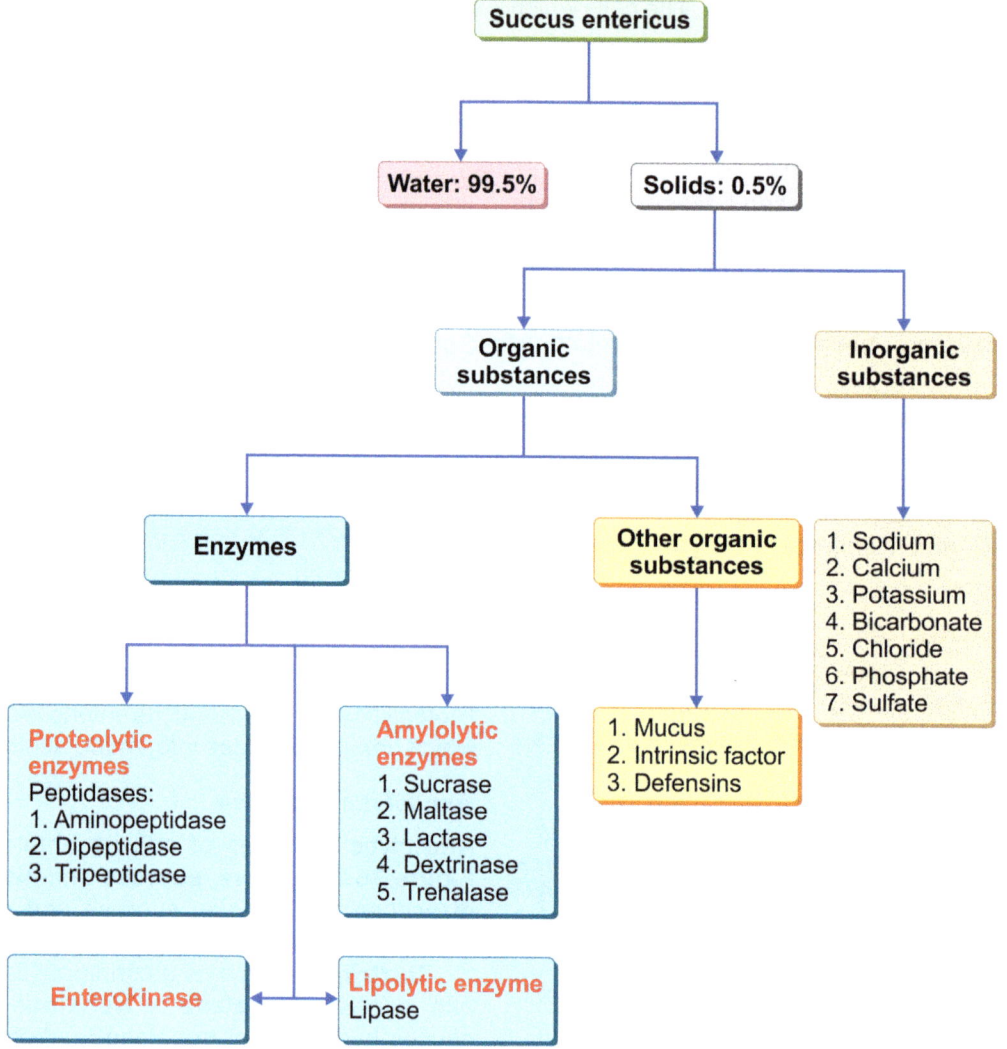

FIGURE 35.2: Composition of succus entericus.

TABLE 35.2: Digestive enzymes of succus entericus.

Enzyme	Substrate	End products
Peptidases	Peptides	Amino acids
Sucrase	Sucrose	Fructose Glucose
Maltase	Maltose Maltotriose	Glucose
Lactase	Lactose	Galactose Glucose
Dextrinase	Dextrin Maltose Maltotriose	Glucose
Trehalase	Trehalose	Glucose
Intestinal lipase	Triglycerides	Fatty acids

5. HYDROLYTIC PROCESS

Intestinal juice helps in all the enzymatic reactions of digestion.

FUNCTIONS OF SMALL INTESTINE

1. MECHANICAL FUNCTION

The mixing movements of small intestine help in the thorough mixing of chyme with the digestive juices like succus entericus, pancreatic juice and bile.

2. SECRETORY FUNCTION

Small intestine secretes succus entericus, enterokinase and the GI hormones.

3. HORMONAL FUNCTION

Small intestine secretes many GI hormones such as secretin, cholecystokinin, etc. These hormones regulate the movement of GI tract and secretory activities of small intestine and pancreas.

4. DIGESTIVE FUNCTION

Refer functions of succus entericus.

5. ACTIVATOR FUNCTION
Refer functions of succus entericus.

6. HEMOPOIETIC FUNCTION
Refer functions of succus entericus.

7. HYDROLYTIC FUNCTION
Refer functions of succus entericus.

8. ABSORPTIVE FUNCTIONS
Presence of villi and microvilli in small intestinal mucosa increases the surface area of the mucosa. This facilitates the absorptive function of intestine.

Digested products of foodstuffs, proteins, carbohydrates, fats and other nutritive substances such as vitamins, minerals and water are absorbed mostly in small intestine. From the lumen of intestine, these substances pass through lacteal of villi, cross the mucosa and enter the blood directly or through lymphatics.

REGULATION OF SECRETION OF SUCCUS ENTERICUS

Secretion of succus entericus is regulated by both the nervous and hormonal mechanisms.

NERVOUS REGULATION
Stimulation of parasympathetic nerves causes vasodilatation and increases the secretion of succus entericus. Stimulation of sympathetic nerves causes vasoconstriction and decreases the secretion of succus entericus. But, the role of these nerves in the regulation of intestinal secretion in physiological conditions is uncertain.

However, the local nervous reflexes play an important role in increasing the secretion of intestinal juice. When chyme enters the small intestine, the mucosa is stimulated by tactile stimuli or irritation. It causes development of local nervous reflexes, which stimulate the glands of intestine.

HORMONAL REGULATION
When the chyme enters the small intestine, the intestinal mucosa secretes enterocrinin, secretin and cholecystokinin which promote the secretion of succus entericus by stimulating the intestinal glands.

APPLIED PHYSIOLOGY: DISORDERS OF SMALL INTESTINE

1. MALABSORPTION
Malabsorption is the failure to absorb nutrients, such as proteins, carbohydrates, fats and vitamins. Malabsorption affects growth and development of the body. It also causes some specific diseases (see below).

2. MALABSORPTION SYNDROME
Malabsorption syndrome is the condition characterized by the failure of digestion and absorption in small intestine.

3. INFLAMMATORY BOWEL DISEASE
Inflammatory bowel disease (IBD) is a group of intestinal disorders characterized by chronic inflammation of digestive tract. Common types of IBD are:

Common Types of Inflammatory Bowel Disease
i. **Crohn's disease** that involves inflammation of small intestine.
ii. **Ulcerative colitis** which involves inflammation of large intestine.

4. TROPICAL SPRUE
Tropical sprue is a malabsorption syndrome affecting the residents of or visitors of tropical areas where the disease is epidemic.

5. STEATORRHEA
Steatorrhea is the condition caused by deficiency of pancreatic lipase resulting in malabsorption of fat. Refer Chapter 33 for details.

6. CELIAC DISEASE
Celiac disease is an autoimmune disease caused by gluten intake and it leads to damage of villi in small intestine resulting in impaired digestion and absorption. It is also known as **gluten-sensitive enteropathy**, **celiac sprue** and **non-tropical sprue**.

Chapter 36: Large Intestine and its Secretion

CHAPTER OUTLINE

- FUNCTIONAL ANATOMY
- SECRETION OF LARGE INTESTINE
- FUNCTIONS OF LARGE INTESTINE
- APPLIED PHYSIOLOGY: DISORDERS OF LARGE INTESTINE

FUNCTIONAL ANATOMY OF LARGE INTESTINE

Large intestine is also known as **colon**. It extends from **ileocecal valve** up to **anus (Fig. 30.1)**.

PARTS OF LARGE INTESTINAL JUICE

Large intestine consists of seven parts:

1. Cecum with appendix.
2. Ascending colon.
3. Transverse colon.
4. Descending colon.
5. Sigmoid colon or pelvic colon.
6. Rectum.
7. Anal canal.

Wall of large intestine is formed by four layers of structures like any other part of the digestive system (Chapter 30).

SECRETION OF LARGE INTESTINE

Large intestinal juice is a watery fluid with pH of 8.0.

COMPOSITION OF LARGE INTESTINAL JUICE

Large intestinal juice contains 99.5% of water and 0.5% of solids. Refer **Figure 36.1** for details.

Digestive enzymes are absent and concentration of bicarbonate is high in large intestinal juice.

FUNCTIONS OF LARGE INTESTINAL JUICE

1. Neutralization of Acids

Strong acids formed by bacterial action in large intestine are neutralized by the alkaline nature of large intestinal juice. Alkalinity of this juice is mainly due to the presence of large quantity of bicarbonate.

2. Lubrication Activity

Mucin present in secretion of large intestine lubricates the mucosa of large intestine and bowel contents, so that the movement of bowel is facilitated.

Mucin also protects mucous membrane of large intestine by preventing the damage caused by mechanical injury or chemical substances.

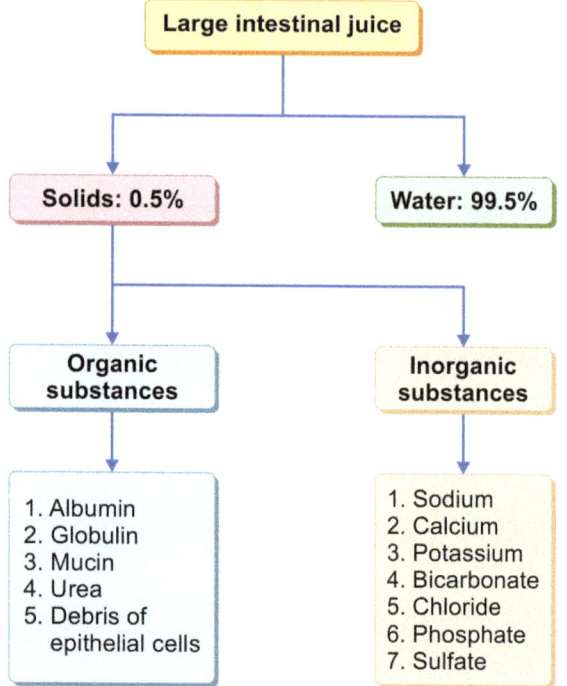

FIGURE 36.1: Composition of large intestinal juice.

FUNCTIONS OF LARGE INTESTINE

1. ABSORPTIVE FUNCTION

Large intestine plays an important role in the absorption of various substances such as water, electrolytes and organic substances like glucose, alcohol and drugs like anesthetic agents, sedatives and steroids.

2. FORMATION OF FECES

After the absorption of nutrients, water and other substances, unwanted substances in the large intestine form feces, which is excreted out.

3. EXCRETORY FUNCTION

Large intestine excretes heavy metals like mercury, lead, bismuth and arsenic through feces.

4. SECRETORY FUNCTION

Large intestine secretes mucin and inorganic substances like chlorides and bicarbonates.

5. SYNTHETIC FUNCTION

Bacterial flora of large intestine synthesizes folic acid, vitamin B_{12} and vitamin K.

By this function, large intestine contributes in erythropoietic activity and blood clotting mechanism.

APPLIED PHYSIOLOGY: DISORDERS OF LARGE INTESTINE

1. DIARRHEA

Diarrhea is the frequent and profuse discharge of intestinal contents in loose and fluid form. It occurs due to the increased movement of intestine. It may be acute or chronic.

Causes of Diarrhea

i. Intake of contaminated water or food, artificial sweeteners found in food, spicy food, etc.
ii. Indigestion.
iii. Infections by bacteria, viruses and parasites.
iv. Reaction to medicines like antibiotics, laxatives.
v. Intestinal diseases.

Features of Diarrhea

Severe diarrhea results in loss of excess water and electrolytes leading to **dehydration** and **electrolyte imbalance**. Chronic diarrhea results in **hypokalemia** and **metabolic acidosis**. Other features of diarrhea are abdominal pain, nausea and **bloating** (a condition in which the subject feels the abdomen full and tight due to excess intestinal gas).

2. CONSTIPATION

Constipation is the failure of voiding of feces, which produces discomfort. It is due to the lack of movements necessary for defecation (Chapter 37). Due to absence of mass movement in colon, feces remain in the large intestine for a longtime resulting in absorption of fluid. So, the feces become hard and dry.

Causes of Constipation

i. Lack of fiber or lack of liquids in diet.
ii. Irregular bowel habit.
iii. Spasm of sigmoid colon.
iv. Many types of diseases.
v. Drugs such as diuretics, pain relievers, antihypertensive drugs antiparkinson drugs, antidepressants and anticonvulsants.
vi. Dysfunction of myenteric plexus in large intestine called megacolon.

3. MEGACOLON

Megacolon is a condition characterized by distension and hypertrophy of colon associated with constipation. It is caused by the absence or damage of ganglionic cells in myenteric plexus, which causes dysfunction of myenteric plexus. It leads to accumulation of large quantity of feces in colon. Colon is distended to a diameter of 4 to 5 inches. It also results in **hypertrophy of colon**.

4. APPENDICITIS

Appendix is a small, finger-like pouch projecting from cecum of ascending colon **(Fig. 30.1)**. Inflammation of appendix is known as appendicitis. It may occur by viral infection of the gastrointestinal (GI) tract or by blockage of connection between appendix and large intestine.

Major symptom of appendicitis is the pain, which starts around the umbilicus and then spreads to the lower right side of the abdomen. This pain becomes severe within 6 to 12 hours. Other features are nausea, vomiting, constipation, diarrhea and abdominal swelling.

If not treated immediately, appendix may rupture and the inflammation will spread to the whole body leading to severe complications, sometimes even death.

Chapter 37: Movements of Gastrointestinal Tract

CHAPTER OUTLINE

- MASTICATION
- DEGLUTITION
- MOVEMENTS OF STOMACH
- FILLING AND EMPTYING OF STOMACH
- VOMITING
- MOVEMENTS OF SMALL INTESTINE
- MOVEMENTS OF LARGE INTESTINE
- DEFECATION

■ MASTICATION

Mastication or **chewing** is the first mechanical process in GI tract by which the food substances are torn or cut into small particles and crushed or ground into a soft **bolus**.

Significances of Mastication

1. Breakdown of foodstuffs into smaller particles.
2. Mixing of saliva with food substances thoroughly.
3. Lubrication and moistening of dry food by saliva so that, the bolus can be easily swallowed.
4. Appreciation of taste of the food.

■ MUSCLES AND THE MOVEMENTS OF MASTICATION

Muscles of Mastication

1. Masseter muscle.
2. Temporal muscle.
3. Pterygoid muscles.
4. Buccinator muscle.

Movements of Mastication

1. Opening and closure of mouth.
2. Rotational movements of jaw.
3. Protraction and retraction of jaw.

■ CONTROL OF MASTICATION

Action of mastication is mostly a reflex process. It is carried out voluntarily also. Center for mastication is situated in medulla and cerebral cortex. Muscles of mastication are supplied by mandibular division of **trigeminal nerve** (V cranial nerve).

■ DEGLUTITION

Definition

Deglutition or **swallowing** is the process by which food passes from mouth into stomach.

Stages of Deglutition

Deglutition occurs in three stages:

I. Oral stage, when food moves from mouth to pharynx.
II. Pharyngeal stage, when food moves from pharynx to esophagus.
III. Esophageal stage, when food moves from esophagus to stomach.

■ I. ORAL STAGE OR FIRST STAGE

Oral stage is a voluntary stage. In this stage, the bolus from oral cavity passes into the pharynx by means of series of actions.

Sequence of Events during Oral Stage

1. Bolus is placed over posterodorsal surface of the tongue. It is called the preparatory position.
2. Anterior part of tongue is retracted and depressed.
3. Posterior part of tongue is elevated and retracted against hard palate. This pushes the bolus backwards into pharynx.
4. Forceful contraction of tongue against the palate produces a positive pressure in the posterior part of

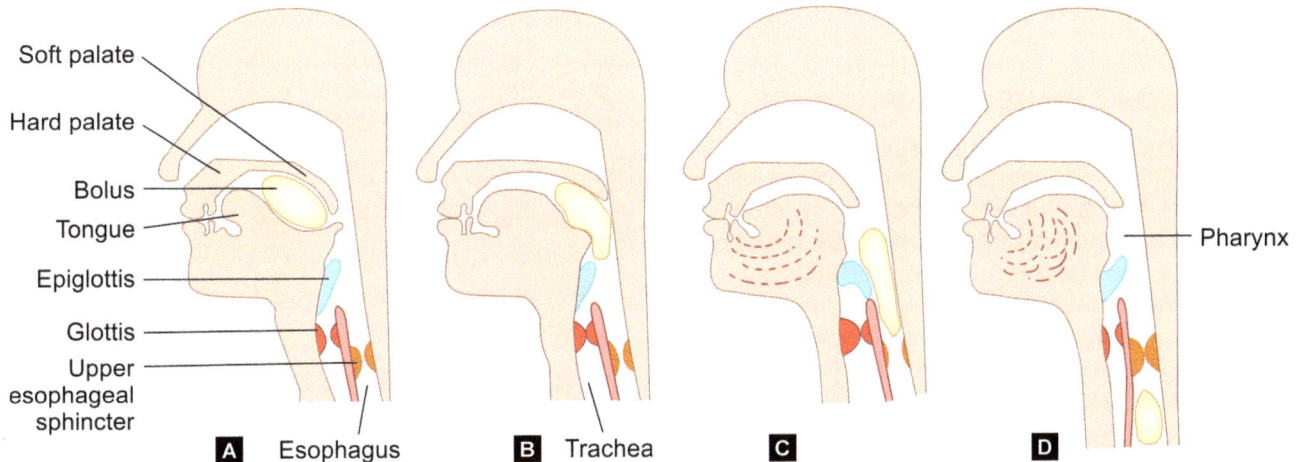

FIGURE 37.1: Stages of deglutition. **A.** Preparatory stage; **B.** Oral stage; **C.** Pharyngeal stage; **D.** Esophageal stage.

oral cavity. This pressure in oral cavity also pushes the food into pharynx **(Fig. 37.1)**.

■ II. PHARYNGEAL STAGE OR SECOND STAGE

Pharyngeal stage is an involuntary stage. In this stage, the bolus is pushed from pharynx into the esophagus. Pharynx is a common passage for food and air. It divides into larynx and esophagus. Larynx lies anteriorly and continues as respiratory passage. Esophagus lies behind the larynx and continues as GI tract. Since pharynx communicates with mouth, nose, larynx and esophagus, during this stage of deglutition, the **bolus** from pharynx can enter into **four paths**:

1. It can come back into mouth.
2. It can go upwards into nasopharynx.
3. It can move forwards into larynx.
4. It can move downwards into esophagus.

However, due to various coordinated movements, bolus is made to enter only into the esophagus. Entrance of bolus through other paths is prevented as follows.

1. Back into Mouth

Return of bolus back into the mouth is prevented by:

   i. Position of tongue against the soft palate (roof of the mouth).
   ii. High intraoral pressure developed by the movement of tongue.

2. Upward into Nasopharynx

Movement of bolus into the nasopharynx from pharynx is prevented by elevation of **soft palate** along with its extension called **uvula**.

3. Forward into Larynx

Movement of bolus into the larynx is prevented by the following actions:

   i. Approximation of the vocal cords.
   ii. Forward and upward movement of larynx.
   iii. Backward movement of epiglottis to seal the opening of the larynx (glottis).

All these movements arrest respiration for a few seconds. It is called deglutition apnea.

Deglutition apnea

Apnea refers to temporary arrest of breathing. Deglutition apnea or **swallowing apnea** is the arrest of breathing during deglutition.

Choking

Choking is the inability to breathe due to obstruction or compression of respiratory passage. Sometimes during second stage of swallowing, solid food particles may enter larynx resulting in obstruction and choking. However, it may be prevented automatically by **gag reflex** (Chapter 93).

4. Entrance of Bolus into Esophagus

Since the other three paths are closed for the bolus, it has to pass only through esophagus. It occurs by the combined effects of various factors:

   i. Upward movement of larynx stretches the opening of esophagus.
   ii. Simultaneously, upper 3 to 4 cm of esophagus relaxes. This part of esophagus is formed by **cricopharyngeal muscle** and it is called **upper esophageal sphincter** or pharyngoesophageal sphincter.
   iii. At the same time, peristaltic contractions start in pharynx due to the contraction of pharyngeal muscles.
   iv. Elevation of larynx also lifts the glottis away from food passage.

All the factors mentioned above act together so that, bolus moves easily into the esophagus. Whole process takes place within 1 to 2 seconds. And this process is purely involuntary.

III. ESOPHAGEAL STAGE OR THIRD STAGE

It is also an involuntary stage. In esophageal stage food from stomach enters esophagus. Function of esophagus is to transport the bolus from pharynx to stomach. Movements of esophagus called **peristaltic waves** are specifically organized for this function. **Peristalsis** means a wave of contraction followed by a wave of relaxation of muscle fibers of GI tract, which travel in aboral direction (away from mouth). By this type of movement, the contents are propelled down along the GI tract.

Role of Lower Esophageal Sphincter

Lower esophageal sphincter is constricted always. When bolus enters this part of the esophagus, this sphincter relaxes so that the contents enter stomach. After entry of bolus into the stomach, this sphincter constricts and closes the lower end of esophagus.

Relaxation and constriction of lower esophageal sphincter occur in sequence with the arrival of peristaltic contractions of esophagus.

DEGLUTITION REFLEX

Though the beginning of swallowing is a voluntary act, later it becomes involuntary and it is carried out by a reflex action called deglutition reflex. This reflex occurs during the pharyngeal and esophageal stages.

Stimulus

When the bolus enters oropharyngeal region, the receptors present in this region are stimulated.

Afferent Fibers

Afferent impulses from the oropharyngeal receptors pass via glossopharyngeal nerve fibers to deglutition center.

Center

Deglutition center is at the floor of fourth ventricle in medulla oblongata of brain.

Efferent Fibers

Impulses from deglutition center travel through glossopharyngeal and vagus nerves (parasympathetic motor fibers) and reach soft palate, pharynx and esophagus. Glossopharyngeal nerve is concerned with pharyngeal stage of swallowing. Vagus nerve is concerned with esophageal stage.

Response

This reflex causes upward movement of soft palate to close nasopharynx and upward movement of larynx to close respiratory passage so that bolus enters the esophagus. Now, peristalsis occurs in esophagus pushing the bolus into stomach.

SWALLOWING IN BABIES

Swallowing hard and solid food by babies below 6 months is prevented by gag reflex or pharyngeal reflex. Gag reflex prevents choking (Chapter 93).

MOVEMENTS OF STOMACH

Movements of the stomach are:

1. Hunger contractions.
2. Receptive relaxation.
3. Peristalsis of stomach.

1. HUNGER CONTRACTIONS

Hunger contractions are the movements of empty stomach. These contractions are related to the sensations of hunger.

Hunger contractions are strong peristaltic contractions associated with hunger pain. This type of peristaltic contractions is different from the **digestive peristaltic contractions** (see below). Digestive peristaltic contractions usually occur in body and pyloric parts of the stomach. But hunger contractions of empty stomach involve the entire stomach.

2. RECEPTIVE RELAXATION

Receptive relaxation is the relaxation of upper portion of stomach when bolus enters the stomach from esophagus. Its significance is to accommodate the food easily without much increase in pressure inside the stomach.

3. PERISTALSIS OF STOMACH

When the food enters the stomach, peristaltic contraction or peristaltic wave appears with a frequency of 3/min. It starts from the lower part of the body of stomach, passes through pylorus till the pyloric sphincter.

Initially, the contraction appears as a slight indentation on the greater and lesser curvatures and travels towards pylorus. Later, the contraction becomes deeper while traveling. Finally, it ends with the constriction of pyloric sphincter. Some of the waves disappear before reaching the sphincter. Each peristaltic wave takes about one minute to travel from point of origin to point of ending.

This type of peristaltic contraction is called **digestive peristalsis** because it is responsible for the grinding of food particles and mixing them with gastric juice for digestive activities.

FILLING AND EMPTYING OF STOMACH

FILLING OF STOMACH

While taking food, it arranges itself in the stomach in different layers. First eaten food is placed against the greater curvature in fundus and body of the stomach. Successive layers of food particles lie nearer the lesser curvature until the last portion of food eaten lies near upper end of lesser curvature, adjacent to cardiac sphincter.

EMPTYING OF STOMACH

Gastric emptying is a process by which chyme from stomach is emptied into intestine. Food that is swallowed enters the stomach and remains there for about 3 hours. During this period, digestion takes place. Partly digested food becomes the chyme.

Chyme

Chyme is a semisolid mass of partially digested food that is formed in the stomach. It is acidic in nature. Acid chyme is emptied from stomach into intestine slowly with the help of peristaltic contractions. It takes about 3 to 4 hours for emptying of the chyme. This slow emptying is necessary to facilitate the final digestion and maximum (about 80%) absorption of digested food materials from small intestine. Gastric emptying occurs due to peristaltic waves in the body and pyloric part of stomach and simultaneous relaxation of pyloric sphincter.

Gastric emptying is influenced by various factors of gastric content and food.

Factors affecting gastric emptying are:

1. Volume of gastric content

Gastric emptying is directly proportional to the volume of gastric content. If the content of stomach is more, a large amount is emptied into the intestine rapidly.

2. Consistency of gastric content

Emptying of stomach depends upon consistency (degree of density) of the contents. Liquids, particularly the inert liquids like water (which do not stimulate the stomach) leave the stomach rapidly. Solids move out of stomach only after being converted into fluid or semifluid. Undigested solid particles are not easily emptied.

3. Chemical composition

Chemical composition of food also plays an important role in the emptying of the stomach. Carbohydrates are emptied rapidly than the proteins. Proteins are emptied rapidly than the fats.

4. pH of the gastric content

Gastric emptying is directly proportional to pH of the chyme.

5. Osmolar concentration of gastric content

Gastric content, which is isotonic to blood, leaves the stomach rapidly than hypotonic or hypertonic content.

VOMITING

Vomiting or emesis is the abnormal emptying of stomach and upper part of intestine through esophagus and mouth.

CAUSES OF VOMITING

Common causes of vomiting are:

1. Any gastrointestinal disorder.
2. Mechanical stimulation of pharynx.
3. Excess intake of alcohol.
4. Nauseating sight, odor or taste.
5. Unusual stimulation of labyrinthine apparatus as in the case of sea sickness, air sickness, car sickness or swinging.
6. Metabolic disturbances such as carbohydrate starvation and ketosis during **pregnancy**, acidosis during **diabetes** and uremia.

MECHANISM OF VOMITING

Nausea

Vomiting is always preceded by nausea. Nausea is unpleasant sensation which induces the desire for vomiting. It is characterized by secretion of large amount of saliva containing more amount of mucus.

Retching

Strong involuntary movements in GI tract start even before actual vomiting and intensify the feeling of vomiting. This condition is called retching (try to vomit). And, vomiting occurs few minutes after this.

Act of Vomiting

Act of vomiting involves series of movements that takes place in GI tract.

Sequence of events

1. Beginning of **antiperistalsis** which runs from ileum towards mouth through intestine pushing the intestinal contents into stomach within few minutes.
2. Deep inspiration followed by temporary cessation of breathing.
3. Closure of glottis.
4. Upward and forward movement of larynx and hyoid bone.
5. Elevation of soft palate.
6. Contraction of diaphragm and abdominal muscles with a characteristic jerk resulting in elevation of intra-abdominal pressure.
7. Compression of stomach between diaphragm and abdominal wall leading to rise in intragastric pressure.
8. Simultaneous relaxation of lower esophageal sphincter, esophagus and upper esophageal sphincter.
9. Forceful expulsion of gastric contents (vomitus) through esophagus, pharynx and mouth.

All the movements during act of vomiting throw the **vomitus** (materials ejected during vomiting) to exterior through mouth. Some movements play important roles by preventing the entry of vomitus through other routes and thereby prevent the adverse effect of the vomitus on many structures.

Such movements are:

1. Closure of glottis and cessation of breathing prevent entry of vomitus into the lungs.

2. Elevation of soft palate prevents entry of vomitus into the nasopharynx.
3. Larynx and hyoid bone move upward and forward and are placed in this position rigidly. This causes dilatation of throat which allows free exit of vomitus.

■ VOMITING REFLEX

Vomiting is a reflex act. Sensory impulses for vomiting arise from the irritated or distended part of GI tract or other organs and are transmitted to vomiting center through vagus and sympathetic fibers.

Vomiting center is situated in medulla oblongata near the nucleus tractus solitarius.

Motor impulses from the vomiting center are transmitted through V, VII, IX, X and XII cranial nerves to the upper part of GI tract; and through spinal nerves to diaphragm and abdominal muscles.

■ MOVEMENTS OF SMALL INTESTINE

Movements of small intestine are essential for mixing the chyme with digestive juices, propulsion of food and absorption.

Movements of small intestine are of four types:
1. Mixing movements:
    i. Segmentation movements.
    ii. Pendular movements.
2. Propulsive movements:
    i. Peristaltic movements.
    ii. Peristaltic rush.
3. Peristalsis in fasting: Migrating motor complex.
4. Movements of villi.

■ MIXING MOVEMENTS

Mixing movements of small intestine are responsible for proper mixing of chyme with digestive juices such as pancreatic juice, bile and intestinal juice. Mixing movements of small intestine are segmentation contractions and pendular movements.

Segmentation Contractions

Segmentation contractions are the common type of movements of small intestine, which occur regularly or irregularly but in a rhythmic fashion. So, these movements are also called rhythmic segmentation contractions.

Contractions occur at regularly spaced intervals along a section of intestine. Segment of the intestine involved in each contraction is about 1 to 5 cm long. Segments of intestine in between the contracted segments are relaxed. Length of the relaxed segments is same as that of the contracted segments. These alternate segments of contraction and relaxation give appearance of rings resembling the chain of sausages.

After sometime, contracted segments are relaxed and the relaxed segments are contracted (Fig. 37.2). Therefore,

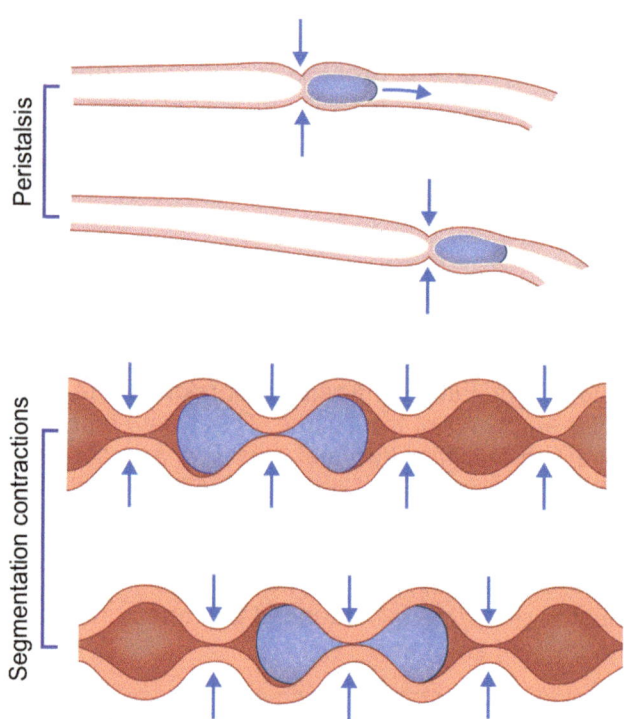

FIGURE 37.2: Movements of small intestine.

segmentation contractions chop the chyme many times. This helps in mixing of chyme with digestive juices.

Pendular Movement

Pendular movement is the sweeping movement of small intestine resembling movements of pendulum of clock. Small portions of intestine (loops) sweep forward and backward or upward and downward. It helps in mixing of chyme with digestive juices.

■ PROPULSIVE MOVEMENTS

Propulsive movements are movements of small intestine which push the chyme in aboral direction through intestine. Propulsive movements are peristaltic movements and peristaltic rush.

Peristaltic Movements

Peristalsis (see above for details) travels from point of stimulation in both directions. But under normal conditions, the progress of contraction in an oral direction is inhibited quickly and the contractions disappear. Only the contraction that travels in an aboral direction persists.

Peristaltic Rush

Sometimes, small intestine shows a powerful peristaltic contraction. It is caused by excessive irritation of intestinal mucosa or extreme distention of the intestine. This type of powerful contraction begins in duodenum and passes through entire length of small intestine and reaches the ileocecal valve within few minutes. This is called peristaltic rush or rush waves.

Peristaltic rush sweeps the contents of intestine into colon. Thus, it relieves the small intestine off either irritants or excessive distention.

■ PERISTALSIS IN FASTING: MIGRATING MOTOR COMPLEX

Peristalsis in fasting or migrating motor complex is a type of peristaltic contraction, which occurs in stomach and small intestine during the periods of fasting for several hours. It is different from regular peristalsis because, a large portion of stomach or intestine is involved in this contraction. Contraction extends to about 20 to 30 cm of the stomach or intestine. This type of movement occurs once in every 1½ to 2 hours.

Significance of Peristalsis in Fasting

Peristalsis in fasting sweeps the excess digestive secretions into colon and prevents the accumulation of secretions in stomach and intestine. It also sweeps the residual undigested materials into colon.

■ MOVEMENTS OF VILLI

Intestinal villi also show movements simultaneously along with intestinal movements. Movements of villi are shortening and elongation, which occur alternatively and help in emptying lymph from the central lacteal into the lymphatic system. Surface area of villi is increased during elongation. This helps absorption of digested food particles from the lumen of intestine.

Movements of villi are caused by local nervous reflexes, which are initiated by the presence of chyme in small intestine.

■ MOVEMENTS OF LARGE INTESTINE

Large intestine shows sluggish movements. Still, these movements are important for mixing, propulsive and absorptive functions. Large intestine shows two types of movements:

■ MIXING MOVEMENTS: SEGMENTATION CONTRACTIONS

Large circular constrictions, which appear in the colon, are called mixing segmentation contractions. The contractions occur at regular distance in colon. Length of the portion of colon involved in each contraction is nearly about 2.5 cm.

■ PROPULSIVE MOVEMENTS: MASS PERISTALSIS

Mass peristalsis or mass movement propels the feces from colon towards anus. Usually, this movement occurs only a few times every day. Duration of mass movement is about 10 minutes in the morning before or after breakfast. This is because of the neurogenic factors like gastrocolic reflex (see below) and parasympathetic stimulation.

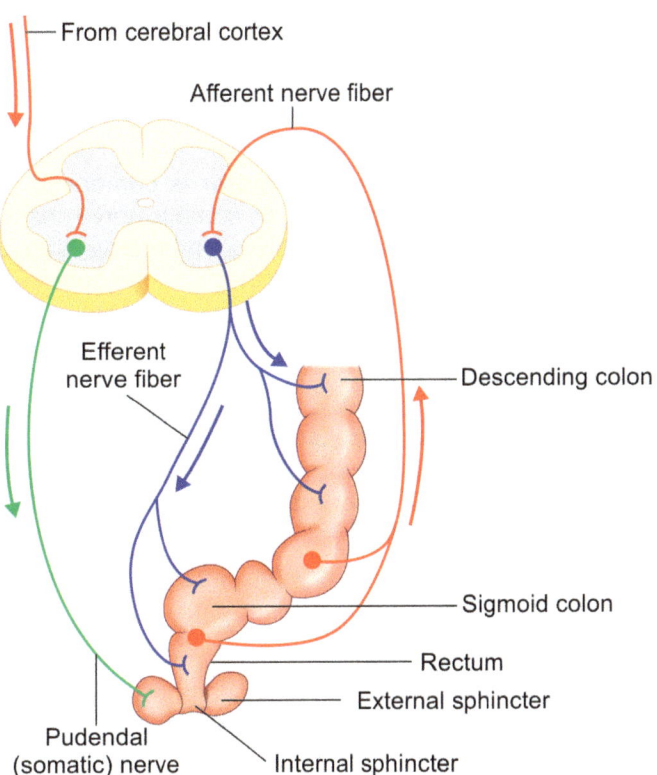

FIGURE 37.3: Defecation reflex. Afferent and efferent fibers of the reflex pass through pelvic (parasympathetic) nerve. Voluntary control of defecation is by pudendal (somatic) nerve. Defecation center is in the sacral segments of spinal cord.

■ DEFECATION

Voiding of feces is known as defecation. **Feces** is formed in the large intestine and stored in **sigmoid colon**. By the influence of an appropriate stimulus, it is expelled out through anus. This is prevented by tonic constriction of anal sphincters, in the absence of the stimulus.

■ DEFECATION REFLEX

Mass movement drives the feces into sigmoid or pelvic colon. In the sigmoid colon, feces is stored. Desire for defecation occurs when some feces enters rectum due to the mass movement. Usually, the desire for defecation is elicited by an increase in **intrarectal pressure** to about 20 to 25 cm H_2O.

Usual stimulus for defecation is intake of liquid like coffee or tea or water. But, it differs from person to person.

Act of Defecation

Act of defecation is preceded by voluntary efforts like assuming an appropriate posture, voluntary relaxation of external sphincter and the compression of abdominal contents by voluntary contraction of abdominal muscles.

Usually, the rectum is empty. During development of mass movement, the feces is pushed into rectum and the defecation reflex is initiated. Process of defecation involves the contraction of rectum and relaxation of internal and external anal sphincters.

Internal anal sphincter is made up of smooth muscle and it is innervated by parasympathetic nerve fibers via pelvic nerve. **External anal sphincter** is composed of skeletal muscle and it is controlled by somatic nerve fibers, which pass through pudendal nerve. Pudendal nerve always keeps the external sphincter constricted and the sphincter can relax only when the pudendal nerve is inhibited.

Gastrocolic Reflex

Gastrocolic reflex is the contraction of rectum followed by desire for defecation caused by distention of stomach by food. It is mediated by intrinsic nerve fibers of GI tract. This reflex causes only a weak contraction of rectum. But it initiates defecation reflex.

Failure of voiding of feces is called **constipation** (Chapter 36).

■ PATHWAY FOR DEFECATION REFLEX

When rectum is distended due to the entry of feces by mass movement, sensory nerve endings are stimulated. Impulses from the nerve endings are transmitted via afferent fibers of pelvic nerve to the defecation center, situated in sacral segments (center) of spinal cord.

The center, in turn sends motor impulses to the descending colon, sigmoid colon and rectum via efferent nerve fibers of pelvic nerve. Motor impulses cause strong contraction of descending colon, sigmoid colon and rectum and relaxation of internal sphincter.

Simultaneously, voluntary relaxation of external sphincter occurs. It is due to the inhibition of pudendal nerve by impulses arising from cerebral cortex **(Fig. 37.3)**.

MODEL QUESTIONS IN DIGESTIVE SYSTEM

■ LONG QUESTIONS

1. What are the different types of salivary glands? Describe the composition, functions and regulation of secretion of saliva.
2. Describe the different phases of gastric secretion with experimental evidences.
3. Explain the composition, functions and regulation of secretion of pancreatic juice.
4. Describe the composition, functions and regulation of secretion of bile. Enumerate the differences between the liver bile and gallbladder bile. Add a note on enterohepatic circulation.

■ SHORT QUESTIONS

1. Enteric nerve supply to GI tract.
2. Properties and composition of saliva.
3. Functions of saliva.
4. Nerve supply to salivary glands.
5. Glands of stomach.
6. Functions of stomach.
7. Properties and composition of gastric juice.
8. Functions of gastric juice.
9. Mechanism of secretion of hydrochloric acid in stomach.
10. Cephalic phase of gastric secretion.
11. Gastrin.
12. Gastritis.
13. Peptic ulcer.
14. Properties and composition of pancreatic juice.
15. Functions of pancreatic juice.
16. Regulation of exocrine function of pancreas.
17. Hormones affecting pancreatic secretion.
18. Composition of bile.
19. Functions of bile.
20. Bile salts/bile pigments.
21. Functions of liver.
22. Differences between liver bile and gallbladder bile.
23. Functions of gallbladder.
24. Jaundice.
25. Gall stones.
26. Properties and composition of succus entericus.
27. Functions of small intestine.
28. Functions of large intestine.
29. Mastication.
30. Swallowing.
31. Movements of stomach.
32. Filling and emptying of stomach.
33. Vomiting.
34. Movements of small intestine.
35. Movements of large intestine.

■ VERY SHORT ANSWER QUESTIONS

1. Functions of digestive system.
2. Functions of sympathetic and parasympathetic nerves on GI tract.
3. Functions of mouth.
4. Classify salivary glands with examples.
5. Structure and duct system of salivary glands.
6. Mention ducts of major salivary glands.
7. Properties of saliva.
8. Enzymes in saliva.
9. Reflexes regulating salivary secretion.
10. Hypersalivation.
11. Hyposalivation.
12. Xerostomia.
13. Drooling.
14. Chorda tympani syndrome.
15. Cells present in glands of stomach and their secretory products.
16. Pavlov's pouch.
17. Sham feeding.
18. Local myenteric reflex.
19. Vagovagal reflex.
20. Enterogastric reflex.
21. Duct system in pancreas.
22. Trypsin/chymotrypsin/peptidase/pancreatic lipase.
23. Neutralizing action of pancreatic juice.
24. Steatorrhea.
25. Secretin.
26. Cholecystokinin.
27. Choleretics and cholagogues.
28. Hepatic lobule and portal triad.
29. Biliary system.
30. Blood supply to liver.
31. Enterohepatic circulation.
32. Properties of bile.
33. Jaundice in newborn babies.
34. Malabsorption and malabsorption syndrome.
35. Parts of large intestine.
36. Deglutition reflex.
37. Deglutition apnea.
38. Choking.
39. Gag reflex.
40. Receptive relaxation.
41. Migrating motor complex.
42. Movements of intestinal villi.
43. Movements of large intestine.
44. Constipation.
45. Diarrhea.

SECTION 5: RENAL PHYSIOLOGY AND SKIN

Chapter 38: Overview of Renal System

CHAPTER OUTLINE

- EXCRETION AND RENAL SYSTEM
- FUNCTIONAL ANATOMY OF KIDNEY
  - DIFFERENT LAYERS OF KIDNEY
  - TUBULAR STRUCTURES OF KIDNEY
- FUNCTIONS OF KIDNEY
  - ROLE IN HOMEOSTASIS
- EXCRETORY FUNCTION
- HEMATOPOIETIC FUNCTION
- ENDOCRINE FUNCTION
- REGULATION OF BLOOD PRESSURE
- REGULATION OF BLOOD CALCIUM LEVEL

EXCRETION AND RENAL SYSTEM

Excretion is the process by which unwanted substances and metabolic wastes are eliminated from the body.

Although various organs such as GI tract, liver, skin and lungs are involved in removal of wastes from the body, their excretory capacity is limited. But the renal system or urinary system has maximum capacity of excretory function.

Renal system includes:

1. A pair of kidneys.
2. Ureters.
3. Urinary bladder.
4. Urethra.

Kidneys produce the urine. **Ureters** transport the urine to **urinary bladder**. Urinary bladder stores urine until it is voided (emptied). Urine is voided from bladder through **urethra** (Fig. 38.1).

FUNCTIONAL ANATOMY OF KIDNEY

Kidney is a compound tubular gland covered by a connective tissue capsule.

There is a depression on the medial border of kidney called **hilum**, through which renal artery, renal veins, nerves and ureter pass.

DIFFERENT LAYERS OF KIDNEY

Components of kidney are arranged in three layers:

1. Outer cortex.
2. Inner medulla.
3. Renal sinus.

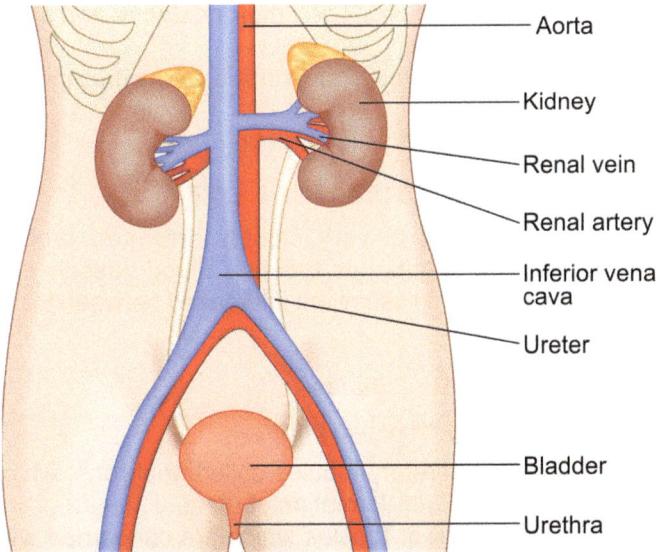

FIGURE 38.1: Urinary system.

1. Outer Cortex

Cortex is dark and granular in appearance. It contains **renal corpuscles** and **convoluted tubules** (Fig. 38.2). At intervals, cortical tissue penetrates medulla in the form of columns, which are called **renal columns** or **columns of Bertin**.

2. Inner Medulla

Medulla contains tubular and vascular structures arranged in parallel radial lines. It is divided into 8 to 18 **Malpighian pyramids** or **medullary pyramids**. Broad base of each

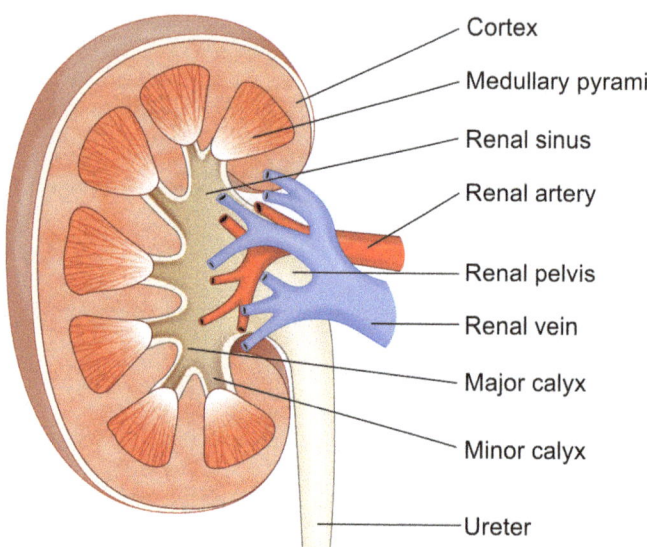

FIGURE 38.2: Longitudinal section of kidney.

pyramid is in contact with cortex and the apex projects into minor calyx.

3. Renal Sinus

Renal sinus consists of the following structures:

i. Upper expanded part of ureter called **renal pelvis**.
ii. Subdivisions of pelvis, 2 or 3 **major calyces** and about 8 **minor calyces**.
iii. Branches of nerves and arteries and tributaries of veins.
iv. Loose connective tissues and fat.

■ TUBULAR STRUCTURES OF KIDNEY

Kidney is made up of very closely arranged tubular structures called uriniferous tubules. Blood vessels and interstitial connective tissues are interposed between these tubules.

Parts of Uriniferous Tubules

Uriniferous tubules have two parts:

1. Terminal or secretary tubules called nephrons, which are concerned with formation of urine.
2. Collecting ducts or tubules which are concerned with transport of urine from nephrons to pelvis of ureter.

Collecting ducts unite to form **ducts of Bellini**, which open into minor calyces through papilla. Other details are given in Chapter 39.

■ FUNCTIONS OF KIDNEY

Kidneys perform several vital functions besides formation of urine. By excreting urine, kidneys play the principal role in homeostasis. Functions of kidneys are detailed below.

■ 1. ROLE IN HOMEOSTASIS

Primary function of kidneys is homeostasis. It is carried out the formation of urine. During the formation of urine, kidneys regulate various activities in the body, which are concerned with homeostasis as detailed below.

i. *Maintenance of Water Balance*

Kidneys are involved in the maintenance of electrolyte balance, especially sodium in relation to water balance. Kidneys retain sodium if the osmolarity of body water decreases and eliminate sodium when osmolarity increases.

ii. *Maintenance of Electrolyte Balance*

Maintenance of electrolyte balance, especially sodium is in relation to water balance. Kidneys retain sodium if the osmolarity of body water decreases and eliminate sodium when osmolarity increases.

iii. *Maintenance of Acid-base Balance*

The pH of blood and body fluids should be maintained within narrow range for healthy living. Body is under constant threat to develop acidosis, because of production of lot of acids during metabolic activities. However, it is prevented by kidneys, lungs and blood buffers, which eliminate these acids. Among these organs, kidneys play major role in preventing acidosis.

■ 2. EXCRETORY FUNCTION

Kidneys excrete the unwanted waste products which are formed during metabolic activities:

i. Urea: End product of amino acid metabolism.
ii. Uric acid: End product of nucleic acid metabolism.
iii. Creatinine: End product of metabolism in muscles.
iv. Bilirubin: End product of hemoglobin degradation.
v. Products of metabolism of other substances.
vi. Harmful foreign chemical substances such as toxins, drugs, heavy metals, pesticides, etc.

■ 3. HEMATOPOIETIC FUNCTION

Kidneys stimulate the production of erythrocytes by secreting **erythropoietin**. Erythropoietin is an important stimulating factor for erythropoiesis (Chapter 9). Kidney also secretes another factor called **thrombopoietin**, which stimulates the production of thrombocytes (Chapter 16).

■ 4. ENDOCRINE FUNCTION

Kidneys secrete many hormonal substances in addition to erythropoietin and thrombopoietin (Chapter 56).

Hormones secreted by kidneys are:

i. Erythropoietin.
ii. Thrombopoietin.
iii. Renin.
iv. 1,25-dihydroxycholecalciferol (calcitriol).
v. Prostaglandins.

■ 5. REGULATION OF BLOOD PRESSURE

Kidneys are involved in long-term regulation of arterial blood pressure (Chapter 71) by two ways by regulating ECF volume and through renin-angiotensin mechanism.

■ 6. REGULATION OF BLOOD CALCIUM LEVEL

Kidneys regulate blood calcium level by activating 1,25-dihydroxycholecalciferol into vitamin D. Vitamin D is necessary for the absorption of calcium from intestine (Chapter 52).

Chapter 39: Nephron

CHAPTER OUTLINE

- **DEFINITION AND PARTS**
- **RENAL CORPUSCLE**
  - SITUATION OF RENAL CORPUSCLE AND TYPES OF NEPHRON
  - STRUCTURE
- **TUBULAR PORTION OF NEPHRON**
  - PROXIMAL CONVOLUTED TUBULE
  - LOOP OF HENLE
  - DISTAL CONVOLUTED TUBULE
- **COLLECTING DUCT**
- **PASSAGE OF URINE**

DEFINITION AND PARTS

Nephron is defined as the structural and functional unit of kidney. Each kidney consists of 1 to 1.3 million nephrons. Number of nephrons decreases in old age.

Each nephron is formed by two parts:
1. A blind end called renal corpuscle or Malpighian corpuscle.
2. A tubular portion called renal tubule.

RENAL CORPUSCLE

Renal corpuscle is also known as **Malpighian corpuscle**. It is a spheroidal and slightly flattened structure with a diameter of about 200 μ (**Fig. 39.1**). Function of renal corpuscle is filtration of blood which forms the first phase of urine formation.

SITUATION OF RENAL CORPUSCLE AND TYPES OF NEPHRON

Renal corpuscle is situated in cortex of kidney either near the periphery or near medulla.

Classification of Nephrons

Based on the situation of renal corpuscle, nephrons are classified into two types:
1. Cortical nephrons or superficial nephrons.
2. Juxtamedullary nephrons.

1. Cortical nephrons

Cortical nephrons are the nephrons, which have their corpuscles in outer cortex of kidney near the periphery (**Fig. 39.2**). In human kidneys 85% nephrons are cortical nephrons.

2. Juxtamedullary nephrons

Juxtamedullary nephrons are the nephrons which have their corpuscles in the inner cortex near medulla or **corticomedullary junction**.

Features of both types of nephrons are given in **Table 39.1**.

STRUCTURE OF RENAL CORPUSCLE

Renal corpuscle is formed by two structures:
1. Glomerulus.
2. Bowman's capsule.

TABLE 39.1: Differences between cortical and juxtamedullary nephrons.

Features	Cortical nephron	Juxtamedullary nephron
Percentage	85%	15%
Situation of renal corpuscle	Outer cortex near the periphery	Inner cortex near medulla
Loop of Henle	Short Hairpin bend penetrates only up to outer zone of medulla	Long Hairpin bend penetrates up to the tip of papilla
Blood supply to tubule	Peritubular capillaries	Vasa recta
Function	Formation of urine	Mainly concentration of urine and also formation of urine

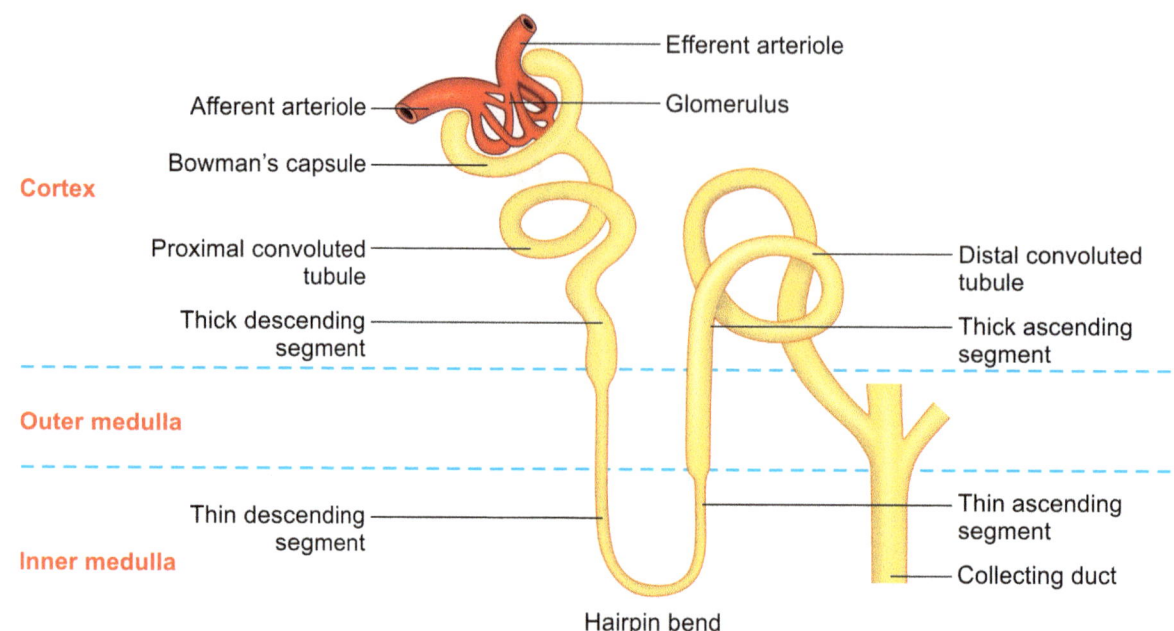

FIGURE 39.1: Structure of nephron.

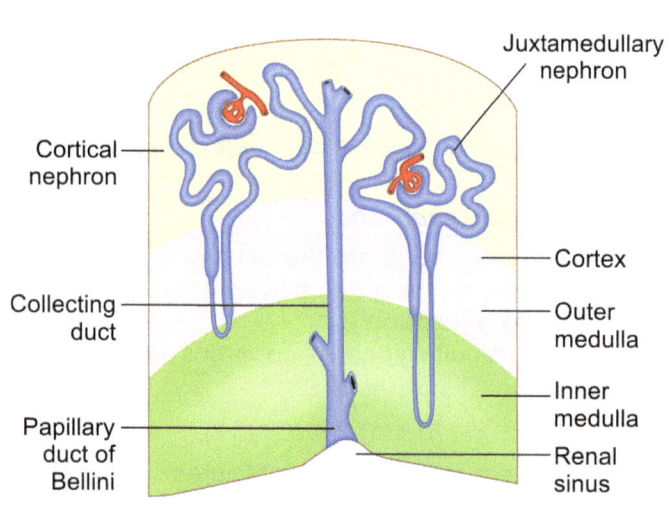

FIGURE 39.2: Types of nephron.

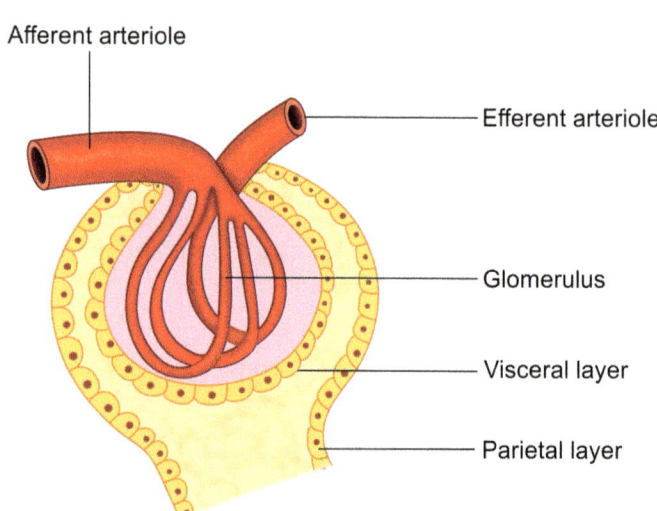

FIGURE 39.3: Renal corpuscle.

1. Glomerulus

Glomerulus is a tuft of capillaries called glomerular capillaries which are enclosed by Bowman's capsule. These capillaries are disposed between afferent arteriole and efferent arteriole. Thus, the vascular system in glomerulus is purely arterial (Fig. 39.3).

After entering Bowman's capsule, afferent arteriole divides into many small capillaries called **glomerular capillaries**. These capillaries arrange themselves as irregular loops and form anastomosis. All the capillaries finally reunite to form **efferent arteriole** which leaves the Bowman's capsule.

Diameter of efferent arteriole is less than that of afferent arteriole. This difference in diameter has functional significance.

Glomerular capillaries are made up of single layer of endothelial cells which are attached to a basement membrane. Endothelium has many pores called **fenestra** or **filtration pores**. Diameter of each pore is 0.1 μ. Presence of the fenestra is evidence of filtration function of the glomerulus.

2. Bowman's Capsule

Bowman's capsule encloses the glomerulus. Structure of Bowman's capsule is similar to a funnel with filter paper. Its diameter is 200 μ.

Bowman's capsule is formed by two layers:

i. Inner visceral layer.
ii. Outer parietal layer.

Visceral layer covers the glomerular capillaries. It is continued as parietal layer at the visceral pole. **Parietal layer** is continued with wall of the tubular portion of nephron. Cleft like space between visceral and parietal layers is continued as the lumen of tubular portion.

Functional histology of Bowman's capsule

Both the layers of Bowman's capsule are composed of a single layer of flattened epithelial cells resting on a basement membrane.

Capillary endothelial layer, basement membrane and epithelium of visceral layer of Bowman's capsule together form the **filtration membrane.** Refer Chapter 42 for structure of filtration membrane.

■ TUBULAR PORTION OF NEPHRON

Tubular portion of nephron is the continuation of Bowman's capsule.

It is made up of three parts:

1. Proximal convoluted tubule.
2. Loop of Henle.
3. Distal convoluted tubule.

■ 1. PROXIMAL CONVOLUTED TUBULE

Proximal convoluted tubule is the coiled portion arising from Bowman's capsule. It is situated in renal cortex. It is continued as descending limb of loop of Henle. Length of proximal convoluted tubule is 14 mm. And its diameter is 55μ.

Functional histology of proximal convoluted tubules

Proximal convoluted tubule is formed by single layer of cuboidal epithelial cells. Special feature of these cells is the presence of hair-like projections directed towards lumen of the tubule. Because of the presence of these projections, epithelial cells are called **brush-borderedcells**.

■ 2. LOOP OF HENLE

Loop of Henle consists of three segments:

i. Descending limb.
ii. Hairpin bend.
iii. Ascending limb.

i. Descending Limb

Descending limb of loop of Henle is made up of thick descending segment and thin descending segment. Thick descending segment is the direct continuation of proximal convoluted tubule. It descends down into medulla. It has a length of 6 mm and a diameter of 55 μ. Thick descending segment of Henle's loop is continued as thin descending segment **(Fig. 39.4)**.

ii. Hairpin Bend

Thin descending segment is continued as hairpin bend of the loop. Hairpin bend is continued as the ascending segment of loop of Henle.

iii. Ascending Limb

Ascending limb of Henle's loop has two parts, thin ascending segment and thick ascending segment. Thin ascending segment is the continuation of hairpin bend.

Total length of thin descending segment, hairpin bend and thin ascending segment of Henle's loop 10 to 15 mm and the diameter is 15 μ **(Table 39.2)**.

Thin ascending segment is continued as thick ascending segment. It is about 9 mm long with a diameter of 30 μ. Thick ascending segment ascends to the cortex and continues as distal convoluted tubule.

Length and Extent of Loop of Henle

Length and extent of the loop of Henle vary in different nephrons:

1. In cortical nephrons, it is short and the hairpin bend penetrates only up to outer medulla.
2. In juxtamedullary nephrons, this is long and the hairpin bend extends deep into the inner medulla. In some nephrons it even runs up to papilla.

■ 3. DISTAL CONVOLUTED TUBULE

Distal convoluted tubule is the continuation of thick ascending segment and it occupies the cortex of kidney. It is continued as collecting duct. Length of the distal convoluted tubule is 14.5 mm to 15 mm. It has a diameter of 22 μ to 50 μ.

Functional Histology

Distal convoluted tubule is lined by single layer of cuboidal epithelial cells without brush border. Epithelial cells in distal convoluted tubule are called **intercalated cells** (I **cells**).

■ COLLECTING DUCT

Distal convoluted tubule continues as the initial or arched collecting duct, which is in cortex. Lower part of the collecting duct lies in medulla. 7 to 10 initial collecting ducts unite to form the straight collecting duct, which passes through medulla.

Length of the collecting duct is 20 mm to 22 mm. Its diameter varies between 40 μ and 200 μ.

Functional Histology

Collecting duct is formed by cuboidal or columnar epithelial cells.

Epithelial cells of collecting duct are of two types:

1. **Principal** or **P cells**.
2. Intercalated or I cells.

■ PASSAGE OF URINE

At the inner zone of medulla, straight **collecting ducts** from each medullary pyramid unite to form **papillary ducts** or **ducts of Bellini** or papillary ducts of Bellini, which open into a 'V-shaped' area called **papilla**. Urine from each medullary pyramid is collected in the papilla. From here it is drained into a **minor calyx.** Three or four minor calyces unite to form one **major calyx.** Each kidney has got about 8 minor calyces and 2 to 3 major calyces.

From minor calyces, urine passes through major calyces, which open into the **pelvis of the ureter** (renal pelvis). Pelvis is the expanded portion of ureter present in the renal sinus.

From **renal pelvis**, urine passes through remaining portion of **ureter** and reaches **urinary bladder**.

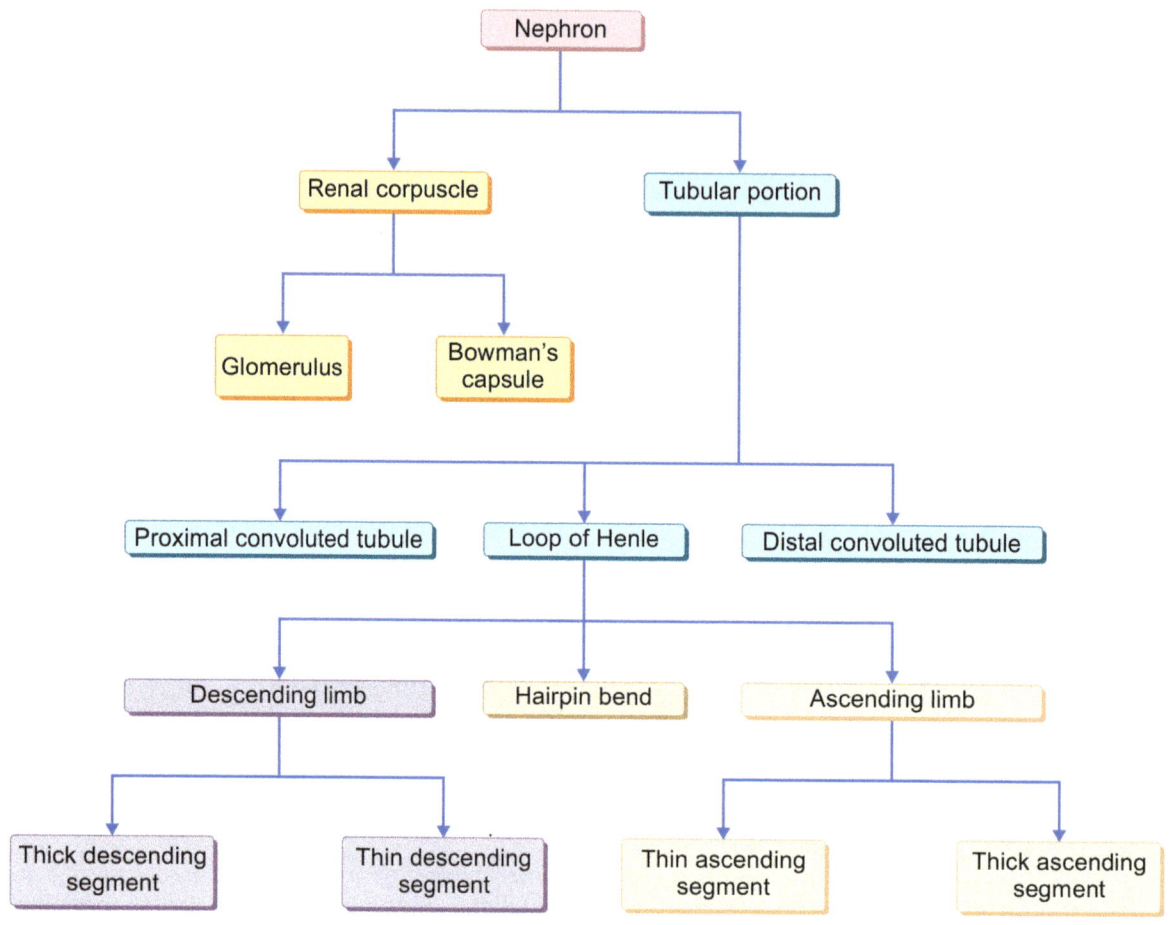

FIGURE 39.4: Parts of nephron.

TABLE 39.2: Epithelium, length and diameter and different parts of nephron and collecting duct.

Segment	Epithelium	Length (mm)	Diameter (μ)
Bowman's capsule	Flattened epithelium	–	200
Proximal convoluted tubule	Cuboidal cells with brush border	14	55
Thick descending segment	Cuboidal cells with brush border	6	55
Thin descending segment, hairpin bend and thin ascending segment	Flattened epithelium	10 to 15	15
Thick ascending segment	Cuboidal epithelium without brush border	9	30
Distal convoluted tubule	Cuboidal epithelium without brush border	14.5 to 15	22 to 50
Collecting duct	Cuboidal epithelium without brush border	20 to 22	40 to 200

Chapter 40: Juxtaglomerular Apparatus

CHAPTER OUTLINE

- **DEFINITION**
- **STRUCTURE**
  - MACULA DENSA
  - EXTRAGLOMERULAR MESANGIAL CELLS
  - JUXTAGLOMERULAR CELLS
- **FUNCTIONS**
  - SECRETION OF HORMONES
  - SECRETION OF OTHER SUBSTANCES
  - REGULATION OF GLOMERULAR BLOOD FLOW AND GLOMERULAR FILTRATION RATE

DEFINITION

Juxtaglomerular apparatus is a specialized organ situated near the glomerulus of each nephron (juxta means near).

STRUCTURE OF JUXTAGLOMERULAR APPARATUS

Juxtaglomerular apparatus is formed by three different structures:

1. Macula densa.
2. Extraglomerular mesangial cells.
3. Juxtaglomerular cells.

1. MACULA DENSA

Macula densa is the terminal portion of thick ascending segment that runs in between afferent and efferent arterioles of the same nephron. Actually, it is very close to afferent arteriole **(Fig. 40.1)**. Macula densa is formed by specialized epithalial cells which are packed closely.

Macula densa plays an important role in tubuloglomerular feedback mechanism. It also secretes **thromboxane A$_2$**.

2. EXTRAGLOMERULAR MESANGIAL CELLS

Extraglomerular cells are situated in the triangular region bound by afferent arteriole, efferent arteriole and macula densa. These cells are also called **agranular cells, lacis cells, Polkissen cells** or **Goormaghtigh cells**.

Extraglomerular mesangial cells secrete **prostaglandin** and **cytokines**.

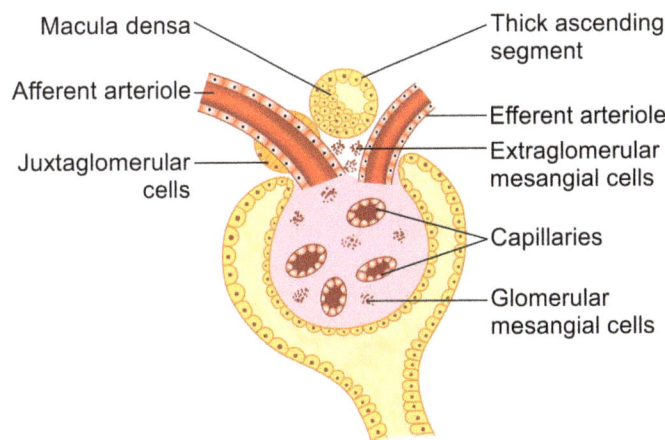

FIGURE 40.1: Juxtaglomerular apparatus.

Glomerular Mesangial Cells

Glomerular mesangial cells or intraglomerular mesangial cells are situated in between glomerular capillaries and form a cellular network which supports the capillary loops. These cells are contractile in nature and play an important role in regulating the glomerular filtration.

Glomerular mesangial cells are also phagocytic and secrete matrix of glomerular interstitium, prostaglandins and cytokines.

3. JUXTAGLOMERULAR CELLS

Juxtaglomerular cells are specialized **smooth muscle cells** situated in the wall of afferent arteriole just before it enters the Bowman's capsule. These smooth muscle cells are mostly present in tunica media and tunica adventitia of the wall of afferent arteriole.

Juxtaglomerular cells are also called **granular cells** because of the presence of secretary granules in their cytoplasm.

Polar Cushion or Polkissen

Juxtaglomerular cells form a thick cuff called **polar cushion** or **Polkissen** around the afferent arteriole before it enters the Bowman's capsule.

■ FUNCTIONS OF JUXTAGLOMERULAR APPARATUS

Primary function of juxtaglomerular apparatus is the secretion of hormonal substances. It also regulates the glomerular blood flow and glomerular filtration rate.

■ 1. SECRETION OF RENIN

Juxtaglomerular cells secrete renin. Renin is a peptide with 340 amino acids. Along with angiotensins, renin forms the renin-angiotensin system which is a hormone system that plays an important role in the maintenance of blood pressure (Chapter 71).

Stimulants for Renin Secretion

Secretion of renin is stimulated by four factors:

1. Fall in arterial blood pressure.
2. Reduction in the ECF volume.
3. Increased sympathetic activity.
4. Decreased load of sodium and chloride in macula densa.

Renin-angiotensin System

When renin is released into the blood, it acts on **angiotensinogen** or renin substrate which is an α_2 globulin and converts it into a decapeptide called **angiotensin I**. Angiotensin I is then converted into **angiotensin II** which is an octapeptide by the activity of **angiotensin-converting enzyme (ACE)** secreted from lungs. Most of the conversion of angiotensin I into angiotensin II takes place in lungs.

Angiotensin II is rapidly degraded into a heptapeptide called **angiotensin III** by **angiotensinases** which are present in RBCs and vascular beds in many tissues. Angiotensin III is converted into **angiotensin IV** which is a **hexapeptide (Fig. 40.2)**.

Actions of Angiotensins

Angiotensin I

Angiotensin I physiologically inactive and serves only as a precursor of angiotensin II.

Angiotensin II

Angiotensin II is the most active form. Its actions are given below:

1. *On blood vessels:*
   i. Angiotensin II increases arterial blood pressure by directly acting on the blood vessels and causing

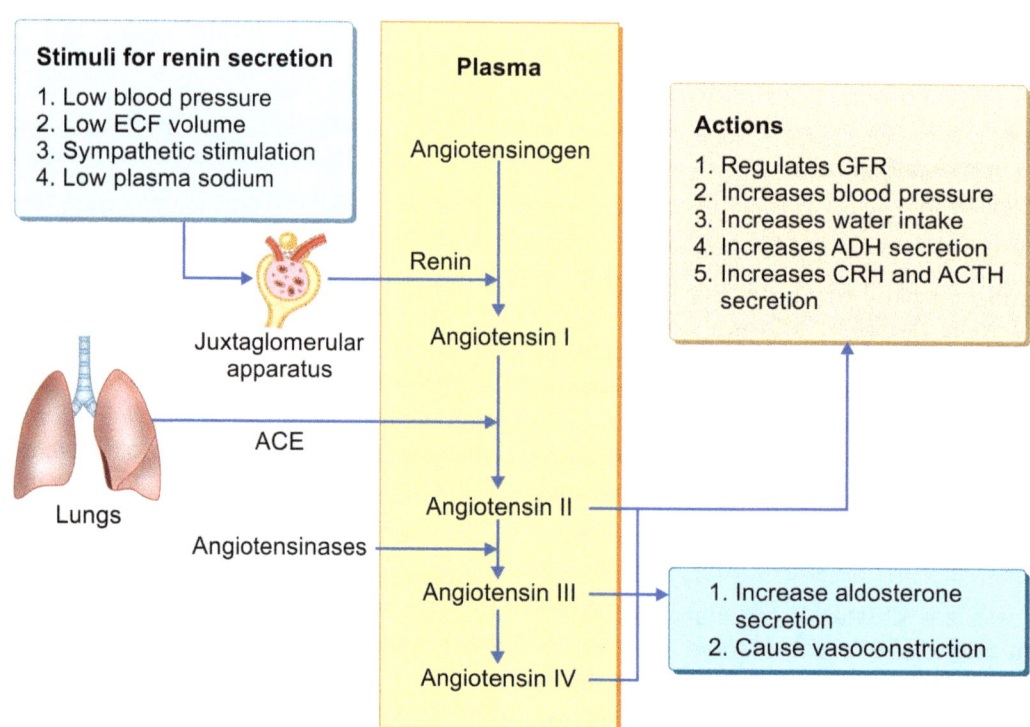

FIGURE 40.2: Renin-angiotensin system.
ECF = Extracellular fluid, ACE = Angiotensin-converting enzyme, GFR = Glomerular filtration rate, ADH = Antidiuretic hormone, CRH = Corticotropin-releasing hormone, ACTH = Adrenocorticotropic hormone.

vasoconstriction. It is a potent constrictor of arterioles. Earlier, when its other actions were not found it was called **hypertensin**.
ii. It increases blood pressure indirectly also by increasing the release of noradrenaline from postganglionic sympathetic fibers. Noradrenaline is a general vasoconstrictor (Chapter 71).

2. *On adrenal cortex:*
Angiotensin II stimulates zona glomerulosa of adrenal cortex to secrete aldosterone. Aldosterone acts on renal tubules and increases retention of sodium. This is also responsible for elevation of blood pressure.

3. *On kidney:*
   i. Angiotensin II regulates glomerular filtration rate by two ways:
      a. It constricts the efferent arteriole which causes decrease in filtration after an initial increase (Chapter 42).
      b. It contracts the glomerular mesangial cells resulting in decrease in surface area of glomerular capillaries resulting in filtration.
   ii. It increases sodium reabsorption from renal tubules. This action is more predominant on proximal tubules.

4. *On brain:*
   i. Angiotensin II inhibits baroreceptor reflex and thereby indirectly increases the blood pressure. Baroreceptor reflex is responsible for decreasing the blood pressure (Chapter 71).
   ii. It increases water intake by stimulating the thirst center.
   iii. It increases the secretion of corticotropin-releasing hormone (CRH) from hypothalamus. CRH in turn increases secretion of adrenocorticotropic hormone (ACTH) from pituitary.
   iv. It increases secretion of antidiuretic hormone (ADH) from hypothalamus.

5. *Other actions:* Angiotensin II acts as a growth factor in heart and it is thought to cause muscular hypertrophy and cardiac enlargement.

Angiotensin III

Angiotensin III increases the blood pressure and stimulates aldosterone secretion from adrenal cortex. It has 100% adrenal cortical stimulating activity and 40% vasopressor activity of angiotensin II.

Angiotensin IV

Angiotensin IV also has adrenal cortical stimulating and vasopressor activities.

■ 2. SECRETION OF OTHER SUBSTANCES

Extraglomerular mesangial cells of juxtaglomerular apparatus secrete prostaglandin (Chapter 56). Macula densa secretes thromboxane A_2.

■ 3. REGULATION OF GLOMERULAR BLOOD FLOW AND GLOMERULAR FILTRATION RATE

Macula densa of juxtaglomerular apparatus plays an important role in the feedback mechanism called tubuloglomerular feedback mechanism, which regulates the renal blood flow and glomerular filtration rate (Chapter 42 for details).

Chapter 41: Renal Circulation

CHAPTER OUTLINE

- RENAL BLOOD FLOW
- RENAL BLOOD VESSELS
- MEASUREMENT OF RENAL BLOOD FLOW
- REGULATION OF RENAL BLOOD FLOW
- SALIENT FEATURES OF RENAL CIRCULATION

■ RENAL BLOOD FLOW

Blood vessels of kidneys are highly specialized to facilitate the functions of nephrons in the formation of urine. Kidneys are supplied by renal arteries.

In adults, during resting conditions both the kidneys receive 1,300 mL of blood per minute or about 26% of cardiac output. Kidneys are the second organs to receive maximum blood flow, the first organ being liver which receives 1,500 mL per minute. Maximum blood supply to kidneys has got the functional significance.

■ RENAL BLOOD VESSELS

Renal Artery

Renal artery arises directly from abdominal aorta and enters the kidney through the hilus.

Segmental Artery

While passing through renal sinus, renal artery divides into many segmental arteries, which subdivide into interlobar arteries **(Fig. 41.1)**.

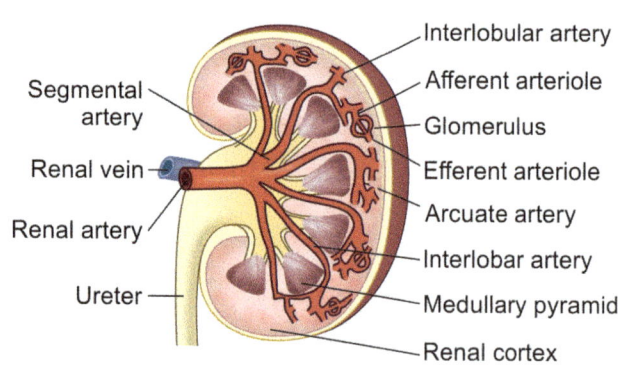

FIGURE 41.1: Renal blood vessels.

Interlobar Artery

Each interlobar artery passes in between the medullary pyramids. At the base of pyramid, it turns and runs parallel to the base of pyramid forming arcuate artery.

Arcuate Artery

Each arcuate artery gives rise to interlobular arteries.

Interlobular Artery

Interlobular arteries run through the renal cortex perpendicular to arcuate artery. From each interlobular artery, numerous afferent arterioles arise.

Afferent Arteriole

Afferent arteriole enters the Bowman's capsule and forms glomerular capillary tuft. After entering the Bowman's capsule, the afferent arteriole divides into 4 or 5 large capillaries.

Glomerular Capillaries

Large capillary divides into small glomerular capillaries, which form the loops. And, **capillary loops** unite to form efferent arteriole, which leaves the Bowman's capsule.

Efferent Arteriole

Efferent arterioles form a second capillary network called peritubular capillaries, which surround the tubular portions of nephrons. Thus, renal circulation forms a **portal system** by the presence of two sets of capillaries, namely glomerular capillaries and peritubular capillaries.

Peritubular Capillaries and Vasa Recta

Peritubular capillaries are found around the tubular portion of cortical nephrons only. Tubular portion of juxtamedullary

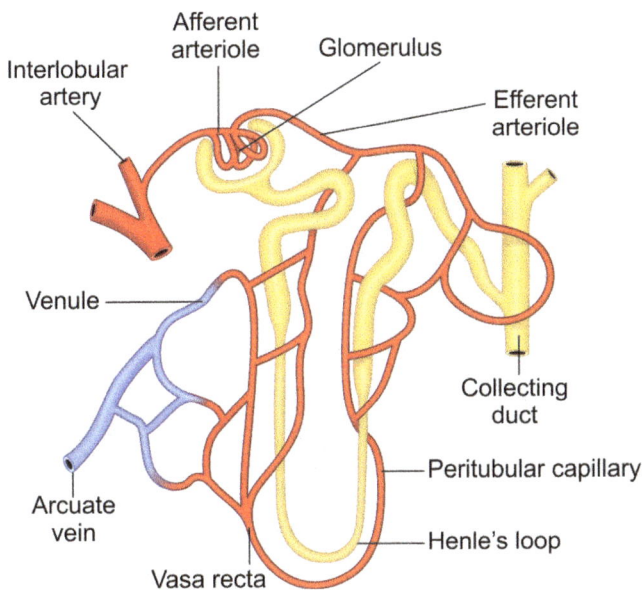

FIGURE 41.2: Renal capillaries.

nephrons is supplied by some specialized capillaries called vasa recta (singular = vas rectum). These capillaries are straight blood vessels hence the name vasa recta. Vasa recta arise directly from efferent arteriole of the juxtamedullary nephrons and run parallel to renal tubule into the medulla and ascend up towards cortex (Fig. 41.2).

Venous System

Peritubular capillaries and vasa recta drain into the venous system. Venous system starts with peritubular venules and continues as interlobular veins, arcuate veins, interlobar veins, segmental veins and finally the renal vein (Fig. 41.3).

Renal vein leaves the kidney through the hilus and joins **inferior vena cava**.

■ MEASUREMENT OF RENAL BLOOD FLOW

Blood flow to kidneys is measured by using plasma clearance of **para-aminohippuric acid** (Chapter 45).

■ REGULATION OF RENAL BLOOD FLOW

Renal blood flow is regulated mostly by autoregulation. Nerves innervating renal blood vessels have no significant role in regulation of blood flow.

■ AUTOREGULATION

Autoregulation is the intrinsic ability of an organ to regulate its own blood flow. Autoregulation is present in some vital organs in the body such as brain, heart and kidneys. It is highly significant and more efficient in kidneys.

Renal Autoregulation

Renal autoregulation is important to maintain the glomerular filtration rate (GFR). Blood flow to kidneys remains normal even when the mean arterial blood pressure varies widely between 60 mm Hg and 180 mm Hg. This helps to maintain normal GFR.

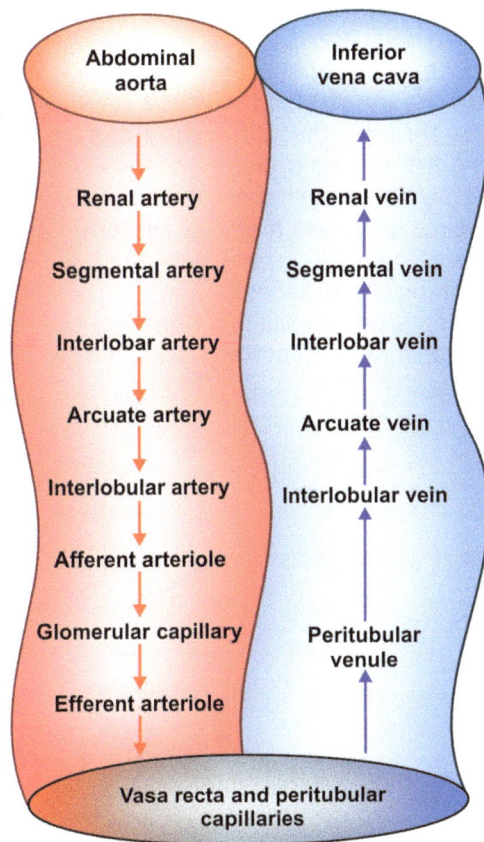

FIGURE 41.3: Schematic diagram showing renal blood flow.

Two mechanisms are involved in renal autoregulation:
1. Myogenic response.
2. Tubuloglomerular feedback.

1. Myogenic Response

Whenever blood flow to kidneys increases, elastic wall of afferent arteriole stretches. Stretch of the vessel wall increases flow of calcium ions from extracellular fluid into the cells. Influx of calcium ions leads to the contraction of smooth muscles in afferent arteriole which causes constriction of afferent arteriole. So, the blood flow is decreased.

2. Tubuloglomerular Feedback

Macula densa plays an important role in tubuloglomerular feedback which controls the renal blood flow and GFR. Refer Chapter 42 for details.

■ SALIENT FEATURES OF RENAL CIRCULATION

Renal circulation has the following special features to cope up with functions of kidneys.

Salient features are:

1. Renal arteries arise directly from the aorta. So, the pressure in aorta is very high and it facilitates a high blood flow to the renal parenchyma.
2. Kidneys receive about 1,300 mL of blood per minute, i.e. about 26% of cardiac output. Kidneys are the

second organs to receive maximum blood flow, the first organ being the liver which receives 1,500 mL per minute, i.e. about 30% of cardiac output.
3. Whole amount of blood which flows to kidney has to pass through the glomerular capillaries before entering the venous system. Because of this, blood is completely filtered at the renal glomeruli.
4. Renal circulation has a **portal system**, i.e. a double network of capillaries namely glomerular capillaries and peritubular capillaries.
5. Renal glomerular capillaries form **high pressure bed** with a pressure of 60 mm Hg to 70 mm Hg. It is much greater than the capillary pressure elsewhere in the body, which is only about 25 mm Hg to 30 mm Hg. High pressure is maintained in the glomerular capillaries because the diameter of afferent arteriole is more than that of efferent arteriole. High capillary pressure augments glomerular filtration.
6. Peritubular capillaries form **low pressure bed** with a pressure of 8 mm Hg to 10 mm Hg. This low pressure helps tubular reabsorption.
7. Autoregulation of renal blood flow is well established.

Chapter 42: Urine Formation

CHAPTER OUTLINE

- **PROCESS OF URINE FORMATION**
- **GLOMERULAR FILTRATION**
  - DEFINITION
  - FILTRATION MEMBRANE
  - PROCESS OF GLOMERULAR FILTRATION
  - GLOMERULAR FILTRATION RATE (GFR)
  - FILTRATION FRACTION
  - PRESSURES DETERMINING FILTRATION
  - FACTORS REGULATING (AFFECTING) GFR
- **TUBULAR REABSORPTION**
  - SELECTIVE REABSORPTION
  - MECHANISM OF REABSORPTION
- **SITE OF REABSORPTION**
- **ROUTES OF REABSORPTION**
- **REGULATION OF TUBULAR REABSORPTION**
- **TRANSPORT MAXIMUM: Tm VALUE**
- **RENAL THRESHOLD**
- **REABSORPTION OF IMPORTANT SUBSTANCES**
- **TUBULAR SECRETION**
  - SUBSTANCES SECRETED IN DIFFERENT SEGMENTS OF RENAL TUBULES
- **SUMMARY OF URINE FORMATION**

PROCESS OF URINE FORMATION

Urine formation is the **blood-cleansing function**. Normally, about 1,300 mL of blood (26% of cardiac output) enters the kidneys. Kidneys excrete the unwanted substances along with water from the blood as urine.

Normal Urinary Output

Urinary output in a normal person is 1 to 1.5 L/day.

Processes of Urine Formation

When blood passes through glomerular capillaries, plasma is filtered into the Bowman's capsule. This process is called **glomerular filtration**.

Filtrate from Bowman's capsule passes through tubular portion of the nephron. While passing through tubule, the filtrate undergoes various changes both in quality and in quantity. Many wanted substances such as glucose, amino acids, water and electrolytes are reabsorbed from the tubules. This process is called **tubular reabsorption**.

And, some unwanted substances are secreted into the tubule from peritubular blood vessels. This process is called **tubular secretion** or excretion (Fig. 42.1).

Thus, urine formation includes three processes:

1. Glomerular filtration.
2. Tubular reabsorption.
3. Tubular secretion.

Among the three processes, filtration is the function of glomerulus. Reabsorption and secretion are the functions of tubular portion of the nephron.

GLOMERULAR FILTRATION

DEFINITION

Glomerular filtration is the process by which blood that passes via glomerular capillaries is filtered through filtration membrane. It is the first process of urine formation. Structure of filtration membrane is well suited for this process.

FILTRATION MEMBRANE

Filtration membrane is formed by three layers:

1. Glomerular Capillary Membrane

Glomerular capillary membrane is formed by single layer of endothelial cells which are attached to the basement membrane. Capillary membrane has many pores called **fenestra** or **filtration pores** with a diameter of 0.1 μ.

2. Basement Membrane

Basement membrane of glomerular capillaries fuses with the basement membrane of visceral layer of Bowman's capsule. Basement membrane separates endothelium of glomerular capillary and epithelium of visceral layer of Bowman's capsule.

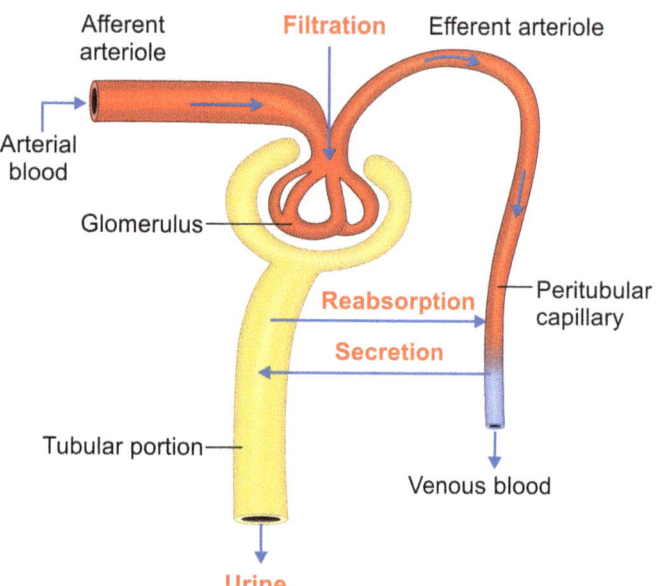

FIGURE 42.1: Events of urine formation.

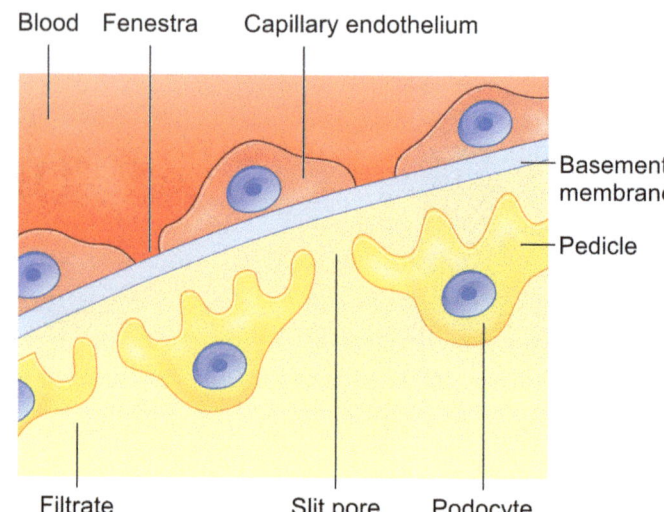

FIGURE 42.2: Filtration membrane in renal corpuscle. It is formed by capillary endothelium on one side (red) and visceral layer of Bowman's capsule (yellow) on the other side.

3. Visceral Layer of Bowman's Capsule

This is composed of a single layer of flattened epithelial cells resting on a basement membrane. Each cell is connected with the basement membrane by cytoplasmic extensions called **pedicles** or feet. Pedicles are arranged in an interdigitating manner leaving small cleft-like spaces in between. Cleft-like space is called **slit pore**. Filtration takes place through these slit pores. Epithelial cells with pedicles are called **podocytes** (Fig. 42.2).

■ PROCESS OF GLOMERULAR FILTRATION

When blood passes through glomerular capillaries, plasma is filtered into the Bowman's capsule. All the substances of plasma are filtered, except the **plasma proteins**. The filtered fluid is called **glomerular filtrate**.

Ultrafiltration

Glomerular filtration is called ultrafiltration because even the minute particles are filtered. But the plasma proteins are not filtered due to their large molecular size. Protein molecules are larger than slit pores present in the endothelium of capillaries. Thus, glomerular filtrate contains all the substances of plasma except the plasma proteins.

■ GLOMERULAR FILTRATION RATE

Glomerular filtration rate (GFR) is defined as the total quantity of filtrate formed in **all nephrons** of **both kidneys** in the given unit of time.

Normal GFR is 125 mL per minute or about 180 L per day.

■ FILTRATION FRACTION

Filtration fraction is the fraction (portion) of renal plasma which becomes filtrate. It is the ratio between renal plasma flow and glomerular filtration rate. It is expressed in percentage.

$$\text{Filtration fraction} = \frac{\text{GFR}}{\text{Renal plasma flow}} \times 100$$

$$= \frac{125 \text{ mL/min}}{650 \text{ mL/min}} \times 100$$

$$= 19.2\%.$$

Normal filtration fraction varies from 15 to 20%.

■ PRESSURES DETERMINING FILTRATION

Glomerular filtration is determined by three types of pressures:

1. Glomerular Capillary Pressure

Glomerular capillary pressure is the pressure exerted by blood in glomerular capillaries. It is about 60 mm Hg, and varies between 45 mm Hg and 70 mm Hg. Glomerular capillary pressure is the highest capillary pressure in the body. This pressure favors glomerular filtration.

2. Colloidal Osmotic Pressure

Colloidal osmotic pressure is exerted by plasma proteins in the glomeruli. Plasma proteins are not filtered through the glomerular capillaries and remain in glomerular capillaries. These proteins develop the colloidal osmotic pressure which is about 25 mm Hg. It opposes glomerular filtration.

3. Hydrostatic Pressure in Bowman's Capsule

Hydrostatic pressure in Bowman's capsule is the pressure exerted by the filtrate in Bowman's capsule. It is also called capsular pressure. It is about 15 mm Hg. It also opposes glomerular filtration.

Net Filtration Pressure

Net filtration pressure is the balance between pressure favoring filtration and pressures opposing filtration. It is otherwise known as **effective filtration pressure** or **essential filtration pressure**.

The net filtration pressure is given by:

$$\text{Glomerular capillary pressure} - \left\{\text{Colloidal osmotic pressure} + \text{Hydrostatic pressure in Bowman's capsule}\right\}$$

= 60 − (25 + 15) = 20 mm Hg.

Normal net filtration pressure is about 20 mm Hg, and it varies between 15 mm Hg and 20 mm Hg.

Starling Hypothesis and Starling Forces of Filtration

Determination of net filtration pressure is based on Starling hypothesis. Starling hypothesis states that the net filtration through capillary membrane is proportional to hydrostatic pressure difference across the membrane minus oncotic pressure difference. Hydrostatic pressure within the glomerular capillaries is the glomerular capillary pressure.

All the pressures involved in determination of filtration are called Starling forces of filtration.

■ FACTORS REGULATING (AFFECTING) GFR

1. Renal Blood Flow

It is the most important factor that is necessary for glomerular filtration. GFR is **directly proportional** to renal blood flow. Renal blood flow itself is controlled by autoregulation. Refer Chapter 41 for details.

2. Tubuloglomerular Feedback

Tubuloglomerular feedback is the mechanism that regulates GFR through renal tubule and macula densa. Macula densa of juxtaglomerular apparatus in the terminal portion of thick ascending limb is sensitive to sodium chloride in the tubular fluid.

When glomerular filtrate passes through the terminal portion of thick ascending segment, macula densa acts like a sensor. It detects the concentration of sodium chloride in tubular fluid and accordingly alters the glomerular blood flow and GFR.

When the concentration of sodium chloride increases in the filtrate

When the concentration of sodium chloride increases in filtrate, macula densa releases **adenosine** from ATP. Adenosine causes constriction of afferent arteriole. So, the blood flow through glomerulus decreases leading to decrease in GFR **(Fig. 42.3)**.

When the concentration of sodium chloride decreases in the filtrate

When the concentration of sodium chloride decreases in the filtrate, macula densa secretes **prostaglandin (PGE$_2$)**, **bradykinin** and **renin**.

PGE$_2$ and bradykinin cause dilatation of afferent arteriole. Renin induces the formation of angiotensin II

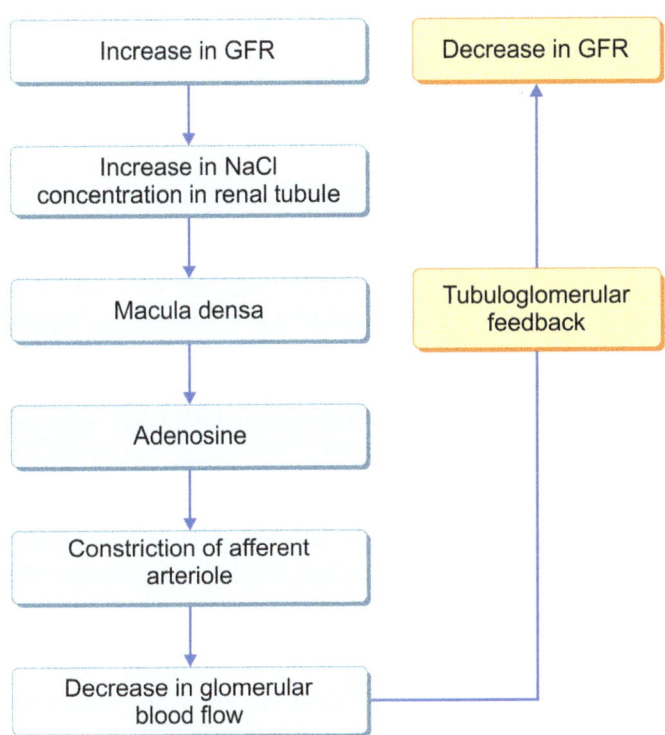

FIGURE 42.3: Tubuloglomerular feedback.
GFR = Glomerular filtration rate, NaCl = Sodium chloride.

which causes constriction of efferent arteriole. Dilatation of afferent arteriole and constriction of efferent arteriole leads to increase in glomerular blood flow and GFR.

3. Glomerular Capillary Pressure

Glomerular filtration rate is **directly proportional** to glomerular capillary pressure. Capillary pressure, in turn depends upon the renal blood flow and arterial blood pressure.

4. Colloidal Osmotic Pressure

GFR is **inversely proportional** to colloidal osmotic pressure which is exerted by plasma proteins in the glomerular capillary blood. When colloidal osmotic pressure increases as in case of dehydration or **hyperproteinemia** (increased plasma protein level), GFR decreases. During **hypoproteinemia**, colloidal osmotic pressure is low and GFR increases.

5. Hydrostatic Pressure in Bowman's Capsule

GFR is **inversely proportional** to this. Hydrostatic pressure in Bowman's capsule increases in conditions like obstruction of urethra and edema of kidney beneath renal capsule.

6. Constriction of Afferent Arteriole

Constriction of afferent arteriole reduces the blood flow to glomerular capillaries which in turn reduces GFR.

7. Constriction of Efferent Arteriole

If efferent arteriole is constricted, initially GFR increases because of stagnation of blood in the capillaries. Later when all the substances are filtered from this blood, further filtration does not occur. This is because the efferent arteriolar constriction prevents outflow of blood from glomerulus and no fresh blood enters the glomerulus for filtration.

8. Systemic Arterial Pressure

Renal blood flow or GFR are not affected till the mean arterial blood pressure is between 60 mm and 180 mm Hg. It is due to the autoregulatory mechanism (Chapter 41). Variation in pressure above 180 mm Hg or below 60 mm Hg affects the renal blood flow and GFR accordingly, because the autoregulatory mechanism fails beyond this range.

9. Sympathetic Stimulation

Afferent and efferent arterioles are supplied by sympathetic nerves. Mild or moderate stimulation of sympathetic nerves does not cause any significant change either in renal blood flow or GFR.

Strong sympathetic stimulation causes severe constriction of the blood vessels by releasing the neurotransmitter substance, **noradrenaline**. Effect is more severe on efferent arterioles than on the afferent arterioles. So, initially there is increase in filtration, but later it decreases. However, if the stimulation is continued for more than 30 minutes, there is recovery of both renal blood flow and GFR. It is because of reduction in sympathetic neurotransmitter.

10. Surface Area of Capillary Membrane

GFR is **directly proportional** to the surface area of the capillary membrane.

If the glomerular capillary membrane is affected as in the cases of some renal diseases, surface area for filtration decreases. So, there is reduction in GFR.

11. Permeability of Capillary Membrane

GFR is **directly proportional** to permeability of glomerular capillary membrane. In many abnormal conditions like hypoxia, lack of blood supply, presence of toxic agents, etc. permeability of the capillary membrane increases. In such conditions, even plasma proteins are filtered and excreted in urine.

12. Contraction of Glomerular Mesangial Cells

Glomerular mesangial cells are situated in between the glomerular capillaries. Contraction of these cells decreases surface area of capillaries resulting in reduction in GFR. Refer Chapter 40 for details.

13. Hormonal and Other Factors

Many hormones and other secretory factors alter GFR by affecting the blood flow through glomerulus.

Factors increasing GFR by vasodilatation

i. Atrial natriuretic peptide.
ii. Brain natriuretic peptide.
iii. Cyclic AMP (cAMP).
iv. Dopamine.
v. Endothelium-derived nitric oxide.
vi. Prostaglandin E_2 (PGE_2).

Factors decreasing GFR by vasoconstriction

i. Angiotensin II.
ii. Endothelin.
iii. Noradrenaline.
iv. Platelet-activating factor.
v. Platelet-derived growth factor.
vi. Prostaglandin F_2 (PGF_2).

TUBULAR REABSORPTION

Tubular reabsorption is the process by which water and other substances are transported from renal tubules back to the blood. When glomerular filtrate flows through the tubular portion of nephron, both quantitative and qualitative changes occur. Large quantity of water (more than 99%), electrolytes and other substances are reabsorbed by the tubular epithelial cells. Reabsorbed substances move into the interstitial fluid of renal medulla. And, from here, the substances move into blood in peritubular capillaries.

Since, the substances are taken back into blood from glomerular filtrate, the entire process is called tubular reabsorption.

SELECTIVE REABSORPTION

Tubular reabsorption is known as selective reabsorption because tubular cells reabsorb only the substances necessary for the body. Essential substances such as glucose, amino acids and vitamins are completely reabsorbed from renal tubule. Whereas the unwanted substances like metabolic waste products are excreted through urine.

MECHANISM OF REABSORPTION

Basic transport mechanisms involved in tubular reabsorption are of **two types**:

1. Active Reabsorption

Active reabsorption is the movement of molecules against the **electrochemical gradient**. It needs liberation of energy which is derived from ATP.

Substances reabsorbed actively

Substances which are reabsorbed actively from the renal tubule are sodium, calcium, potassium, phosphates, sulfates, bicarbonates, glucose, amino acids, ascorbic acid, uric acid and ketone bodies.

2. Passive Reabsorption

Passive reabsorption is the movement of molecules along the electrochemical gradient. This process does not need energy.

Substances reabsorbed passively

Substances which are reabsorbed passively are chloride, urea and water.

■ SITE OF REABSORPTION

Reabsorption of the substances occurs in almost all the segments of tubular portion of nephron.

1. Substances Reabsorbed from Proximal Convoluted Tubule

About 7/8 of the filtrate (about 88%) is reabsorbed in proximal convoluted tubule. Brush border of the epithelial cell in proximal convoluted tubule increases the surface area and facilitates reabsorption.

Substances reabsorbed from proximal convoluted tubule are glucose, amino acids, sodium, potassium, calcium, bicarbonates, chlorides, phosphates, uric acid and water.

2. Substances Reabsorbed from Loop of Henle

Substances reabsorbed from loop of Henle are sodium and chloride.

3. Substances Reabsorbed from Distal Convoluted Tubule

Sodium, calcium, bicarbonate and water are reabsorbed from distal convoluted tubule.

■ ROUTES OF REABSORPTION

Reabsorption of substances from tubular lumen into the peritubular capillary occurs by **two routes**:

1. Transcellular Route

In this route, the substances move through the cell.

It includes transport of substances:

i. From tubular lumen into tubular cell through apical (luminal) surface of the cell membrane
ii. Tubular cell into interstitial fluid
iii. Interstitial fluid into capillary.

2. Paracellular Route

In this route, the substances move through intercellular space.

It includes transport of substances:

i. From tubular lumen into interstitial fluid present in lateral intercellular space through highly permeable tight junction between the cells.
ii. From interstitial fluid into capillary **(Fig. 42.4)**.

■ REGULATION OF TUBULAR REABSORPTION

Tubular reabsorption is regulated by three factors:

1. Glomerulotubular Balance

Glomerulotubular balance is the balance between filtration and reabsorption of solutes and water in kidney. When GFR increases, the tubular load of solutes and water in proximal convoluted tubule is increased. It is followed by increase in the reabsorption of solutes and water.

This process helps in constant reabsorption of solute, particularly sodium and water from renal tubule.

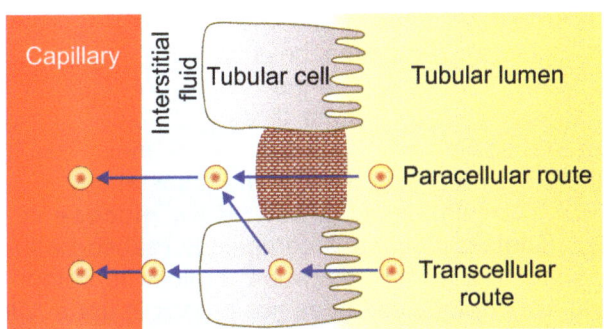

FIGURE 42.4: Routes of reabsorption.

TABLE 42.1: Hormones regulating tubular reabsorption.

Hormone	Action
1. Aldosterone	Increases sodium reabsorption in ascending limb, distal convoluted tubule and collecting duct
2. Angiotensin II	Increases sodium reabsorption in proximal tubule, thick ascending limb, distal tubule and collecting duct (mainly in proximal convoluted tubule)
3. Antidiuretic hormone	Increases water reabsorption in distal convoluted tubule and collecting duct
4. Atrial natriuretic factor	Decreases sodium reabsorption
5. Brain natriuretic factor	Decreases sodium reabsorption
6. Parathormone	Increases reabsorption of calcium, magnesium and hydrogen Decreases phosphate reabsorption
7. Calcitonin	Decreases calcium reabsorption

2. Hormonal Factors

Hormones which regulate tubular absorption are listed in **Table 42.1**.

3. Nervous Factor

Activation of sympathetic nervous system increases the tubular reabsorption (particularly of sodium) from renal tubules. It also increases the tubular reabsorption indirectly by stimulating secretion of renin from juxtaglomerular cell. Renin causes formation of angiotensin II which increases the sodium reabsorption (Chapter 40).

■ TRANSPORT MAXIMUM: Tm VALUE

Tubular transport maximum or Tm is the rate at which a substance is reabsorbed from renal tubule. For example, **transport maximum for glucose (TmG)**, is 375 mg/minute in adult males and about 300 mg/minute in adult females.

■ RENAL THRESHOLD

Renal threshold is the plasma concentration at which a substance appears first in urine. Every substance has a threshold level in plasma or blood. Below that threshold level, the substance is completely reabsorbed and does not appear in urine. When concentration of that substance reaches the threshold, excess amount is not reabsorbed and, so it appears in urine. This level is called the renal threshold of that substance.

For example, **renal threshold for glucose** is 180 mg/dL. That is, glucose is completely reabsorbed from tubular fluid, if its concentration in blood is below 180 mg/dL. So, the glucose does not appear in urine. When the blood level of glucose reaches 180 mg/dL, it is not reabsorbed completely and appears in urine.

■ REABSORPTION OF IMPORTANT SUBSTANCES

1. Reabsorption of Sodium

From the glomerular filtrate, 99% of sodium is reabsorbed. Two thirds of sodium are reabsorbed in proximal convoluted tubule and remaining one-third in other segments (except descending limb) and collecting duct.

Sodium reabsorption occurs in three steps:

i. Transport from lumen of renal tubules into the tubular epithelial cells.
ii. Transport from tubular cells into the interstitial fluid.
iii. Transport from interstitial fluid to the blood.

2. Reabsorption of Water

Reabsorption of water occurs from proximal and distal convoluted tubules and in collecting duct.

Reabsorption of water from proximal convoluted tubule: Obligatory water reabsorption

Obligatory reabsorption is the type of water reabsorption in proximal convoluted tubule, which is secondary (obligatory) to sodium reabsorption. When sodium is reabsorbed from the tubule, osmotic pressure decreases. It causes osmosis of water from renal tubule.

Reabsorption of water from distal convoluted tubule and collecting duct: Facultative water reabsorption

Facultative reabsorption is the type of water reabsorption in distal convoluted tubule and collecting duct that occurs by the activity of antidiuretic hormone (ADH). Normally, distal convoluted tubule and the collecting duct are not permeable to water. But antidiuretic hormone (ADH), makes these segments become permeable to water and so it is reabsorbed.

Mechanism of action of antidiuretic hormone

Antidiuretic hormone (ADH) combines with **V_2 receptors** in tubular epithelial membrane and activates adenyl cyclase, to form cyclic AMP. This cyclic AMP increases the permeability of the tubules for water by activating aquaporins which form the water channels.

Aquaporins

Aquaporins (AQP) are the membrane proteins which function as water channels. ADH increases water reabsorption in distal convoluted tubules and collecting ducts by regulating the aquaporins.

3. Reabsorption of Glucose

Glucose is completely reabsorbed in the proximal convoluted tubule. It is transported by secondary active transport (sodium cotransport) mechanism. Glucose and sodium bind to a common carrier protein in the luminal membrane of tubular epithelium and enter the cell. Carrier protein is called **sodium-dependent glucose transporter 2 (SGLT2)**. From tubular cell glucose is transported into medullary interstitium by another carrier protein called **glucose transporter 2 (GLUT2)**.

Renal threshold for glucose

Renal threshold for glucose is 180 mg/dL in venous blood. When the blood level reaches 180 mg/dL glucose is not reabsorbed completely and appears in urine.

Tubular maximum for glucose (TmG)

In adult male, TmG is 375 mg/minute and in adult females, it is about 300 mg/minute (see above).

4. Reabsorption of Bicarbonates

Most of the bicarbonate ions are reabsorbed actively, in proximal tubule (Chapter 44). It is reabsorbed in the form of carbon dioxide.

Bicarbonate is mostly present as sodium bicarbonate in the filtrate. Sodium bicarbonate dissociates into sodium and bicarbonate ions in the tubular lumen.

Sodium diffuses into tubular cell in exchange of hydrogen. Bicarbonate combines with hydrogen to form carbonic acid. Carbonic acid dissociates into carbon dioxide and water in the presence of carbonic anhydrase. Carbon dioxide and water enter the tubular cell.

In the tubular cells, carbon dioxide combines with water to form carbonic acid. It immediately dissociates into hydrogen and bicarbonate. Bicarbonate from the tubular cell enters the interstitium. There it combines with sodium to form sodium bicarbonate **(Fig. 44.1)**.

5. Reabsorption of Amino Acids

Amino acids are also reabsorbed completely in proximal convoluted tubule. Amino acids are reabsorbed actively by the secondary active transport mechanism along with sodium.

■ TUBULAR SECRETION

Tubular secretion is the process by which the substances are transported from blood into renal tubules. It is also called tubular excretion.

■ SUBSTANCES SECRETED IN DIFFERENT SEGMENTS OF RENAL TUBULES

1. Potassium is secreted actively by sodium-potassium pump in proximal and distal convoluted tubules and collecting ducts.
2. Ammonia is secreted in the proximal convoluted tubule.
3. Hydrogen ions are secreted in the proximal and distal convoluted tubules. Maximum hydrogen ion secretion occurs in proximal tubule.

Thus, urine is formed in the nephron by the processes of glomerular filtration, selective reabsorption and tubular secretion.

SUMMARY OF URINE FORMATION

Urine formation takes place in three processes.

1. Glomerular Filtration

Plasma is filtered in glomeruli and the substances reach the renal tubules along with water as filtrate.

2. Tubular Reabsorption

About 99% of filtrate is reabsorbed in different segments of renal tubules.

3. Tubular Secretion

Some substances are secreted from blood into the renal tubule.

With all these changes filtrate becomes urine.

Chapter 43: Concentration of Urine

CHAPTER OUTLINE

- **OSMOLARITY OF URINE**
  - FORMATION OF DILUTE URINE
  - FORMATION OF CONCENTRATED URINE
- **MEDULLARY GRADIENT**
  - MEDULLARY HYPEROSMOLARITY
  - DEVELOPMENT AND MAINTENANCE OF MEDULLARY GRADIENT
- **COUNTERCURRENT MECHANISM**
  - COUNTERCURRENT FLOW
  - COUNTERCURRENT MULTIPLIER
  - COUNTERCURRENT EXCHANGER
- **ROLE OF ADH**
- **SUMMARY OF URINE CONCENTRATION**
- **APPLIED PHYSIOLOGY**

OSMOLARITY OF URINE

Everyday 180 L of glomerular filtrate is formed with large quantity of water. If this much of water is excreted in urine, body will face serious threats. So, the concentration of urine is very essential.

Osmolarity of glomerular filtrate is same as that of plasma and it is 300 mOsm/L. But normally urine is concentrated and its osmolarity is four times more than that of plasma, i.e. 1,200 mOsm/L.

Factors Determining Osmolarity of Urine

Osmolarity of urine depends upon two factors, **water content** in the body and **antidiuretic hormone (ADH)**.

Mechanism of urine formation is the same for **dilute urine** and **concentrated urine** till the fluid reaches distal convoluted tubule. However, dilution or concentration of urine depends upon water content of the body.

FORMATION OF DILUTE URINE

When, water content in the body increases, kidney excretes dilute urine. This is achieved by **inhibition of ADH** secretion from posterior pituitary (Chapter 50). So, water reabsorption from renal tubules does not take place leading to excretion of large amount of water. This makes the urine dilute.

FORMATION OF CONCENTRATED URINE

When the water content in body decreases, kidney retains water and excretes concentrated urine. Formation of concentrated urine is not as simple as that of dilute urine.

It involves two processes:

1. Development and maintenance of medullary gradient by countercurrent system
2. Secretion of ADH.

MEDULLARY GRADIENT

MEDULLARY HYPEROSMOLARITY

Interstitial fluid in renal cortex is isotonic to plasma with the osmolarity of 300 mOsm/L. Osmolarity interstitial fluid in medulla near the cortex also is 300 mOsm/L.

However, while proceeding from outer part towards the inner part of medulla, osmolarity increases gradually and, reaches the maximum at the inner most part of medulla near renal sinus. Here, it is 1,200 mOsm/L **(Fig. 43.1)**.

This type of gradual increase in osmolarity of the medullary interstitial fluid is called the medullary gradient. It plays an important role in the concentration of urine.

DEVELOPMENT AND MAINTENANCE OF MEDULLARY GRADIENT

Kidney has some unique anatomical arrangements called countercurrent system, which are responsible for the development and maintenance of medullary gradient and hyperosmolarity of interstitial fluid in the inner medulla.

COUNTERCURRENT MECHANISM

COUNTERCURRENT FLOW

A **countercurrent system** is a system of 'U' shaped tubules (tubes) in which, the flow of fluid is in opposite direction in two limbs of the U-shaped tubules.

Events During Development of Medullary Gradient by Countercurrent Multiplier

1. Hyperosmolarity of medullary interstitial fluid is due to active reabsorption of sodium chloride and other solutes from ascending limb of Henle's loop into the medullary interstitium. These solutes accumulate in the medullary interstitium and increase the osmolarity.
2. Now, due to the concentration gradient, sodium and chloride ions diffuse from medullary interstitium into the descending limb of Henle's loop. Then it reaches ascending limb again via hairpin bend.
   Thus, the sodium and chlorine ions are repeatedly **recirculated** between descending limb and ascending limb of Henle's loop through medullary interstitial fluid leaving a small portion to be excreted in the urine.
3. Apart from this, there is regular addition of more and more new sodium and chlorine ions into descending limb by constant filtration.
4. Thus, the reabsorption of sodium chloride from ascending limb and addition of new sodium chlorine ions into filtrate multiply the osmolarity of medullary interstitial fluid and medullary gradient. Hence, it is called countercurrent multiplier.

In addition, recycling of urea also is involved in hyperosmolarity of medullary interstitial fluid:

Recirculation of urea

Urea is completely filtered in the glomeruli. As it is a waste product, it is not reabsorbed from the renal tubule. So, all the filtered urea reach collecting duct. Now, due to concentration gradient, urea diffuses from collecting duct into the inner medullary interstitium. So, the osmolarity increases in the inner medulla.

Again, by concentration gradient, urea enters the ascending limb. From here, it passes through distal convoluted tubule and reaches the collecting duct. From here, urea enters medullary interstitium and the cycle repeats. By this way urea recirculates repeatedly, and helps to maintain the hyperosmolarity in the inner medullary interstitium. Only a small amount of urea is excreted in urine.

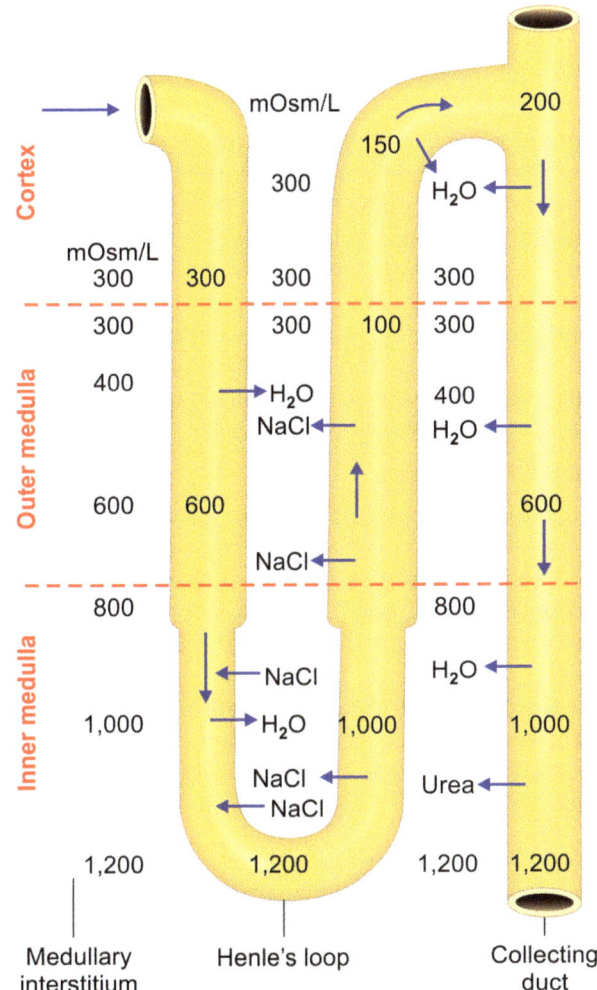

FIGURE 43.1: Countercurrent multiplier. Numerical indicate osmolarity (mOsm/L).

In kidney, the structures, which form countercurrent system, are loop of Henle and vasa recta. In both, the direction of flow of fluid in the descending limb is just opposite to that in the ascending limb.

Divisions of Countercurrent System in Kidney

In kidney, countercurrent system has two divisions:

1. Countercurrent multiplier formed by loop of Henle.
2. Countercurrent exchanger formed by vasa recta.

■ COUNTERCURRENT MULTIPLIER

Loop of Henle

Loop of Henle functions as countercurrent multiplier. It is responsible for the development of hyperosmolarity of medullary interstitial fluid and medullary gradient.

Role of Loop of Henle in Development of Medullary Gradient

Loop of Henle of juxtamedullary nephrons plays a major role as countercurrent multiplier. It is because the loop of juxtamedullary nephrons is long and extends up to the deeper parts of medulla.

■ COUNTERCURRENT EXCHANGER

Vasa Recta

Vasa recta functions as countercurrent exchanger. It is responsible for the maintenance of hyperosmolarity of medullary interstitial fluid and the medullary gradient developed by countercurrent multiplier **(Fig. 43.2)**.

Role of Vasa Recta in the Maintenance of Medullary Gradient

Vasa recta act like countercurrent exchanger because of its position. It is also 'U' shaped tubule with a descending limb, hairpin bend and an ascending limb. Vasa recta runs parallel to loop of Henle. Its descending limb runs along the ascending limb of Henle's loop and its ascending limb runs along with descending limb of Henle's loop.

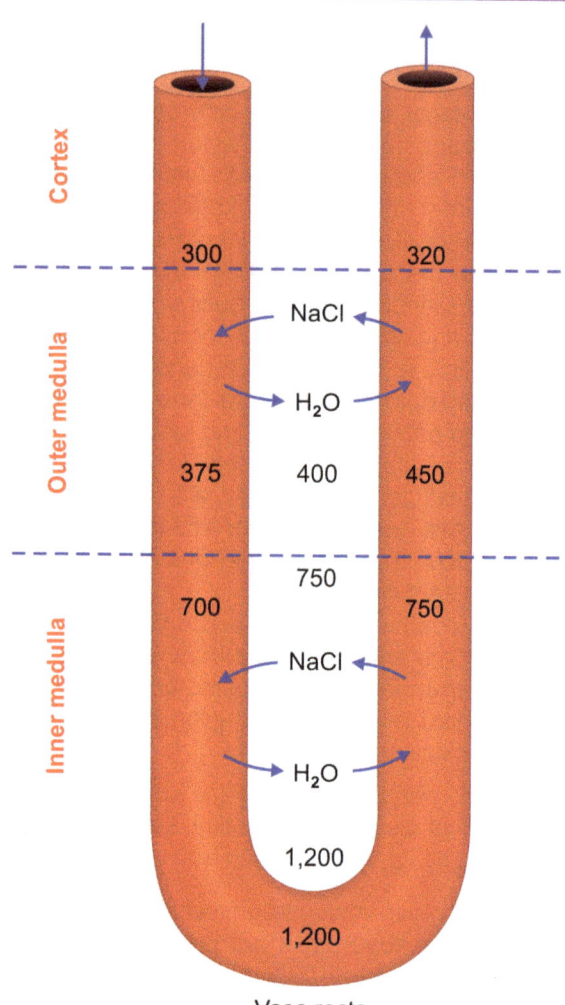

FIGURE 43.2: Countercurrent exchanger. Numerical indicate osmolarity (mOsm/L).

Events during Maintenance of Medullary Gradient by Countercurrent Exchanger

1. Sodium chloride is reabsorbed from ascending limb of Henle's loop enters the medullary interstitium. From here it enters the descending limb of vasa recta.
2. Simultaneously water diffuses from descending limb of vasa recta into medullary interstitium.
3. Blood flows very slowly through vasa recta. So, a large quantity of sodium chloride accumulates in descending limb of vasa recta and flows slowly towards ascending limb.
4. By the time the blood reaches the ascending limb of vasa recta, the concentration of sodium chloride increases very much.
5. This causes diffusion of sodium chloride into the medullary interstitium.
6. Simultaneously, water from medullary interstitium enters the ascending limb of vasa recta. And the cycle is repeated.

If the vasa recta would be a straight vessel without hairpin arrangement, blood would leave the kidney quickly at renal papillary level. In that case, the blood would remove all the sodium chloride from medullary interstitium and thereby the hyperosmolarity will be decreased. However, this does not happen, since the vasa recta has a hairpin bend.

Therefore, when blood passes through the ascending limb of vasa recta, sodium chloride diffuses out of blood and enters the interstitial fluid of medulla and, water diffuses into the blood.

Thus, vasa recta retain sodium chloride in the medullary interstitium and removes water from it. So, the hyperosmolarity of medullary interstitium is maintained. Blood passing through the ascending limb of vasa recta may carry very little amount of sodium chloride from the medulla.

Recirculation of urea

Recirculation of urea also occurs through vasa recta. From medullary interstitium, along with sodium chloride, urea also enters the descending limb of vasa recta. When blood passes through ascending limb of vasa recta, urea diffuses back into the medullary interstitium along with sodium chloride.

Thus, **sodium chloride** and **urea** are **exchanged for water** between the ascending and descending limbs of vasa recta, hence this system is called countercurrent exchanger.

ROLE OF ANTIDIURETIC HORMONE

Final concentration of urine is achieved by antidiuretic hormone (ADH). Normally, distal convoluted tubule and the collecting duct are not permeable to water. In the presence of ADH, distal convoluted tubule and collecting duct become permeable to water resulting in water reabsorption. The water reabsorption induced by ADH is called **facultative reabsorption** of water (Chapter 42).

A large quantity of water is removed from the fluid while passing through distal convoluted tubule and collecting duct. So, the urine becomes hypertonic with an osmolarity of 1,200 mOsm/L **(Fig. 43.3)**.

SUMMARY OF URINE CONCENTRATION

When the glomerular filtrate passes through renal tubule, its osmolarity is altered in different segments as described below **(Fig. 43.4)**.

1. BOWMAN'S CAPSULE

Glomerular filtrate collected at the Bowman's capsule is **isotonic to plasma**. This is because it contains all the substances of plasma except proteins. Osmolarity of the filtrate at Bowman's capsule is 300 mOsm/L.

2. PROXIMAL CONVOLUTED TUBULE

When the filtrate flows through proximal convoluted tubule, there is active reabsorption of sodium and chloride followed by obligatory reabsorption of water. So, osmolarity of fluid remains the same as in the case of Bowman's capsule, i.e. 300 mOsm/L. Thus, in proximal convoluted tubules, the fluid is **isotonic to plasma**.

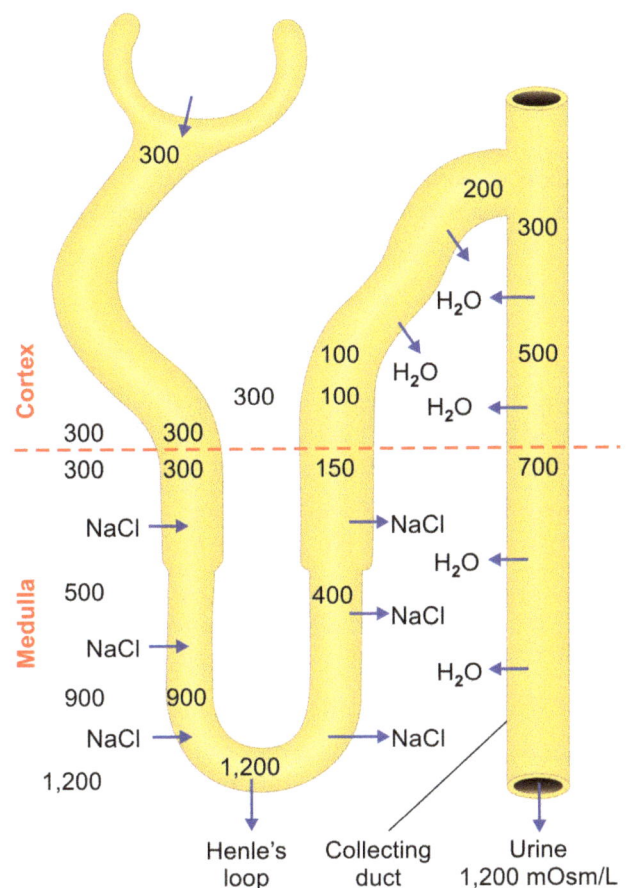

FIGURE 43.3: Role of ADH in the formation of concentrated urine. ADH increases the permeability for water in distal convoluted tubule and collecting duct.

■ 3. THICK DESCENDING SEGMENT

When the fluid passes from proximal convoluted tubule into thick descending segment, water is reabsorbed from the tubule into outer medullary interstitium by means of osmosis. It is due to the increased osmolarity in the medullary interstitium, i.e. outside the thick descending tubule. Osmolarity of the fluid inside this segment is between 450 and 600 mOsm/L. That means the fluid is **slightly hypertonic to plasma (Table 43.1)**.

■ 4. THIN DESCENDING SEGMENT OF HENLE'S LOOP

As the thin descending segment of Henle's loop passes through inner medullary interstitium (which is increasingly hypertonic) more water is reabsorbed.

This segment is highly permeable to water, and so the osmolarity of tubular fluid becomes equal to that of the surrounding medullary interstitium.

In the short loops of cortical nephrons, osmolarity of fluid at the hairpin bend of loop becomes 600 mOsm/L. And, in the long loops of juxtamedullary nephrons, at the hairpin bend, osmolarity is 1,200 mOsm/L. Thus, in this segment the fluid is **hypertonic to plasma**.

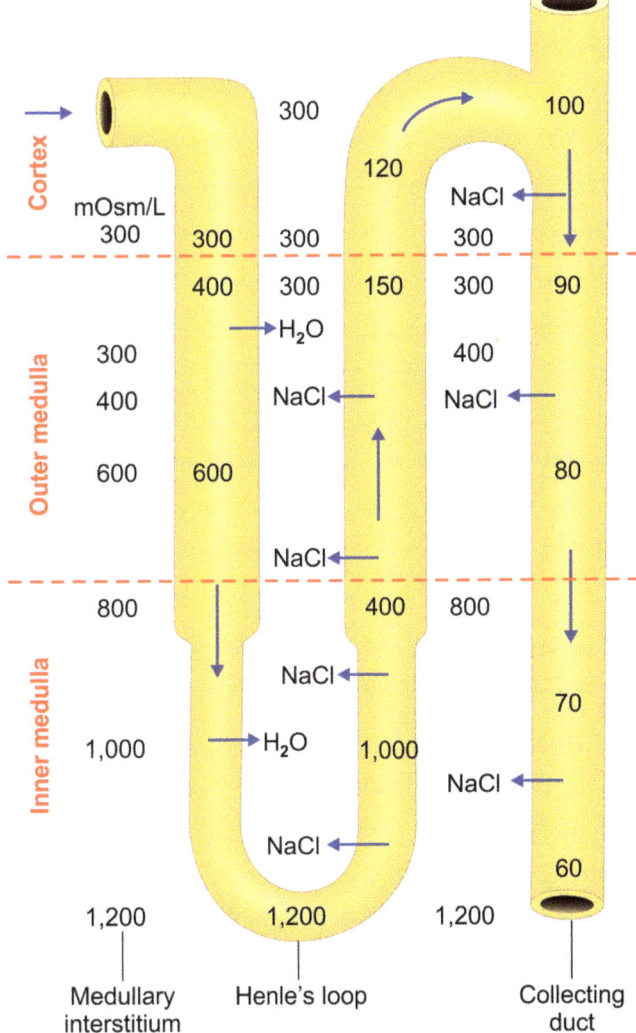

FIGURE 43.4: Mechanism for the formation of dilute urine. Numerical indicate osmolarity (mOsm/L).

TABLE 43.1: Osmolarity of fluid at different parts of nephron.

Parts of nephron	Osmolarity of fluid (mOsm/L)	Comparison to plasma
Bowman's capsule (glomerular filtrate)	300	Isotonic
Proximal convoluted tubule	300	Isotonic
Thick descending segment	450 to 600	Hypertonic
Thin descending segment of Henle's loop (short loop of cortical nephron)	600	Hypertonic
Thin descending segment of Henle's loop (long loop of juxtamedullary nephron)	1,200	Hypertonic
Thin ascending segment of Henle's loop	400	Hypertonic
Thick ascending segment	150 to 200	Hypotonic
While entering distal convoluted tubule	200	Hypotonic
While leaving collecting duct (urine)	1,200	Hypertonic

5. THIN ASCENDING SEGMENT OF HENLE'S LOOP

When the thin ascending segment of loop ascends upwards through the medullary region, osmolarity decreases gradually.

Due to concentration gradient, sodium chloride diffuses out of tubular fluid and osmolarity decreases to 400 mOsm/L. Fluid in this segment is **slightly hypertonic to plasma**.

6. THICK ASCENDING SEGMENT

This segment is impermeable to water. But there is active reabsorption of sodium and chloride from this. Reabsorption of sodium decreases the osmolarity of tubular fluid to a greater extent. The osmolarity is between 150 mOsm/L and 200 mOsm/L. The fluid inside becomes **hypotonic to plasma**.

7. DISTAL CONVOLUTED TUBULE AND COLLECTING DUCT

In the presence of ADH, distal convoluted tubule and collecting duct become permeable to water resulting in water reabsorption and final concentration of urine.

Reabsorption of large quantity of water increases the osmolarity to 1,200 mOsm/L **(Fig. 43.3)**. The urine becomes **hypertonic to plasma**.

APPLIED PHYSIOLOGY

1. DIURESIS

Diuresis is the excretion of large quantity of water through urine.

Diuresis is classified into two types:
1. Osmotic diuresis.
2. Water diuresis.

1. *Osmotic Diuresis*

Osmotic diuresis is the diuresis induced by presence of some osmotically active substances such as glucose in renal tubule. Such substances increase osmotic pressure in renal tubules and reduce reabsorption of water resulting in excretion of water through urine.

Osmotic diuresis is common in diabetes mellitus because of high blood glucose level (Chapter 53).

2. *Water Diuresis*

Osmotic diuresis is the diuresis due to decreased reabsorption of water in renal tubules particularly distal convoluted tubule and collecting duct. It is caused by deficiency of antidiuretic hormone.

Water diuresis is common in diabetes insipidus (Chapter 50).

2. POLYURIA

Polyuria is the increased urinary output with frequent voiding. It is due to osmotic diuresis as in diabetes mellitus or water diuresis as in diabetes insipidus (see above).

3. SYNDROME OF INAPPROPRIATE HYPERSECRETION OF ADH (SIADH)

It is a pituitary disorder characterized by hypersecretion of ADH. Excess ADH causes water retention, which decreases osmolarity of ECF (Chapter 50).

4. NEPHROGENIC DIABETES INSIPIDUS

Sometimes ADH secretion is normal, but the renal tubules fail to give response to ADH resulting in polyuria. This condition is called nephrogenic diabetes insipidus.

5. BARTTER'S SYNDROME

Bartter's syndrome is a genetic disorder characterized by dysfunction of thick ascending segment and distal convoluted tubule resulting in loss of sodium, potassium, chloride and calcium lost through urine.

6. OLIGURIA

Oliguria is the condition with decreased output of urine. Urine output is less than 500 mL per day in this condition. It is different from another condition called **anuria** in which urine output is less than 50 mL per day. Anuria means absence of urine output.

Oliguria occurs in many conditions including acute renal failure, obstruction in urinary tract, infection or trauma of kidneys.

Chapter 44: Acidification of Urine and Role of Kidney in Acid-base Balance

CHAPTER OUTLINE

- INTRODUCTION
- REABSORPTION OF BICARBONATE IONS
- SECRETION OF HYDROGEN IONS
  - SODIUM-HYDROGEN ANTIPORT PUMP
  - ATP-DRIVEN PROTON PUMP
- REMOVAL OF HYDROGEN IONS AND ACIDIFICATION OF URINE
  - BICARBONATE MECHANISM
  - PHOSPHATE MECHANISM
- AMMONIA MECHANISM
- APPLIED PHYSIOLOGY: DISTURBANCES OF ACID-BASE STATUS
  - ACIDOSIS
  - ALKALOSIS
  - RESPIRATORY ACIDOSIS
  - RESPIRATORY ALKALOSIS
  - METABOLIC ACIDOSIS
  - METABOLIC ALKALOSIS

INTRODUCTION

Kidney plays an important role in maintenance of acid-base balance by excreting hydrogen ions and retaining bicarbonate ions.

Normally, urine is acidic in nature with a pH of 4.5 to 6. Metabolic activities in the body produce large quantity of acids (with lot of hydrogen ions), which threaten to push the body towards acidosis. However, kidneys prevent this.

Kidneys prevent acidosis by two ways:

1. Reabsorption of bicarbonate ions (HCO_3^-)
2. Secretion of hydrogen ions (H^+).

REABSORPTION OF BICARBONATE IONS

About 4,320 mEq of HCO_3^- is filtered by the glomeruli every day. It is called **filtered load** of HCO_3^-. Excretion of this much HCO_3^- in urine will affect the acid-base balance of body fluids. So, HCO_3 must be taken back from the renal tubule by reabsorption.

SECRETION OF HYDROGEN IONS

Reabsorption of filtered HCO^- occurs by the secretion of H^+ in the renal tubules. About 4,380 mEq of H^+ appear every day in the renal tubule by means of filtration and secretion. Not all the H^+ are excreted in urine. Out of 4,380 mEq, about 4,280 to 4,330 mEq of H^+ is utilized for the reabsorption of filtered HCO_3^-. Only the remaining 50 to 100 mEq is excreted. It results in the **acidification of urine**.

Secretion of H^+ into the renal tubules occurs by the formation of **carbonic acid**. Carbon dioxide formed in the tubular cells or derived from tubular fluid combines with water to form carbonic acid in the presence of **carbonic anhydrase**. This enzyme is available in large quantities in the epithelial cells of the renal tubules. Carbonic acid immediately dissociates into H^+ and HCO_3^- **(Fig. 44.1)**.

H^+ is secreted into the lumen of proximal convoluted tubule, distal convoluted tubule and collecting duct. Distal convoluted tubule and collecting duct have a special type of cells called **intercalated cells (I cells)**. I cells are involved in handling hydrogen and bicarbonate ions.

Secretion of hydrogen ions occurs by two pumps:

1. Sodium-hydrogen antiport pump.
2. ATP-driven proton pump.

SODIUM-HYDROGEN ANTIPORT PUMP

When sodium ion (Na^+) is reabsorbed from the tubular fluid into the tubular cell, H^+ is secreted from the cell into the tubular fluid in exchange for Na^+. The sodium-hydrogen antiport pump present in the tubular cells is responsible for the exchange of Na^+ and H^+. This type of sodium-hydrogen counter transport occurs predominantly in distal convoluted tubule **(Table 44.1)**.

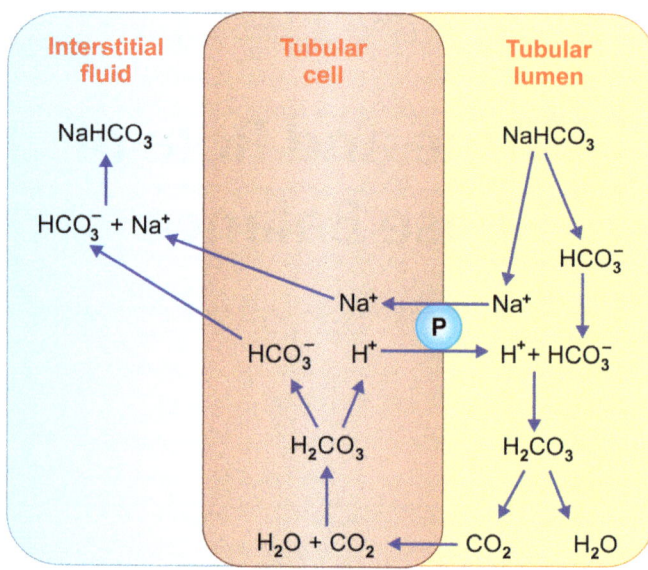

FIGURE 44.1: Reabsorption of bicarbonate ions by secretion of hydrogen ions in renal tubule.
P = Sodium-hydrogen antiport pump.

TABLE 44.1: Mechanisms involved in secretion of hydrogen ions in renal tubule.

Mechanism	Segment of renal tubule
Sodium-hydrogen pump	Distal convoluted tubule
ATP-driven proton pump	Distal convoluted tubule Collecting duct
Bicarbonate mechanism	Proximal convoluted tubule Henle's loop Distal convoluted tubule
Phosphate mechanism	Distal convoluted tubule Collecting duct
Ammonia mechanism	Proximal convoluted tubule

ATP-DRIVEN PROTON PUMP

This is an additional mechanism of H⁺ secretion in distal convoluted tubule and collecting duct. This pump is operated by obtaining energy from ATP.

REMOVAL OF HYDROGEN IONS AND ACIDIFICATION OF URINE

Kidney plays an important role in preventing metabolic acidosis by excreting H⁺.

Excretion of hydrogen ions occurs by three mechanisms:
1. Bicarbonate mechanism.
2. Phosphate mechanism.
3. Ammonia mechanism.

BICARBONATE MECHANISM

All the HCO_3^- filtered into the renal tubules is reabsorbed. About 80% of it is reabsorbed in proximal convoluted tubule; 15% in Henle's loop and 5% in distal convoluted tubule and collecting duct. Reabsorption of HCO_3^- utilizes the H⁺ secreted into the renal tubules.

The H⁺ secreted into the renal tubule, combines with filtered HCO_3^- forming carbonic acid. Carbonic acid dissociates into carbon dioxide and water in the presence of carbonic anhydrase. Carbon dioxide and water enter the tubular cell.

In tubular cells, carbon dioxide combines with water to form carbonic acid. It immediately dissociates into H⁺ and HCO_3^-. HCO_3^- from the tubular cell enters the interstitium. Simultaneously Na⁺ is reabsorbed from the renal tubule under the influence of **aldosterone**. HCO_3^- combines with Na⁺ to form $NaHCO_3$. Now, the H⁺ is secreted into the tubular lumen from the cell in exchange for Na⁺ **(Fig. 44.1)**.

Thus, for every hydrogen ion secreted into lumen of tubule, one bicarbonate ion is reabsorbed from the tubule. In this way, kidneys conserve the HCO_3^-. Reabsorption of filtered HCO_3^- is an important factor in maintaining pH of the body fluids.

PHOSPHATE MECHANISM

In the tubular cells, carbon dioxide combines with water to form **carbonic acid**. It immediately dissociates into H⁺ and HCO_3^-. HCO_3^- from the tubular cell enters the interstitium. Simultaneously, Na⁺ is reabsorbed from renal tubule under the influence of aldosterone. Na⁺ enters the interstitium and combines with HCO_3^-. The H⁺ is secreted into the tubular lumen from the cell in exchange for Na⁺ **(Fig. 44.2)**.

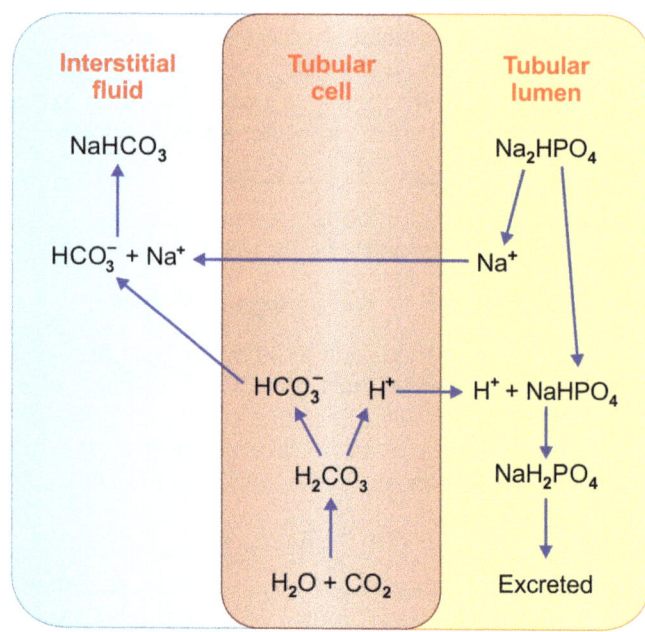

FIGURE 44.2: Excretion of hydrogen ions in combination with phosphate ions.

The H⁺, which is secreted into renal tubules, reacts with **phosphate buffer system**. It combines with sodium-hydrogen phosphate to form sodium-dihydrogen phosphate. Sodium-dihydrogen phosphate is excreted in urine. The H⁺, which is added to urine, makes it acidic. It happens mainly in distal tubule and collecting duct because of the presence of large quantity of sodium-hydrogen phosphate in these segments.

AMMONIA MECHANISM

This is the most important mechanism by which kidneys excrete H⁺ and make the urine acidic. In the tubular epithelial cells, ammonia is formed when the amino acid **glutamine** is converted into **glutamic acid** in the presence of enzyme **glutaminase**. Ammonia is also formed by the deamination of some of the amino acids such as **glycine** and **alanine (Fig. 44.3)**.

Ammonia (NH_3) formed in tubular cells is secreted into tubular lumen in exchange for sodium ion. Here, it combines with H⁺ to form **ammonium** (NH_4). Tubular cell membrane is not permeable to ammonium. Therefore, it remains in the lumen and combines with **sodium acetoacetate** to form **ammonium acetoacetate**. Ammonium acetoacetate is excreted through urine. Thus, H⁺ is added to urine in the form of ammonium compounds resulting in acidification of urine.

This process takes place mostly in the proximal convoluted tubule because glutamine is converted into ammonia in the cells of this segment.

Thus, by excreting H⁺ and conserving HCO_3^-, kidneys produce acidic urine and help to maintain the acid-base balance of body fluids.

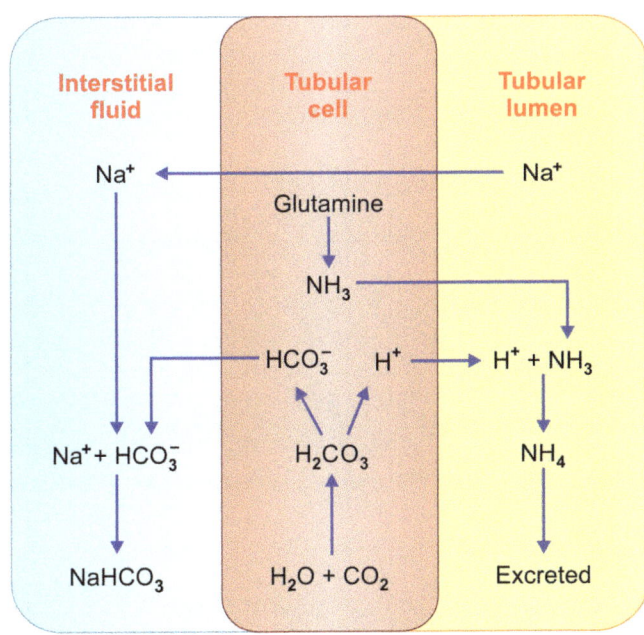

FIGURE 44.3: Excretion of hydrogen in combination with ammonia.

APPLIED PHYSIOLOGY: DISTURBANCES OF ACID-BASE STATUS

ACIDOSIS

Acidosis is the condition characterized by abnormal increase in acidity of blood and body fluids with reduction in pH below normal range.

Acidosis is produced by:

1. Increase in partial pressure of **carbon dioxide** in the body fluids particularly in arterial blood.
2. Decrease in **bicarbonate** concentration.

ALKALOSIS

Alkalosis is the condition characterized by abnormal increase in alkalinity of blood and body fluids with increase in pH above the normal range.

Alkalosis is produced by:

1. Decrease in partial pressure of **carbon dioxide** in the arterial blood.
2. Increase in **bicarbonate** concentration.

Since the partial pressure of carbon dioxide in arterial blood is controlled by lungs, the acid-base disturbances produced by the change in arterial carbon dioxide are called **respiratory disturbances**.

On the other hand, the disturbances in acid-base status produced by the change in bicarbonate concentration are called **metabolic disturbances**.

Thus acid-base disturbances are:

1. Respiratory acidosis
2. Respiratory alkalosis
3. Metabolic acidosis
4. Metabolic alkalosis.

1. RESPIRATORY ACIDOSIS

Respiratory acidosis is the acidosis that is caused by alveolar hypoventilation. During hypoventilation, the lungs fail to expel carbon dioxide, which is produced in the tissues. Carbon dioxide is the major end product of oxidation of carbohydrates, proteins and fats.

Carbon dioxide accumulates in blood where it reacts with water to form carbonic acid, which is called **respiratory acid**. Carbonic acid dissociates into hydrogen and bicarbonate. Increased hydrogen concentration in blood leads to decrease in pH and acidosis.

2. RESPIRATORY ALKALOSIS

Respiratory alkalosis is the alkalosis that is caused by alveolar hyperventilation. Hyperventilation causes excess loss of carbon dioxide from the body. Loss of carbon dioxide leads to decreased formation of carbonic acid and decreased release of hydrogen ions. Decreased hydrogen ion concentration increases the pH leading to respiratory alkalosis **(Table 44.2)**.

TABLE 44.2: Biochemical changes in arterial blood during acid-base disturbance.

Parameters	Acidosis		Alkalosis	
	Respiratory acidosis	Metabolic acidosis	Respiratory alkalosis	Metabolic alkalosis
H^+	Increases	Increases	Decreases	Decreases
pH	Decreases	Decreases	Increases	Increases
pCO_2	Increases	Decreases	Decreases	Increases
HCO_3^-	Increases slightly	Decreases very much	Decreases slightly	Increases very much

3. METABOLIC ACIDOSIS

Metabolic acidosis is the acid-base imbalance characterized by excess accumulation of **organic acids** in the body, which is caused by abnormal metabolic processes. Organic acids such as lactic acid, ketoacids and uric acid are formed by normal metabolism. The quantity of these acids increases due to abnormality in the metabolism.

4. METABOLIC ALKALOSIS

Metabolic alkalosis is the acid-base imbalance caused by loss of excess hydrogen ions resulting in increased bicarbonate concentration. Some of the endocrine disorders, renal tubular disorders, etc. cause metabolic disorders leading to loss of hydrogen ions. It increases bicarbonate ions and pH in the body leading to metabolic alkalosis.

Chapter 45: Renal Function Tests, Renal Failure, Dialysis and Diuretics

CHAPTER OUTLINE

- **PROPERTIES AND COMPOSITION OF NORMAL URINE**
  - PROPERTIES OF URINE
  - COMPOSITION OF URINE
- **RENAL FUNCTION TESTS**
  - EXAMINATION OF URINE: URINALYAIS
  - EXAMINATION OF BLOOD
  - EXAMINATION OF BLOOD AND URINE
- **RENAL FAILURE**
  - ACUTE RENAL FAILURE
  - CHRONIC RENAL FAILURE
- **DIALYSIS AND ARTIFICIAL KIDNEY**
- **KIDNEY TRANSPLANTATION**
- **DIURETICS**
  - USES OF DIURETICS
  - TYPES OF DIURETICS

■ PROPERTIES AND COMPOSITION OF NORMAL URINE

■ PROPERTIES OF URINE

Volume	:	1,000 to 1,500 mL/day
Appearance	:	Clear
Reaction	:	Slightly acidic with pH of 4.5 to 6
Specific gravity	:	1.010 to 1.025
Color	:	Normally, urine is straw colored
Odor	:	Fresh urine has light aromatic odor. If stored for some time, the odor becomes stronger due to bacterial decomposition.

■ COMPOSITION OF URINE

Urine consists of water and solids. Solids include organic and inorganic substances (**Fig. 45.1**).

■ RENAL FUNCTION TESTS

Renal function tests are the group of tests that are performed to assess the functions of kidney.

Renal function tests are of three types:

I. Examination of urine alone.
II. Examination of blood alone.
III. Examination of blood and urine.

■ EXAMINATION OF URINE: URINALYSIS

Routine examination of urine or urinalysis is a group of diagnostic tests performed on the sample of urine.

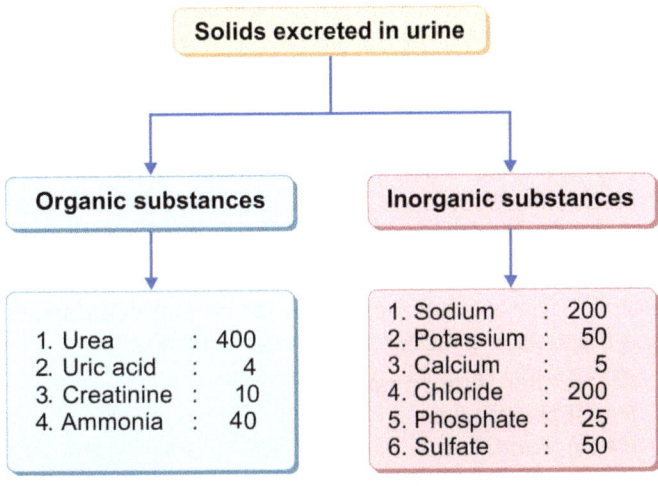

FIGURE 45.1: Quantity of solids excreted in urine (mMol/day).

Urinalysis is done by:

1. Physical examination.
2. Microscopic examination
3. Chemical analysis.

1. *Physical Examination of Urine*

i. Volume.
ii. Appearance.
iii. Reaction.
iv. Specific gravity.

v. Color.
vi. Odor.

2. Microscopic Examination of Urine

Microscopic examination reveals the presence of red blood cells, pus cells, epithelial cells, casts and crystals which suggests the renal pathology.

3. Chemical Analysis of Urine

Chemical analysis of urine helps to determine the presence of abnormal constituents of urine or presence of normal constituents in abnormal quantity. Both the findings reveal the presence of renal abnormality.

Chemical analysis is done to determine the following substances:

 i. Glucose.
 ii. Protein, particularly albumin.
 iii. Ketone bodies.
 iv. Bilirubin.
 v. Urobilinogen.
 vi. Bile salts.
 vii. Blood
 viii. Hemoglobin
 ix. Nitrite

■ EXAMINATION OF BLOOD

Level of plasma proteins, urea, uric acid and creatinine are determined in blood. Blood level of these substances is altered in renal failure.

■ EXAMINATION OF BLOOD AND URINE

Plasma Clearance

Plasma clearance is defined as the amount of plasma that is cleared off a substance in a given unit of time. It is also known as **renal clearance**. It is based on **Fick's principle** (Chapter 69).

Determination of clearance value for certain substances helps in assessing the following renal functions:

1. Glomerular filtration rate.
2. Renal plasma flow.
3. Renal blood flow.

To determine the plasma clearance of a particular substance, measurement of the following factors is required:

 i. Volume of urine excreted.
 ii. Concentration of the substance in urine.
 iii. Concentration of the substance in blood.

Formula to calculate clearance value is:

$$C = \frac{UV}{P}$$

Where,
 C = Clearance.
 U = Concentration of the substance in urine.
 V = Volume of urine flow.
 P = Concentration of the substance in plasma.

1. Measurement of Glomerular Filtration Rate

A substance that is completely filtered but neither reabsorbed nor secreted should be used to measure glomerular filtration rate (GFR). Inulin is a substance that is completely filtered. And, it is neither reabsorbed nor secreted. So, **inulin** is the ideal substance used to measure GFR.

Inulin clearance

A known amount of inulin is injected into the body. After sometime, the concentration of inulin in plasma and urine and the volume of urine excreted are estimated.

For example,
 Concentration of inulin in urine = 125 mg/dL
 Plasma concentration = 1 mg/dL
 Volume of urine output = 1 mL/min
Thus,

$$\text{Glomerular filtration rate} = \frac{UV}{P}$$
$$= \frac{125 \times 1}{1}$$
$$= 125 \text{ mL/min}$$

2. Measurement of Renal Plasma Flow

To measure renal plasma flow, a substance, which is filtered and secreted but not reabsorbed, should be used. Such a substance is **para-aminohippuric acid (PAH)**. PAH clearance indicates the amount of plasma passed through kidneys.

A known amount of PAH is injected into the body. After sometime, the concentration of PAH in plasma and urine and the volume of urine excreted are estimated.

For example,
 Concentration of PAH in urine = 66 mg/dL
 Plasma concentration = 0.1 mg/dL
 Volume of urine output = 1 mL/min
Thus,

$$\text{Renal plasma flow} = \frac{UV}{P}$$
$$= \frac{66 \times 1}{0.1}$$
$$= 660 \text{ mL/min}$$

3. Measurement of Renal Blood Flow

To determine renal blood flow, value of the following two factors is necessary:

 i. Renal plasma flow.
 ii. Percentage of plasma volume in the blood.

i. Renal plasma flow

Renal plasma flow is measured by using PAH clearance.

ii. Percentage of plasma volume in the blood

Percentage of plasma volume is indirectly determined by using PCV. For example, if PCV is 45%, the plasma volume in the blood is 100 − 45 = 55%, i.e. 55 mL of plasma is present in every 100 mL of blood.

Renal blood flow is calculated with the values of renal plasma flow and % of plasma in blood by using a formula given below:

$$\text{Renal blood flow} = \frac{\text{Renal plasma flow}}{\text{\% of plasma in blood}}$$

For example,

Renal plasma flow = 660 mL/min
Amount of plasma in blood = 55%

$$\text{Renal blood flow} = \frac{660}{55/100}$$
$$= \frac{660 \times 100}{55}$$
$$= 1{,}200 \text{ mL/min}$$

■ RENAL FAILURE

Renal failure refers to failure of functions of kidney.

Renal failure is of two types:

I. Acute renal failure.
II. Chronic renal failure.

■ ACUTE RENAL FAILURE

Acute renal failure is the temporary loss of kidney function. It occurs abruptly or suddenly. It is often reversible within few days to few weeks. Acute renal failure may result in sudden life-threatening reactions in the body with the need for emergency treatment.

Causes of Acute Renal Failure

Common causes of acute renal failure are:

1. **Pyelonephritis**: Inflammation of kidney involving glomeruli, tubules and insterstitium.
2. Acute **glomerulonephritis**: Inflammation of glomeruli.
3. Renal ischemia: Inadequate blood supply to kidney.
4. Acute tubular necrosis: Necrosis of tubular cells in kidney.
5. Severe transfusion reactions: Refer Chapter 19 for transfusion reactions.
6. Sudden fall in blood pressure: Due to conditions such as hemorrhage, diarrhea, severe burns and cholera.
7. **Blockage of ureter**: Caused by the formation of calculi (renal stone) or tumor.

Treatment for Acute Renal Failure

Acute renal failure can be treated in most of the cases if diagnosed earlier. Cause of the condition is determined and treatment is carried on accordingly. Treatment involves use of medications, change in diet and dialysis if necessary.

■ CHRONIC RENAL FAILURE

Chronic renal failure is the progressive, long standing and irreversible impairment of renal functions. Last stage of chronic renal failure is called **end stage renal disease (ESRD)**.

Causes of Chronic Renal Failure

1. Chronic glomerulonephritis: Long-term inflammation of glomeruli.
2. **Polycystic kidney disease (PKD)**: Development of clusters of cysts in kidneys.
3. Renal calculi.
4. Urethral constriction.
5. Hypertension.
6. Atherosclerosis.
7. Tuberculosis.
8. Slow poisoning by drugs or metals.

Treatment for Chronic Renal Failure

Chronic renal failure is treated by dialysis or kidney transplant.

■ DIALYSIS AND ARTIFICIAL KIDNEY

Dialysis is the procedure to remove waste materials and toxic substances and to restore normal volume and composition of body fluid in severe **renal failure**. It is also called **hemodialysis**.

Principle of artificial kidney is the diffusion of solutes from an area of higher concentration to the area of lower concentration, through a semipermeable membrane. Artificial kidney is a machine that is used to carry out hemodialysis during renal failure.

Patient's arterial blood is passed continuously or intermittently through the artificial kidney and then back to the body through the vein.

Dialysis is used to treat the patients suffering from acute or chronic renal failure.

In some cases, patient's peritoneal membrane is used as a semipermeable membrane. This technique is called **peritoneal dialysis**. It is also used to treat the patients suffering from renal failure.

■ KIDNEY TRANSPLANTATION

Kidney or renal transplantation is the surgical procedure to place the healthy kidney into the renal failure patients. Transplanted kidney takes over the functions of diseased kidney and the patient needs no further dialysis. Healthy kidney is taken from either a live donor or a deceased donor.

Kidney transplantation is the treatment of choice for patients suffering from **end stage renal disease (ESRD)**.

DIURETICS

Diuretics or **diuretic agents** are the substances which enhance the urine formation and output. These substances increase the excretion of water, sodium and chloride through urine. Diuretic agents increase the urine formation, by influencing any of the processes involved in urine formation. Diuretics are commonly called '**water pills**'.

USES OF DIURETICS

Diuretics are generally used for the treatment of disorders involving increase in extracellular fluid volume such as:

1. Hypertension.
2. Congestive cardiac failure.
3. Edema.

Diuretic agents prevent the above disorders by increasing the urinary output and reducing extracellular fluid (ECF) volume.

TYPES OF DIURETICS

1. Osmotic Diuretics

Osmotic diuretics are the substances that induce **osmotic diuresis.** When injected in large quantities into the body, these substances increase the osmotic pressure in the tubular fluid. Increased osmotic pressure in the tubular fluid, in turn reduces water reabsorption. It leads to excretion of excess of water through urine. Elevated blood sugar level in diabetes can also cause osmotic diuresis in the same manner.

Examples of osmotic diuretics are urea, mannitol, sucrose and glucose.

2. Diuretics which Inhibit Reabsorption of Electrolytes

Diuretics of this type inhibit the active reabsorption of electrolytes like sodium and potassium from the renal tubular fluid. Inhibition of electrolyte reabsorption causes osmotic diuresis. Common diuretics of this category are loop diuretics

Loop diuretics

Loop diuretics are the substances that inhibit electrolyte reabsorption in **Henle's loop.** These diuretics inhibit the sodium and chloride reabsorption from thick ascending limb of Henle's loop. So, the osmotic pressure in tubular fluid increases, leading to diuresis.

Examples are furosemide and torasemide.

3. Diuretics which Inhibit Action of Aldosterone

Some diuretics inhibit sodium reabsorption and potassium excretion in the distal convoluted tubule and collecting duct, by inhibiting the action of aldosterone. These substances are also called the **potassium-retaining diuretics** or **aldosterone antagonists.**

Examples are spironolactone and eplerenone.

4. Diuretics which Inhibit Activity of Carbonic Anhydrase

Some diuretics inhibit the activity of carbonic anhydrase in proximal convoluted tubules and prevent reabsorption of bicarbonate from renal tubules, resulting in osmotic diuresis. Such diuretic agents are called **carbonic anhydrase inhibitors.**

Acetazolamide is a carbonic anhydrase inhibitor.

5. Diuretics which Increase Glomerular Filtration Rate

Some xanthines (alkaloids, used as mild stimulants) cause diuresis by increasing the glomerular filtration rate and to some extent by decreasing the sodium reabsorption.

Examples are caffeine and theophylline.

6. Diuretics which Inhibit Secretion of ADH

Some diuretics produce diuresis by inhibiting the secretion of ADH.

Examples are water and ethanol.

7. Diuretics which Inhibit ADH Receptors

The antagonists of V2 receptors cause diuresis by inhibiting the receptors of antidiuretic hormone, thereby preventing the activity of this hormone.

Chapter 46

Micturition

CHAPTER OUTLINE

- DEFINITION
- FUNCTIONAL ANATOMY OF URINARY BLADDER AND URETHRA
  - URINARY BLADDER
  - URETHRA
  - URETHRAL SPHINCTERS
- NERVE SUPPLY TO URINARY BLADDER AND SPHINCTERS
  - SYMPATHETIC NERVE SUPPLY
  - PARASYMPATHETIC NERVE SUPPLY
  - SOMATIC NERVE SUPPLY
- FILLING OF URINARY BLADDER
  - PROCESS OF FILLING
  - CYSTOMETROGRAM
- MICTURITION REFLEX
- APPLIED PHYSIOLOGY: ABNORMALITIES OF MICTURITION
  - ATONIC BLADDER
  - ATOMATIC BLADDER
  - UNINHIBITED NEUROGENIC BLADDER
  - NOCTURNAL MICTURITION

DEFINITION

Micturition is defined as a process by which urine is voided from the urinary bladder. It is a reflex process. However, in grown up children and adults, it can be controlled voluntarily to some extent.

Knowledge of functional anatomy and nerve supply of urinary bladder, urethra and sphincters is essential to understand the process of micturition.

FUNCTIONAL ANATOMY OF URINARY BLADDER AND URETHRA

URINARY BLADDER

Urinary bladder consists of the body, neck and internal urethral sphincter. Smooth muscle forming the body of bladder is called **detrusor muscle**. At the posterior surface of the bladder wall, there is a triangular area called **trigone**. At the upper angles of this trigone, two ureters enter the bladder.

Lower part of bladder is narrow and forms the neck. Distal end of the bladder is guarded by **internal urethral sphincter**. This sphincter is made up of detrusor muscle. It opens towards urethra. At the distal end of urethra, there is **external urethral sphincter**. It is made up of skeletal muscle fibers. Therefore, it is responsible for voluntary control of micturition.

URETHRA

Male urethra has both urinary function and reproductive function. It transports urine and semen. Female urethra has only urinary function and it transports only urine. So, male urethra is structurally different from female urethra.

Male Urethra

Male urethra is about 20 cm long. After taking origin from bladder it traverses the prostate gland and then runs through penis **(Fig. 46.1)**. Throughout its length, the urethra has mucus glands called **glands of Littre**.

Male urethra is divided into three parts:

1. Prostatic urethra.
2. Membranous urethra.
3. Spongy urethra.

Female Urethra

Female urethra is narrower and shorter than male urethra. It is about 3.5 cm to 4 cm long. After arising from bladder, it traverses through urogenital diaphragm and runs along anterior wall of vagina. Then, it terminates at external orifice of urethra which is located between clitoris and vaginal opening **(Fig. 46.2)**.

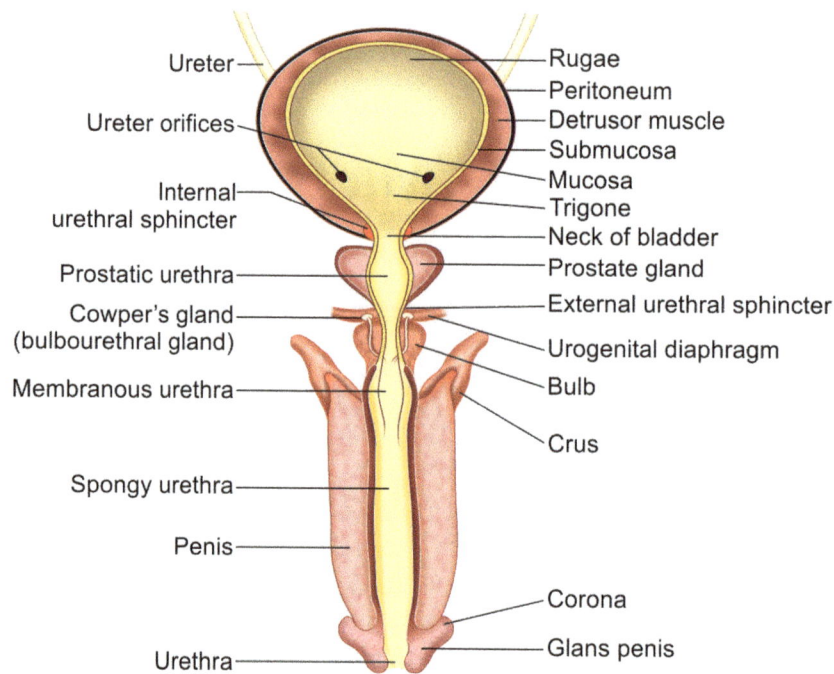

FIGURE 46.1: Urinary bladder and urethra in male.

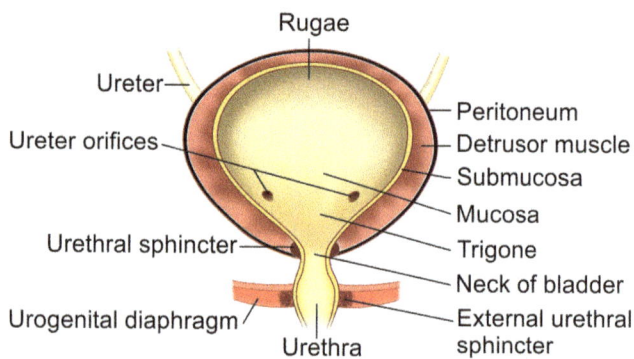

FIGURE 46.2: Urinary bladder and urethra in female.

URETHRAL SPHINCTERS

Urinary tract has two urethral sphincters:
1. Internal urethral sphincter
2. External urethral sphincter.

1. Internal Urethral Sphincter

This sphincter is situated between neck of the bladder and upper end of urethra. It is made up of smooth muscle fibers and formed by thickening of detrusor muscle.

2. External Urethral Sphincter

External sphincter is located in the urogenital diaphragm. This sphincter is made up of circular skeletal muscle fibers.

NERVE SUPPLY TO URINARY BLADDER AND SPHINCTERS

Urinary bladder and the internal sphincter are supplied by sympathetic and parasympathetic divisions of autonomic nervous system whereas, the external sphincter is supplied by the somatic nerve fibers **(Fig. 46.3)**.

SYMPATHETIC NERVE SUPPLY

Preganglionic fibers of sympathetic nerve arise from first two lumbar segments (L1 and L2) of spinal cord. After leaving spinal cord, the fibers pass through lateral sympathetic chain without any synapse in the sympathetic ganglia and finally terminate in **hypogastric ganglion**. Postganglionic fibers arising from this ganglion form the **hypogastric nerve**, which supplies detrusor muscle and internal sphincter.

Function of Sympathetic Nerve

Sympathetic nerve causes relaxation of detrusor muscle and constriction of the internal sphincter. It results in filling of urinary bladder and so, the sympathetic nerve is called **nerve of filling**.

PARASYMPATHETIC NERVE SUPPLY

Preganglionic fibers of parasympathetic nerve form the **pelvic nerve** or **nervous erigens**. Pelvic nerve fibers arise from second, third and fourth sacral segments (S2, S3 and S4) of spinal cord. These fibers run through **hypogastric ganglion** and synapse with postganglionic neurons situated in close relation to urinary bladder and internal sphincter **(Table 46.1)**.

Function of Parasympathetic Nerve

Pelvic (parasympathetic) nerve causes contraction of detrusor muscle and relaxation of the internal sphincter leading to emptying of urinary bladder **(Table 46.2)**. So, the parasympathetic nerve is called the **nerve of emptying** or **nerve of micturition**.

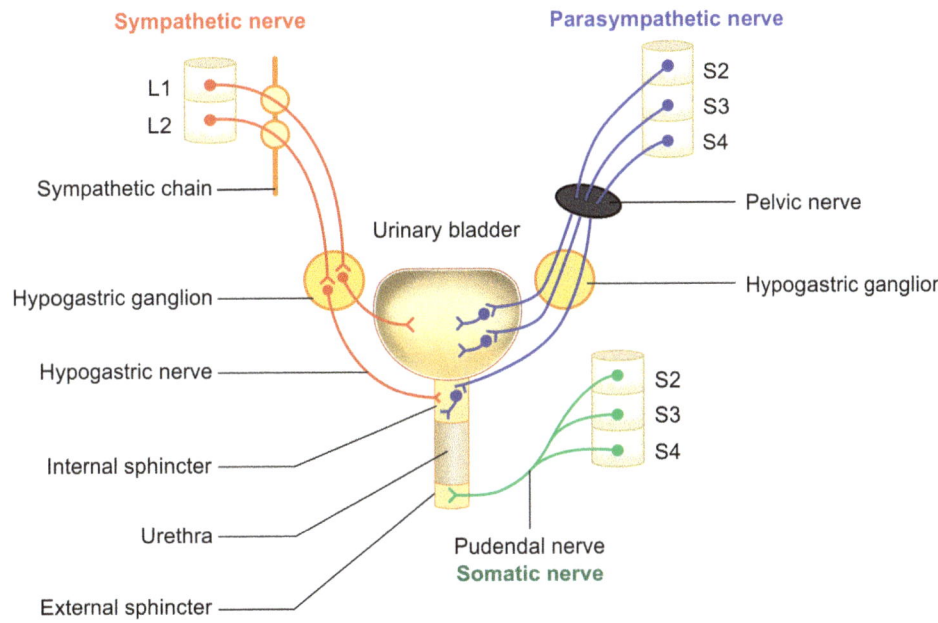

FIGURE 46.3: Nerve supply to urinary bladder and urethra.

TABLE 46.1: Functions of nerves supplying urinary bladder and sphincters.

Nerve	On detrusor muscle	On internal sphincter	On external sphincter	Function
Sympathetic nerve (hypogastric nerve)	Relaxation	Constriction	Not supplied	Filling of urinary bladder
Parasympathetic nerve (pelvic nerve)	Contraction	Relaxation	Not supplied	Emptying of urinary bladder (micturition)
Somatic nerve (pudendal nerve)	Not supplied	Not supplied	Constriction	Voluntary control of micturition

TABLE 46.2: Urethral sphincters.

Features	Internal urethral sphincter	External urethral sphincter
Situation	Between neck of bladder and upper end of urethra	In urogenital diaphragm
Muscle involved	Made up of smooth muscle fibers: Detrusor muscle	Made up of circular skeletal muscle fibers

Nerve supply	Supplied by autonomic nerves
	  Sympathetic: Hypogastric nerve
	  Parasympathetic: Pelvic nerve
		Supplied by somatic nerve: Pudendal nerve

Pelvic nerve has also the sensory fibers which carry impulses from **stretch receptors** present on the wall of the urinary bladder and urethra to the central nervous system.

■ SOMATIC NERVE SUPPLY

External sphincter is innervated by the somatic nerve called the **pudendal nerve**. It arises from second, third and fourth sacral segments of the spinal cord.

Function of Pudendal Nerve

It maintains the tonic contraction of skeletal muscle fibers of external sphincter and keeps the external sphincter constricted always.

During micturition, this nerve is inhibited. It causes relaxation of external sphincter leading to voiding of urine.

Thus, the pudendal nerve is responsible for voluntary control of micturition.

■ FILLING OF URINARY BLADDER

■ PROCESS OF FILLING

Urine is continuously formed in nephrons and it is transported drop by drop through the ureters into the urinary bladder. **Peristaltic waves** push the urine from pelvis of ureter into bladder through ureter.

A reasonable volume of urine can be stored in urinary bladder without any discomfort and without much increase in pressure inside the bladder (**intravesical pressure**). It is due to the adaptation of detrusor muscle. Relationship between the volume of urine and pressure in urinary bladder is studied by cystometrogram.

CYSTOMETROGRAM

Definition

Cystometrogram is the graphical registration (recording) of pressure changes in urinary bladder in relation to volume of urine collected in it.

Method of Recording Cystometrogram

A **double lumen catheter** is introduced into the urinary bladder. One lumen is used to infuse fluid into the bladder and the other one is used to record the pressure changes by connecting it to a suitable recording instrument.

First, bladder is emptied completely. Then, a known quantity of fluid is introduced into the bladder at regular intervals. Intravesical pressure developed by the fluid is recorded continuously. A graph is obtained by plotting all the values of volume and the pressure. This graph is the cystometrogram **(Fig. 46.4)**.

Segments of Cystometrogram

Cystometrogram shows three segments.

Segment I

Initially, when urinary bladder is empty, the intravesical pressure is 0. When about 100 mL of fluid is collected, the pressure rises sharply to about 10 cm H_2O.

Segment II

This segment shows the plateau, i.e. the intravesical pressure remains more or less at 10 cm H_2O (level of segment I) without any change even after introducing 300 mL to 400 mL of fluid. It is because of adaptation of urinary bladder by relaxation. It is in accordance with law of Laplace.

Law of Laplace

According to this law, pressure in a spherical organ is inversely proportional to its radius, the tone remaining constant. That is, if radius is more, the pressure is less and if radius is less the pressure is more, provided tone remains constant.

Urinary bladder obeys Laplace law. In urinary bladder, the tension increases as urine is filled. At the same time, radius also increases due to relaxation of detrusor muscle. Because of this, the pressure rise is almost zero.

When about 100 mL of urine is collected, the pressure rises to about 10 cm H_2O and now, the desire for micturition occurs. The desire for micturition is associated with a vague feeling in the perineum. An additional volume of about 200 mL to 300 mL of urine can be collected in bladder without much increase in pressure. However, when total volume rises beyond 400 mL, the pressure rises sharply and the **urge for micturition** starts. Still **voluntary control of micturition** is possible. And, beyond 600 mL to 700 mL of urine, voluntary control starts failing.

Segment III

As pressure increases with collection of 300 mL to 400 mL of fluid, the contraction of detrusor muscle becomes intense, increasing the consciousness and urge for micturition. Still, voluntary control is possible. Voluntary control is possible up to volume of 600 mL to 700 mL at which the pressure rises to about 35 cm H_2O to 40 cm H_2O.

When intravesical pressure rises above 40 cm water, the contraction of detrusor muscle becomes still more intense. And, voluntary control of micturition is not possible. Now, pain sensation develops and micturition should take place.

MICTURITION REFLEX

It is a reflex by which micturition occurs. This reflex is elicited by stimulation of **stretch receptors** situated on the wall of urinary bladder and urethra. When about 300 mL to 400 mL of urine is collected in bladder, the pressure inside bladder increases. This stretches the wall of bladder resulting in stimulation of stretch receptors and generation of sensory impulses.

Sensory (afferent) impulses from receptors reach the sacral segments of spinal cord via sensory fibers of pelvic (parasympathetic) nerve. Motor (efferent) impulses produced in spinal cord, travel through motor fibers of pelvic nerve towards bladder and internal sphincter. These motor impulses cause contraction of detrusor muscle and relaxation of internal sphincter so that, urine enters the urethra from bladder **(Fig. 46.5)**.

Once urine enters urethra, stretch receptors in the urethra are stimulated and send afferent impulses to spinal cord via pelvic nerve fibers. These impulses inhibit

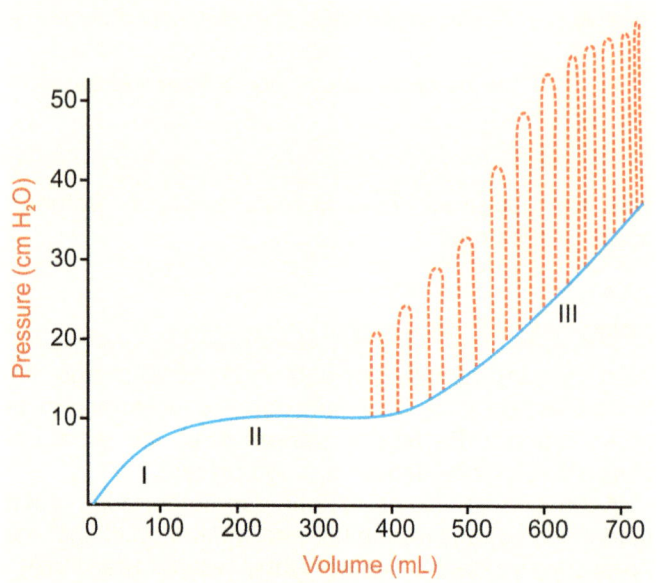

FIGURE 46.4: Cystometrogram. Dotted lines = Contraction of detrusor muscle.

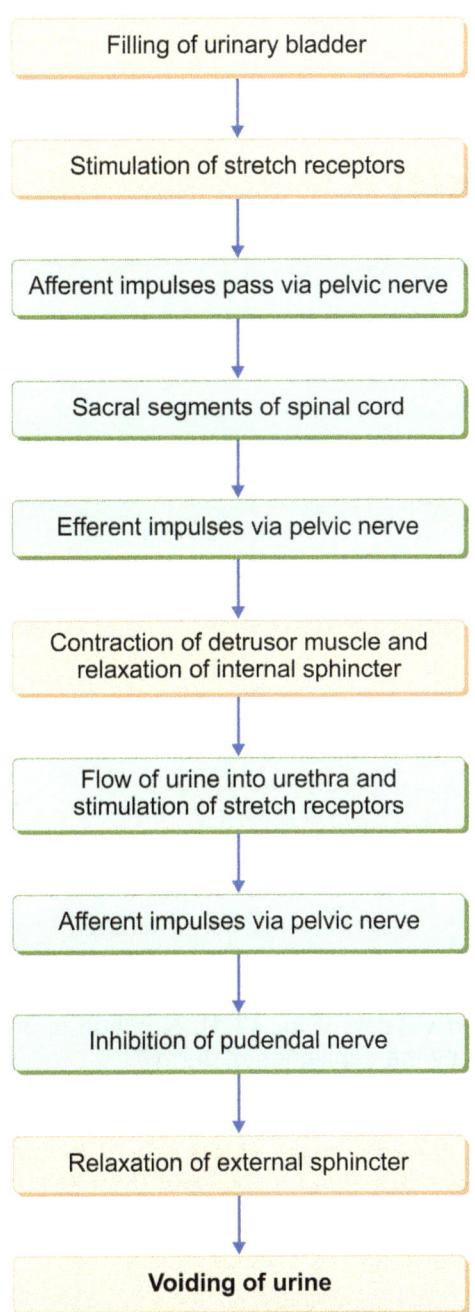

FIGURE 46.5: Micturition reflex.

pudendal nerve. So, the external sphincter relaxes and micturition occurs.

Once a micturition reflex begins, it is **self-regenerative**, i.e. initial contraction of bladder further activates the receptors to cause still further increase in sensory impulses from the bladder and urethra. These impulses, in turn cause further increase in reflex contraction of bladder. This cycle continues repeatedly until force of contraction of bladder reaches the maximum and urine is voided out completely.

During micturition, the flow of urine is facilitated by increase in abdominal pressure due to the voluntary contraction of abdominal muscles.

Higher Centers for Micturition

Spinal centers for micturition are present in sacral and lumbar segments. Spinal centers are regulated by higher centers.

Higher centers are of two types:

1. **Inhibitory centers** which are situated in midbrain and cerebral cortex.
2. **Facilitatory centers** which are situated in pons and cerebral cortex.

■ APPLIED PHYSIOLOGY: ABNORMALITIES OF MICTURITION

■ 1. ATONIC BLADDER: EFFECT OF DESTRUCTION OF SENSORY NERVE FIBERS

Atonic bladder is the urinary bladder with loss of tone in detrusor muscle. It is caused by destruction of sensory (pelvic) nerve fibers of urinary bladder.

Due to destruction of sensory nerve fibers, urinary bladder is filled up without any stretch signals to spinal cord. Detrusor muscle loses the tone and becomes flaccid. So, micturition does not occur and bladder is completely filled with urine. Later, overflow occurs in drops as and when urine enters the bladder. It is called **overflow incontinence** or **overflow dribbling**. It occurs in spinal injury and syphilis.

■ 2. AUTOMATIC BLADDER

Automatic bladder is the urinary bladder characterized by **hyperactive micturition reflex** with loss of voluntary control. So, even with small amount of urine collected in the bladder, micturition reflex occurs resulting in emptying of bladder. This occurs in transaction of spinal cord above the sacral segments.

■ 3. UNINHIBITED NEUROGENIC BLADDER

It is the urinary bladder with frequent and **uncontrollable micturition.** It is caused by lesion in midbrain.

Lesion in midbrain causes continuous excitation of spinal micturition centers resulting in frequent and uncontrollable micturition. Even a small quantity of urine collected in bladder will elicit the micturition reflex.

■ 4. NOCTURNAL MICTURITION

Nocturnal micturition is the involuntary voiding of urine during night. It is otherwise known as **enuresis** or **bedwetting**. It occurs due to the absence of voluntary control of micturition. It is a common and normal process in infants and children below 3 years. It is because of incomplete myelination of motor nerve fibers of the bladder. When myelination is complete, voluntary control of micturition develops and bedwetting stops.

Nocturnal micturition occurs after 3 years of age because of neurological disorders such as lumbosacral vertebral defects and impairment of motor area of cerebral cortex.

Chapter 47: Skin

CHAPTER OUTLINE

- **STRUCTURE OF SKIN**
  - EPIDERMIS
  - DERMIS
  - APPENDAGES OF SKIN
  - COLOR OF SKIN
- **GLANDS OF SKIN**
  - SEBACEOUS GLANDS
  - SWEAT GLANDS
- **FUNCTIONS OF SKIN**
  - PROTECTIVE FUNCTION
- SENSORY FUNCTION
- STORAGE FUNCTION
- SYNTHETIC FUNCTION
- REGULATION OF BODY TEMPERATURE
- REGULATION OF WATER AND ELECTROLYTE BALANCE
- EXCRETORY FUNCTION
- ABSORPTIVE FUNCTION
- SECRETORY FUNCTION

STRUCTURE OF SKIN

Skin forms largest organ of the body. It is not uniformly thick. At some places, it is thick and in some places it is thin. Average thickness of the skin is about 1 to 2 mm. In sole of foot, palm of the hand and in the interscapular region, it is considerably thick, measuring about 5 mm. In other areas of the body, skin is thin. It is thinnest over eyelids and penis measuring about 0.5 mm only.

Layers of Skin

Skin is made up of two layers:

1. Outer epidermis.
2. Inner dermis.

EPIDERMIS

Epidermis is the outer layer of skin. It is formed by stratified epithelium.

Epidermis is formed by five layers of structures:

1. Stratum corneum.
2. Stratum lucidum.
3. Stratum granulosum.
4. Stratum spinosum.
5. Stratum germinativum.

Important feature of epidermis is that, it does not have blood vessels (**Fig. 47.1**). Nutrition is provided to epidermis by the capillaries of dermis.

DERMIS

Dermis is the inner layer of the skin. It is a connective tissue layer made up of dense and stout collagen fibers, fibroblasts and histiocytes.

Dermis is made up of 2 layers:

1. Superficial papillary layer.
2. Deeper reticular layer.

APPENDAGES OF SKIN

Hair follicles with hairs, nails, sweat glands, sebaceous glands and mammary glands are considered as appendages of the skin.

COLOR OF THE SKIN

Color of the skin depends upon two important factors:

1. Pigmentation of skin.
2. Hemoglobin in the blood.

1. Pigmentation of the Skin

Cells of the skin contain a brown pigment called melanin. Melanin is synthesized by **melanocytes** which are present

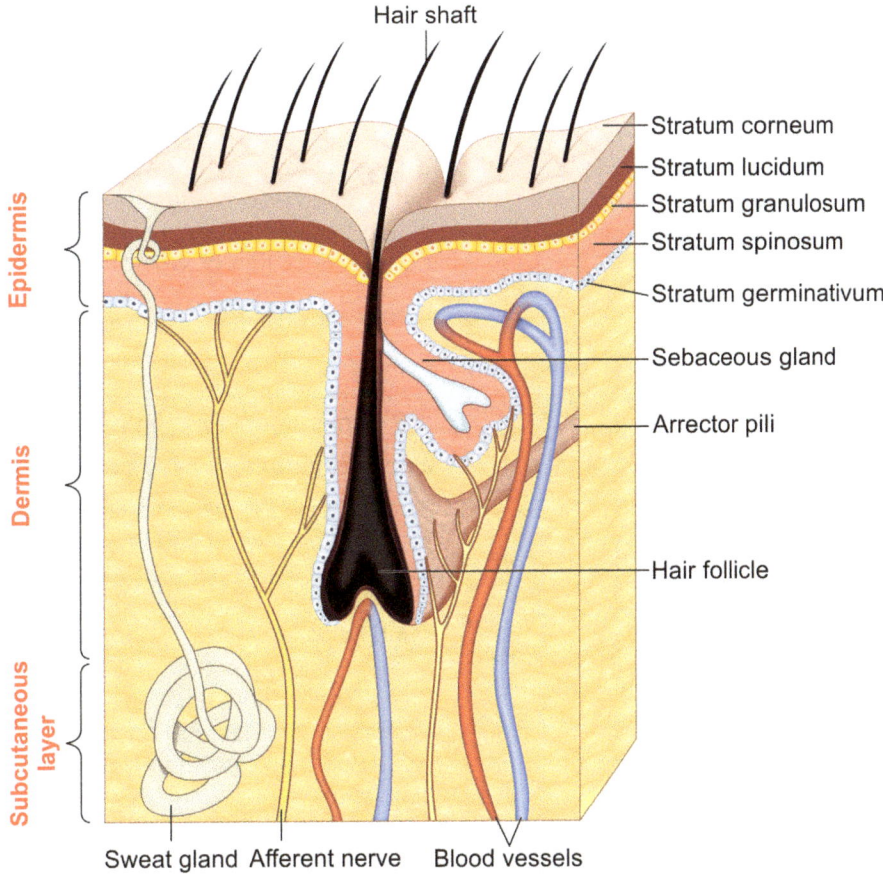

FIGURE 47.1: Structure of skin.
(*Courtesy:* JS Pascricha and Ramji Gupta)

mainly in the stratum germinativum and stratum spinosum of epidermis. After synthesis, this pigment spreads to cells of other layers.

Melanin

Melanin is the skin pigment and it forms the major color determinant of human skin. Skin becomes dark when melanin content increases. It is protein in nature and it is synthesized from the amino acid **tyrosine** via **dihydroxy phenylalanine (DOPA)**.

2. Hemoglobin in Blood

Amount and nature of hemoglobin that circulates in the cutaneous blood vessels play an important role in coloration of the skin.

Skin becomes:

i. Pale when hemoglobin content decreases.
ii. Pink when blood rushes to skin due to cutaneous vasodilatation (blushing).
iii. Bluish during cyanosis which is caused by excess amount of reduced hemoglobin.

■ GLANDS OF SKIN

Skin contains two types of glands, sebaceous glands and the sweat glands.

■ SEBACEOUS GLANDS

Sebaceous glands are simple or branched alveolar glands situated in the dermis of the skin.

These glands are ovoid or spherical in shape and open into the neck of the hair follicle through a duct. In some areas like face, lips, nipple, glans penis and labia minora the sebaceous glands open directly into the exterior.

Sebaceous glands secrete an oily substance called sebum.

Composition of Sebum

Sebum contains:

1. Free fatty acids.
2. Triglycerides.
3. Squalene.
4. Sterols.
5. Waxes.
6. Paraffin.

Functions of Sebum

1. Free fatty acid content of the sebum has antibacterial and antifungal actions. Thus, it prevents the infection of skin by bacteria or fungi.

2. Lipid nature of sebum keeps the skin smooth and oily. It protects the skin from unnecessary desquamation and injury caused by dryness.
3. Lipids of the sebum prevent heat loss from the body. It is particularly useful in cold climate.

Activation of Sebaceous Glands at Puberty

Sebaceous glands are inactive till puberty. At the time of puberty these glands are activated by sex hormones in both males and females.

At the time of puberty particularly in males, due to increased secretion of sex hormones especially dehydroepiandrosterone, the sebaceous glands are stimulated suddenly. It leads to development of acne on the face.

Acne

Acne is the localized inflammatory condition of skin characterized by pimples on face, chest and back. It occurs because of over activity of sebaceous glands. **Acne vulgaris** is the common type of acne that is developed during adolescence. Acne disappears within few years when the sebaceous glands become adapted to the sex hormones.

■ SWEAT GLANDS

Sweat glands are of two types:
1. Eccrine glands.
2. Apocrine glands.

Eccrine Glands

Eccrine glands are tubular glands distributed throughout the body **(Table 47.1)**. These glands open out through the sweat pore.

Secretory activity of eccrine glands

Eccrine glands function throughout life since birth. These glands secrete a clear watery sweat. The secretion increases during increase in temperature and emotional conditions.

Eccrine glands play important role in regulating the body temperature by secreting sweat. Sweat contains water, sodium chloride, urea and lactic acid.

Control of eccrine glands

Eccrine glands are under nervous control and are supplied by sympathetic postganglionic cholinergic nerve fibers, which secrete acetylcholine. Stimulation of these nerves causes secretion of sweat.

Apocrine Glands

Apocrine glands are situated only in certain areas of the body like axilla, pubis, areola and umbilicus. These glands are also tubular in nature but open into the hair follicles.

Secretory activity of apocrine glands

Apocrine sweat glands are nonfunctional till puberty and start functioning only at the time of puberty. In old age, the function of these glands gradually declines.

Secretion of the apocrine glands is thick and milky. At the time of secretion, it is odorless. When microorganisms grow in this secretion, a characteristic odor develops in the regions where apocrine glands are present. Secretion increases in emotional conditions.

Apocrine glands do not play any role in temperature regulation.

Control of apocrine glands

Apocrine glands are innervated by sympathetic adrenergic nerve fibers. But the secretory activity is not under nervous control. However, adrenaline from adrenal medulla causes secretion by apocrine glands.

Glands of eyelids, glands of external auditory meatus and mammary glands are the modified apocrine glands.

Pheromones

Pheromones or **vomeropherins** are substances secreted by apocrine glands. It is observed that the pheromones excreted in axilla of a woman affects the menstrual cycle of her room-mate or another woman living with her. These substances stimulate receptors of vomeronasal receptors.

TABLE 47.1: Differences between eccrine and apocrine sweat glands.

Features	Eccrine glands	Apocrine glands
1. Distribution	Throughout the body	Only in limited areas like axilla, pubis, areola and umbilicus
2. Opening	Exterior through sweat pore	Into the hair follicle
3. Period of functioning	Function throughout life	Start functioning only at puberty
4. Secretion	Clear and watery	Thick and milky
5. Regulation of body temperature	Play important role in temperature regulation	Do not play any role in temperature regulation
6. Conditions when secretion increases	During increased temperature and emotional conditions	During emotional conditions
7. Control of secretory activity	Under nervous control	Under hormonal control
8. Nerve supply	Sympathetic cholinergic fibers	Sympathetic adrenergic fibers

Vomeronasal receptors detect the odor of pheromones. Impulses from these receptors are transmitted to hypothalamus, which influences the menstrual cycle via pituitary gonadal axis. Effect of pheromones on the menstrual cycle of other individuals is called **dormitory effect.** Refer Chapter 120 for details of vomeronasal organ and its receptors.

FUNCTIONS OF THE SKIN

Primary function of skin is the protection of organs. However, it has many other important functions also.

1. PROTECTIVE FUNCTION

Skin forms covering of all organs of the body and protects these organs from the following factors:

i. Bacteria and toxic substances.
ii. Mechanical blow.
iii. Ultraviolet rays.

i. Protection from Bacteria and Toxic Substances

Skin covers and protects the organs from having direct contact with external environment. Thus, it prevents the bacterial infection.

Lysozyme secreted in skin destroys the bacteria. Stratum corneum of epidermis is responsible for the protective function of skin. This layer also offers resistance against toxic chemicals like acids and alkalis.

ii. Protection from Mechanical Blow

Skin is not tightly placed over the underlying organs or tissues. It is somewhat loose and moves over the underlying subcutaneous tissues. So, the mechanical impact of any blow to skin is not transmitted to underlying tissues.

iii. Protection from Ultraviolet Rays

Skin protects the body from ultraviolet rays of sunlight. Exposure to sunlight or to any other source of ultraviolet rays increases the production of melanin pigment in skin. Melanin absorbs ultraviolet rays. At the same time, the thickness of stratum corneum increases. This layer of epidermis also absorbs the ultraviolet rays.

2. SENSORY FUNCTION

Skin is considered as the largest sense organ in the body. It has many nerve endings, which form the specialized cutaneous receptors (Chapter 91).

These receptors are stimulated by the sensations of touch, pain, pressure or temperature sensation and convey these sensations to the brain via afferent nerves. At the brain level, perception of different sensations occurs.

3. STORAGE FUNCTION

Skin stores fat, water, chloride and sugar. It can also store blood by the dilatation of the cutaneous blood vessels.

4. SYNTHETIC FUNCTION

Vitamin D_3 is synthesized in skin by the action of ultraviolet rays from sunlight on cholesterol (Chapter 52).

5. REGULATION OF BODY TEMPERATURE

Skin plays an important role in the regulation of body temperature. Excess heat is lost from the body through skin by radiation, conduction, convection and evaporation. Sweat glands of the skin play active part in heat loss by secreting sweat. The lipid content of sebum prevents loss of heat from the body in cold environment. More details are given in Chapter 48.

6. REGULATION OF WATER AND ELECTROLYTE BALANCE

Skin regulates water balance and electrolyte balance by excreting water and salts through sweat.

7. EXCRETORY FUNCTION

Skin excretes small quantities of waste materials like urea, salts and fatty substance.

8. ABSORPTIVE FUNCTION

Skin absorbs the fat-soluble substances and some ointments.

9. SECRETORY FUNCTION

Skin secretes sweat through sweat glands and sebum through sebaceous glands. By secreting sweat, skin regulates body temperature and water balance. Sebum keeps the skin smooth and moist.

Chapter 48: Body Temperature

CHAPTER OUTLINE

- **BODY TEMPERATURE**
  - NORMAL BODY TEMPERATURE
  - TEMPERATURE AT DIFFERENT PARTS OF THE BODY
  - VARIATIONS OF BODY TEMPERATURE
- **HEAT BALANCE**
  - HEAT GAIN OR HEAT PRODUCTION IN THE BODY
  - HEAT LOSS FROM THE BODY
- **REGULATION OF BODY TEMPERATURE**
  - HOMEOTHERMIC ANIMALS
  - POIKILOTHERMIC ANIMALS
  - HEAT LOSS CENTER
  - HEAT GAIN CENTER
  - ROLE OF HYPOTHALAMUS
  - MECHANISM OF TEMPERATURE REGULATION
- **APPLIED PHYSIOLOGY: THERMOREGULATORY DISORDERS**
  - HYPERTHERMIA: FEVER
  - HYPOTHERMIA

■ BODY TEMPERATURE

Body temperature can be measured by placing the clinical thermometer in different parts of the body such as:

1. Mouth (oral temperature).
2. Axilla (axillary temperature).
3. Rectum (rectal temperature).
4. Over the skin (surface temperature).

■ NORMAL BODY TEMPERATURE

Normal body temperature in human is 37°C (98.6°F) when measured by placing clinical thermometer in the mouth (**oral temperature**). It varies between 35.8°C and 37.3°C (96.4°F and 99.1°F).

■ TEMPERATURE AT DIFFERENT PARTS OF THE BODY

Axillary temperature is 0.3 to 0.6°C (0.5 to 1°F) lower than the oral temperature. And, the **rectal temperature** is 0.3 to 0.6°C (0.5 to 1°F) higher than oral temperature. The **surface temperature** (skin or **superficial temperature**) varies between 29.5°C and 33.9°C (85.1°F and 93°F). Surface temperature is slightly less than oral temperature.

Core Temperature

Core temperature is the average temperature of structures present in deeper part of the body. Core temperature is always more than oral or rectal temperature. Temperature at different parts of the body are given in **Table 48.1**.

TABLE 48.1: Temperature at different parts of the body.

Parts	Temperature	
	Fahrenheit	Celsius
Oral temperature	98.6° (96.4 to 99.1°)	37.0° (35.8 to 37.3°)
Surface temperature	85.1 to 93°	29.5 to 33.9°
Axillary temperature	0.5 to 1° Lower than the oral temperature	0.3 to 0.6°
Rectal temperature	0.5 to 1° Higher than oral temperature	0.3 to 0.6°
Core temperature	100°	37.8°

■ VARIATIONS OF BODY TEMPERATURE

Physiological Variations

1. Age

In infants, the body temperature varies in accordance to environmental temperature for the first few days after birth. It is because the temperature regulating system does not function properly during infancy. In children the temperature is slightly (0.5°C) more than in adults because of more physical activities. In old age, since the heat production is less, the body temperature decreases slightly.

2. Sex

In females, body temperature is less because of low basal metabolic rate when compared to that of males. During menstrual phase it decreases slightly.

3. Diurnal variation

In early morning, temperature is 1°C less. In the afternoon, it reaches the maximum (about 1°C more than normal).

4. After meals

Body temperature rises slightly (0.5°C) after meals.

5. Exercise

During exercise, the temperature raises due to production of heat in muscles.

6. Sleep

During sleep, body temperature decreases by 0.5°C.

7. Emotion

During emotional conditions, body temperature increases.

8. Menstrual cycle

In females, immediately after ovulation, temperature rises (0.5°C to 1°C) sharply. It decreases (0.5°C) during menstrual phase.

Pathological Variations

Abnormal increase in body temperature is called hyperthermia or fever and decreased body temperature is called hypothermia. Refer Applied Physiology in this Chapter.

HEAT BALANCE

Regulation of body temperature depends upon the balance between heat produced in body and heat lost from the body.

HEAT GAIN OR HEAT PRODUCTION IN THE BODY

Various mechanisms are involved in production of heat in the body.

1. Metabolic Activities

Major portion of heat produced in the body is due to metabolism of foodstuffs. Heat production is more during metabolism of fat. About 9 calories of heat is produced during metabolism of fats, when 1 liter of oxygen is utilized. For the same amount of oxygen, carbohydrate metabolism produces 4.7 calories of heat. Protein metabolism produces 4.5 Cal/L. Liver is the organ in which maximum heat is produced due to metabolic activity.

2. Muscular Activity

Heat is produced in the muscle both at rest and during activities. During rest, heat is produced by muscle tone. About 80% of heat of activity is produced by the activity of skeletal muscles.

3. Role of Hormones

Thyroxine and adrenaline increase the heat production by accelerating metabolic activities.

4. Radiation of Heat from the Environment

Body gains heat by radiation. It occurs when environmental temperature is higher than the body temperature.

5. Shivering

Shivering is the shaking of body caused by rapid involuntary contraction or twitching of muscles during exposure to cold. It is a compensatory physiological mechanism in the body, during which enormous heat is produced.

6. Brown Fat Tissue

Brown fat or **brown adipose tissue** is one of the two types of adipose tissues, the other being white adipose tissue. Brown fat produces enormous body heat, particularly in infants.

HEAT LOSS FROM THE BODY

Maximum heat is lost from the body through skin and small amount of heat is lost through respiratory system, kidney and GI tract. When environmental temperature is less than body temperature, heat is lost from the body. Heat loss occurs by the following methods:

1. Conduction

Heat is lost from the surface of the body to other objects such as chair or bed by means of conduction.

2. Radiation

Sixty percent of heat is lost by means of radiation, i.e. transfer of heat by infrared electromagnetic radiation from body to other objects through the surrounding air.

3. Convection

Heat is conducted to the air surrounding the body and then carried away by air currents, i.e. convection.

4. Evaporation: Insensible Perspiration

When body temperature increases sweating occurs. During sweating, water evaporates from sweat and heat is lost from the body. About 22% of heat is lost through evaporation of water.

Perspiration

Perspiration means formation of sweat from which water is lost by means of evaporation.

Insensible perspiration

Insensible perspiration is the perspiration which occurs before it is being perceived or sensed, i.e., we are not aware of perspiration. In addition to loss of water through sweat, insensible perspiration includes evaporation of water through lungs also. Usually insensible perspiration is about 400 mL to 600 mL per day.

5. Panting

Panting is the rapid shallow breathing associated with dribbling of more saliva. In some animals such as dogs, which do not have sweat glands, heat is lost by evaporation of water from lungs and saliva by means of panting.

■ REGULATION OF BODY TEMPERATURE

Living organisms are classified into two groups depending upon the maintenance (regulation) of body temperature:
1. Homeothermic animals.
2. Poikilothermic animals.

■ HOMEOTHERMIC ANIMALS

Homeothermic animals are the animals whose body temperature is maintained at a constant level irrespective of the environmental temperature. Birds and mammals including man belong to this category. They are also called **warm-blooded animals**.

■ POIKILOTHERMIC ANIMALS

Poikilothermic animals are the animals whose body temperature is not constant. It varies according to environmental temperature. Amphibians and reptiles are the poikilothermic animals. These animals are also called **cold-blooded animals**.

Set Point for Body Temperature

In homeothermic animals, body temperature is regulated by hypothalamus, which sets the normal range of body temperature. The set point for body temperature under normal physiological conditions is 37°C.

Hypothalamus has two centers which regulate the body temperature:
1. Heat loss center.
2. Heat gain center.

■ HEAT LOSS CENTER

This center is situated in **preoptic nucleus** of anterior hypothalamus. Neurons in preoptic nucleus are heat-sensitive nerve cells which are called **thermoreceptors**. Stimulation of preoptic nucleus results in cutaneous vasodilatation and sweating. Removal or lesion of this nucleus increases the body temperature.

■ HEAT GAIN CENTER

It is otherwise known as heat production center. It is situated in posterior hypothalamic nucleus. Stimulation of posterior hypothalamic nucleus causes shivering. Removal or lesion of this nucleus leads to fall in body temperature.

■ MECHANISM OF TEMPERATURE REGULATION

When Body Temperature Increases

When body temperature increases, blood temperature also increases. When blood with increased temperature passes through hypothalamus, it stimulates the thermoreceptors present in the heat loss center in preoptic nucleus (Fig. 48.1).

Now, the heat loss center brings temperature back to normal by two mechanisms:
1. Promotion of heat loss.
2. Prevention of heat production.

1. Promotion of heat loss

Heat loss center promotes heat loss from the body by:
 i. Increasing the secretion of sweat. When sweat secretion increases, more water is lost from skin along with heat.
 ii. Inhibiting the sympathetic centers in posterior hypothalamus. This causes cutaneous vasodilatation. Now, blood flow through skin increases causing excess sweating. It increases the heat loss through sweat leading to decrease in body temperature.

2. Prevention of heat production

Heat loss center prevents heat production in the body by inhibiting mechanisms involved in heat production such as shivering and chemical (metabolic) reactions.

When Body Temperature Decreases

When the body temperature decreases it is brought back to normal by two mechanisms:
1. Prevention of heat loss.
2. Promotion of heat production.

1. Prevention of heat loss

When body temperature decreases, the preoptic thermoreceptors are not activated. So, the posterior hypothalamus is not inhibited. This causes cutaneous vasoconstriction. The blood flow to skin decreases and so the heat loss is prevented.

2. Promotion of heat production

Heat production is promoted by two ways:
 i. *Shivering:* Primary motor center for shivering is situated in posterior hypothalamus near the wall of the III ventricle. When body temperature is low, this center is activated by heat gain center and, shivering occurs. Enormous heat is produced during shivering due to severe muscular activities.
 ii. *Increased metabolic reactions:* Sympathetic centers, which are activated by heat gain center, stimulate secretion of adrenaline and noradrenaline. These hormones, particularly adrenaline increase heat production by accelerating cellular metabolic activities.

Simultaneously, hypothalamus secretes thyrotropin-releasing hormone. It causes release of thyroid stimulating hormone from pituitary. It in turn increases release of thyroxine from thyroid. Thyroxine accelerates the metabolic activities in the body and increases heat production.

Chemical thermogenesis

It is the process in which heat is produced in the body by metabolic activities induced by hormones.

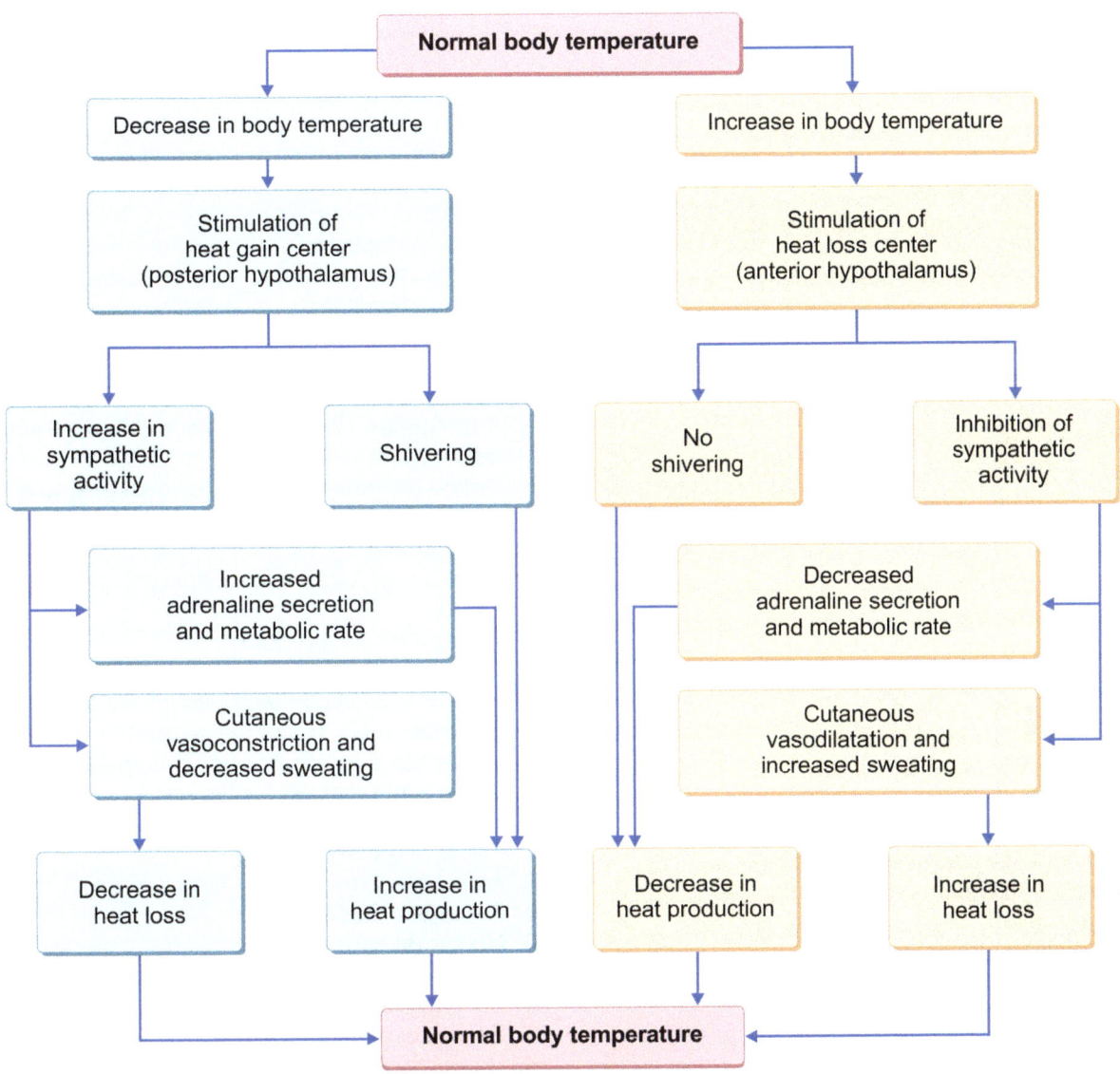

FIGURE 48.1: Regulation of body temperature.

■ APPLIED PHYSIOLOGY: THERMOREGULATORY DISORDERS

■ HYPERTHERMIA: FEVER

Elevation of body temperature above the set point is called hyperthermia, fever or **pyrexia**. Fever itself is not an illness. But it is an important sign of something going wrong in the body. It is the part of body's response to disease. Fever may be beneficial to body and on many occasions, it plays an important role in helping the body fight diseases, particularly the infections.

Hyperpyrexia

Hyperpyrexia is the rise in body temperature beyond 107.6°F (42°C). Hyperpyrexia results in damage of body tissues. Further increase in temperature becomes life threatening.

Causes of Fever

1. *Infection:* Certain substances **(pyrogens)** released from bacteria or parasites affect the heat regulating system in hypothalamus, resulting in the production of excess heat and fever.
2. *Hyperthyroidism:* Increased basal metabolic rate during hyperthyroidism causes fever.
3. *Brain lesions:* When lesion involves temperature regulating centers, fever occurs.
4. *Diabetes insipidus:* In this condition, fever occurs without any apparent cause.

■ HYPOTHERMIA

Decrease in body temperature below 95°F (35°C) is called hypothermia. It is considered as the clinical state of subnormal body temperature, when the body fails to produce enough heat to maintain the normal activities. Major setback of this condition is the impairment of metabolic activities of the body. When the temperature drops below 87.8°F (31°C), it becomes fatal. Elderly persons are more susceptible for hypothermia.

MODEL QUESTIONS IN RENAL PHYSIOLOGY AND SKIN

■ LONG QUESTIONS

1. Describe the process of urine formation.
2. What are the different stages of urine formation? Explain glomerular filtration.
3. Give an account of role of renal tubules in the process of urine formation.
4. What is countercurrent mechanism? Describe the anatomical and physiological basis of countercurrent mechanism in kidney.
5. Describe the mechanism involved in concentration of urine.
6. Give an account of micturition.
7. What is normal body temperature? Explain heat balance and regulation of body temperature. Add a note on fever.

■ SHORT QUESTIONS

1. Functions of kidney.
2. Structure of nephron.
3. Juxtaglomerular apparatus.
4. Renin-angiotensin system.
5. Salient features of renal circulation.
6. Autoregulation of renal circulation.
7. Glomerular filtration rate.
8. Factors regulating glomerular filtration rate.
9. Effective filtration pressure in kidney.
10. Reabsorption of water in renal tubule.
11. Tubular secretion.
12. Renal medullary gradient.
13. Countercurrent multiplier.
14. Countercurrent exchanger.
15. Actions of hormones on renal tubules.
16. Acidification of urine.
17. Plasma clearance.
18. Nerve supply to urinary bladder and sphincters.
19. Cystometrogram.
20. Micturition reflex.
21. Structure of skin.
22. Sweat glands.
23. Functions of skin.
24. Regulation of body temperature.
25. Heat balance.

■ VERY SHORT ANSWER QUESTIONS

1. Renal corpuscle.
2. Differences between two types of nephron.
3. List the substances secreted by juxtaglomerular apparatus.
4. Renal blood vessels.
5. Autoregulation of renal blood flow.
6. Filtration membrane in glomerulus.
7. Ultrafiltration.
8. GFR.
9. Filtration fraction.
10. Net filtration pressure.
11. Starling hypothesis and Starling forces of filtration.
12. Tubuloglomerular feedback.
13. Hormones affecting GFR.
14. Selective reabsorption.
15. Substances reabsorbed from different segments of renal tubule.
16. Define tubular maximum and give example.
17. Define renal threshold and give example.
18. Aquaporins.
19. Substances secreted in different segments of renal tubule.
20. Renal medullary gradient.
21. Recycling of urea in renal medulla.
22. Role of ADH in concentration of urine.
23. Diuresis.
24. Properties and composition of urine.
25. Urethra in males and females.
26. Urethral sphincters.
27. Filling of urinary bladder.
28. Atonic bladder.
29. Automatic bladder.
30. Nocturnal enuresis.
31. Apocrine glands.
32. Eccrine glands.
33. Sebaceous glands/Sebum.
34. Homeothermic and poikilothermic animals.
35. Temperature at different parts of the body and core temperature.
36. Heat loss center.
37. Heat gain center.
38. Perspiration and insensible perspiration.
39. Fever.
40. Hypothermia.

SECTION 6: ENDOCRINOLOGY

Chapter 49: Overview of Endocrine System

CHAPTER OUTLINE

- **ENDOCRINE SYSTEM**
  - CELL-TO-CELL SIGNALING
  - CHEMICAL MESSENGERS
- **ENDOCRINE GLANDS**
- **CLASSIFICATION OF HORMONES**
- **HORMONAL ACTION**
  - HORMONE RECEPTORS
  - MECHANISM OF HORMONAL ACTION

ENDOCRINE SYSTEM

All physiological activities of the body are regulated by two major controlling systems in the body:

1. Nervous system.
2. Endocrine system.

Both the systems interact with one another and regulate the body functions. This section deals with endocrine system and Section 10 deals with nervous system. Endocrine system functions by secreting some chemical substances called **hormones**.

CELL-TO-CELL SIGNALING

Cell-to-cell signaling is the transfer of information from one cell to another. It is also called **cell signaling** or **intercellular communication**. Cell signaling occurs chemical messengers.

CHEMICAL MESSENGERS

Chemical messengers are the substances involved in cell signaling. Most of the chemical messengers are secreted by endocrine glands. Some of them are secreted by nerve endings and the cells of other tissues.

All the chemical messengers carry the message (signal) from **signaling cells (controlling cells)** to target **cells**.

Classification of Chemical Messengers

Chemical messengers are classified into four types:

1. Endocrine messengers.
2. Paracrine messengers.
3. Autocrine messengers.
4. Neurocrine messengers.

1. *Endocrine Messengers*

Endocrine messengers are the classical hormones secreted by endocrine glands. **Classical hormone** is defined as a chemical messenger, synthesized by endocrine gland and transported by blood to the target organs or tissues (site of action).

Examples are growth hormone and insulin.

2. *Paracrine Messengers*

Paracrine messengers are the chemical messengers, which diffuse from control cells to the target cells through interstitial fluid **(Fig. 49.1)**.

Juxtacrine messengers or local hormones

Juxtacrine messengers or **local hormones** are some of the paracrine messengers which directly enter the neighboring target cells through gap junctions.

Examples are prostaglandins and histamine.

3. *Autocrine Messengers*

Autocrine messengers are the chemical messengers that control the source cells which secrete them. So, these messengers are also called **intracellular chemical mediators**.

Examples are leukotrienes.

4. *Neurocrine or Neural Messengers*

Neurocrine or neural messengers are of two types:

1. *Neurotransmitter*. Neurotransmitter is the chemical messenger that carries information form a nerve cell to another nerve cell or muscle or another tissue. Examples are acetylcholine and dopamine.

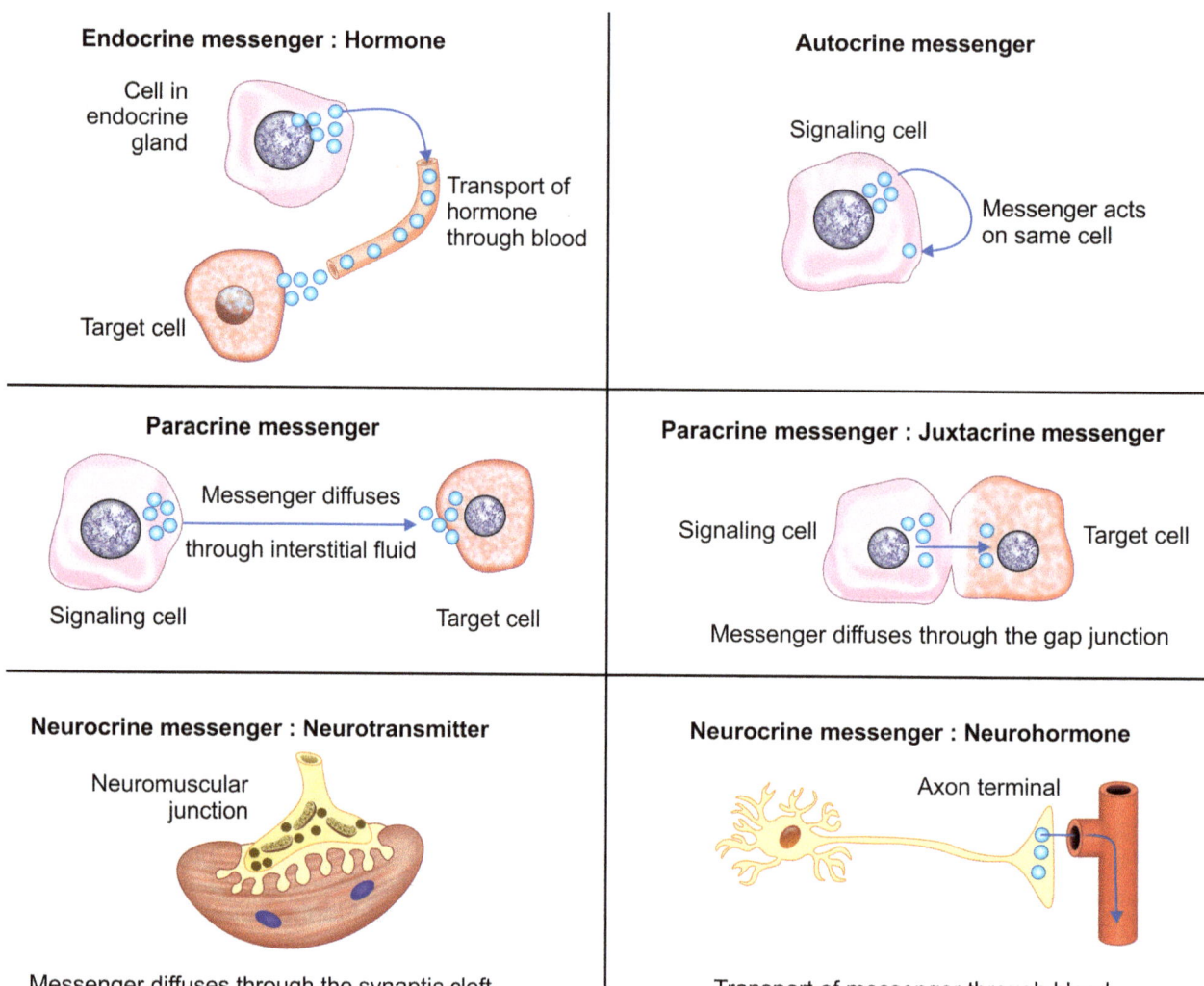

FIGURE 49.1: Chemical messengers.

2. *Neurohormone*: Neurohormone is a chemical messenger that is released by the nerve cell directly into the blood and transported to the distant target cells.

Examples are oxytocin, antidiuretic hormone and hypothalamic releasing hormones.

■ ENDOCRINE GLANDS

Endocrine glands are the glands which synthesize and release the classical hormones into the blood. Endocrine glands are also called **ductless glands** because the hormones secreted by them are released directly into blood without any duct.

Major endocrine glands: **Figure 49.2**.
Hormones secreted by endocrine glands: **Table 49.1**.
Hormones secreted by gonads: **Table 49.2**.
Hormones secreted by other organs: **Table 49.3**.
Local hormones: **Box 49.1**.

■ CLASSIFICATION OF HORMONES

Based on chemical nature, hormones are classified into three types:

1. Steroid hormones which are synthesized from cholesterol or its derivatives.
2. Protein hormones which are peptides in nature.
3. Hormones derived from amino acid tyrosine.

Classification of hormones depending upon their chemical nature is given in **Table 49.4**.

■ HORMONAL ACTION

Hormone does not act directly on the cellular structures. It combines with receptors present on the target cells and forms a hormone-receptor complex. This **hormone-receptor complex** induces various changes or reactions in the target cells.

■ HORMONE RECEPTORS

Hormone receptors are the large **proteins** present in the target cells to which the hormones bind to execute their actions.

Each cell has thousands of receptors. Important characteristic feature of the receptors is that, each receptor is specific for one single hormone, i.e. each receptor can combine with only one hormone.

Chapter 49: Overview of Endocrine System

TABLE 49.1: Hormones secreted by major endocrine glands.

Endocrine gland	Hormones	Endocrine gland	Hormones
Anterior pituitary	1. Growth hormone (GH) 2. Thyroid-stimulating hormone (TSH) 3. Adrenocorticotropic hormone (ACTH) 4. Follicle-stimulating hormone (FSH) 5. Luteinizing hormone (LH) 6. Prolactin	Adrenal cortex	Mineralocorticoids 1. Aldosterone 2. 11-deoxycorticosterone Glucocorticoids 1. Cortisol 2. Corticosterone Sex hormones 1. Androgens 2. Estrogen 3. Progesterone
Posterior pituitary	1. Antidiuretic hormone (ADH) 2. Oxytocin		
Thyroid gland	1. Thyroxine (T$_4$) 2. Triiodothyronine (T$_3$) 3. Calcitonin		
Parathyroid gland	1. Parathormone	Adrenal medulla	Catecholamines 1. Adrenaline (epinephrine) 2. Noradrenaline (norepinephrine) 3. Dopamine
Pancreas: Islets of Langerhans	1. Insulin 2. Glucagon 3. Somatostatin 4. Pancreatic polypeptide		

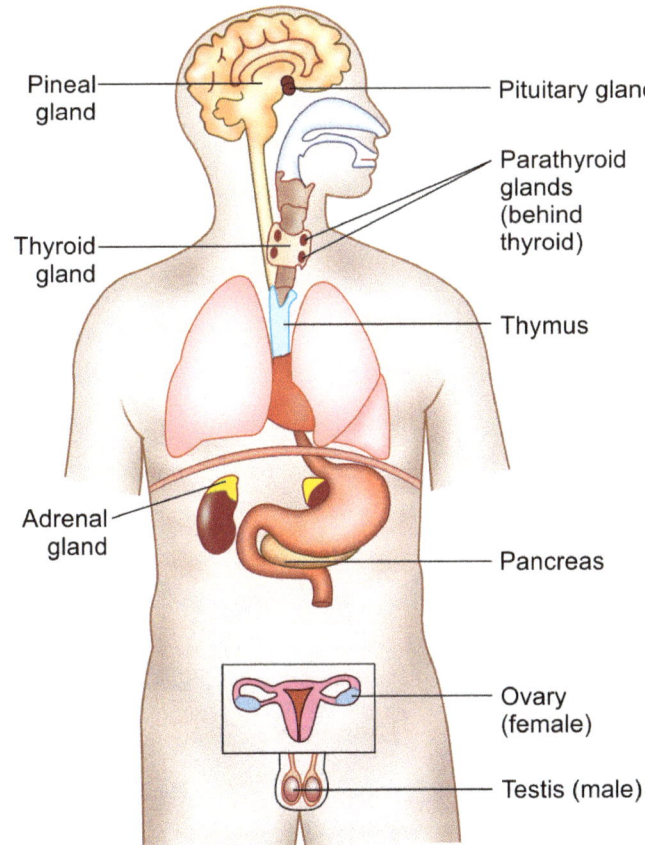

FIGURE 49.2: Diagram showing major endocrine glands.

TABLE 49.2: Hormones secreted by gonads.

Gonad	Hormones
Testis	1. Testosterone 2. Dihydrotestosterone 3. Androstenedion
Ovary	1. Estrogen 2. Progesterone

TABLE 49.3: Hormones secreted by other organs.

Organ	Hormones
Pineal gland	1. Melatonin
Thymus	1. Thymosin 2. Thymin
Kidney	1. Erythropoietin 2. Thrombopoietin 3. Renin 4. 1,25-dihydroxycholecalciferol (calcitriol) 5. Prostaglandins
Heart	1. Atrial natriuretic peptide 2. Brain natriuretic peptide 3. C-type natriuretic peptide
Placenta	1. Human chorionic gonadotropin (HCG) 2. Human chorionic somatomammotropin 3. Estrogen 4. Progesterone

BOX 49.1: Local hormones.

1. Prostaglandins
2. Thromboxanes
3. Prostacyclin
4. Leukotrienes
5. Lipoxins
6. Acetylcholine
7. Serotonin
8. Histamine
9. Substance P
10. Heparin
11. Bradykinin
12. Gastrointestinal hormones

Thus, a hormone can act on a target cell, only if the target cell has the receptor for that particular hormone.

Situation of the Hormone Receptors

Hormone receptors are situated in any of the following parts of a cell:

TABLE 49.4: Classification of hormones depending upon chemical nature.

Chemical nature	Hormones	Source of secretion
Steroids	1. Aldosterone 2. 11-deoxycorticosterone 3. Cortisol 4. Corticosterone	Adrenal cortex
	1. Estrogen 2. Progesterone	Ovary Adrenal cortex
	1. Testosterone 2. Dihydrotestosterone 3. Dehydroepiandrosterone	Testis Adrenal cortex
Proteins	1. Growth hormone (GH) 2. Thyroid-stimulating hormone (TSH) 3. Adrenocorticotropic hormone (ACTH) 4. Follicle-stimulating hormone (FSH) 5. Luteinizing hormone (LH) 6. Prolactin	Anterior pituitary gland
	1. Antidiuretic hormone 2. Oxytocin	Posterior pituitary gland
	1. Insulin 2. Glucagon 3. Somatostatin 4. Pancreatic polypeptide	Pancreas (Islets of Langerhans)
	1. Human chorionic gonadotropin (HCG) 2. Human chorionic somatomammotropin	Placenta
	1. Parathormone	Parathyroid gland
	1. Calcitonin	Thyroid gland
Derivatives of tyrosine	1. Thyroxine (T_4) 2. Triiodothyronine (T_3)	
	1. Adrenaline (epinephrine) 2. Noradrenaline (norepinephrine) 3. Dopamine	Adrenal medulla

1. Cell membrane

Receptors of protein hormones and adrenal medullary hormones (catecholamines) are situated in the cell membrane **(Fig. 49.3)**.

2. Cytoplasm

Receptors of steroid hormones are situated in cytoplasm of the cells.

3. Nucleus

Receptors of thyroid hormones are in the nucleus of the cell.

MECHANISM OF HORMONAL ACTION

On the target cell, the hormone-receptor complex acts by any one of the following mechanisms:

1. By altering permeability of cell membrane.
2. By activating intracellular enzyme.
3. By activating gene.

1. By Altering Permeability of Cell Membrane

Neurotransmitter substances in a synapse or neuromuscular junction act by altering the permeability of postsynaptic membrane.

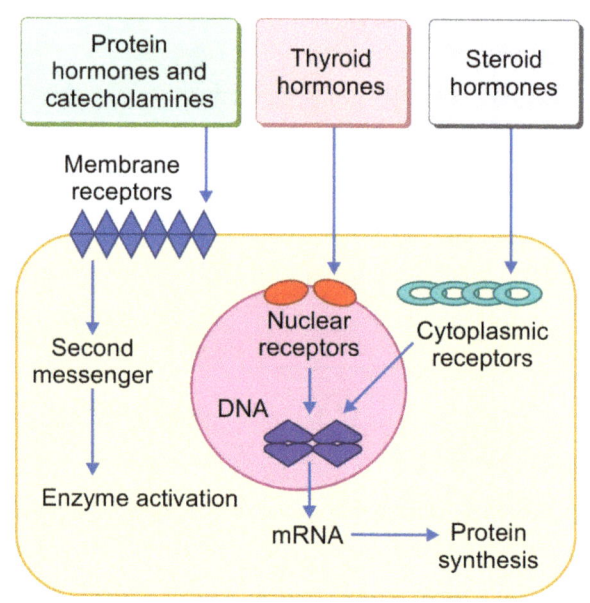

FIGURE 49.3: Situation of hormonal receptors.

For example, in a **neuromuscular junction**, when an impulse (action potential) reaches the axon terminal of motor nerve, acetylcholine is released from synaptic vesicles. **Acetylcholine** increases permeability of postsynaptic membrane by opening the **ligand gated sodium channels**. So, sodium ions enter the neuromuscular junction from ECF through channels. Sodium ions alter the resting membrane potential so that, endplate potential is developed.

2. By Activating Intracellular Enzyme

Protein hormones and the catecholamines act by activating the intracellular enzymes.

A hormone which acts on a target cell is called **first messenger** or chemical mediator. It combines with the receptor and forms hormone-receptor complex.

Hormone-receptor complex activates the enzymes of the cell and causes the formation of a second messenger.

Second messenger is a substance through which the hormonal actions are executed. Second messenger produces the effects of hormone inside the cells. Protein hormones and the catecholamines act through second messenger. Most common second messenger is cyclic AMP.

Cyclic AMP

Cyclic AMP or cAMP or cyclic adenosine 3'5'-monophosphate acts as second messenger for protein hormones and catecholamines.

Formation of cAMP: Role of G proteins

G proteins is necessary for the formation of cAMP. G proteins or guanosine nucleotide-binding proteins are the membrane proteins situated on inner surface of cell membrane.

Each G protein molecule has three subunits called α, β and γ subunits. The α-subunit has the biological actions. It is bound with guanosine diphosphate (GDP) and forms α-GDP unit. The α-subunit is also having the intrinsic enzyme activity called GTPase activity. The β and γ subunits always bind together to form the β-γ dimmer which also bring about some actions. In inactivated G protein, both α-GDP unit and β-γ dimmer are united (**Fig. 49.4**: Stage 1).

Sequence of events in the formation of cAMP

i. Hormone binds with receptor and forms hormone-receptor complex and activates the G protein.
ii. G protein releases GDP from α-GDP unit. The α-subunit now binds with a new molecule of GTP, i.e. the GDP is exchanged for GTP.
iii. This exchange triggers the dissociation of α-GTP unit and β-γ dimmer from the receptor.
iv. Both α-GTP unit and β-γ dimmer now activate the second messenger pathways (**Fig. 49.4**: Stage 2).
v. The α-GTP unit activates the enzyme **adenyl cyclase**.
vi. Activated adenyl cyclase converts the adenosine triphosphate (ATP) into **cyclic adenosine monophosphate (cAMP)**.
vii. When the action is over, α-subunit reunites with β-γ dimmer and commencing a new cycle as in **Figure 49.4**: Stage 1.

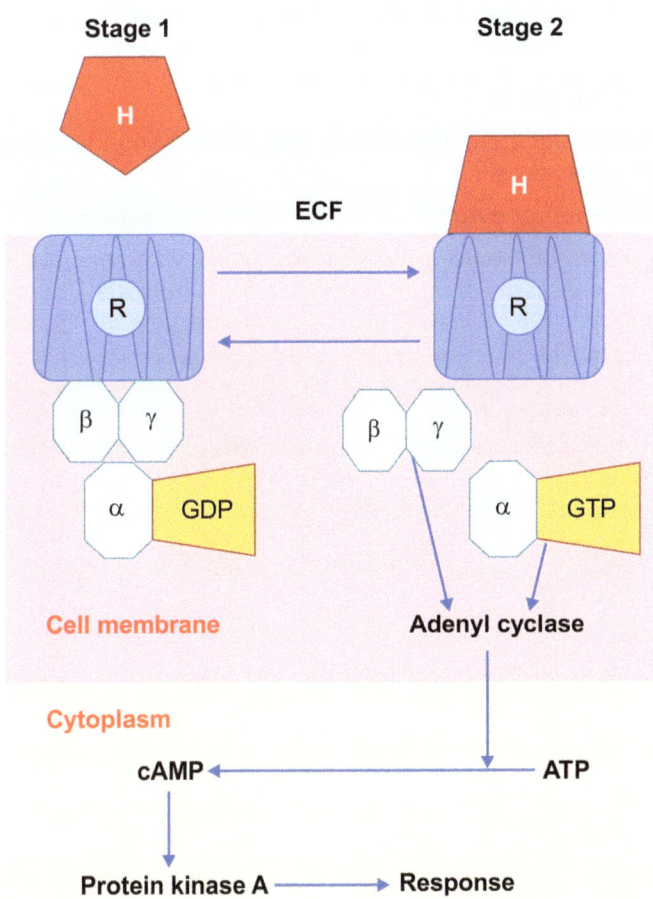

FIGURE 49.4: Mode of action of protein hormones and catecholamines.
H = Hormone, R = Receptor, α, β, γ = G protein, GDP = Guanosine diphosphate, GTP = Guanosine triphosphate, ECF = Extracellular fluid, cAMP = Cyclic adenosine 3'5'-monophosphate, ATP = Adenosine triphosphate.

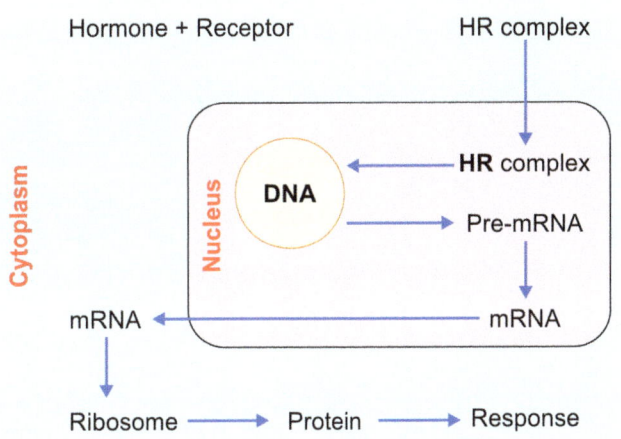

FIGURE 49.5: Mode of action of steroid hormones. Thyroid hormones also act in the similar way but their receptors are in the nucleus.
HR = Hormone-receptor complex.

Actions of cAMP

Cyclic AMP executes the actions of hormone inside the cell by stimulating the enzymes such as protein kinase A.

3. By Acting on Genes

Thyroid and steroid hormones act by activating the genes of the target cells.

Sequence of events during activation of genes

i. Hormone enters the cell and binds with receptor in cytoplasm (steroid hormone) or in nucleus (thyroid hormone) and forms hormone-receptor complex. This complex binds to DNA and increases transcription of mRNA.

ii. The mRNA moves out of nucleus and reaches ribosomes and activates them.

iii. Activated ribosomes produce large quantities of proteins which produce the physiological responses in the target cells **(Fig. 49.5)**.

Chapter 50: Pituitary Gland

CHAPTER OUTLINE

- **PITUITARY GLAND**
  - **DIVISIONS**
  - **HYPOTHALAMO-HYPOPHYSEAL RELATIONSHIP**
- **ANTERIOR PITUITARY OR ADENOHYPOPHYSIS**
  - **PARTS**
  - **FUNCTIONAL HISTOLOGY**
  - **REGULATION**
  - **HORMONES**
  - **GROWTH HORMONE**
  - **OTHER HORMONES**
- **POSTERIOR PITUITARY OR NEUROHYPOPHYSIS**
  - **PARTS**
- **FUNCTIONAL HISTOLOGY**
  - **HORMONES**
  - **ANTIDIURETIC HORMONE**
  - **OXYTOCIN**
- **APPLIED PHYSIOLOGY: DISORDERS OF PITUITARY GLAND**
  - **HYPERACTIVITY OF ANTERIOR PITUITARY**
  - **HYPOACTIVITY OF ANTERIOR PITUITARY**
  - **HYPERACTIVITY OF POSTERIOR PITUITARY**
  - **HYPOACTIVITY OF POSTERIOR PITUITARY**
  - **HYPOACTIVITY OF ANTERIOR AND POSTERIOR PITUITARY**

■ PITUITARY GLAND

Pituitary gland is also known as **hypophysis**. It is a small gland that lies at the base of brain. It is connected with the hypothalamus by **pituitary stalk** or **hypophyseal stalk**.

■ DIVISIONS OF PITUITARY GLAND

Pituitary gland is divided into two portions:

1. Anterior pituitary or **adenohypophysis**.
2. Posterior pituitary or **neurohypophysis**.

Even though anterior pituitary and posterior pituitary are situated in close approximation, both are entirely different in their development, structure and function.

■ HYPOTHALAMO-HYPOPHYSEAL RELATIONSHIP

Relationship between hypothalamus and pituitary gland is called hypothalamo-hypophyseal relationship. Hormones secreted by hypothalamus are transported to anterior pituitary and posterior pituitary. But, the mode of transport of these hormones is different.

Hormones from hypothalamus are transported to anterior pituitary through hypothalamo-hypophyseal portal blood vessels. But, the hormones from hypothalamus to posterior pituitary are transported by nerve fibers of hypothalamo-hypophyseal tract (see below for details).

■ ANTERIOR PITUITARY

■ PARTS OF ANTERIOR PITUITARY

Anterior pituitary consists of three divisions **(Fig. 50.1)**:

1. Pars distalis.
2. Pars tuberalis.
3. Pars intermedia.

■ FUNCTIONAL HISTOLOGY OF ANTERIOR PITUITARY

Depending upon staining property, the cells of anterior pituitary are classified into two types:

I. **Chromophobe cells** which do not have granules and stain poorly. These cells are not secretory in nature.
II. **Chromophil cells** which contain large granules and are stained darkly. These cells are secretory in nature.

Classification of Chromophil Cells

Chromophil cells are classified by two methods:

1. On the basis of staining property

On the basis of staining property, chromophil cells are divided into two types.

i. **Acidophilic cells** or α-cells.
ii. **Basophilic cells** or β-cells.

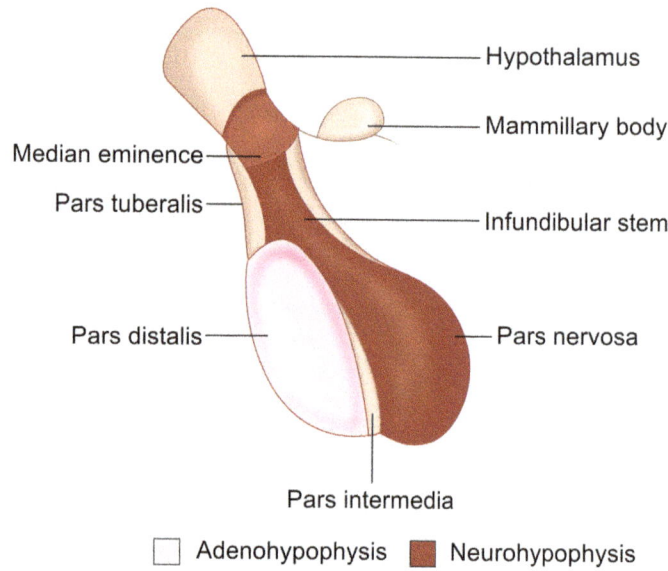

FIGURE 50.1: Parts of pituitary gland.

2. On the basis of secretory function

Depending upon the secretory function, chromophil cells are classified into five types:

i. **Somatotrophs** which secrete growth hormone.
ii. **Corticotrophs** which secrete adrenocorticotropic hormone.
iii. **Thyrotrophs** which secrete thyroid stimulating hormone.
iv. **Gonadotrophs** which secrete follicle stimulating hormone and luteinizing hormone.
v. **Lactotrophs** which secrete prolactin.

Somatotrophs and lactotrophs are acidophilic cells, whereas others are basophilic cells.

REGULATION OF SECRETION OF ANTERIOR PITUITARY HORMONES

Secretion of anterior pituitary hormones is regulated by hypothalamus. Hypothalamus secretes some releasing and inhibitory hormones (factors) which are transported from hypothalamus to anterior pituitary through hypothalamo-hypophyseal portal vessels.

Releasing and Inhibitory Hormones Secreted by Hypothalamus

1. Growth hormone-releasing hormone (GHRH): Stimulates the release of GH.
2. Growth hormone-releasing polypeptide (GHRP): Stimulates the release of GHRH and GH.
3. Growth hormone-inhibitory hormone (GHIH) or somatostatin: Inhibits GH release.
4. Thyrotropin-releasing hormone (TRH): Stimulates the release of TSH.
5. Corticotropin-releasing hormone (CRH): Stimulates the release of ACTH.
6. Gonadotropin-releasing hormone (GnRH): Stimulates the release of the gonadotropins, FSH and LH.
7. Prolactin-inhibitory hormone (PIH): Inhibits prolactin secretion.

HORMONES SECRETED BY ANTERIOR PITUITARY

Anterior pituitary is also known as the **master gland** because it regulates many other endocrine glands.

Six hormones are secreted by the anterior pituitary:

1. Growth hormone (GH) or somatotropic hormone (STH).
2. Thyroid-stimulating hormone (TSH) or thyrotropic hormone.
3. Adrenocorticotropic hormone (ACTH).
4. Follicle stimulating hormone (FSH).
5. Luteinizing hormone (LH) in females or interstitial cell stimulating hormone (ICSH) in males.
6. Prolactin.

Recently, the hormone β-lipotropin is found to be secreted by anterior pituitary.

Tropic Hormones

First five hormones of anterior pituitary stimulate the other endocrine glands. Growth hormone also stimulates the secretory activity of liver and other tissues. Therefore, these five hormones are called tropic hormones. Prolactin is concerned with milk secretion.

Gonadotropic Hormones

FSH and LH are together called gonadotropic hormones or gonadotropins because of their action on the gonads.

GROWTH HORMONE

Growth hormone (GH) is secreted by **somatotrophs** which are acidophils of anterior pituitary.

GH is a protein having a single chain polypeptide with 191 amino acids. GH is transported in blood by **GH-binding proteins (GHBP)**.

Basal level of GH concentration in blood of the normal adult is up to 300 g/dL and in children it is about 500 ng/dL. It's daily output in adults is 0.5 to 1.0 mg.

Actions of Growth Hormone

Growth hormone is responsible for the growth of almost all tissues of the body, which are capable of growing. It actually increases size and also the number of cells by increasing the mitotic division. GH also causes specific differentiation of certain types of cells like bone cells and muscle cells.

GH also acts on the metabolism of all the three major types of foodstuffs in the body, viz. proteins, fats and carbohydrates.

GH increases the synthesis of proteins, mobilization of lipids and conservation of carbohydrates.

1. Action on metabolism

a. On protein metabolism

GH accelerates synthesis of proteins by:

i. Increasing amino acid transport through cell membrane.

ii. Increasing ribonucleic acid (RNA) translation: Because of this, ribosomes are activated and more proteins are synthesized.
iii. Increasing transcription of DNA to RNA: RNA, in turn accelerates the synthesis of proteins in the cells.
iv. Decreasing catabolism of protein: GH inhibits the breakdown of cellular protein. It helps in the building up of tissues.
v. Promoting **anabolism of proteins** indirectly by causing release of insulin from β-cells of islets in pancreas, which has anabolic effect on proteins.

b. On fat metabolism

GH mobilizes fats from adipose tissue. Because of this, the concentration of fatty acids increases in the body fluids. Fatty acids are used for production of energy by the cells. So, proteins are spared.

During the utilization of fatty acids for production of energy, lot of acetoacetic acid is produced by the liver and released into the body fluids leading to **ketosis**. Sometimes excess mobilization of fat from the adipose tissue causes accumulation of fat in liver, resulting in **fatty liver**.

c. On carbohydrate metabolism

Major action of GH on carbohydrates is the conservation of glucose.

Effects of GH on the carbohydrate metabolism are:

i. Decrease in peripheral utilization of glucose for the production of energy.
ii. Increase in deposition of glycogen in the cells. Since, glucose is not utilized for energy production by the cells, it is converted into glycogen which is deposited in the cells.
iii. Decrease in uptake of glucose by the cells. As the deposition of glycogen increases, cells become saturated with glycogen. Because of this, no more glucose can enter the cells. So, the blood glucose level increases.

Diabetogenic effect of GH

Hypersecretion of GH increases blood glucose level enormously. Increased blood sugar stimulates the β-cells in the islets of Langerhans in pancreas continuously and increases insulin secretion. In addition to this, the GH also stimulates the β-cells of islets in pancreas directly and causes secretion of insulin. Because of excess stimulation, the β-cells are burnt out at one stage. This causes deficiency of insulin, which leads to true diabetes mellitus or full-blown diabetes mellitus. This is called the diabetogenic effect of GH.

2. Action on bones

In embryonic stage, GH is responsible for the differentiation and development of bone cells. In later stages, GH increases growth of the skeleton. It increases both length as well as thickness of the bones.

In bones, GH increases:

i. Protein synthesis by **chondrocytes** and **osteogenic cells**.
ii. Multiplication of chondrocytes and osteogenic cells.
iii. Formation of new bones by converting chondrocytes into osteogenic cells.
iv. Increases the calcium absorption from intestine. By this GH enhances the availability of calcium for mineralization of bone matrix.

GH increases length of the bones until epiphysis fuses with shaft of bone. Usually fusion occurs at puberty. After **epiphyseal fusion**, length of the bones cannot be increased. However, GH stimulates the osteoblasts strongly. So, the bone continues to grow in thickness throughout life. Particularly, the membranous bones such as jaw bone and skull bones become thicker under the influence of GH.

Mode of Action of GH on Bones and Metabolism

GH acts on bones, growth and protein metabolism through a substance called somatomedin, which is secreted by liver. GH stimulates the liver to secrete somatomedin. Sometimes, in spite of normal secretion of GH, growth is arrested (dwarfism) due to the absence or deficiency of somatomedin.

Somatomedin

Somatomedin is a polypeptide. It is of two types:

1. **Insulin like growth factor - I (IGF-I)**, which is also called **somatomedin C**.
2. **Insulin like growth factor - II**.

Among the two somatomedins, somatomedin C (IGF-I) is responsible for the action of bones on bones and metabolism.

Regulation of GH Secretion

Secretion of GH is regulated by hypothalamus and feedback control.

Role of hypothalamus in the secretion of GH

Hypothalamus regulates GH secretion by releasing three hormones:

1. **Growth hormone releasing hormone (GHRH)** that increases secretion of GH by stimulating the somatotrophs of anterior pituitary.
2. **Growth hormone releasing polypeptide (GHRP)** that promotes release of GHRH from hypothalamus and GH from pituitary.
3. **Growth hormone inhibitory hormone (GHIH) or somatostatin** which inhibits secretion of GH.

These three hormones are transported from hypothalamus to anterior pituitary by hypothalamo-hypophyseal portal blood vessels.

Hypothalamus is in turn influenced by many factors which cause increase or decrease in GH secretion.

Factors which increase the GH secretion:

1. Hypoglycemia.
2. Fasting.
3. Starvation.
4. Exercise.
5. Stress and trauma.
6. Initial stages of sleep.

Factors which decrease the GH secretion:

1. Hyperglycemia.
2. Increase in free fatty acids in blood.
3. Later stages of sleep.

Feedback control

GH secretion is under negative feedback control (Chapter 4). Hypothalamus releases GHRH and GHRP, which in turn promote the release of GH from anterior pituitary. GH acts on various tissues. It also activates the liver cells to secrete somatomedin C (IGF-I).

Now, the somatomedin C acts in three ways:

i. It increases release of GHIH from hypothalamus. GHIH in turn inhibits release of GH from pituitary.
ii. Somatomedin also inhibits release of GHRP from hypothalamus.
iii. It acts on pituitary directly and inhibits the secretion of GH **(Fig. 50.2)**.

GH inhibits its own secretion by stimulating the release of GHIH from hypothalamus. This type of feedback is called **short-loop feedback control**. Similarly, GHRH inhibits its own release by short- loop feedback control.

Whenever, blood level of GH decreases, GHRH is secreted from the hypothalamus. It in turn causes secretion of GH from pituitary.

■ OTHER HORMONES OF ANTERIOR PITUITARY

Thyroid-stimulating Hormone (TSH)

TSH is necessary for growth and secretory activity of the thyroid gland. Refer chapter 51 for details of TSH.

Adrenocorticotropic Hormone (ACTH)

ACTH is necessary for structural integrity and the secretory activity of adrenal cortex. Refer chapter 54 for details of ACTH.

Follicle-stimulating Hormone (FSH)

Actions in males

In males, FSH acts along with testosterone and accelerates the process of spermiogenesis.

Actions in females

1. It is responsible for the development of graafian follicle from primordial follicle.
2. It stimulates the theca cells of graafian follicle and causes secretion of estrogen.
3. Promotes aromatase activity in granulosa cells resulting in conversion of androgens into estrogen.

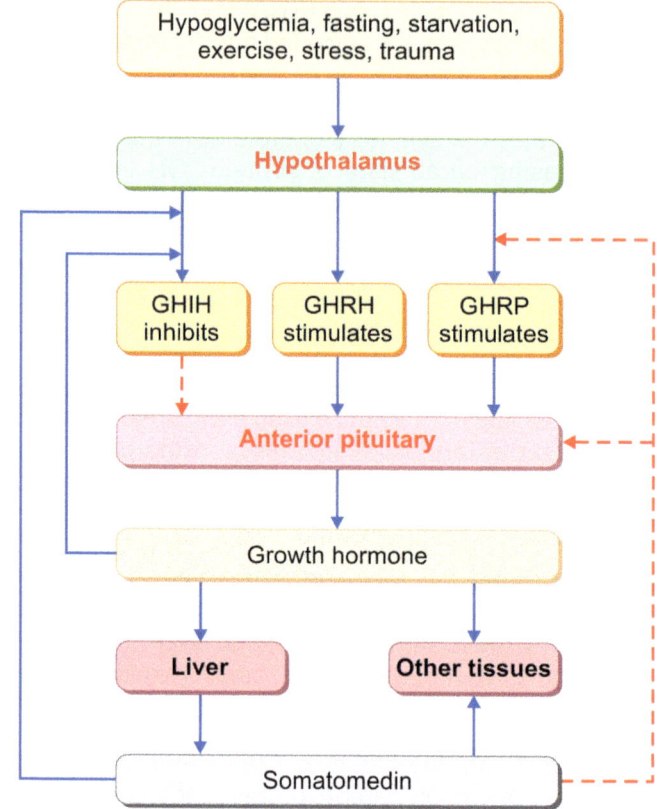

FIGURE 50.2: Regulation of GH secretion.
GHIH = Growth hormone-inhibitory hormone, GHRH = Growth hormone-releasing hormone, GHRP = Growth hormone-releasing polypeptide. Growth hormone and somatomedin stimulate hypothalamus to release GHIH. Somatomedin inhibits anterior pituitary directly. Solid blue line = Stimulation/Secretion. Dashed red line = Inhibition.

Luteinizing Hormone (LH)

Actions in males

In males, LH is known as **interstitial cell stimulating hormone (ICSH)** because it stimulates the interstitial cells of Leydig in testes. This hormone is essential for the secretion of testosterone from Leydig cells.

Actions in females

1. LH causes maturation of vesicular follicle into graafian follicle along with follicle stimulating hormone.
2. It induces synthesis of androgens from theca cells of growing follicle.
3. It is responsible for ovulation.
4. It is necessary for the formation of corpus luteum.
5. It activates the secretory functions of corpus luteum.

Prolactin

Prolactin is necessary for the final preparation of mammary glands for production and secretion of milk.

β-lipotropin

It mobilizes fat from adipose tissue and promotes lipolysis.

POSTERIOR PITUITARY

PARTS OF POSTERIOR PITUITARY

Posterior pituitary consists of three divisions:

1. Pars nervosa or infundibular process.
2. Nural stalk or infundibular stem.
3. Median eminence.

Pars tuberalis of anterior pituitary and the neural stalk of posterior pituitary together form the **hypophyseal stalk**.

FUNCTIONAL HISTOLOGY OF POSTERIOR PITUITARY

Posterior pituitary is made up of nerve cells called **pituicytes** and unmyelinated nerve fibers. Pituicytes act as supporting cells and do not secrete any hormone. Posterior pituitary also has numerous blood vessels, hyaline bodies, neuroglial cells and mast cells.

HORMONES OF POSTERIOR PITUITARY

Posterior pituitary hormones are:

1. Antidiuretic hormone (ADH) or vasopressin.
2. Oxytocin.

Source of Secretion of Posterior Pituitary Hormones

Actually, the posterior pituitary does not secrete any hormone. ADH and oxytocin are synthesized in the hypothalamus. From hypothalamus, these two hormones are transported to the posterior pituitary through the nerve fibers of **hypothalamo-hypophyseal tract (Fig. 50.3)**, by means of axonic flow.

In the posterior pituitary, these hormones are stored at the nerve endings. Whenever, the impulses from hypothalamus reach the posterior pituitary, these hormones are released from the nerve endings into the circulation. Hence, these two hormones are called **neurohormones.**

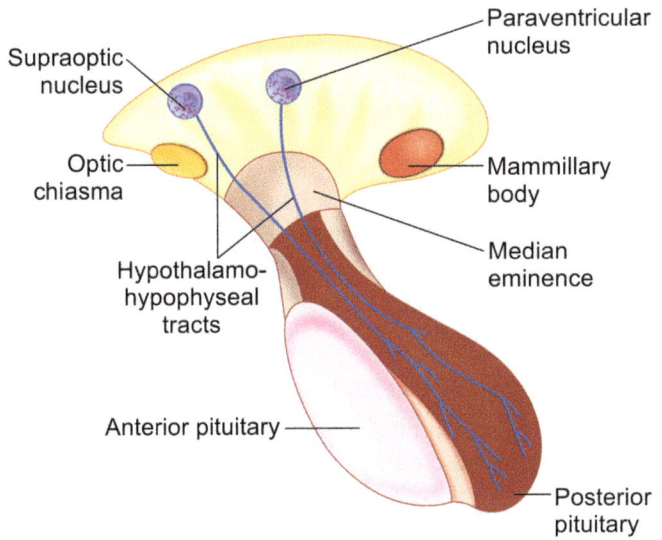

FIGURE 50.3: Hypothalamo-hypophyseal tracts.

ANTIDIURETIC HORMONE

ADH is secreted mainly by **supraoptic nucleus** of hypothalamus and in small quantity by paraventricular nucleus. From here, this hormone is transported to the posterior pituitary through the nerve fibers of hypothalamo-hypophyseal tract by means of **axonic flow (Fig. 50.3)**.

Antidiuretic hormone is a polypeptide, containing 9 amino acids.

Actions of ADH

Major function of ADH is **retention of water** by acting on kidneys. It increases **facultative reabsorption of water** from distal convoluted tubule and collecting duct in the kidneys (Chapter 42).

ADH increases water reabsorption in the tubular epithelial membrane by regulating water channel proteins called **aquaporins** through **V2 receptors** (Chapter 42).

Vasopressor Action

In large amount, ADH shows vasoconstrictor action in all parts of the body. Due to vasoconstriction, the blood pressure increases. ADH acts on blood vessels through **V1A receptors**.

Regulation of Secretion

Secretion of ADH depends upon volume of body fluid and osmolarity of the body fluids.

Potent stimulants for ADH secretion are:

1. Decrease in ECF volume.
2. Increase in osmolar concentration in ECF.

Role of osmoreceptors

Osmoreceptors are the receptors, which give response to change in osmolar concentration of the blood. Osmoreceptors are situated in the hypothalamus near supraoptic and paraventricular nuclei. When osmolar concentration of blood increases, the osmoreceptors are activated. In turn, the osmoreceptors stimulate supraoptic and paraventricular nuclei. These two nuclei send motor impulses to posterior pituitary through the nerve fibers and cause release of ADH. ADH causes reabsorption of water from the renal tubules. This increases volume of ECF and restores the normal osmolarity.

OXYTOCIN

Oxytocin is secreted mainly by the **paraventricular nucleus** and a small quantity is secreted by the supra-optic nucleus in the hypothalamus. And it is transported from hypothalamus to posterior pituitary through the nerve fibers of hypothalamo-hypophyseal tract.

In the posterior pituitary, oxytocin is stored in nerve endings of hypothalamo-hypophyseal tract. When suitable stimuli reach the posterior pituitary from hypothalamus, oxytocin is released into the blood. Oxytocin is secreted in both males and females.

Oxytocin is a polypeptide, having 9 amino acids.

Actions in Females

In females, oxytocin acts on mammary glands and uterus.

Action of oxytocin on mammary glands

It causes ejection of milk from the mammary glands. Ducts of the mammary glands are lined by myoepithelial cells. Oxytocin causes contraction of myoepithelial cells and squeezes the milk from alveoli of mammary glands to the exterior through duct system and nipple. The process by which milk is ejected from the alveoli of mammary glands is called milk ejection reflex or **milk let-down reflex**.

Milk ejection reflex

Plenty of **touch receptors** are present on the mammary glands, particularly around nipple. When the infant suckles mother's nipple, touch receptors are stimulated and impulses are discharged. Impulses from here are carried by the somatic afferent nerve fibers and reach the paraventricular and supraoptic nuclei of hypothalamus.

Now, hypothalamus in turn, sends impulses to the posterior pituitary through hypothalamo-hypophyseal tract and cause release of oxytocin into the blood. When the hormone reaches mammary gland, it causes contraction of **myoepithelial cells** resulting in ejection of milk from mammary glands **(Fig. 50.4)**.

As this reflex is initiated by nervous factors and completed by the hormonal action, it is called a **neuroendocrine reflex**. During this reflex, large amount of oxytocin is released by **positive feedback mechanism**.

Action of oxytocin on uterus

Oxytocin acts on pregnant uterus and nonpregnant uterus.

Action on pregnant uterus

Throughout the period of pregnancy, oxytocin secretion is inhibited by estrogen and progesterone. At the end of pregnancy, secretion of these two hormones decreases suddenly and the secretion of oxytocin increases. Oxytocin causes **contraction of uterus** and helps in **expulsion of fetus**.

During **labor**, large quantity of oxytocin is released by means of **positive feedback mechanism**, i.e. oxytocin induces contraction of uterus, which in turn causes release of more amount of oxytocin **(Fig. 4.5)**.

Contraction of uterus during labor is also a neuroendocrine reflex. Oxytocin also stimulates the release of prostaglandins in placenta. Prostaglandins intensify the uterine contraction induced by oxytocin.

Action on non-pregnant uterus

Action of oxytocin on non-pregnant uterus is to facilitate the transport of sperms through female genital tract up to fallopian tube by producing the uterine contraction during sexual intercourse.

During sexual intercourse, the receptors in vagina are stimulated. Vaginal receptors generate the impulses, which are transmitted by somatic afferent nerves to

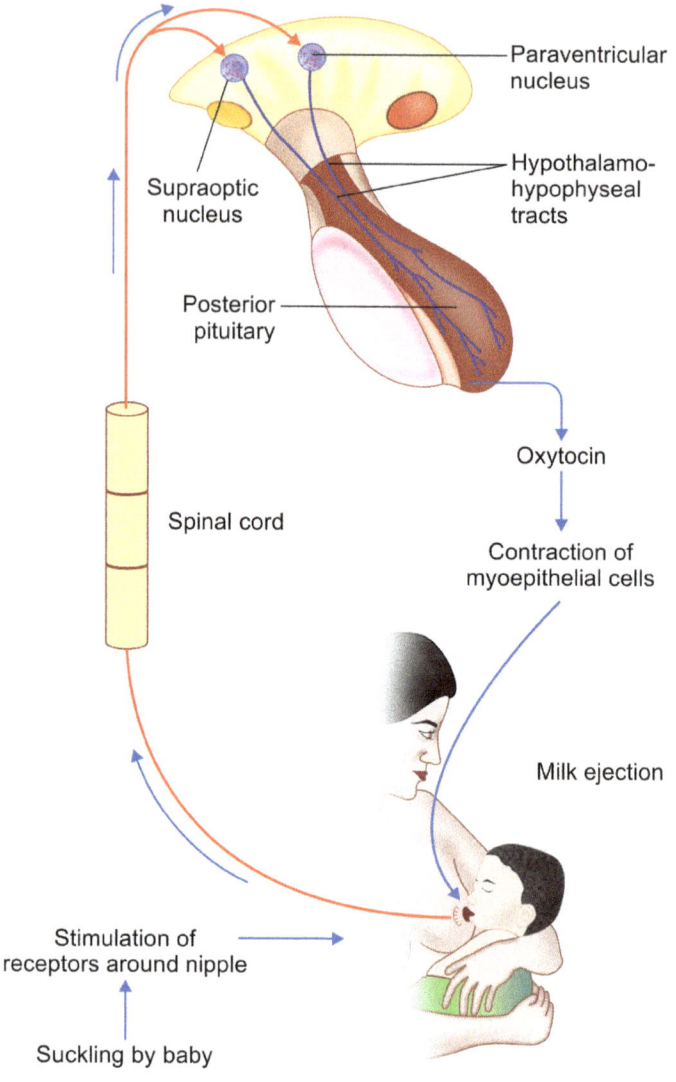

FIGURE 50.4: Milk ejection reflex.

paraventricular and supraoptic nuclei of hypothalamus. When, these two nuclei are stimulated, oxytocin is released, and transported by blood. While reaching the female genital tract, the hormone causes antiperistaltic contractions of uterus towards the fallopian tube which accelerate transport of sperms. It is also a neuroendocrine reflex.

Action in Males

In males, release of oxytocin increases during ejaculation. It facilitates release of sperm into urethra by causing contraction of smooth muscle fibers in reproductive tract particularly vas deferens.

Mode of Action of Oxytocin

Oxytocin acts on mammary glands and uterus by activating G protein-coupled oxytocin receptor.

■ APPLIED PHYSIOLOGY: DISORDERS OF PITUITARY GLAND

Disorders of pituitary gland are given in **Table 50.1**.

TABLE 50.1: Disorders of pituitary gland.

Parts involved	Hyperactivity	Hypoactivity
Anterior pituitary	Gigantism Acromegaly Acromegalic gigantism Cushing's disease	Dwarfism Acromicria Simmonds' disease
Posterior pituitary	Syndrome of inappropriate hypersecretion of ADH (SIADH)	Diabetes insipidus
Anterior and posterior pituitary	–	Dystrophia adiposogenitalis Panhypopituitarism

■ HYPERACTIVITY OF ANTERIOR PITUITARY

1. Gigantism

Gigantism is a pituitary disorder characterized by excess growth of the body. The affected subjects look like **giants** with average height of about 7 to 8 feet.

Causes of gigantism

Gigantism is due to hypersecretion of GH in childhood or preadult life **before fusion of epiphysis** of bone with shaft. It occurs due to **pituitary tumors**.

Signs and symptoms of gigantism

i. General overgrowth of the person leads to development of a **huge stature** with a height of more than 7 or 8 feet. Limbs are disproportionately long.
ii. Giants are hyperglycemic and they develop glycosuria and **pituitary diabetes**. Hyperglycemia causes constant stimulation of β-cells of islets of Langerhans in the pancreas and release of insulin. However, the over activity of β-cells of Langerhans in pancreas leads to degeneration of these cells and deficiency of insulin. And, ultimately diabetes mellitus is developed.
iii. Pituitary tumor itself causes constant headache.
iv. Pituitary tumor also causes **visual disturbances**. It compresses the lateral fibers of optic chiasma leading to bitemporal hemianopia (Chapter 112).

2. Acromegaly

Acromegaly is the pituitary disorder characterized by enlargement, thickening and broadening of bones, particularly in the extremities of the body.

Cause of acromegaly

Acromegaly is due to hypersecretion of GH in adults **after fusion of epiphysis** with shaft of the bone. Hypersecretion of GH is due to **adenomatous tumor** of anterior pituitary involving the acidophil cells.

Signs and symptoms of acromegaly

i. Striking facial features such as protrusion of supraorbital ridges, broadening of nose, thickening of lips, thickening and wrinkles formation on forehead, and **prognathism** (protrusion of lower jaw) are developed.

Face with these features is called **acromegalic** or **guerrilla face (Fig. 50.5)**.

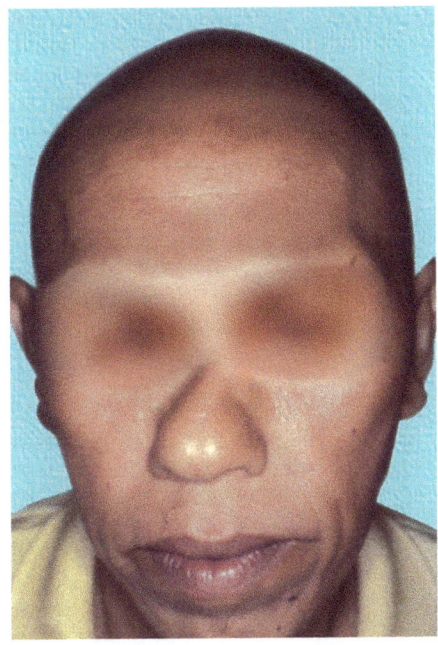

Guerrilla face: Protrusion of supraorbital ridges, broad nose, thickened lips and protrusion of lower jaw

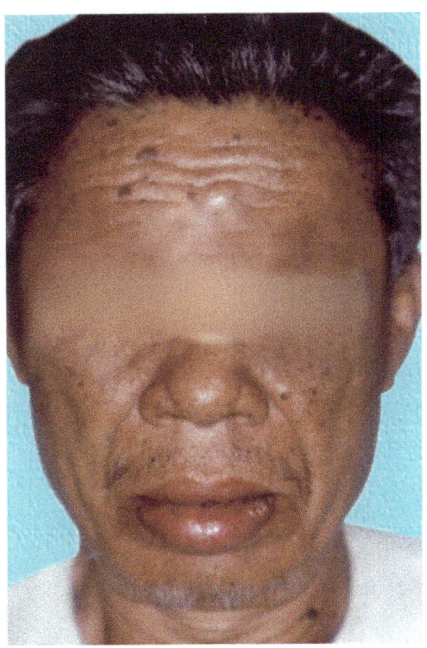

Wrinkled forehead, with other features of acromegalic face

FIGURE 50.5: Acromegaly. (*Courtesy:* Prof Mafauzy Mohamed).

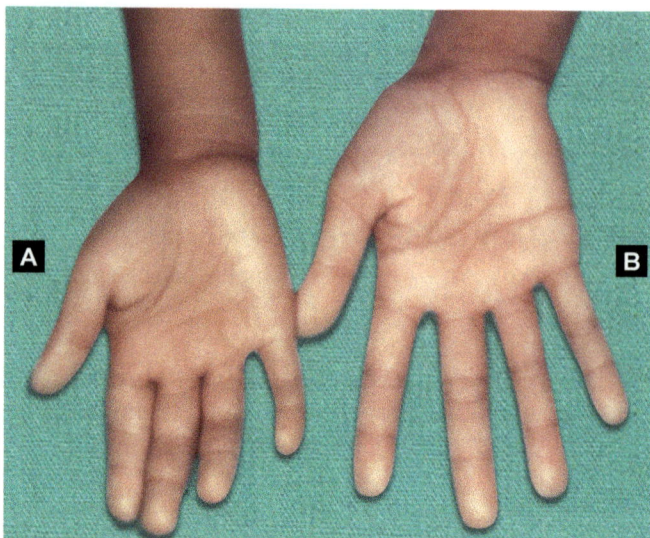

FIGURE 50.6: **A.** Normal hand, **B.** Acromegalic hand.
(*Courtesy:* Prof Mafauzy Mohamed).

ii. Hands and feet are enlarged **(Fig. 50.6)** with **kyphosis** (bowing of spine).
iii. Scalp is thickened and thrown into folds or wrinkles like **bulldog scalp**. There is general overgrowth of body hair.
iv. Visceral organs such as lungs, heart, liver and spleen are enlarged.
v. Thyroid gland, parathyroid glands and the adrenal glands show hyperactivity.
vi. Hyperglycemia and glucosuria occur resulting **in diabetes mellitus**.
vii. Hypertension.
viii. Headache.
ix. Visual disturbance (bitemporal hemianopia) is developed.

3. Acromegalic Gigantism

It is a rare disorder with symptoms of both gigantism and acromegaly. Hypersecretion of GH in children, before the fusion of epiphysis with shaft of the bones causes gigantism. And, if hypersecretion of GH is continued even after the fusion of epiphysis, the symptoms of acromegaly also appear.

4. Cushing's Disease

It is also a rare disorder characterized by obesity. Details of this disorder are given in Chapter 54.

■ HYPOACTIVITY OF ANTERIOR PITUITARY

1. Dwarfism

It is a pituitary disorder in children characterized by stunted growth.

Causes of dwarfism

Hyposecretion of GH in infancy or early childhood causes dwarfism.

Hyposecretion of GH occurs in the following conditions:
i. Deficiency of GHRH from hypothalamus.
ii. Deficiency of somatomedin C.
iii. Atrophy or degeneration of acidophilic cells in the anterior pituitary.
iv. Tumor of chromophobes: It is a nonfunctioning tumor, which compresses and destroys the normal GH secreting cells.
v. Panhypopituitarism: It is the endocrine disorder characterized by hyposecretion of all the hormones of anterior pituitary gland. Dwarfism due to this disorder is associated with other symptoms which occur due to the deficiency of other anterior pituitary hormones.

Signs and symptoms of dwarfism

i. Primary symptom of hypopituitarism in children is the **stunted skeletal growth**. Maximum height of anterior pituitary dwarf at the adult age is only about 3 feet.
ii. But, proportions of different parts of the body are almost normal. Only, head becomes slightly larger in relation to the body.
iii. Pituitary dwarfs do not show any deformity and their mental activity is normal with no mental retardation.
iv. Reproductive function is not affected, if there is only GH deficiency. However, in panhypopituitarism (see below), dwarfs do not obtain puberty due to deficiency of gonadotropic hormones.

Other types of dwarfism

Other types of dwarfism are given in **Box 50.1**.

BOX 50.1: Different types of dwarfism.

Pituitary dwarfism
Caused by hyposecretion of GH in infancy or early childhood
Laron dwarfism
Laron dwarfism or Laron syndrome is due to mutations in genes of growth hormone receptor (GHR)
GH secretion is normal or high. Since, the hormone cannot stimulate growth because of abnormal GHR, dwarfism occurs
Psychosocial dwarfism
Psychosocial or stress dwarfism is a pituitary disorder that occurs due deficiency of GH caused by exposure of the child to extreme emotional deprivation or stress
Dwarfism in dystrophia adiposogenitalis
Dystrophia adiposogenitalis or Fröhlich syndrome is a pituitary disorder caused by hypoactivity of both anterior and posterior pituitary. In children it results in dwarfism
Dwarfism in panhypopituitarism
Panhypopituitarism a pituitary disorder caused by hyposecretion of all hormones of anterior pituitary. It results in dwarfism if it affects children
Cretinism
Cretinism is the hypothyroid condition characterized by stunted growth (Chapter 51)

2. Acromicria

It is a rare pituitary disorder in adults characterized by atrophy of the extremities of the body.

Causes of acromicria

Hyposecretion of GH in adults causes acromicria.

Hyposecretion of GH occurs in the following conditions:

   i. Deficiency of GH releasing hormone from hypothalamus.
   ii. Atrophy or degeneration of acidophilic cells in the anterior pituitary.
   iii. Tumor of chromophobes: It is a nonfunctioning tumor, which compresses and destroys the normal cells secreting the GH.
   iv. **Panhypopituitarism**: In this condition, there is reduction in the secretion of all the hormones of anterior pituitary gland. Acromicria is associated with other symptoms due to the deficiency of other anterior pituitary hormones.

Signs and symptoms of acromicria

   i. Atrophy and thinning of extremities of body, (hands and feet) are the major symptoms in acromicria.
   ii. Acromicria is mostly associated with hypothyroidism and hyposecretion of adrenocortical hormones.
   iii. Affected person becomes lethargic and obese.
   iv. Sexual functions are lost.

3. Simmond's Disease

Simmond's disease is a rare pituitary disease. It is also called **pituitary cachexia**.

Cause of Simmond's disease

Simmonds disease occurs mostly in panhypopituitarism.

Symptoms of Simmond's disease

   i. A major feature of Simmonds' disease is the rapidly developing **senile decay**. Thus, a 30 years old person looks like a 60 years old person.
   ii. There is loss of hair over the body and loss of teeth.
   iii. Skin over face becomes dry and wrinkled. So, there is shrunken appearance of facial features. It is the most common feature of this disease.

■ HYPERACTIVITY OF POSTERIOR PITUITARY

Syndrome of Inappropriate Hypersecretion of Antidiuretic Hormone (SIADH)

SIADH is the disease characterized by loss of sodium through urine due to hypersecretion of ADH.

Cause of SIADH

SIADH occurs due to cerebral tumors, lung tumors and lung cancers because the tumor cells and cancer cells secrete ADH.

In normal conditions ADH decreases the urine output by facultative reabsorption of water in distal convoluted tubule and collecting duct. So, concentrated urine is formed with more sodium and other ions and less water. This decreases the osmolarity of plasma making it hypotonic. Hypotonic plasma inhibits ADH secretion resulting in restoration of plasma osmolarity.

However, ADH secreted from tumor or cancer cells is not inhibited by hypotonic plasma. So, there is continuous loss of sodium resulting in **persistent plasma hypotonicity**.

Signs and symptoms of SIADH

1. Loss of appetite.
2. Weight loss.
3. Nausea and vomiting.
4. Headache.
5. Muscle weakness, spasm and cramps.
6. Fatigue.
7. Restlessness and irritability.

In severe conditions, the patients die because of convulsions and coma.

■ HYPOACTIVITY OF POSTERIOR PITUITARY

Diabetes Insipidus

Diabetes insipidus is a posterior pituitary disorder characterized by excess excretion of water through urine **(Table 50.1)**.

Causes of diabetes insipidus

This disorder develops due to the deficiency ADH which occurs in the following conditions:

1. Lesion (injury) or degeneration of supraoptic and paraventricular nuclei of hypothalamus.
2. Lesion in hypothalamo-hypophyseal tract.
3. Atrophy of posterior pituitary.
4. Inability of renal tubules to give response to ADH. Such condition is called **nephrogenic diabetic insipidus**.

Signs and symptoms of diabetes insipidus

1. **Polyuria**: Polyuria is the increased urinary output with frequent voiding. It is due to water diuresis. Daily output of urine varies between 4 and 12 liters. In the absence of ADH, water is not reabsorbed from the renal tubule and collecting duct leading to loss of water through urine.
2. **Polydipsia**: Polydipsia is intake of excess water. Loss of water due to polyuria stimulates the thirst center in hypothalamus resulting in intake of large quantity of water.
3. **Dehydration**: In some cases, thirst center in the hypothalamus is also affected by lesion. Water intake decreases in these patients and, the loss of water through urine is not compensated. So, dehydration develops which may lead to death.

■ HYPOACTIVITY OF ANTERIOR AND POSTERIOR PITUITARY

Dystrophia Adiposogenitalis

Dystrophia adiposogenitalis is a disease characterized by obesity and hypogonadism affecting mainly the adolescent boys. It is also called Fröhlich's syndrome or hypothalamic eunuchism.

Causes of dystrophia adiposogenitalis

It is due to hypoactivity of both anterior pituitary and posterior pituitary. Common cause of this disease is the tumor in pituitary gland and hypothalamic regions concerned with food intake and gonadal development.

Symptoms of dystrophia adiposogenitalis

Obesity is the common feature of this disorder. Due to abnormal stimulation of feeding center, the person overeats and becomes obese. Obesity is accompanied by **sexual infantilism** (failure to develop secondary sexual characters) or **eunuchism**. Dwarfism occurs if the disease starts in growing age. In children, it is called infantile or prepubertal type of **Fröhlich's syndrome**.

This disease develops in adults also. When it occurs in adults, it is called adult type of Fröhlich's syndrome. In adults, the major symptoms are obesity and atrophy of sex organs.

Chapter 51: Thyroid Gland

CHAPTER OUTLINE

- MORPHOLOGY OF THYROID GLAND
- FUNCTIONAL HISTOLOGY
- HORMONES
- SYNTHESIS OF THYROID HORMONES
- STORAGE OF THYROID HORMONES
- RELEASE OF THYROID HORMONES
- TRANSPORT OF THYROID HORMONES IN THE BLOOD
- FUNCTIONS OF THYROID HORMONES
- MODE OF ACTION OF THYROID HORMONES
- REGULATION OF SECRETION OF THYROID HORMONES
- APPLIED PHYSIOLOGY: DISORDERS OF THYROID GLAND
- TREATMENT FOR THYROID DISORDERS
- THYROID FUNCTION TESTS

MORPHOLOGY OF THYROID GLAND

Thyroid is an endocrine gland situated at the root of neck on either side of trachea. It has two lobes, which are connected in the middle by an isthmus **(Fig. 51.1)**. It weighs about 20 to 40 g in adults. Thyroid is larger in females than in males. Structure and function of the thyroid gland change in different stages of the sexual cycle in females. Activity of thyroid gland increases slightly during pregnancy and lactation, and decreases during menopause.

FUNCTIONAL HISTOLOGY OF THYROID GLAND

Thyroid gland is composed of large number of closed follicles called **thyroid follicles**. Each follicle is formed by cuboidal epithelial cells namely the **follicular cells** around the follicular cavity **(Fig. 51.2)**. **Follicular cavity** is filled with a colloidal substance known as **thyroglobulin** which is secreted by the follicular cells. Follicular cells also secrete tetraiodothyronine (T_4) or thyroxine and triiodothyronine (T_3). In between the follicles, are the **parafollicular cells** or **clear cells** or **C cells**, which secrete calcitonin.

HORMONES OF THYROID GLAND

Thyroid gland secretes three hormones:

1. **Tetraiodothyronine (T_4) or thyroxine**.
2. **Triiodothyronine (T_3)**.
3. **Calcitonin**.

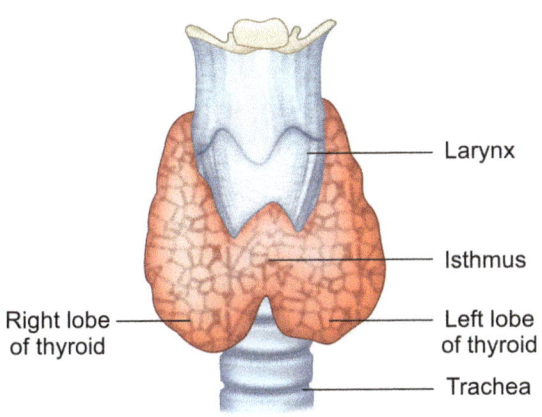

FIGURE 51.1: Thyroid gland.

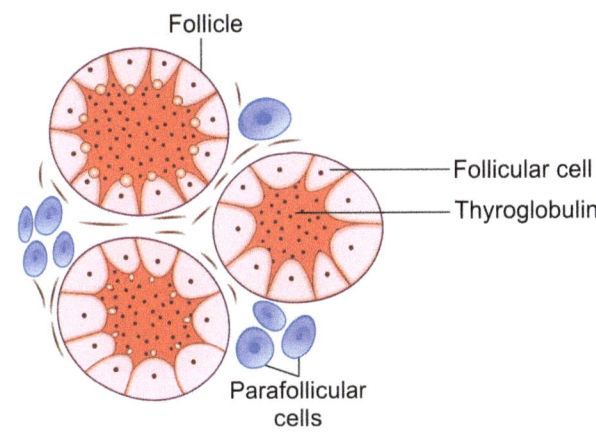

FIGURE 51.2: Histology of thyroid gland.

T_4 is forms about 90% of the total secretion, whereas, T_3 is only 9 to 10%. But the potency of T_3 is four times more than that of T_4. Calcitonin is described in Chapter 52.

■ SYNTHESIS OF THYROID HORMONES

Synthesis of thyroid hormones takes place in thyroglobulin present in follicular cavity. **Iodine** and **tyrosine** are essential for the formation of thyroid hormones. Iodine which is consumed through diet is converted into **iodide** and absorbed from GI tract. Tyrosine is also consumed through diet and is absorbed from the GI.

For the synthesis of normal quantities of thyroid hormones, approximately 1 mg of iodine is required per week or about 50 mg per year. To prevent iodine deficiency, common table salt is iodized with one part of sodium iodide to every 100,000 parts of sodium chloride.

■ STAGES OF SYNTHESIS OF THYROID HORMONES

Synthesis of thyroid hormones takes place in five stages:
1. Thyroglobulin synthesis.
2. Iodide trapping or iodide pump.
3. Oxidation of iodide.
4. Iodination of tyrosine.
5. Coupling reactions.

1. Thyroglobulin Synthesis

Endoplasmic reticulum and Golgi apparatus in the follicular cells of thyroid gland synthesize thyroglobulin continuously. Each thyroglobulin molecule contains 140 tyrosine molecules. After synthesis, the thyroglobulin is stored in the follicle.

2. Iodide Trapping or Iodide Pump

Iodide is transported actively from the blood into follicular cell against electrochemical gradient by a process called iodide trapping. Iodide is pumped with sodium into the follicular cell by **sodium-iodide symport pump**. From here, iodide is transported into the follicular cavity by an **iodide-chloride pump**.

3. Oxidation of the Iodide

Iodide must be oxidized to elementary iodine because only iodine is capable of combining with tyrosine to form thyroid hormones. Oxidation of iodide into iodine occurs inside the follicular cells in the presence of **thyroid peroxidase**.

4. Iodination of Tyrosine

Combination of iodine with tyrosine is known as iodination. It takes place in the follicle within thyroglobulin. First, iodine is released from follicular cells into the follicular cavity where it binds with thyroglobulin. This process is called **organification of thyroglobulin**. In the thyroglobulin, iodine combines with tyrosine which is already present there.

Binding of iodine (I) with tyrosine is accelerated by the enzyme **iodinase** which is secreted by the follicular cells **(Fig. 51.3)**. Iodination of tyrosine occurs in several stages. Tyrosine is iodized first into **monoiodotyrosine (MIT)** and later into **diiodo- tyrosine (DIT)**. MIT and DIT are called the **iodotyrosine residues**.

5. Coupling Reactions

Iodotyrosine residues get coupled with one another through coupling reactions. Coupling occurs in different configurations to give rise to different thyroid hormones.

Coupling reactions are:

i. One molecule of DIT and one molecule of MIT combine to form triiodothyronine (T_3).

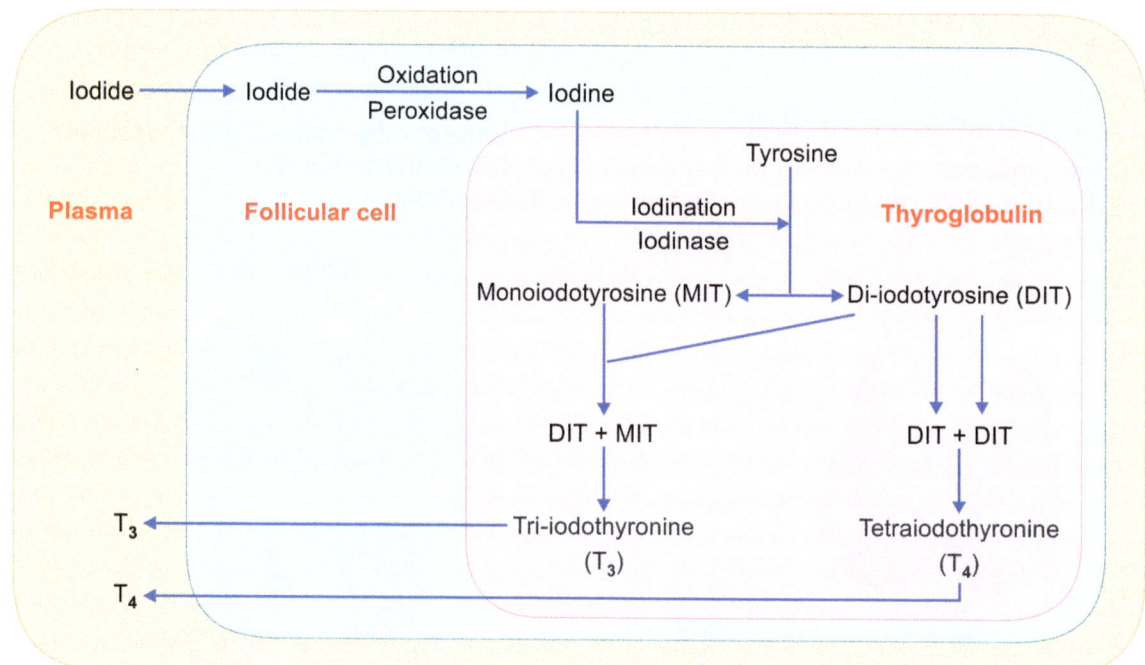

FIGURE 51.3: Synthesis of thyroid hormones.

ii. Sometimes one molecule of MIT and one molecule of DIT combine to produce another form of T_3 called reverse T_3 or rT_3. **Reverse T_3** is only 1% of thyroid output.
iii. Two molecules of DIT combine to form tetraiodothyronine (T_4) which is thyroxine:

  Tyrosine + I = Monoiodotyrosine (MIT)
  MIT + I = Diiodotyrosine (DIT)
  DIT + MIT = Triiodothyronine (T_3)
  MIT + DIT = Reverse T_3
  DIT + DIT = Tetraiodothyronine or Thyroxine (T_4)

STORAGE OF THYROID HORMONES

After synthesis, thyroid hormones remain in the form of vesicles within thyroglobulin. In combination with thyroglobulin, thyroid hormones can be stored for several months. And, thyroid gland is unique in this, as it is the only endocrine gland that can store its hormones for a long period of about 4 months. So, when the synthesis of thyroid hormone stops, signs and symptoms of deficiency do not appear for about 4 months.

RELEASE OF THYROID HORMONES FROM THE THYROID GLAND

Thyroglobulin itself is not released into the bloodstream. On the other hand, the hormones are first cleaved from thyroglobulin.

Only T_3 and T_4 are released into the blood. In the peripheral tissues T_4 is converted into T_3. A small amount of reverse T_3 is also formed. But reverse T_3 is biologically inactive.

The MIT and DIT are not released into blood. These iodotyrosine residues are deiodinated by an enzyme called **iodotyrosine deiodinase** resulting in release of iodine. This iodine is reutilized by the follicular cells for synthesis of thyroid hormones. During congenital absence of iodotyrosine deiodinase, MIT and DIT are excreted in urine and the symptoms of iodine deficiency develop.

TRANSPORT OF THYROID HORMONES IN THE BLOOD

Thyroid hormones are transported in the blood in combination with three types of plasma proteins:

1. **Thyroxine-binding globulin (TBG)**.
2. **Thyroxine-binding prealbumin (TBPA)**.
3. Albumin.

Normal Plasma Level of Thyroid Hormones

  Total T_3 = 0.12 µg/dL.
  Total T_4 = 8 µg/dL.

FUNCTIONS OF THYROID HORMONES

Thyroid hormones have two major functions:
  I. Stimulation of overall metabolic rate in the body.
  II. Stimulation of growth in children.

Actions of thyroid hormones are detailed below.

1. ON BASAL METABOLIC RATE

Thyroxine increases the metabolic activities of almost all tissues of the body except brain, retina, spleen, testes and lungs. It increases the basal metabolic rate (BMR) by increasing the oxygen consumption of the tissues. Action that increases the BMR is called calorigenic action. Basal metabolic rate is defined as the energy (number of calories) required for body functions at rest.

2. ON PROTEIN METABOLISM

Thyroid hormones increase synthesis of proteins. Thyroxine accelerates protein synthesis by the following ways:
  i. By increasing translation of RNA in the cells.
  ii. By increasing transcription of DNA to RNA.
  iii. By increasing activity of mitochondria.
  iv. By increasing activity of cellular enzymes.

Though thyroxine increases protein synthesis, it also causes catabolism of proteins.

3. ON CARBOHYDRATE METABOLISM

Thyroxine stimulates almost all processes involved in the metabolism of carbohydrate.

Thyroxine:
  i. Increases absorption of glucose from GI tract.
  ii. Enhances glucose uptake by the cells, by accelerating transport of glucose through cell membrane.
  iii. Accelerates breakdown of glycogen into glucose.
  iv. Stimulates gluconeogenesis.

4. ON FAT METABOLISM

Thyroxine decreases the fat storage by mobilizing it from adipose tissues and fat depots. Mobilized fat is converted into free fatty acid and transported by blood. Thus, thyroxine increases the free fatty acid level in blood.

5. ON PLASMA AND LIVER FATS

Even though there is increase in the blood level of free fatty acids, thyroxine specifically decreases the cholesterol, phospholipids and triglyceride levels in the plasma. So, in hyposecretion of thyroxine, the cholesterol level in plasma increases resulting in **atherosclerosis**.

Thyroxine also increases deposition of fats in the liver resulting in **fatty liver**. Thyroxine decreases plasma cholesterol level by increasing its excretion from liver cells into bile. Cholesterol enters the intestine through bile and, then it is excreted through the feces.

6. ON VITAMIN METABOLISM

Thyroxine increases the formation of many enzymes. Since, the vitamins form the essential parts of the enzymes it is believed that the vitamins may be utilized during the formation of the enzymes. Hence, vitamin deficiency is possible during hypersecretion of thyroxine.

7. ON BODY TEMPERATURE

Thyroid hormone increases the heat production in the body by accelerating various cellular metabolic processes and increasing BMR.

8. ON GROWTH

Thyroid hormones have general and specific effects on growth. Increase in thyroxine secretion accelerates the growth of the body, especially in growing children. Lack of thyroxine arrests the growth. At the same time, thyroxine causes early closure of epiphysis. So, the height of the individual may be slightly less in hypothyroidism.

Thyroxine is more important to promote growth and development of brain during fetal life and first few years of postnatal life. Deficiency of thyroid hormones during this period leads to **mental retardation**.

9. EFFECT ON BODY WEIGHT

Thyroxine is essential for maintaining body weight. Increase in thyroxine secretion decreases the body weight and fat storage. Decrease in thyroxine secretion increases the body weight because of fat deposition.

10. EFFECT ON BLOOD

Thyroxine increases production of RBCs. It is one of the important general factors necessary for erythropoiesis. Thus, thyroxine increases erythropoietic activity and blood volume.

11. ON CARDIOVASCULAR SYSTEM

Thyroxine increases overall activity of cardiovascular system.

i. On Heart

Thyroxine acts directly on heart and increases rate and force of contraction.

ii. On Blood Vessels

Thyroxine causes vasodilatation by increasing the metabolic activity. During metabolic activity, production of metabolites is increased. These metabolites cause vasodilatation and increase the blood flow.

iii. On Arterial Blood Pressure

Thyroxine increases systolic blood pressure by increasing rate and force of contraction of the heart, blood volume and cardiac output. At the same time, it decreases diastolic pressure by its vasodilator effect. So only the pulse pressure increases and the mean pressure is not altered.

12. EFFECT ON RESPIRATION

Thyroxine increases the rate and force of respiration indirectly. Increased metabolic rate (caused by thyroxine) increases the demand for oxygen and formation of excess carbon dioxide. These two factors stimulate the respiratory centers to increase the rate and force of respiration.

13. ON GASTROINTESTINAL TRACT

Generally, thyroxine increases the appetite and food intake. It also increases the secretions and movements of GI tract.

14. ON CENTRAL NERVOUS SYSTEM

Thyroxine is very essential for the development and maintenance of normal functioning of the central nervous system.

1. Action on Development of Central Nervous System

Thyroxine is very important to promote growth and development of the brain during fetal life and during the first few years of postnatal life. Thyroid deficiency in infants results in mental retardation.

2. Action on the Normal Function of Central Nervous System

Thyroxine is a stimulating factor for the brain, So, normal functioning of brain needs the presence of thyroxine. Thyroxine also increases the blood flow to brain.

Thus, during hypersecretion of thyroxine, there is excess stimulation of the central nervous system. So, the person is likely to have extreme nervousness and may develop psychoneurotic problems such as anxiety complexes, excess worries.

Hyposecretion of thyroxine leads to lethargy and **somnolence** (sleepiness).

15. ON SKELETAL MUSCLE

Thyroxine is essential for the normal activity of the skeletal muscles. Slight increase in thyroxine level makes the muscles to work with more vigor. But, hypersecretion of thyroxine causes weakness of the muscles due to the catabolism of proteins. Lack of thyroxine makes the muscles more sluggish.

16. ON SLEEP

Normal thyroxine level is essential to maintain normal sleep. Hypersecretion of thyroxine causes excessive stimulation of the muscles and central nervous system. So, the person feels tired, exhausted, and feels like sleeping. But the person cannot sleep because of the stimulatory effect of thyroxine on neurons. On the other hand, hyposecretion of thyroxine causes somnolence.

17. ON SEXUAL FUNCTION

Normal thyroxine level is essential for normal sexual function. In men, hypothyroidism leads to complete loss of **libido** (sexual drive). And hyperthyroidism leads to **impotence**.

In women, hypothyroidism causes **menorrhagia** and **polymenorrhea** (Chapter 60). In some women, it causes irregular menstruation and occasionally **amenorrhea**. Hyperthyroidism in women leads to **oligomenorrhea** and sometimes **amenorrhea** (Chapter 60).

18. ON OTHER ENDOCRINE GLANDS

Because of its metabolic effects, thyroxine increases the demand for secretion of other endocrine glands.

MODE OF ACTION OF THYROID HORMONES

Thyroid hormones act by activating the genes (Chapter 49).

REGULATION OF SECRETION OF THYROID HORMONES

The secretion of thyroid hormones is controlled by anterior pituitary and hypothalamus through feedback mechanism **(Fig. 51.4)**.

ROLE OF PITUITARY GLAND

Thyroid-stimulating Hormone

Thyroid-stimulating hormone (TSH) secreted by anterior pituitary is the major factor regulating the synthesis and release of thyroid hormones.

TSH is a peptide hormone with one α-chain and one β-chain. Normal plasma level of TSH is approximately 2 U/mL.

Actions of TSH

Immediate effect of TSH is proteolysis of the thyroglobulin, by which thyroxine is released within 30 minutes. Effect of TSH on thyroxine synthesis takes place after some hours, days or weeks.

TSH accelerates thyroxine synthesis by the following ways:

1. Increases number of follicular cells of thyroid.
2. Accelerates development of thyroid follicles by converting cuboidal cells in thyroid gland into columnar cells.
3. Increases the size and secretory activity of follicular cells.
4. Activates iodide pump and iodide trapping in follicular cells.
5. Increases thyroglobulin secretion into follicles.
6. Increases iodination of tyrosine and coupling to form the hormones.
7. Increases proteolysis of the thyroglobulin, and release of hormones.

Mode of Action of TSH

TSH acts through cyclic AMP mechanism.

ROLE OF HYPOTHALAMUS

Hypothalamus regulates thyroid secretion by inducing release of TSH by thyrotropin-releasing hormone (TRH). From hypothalamus, TRH is transported through hypothalamo-hypophyseal portal vessels to the anterior pituitary. After reaching the pituitary gland, the TRH causes the release of TSH.

FEEDBACK CONTROL

Thyroid hormones regulate their own secretion through negative feedback control by inhibiting the release of TRH from hypothalamus and TSH from anterior pituitary **(Fig. 51.4)**.

ROLE OF IODIDE

Iodide is an important factor regulating the synthesis of thyroid hormones. When the dietary level of iodine is moderate, blood level of thyroid hormones is normal. However, when iodine intake is high, the enzymes necessary for synthesis of thyroid hormones are inhibited by iodide itself resulting in suppression of hormone synthesis.

APPLIED PHYSIOLOGY: DISORDERS OF THYROID GLAND

Disorders of thyroid glands are:

I. Hyperthyroidism.
II. Hypothyroidism.
III. Goiter.

HYPERTHYROIDISM: THYROTOXICOSIS

Hyperthyroidism refers to excess synthesis and release of thyroid hormones by thyroid gland resulting in increased level of hormones in blood.

Thyrotoxicosis is defined as high level of thyroid hormones in blood. It is the condition caused by not only

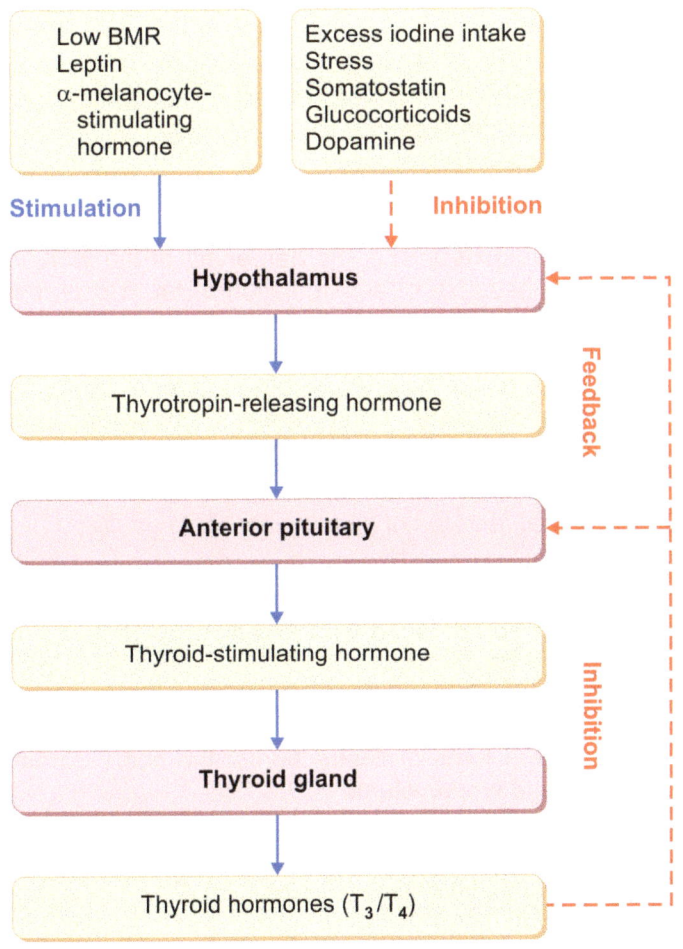

FIGURE 51.4: Regulation of secretion of thyroid hormones.

excess secretion by thyroid glands, but also release of stored hormones.

Causes for Hyperthyroidism

Hyperthyroidism is caused by:

1. Graves' disease.
2. Thyroid adenoma.

1. Graves' disease

Graves' disease is an autoimmune disease characterized by hypersecretion of thyroid hormones. Normally, thyroid-stimulating hormone (TSH) combines with surface receptors of thyroid cells and causes the synthesis of thyroid hormones. In Graves' disease the B lymphocytes (plasma cells) produce autoimmune antibodies called **thyroid stimulating hormone receptor antibodies** (TSHRAb). These antibodies act like TSH by binding with membrane receptors of TSH and activating cAMP system of the thyroid follicular cells. This results in hypersecretion of thyroid hormones.

2. Thyroid adenoma

Sometimes, a localized tumor develops in the thyroid tissue. It is known as thyroid adenoma and it secretes large quantities of thyroid hormones.

Signs and Symptoms of Hyperthyroidism

1. **Intolerance to heat** because of production of more heat during increased basal metabolic rate caused by hyperthyroidism.
2. Increased sweating due to vasodilatation.
3. Decreased body weight due to fat mobilization.
4. Diarrhea due to increased motility of GI tract.
5. Muscular weakness due to excess protein catabolism.
6. Neuronal disturbances such as nervousness, extreme fatigue, inability to sleep, mild tremor in hands and psychoneurotic symptoms such as hyperexcitability, extreme anxiety or worry.
7. Toxic goiter.
8. Oligomenorrhea or amenorrhea.
9. Exophthalmos.
10. Polycythemia.
11. Tachycardia and atrial fibrillation.
12. Systolic hypertension.
13. Cardiac failure.

Exophthalmos

Protrusion of eyeballs is called exophthalmos. Most, but not all hyperthyroid patients develop some degree of protrusion of eyeballs.

Causes for exophthalmos

Exophthalmos in hyperthyroidism is due to the edematous swelling of the retro-orbital tissues and degenerative changes in the extraocular muscles.

Effect of exophthalmos on vision

Severe exophthalmic conditions lead to blindness because of two reasons:

1. Protrusion of the eyeball stretches and damages the optic nerve resulting in blindness.
2. Due to the protrusion of eyeballs, eyelids cannot be closed completely while blinking or during sleep. So, the constant exposure of eyeball to atmosphere causes dryness of the cornea leading to irritation and infection. It finally results in ulceration of the cornea leading to blindness.

■ HYPOTHYROIDISM

Decreased secretion of thyroid hormones is called hypothyroidism. Hypothyroidism leads to myxedema in adults and cretinism in children.

Myxedema

It is the hypothyroidism in adults characterized by generalized edematous appearance.

Causes for myxedema

1. Diseases of thyroid gland.
2. Genetic disorder.
3. Iodine deficiency.
4. Deficiency of thyroid-stimulating hormone or thyrotropin-releasing hormone.
5. Autoimmune disease called **Hashimoto's thyroiditis**.

Signs and symptoms of myxedema

Typical feature myxedema is an edematous appearance throughout the body.

It is associated with following symptoms:

1. Swelling of the face.
2. Bagginess under the eyes.
3. Non-pitting type of edema, i.e. when pressed, it does not make pits and the edema is hard.
4. **Atherosclerosis**: It is the hardening of the walls of arteries because of accumulation of fat. It occurs in myxedema because of increased plasma level of cholesterol which leads to deposition of cholesterol on walls of the arteries. Atherosclerosis produces **arteriosclerosis** which means thickening and stiffening of arterial wall. Arteriosclerosis causes hypertension.

Other general features of hypothyroidism in adults:

1. Anemia.
2. Fatigue and muscular sluggishness.
3. Extreme somnolence with sleeping up to 14 to 16 hours per day.
4. Menorrhagia and polymenorrhea.
5. Decreased cardiovascular functions such as reduction in rate and force of contraction of the heart, cardiac output and blood volume.
6. Increase in body weight.
7. Constipation.
8. Mental sluggishness.
9. Depressed hair growth.
10. Scaliness of the skin.
11. **Frog-like husky voice**.
12. **Intolerance to cold**.

Cretinism

Cretinism is the hypothyroidism in children characterized by stunted growth.

Causes for cretinism

Cretinism occurs due to congenital absence of thyroid gland, genetic disorder or lack of iodine in the diet.

Features of cretinism

1. A newborn baby with thyroid deficiency may appear normal at the time of birth because thyroxine might have been supplied from mother. But a few weeks after birth, the baby starts developing the signs like sluggish movements and croaking sound while crying. Unless treated immediately, the baby will be mentally retarded permanently.
2. Skeletal growth is more affected than the soft tissues. So, there is **stunted growth.** Abdominal bloating is common in cretins **(Fig. 51.5)**. Tongue becomes so big, that it hangs down with dripping of saliva. The big tongue obstructs swallowing and breathing. Tongue produces characteristic **guttural breathing** that may sometimes choke the baby.

Cretin vs dwarf

A cretin is different from pituitary dwarfism. Differences between cretinism and dwarfism are listed in **Table 51.1**.

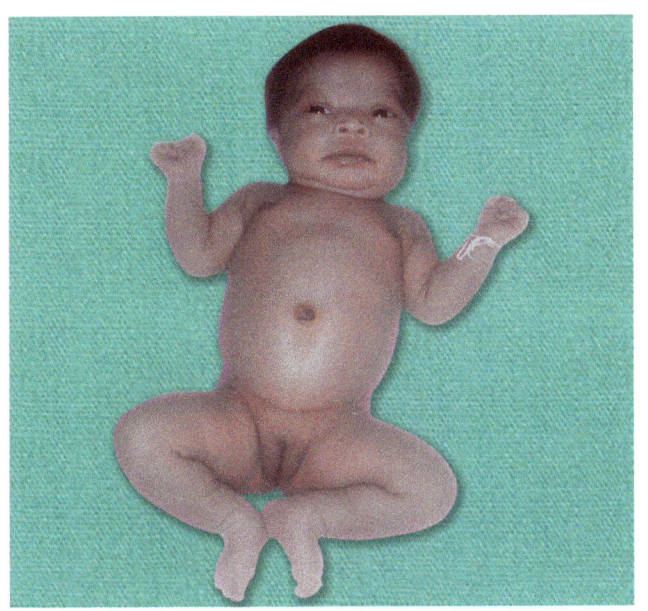

FIGURE 51.5: Cretinism (3-month-old baby).
(*Courtesy:* Prof Mafauzy Mohamed)

■ GOITER

Goiter means enlargement of the thyroid gland. It occurs both in hypothyroidism and hyperthyroidism.

Goiter in Hyperthyroidism: Toxic Goiter

Toxic goiter is the enlargement of thyroid gland with increased secretion of thyroid hormones caused by thyroid tumor.

Goiter in Hypothyroidism: Non-toxic Goiter

Non-toxic goiter is the enlargement of thyroid gland without increase in hormone secretion. It is also called **hypothyroid goiter (Fig. 51.6)**. Based on the cause, the nontoxic hypothyroid goiter is classified into two types:

1. Endemic colloid goiter.
2. Idiopathic non-toxic goiter.

1. Endemic colloid goiter

It is the non-toxic goiter caused by iodine deficiency. It is also called **iodine deficiency goiter**. Iodine deficiency occurs when intake is less than 50 μg/day. Lack of iodine leads to stoppage of formation of thyroid hormones. By feedback mechanism, hypothalamus and anterior pituitary are stimulated. It increases the secretion of TRH and TSH. Excess TSH causes thyroid cells to secrete tremendous amounts of thyroglobulin into the follicle. As there are no hormones to be cleaved, the thyroglobulin remains as it is, and gets accumulated in the follicles of gland. This increases the size of gland.

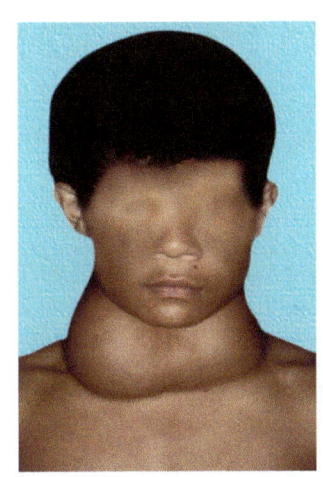 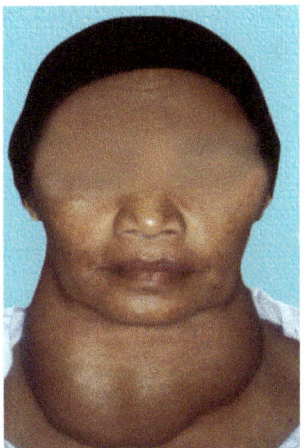

FIGURE 51.6: Non-toxic goiter.
(*Courtesy:* Prof Mafauzy Mohamed)

TABLE 51.1: Differences between cretinism and dwarfism.

Factor	Cretinism	Dwarfism
Cause	Hyposecretion of thyroxine	Hyposecretion of growth hormone
Different parts of the body	Disproportionate	Proportionate
Development of nervous system	Affected	Normal
Mental retardation	Present	Absent
Reproductive system	Affected	Normal

2. Idiopathic non-toxic goiter

It is the goiter due to unknown cause. Enlargement of thyroid gland occurs even without iodine deficiency. The exact cause is not known.

Some foodstuffs contain **goitrogens** (goitrogenic substances) such as **goitrin**. These substances contain antithyroid substances like **propylthiouracil**. Goitrogens suppress the synthesis of thyroid hormones. Therefore, TSH secretion increases resulting in enlargement of the gland. Such goitrogens are found in vegetables such as turnips and cabbages. Soybean also contains some amount of goitrogens.

Goitrogens become active only during low iodine intake.

TREATMENT FOR THYROID DISORDERS

TREATMENT FOR HYPERTHYROIDISM

Hyperthyroidism is treated by two methods:

1. By antithyroid substances such as **thiocyanate**, **thioureylenes** and high concentration of inorganic iodides.
2. By surgical removal.

TREATMENT FOR HYPOTHYROIDISM

Only treatment for hypothyroidism is the administration of thyroid extract or ingestion of pure thyroxine in the form of tablets, orally.

THYROID FUNCTION TESTS

Functional status of thyroid gland is assessed by the following tests:

1. Measurement of concentration of T_3 and T_4 in plasma.
2. Measurement of TRH and TSH in plasma.
3. Measurement of basal metabolic rate.

Chapter 52: Parathyroid Glands and Physiology of Bone

CHAPTER OUTLINE

- MORPHOLOGY OF PARATHYROID GLANDS
- PARATHORMONE
- APPLIED PHYSIOLOGY: DISORDERS OF PARATHYROID GLANDS
- PARATHYROID FUNCTION TESTS
- CALCITONIN
- CALCIUM METABOLISM
- PHOSPHATE METABOLISM
- PHYSIOLOGY OF BONE

■ MORPHOLOGY OF PARATHYROID GLANDS

There are four parathyroid glands located immediately behind thyroid gland at the upper and lower poles (Fig. 52.1). Parathyroid glands are very small in size measuring about 6 mm long, 3 mm wide and 2 mm thick with dark brown color.

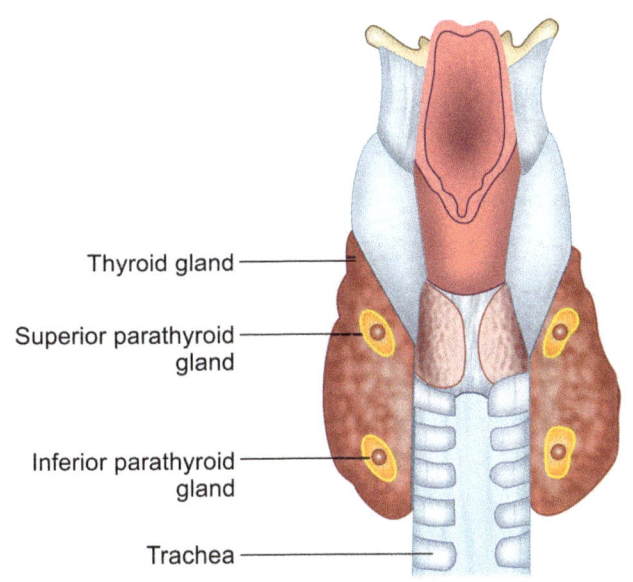

FIGURE 52.1: Parathyroid glands on the posterior surface of thyroid gland.

■ FUNCTIONAL HISTOLOGY OF PARATHYROID GLANDS

Each parathyroid gland is made up of **chief cells** and **oxyphil cells**. Chief cells secrete parathormone but, function of the oxyphil cell is not known. It is believed that oxyphil cells are the degenerated chief cells.

■ PARATHORMONE

Parathormone is secreted by parathyroid gland. It is essential for the maintenance of **blood calcium level**.

■ SOURCE, CHEMISTRY AND PLASMA LELVEL

Parathormone (PTH) is secreted by the chief cells of the parathyroid glands. It is protein in nature having 84 amino acids. Normal plasma level of PTH is about 1.5 to 5.5 ng/dL.

■ ACTIONS OF PARATHORMONE

Parathormone maintains the blood calcium level and blood phosphate level.

Action of PTH on Blood Calcium Level

Primary action of PTH is to maintain the blood calcium level within the critical range of 9 to 11 mg/dL. Blood calcium level has to be maintained critically because, it is very important for many activities in the body.

PTH maintains the blood calcium level by acting on:

1. Bones.
2. Kidneys.
3. GI tract.

1. Effect on bones

i. Parathormone increases **osteoclastic activity** (resorption of calcium from the bones) by acting on **osteoclasts** of the bone.
ii. Parathormone also stimulates the proliferation of osteoclasts.
iii. PTH increases the permeability of membranes of osteoblasts for calcium ions. So, calcium ions move from these bone cells into the blood.
iv. PTH stimulates osteoclasts and causes release of proteolytic enzymes and some acids such as citric acid and lactic acid. All these substances digest or dissolve the organic matrix of bone, releasing calcium ions into plasma.

2. Effect on kidneys

Parathormone increases reabsorption of calcium from distal convoluted tubule and proximal part of collecting duct into the plasma. It also increases the formation of **1,25-dihydroxycholecalciferol** (activated form of vitamin D) from **25-hydroxycholecalciferol** in kidneys. **Activated vitamin D** is necessary for absorption of calcium form GI tract.

3. Effect on gastrointestinal tract (GI)

PTH increases **absorption of calcium** from GI tract by increasing the formation of 1,25-dihydroxycholecalciferol in kidneys.

Role of PTH on activation of vitamin D

Vitamin D is in different forms. But, the most important one is **vitamin D_3**. It is also known as **cholecalciferol**. Vitamin D_3 is synthesized in the skin from **7-dehydrocholesterol** by the action of ultraviolet rays from sunlight. It is also obtained from dietary sources activation of vitamin D_3 occurs in two steps **(Fig. 52.2)**.

In the first step, cholecalciferol (vitamin D_3) is converted into **25-hydroxycholecalciferol** in the liver. This process is limited and it is inhibited by 25-hydroxycholecalciferol itself by feedback mechanism.

In the second step, 25-hydroxycholecalciferol is converted into **1,25-dihydroxycholecalciferol** (**calcitriol**) in kidney. And, it is the active form of vitamin D_3. This step needs the presence of PTH.

The 1,25-dihydroxycholecalciferol increases absorption of calcium and phosphate from intestine.

Action of PTH on Blood Phosphate Level

PTH decreases blood level of phosphate by increasing its urinary excretion. It also acts on bone and GI tract.

1. Effect on bone

Along with calcium resorption, PTH also increases phosphate absorption from the bones.

2. Effect on kidneys: Phosphaturic action

Phosphaturic action is excretion of phosphate through urine. PTH inhibits reabsorption of phosphate from renal tubules so that excretion of phosphate through urine increases.

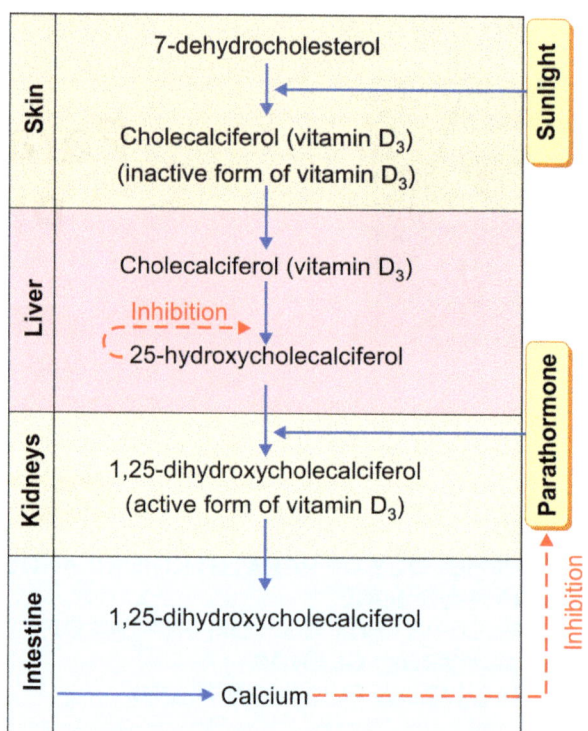

FIGURE 52.2: Schematic diagram showing activation of vitamin D.

3. Effect on gastrointestinal tract

PTH increases the formation of 1,25-dihydroxycholecalciferol in the kidneys. This vitamin in turn increases the absorption of phosphate along with calcium.

■ MODE OF ACTION OF PARATHORMONE

On the target cells, PTH binds with **parathormone receptor** which is coupled to G protein and forms hormone-receptor complex. Hormone-receptor complex causes formation of cAMP, which acts as a second messenger for the hormone.

■ REGULATION OF PARATHORMONE SECRETION

Blood level of calcium is the main factor that regulates the secretion of PTH. Blood phosphate level also influences PTH secretion.

Role of Blood Level of Calcium

PTH secretion is **inversely proportional** to blood calcium level. Increase in blood calcium level decreases PTH secretion.

Role of Blood Level of Phosphate

PTH secretion is **directly proportional** to blood phosphate level. Whenever the blood level of phosphate increases, it combines with ionized calcium to form of calcium hydrogen phosphate. This decreases ionized calcium level in blood which stimulates PTH secretion.

APPLIED PHYSIOLOGY: DISORDERS OF PARATHYROID GLANDS

Disorders of parathyroid glands are of two types:

I. Hypoparathyroidism.
II. Hyperparathyroidism.

HYPOPARATHYROIDISM: HYPOCALCEMIA

Hypoparathyroidism leads to hypocalcemia (decrease in blood calcium level).

Causes for Hypoparathyroidism

1. Surgical removal of parathyroid glands (**parathyroidectomy**).
2. Removal of parathyroid glands during surgical removal of thyroid gland (**thyroidectomy**).
3. Autoimmune disease.
4. Deficiency of receptors for PTH in the target cells. In this, the PTH secretion is normal or increased but the hormone cannot act on the target cells. This condition is called **pseudohypoparathyroidism**.

Hypocalcemia

Hypoparathyroidism causes hypocalcemia by decreasing the resorption of calcium from bones. Hypocalcemia causes neuromuscular hyperexcitability resulting in hypocalcemic tetany.

Hypocalcemic Tetany

Tetany is an abnormal condition characterized by painful muscular spasm (involuntary contraction of muscle or group of muscles) particularly in feet and hand. It is because of hyperexcitability of nerves and skeletal muscles due to calcium deficiency.

Tetany occurs when blood calcium level falls below 6 mg/dL.

Signs and symptoms of hypocalcemic tetany

1. *Hyperreflexia and convulsions*

Increased neural excitability results in hyperreflexia (overactive reflex actions) and convulsive muscular contractions.

2. *Carpopedal spasm*

Carpopedal spasm is the **spasm** (violent and painful muscular contraction) in hand and feet that occurs due to hypocalcemia. During carpopedal spasm, hand shows a peculiar attitude with flexion at wrist joint and metacarpophalangeal joints, adduction of the thumb, and extension of interphalangeal joints **(Fig. 52.3)**.

3. *Laryngeal stridor*

Stridor means noisy breathing. Laryngeal stridor means a loud crowing sound during inspiration which occurs mainly due to laryngospasm (involuntary contraction of laryngeal muscles). Laryngeal stridor is a common feature of hypocalcemic tetany.

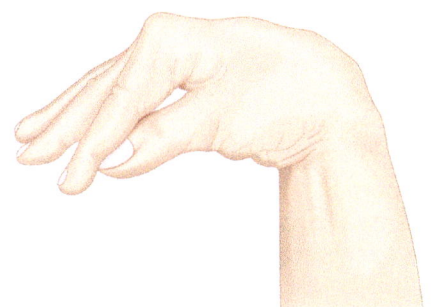

FIGURE 52.3: Carpopedal spasm.

4. *Cardiovascular changes*

   i. Dilatation of the heart.
   ii. Prolonged duration of ST segment and QT interval in ECG.
   iii. Arrhythmias (irregular heartbeat).
   iv. Hypotension.
   v. Heart failure.

Other features

   i. Decreased permeability of the cell membrane.
   ii. Dry skin with brittle nails.
   iii. Hair loss.
   iv. Seizures.
   v. Signs of mental retardation in children or dementia in adults (Chapter 107).

It becomes fatal when the calcium level falls below 4 mg/dL. During such severe hypocalcemic conditions, tetany occurs so quickly that a person develops spasm of different groups of muscles in the body. Worst affected are the laryngeal and bronchial muscles which develop respiratory arrest resulting in death.

Latent Tetany or Subclinical Tetany

Latent or subclinical tetany is the neuromuscular hyperexcitability due to hypocalcemia that develops before the onset of tetany. It is characterized by general weakness and cramps in feet and hand. Hyperexcitability in these patients is detected by some signs, which do not appear in normal persons.

1. Trousseau's sign

It is the spasm of hand that is developed after 3 minutes of arresting the blood flow to lower arm and hand. Blood flow to lower arm and hand is arrested by inflating blood pressure cuff 20 mm Hg above the patient's systolic pressure.

2. Chvostek's sign

Chvostek's sign is the twitch of facial muscles caused by a gentle tap over the facial nerve in front of ear. It is due to the hyperirritability of facial nerve.

3. Erb's sign

Hyperexcitability of the skeletal muscles even to a mild electrical stimulus is called Erb's sign. It is also called **Erb-Westphal sign**.

HYPERPARATHYROIDISM: HYPERCALCEMIA

Hyperparathyroidism results in hypercalcemia (increase in blood calcium level).

Causes of Hyperparathyroidism

1. Tumor in parathyroid glands.
2. Compensatory hypertrophy of parathyroid glands in response to hypocalcemia which occurs due to other pathological conditions such as chronic renal failure, vitamin D deficiency and rickets.
3. **Hyperplasia** (abnormal increase in the number of cells) of all the parathyroid glands.

Hypercalcemia

Hypercalcemia is the increase in plasma calcium level. It occurs in hyperparathyroidism because of increased resorption of calcium from bones.

Common signs and symptoms of hypercalcemia:

1. Depression of the nervous system.
2. Sluggishness of reflex activities.
3. Reduced ST segment and QT interval in ECG.
4. Lack of appetite.
5. Constipation.

Depressive effects of hypercalcemia are noticed when the blood calcium level increases to 12 mg/dL. The condition becomes severe with 15 mg/dL and it becomes lethal when blood calcium level reaches 17 mg/dL.

Other effects of hypercalcemia:

1. **Bone diseases**: Development of bone diseases such as **osteitis fibrosa cystica** (disorder characterized by weak and fragile bone).
2. **Parathyroid poisoning**: It is the condition characterized by severe manifestations that occur when blood calcium level rises above 15 mg/dL along with increase in phosphate level leading to formation of **calcium-phosphate crystals**. The calcium-phosphate crystals may be deposited in the tubules of the kidneys, thyroid gland, alveoli of lungs, gastric mucosa and in the wall of the arteries. Calcium deposition results in dysfunction of these organs. **Renal stones** are formed when it is deposited in kidney.

PARATHYROID FUNCTION TESTS

Functions of parathyroid glands are assessed by the following tests:

1. Measurement of blood calcium level.
2. Chvostek's sign and Trousseau's sign for hypoparathyroidism.

CALCITONIN

SOURCE OF CHEMISTRY AND PLASMA LEVEL OF CALCITONIN

Calcitonin is secreted by the **parafollicular cells** or **clear cells (C cells)** situated amongst the follicles in **thyroid gland**.

It is a polypeptide chain with 32 amino acids. Its molecular weight is about 3,400. Plasma level of calcitonin it 1 to 2 ng/dL.

ACTIONS OF CALCITONIN

1. Action of Calcitonin on Blood Calcium Level

Calcitonin decreases the blood calcium level and thereby counteracts parathormone.

Calcitonin decreases blood calcium level by acting on:

i. Bones.
ii. Kidneys.
iii. Intestine.

i. Effect on bones

Calcitonin stimulates **osteoblastic activity** and facilitates the deposition of calcium on bones. At the same time, it suppresses the activity of osteoclasts and inhibits the resorption of calcium from bones. It inhibits even the development of new osteoclasts in bones.

ii. Effect on kidneys

Calcitonin increases the excretion of calcium through urine, by inhibiting the reabsorption of calcium from the renal tubules.

iii. Effect on intestine

It prevents the absorption of calcium from intestine into the blood.

Action of Calcitonin on Blood Phosphate Level

With respect to calcium, calcitonin is an antagonist to PTH. But, it has similar actions of PTH with respect to phosphate.

Calcitonin decreases blood level of phosphate by acting on:

i. Bones.
ii. Kidneys.

i. Effect on bones

Calcitonin inhibits the resorption of phosphate from bone and stimulates deposition of phosphate on bones.

ii. Effect on kidneys

Calcitonin increases the excretion of phosphate through urine, by inhibiting the reabsorption of calcium from the renal tubules.

REGULATION OF CALCITONIN SECRETION

High calcium content in plasma stimulates the calcitonin secretion through a **calcium receptor** in parafollicular cells. Gastrin also is known to stimulate release of calcitonin.

CALCIUM METABOLISM

IMPORTANCE OF CALCIUM

Calcium is very essential for many activities in the body such as:

1. Bone and teeth formation.
2. Neuronal activity.

3. Skeletal muscle activity.
4. Cardiac activity.
5. Smooth muscle activity.
6. Secretory activity of the glands.
7. Cell division and growth.
8. Coagulation of blood.

■ NORMAL VALUE OF CALCIUM LEVEL

In a normal young healthy adult, there is about 1,100 g of calcium in the body. It forms about 1.5% of total body weight. Ninety nine percent of calcium is present in the bones and teeth and the rest is present in the plasma.

Normal **blood calcium level** ranges between 9 and 11 mg/dL.

■ TYPES OF CALCIUM

Types of Calcium in Plasma

Calcium is present in three forms in plasma:

1. Ionized or diffusible calcium.
2. Non-ionized or non-diffusible calcium.
3. Calcium bound to albumin.

Ionized calcium is found freely in plasma and it forms about 50% of plasma calcium. It is essential for the vital functions such as neuronal activity, muscle contraction, cardiac activity, secretions in the glands, blood coagulation, etc. About 8 to 10% of plasma calcium is present in nonionic form such as calcium bicarbonate. About 40 to 42% of calcium is bound with plasma protein particularly, albumin.

Calcium in Bones

Calcium is constantly removed from bone and deposited in bone. Process of calcium metabolism is explained schematically in **Figure 52.4**.

■ SOURCE OF CALCIUM

1. Dietary Source

Calcium is available in several foodstuffs such as milk, cheese, vegetables, meat, egg, grains, sugar, coffee, tea, chocolate, etc.

2. From Bones

Besides dietary calcium, blood also gets calcium from bone by resorption.

■ DAILY REQUIREMENTS OF CALCIUM

1 to 3 years	= 500 mg
4 to 8 years	= 800 mg
9 to 18 years	= 1,300 mg
19 to 50 years	= 1,000 mg
51 years and above	= 1,200 mg
Pregnant women and lactating mothers	= 1,300 mg

■ ABSORPTION AND EXCRETION OF CALCIUM

Calcium taken through dietary sources is absorbed from the GI tract into blood and distributed to various parts of the body. Depending upon the blood level, the calcium is either deposited in the bone or removed from the bone (resorption). Calcium is excreted from the body through urine and feces.

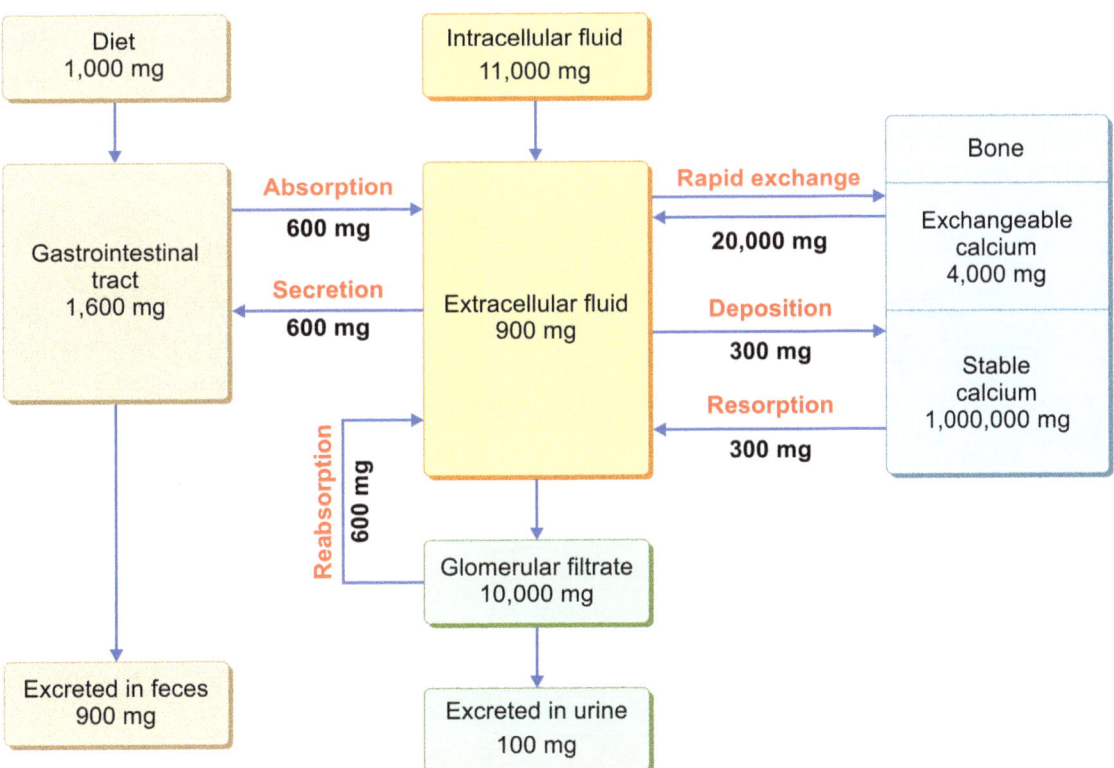

FIGURE 52.4: Schematic diagram showing calcium metabolism. Values belong to adults.

Absorption of Calcium from GI Tract

Calcium is absorbed from duodenum by carrier mediated active transport and from the rest of the small intestine by facilitated diffusion. **Vitamin D** is essential for the absorption of calcium from GI tract.

Excretion of Calcium

While passing through the kidney, large quantity of calcium is filtered in the glomerulus. From the filtrate, 98 to 99% of calcium is reabsorbed from renal tubules into the blood. And only small quantity is excreted through urine.

Most of the filtered calcium is reabsorbed in the distal convoluted tubules and proximal part of collecting duct. In distal convoluted tubule parathormone increases the reabsorption. In collecting duct vitamin D increases the reabsorption and calcitonin decreases reabsorption.

About 1,000 mg of calcium is excreted daily. Out of this 900 mg is excreted through feces and 100 mg through urine.

■ REGULATION OF BLOOD CALCIUM LEVEL

Calcium metabolism is regulated mainly by three hormones **(Figs. 52.5 and 52.6)**:

1. Parathormone.
2. 1,25-dihydroxycholecalciferol (calcitriol).
3. Calcitonin.

1. Role of Parathormone

It is protein hormone secreted by parathyroid gland and its main function is to increase the blood calcium level by bone resorption (mobilization of calcium from bone: see above for details).

2. Role of 1,25-dihydroxycholecalciferol: Calcitriol

It is a steroid hormone synthesized in kidney. It is the activated form of vitamin D. Its main action is to increase the blood calcium level by increasing the calcium absorption from small intestine (see above for details).

3. Role of Calcitonin

It is a protein hormone secreted by parafollicular cells of thyroid gland. It is a calcium lowering hormone. It reduces the blood calcium level mainly by decreasing bone resorption (see above for details).

Role of Other Hormones

In addition to the above mentioned three hormones, growth hormone and glucocorticoids also influence the calcium level.

1. Growth hormone

It increases the blood calcium level by increasing the intestinal calcium absorption.

2. Glucocorticoids

Glucocorticoids (cortisol) decrease blood calcium by inhibiting intestinal absorption and increasing the renal excretion of calcium.

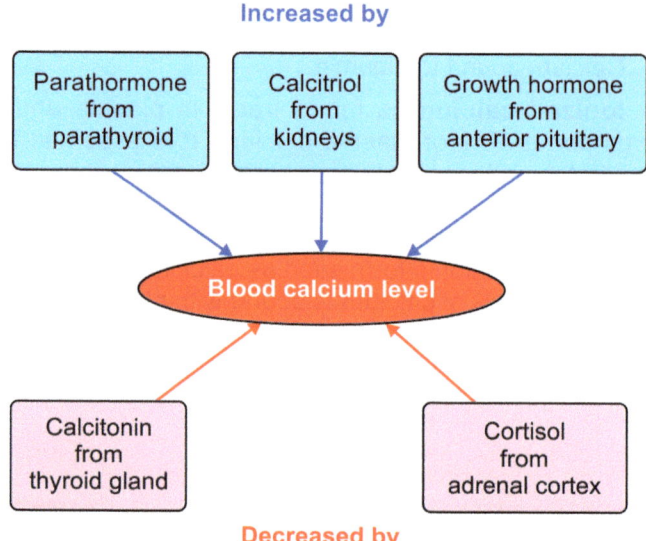

FIGURE 52.6: Effect of hormones on blood calcium level.

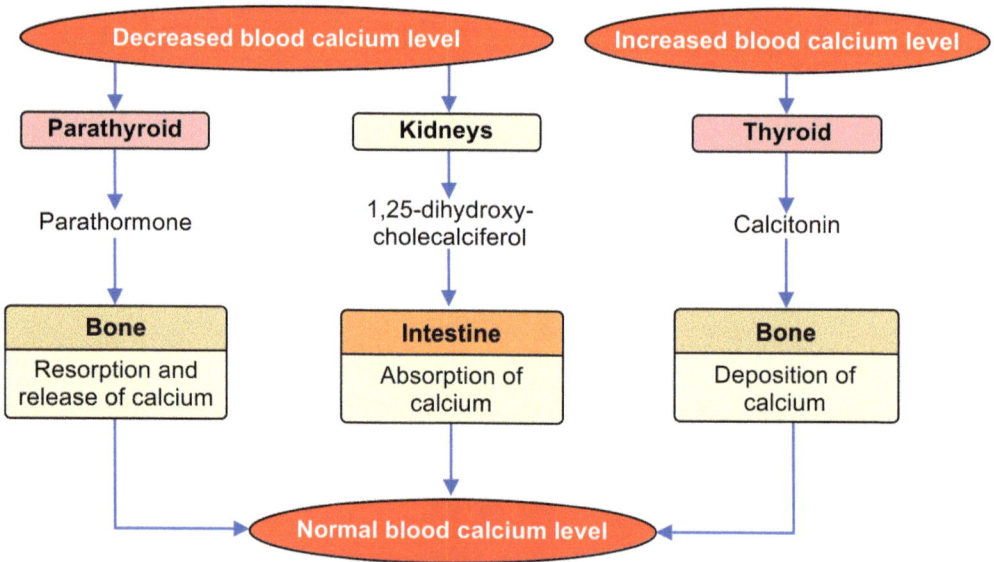

FIGURE 52.5: Schematic diagram showing regulation of blood calcium level.

PHOSPHATE METABOLISM

Phosphorus (P) is an essential mineral that is required by every cell in the body for normal function. Phosphorus is present in many food substances, such as peas, dried beans, nuts, milk, cheese and butter. **Inorganic phosphorus (Pi)** is in the form of the **phosphate (PO_4)**. Majority of the phosphorus in the body is found as phosphate. In the body, phosphate is the most abundant intracellular anion.

IMPORTANCE OF PHOSPHATE

1. Phosphate is an important component of many organic substances such as, ATP, DNA, RNA and many intermediates of metabolic pathways.
2. Along with calcium it forms an important constituent of bone and teeth.
3. It forms a buffer in the maintenance of acid-base balance.

NORMAL VALUE OF PHOSPHATE LEVEL

Total amount of phosphate in the body is 500 g to 800 g. Though it is present in every cell of the body, 85 to 90% of body's phosphate is found in the bones and teeth.

Normal plasma level of phosphate is 4 mg/dL.

REGULATION OF PHOSPHATE LEVEL

Phosphorous is taken through dietary sources. It is absorbed from the GI tract into blood and distributed to various parts of the body. While passing through the kidney, large quantity of phosphate is excreted through urine.

Regulation of phosphate level depends upon three processes:

1. Absorption from gastrointestinal tract.
2. Resorption from bone.
3. Excretion through urine.

All the three processes are regulated by three hormones:

1. Parathormone.
2. Calcitonin.
3. 1,25-dihydroxycholecalciferol (calcitriol).

1. Role of Parathormone

Parathormone stimulates resorption of phosphate from bone, but increases its urinary excretion. It also increases the absorption of phosphate from gastrointestinal tract through calcitriol. The overall action of parathormone is to decrease the plasma level of phosphate.

2. Role of Calcitonin

Calcitonin also decreases the plasma level of phosphate by inhibiting bone resorption and stimulating urinary excretion.

3. 1,25-dihydroxycholecalciferol: Calcitriol

This hormone increases absorption of phosphate from small intestine **(Fig. 52.7)**.

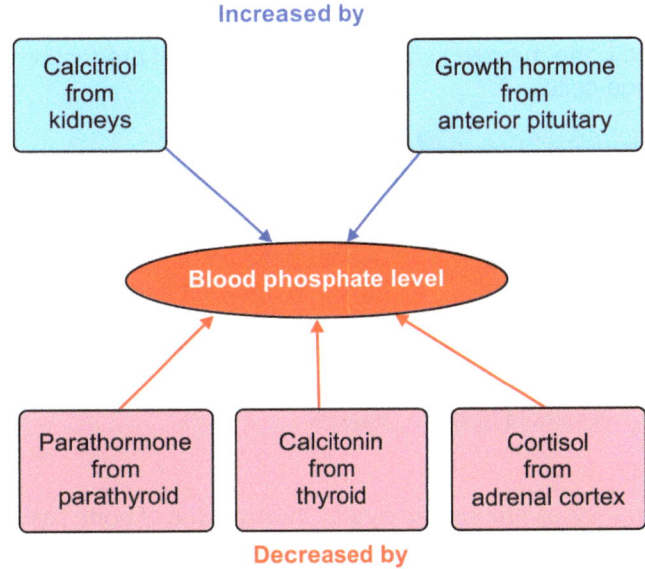

FIGURE 52.7: Effect of hormones on blood phosphate level.

Effects of Other Hormones

In addition to the above mentioned three hormones, growth hormone, and glucocorticoids also influence the phosphate level.

1. Growth hormone

It increases the blood phosphate level by increasing the intestinal phosphate absorption.

2. Glucocorticoids

Glucocorticoids (cortisol) decrease blood phosphate by inhibiting intestinal absorption and increasing the renal excretion of phosphate.

PHYSIOLOGY OF BONE

Bone or **osseous tissue** is a specialized rigid connective tissue that forms the skeleton. It consists of special type of cells and tough intercellular matrix of ground substance. **Matrix** is formed by organic substances like collagen. And it is strengthened by deposition of mineral salts such as calcium phosphate and calcium carbonate. Throughout life, bone is renewed by the process of bone formation and bone resorption.

FUNCTIONS OF BONE

1. Protective Function

Bone protects soft tissues and vital organs of the body.

2. Mechanical Function

It supports the body and brings out various movements of the body.

3. Metabolic Function

It is responsible for metabolism and homeostasis of calcium and phosphate in the body.

4. Hematopoietic Function

Red bone marrow in the bones is the site of production of blood cells.

■ CLASSIFICATION OF BONE

Bones are classified into five types depending upon the size and shape:

1. Long bones   : Bones of the limbs.
2. Short bones   : Bones in the wrist and ankle.
3. Flat bones   : Skull bones, mandible, scapula, etc.
4. Irregular bones : Vertebra.
5. Sesamoid bones : Patella.

■ PARTS OF BONE

Long bones are formed by a cylindrical tube of bone tissue, which has three portions:

1. **Diaphysis**: Midportion or midshaft.
2. **Epiphysis**: Wider extremity or the head on either end.
3. **Metaphysis**: Portion between the diaphysis and epiphysis **(Fig. 52.8)**.

In growing age, a layer of cartilage called **epiphyseal cartilage** or **epiphyseal plate** or **growth plate** is present in between epiphysis and metaphysis. Epiphyseal plate is responsible for the longitudinal growth of the bones.

■ STRUCTURE OF BONE

Bone is covered by an outer white fibrous connective layer called **periosteum** and an inner dense fibrous membrane called **endosteum**. Tendons from the muscles are attached to **periosteum**. Heads (epiphysis) of bone are covered by a **hyaline cartilage**. It forms the synovial joint with adjoining bones.

Bones have two layers of structures:

1. Outer compact bone.
2. Inner spongy bone.

In most of the bones, both compact and spongy forms are present. However, the thickness of each type varies in different regions. Epiphysis contains large amount of spongy bone and outer thin compact bone. In diaphysis, the amount of compact bone is more and spongy bone is very thin.

■ TYPES OF CELLS IN BONE

Bone has three major types of cells:

1. Osteoblasts.
2. Osteocytes.
3. Osteoclasts.

1. Osteoblasts

Osteoblasts are the bone cells that are concerned with bone formation. These cells are situated in the outer surface of bone, marrow cavity and epiphyseal plate. Osteoblasts arise from the giant multinucleated primitive cells called the **osteoprogenitor cells**.

Functions of osteoblasts

Osteoblasts:

i. Are responsible for the synthesis of bone matrix.
ii. Are rich in alkaline phosphatase, which is necessary for **calcification** (deposition of calcium in the bone matrix).
iii. Synthesize of the proteins called **matrix Gla-protein** and **osteopontin**, which are involved in the calcification.

Fate of osteoblasts

After taking part in bone formation, the osteoblasts differentiate into osteocytes, which are trapped inside lacunae of calcified bone.

2. Osteocytes

Osteocytes are the cells concerned with maintenance of bone. Osteocytes are small flattened and rounded cells embedded in the bone lacunae. These bone cells are the main cells of developed bone and are derived from the matured osteoblasts.

Functions of osteocytes

Osteocytes:

i. Help to maintain the bone as living tissue because of their metabolic activity.
ii. Maintain the exchange of calcium between the bone and ECF.

3. Osteoclasts

Osteoclasts are the bone cells that are concerned with bone resorption. Osteoclasts are the giant phagocytic

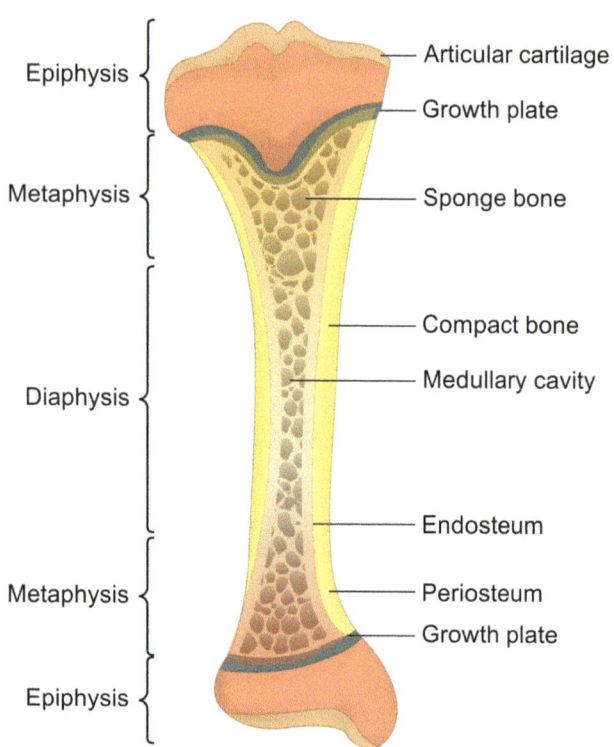

FIGURE 52.8: Parts of long bone.

multinucleated cells found in the lacunae of bone matrix. These bone cells are derived from hematopoietic stem cells via monocytes (CFU-M).

Functions of osteoclasts

Osteoclasts:

i. Are responsible for bone resorption during bone remodeling.
ii. Are responsible for synthesis and release of **lysosomal enzymes** necessary for bone resorption into the bone resorbing compartment.

■ BONE REMODELING

Bone remodeling is a dynamic lifelong process in which old bone is resorbed and new bone is formed. Usually, it takes place in groups of bone cells called the **basic multicellular units (BMU)**. Entire process of remodeling extends for about 100 days in compact bone and about 200 days in spongy bone.

Bone remodeling includes two processes:

1. *Bone resorption:* **Osteoclastic activity** (destruction of entire bone matrix and removal of calcium). Osteoclasts are responsible for this.
2. *Bone formation:* **Osteoblastic activity** (development and mineralization of new matrix). Osteoblasts are responsible for this.

Significance of Bone Remodeling

In children:

1. Thickness of bone increases.
2. Bone obtains strength in proportion to the growth.
3. Shape of bone is realtered in relation to growth of the body.

In adults:

1. Maintenance of toughness of bone.
2. Mechanical integrity of skeleton throughout life.
3. Calcium homeostasis.

■ APPLIED PHYSIOLOGY: DISEASES OF BONE

1. Osteoporosis

Osteoporosis is a bone disease characterized by the loss of bone matrix and minerals. Osteoporosis means '**porous bones**'. It occurs due to excessive bone resorption and decreased bone formation.

Loss of bone matrix and minerals leads to loss of bone strength associated with architectural deterioration of bone tissue. Ultimately, the bones become fragile with **high-risk of fracture**. Commonly affected bones are vertebrae and hip. Osteoporosis is common in women after 60 years.

2. Rickets

Rickets is the bone disease in children characterized by inadequate mineralization of bone matrix. It occurs due to vitamin D deficiency. Vitamin D deficiency develops due to insufficiency in diet or due to inadequate exposure to sunlight.

Deficiency of vitamin D affects the reabsorption of calcium and phosphorus from renal tubules resulting in calcium deficiency. It causes inadequate mineralization of epiphyseal growth plate in growing bones. This defect produces various manifestations.

Manifestations of rickets

i. Collapse of chest wall: Due to the flattening of sides of thorax with projecting sternum called **pigeon chest**, **chicken chest** or **pectus carinatum**.
ii. **Rachitic rosary**: A visible swelling where the ribs join their cartilages.
iii. **Kyphosis**: Excess curvature of upper back-bone with convexity backward (forward bending or forward curvature).
iv. **Lordosis**: Excess forward curvature of back-bone in lumbar region.
v. **Scoliosis**: Lateral curvature of spine.
vi. Bowing of hands and legs.
vii. Enlargement of liver and spleen.
viii. Tetany in advanced stages. The patient may die because of tetany involving the respiratory muscles.

3. Osteomalacia

Rickets in adults is called osteomalacia or **adult rickets**. It occurs because of deficiency of vitamin D. It also occurs due to prolonged damage of kidney (**renal rickets**).

Characteristic features of osteomalacia are:

i. Vague pain.
ii. Tenderness in bones and muscles.
iii. **Myopathy** leading to **waddling gait** (gait means the manner of walking). In waddling gait, the feet are wide apart and walk resembles that of a duck.
iv. Occasional hypoglycemic tetany.

Chapter 53: Endocrine Functions of Pancreas

CHAPTER OUTLINE

- ISLETS OF LANGERHANS
- INSULIN
- GLUCAGON
- SOMATOSTATIN
- PANCREATIC POLYPEPTIDE
- REGULATION OF BLOOD SUGAR LEVEL
- APPLIED PHYSIOLOGY: DISORDERS OF PANCREAS

■ ISLETS OF LANGERHANS

Endocrine function of pancreas is performed by the islets of Langerhans **(Fig. 53.1)**. Human pancreas contains about 1 to 2 million islets.

Islets of Langerhans consist of four types of cells:

1. A cells or α-cells which secrete glucagon.
2. B cells or β-cells which secrete insulin.
3. D cells or γ-cells which secrete somatostatin.
4. F cells or PP cells which secrete pancreatic polypeptide.

■ INSULIN

■ SOURCE, CHEMISTRY AND BLOOD LEVEL OF INSULIN

Insulin is secreted by B cells or the **β-cells** in islets of Langerhans of pancreas.

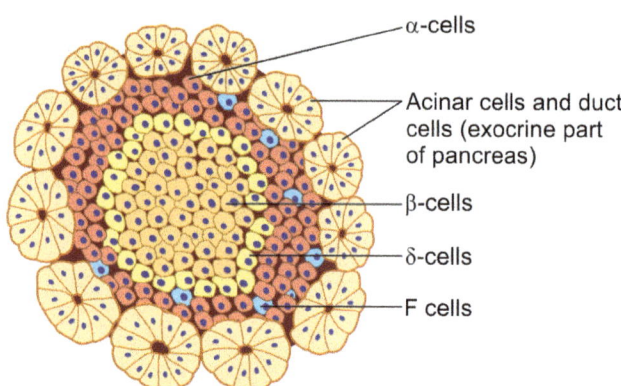

FIGURE 53.1: Islets of Langerhans.

Insulin is a polypeptide with 51 amino acids. It has two amino acid chains called α- and β-chains which are linked by **disulfide bridges**. The α-chain of insulin contains 21 amino acids, and β-chain contains 30 amino acids.

Basal level of insulin in plasma is 10 µU/mL.

■ ACTIONS OF INSULIN

Insulin is the important hormone that is concerned with regulation of carbohydrate metabolism and blood sugar level. It is also concerned with metabolism of proteins and fats.

1. *Action on Carbohydrate Metabolism*

Insulin is the only **antidiabetic hormone** secreted in the body, i.e. it is the only hormone in body that reduces blood sugar level. Insulin reduces the blood sugar level by its following actions on carbohydrate metabolism.

i. *By facilitating transport and uptake of glucose by the cells*

Insulin facilitates transport of glucose from the blood into cells by increasing the permeability of cell membrane to glucose. Insulin stimulates the rapid uptake of glucose by all the tissues particularly liver, muscle and adipose tissues. However, insulin is not required for glucose uptake in some tissues such as brain (except hypothalamus), renal tubules, mucous membrane of intestine and RBCs. Insulin also increases the number of glucose transporters called **GLUT4** in cell membrane.

ii. *By increasing peripheral utilization of glucose*

Insulin promotes the peripheral utilization of glucose. In the presence of insulin, glucose which enters the cell is oxidized immediately. The rate of utilization depends upon intake of glucose.

iii. By increasing storage of glucose: Glycogenesis

Insulin promotes the rapid conversion of glucose into glycogen (glycogenesis), which is stored in muscle and liver. Thus, glucose is stored in these two organs in the form of glycogen. Insulin activates the enzymes, which are necessary for glycogenesis. In liver, when glycogen content increases beyond its storing capacity, insulin causes conversion of glucose into fatty acids.

iv. By inhibiting of glycogenolysis

Insulin inhibits glycogenolysis, i.e. the breakdown of glycogen into glucose in muscle and liver.

v. By inhibiting of gluconeogenesis

Insulin inhibits gluconeogenesis, i.e. the formation of glucose from proteins.

2. Action on Protein Metabolism

Insulin facilitates the synthesis and storage of proteins, and inhibits the cellular utilization of proteins by:

i. Facilitating the transport of amino acids into cell from blood. Insulin actually, increases the permeability of cell membrane for amino acids.
ii. Accelerating the synthesis of proteins by influencing the transcription of DNA and by increasing the translation of mRNA.
iii. Preventing catabolism of proteins by decreasing the activity of cellular enzymes, which act on proteins.
iv. Preventing conversion of proteins into glucose.

Thus, insulin is responsible for **protein conservation** (**protein sparing effect**) and synthesis and storage (**anabolic effect**) of proteins in the body.

3. Action on Fat Metabolism

Insulin stimulates the synthesis of fat. It also increases the storage of fat in the adipose tissue.

Actions of insulin on fat metabolism are:

i. Synthesis of fatty acids and triglycerides

Insulin promotes the transport of excess glucose into cells, particularly the liver cells. This glucose is utilized for the synthesis of fatty acids and triglycerides. Insulin promotes the synthesis of lipids by activating the enzymes which convert:

a. Glucose into fatty acids.
b. Fatty acids into triglycerides.

ii. Transport of fatty acids into adipose tissue

Insulin facilitates the transport of fatty acids into the adipose tissue.

iii. Storage of fat

Insulin promotes the storage of fat in adipose tissue by inhibiting the enzymes, which degrade the triglycerides.

4. Action on Growth

Along with growth hormone, insulin promotes growth of body by its **anabolic action** on proteins. It enhances the transport of amino acids into the cell and synthesis of proteins in the cells. It also has the **protein sparing effect**, i.e. it causes conservation of proteins by increasing the glucose utilization by the tissues.

■ MODE OF ACTION OF ACTION OF INSULIN

On the target cells, insulin binds with **insulin receptor** and forms insulin-receptor complex. This complex executes the action by activating intracellular enzyme system.

Insulin Receptor

Insulin receptor is a glycoprotein and it is present in almost all the cells of body.

Insulin receptor is formed by four glycoprotein subunits (two α-subunits and two β-subunits). The α-subunits protrude out of the cell and β-subunits protrude inside the cell (**Fig. 53.2**). The α- and β-subunits are linked to each other by disulfide bonds. Intracellular surfaces of α-subunits have the enzyme activity, protein kinase (tyrosine kinase) activity.

When insulin binds with α-subunits of the receptor protein, **tyrosine kinase** at the β-subunit (that protrudes into the cell) is activated by means of **autophosphorylation**.

Activated tyrosine kinase acts on many intracellular enzymes. It activates some of the enzymes and inactivates

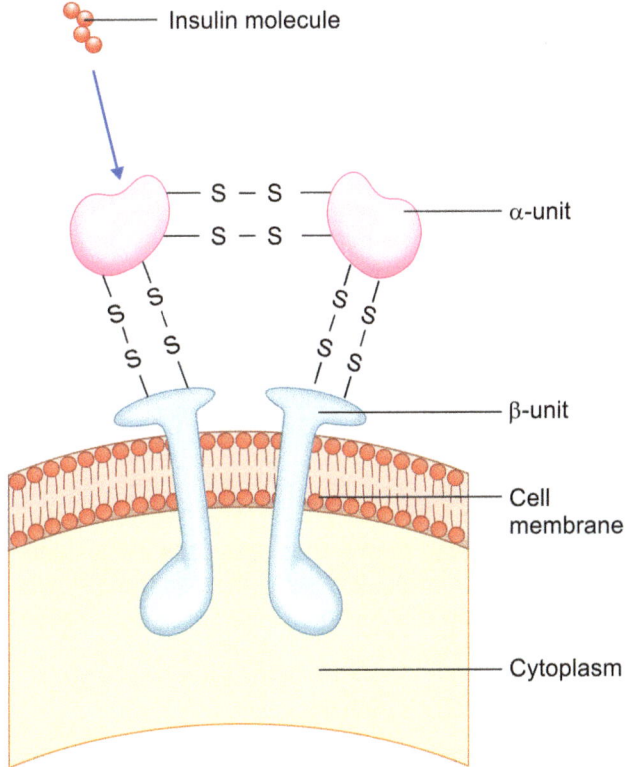

FIGURE 53.2: Diagram showing the structure of insulin receptor. S – S = Disulfide bond.

other enzymes. Thus, insulin action is exerted on the target cells by the activation of some intracellular enzymes and by the inactivation of other enzymes.

REGULATION OF SECRETION OF INSULIN

Insulin secretion is mainly regulated by blood glucose level. In addition, other factors like amino acids, lipid derivatives, gastrointestinal and endocrine hormones, and autonomic nerve fibers also stimulate insulin secretion.

1. Role of Blood Glucose Level

When blood glucose level is normal (80 mg to 100 mg/dL), the rate of insulin secretion is low (up to 10 µU/minute). When blood glucose level increases between 100 mg and 120 mg/dL, the rate of insulin secretion rises rapidly to 100 µU/minute. When the blood glucose level rises above 200 mg/dL, the rate of insulin secretion also rises very rapidly up to 400 µU/minute.

2. Role of Proteins

Excess amino acids in blood also stimulate insulin secretion.

3. Role of Lipid Derivatives

The **β-ketoacids** such as **acetoacetate** also stimulate insulin secretion.

4. Role of Gastrointestinal Hormones

Insulin secretion is increased by some of the gastrointestinal hormones such as gastrin, secretin, cholecystokinin and gastric inhibitory peptide (GIP).

5. Role of Endocrine Hormones

Diabetogenic hormones such as glucagon, growth hormone and cortisol increase the blood sugar level which, in turn stimulate insulin secretion indirectly. Prolonged hypersecretion of these hormones causes exhaustion of β-cells resulting in diabetes mellitus.

6. Role of Autonomic Nerves

Stimulation of parasympathetic nerve to the pancreas (right vagus) increases insulin secretion.

GLUCAGON

SOURCE AND CHEMISTRY OF GLUCAGON

Glucagon is secreted from A cells or **α-cells** in the islets of Langerhans of pancreas. It is also secreted from A cells of stomach and L cells of intestine. Glucagon is a polypeptide with 29 amino acids.

ACTIONS OF GLUCAGON

Actions of glucagon are **antagonistic to insulin** actions. It increases the blood sugar level and peripheral utilization of lipids, and facilitates the conversion of proteins into glucose.

1. Action on Carbohydrate Metabolism

Glucagon increases the blood glucose level by increasing **glycogenolysis** and **gluconeogenesis** in liver and releasing glucose into the blood.

2. Action on Protein Metabolism

Glucagon increases transport of amino acids into liver cells. The amino acids are utilized for gluconeogenesis.

3. Action on Fat Metabolism

Glucagon shows lipolytic and ketogenic actions. It increases lipolysis by increasing the release of free fatty acids from adipose tissue and making them available for peripheral utilization. **Lipolytic activity** of glucagon, in turn promotes **ketogenesis** (formation of ketone bodies) in liver.

4. Other Actions of Glucagon

Glucagon:
i. Inhibits secretion of gastric juice.
ii. Increases secretion of bile from liver.

MODE OF ACTION OF GLUCAGON

On target cells, glucagon causes formation of cyclic AMP which brings out the actions of glucagon.

REGULATION OF SECRETION OF GLUCAGON

Secretion of glucagon is controlled mainly by blood glucose and amino acid levels in the blood.

1. Role of Blood Glucose Level

Important factor that regulates secretion of glucagon is the decrease in blood glucose level. When blood glucose level decreases below 80 mg/dL of blood, α-cells of islets of Langerhans are stimulated and more glucagon is released. Glucagon in turn increases the blood glucose level. On the other hand, when blood sugar level increases, α-cells are inhibited and the secretion of glucagon decreases.

2. Role of Amino Acid Level in Blood

Increase in amino acid level in blood stimulates the secretion of glucagon. Glucagon, in turn converts the amino acids into glucose.

3. Role of Other Factors

Factors which increase glucagon secretion:
i. Exercise.
ii. Stress.
iii. Gastrin.
iv. Cholecystokinin.
v. Cortisol.

Factors which inhibit glucagon secretion:
i. Somatostatin.
ii. Insulin.
iii. Free fatty acids.
iv. Ketones.

SOMATOSTATIN

SOURCE AND CHEMISTRY OF SOMATOSTATIN

Somatostatin is secreted from **D cells (δ-cells)** in islets of Langerhans of pancreas, hypothalamus, and D cells in stomach and upper part of small intestine. Somatostatin is a polypeptide.

ACTIONS OF SOMATOSTATIN

1. Somatostatin acts within islets of Langerhans, and inhibits α- and β-cells, i.e. it inhibits the secretion of both glucagon and insulin.
2. It decreases the motility of stomach, duodenum and gallbladder.
3. Somatostatin reduces the secretion of gastrointestinal hormones gastrin, cholecystokinin, gastric inhibitory peptide and vasoactive intestinal polypeptide.
4. Hypothalamic somatostatin inhibits secretion of GH and TSH from anterior pituitary. That is why, it is also called growth hormone inhibitory hormone (GHIH).

MODE OF ACTION OF SOMATOSTATIN

Somatostatin brings out its actions through cAMP.

REGULATION OF SECRETION OF SOMATOSTATIN

Pancreatic Somatostatin

Secretion of pancreatic somatostatin is stimulated by glucose, amino acids and CCK. Tumor of D cells in islets of Langerhans causes hypersecretion of somatostatin. It leads to hyperglycemia and other symptoms of diabetes mellitus.

Gastrointestinal Tract Somatostatin

Secretion of somatostatin in GI tract is increased by the presence of chyme-containing glucose and proteins in stomach and small intestine.

PANCREATIC POLYPEPTIDE

SOURCE AND CHEMISTRY OF PANCREATIC POLYPEPTIDE

Pancreatic polypeptide is secreted by **F cells** or **PP cells** in the islets of Langerhans of pancreas. It is also found in small intestine. It is a polypeptide with 36 amino acids.

ACTIONS OF PANCREATIC POLYPEPTIDE

Exact physiological action of pancreatic polypeptide is not known. It is believed to increase the secretion of glucagon from α-cells in islets of Langerhans.

MODE OF ACTION OF PANCREATIC POLYPEPTIDE

Pancreatic polypeptide brings out its actions through cAMP.

REGULATION OF SECRETION OF PANCREATIC POLYPEPTIDE

Secretion of pancreatic polypeptide is stimulated by the presence of chyme containing more proteins in small intestine.

REGULATION OF BLOOD SUGAR LEVEL (BLOOD GLUCOSE LEVEL)

NORMAL BLOOD SUGAR LEVEL

In normal persons, blood sugar level is controlled within a narrow range. In early morning after overnight fasting, the **fasting blood sugar** level is low ranging between 70 and 110 mg/dL of blood. Between 1st and 2nd hour after meals **postprandial blood sugar level** rises from 100 to 140 mg/dL. Sugar level in the blood is brought back to normal at the end of 2nd hour after the meals.

Blood sugar-regulating mechanism is operated through liver and muscle by the influence of pancreatic hormones insulin and glucagon. Many other hormones are also involved in the regulation of blood sugar level.

Among all the hormones, insulin is the only hormone that reduces blood sugar level and it is called **antidiabetogenic hormone**. Hormones, which increase blood sugar level are called diabetogenic hormones or **anti-insulin hormones**.

Necessity of Regulation of Blood Glucose Level

Regulation of blood sugar (glucose) level is very essential, because glucose is the only nutrient that is utilized for energy by many tissues such as brain tissues, retina and germinal epithelium of the gonads.

ROLE OF LIVER IN THE MAINTENANCE OF BLOOD SUGAR LEVEL

Liver serves as an important **glucose buffer system**. When blood sugar level increases after a meal, the excess glucose is converted into glycogen and stored in liver. Afterwards, when blood sugar level falls, the glycogen in liver is converted into glucose and released into the blood. Storage of glycogen and release of glucose from liver are mainly regulated by insulin and glucagon.

ROLE OF INSULIN IN THE MAINTENANCE OF BLOOD SUGAR LEVEL

Insulin decreases blood sugar level and it is the only antidiabetic hormone available in the body. Refer the actions on insulin on carbohydrate metabolism in this Chapter.

ROLE OF GLUCAGON IN THE MAINTENANCE OF BLOOD SUGAR LEVEL

Glucagon increases the blood sugar level. Refer actions of glucagon on carbohydrate metabolism in this Chapter.

ROLE OF OTHER HORMONES IN THE MAINTENANCE OF BLOOD SUGAR LEVEL

Other hormones which increase the blood sugar level are:

1. Growth hormone (Chapter 50).
2. Thyroxine (Chapter 51).
3. Cortisol (Chapter 54).
4. Adrenaline (Chapter 55).

Thus, liver helps to maintain the blood sugar level by storing glycogen, when blood glucose level is high after meals; and by releasing glucose, when blood sugar level is low after 2 to 3 hours of food intake. Insulin helps to control blood sugar level, especially after meals. Glucagon and other hormones help to maintain the blood sugar level by raising it in between the meals.

APPLIED PHYSIOLOGY: DISORDERS OF PANCREAS

HYPOACTIVITY: DIABETES MELLITUS

Diabetes mellitus is a metabolic disorder characterized by high blood sugar (glucose) level associated with other manifestations. In most of the cases, the diabetes mellitus develops due to the **deficiency of insulin**.

Classification of Diabetes Mellitus

Diabetes mellitus is of two types, type I and type II. Differences between the two types are given in **Table 53.1**.

Type I Diabetes Mellitus

Type I diabetes mellitus is due to the deficiency of **insulin**. So, it is also called **insulin dependent diabetes mellitus (IDDM)**. Type I diabetes mellitus may occur at any age of life. But, it usually occurs before 40 years of age. When it occurs at infancy (due to congenital disorder) or in childhood, it is called **juvenile diabetes**.

Causes of type I diabetes mellitus

1. Degeneration of β-cells in the islets of Langerhans of pancreas.
2. Destruction of β-cells by viral infection.
3. Congenital disorder of β-cells.
4. Destruction of β-cells during autoimmune diseases.

Other forms of Type I Diabetes Mellitus

1. **Latent autoimmune diabetes in adults (LADA)**: LADA or slow onset diabetes has slow onset and slow progress than IDDM and it occurs in later life after 35 years. It may be difficult to distinguish LADA from type II diabetes mellitus, since pancreas takes longer period to stop secreting insulin.
2. **Maturity onset diabetes in young individuals (MODY)**: It is a rare inherited form of diabetes mellitus that occurs before 25 years. It is due to hereditary defects in insulin secretion.

Type II Diabetes Mellitus

It is due to the absence or deficiency of **insulin receptors**. It usually occurs after 40 years; hence, it is called maturity onset diabetes mellitus. This type of diabetes mellitus is also called **non-insulin-dependent diabetes mellitus (NIDDM)**.

Causes for type II diabetes mellitus

In this type of diabetes, structure and function of β-cells and blood level of insulin are normal. But insulin receptors may be less, absent or abnormal, resulting in insulin resistance.

Common causes of insulin resistance are:

1. Genetic disorders (significant factors causing type II diabetes mellitus).
2. Lifestyle changes such as bad eating habits and physical inactivity, leading to obesity.
3. Stress.

Diabetes Mellitus Associated with Other Endocrine Disorders

Diabetes is very common in some of the endocrine disorders such as gigantism, acromegaly and Cushing's syndrome. Hyperglycemia in these conditions causes excess stimulation of β-cells. Constant and excess stimulation, in turn causes burning out and degeneration of β-cells. The β-cell exhaustion leads to permanent diabetes mellitus. This type of diabetes mellitus is called **secondary diabetes**.

TABLE 53.1: Differences between type I and type II diabetes mellitus.

Features	Type I (IDDM)	Type II (NIDDM)
Age of onset	Usually before 40 years	Usually after 40 years
Major cause	Lack of insulin	Lack of insulin receptor
Insulin deficiency	Yes	Partial deficiency
Immune destruction of β-cells	Yes	No
Involvement of other endocrine disorders	No	Yes
Hereditary cause	Yes	May or may not be
Need for insulin	Always	Not in initial stage. May require in later stage
Insulin resistance	No	Yes
Control by oral hypoglycemic agents	No	Yes
Symptoms appear	Rapidly	Slowly
Body weight	Usually thin	Usually overweight
Stress-induced obesity	No	Yes
Ketosis	Yes	May or may not be

Signs and Symptoms of Diabetes Mellitus

Various manifestations of diabetes mellitus develop because of three major setbacks of insulin deficiency:

1. Increased blood sugar level (300 to 400 mg/dL) due to reduced utilization by tissue.
2. Mobilization of fats from adipose tissue for energy purpose, leading to elevated fatty acid content in blood. This causes deposition of fat on the wall of arteries and development of atherosclerosis.
3. Depletion of proteins from the tissues.

Following are the signs and symptoms of diabetes mellitus:

1. Glucosuria

Loss of glucose in urine is known as glucosuria. Normally glucose does not appear in urine. When glucose level rises above 180 mg/dL in blood, glucose appears in urine. It is the **renal threshold** level for glucose.

2. Osmotic diuresis

Diuresis due to osmotic effects is called **osmotic diuresis**. Excess glucose in the renal tubules develops osmotic effect. Osmotic effect decreases the reabsorption of water from renal tubules resulting in diuresis. It leads to polyuria and polydipsia.

3. Polyuria

Excess urine formation with increase in frequency of voiding urine is called polyuria. It is due to the osmotic diuresis caused by increase in blood sugar level.

4. Polydipsia

Polydipsia is the increase in water intake. Excess loss of water decreases water content and increases salt content in the body. This stimulates the thirst center in hypothalamus. Thirst center in turn induces water intake.

5. Polyphagia

Polyphagia means the intake of excess food. It is very common in diabetes mellitus.

6. Asthenia

Asthenia is the loss of strength. Body becomes very weak. There is loss of energy. Asthenia is because of **protein depletion** which is caused by lack of insulin.

7. Acidosis

During insulin deficiency, glucose cannot be utilized by the peripheral tissues for energy. So, a large amount of fat is broken down to release energy. It causes the formation of **excess ketoacids** leading to **acidosis**.

8. Acetone breathing

In cases of severe ketoacidosis, acetone is expired in the expiratory air, giving the characteristic **acetone breath odor** or **fruity breath odor**. It is a life-threatening condition of severe diabetes.

9. Kussmaul breathing

Kussmaul breathing is the increase in rate and depth of respiration caused by severe acidosis.

10. Circulatory shock

Osmotic diuresis leads to dehydration, which causes circulatory shock. It occurs only in severe diabetes.

11. Coma

Due to Kussmaul breathing, large amount of carbon dioxide is lost during expiration. It leads to drastic reduction in the concentration of bicarbonate ions causing severe acidosis and coma. It occurs in severe cases of diabetes mellitus.

Increase in blood sugar level develops hyperosmolarity of plasma which also leads to coma. It is called **hyperosmolar coma**.

Complications of Diabetes Mellitus

Prolonged hyperglycemia in diabetes mellitus causes dysfunction and injury of many tissues resulting in some complications such as:

1. Cardiovascular complications such as **hypertension** and **myocardial infarction**.
2. Degenerative changes in retina called **diabetic retinopathy**.
3. Degenerative changes in kidney known as **diabetic nephropathy**.
4. Degeneration of autonomic and peripheral nerves called **diabetic neuropathy**.

Diagnostic Tests for Diabetes Mellitus

Diagnosis of diabetes mellitus includes the determination of:

1. Fasting blood sugar.
2. Postprandial blood sugar.
3. Glucose tolerance test (GTT).
4. Hemoglobin A1c (HbA1c) or Glycosylated (glycated) hemoglobin test.

Determination of HbA1c is commonly done to monitor the glycemic control of the persons already diagnosed with diabetes mellitus.

■ HYPERACTIVITY: HYPERINSULINISM

Hyperinsulinism is the hypersecretion of insulin.

Cause of Hyperinsulinism

Hyperinsulinism occurs due to the tumor of β-cells in the islets of Langerhans.

Signs and Symptoms of Hyperinsulinism

1. Hypoglycemia

Blood sugar level falls below 50 mg/dL.

2. Manifestations of central nervous system

Manifestations of central nervous system occur when the blood sugar level decreases. All the manifestations are together called **neuroglycopenic symptoms**.

Initially, the activity of neurons increases resulting in nervousness, tremor all over the body and sweating. If not treated immediately, it leads to clonic convulsions and unconsciousness. Slowly, the convulsions cease and coma occurs due to damage of neurons.

Chapter 54: Adrenal Cortex

CHAPTER OUTLINE

- IMPORTANCE OF ADRENAL GLANDS
- FUNCTIONAL ANATOMY OF ADRENAL GLANDS
- FUNCTIONAL HISTOLGY OF ADRENAL CORTEX
- HORMONES SECRETED BY ADRENAL CORTEX
- MINERALOCORTICOIDS
- GLUCOCORTICOIDS
- ADRENAL SEX HORMONES
- APPLIED PHYSIOLOGY: DISORDERS OF ADRENAL CORTEX

IMPORTANCE OF ADRENAL GLANDS

Adrenal glands are called the **life-saving glands** or **essential endocrine glands.** It is because the absence of adrenocortical hormones causes death within a week and absence of adrenomedullary hormones, drastically decreases the resistance to mental and physical stress.

FUNCTIONAL ANATOMY OF ADRENAL GLANDS

There are two adrenal glands. Each gland is situated on the upper pole of each kidney. Because of their situation, adrenal glands are otherwise called **suprarenal glands**.

PARTS OF ADRENAL GLAND

Adrenal gland **(Fig. 54.1)** is made of two distinct parts:

1. Adrenal cortex: Outer portion, constituting 80% of the gland.
2. Adrenal medulla: Central portion, constituting 20% of the gland.

Each part of the gland is different from other one in development, structure and functions.

FUNCTIONAL HISTOLOGY OF ADRENAL CORTEX

Adrenal cortex is formed by three distinct layers of structures:

1. **Zona glomerulosa** or outer layer.
2. **Zona fasciculata** or middle layer.
3. **Zona reticularis** or inner layer.

HORMONES SECRETED BY ADRENAL CORTEX

Hormones secreted by adrenal cortex are collectively known as **adrenocortical hormones** or **corticosteroids**. Based on their functions, the corticosteroids are classified into three groups:

I. Mineralocorticoids.
II. Glucocorticoids.
III. Sex hormones.

MINERALOCORTICOIDS

Mineralocorticoids are the corticosteroids which act on minerals (electrolytes), particularly sodium and potassium. Mineralocorticoids are secreted by zona glomerulosa of adrenal cortex **(Table 54.1)**.

Mineralocorticoids are:

1. Aldosterone.
2. 11-deoxycorticosterone.

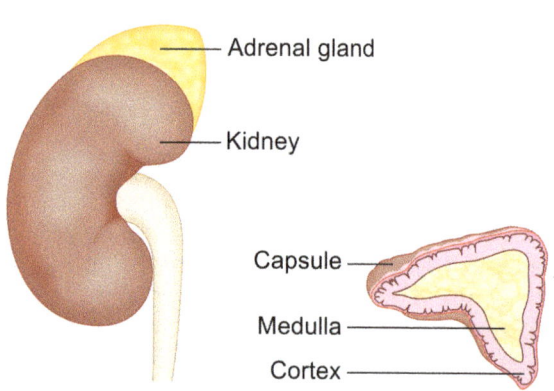

FIGURE 54.1: Adrenal gland.

TABLE 54.1: Hormones secreted by different layers of adrenal cortex.

Layer	Hormones
Zona glomerulosa	Mineralocorticoids 1. Aldosterone 2. 11-deoxycorticosterone
Zona fasciculata	Glucocorticoids 1. Cortisol 2. Corticosterone 3. Cortisone Small quantity of sex hormones
Zona reticularis	Sex hormones 1. Dehydroepiandrosterone 2. Androstenedione 3. Testosterone 4. Estrogen 5. Progesterone Small quantity of glucocorticoids

Mineralocorticoids are C_{21} steroids having 21 carbon atoms. Plasma level of aldosterone and 11-deoxycorticosterone is 0.006 μg/dL.

■ FUNCTIONS OF MINERALOCORTICOIDS

Ninety percent of mineralocorticoid activity is provided by aldosterone.

Life-saving Hormone

Aldosterone is very essential for life and it is usually called **life-saving hormone**, because the absence of this hormone causes death within a week. It is mainly because of loss of mineralocorticoids which are essential to maintain the osmolarity and volume of ECF. Actions of aldosterone are explained below.

1. Action on Sodium Ions

Aldosterone increases reabsorption of sodium from distal convoluted tubule and collecting duct in the kidney. Aldosterone helps conservation of sodium in the body.

2. Action on Extracellular Fluid Volume

When sodium ions are reabsorbed from the renal tubules, almost an equal amount of water is also reabsorbed. So, the net result is increase in ECF volume.

Even though aldosterone increases the sodium reabsorption from renal tubules, concentration of sodium in the body does not increase very much because of simultaneous reabsorption of water.

But still, there is possibility for mild increase in concentration of sodium in the blood (**mild hypernatremia**). It induces thirst, leading to intake of water which again increases the ECF volume and blood volume.

3. Action on Blood Pressure

Increase in ECF volume and blood volume finally leads to increase in blood pressure.

Aldosterone escape or escape phenomenon

Aldosterone escape means escape of the kidney from **salt-retaining effect** of excess of aldosterone as in the case of primary hyperaldosteronism.

Mechanism of aldosterone escape

When aldosterone level increases, there is excess retention of sodium and water. This increases the ECF volume and blood pressure.

Aldosterone-induced high blood pressure decreases the ECF volume through two types of reactions:

i. It stimulates secretion of **atrial natriuretic peptide (ANP)** from atrial muscles of the heart. ANP causes excretion of sodium in spite of increase in aldosterone secretion.

ii. It causes **pressure diuresis** (excretion of excess salt and water by high blood pressure) through urine. This decreases the salt and water content in ECF in spite of hypersecretion of aldosterone (**Fig. 54.2**).

Significance of aldosterone escape

Because of aldosterone escape, edema does not occur in primary hyperaldosteronism.

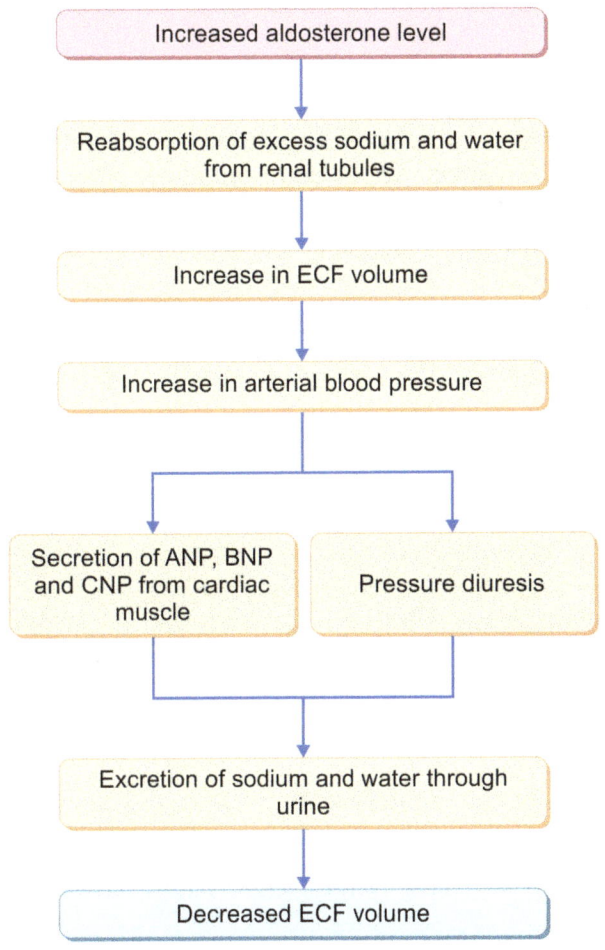

FIGURE 54.2: Aldosterone escape.
ANP = Atrial natriuretic peptide, BNP = Brain natriuretic peptide, CNP = C-type natriuretic peptide, ECF = Extracellular fluid.

4. Action on Potassium Ions

Aldosterone increases the potassium excretion through renal tubules.

5. Action on Hydrogen Ion Concentration

While increasing the sodium reabsorption from the renal tubules, aldosterone causes tubular secretion of hydrogen ions which is essential to maintain acid-base balance in the body.

6. Action on Sweat Glands and Salivary Glands

Aldosterone has almost similar effect on sweat glands and salivary glands as it shows on renal tubules. Sodium is reabsorbed from sweat glands under the influence of aldosterone, thus loss of sodium from the body is prevented. Same effect is shown on saliva also.

7. Action on Intestine

Aldosterone increases sodium absorption from the intestine, especially in colon and prevents loss of sodium through feces.

MODE OF ACTION OF MINERALOCORTICOIDS

Mineralocorticoids act through the messenger RNA mechanism.

REGULATION OF SECRETION OF MINERALOCORTICOIDS

Aldosterone secretion is regulated by four important factors **(Fig. 54.3)**. Factors stimulating secretion of aldosterone are given below in the order of their potency:

1. Increase in potassium ion concentration in ECF.
2. Decrease in sodium ion concentration in ECF.
3. Decrease in ECF volume.
4. Adrenocorticotropic hormone.

Increase in the concentration of potassium ions is the most effective stimulant for aldosterone secretion. It acts directly on the zona glomerulosa and increases the secretion of aldosterone. Decrease in sodium ion concentration and ECF volume stimulates aldosterone secretion through rennin-angiotensin mechanism.

Renin secreted from juxtaglomerular apparatus of kidney acts on angiotensinogen in the plasma and converts it into angiotensin I, which is converted into angiotensin II by converting enzyme (ACE) secreted by lungs. Angiotensin II acts on the zona glomerulosa to secrete more aldosterone. Aldosterone in turn, increases the retention of sodium and water and excretion of potassium leading to increase in the sodium ion concentration and ECF volume.

Now, increased sodium ion concentration and the ECF volume inhibit juxtaglomerular apparatus and stop the release of renin. So, angiotensin II is not formed and release of aldosterone from adrenal cortex is stopped.

Adrenocorticotropic hormone mainly stimulates the secretion of glucocorticoids. It has only a mild stimulating effect on aldosterone secretion.

GLUCOCORTICOIDS

Glucocorticoids are the corticosteroids which act mainly on glucose metabolism. Glucocorticoids are secreted mainly by zona fasciculata of adrenal cortex. A small quantity of glucocorticoids is also secreted by zona reticularis.

Glucocorticoids are:

1. Cortisol.
2. Corticosterone.
3. Cortisone.

Glucocorticoids are having 21 carbon atoms. Plasma level of cortisol is 13.9 µg/dL and that of corticosterone is 0.4 µg/dL.

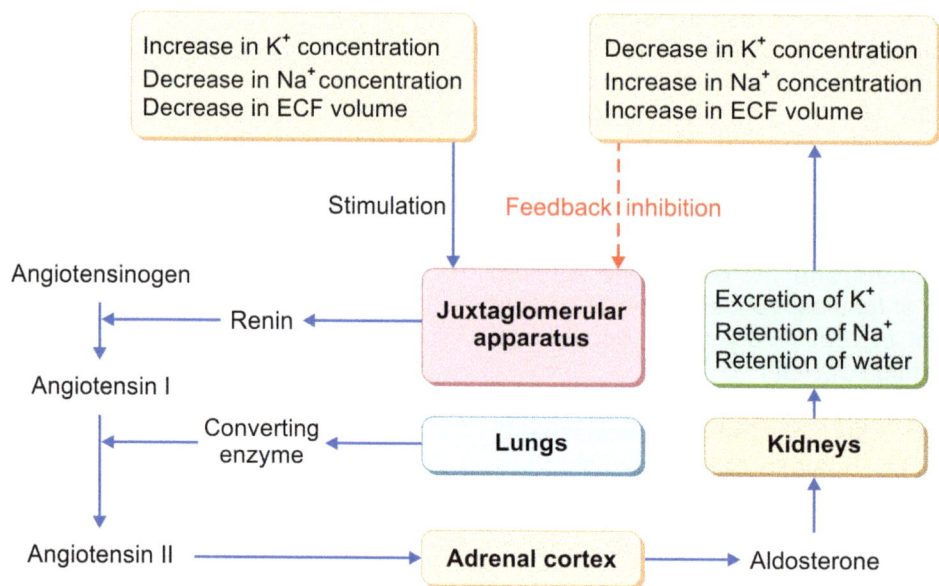

FIGURE 54.3: Regulation of aldosterone secretion.

FUNCTIONS OF GLUCOCORTICOIDS

Cortisol is more potent and it has 95% of glucocorticoid activity. Corticosterone is less potent showing only 4% of glucocorticoid activity. Cortisone with 1% activity is secreted in minute quantity.

Life-protecting Hormone

Like aldosterone, cortisol is also essential for life, but in a different way. Aldosterone is a life-saving hormone, whereas cortisol is a life protecting hormone, because it helps to withstand the stress and trauma in life.

Glucocorticoids have metabolic effects on carbohydrates, proteins, fats and water. These hormones also show mild mineralocorticoid effect.

1. Action on Carbohydrate Metabolism

Glucocorticoids increase the blood glucose level by two ways:

i. By promoting gluconeogenesis in liver from amino acids.
ii. By inhibiting glucose uptake and utilization by peripheral cells.

2. Action on Protein Metabolism

Glucocorticoids promote catabolism of proteins leading to decrease in cellular proteins, and increase in plasma amino acids and protein content in liver by the following methods:

i. Glucocorticoids decrease the protein in body cells, except liver cells by accelerating protein catabolism and release of amino acids from the tissues.
ii. Glucocorticoids increase the transport of amino acids into hepatic cells. In hepatic cells, the amino acids are used for synthesis of proteins, plasma proteins and for gluconeogenesis.

Thus, glucocorticoids cause mobilization of proteins from tissues other than liver.

3. Action on Fat Metabolism

Glucocorticoids cause mobilization and redistribution of fats.

Actions on fats are:

i. Mobilization of fatty acids from adipose tissue.
ii. Increasing the concentration of fatty acids in blood.
iii. Increasing the utilization of fat for energy.

By increasing the utilization of fats for energy release, glucocorticoids cause the formation of a large amount of ketone bodies. It is called ketogenic effect of glucocorticoids.

4. Action on Water Metabolism

Glucocorticoids accelerate the excretion of water and play important role in the maintenance of water balance.

5. Action on Mineral Metabolism

Glucocorticoids enhance the retention of sodium and to lesser extent, increase the excretion of potassium. Glucocorticoids decrease blood calcium by inhibiting absorption of calcium from intestine and increasing the excretion of calcium through urine.

6. Action on Bone

Glucocorticoids stimulate osteoclastic activity (bone resorption) and inhibit osteoblastic activity (bone formation and mineralization).

7. Action on Muscles

Glucocorticoids cause catabolism of proteins from muscle.

8. Action Blood Cells

Glucocorticoids decrease the number of circulating eosinophils by increasing the destruction of eosinophils in reticuloendothelial cells. These hormones also decrease the number of basophils and lymphocytes, and increase the number of circulating neutrophils, RBCs and platelets.

9. Action on Vascular Response

Presence of glucocorticoids is essential for the constrictor action of catecholamines (adrenaline and noradrenaline). In adrenal insufficiency, the blood vessels fail to respond to adrenaline and noradrenaline leading to vascular collapse.

10. Action on Central Nervous System

Glucocorticoids are essential for normal functioning of nervous system. Insufficiency of these hormones causes personality changes like irritability and lack of concentration.

11. Permissive Action of Glucocorticoids

Permissive action of glucocorticoids is the execution of actions of some hormones only in the presence of glucocorticoids.

Examples are:

i. Calorigenic effects of glucagon.
ii. Lipolytic effects of catecholamines.
iii. Pressor effects of catecholamines.
iv. Bronchodilator effect of catecholamines.

12. Action on Resistance to Stress

Exposure to any type of stress, either physical or mental, increases the secretion of adrenocorticotropic hormone (ACTH). ACTH in turn increases glucocorticoid secretion. Increase in glucocorticoid level is very essential for survival, as it offers high resistance to body against stress.

Glucocorticoids enhance the resistance by the following ways:

i. Immediate release and transport of amino acids from tissues to liver cells for synthesis of new proteins and other substances which are essential to withstand the stress.
ii. Release of fatty acids from cells for production of more energy during stress.
iii. Enhancement of vascular reactivity to catecholamines and fatty acid mobilizing action of catecholamines, which are necessary to withstand the stress.

iv. Prevention of severity of other changes in the body caused by stress.

13. Anti-inflammatory Effects

Inflammation is defined as a localized protective response induced by injury or destruction of tissues. When tissue is injured by mechanical or chemical factors, some substances are released from the affected area, which produce series of changes in the affected area.

Glucocorticoids prevent the inflammatory changes in injured or infected tissues by:

i. Inhibiting the release of proteolytic enzymes responsible for inflammation.
ii. Preventing rush of blood to the injured area by enhancing vasoconstrictor action of catecholamines.
iii. Inhibiting migration of leukocytes into the affected area.
iv. Preventing loss of fluid from plasma into the affected tissue by decreasing the permeability of capillaries.
v. Reducing the reactions of tissues by suppressing T cells and other leukocytes.

In addition to preventing inflammatory reactions, if inflammation has already started, the glucocorticoids cause an early resolution of inflammation and rapid healing.

14. Antiallergic Actions

Corticosteroids prevent the various reactions in allergic conditions as in the case of inflammation.

15. Immunosuppressive Action

Glucocorticoids suppress the immune system of body by decreasing the number of circulating T lymphocytes. It is done by suppressing lymphoid tissues (lymph nodes and thymus) and proliferation of T cells. Glucocorticoids also prevent release of interleukin-2 by T cells.

Thus, hypersecretion or excess use of glucocorticoids decreases the immune reactions against all foreign bodies entering the body. It leads to severe infection causing death.

Immunological reactions, which are common during organ transplantation, may cause rejection of the transplanted tissues. So, glucocorticoids are administered to suppress the immunological reactions, because of their immunosuppressive action.

■ MODE OF ACTION OF GLUCOCORTICOIDS

Glucocorticoids act through the messenger RNA mechanism.

■ REGULATION OF SECRETION OF GLUCOCORTICOIDS

Anterior pituitary regulates glucocorticoid secretion by secreting adrenocorticotropic hormone (ACTH).

ACTH secretion is in turn regulated by hypothalamus through corticotropin releasing factor (CRF).

Role of Anterior Pituitary: ACTH

Anterior pituitary controls the activities of adrenal cortex by secreting ACTH. ACTH is secreted by the basophilic chromophilic cells of anterior pituitary. It is a single chained polypeptide with 39 amino acids. Its concentration in plasma is 3 ng/dL.

ACTH is mainly concerned with regulation of cortisol secretion. It plays only a minor role in the regulation of mineralocorticoid secretion.

Actions of ACTH

ACTH is necessary for structural integrity and the secretory activity of adrenal cortex. It has other functions also.

Adrenal actions of ACTH on adrenal cortex

1. Maintenance of structural integrity, and vascularization of zona fasciculata and zona reticularis of adrenal cortex. In hypophysectomy, these two layers in the adrenal cortex are atrophied.
2. Conversion of cholesterol into pregnenolone, which is the precursor of glucocorticoids. Thus, adrenocorticotropic hormone is responsible for synthesis of glucocorticoids.
3. Release of glucocorticoids.
4. Prolongation of glucocorticoid action on various cells.

Other (nonadrenal) actions of ACTH

1. Mobilization of fats from tissues.
2. Melanocyte stimulating effect. Because of structural similarity with **melanocyte stimulating hormone**, ACTH shows melanocyte stimulating effect. It causes darkening of skin by acting on melanophores which are the cutaneous pigment cells containing melanin.

Mode of action of ACTH

ACTH acts by the formation of cyclic AMP.

Role of Hypothalamus

Hypothalamus also plays an important role in the regulation of cortisol secretion by controlling the ACTH secretion through corticotropin releasing factor (CRF). It is also called corticotropin releasing hormone. CRF reaches the anterior pituitary through the hypothalamo-hypophyseal portal vessels.

CRF stimulates the corticotrophs of anterior pituitary and causes synthesis and release of ACTH.

CRF secretion is induced by several factors such as emotion, stress, trauma and circadian rhythm. CRF in turn, causes release of ACTH, which induces glucocorticoid secretion.

Feedback Control

Cortisol regulates its own secretion through negative feedback control by inhibiting the release of CRF from hypothalamus and ACTH from anterior pituitary **(Fig. 54.4)**.

■ ADRENAL SEX HORMONES

Adrenal sex hormones are secreted mainly by zona reticularis. Zona fasciculata secretes small quantities of sex hormones. Most of the hormones are **androgens** (male sex hormones) androgens. But small quantity of estrogen and progesterone are also secreted by adrenal cortex.

Chapter 54: Adrenal Cortex **271**

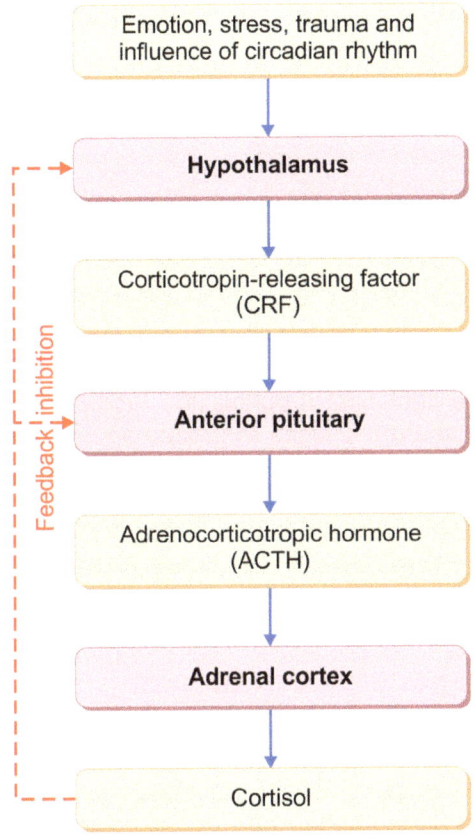

FIGURE 54.4: Regulation of cortisol secretion.

Androgens secreted by adrenal cortex are:

1. Dehydroepiandrosterone.
2. Androstenedione.
3. Testosterone.

Dehydroepiandrosterone is the most active adrenal androgen.

Androgens, in general, are responsible for masculine features of the body (Chapter 58). But in normal conditions, the adrenal androgens have insignificant physiological effects, because of the low amount of secretion both in males and females.

In congenital **hyperplasia of adrenal cortex** or tumor of zona reticularis, an excess quantity of androgens is secreted. In males, it does not produce any special effect, because large quantity of androgens is produced by testes also. But in females, adrenal androgens produce masculine features. Some of the androgens are converted into testosterone. Testosterone is responsible for the androgenic activity in adrenogenital syndrome or congenital adrenal hyperplasia.

■ **APPLIED PHYSIOLOGY: DISORDERS OF ADRENAL CORTEX**

■ **HYPERACTIVITY OF ADRENAL CORTEX**

Hypersecretion of adrenocortical hormones leads to the following conditions:

1. Cushing's syndrome.
2. Hyperaldosteronism.
3. Adrenogenital syndrome.

■ **1. CUSHING'S SYNDROME**

Cushing's syndrome is a disorder characterized by obesity **(Fig. 54.5)**.

Causes of Cushing's Syndrome

Cushing's syndrome is due to the hypersecretion of glucocorticoids, particularly cortisol. It may be either due to pituitary origin or adrenal origin.

If it is due to pituitary origin, it is known as **Cushing's disease**. If it is due to adrenal origin, it is called **Cushing's syndrome**. Generally, these two terms are used interchangeably.

Cushing's disease by pituitary origin

Increased secretion of ACTH causes hyperplasia of adrenal cortex leading to hypersecretion of cortisol.

Cushing's syndrome by adrenal origin

Cortisol secretion is increased by:

i. Tumor or carcinoma in zona fasciculata of adrenal cortex.
ii. Prolonged treatment with exogenous glucocorticoids.
iii. Prolonged treatment with high dose of ACTH.

Signs and Symptoms of Cushing's Syndrome

Signs and symptoms developed during Cushing's syndrome are listed in **Box 54.1**.

Tests for Cushing's Syndrome

i. Observation of external features.
ii. Determination of blood sugar and cortisol levels.
iii. Analysis of urine for 17-hydroxysteroids.

■ **2. HYPERALDOSTERONISM**

Increased secretion of aldosterone is called hyperaldosteronism.

Types and Causes of Hyperaldosteronism

Depending upon the causes, hyperaldosteronism is classified into two types:

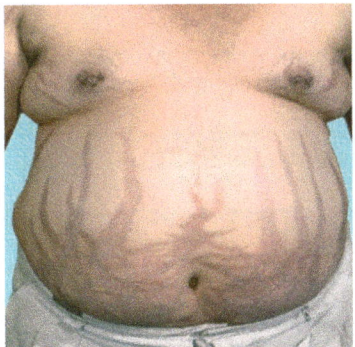

Pot belly with purple striae

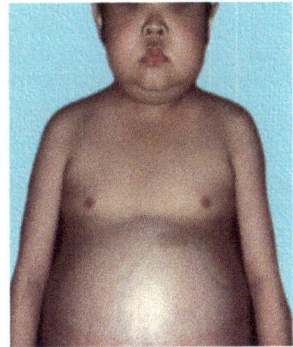

Fat deposition in upper abdomen, thorax and face (moon face) with thin hands

FIGURE 54.5: Cushing's syndrome.
(*Courtesy: Prof Mafauzy Mohamed*)

BOX 54.1: Signs and symptoms of Cushing's syndrome.

1. Abnormal features due to disproportionate distribution of fat

a. Moon face: Edematous facial appearance due to accumulation of fat and retention of water and salt
b. Torso: Fat accumulation in the chest and abdomen. Torso means trunk.
c. Buffalo hump: Fat deposit on the back of neck and shoulder
d. Pot belly: Fat accumulation in upper abdomen

2. Purple striae

Reddish purple stripes on abdomen due to:
a. Stretching of abdominal wall by excess subcutaneous fat
b. Rupture of subdermal tissues due to stretching
c. Deficiency of collagen fibers due to protein depletion

3. Thinning of extremities

Due to protein depletion

4. Thinning of skin and subcutaneous tissue

Due to protein depletion

5. Acanthosis

Skin disease characterized by dark patches in axilla, neck and groin

6. Pigmentation of skin

Due to melanocyte-stimulating effect of ACTH

7. Facial plethora

Redness of face

8. Hirsutism

Heavy growth of hair on body and face

9. Weakening of muscles

Because of protein depletion

10. Susceptibility of bone for fracture

Due to bone resorption and osteoporosis

11. Hyperglycemia and glucosuria

Due to gluconeogenesis and inhibition of peripheral utilization of glucose
In severe conditions adrenal diabetes develops

12. Hypertension

Caused by mineralocorticoid effects of glucocorticoids:
Retention of sodium and water resulting in increase in ECF volume and blood volume

13. Susceptibility for infection

Due to immunosuppression

14. Poor wound healing

Prevention of wound healing due to hypersecretion of cortisol

---

i. **Primary hyperaldosteronism** which occurs due to tumor in zona glomerulosa of adrenal cortex. It is otherwise known as **Conn's syndrome**. It develops due to tumor in zona glomerulosa of adrenal cortex. In primary hyperaldosteronism, edema does not occur because of escape phenomenon.

ii. **Secondary hyperaldosteronism** which occurs due to extra adrenal causes such as:
   a. Congestive cardiac failure.
   b. Nephrosis.
   c. Toxemia of pregnancy.
   d. Cirrhosis of liver.

Signs and Symptoms of Hyperaldosteronism

i. Increase in ECF volume and blood volume.
ii. Hypertension due to increase in ECF volume and blood volume.
iii. Severe depletion of potassium. Prolonged **depletion of potassium** causes renal damage. Kidneys fail to produce concentrated urine. It leads to polyuria and polydipsia.
iv. Muscular weakness due to potassium depletion.
v. Metabolic alkalosis due to secretion of large amount of hydrogen ions into renal tubules. Metabolic alkalosis reduces blood calcium level causing tetany.

■ 3. ADRENOGENITAL SYNDROME

Adrenogenital syndrome is a group of diseases caused by secretion of abnormal quantities of adrenal androgens.

Under normal conditions, adrenal cortex secretes small quantities of androgens which do not have any significant effect on sex organs or sexual function. However, secretion of abnormal quantities of adrenal androgens develops adrenogenital syndrome.

Causes of Adrenogenital Syndrome

It is due to the tumor of zona reticularis in adrenal cortex.

Symptoms of Adrenogenital Syndrome

Adrenogenital syndrome is characterized by the tendency for the development of secondary sexual character of opposite sex.

In females, increased secretion of androgens causes development of male secondary sexual characters. The condition is called adrenal **virilism**.

In males, the tumor of estrogen-secreting cells produces more than normal quantity of estrogens resulting in symptoms such as **feminization**, **gynecomastia** (enlargement of breast) and **atrophy of testes**.

■ HYPOACTIVITY OF ADRENAL CORTEX

Hyposecretion of adrenocortical hormones leads to the following conditions:
1. Addison's disease or chronic adrenal insufficiency.
2. Congenital adrenal hyperplasia.

■ 1. ADDISON'S DISEASE OR CHRONIC ADRENAL INSUFFICIENCY

Addison's disease is an endocrine disorder caused by failure of adrenal cortex to secrete corticosteroids **(Box 54.2)**.

BOX 54.2: Disorders of adrenal cortex.

During hyperactivity
1. Cushing's syndrome
2. Hyperaldosteronism
3. Adrenogenital syndrome

During hypoactivity
1. Addison's disease
2. Congenital adrenal hyperplasia
   In boys: Macro-genitosomia praecox
   In girls: Virilism or Pseudohermaphroditism

Types of Addison's Disease

Addison's disease is classified into three types:
  i. Primary Addison's disease that occurs due to adrenal cause.
  ii. Secondary Addison's disease which is due to failure of anterior pituitary to secrete ACTH.
  iii. Tertiary Addison's disease which is due to failure of hypothalamus to secrete CRF.

Causes for Primary Addison's Disease

  i. Atrophy or destruction of adrenal cortex.
  ii. Malignancy of adrenal cortex.
  iii. Congenital failure to secrete cortisol.
  iv. Adrenalectomy and failure to take hormone therapy.

Signs and Symptoms

Signs and symptoms develop in Addison's disease because of deficiency of both cortisol and aldosterone.

Common signs and symptoms are:
  i. Pigmentation of skin and mucous membrane.
  ii. Muscular weakness.
  iii. Dehydration with loss of sodium.
  iv. Hypotension.
  v. Decrease in size of the heart.
  vi. Hypoglycemia.
  vii. Nausea, vomiting and diarrhea.
  viii. Loss of body weight.
  ix. Susceptibility to any type of infection.
  x. Inability to withstand any stress resulting in Addisonian crisis (see below).

Addisonian Crisis or Adrenal Crisis or Acute Adrenal Insufficiency

It is a common symptom of Addison's disease characterized by sudden collapse associated with an increase in need for large quantities of glucocorticoids. The condition becomes fatal, if not treated in time.

Causes of Addisonian Crisis

  i. Exposure to even mild stress.
  ii. Hypoglycemia due to fasting.
  iii. Trauma.
  iv. Surgical operation.
  v. Sudden withdrawal of glucocorticoid treatment.

■ 2. CONGENITAL ADRENAL HYPERPLASIA

It is a congenital disorder characterized by increase in size of adrenal cortex. Size increases due to abnormal increase in the number of steroid-secreting cortical cells resulting in hypersecretion of adrenal androgens.

Causes of Congenital Adrenal Hyperplasia

Even though the size of the gland increases, cortisol secretion decreases. It is because of congenital deficiency of enzymes necessary for the synthesis of cortisol, particularly the enzyme called 21-hydroxylases.

Lack of this enzyme reduces the synthesis of cortisol. It in turn, increases the secretion of ACTH from pituitary by feedback mechanism. ACTH stimulates the adrenal cortex causing hyperplasia with the accumulation of lipid droplets. Cortisol cannot be synthesized because of lack of 21-hydroxylase. Therefore, due to the constant simulation of adrenal cortex by ACTH, the secretion of androgens increases. It results in sexual abnormalities such as virilism.

Symptoms of Congenital Adrenal Hyperplasia

Characteristic features of adrenal hyperplasia are virilism and excess body growth.

In boys

Adrenal hyperplasia produces a condition known as **macrogenitosomia praecox (Fig. 54.6)**.

Features of this condition are:
  i. Precocious body growth, causing stocky appearance called **infant Hercules**.
  ii. Precocious sexual development with enlarged penis even at age of 4 years.

In girls

In girls, adrenal hyperplasia produces **masculinization**. It is otherwise called **virilism**. In some cases of genetic disorders, the female child is born with external genitalia of male type. This condition is called **pseudohermaphroditism**.

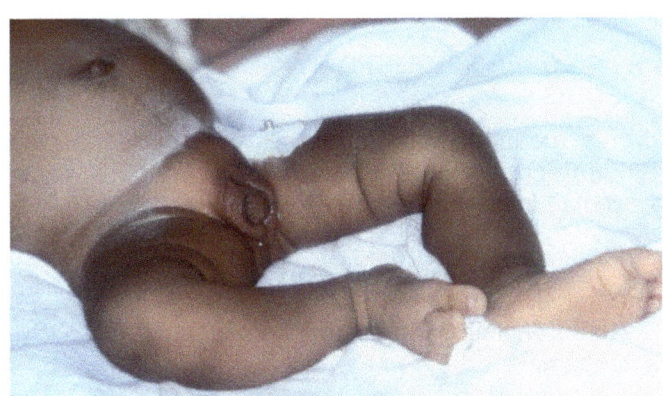

FIGURE 54.6: Congenital adrenal hyperplasia (macrogenitosomia praecox).
(*Courtesy:* Prof Mafauzy Mohamed).

Chapter 55: Adrenal Medulla

CHAPTER OUTLINE

- FUNCTIONAL HISTOLOGY OF ADRENAL MEDULLA
- HORMONES SECRETED BY ADRENAL MEDULLA
- PLASMA LEVEL OF CATECHOLAMINES
- SYNTHESIS OF CATECHOLAMINES
- METABOLISM OF CATECHOLAMINES
- ACTIONS OF ADRENALINE AND NORADRENALINE
- REGULATION OF SECRETION OF ADRENALINE AND NORADRENALINE
- DOPAMINE
- APPLIED PHYSIOLOGY: PHEOCHROMOCYTOMA

■ FUNCTIONAL HISTOLOGY OF ADRENAL MEDULLA

Medulla is the inner part of adrenal gland and it forms 20% of mass of adrenal gland.

Adrenal medulla is made up of interlacing cords of cells known as **chromaffin cells** or **pheochrome cells**. These cells contain fine granules which are stained brown by potassium dichromate.

Types of Chromaffin Cells in Adrenal Medulla

Chromaffin cells present adrenal medulla are of two types:

1. Adrenaline secreting cells (90%).
2. Noradrenaline secreting cells (10%).

■ HORMONES SECRETED BY ADRENAL MEDULLA

Adrenal medullary hormones are the amines derived from catechol and so these hormones are called catecholamines.

Catecholamines Secreted by Adrenal Medulla

1. Adrenaline or epinephrine.
2. Noradrenaline or norepinephrine.
3. Dopamine.

■ PLASMA LEVEL OF CATECHOLAMINES

1. Adrenaline : 3 µg/dL
2. Noradrenaline : 30 µg/dL
3. Dopamine : 3.5 µg/dL

■ SYNTHESIS OF CATECHOLAMINES

Catecholamines are synthesized from amino acid **tyrosine** in the chromaffin cells of adrenal medulla. First dopamine is synthesized. Then noradrenaline is derived from dopamine. And finally, adrenaline is derived from noradrenaline (Fig. 55.1).

Stages of Synthesis of Catecholamines

1. Formation of tyrosine from phenylalanine in the presence of enzyme **phenylalanine hydroxylase**.
2. Uptake of tyrosine from blood into the chromaffin cells of adrenal medulla by active transport.
3. Conversion of tyrosine into **dihydroxyphenylalanine (DOPA)** by hydroxylation in the presence of **tyrosine hydroxylase**.
4. Decarboxylation of DOPA into **dopamine** by **DOPA decarboxylase**.
5. Entry of dopamine into granules of chromaffin cells.
6. Hydroxylation of dopamine into **noradrenaline** by the enzyme **dopamine beta-hydroxylase**.
7. Release of noradrenaline from granules into the cytoplasm.
8. Methylation of noradrenaline into **adrenaline** by the most important enzyme called **phenylethanolamine-N-methyltransferase (PNMT)**. PNMT is present in chromaffin cells.

■ METABOLISM OF CATECHOLAMINES

Eighty five percent of noradrenaline is taken up by the sympathetic adrenergic neurons. Remaining 15% of noradrenaline and adrenaline are degraded (Fig. 55.2).

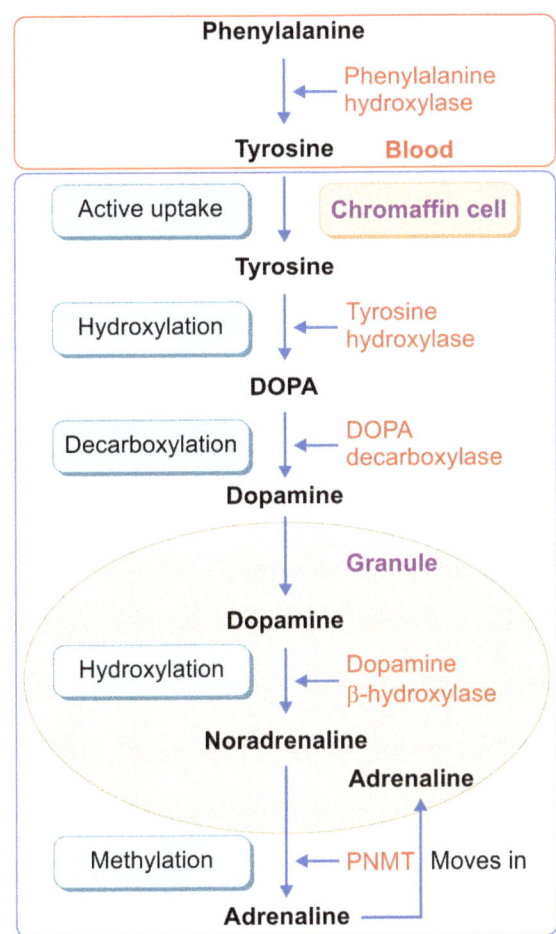

FIGURE 55.1: Synthesis of catecholamines.
PNMT = Phenyl-ethanolamine-N-methyl-transferase,
DOPA = Dihydroxyphenylalanine.

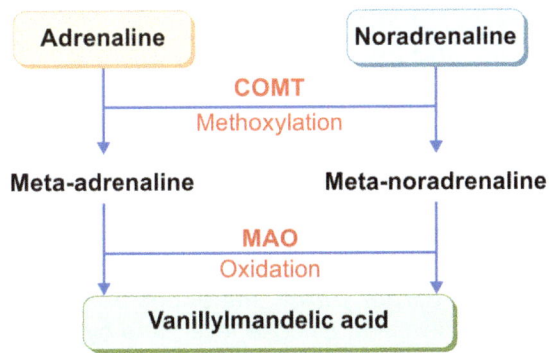

FIGURE 55.2: Metabolism of catecholamines.
COMT = Catechol-O-methyltransferase,
MAO = Monoamine oxidase.

Stages of Metabolism of Catecholamines

1. Adrenaline is methoxylated into **meta-adrenaline**. Noradrenaline is methoxylated into **meta-noradrenaline**. Methoxylation occurs in the presence of **catechol-O-methyltransferase (COMT)**. Meta-adrenaline and metanoradrenaline are together called **metanephrines**.
2. Then, oxidation of metanephrines into **vanillylmandelic acid (VMA)** occurs by **monoamine oxidase (MAO)**.

Removal of Catecholamines

Catecholamines are removed from body through urine in three forms:

1. 15% as free adrenaline and free noradrenaline.
2. 50% as free or conjugated meta-adrenaline and meta-noradrenaline.
3. 35% as VMA.

▪ ACTIONS OF ADRENALINE AND NORADRENALINE

Adrenaline and noradrenaline stimulate the nervous system. Adrenaline has significant effects on metabolic functions and both adrenaline and noradrenaline have significant effects on cardiovascular system.

▪ MODE OF ACTION OF ADRENALINE AND NORADRENALINE: ADRENERGIC RECEPTORS

Actions of adrenaline and noradrenaline are executed by binding with receptors called adrenergic receptors which are present in the target organs.

Types of Adrenergic Receptors

Adrenergic receptors are of two types:

1. **Alpha-adrenergic receptors**.
2. **Beta-adrenergic receptors**.

Alpha receptors and, beta receptors are divided into beta-1 and beta-2 receptors. Refer **Table 55.1** for their mode of action and response.

▪ SPECIFIC ACTIONS OF ADRENALINE AND NORADRENALINE

Actions of adrenaline and noradrenaline on various target organs depend upon the type of receptors present in cells of the organs. Adrenaline acts through both alpha and beta receptors equally. Noradrenaline acts mainly through alpha receptors and occasionally through beta receptors.

TABLE 55.1: Adrenergic receptors.

Receptor	Mode of action	Response
Alpha-1 receptor	Activates IP$_3$ through phospholipase C	Give more response to noradrenaline than to adrenaline
Alpha-2 receptor	Inhibits adenyl cyclase and cAMP	
Beta-1 receptor	Activates adenyl cyclase and cAMP	Gives equal response to adrenaline and noradrenaline
Beta-2 receptor	Activates adenyl cyclase and cAMP	Gives more response to adrenaline than to noradrenaline

1. **Actions on Metabolism
   (via Alpha and Beta Receptors)**

Adrenaline influences the metabolic functions more than noradrenaline:

   i. *Action on general metabolism:* Adrenaline increases oxygen consumption and carbon dioxide removal. It increases basal metabolic rate. So, it is said to be a **calorigenic hormone**.
   ii. *Action on carbohydrate metabolism:* Adrenaline increases the blood glucose level. It is by increasing the glycogenolysis in liver and muscle. So, a large quantity of glucose enters the circulation.
   iii. *Action on fat metabolism:* Adrenaline causes mobilization of free fatty acids from adipose tissues. Catecholamines need the presence of glucocorticoids for this action.

2. **Action on Blood (via Beta Receptors)**

Adrenaline decreases blood coagulation time. It increases RBC count in blood by contracting smooth muscles of splenic capsule and releasing RBCs from spleen into circulation.

3. **Action on Heart (via Beta Receptors)**

Adrenaline has stronger effects on heart than noradrenaline. It increases overall activity of the heart, i.e.:

   i. Heart rate (chronotropic effect).
   ii. Force of contraction (inotropic effect).
   iii. Excitability of heart muscle (bathmotropic effect).
   iv. Conductivity in heart muscle (dromotropic effect).

4. **Action on Blood Vessels
   (via Alpha and Beta-2 Receptors)**

Noradrenaline has strong effects on blood vessels. It causes constriction of all blood vessels throughout the body via alpha receptors. So, it is called '**General vasoconstrictor**'. Vasoconstrictor effect of noradrenaline increases total peripheral resistance.

Adrenaline also causes constriction of blood vessels. However, it causes dilatation of blood vessels in skeletal muscle, liver and heart through beta-2 receptors. So, the total peripheral resistance is decreased by adrenaline.

5. **Action on Blood Pressure
   (via Alpha and Beta Receptors)**

Adrenaline increases systolic blood pressure by increasing the force of contraction of the heart and cardiac output. But, it decreases diastolic blood pressure by reducing the total peripheral resistance.

Noradrenaline increases diastolic pressure due to general vasoconstrictor effect by increasing the total peripheral resistance. It also increases the systolic blood pressure to a slight extent by its actions on heart. Action of catecholamines on blood pressure needs the presence of glucocorticoids.

Thus, hypersecretion of catecholamines leads to hypertension.

6. **Action on Respiration (via Beta-2 Receptors)**

Adrenaline increases rate and force of respiration. Adrenaline injection produces apnea, which is known as **adrenaline apnea**. It also causes **bronchodilation**.

7. **Action on Skin (via Alpha and Beta-2 Receptors)**

Adrenaline causes contraction of arrector pili. It also increases the secretion of sweat.

8. **Action on Skeletal Muscle
   (via Alpha and Beta-2 Receptors)**

Adrenaline causes severe contraction and quick fatigue of skeletal muscle. It increases glycogenolysis and release of glucose from muscle into blood. It also causes vasodilatation in skeletal muscles.

9. **Action on Smooth Muscle
   (via Alpha and Beta Receptors)**

Catecholamines cause contraction of smooth muscles in the following organs:

   i. Splenic capsule.
   ii. Sphincters of GI tract.
   iii. Arrector pili of skin.
   iv. Gallbladder.
   v. Uterus.
   vi. Dilator pupillae of iris.

Catecholamines cause relaxation of smooth muscles in the following organs:

   i. Nonsphincteric part of GI tract (esophagus, stomach and intestine).
   ii. Bronchioles.
   iii. Urinary bladder.

10. **Action on Central Nervous System
    (via Beta Receptors)**

Adrenaline increases the activity of brain. Adrenaline secretion increases during **fight or flight reactions** after exposure to stress. It enhances the cortical arousal and other facilitatory functions of central nervous system.

11. **Other Actions of Catecholamines**

    i. On salivary glands (via alpha and beta-2 receptors): Cause vasoconstriction in salivary gland leading to mild increase in salivary secretion.
    ii. On sweat glands (via beta-2 receptors): Increase the secretion of apocrine sweat glands.
    iii. On lacrimal glands (via alpha receptors): Increase the secretion of tears.
    iv. On ACTH secretion (via alpha receptors): Adrenaline increases ACTH secretion.
    v. On nerve fibers (via alpha receptors): Adrenaline decreases the latency of action potential in the nerve fibers, i.e. electrical activity is accelerated.
    vi. On renin secretion (via beta receptors): Increase the secretion of renin from juxtaglomerular apparatus of the kidney.

REGULATION OF SECRETION OF ADRENALINE AND NORADRENALINE

Adrenaline and noradrenaline are secreted from adrenal medulla in small quantities even during rest. During stress conditions, due to sympathoadrenal discharge, a large quantity of catecholamines is secreted. These hormones prepare the body for fight or flight reactions.

Catecholamine secretion increases in exposure to cold and hypoglycemia also.

DOPAMINE

Dopamine is secreted by adrenal medulla. Type of cells secreting this hormone is not known. Dopamine is also secreted by **dopaminergic neurons** in some areas of brain particularly, **basal ganglia**. In brain, this hormone acts as a neurotransmitter.

Injected dopamine produces following effects:

1. Vasoconstriction by releasing norepinephrine.
2. Vasodilatation in mesentery.
3. Increase in heart rate via beta receptors.
4. Increase in systolic blood pressure. Dopamine does not affect diastolic blood pressure.

Deficiency of dopamine in basal ganglia produces nervous disorder called Parkinsonism (Chapter 100).

APPLIED PHYSIOLOGY: PHEOCHROMOCYTOMA

Pheochromocytoma is a condition characterized by hypersecretion of catecholamines.

Cause of Pheochromocytoma

Pheochromocytoma is caused by tumor of pheochrome cells in adrenal medulla

Signs and Symptoms of Pheochromocytoma

Characteristic feature of pheochromocytoma is hypertension. This type of hypertension is known as endocrine or **secondary hypertension**.

Other common features of pheochromocytoma:

1. Chest pain.
2. Palpitation and tachycardia.
3. Fever.
4. Headache.
5. Metabolic disorders.
6. Nausea and vomiting.
7. Sweating and flushing.
8. Weight loss.

Chapter 56: Endocrine Functions of Other Organs

CHAPTER OUTLINE

- **PINEAL GLAND**
  - SITUATION AND STRUCTURE
  - FUNCTIONS
- **THYMUS**
  - SITUATION AND STRUCTURE
  - FUNCTIONS
- **KIDNEYS**
  - ERYTHROPOIETIN
  - THROMBOPOIETIN
- RENIN
- 1,25-DIHYDROXYCHOLECALCIFEROL: CALCITRIOL
- PROSTAGLANDINS
- **HEART**
  - ATRIAL NATRIURETIC PEPTIDE
  - BRAIN NATRIURETIC PEPTIDE
  - C-TYPE NATRIURETIC PEPTIDE

■ PINEAL GLAND

■ SITUATION AND STRUCTURE OF PINEAL GLAND

Pineal gland is otherwise called **epiphysis of cerebri**. It is a small cone-shaped structure. In human, it is about 10 mm long. Pineal gland is located in diencephalic area of brain above the hypothalamus.

Pineal gland has two types of cells:

1. Parenchymal cells, which are large epithelial cells.
2. Neuroglial cells.

In adults, the pineal gland is **calcified**. But the **parenchymal cells** (epithelial cells) exist and secrete the hormonal substance.

■ FUNCTIONS OF PINEAL GLAND

Pineal gland has two functions:

1. It controls the sexual activities in animals by regulating **seasonal fertility**. However, the pineal gland plays little role in regulating the sexual functions in human being.
2. Pineal gland secrete a hormonal substance called melatonin.

Melatonin

Melatonin is secreted by parenchymal cells of pineal gland. It is an **indole** (N-acetyl-5-methoxytryptamine).

Actions of melatonin

Melatonin acts mainly on gonads. Its action differs from species to species. In some animals, it stimulates the gonads while in other animals it inhibits the gonads.

In humans, melatonin inhibits the onset of puberty by inhibiting the gonads.

Diurnal variation in melatonin secretion

Melatonin secretion is more in darkness than in daylight. Secretion of melatonin varies according to activities in different periods of the day, i.e. **circadian rhythm**. Hypothalamus is responsible for the circadian fluctuations of melatonin secretion.

■ THYMUS

■ SITUATION AND STRUCTURE OF THYMUS

It is situated in front of trachea below the thyroid gland. Thymus is small in newborn infants and gradually enlarges till puberty, and then decreases in size.

Thymus is formed by two **lobes**. Each lobe is divided into many **lobules**. Each lobule has two layers of structures namely outer cortex and inner medulla.

Cortex consists of large number of T lymphocytes and supporting reticular cells. **Medulla** contains large number of reticular cells and a smaller number of T lymphocytes. In addition, medulla has **Hassall corpuscles**. Each Hassall corpuscle has central portion of degenerated cells which are surrounded in concentric layers of flattened cells. Function of these corpuscles is not known.

FUNCTIONS OF THYMUS

Thymus has lymphoid function and endocrine function. It is responsible for development of immunity in the body.

Thymus has two functions:
1. Processing of T lymphocytes.
2. Endocrine function.

1. Processing of T Lymphocytes

Thymus plays an essential role in the development of immunity by processing the T lymphocytes (Chapter 15). Lymphocytes, produced in bone marrow, are processed in thymus into T lymphocytes. It occurs during the period between 3 months before birth and 3 months after birth. So, the removal of thymus 3 months after birth will not affect cell-mediated immunity.

2. Endocrine Function of Thymus

Thymus secretes two hormones:
  i. Thymosin.
  ii. Thymin.

Thymosin

Thymosin is a peptide. It accelerates lymphopoiesis and proliferation of T lymphocytes.

Thymin

It is also called **thymopoietin**. It suppresses the neuromuscular activity by inhibiting acetylcholine release.

Hyperactivity of thymus causes **myasthenia gravis**.

KIDNEYS

Kidneys secrete five hormonal substances:
1. Erythropoietin.
2. Thrombopoietin.
3. Renin.
4. 1,25-dihydroxycholecalciferol (calcitriol).
5. Prostaglandins.

Recently, it is discovered that kidney secretes small quantity of C-type natriuretic peptide (see below).

1. ERYTHROPOIETIN

Erythropoietin is secreted by endothelial cells of peritubular capillaries in the kidney. It is a glycoprotein with 165 amino acids.

Erythropoietin stimulates the bone marrow and causes erythropoiesis. More details are given in Chapter 9.

2. THROMBOPOIETIN

Thrombopoietin is a glycoprotein. It is secreted by kidneys and liver. It stimulates production of platelets.

3. RENIN

Renin is secreted by granular cells of juxtaglomerular apparatus of the kidney.

Actions of Renin

When renin is released into the blood, it acts on a specific plasma protein called alpha-2 globulin. It is also called angiotensinogen or renin substrate.

Renin converts angiotensinogen into angiotensin I which is converted into angiotensin II by a converting enzyme. Other details of renin and angiotensin II are given in Chapter 40.

4. 1,25-DIHYDROXYCHOLECALCIFEROL: CALCITRIOL

Formation of 1,25-dihydroxycholecalciferol

1,25-dihydroxycholecalciferol is otherwise known as **calcitriol** or **activated vitamin D**. It is formed from **cholecalciferol** (vitamin D_3) which is present in skin and intestine. **Cholecalciferol** is converted into **25-hydroxycholecalciferol** in liver. This in turn, is activated into **1,25-dihydroxycholecalciferol** by parathormone in kidney (Chapter 52).

Action of 1,25-dihydroxycholecalciferol

Activated vitamin D plays an important role in the maintenance of blood calcium level. It acts on the intestinal epithelium and enhances absorption of calcium from intestine into the blood. Details are given in Chapter 52.

5. PROSTAGLANDINS

Kidney secretes prostaglandins PGA_2 and PGE_2. These hormones are secreted by juxtaglomerular cells and type I interstitial cells present in medulla of kidney.

Prostaglandins decrease the blood pressure by systemic vasodilatation, diuresis and natriuresis. Details of prostaglandins are given in Chapter 57.

HEART

Heart secretes the hormones atrial natriuretic peptide and brain natriuretic peptide. Recently another peptide called C-type natriuretic peptide is found in heart.

1. ATRIAL NATRIURETIC PEPTIDE

Atrial natriuretic peptide (ANP) is a polypeptide with 28 amino acids. It is secreted by atrial musculature of the heart. Recently, it is found in hypothalamus of brain also. However, its action in brain is not known.

ANP is secreted during overstretching of atrial muscles in conditions like increase in blood volume. ANP in turn increases excretion of sodium (followed by water excretion) through urine and helps in the maintenance of ECF volume and blood volume. It also lowers blood pressure.

Effect of ANP on Sodium Excretion

ANP increases excretion of sodium ions through urine by:

i. Increasing glomerular filtration rate.
ii. Inhibiting sodium reabsorption from distal convoluted tubules and collecting ducts.
iii. Increasing the secretion of sodium into the renal tubules.

Escape phenomenon

Thus, ANP is responsible for escape phenomenon, and prevention of edema in primary hyperaldosteronism in spite of increased ECF volume. Refer Chapter 54 for details.

Effect of ANP on Blood Pressure

ANP decreases the blood pressure by:

i. Vasodilatation.
ii. Inhibiting renin secretion from juxtaglomerular apparatus.
iii. Inhibiting vasoconstrictor effect of angiotensin II.
iv. Inhibiting vasoconstrictor effects of catecholamines.

2. BRAIN NATRIURETIC PEPTIDE

Brain natriuretic peptide (BNP) is also called **B-type natriuretic peptide**. It is a polypeptide with 32 amino acids. It is secreted by the cardiac muscle. It is also secreted in some parts of brain. Stimulant for its secretion is not known.

BNP has same actions of ANP (see above). On brain, its actions are not known.

3. C-TYPE NATRIURETIC PEPTIDE

C-type natriuretic peptide (CNP) is a peptide with 22 amino acid. Initially, it was identified in brain. Now, it is known to be secreted by several tissues which include myocardium, endothelium of blood vessels, gastrointestinal tract and kidneys. Its function is similar to that of atrial natriuretic peptide.

Chapter 57: Local Hormones

CHAPTER OUTLINE

- **DEFINITION AND CLASSIFICATION**
- **LOCAL HORMONES SYNTHESIZED IN TISSUES**
- **LOCAL HORMONES PRODUCED IN BLOOD**

DEFINITION AND CLASSIFICATION

Local hormones are the substances which act on same area of their secretion or in immediate neighborhood. Endocrine hormones are secreted in one place but execute their actions on some other remote place.

Local hormones are produced in tissues and blood. These hormones are usually released in an inactive form and are activated by some conditions or substances.

Local hormones are classified into two types:

I. Hormones synthesized in tissues.
II. Hormones synthesized in blood.

LOCAL HORMONES SYNTHESIZED IN TISSUES

Local hormones synthesized in the tissues are of two types:

A. Prostaglandins and related substances.
B. Other local hormones synthesized in tissues.

PROSTAGLANDINS AND ITS RELATED HORMONES: EICOSANOIDS

Prostaglandins and other hormones which are derived from arachidonic acid are collectively called eicosanoids.

Eicosanoids are:

1. Prostaglandins.
2. Thromboxanes.
3. Prostacyclin.
4. Leukotrienes.
5. Lipoxins.

1. *Prostaglandins*

Prostaglandins were first discovered and isolated from human **semen**. However, now it is believed that almost all tissues of the body including renal tissues synthesize prostaglandins. Prostaglandins are unsaturated fatty acids with a cyclopentane ring and 20 carbon atoms.

Types of prostaglandins

A variety of prostaglandins are identified. Active forms of prostaglandins are PGA_2, PGD_2, PGE_2, and PGF_2.

Actions of prostaglandins

i. *Action on blood:* Prostaglandins accelerate the capacity of RBCs to pass through minute blood vessels.
ii. *Action on blood vessels:* PGE_2 causes **vasodilatation**.
iii. *Action on GI tract:* Prostaglandins reduce gastric secretion.
iv. *Action on respiratory system:* PGE_2 causes **bronchodilatation**.
v. *Action on lipids:* Some of the prostaglandins inhibit the release of free fatty acids from adipose tissue.
vi. *Action on nervous system:* Prostaglandins control or alter the actions of neurotransmitters.
vii. *Action on reproduction:* Prostaglandins play an important role in regulating the reproductive cycle. Prostaglandins also cause degeneration of corpus luteum **(luteolysis).** Prostaglandins increase the receptive capacity of cervical mucosa for sperms and cause **reverse peristaltic movement** of uterus and fallopian tubes during coitus. This in turn, increases the velocity of sperm transport in female genital tract.

Prostaglandins (PGE_2) play an important role during **parturition** and facilitate **labor** by increasing the force of uterine contractions.

When injected intra-amniotically during pregnancy, prostaglandins induce **abortion**. When injected during last stages of pregnancy, the prostaglandins induce **labor**.

viii. *Action on kidney:* Prostaglandins stimulate juxtaglomerular apparatus and enhance the secretion of renin, diuresis and natriuresis.

2. Thromboxanes

Thromboxanes are derived from **arachidonic acid**.

Thromboxanes are of two types:

i. Thromboxane A_2 which is secreted in platelets.
ii. Thromboxane B_2 the metabolite of thromboxane A_2.

Actions of thromboxane A_2

Thromboxane A_2

i. Causes vasoconstriction.
ii. Plays an important role in **hemostasis** by accelerating aggregation of platelets.
iii. Accelerates the clot formation.

3. Prostacyclin

Prostacyclin is also a derivative of arachidonic acid. It is produced in the endothelial cells and smooth muscle cells of blood vessels.

Actions of prostacyclin

Prostacyclin causes vasodilatation and inhibits platelet aggregation.

4. Leukotrienes

Leukotrienes are derived from arachidonic acid via 5-hydroperoxy eicosatetraeonic acid (5-HETE). Leukotrienes are the mediators of allergic responses. These hormones also promote inflammatory reactions.

Release of leukotrienes increases when some allergic agents combine with antibodies like IgE.

Actions of leukotrienes

Leukotrienes cause:

i. Bronchiolar constriction.
ii. Arteriolar constriction.
iii. Vascular permeability.
iv. Attraction of neutrophils and eosinophils towards the site of inflammation.

5. Lipoxins

Lipoxins are also derived from arachidonic acid via 15-hydroperoxy eicosatetraenoic acid (15-HETE). Lipoxins are of two types namely, Lipoxin A and Lipoxin B.

Actions of lipoxins

Lipoxin A causes dilation of minute blood vessels. Both the types inhibit the cytotoxic effects of killer T cells.

■ OTHER LOCAL HORMONES SYNTHESIZED IN TISSUES

In addition to prostaglandins and related hormonal substances, tissues secrete some more hormones which are listed below:

1. Acetylcholine.
2. Serotonin.
3. Histamine.
4. Substance P.
5. Heparin.
6. Leptin.
7. GI hormones.

1. Acetylcholine

Acetylcholine is the **cholinergic neurotransmitter** (Chapter 92). It is the transmitter substance at neuromuscular junction. It is also secreted by other nerve endings and other cells.

Source of secretion of acetylcholine

i. Presynaptic terminals.
ii. Preganglionic parasympathetic nerve.
iii. Postganglionic parasympathetic nerve.
iv. Preganglionic sympathetic nerve.
v. Postganglionic sympathetic cholinergic nerves, such as:
   a. Nerves supplying eccrine sweat glands.
   b. Sympathetic vasodilator nerves in skeletal muscle.
vi. Nerves in amacrine cells of retina.
vii. Mast cell.
viii. Gastric mucosa.
ix. Lungs.
x. Many regions of brain.

Actions of acetylcholine

Acetylcholine:

i. Is an **excitatory neurotransmitter**.
ii. Produces excitatory function of synapse by opening the sodium channels.
iii. Activates smooth muscles in GI tract and urinary tract.
iv. Activates skeletal muscles.
v. Inhibits cardiac function.
vi. Dilates blood vessels.

Destruction of acetylcholine

Acetylcholine is very quick in action. Immediately after executing the action, it is destroyed by acetylcholinesterase. This enzyme is present in basal lamina of the synaptic cleft.

2. Serotonin or 5-HT

Source of secretion of serotonin

Serotonin or 5-hydroxy-tryptamine is secreted in the following structures:

i. Hypothalamus.
ii. Limbic system.
iii. Cerebellum.
iv. Spinal cord.
v. Retina.
vi. GI tract.
vii. Lungs.
viii. Platelets.

Actions of serotonin

Serotonin:

i. Is an inhibitory neurotransmitter (Chapter 92).
ii. Inhibits impulses of pain sensation in posterior gray horn of spinal cord.

iii. Causes mood depression and induces sleep (Chapter 106).
iv. Causes vasoconstriction.

3. Histamine

Source of secretion of histamine

Histamine is secreted in nerve endings of hypothalamus, limbic cortex and other parts of cerebral cortex, spinal cord and gastrointestinal tract. Histamine is also released from tissues during allergic condition, inflammation or damage.

Actions of histamine

i. It is an excitatory neurotransmitter.
ii. Histamine released from tissues causes vasodilatation and enhances the capillary permeability for fluid and plasma proteins from blood into the affected tissues. So, the accumulation of fluid with proteins develops local edema.
iii. In GI tract, histamine increases the motility.

4. Substance P

Source of secretion of substance P

i. Nerve endings (first order neurons of pain pathway) in spinal cord and retina.
ii. GI tract (by the presence of chyme).

Actions of substance P

i. Substance P is the neurotransmitter for pain sensation.
ii. It is also the neurotransmitter substance in GI tract. In GI tract, it increases the mixing and propulsive movements of small intestine.

5. Heparin

Source of secretion of heparin

i. Mast cells.
ii. Basophils.

Actions of heparin

Heparin is a naturally produced anticoagulant. Refer Chapter 18 for other details.

6. Leptin

Leptin (in Greek, leptin means thin) is a protein hormone with 167 amino acids.

Source of secretion of leptin

Leptin is secreted by adipocytes in adipose tissues.

Actions of leptin

Leptin controls food intake and adipose tissue. Leptin acts on hypothalamus and inhibits the feeding center resulting in stoppage of food intake (Chapter 98). At the same time, it also stimulates the metabolic reactions involved in utilization of fat stored in adipose tissue for energy. Thus, the circulating leptin level informs the brain about energy storage and necessity to regulate metabolic reactions, food intake and body weight.

7. Gastrointestinal Hormones

i. Gastrin (Chapter 32).
ii. Secretin (Chapter 33).
iii. Cholecystokinin (Chapter 33).
iv. Gastric inhibitory peptide (GIP) (Chapter 32).
v. Vasoactive intestinal polypeptide (VIP) (Chapter 32).
vi. Pancreatic polypeptide (Chapter 33).
vii. Somatostatin (Chapter 33).
viii. Peptide YY (Chapter 33).

■ LOCAL HORMONES SYNTHESIZED IN BLOOD

Local hormones produced in the blood are:

1. Serotonin.
2. Angiotensinogen.
3. Kinins.

Serotonin is described above. Angiotensinogen is explained in Chapter 40.

Kinins are protein hormones circulating in blood. Kinins dilates blood vessels and decreases the blood pressure and increase blood flow throughout the body. Kinins also increases permeability of capillaries during inflammatory conditions resulting in edema in the affected area.

MODEL QUESTIONS IN ENDOCRINOLOGY

■ LONG QUESTIONS

1. Enumerate the hormones secreted by pituitary gland. Describe actions and regulation of secretion of growth hormone. Write in brief about effects of hypersecretion of anterior pituitary gland.
2. Describe the synthesis, storage, release, transport, functions and regulation of secretion of thyroid hormones.
3. Explain the functions and regulation of secretion of parathormone. Add a note on the disorders of parathormone secretion.
4. List the hormones secreted by pancreas. Explain functions and regulation of secretion of insulin.
5. Describe in detail the regulation of blood sugar level.
6. Classify the hormones secreted by adrenal cortex. Explain actions and regulation of secretion of cortisol.
7. Enumerate the corticosteroids. Describe actions and regulation of secretion of aldosterone.
8. What are catecholamines? Explain the synthesis, metabolism, actions and regulation of secretion of catecholamines.

■ SHORT QUESTIONS

1. Growth hormone.
2. Thyroid stimulating hormone.
3. Adrenocorticotropic hormone.
4. Oxytocin.
5. Antidiuretic hormone.
6. Milk ejection/Neuroendocrine reflex.
7. Gigantism.
8. Dwarfism.
9. Disorders of posterior pituitary gland.
10. Thyroxine.
11. Hyperthyroidism/hypothyroidism.
12. Goiter.
13. Cretinism.
14. Myxedema.
15. Parathormone.
16. Tetany.
17. Hypercalcemia/Hypocalcemia.
18. Insulin.
19. Glucagon.
20. Diabetes mellitus.
21. Hyperinsulinism.
22. Cortisol.
23. Non-metabolic actions of cortisol.
24. Aldosterone.
25. Cushing's syndrome or disease.
26. Hyperaldosteronism.
27. Adrenogenital syndrome.
28. Addison's disease.
29. Synthesis of catecholamines.
30. Actions of catecholamines.
31. Prostaglandins.
32. Acetylcholine.

■ VERY SHORT ANSWER QUESTIONS

1. Any hormone.
2. Any endocrine disorder.
3. Cell-to-cell signaling.
4. Define classical hormone, neurotransmitter and neurohormone. Give examples.
5. Classify classical hormone.
6. Hormonal receptors.
7. Cyclic AMP.
8. G proteins.
9. Hypothalamo-hypophyseal relationship.
10. Parts and cell types in anterior pituitary. Name the hormone secreted by each cell type.
11. Mode of action of GH/Somatomedin.
12. Gonadotropins.
13. Feedback control of regulation GH secretion.
14. Diabetogenic effect of growth hormone.
15. Parts and cell types in posterior pituitary.
16. Role of osmoreceptors in regulations of ADH secretion.
17. Acromegaly/Acromegalic gigantism.
18. Acromicria.
19. Simmond's disease.
20. Fröhlich's syndrome.
21. SIADH.
22. Diabetes insipidus.
23. Thyroglobuilin.
24. Exophthalmos.
25. Graves' disease.
26. Cretin vs dwarf.
27. Treatment for thyroid disorders.
28. Thyroid function tests.
29. Non-toxic or endemic colloid goiter.
30. Activation of vitamin D.
31. Carpopedal spasm.
32. Trousseau's sign and Chvostek's sign.
33. Importance of calcium.
34. Effect of parathormone and calcitonin on blood calcium level.
35. Osteoporosis.
36. Rickets.
37. Cells of islets of Langerhans and their secretions.
38. Somatostatin.
39. Pancreatic polypeptide.
40. Complications of prolonged diabetes mellitus.
41. Aldosterone escape.
42. Action of ACTH on adrenal cortex.
43. Adrenal androgens.
44. Adrenergic receptors.
45. Dopamine.
46. Pheochromocytoma.
47. Functions of pineal gland.
48. Functions of thymus.
49. Endocrine function of heart.
50. Serotonin.
51. Histamine.
52. Substance P.

SECTION 7: REPRODUCTIVE SYSTEM

Chapter 58: Male Reproductive System

CHAPTER OUTLINE

- REPRODUCTIVE SYSTEM
- MALE REPRODUCTIVE ORGANS
- FUNCTIONAL ANATOMY OF TESTES
- ACCESSORY SEX ORGANS IN MALES
- SEMINAL VESICLES
- PROSTATE GLAND
- URETHRA
- PENIS
- FUNCTIONS OF TESTIS
- GAMETOGENIC FUNCTIONS OF TESTIS: SPERMATOGENESIS
- ENDOCRINE FUNCTIONS OF TESTIS
- SEMEN
- MALE CLIMACTERIC
- APPLIED PHYSIOLOGY

■ REPRODUCTIVE SYSTEM

Reproductive system ensures the continuation of species. **Gonads** are the **primary reproductive organs** which produce the gametes. Gametes are the sperms and ova. Sperms are produced in males by a pair of testes. And, ova are produced in females by a pair of ovaries.

Normally, most of the animals including humans are either definite males or definite females. However, in some organisms like earthworms and snails, both sexes may be present in the same organism and this condition is known as **hermaphroditism**.

In humans and most of the higher animals, reproduction occurs sexually, i.e. by mating. However, there are some species like insects which can produce offspring without mating.

■ MALE REPRODUCTIVE ORGANS

Male reproductive organs include:

1. Primary sex organs.
2. Accessory sex organs.

Primary Sex Organs

Testes are the primary sex organs or gonads in males.

Accessory Sex Organs

Accessory sex organs in males are:

1. Seminal vesicles.
2. Prostate gland.
3. Urethra.
4. Penis.

See below for details of accessary sex organs in males.

■ FUNCTIONAL ANATOMY OF TESTES

There are two testes in almost all the species (singular = **testis**). Testes are ovoid or walnut-shaped bodies located in the sac-like structure called **scrotum (Fig. 58.1)**.

■ COVERINGS OF TESTIS

Each testis is enclosed by three coverings:

1. Tunica Vasculosa

Tunica vasculosa is the innermost covering of testis. It is made up of connective tissue. And it is rich in blood vessels.

2. Tunica Albuginea

This is the middle covering and it is a dense fibrous capsule.

3. Tunica Vaginalis

Tunica vaginalis is the outermost covering and it is formed by visceral and parietal layers.

■ PARENCHYMA OF TESTIS

Lobules of Testis

Tunica albuginea on the posterior surface of testis is thickened to form **mediastinum testis**. From this, the connective tissue septa called **septula testis** radiate

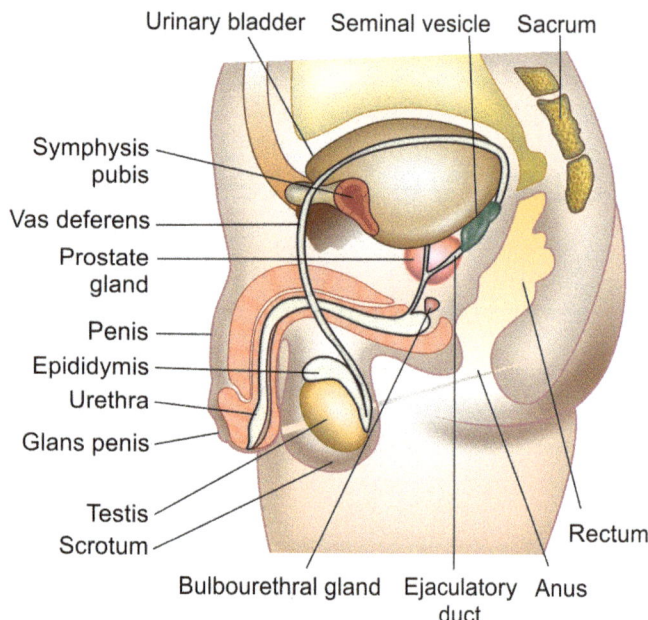

FIGURE 58.1: Male reproductive system and other organs of pelvis.

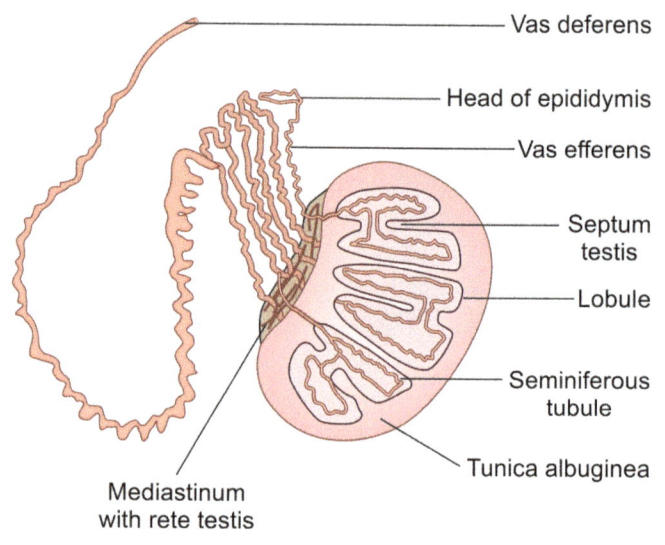

FIGURE 58.2: Structure of testis.

into testis and bind with tunica albuginea at various points. Because of this, testis is divided into a number of **pyramidal lobules**, with bases directed towards the periphery and the apices towards mediastinum **(Fig. 58.2)**.

Each testis has about 200 to 300 lobules. Each lobule contains 1 to 4 coiled tubules known as the seminiferous tubules.

Seminiferous Tubules

Seminiferous tubules are thread-like convoluted tubular structures in which the spermatozoa or sperms are produced. There are about 400 to 600 seminiferous tubules in each testis. Length of each seminiferous tubule is between 30 cm and 70 cm. Its diameter is between 150 μ and 300 μ.

Wall of seminiferous tubule is formed by three layers:

1. Outer capsule or tunica propria, formed by fibroelastic connective tissue.
2. Thin homogeneous basement membrane.
3. Stratified epithelium, which consists of two types of cells:
   i. Spermatogenic cells or germ cells.
   ii. Sertoli cells or supporting cells.

Spermatogenic cells

Spermatogenic cells or **germ cells** present in seminiferous tubules are the precursor cells of spermatozoa. These cells lie in between Sertoli cells. Spermatogenic cells are attached to Sertoli cells by means of cytoplasmic connection.

In children, spermatogenic cells are in the primitive stage called **spermatogonia**. With onset of puberty, spermatogonia develop into sperms through different stages.

Sertoli cells

Sertoli cells or **supporting cells** are large and tall irregular columnar cells present in seminiferous tubule.

Spermatogenic cells are attached to Sertoli cells by means of cytoplasmic connection.

Functions of Sertoli cells

Sertoli cells:

1. Support and nourish the spermatogenic cells till spermatozoa are released from them.
2. Secrete the enzyme **aromatase** which converts androgens into estrogen.
3. Secrete **androgen-binding protein (ABP)** which is essential for testosterone activity particularly during spermatogenesis.
4. Secrete **estrogen-binding protein (EBP)**.
5. Secrete **inhibin** which inhibits the release of follicle stimulating hormone (FSH) from anterior pituitary.
6. Secrete **activin** which increases FSH release.
7. Secrete **Müllerian regression factor (MRF)** in fetal testes. MRF is also called **Müllerian inhibiting substance (MIS)**. MRF is responsible for the regression of Müllerian duct during sex differentiation in fetus (see below).
8. Tight junctions between Sertoli cells form blood-testis barrier.

Blood-testis Barrier

Blood-testis barrier is a mechanical barrier that separates blood from seminiferous tubules of the testes. It is formed by **tight junctions** between the adjacent Sertoli cells near the basal membrane of seminiferous tubule.

Blood-testis barrier protects the seminiferous tubules and spermatogenic cells by preventing the entry of toxic substances from blood into testis. At the same time, it permits nutritive and other essential substances necessary for spermatogenic cells.

Rete Testis, Vas Efferens, Epididymis and Vas Deferens

Each seminiferous lobule opens into a network of thin walled channels called the **rete testis**. From rete testis, 8 to 15 tubules called **vas efferens** arise. Vas efferens join together and form the **head of epididymis** and then converge to form **duct of epididymis (Fig. 58.3)**.

Duct of epididymis is an enormously convoluted tubule with a length of about 4 meters. It begins at head, where it receives vas efferens. At the caudal pole of testis, epididymis turns sharply upon itself and continues as **vas deferens** without any definite demarcation.

Interstitial Cells of Leydig

Interstitial cells of Leydig are the hormone secreting cells in testes. These cells are situated in between the seminiferous tubules.

ACCESSORY SEX ORGANS IN MALES

Accesory sex organs in males viz. seminal vesicles, prostate gland, urethra and penis are explained below.

SEMINAL VESICLES

Seminal vesicles are paired glands situated in lower abdomen on either side of the prostate gland behind urinary bladder. Each seminal vesicle is a hollow sac of irregular shape. It is lined by complexly folded mucous membrane which secretes seminal fluid.

SEMINAL FLUID

Seminal fluid from each seminal vesicle is added to semen in the **ejaculatory duct** through **ampulla of vas deferens**. Ejaculatory duct opens into urethra.

Seminal fluid is mucoid and viscous in nature. It is neutral or slightly alkaline in reaction. It adds to the bulk of semen as it forms 60% of total semen. Seminal vesicles secrete several important substances. Refer **Figure 58.7** for the products secreted by seminal vesicles.

FUNCTIONS OF SEMINAL FLUID

1. Nutrition to Sperms

Fructose and other nutritive substances present in seminal fluid are utilized by sperms after being ejaculated into female genital tract.

2. Clotting of Semen

As soon as semen is ejaculated it is clotted because of conversion of **fibrinogen** of seminal fluid into **fibrin**. Clotting of semen is essential for holding the sperms in uterine cervix.

3. On Fertilization

Prostaglandin of seminal fluid enhances fertilization of ovum by the following processes:
  i. Increasing the receptive capacity of cervical mucosa for sperms.
  ii. Causing **reverse peristalsis** in uterus and fallopian tubes. This, in turn, increases the rate of transport of sperms in female genital tract during coitus (oxytocin is also responsible for this process).

PROSTATE GLAND

Prostate gland weighs about 40 g. It is formed by 20 to 30 separate secretory glands, which open separately into the urethra. Prostate secretes prostatic fluid.

PROSTATIC FLUID

Prostatic fluid is a thin, milky and alkaline fluid. It forms 30% of total semen. Refer **Figure 58.7** for the products secreted by prostate gland.

FUNCTIONS OF PROSTATIC FLUID

1. Maintenance of Sperm Motility

Prostatic fluid provides optimum pH for the motility of sperms. Generally, sperms are nonmotile at a pH of less than 6.0. There are some factors which decrease the pH and motility of sperm both in vas deferens and female genital tract.

In vas deferens

End products of metabolic activities in the sperm make the fluid in vas deferens acidic, so that the sperms are nonmotile.

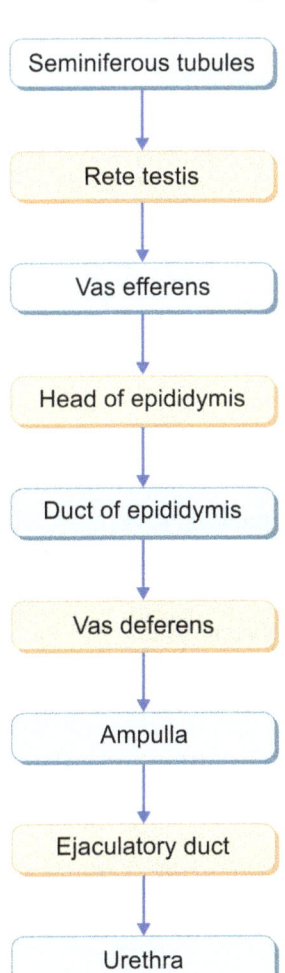

FIGURE 58.3: Pathway for passage of sperms.

In female genital tract

Vaginal secretions in females are highly acidic with a pH of 3.5 to 4.0. So, when semen is ejaculated into female genital tract at coitus, sperms are nonmotile initially.

However, the alkaline prostatic secretion which is also present in semen, neutralizes the acidity in vagina and maintains a pH of 6.0 to 6.5. At this pH, the sperms become motile and chances of fertilization are enhanced.

2. Clotting of Semen

Clotting enzymes present in prostatic fluid convert fibrinogen (from seminal vesicles) into clot.

3. Lysis of Clot

The clot is dissolved by fibrinolysin of the prostatic fluid so that, the sperms become motile.

URETHRA

Male urethra is about 20 cm long. After origin from bladder it traverses the prostate gland, which lies below the bladder and then runs through the penis. Ejaculatory duct opens into urethra. Other details of urethra are given in Chapter 46.

Internal urethra passes through penis as **external urethra**. Urethra contains mucus glands throughout its length, which are called **glands of Littre**. Bilateral **bulbourethral glands** also open into the urethra.

PENIS

Penis is the male genital organ. Urethra passes through penis and opens to the exterior. Penis is formed by three erectile tissue masses, i.e. a paired **corpora cavernosa** and an unpaired **corpus spongiosum**. Corpus spongiosum surrounds the urethra and terminates distally to form **glans penis**.

FUNCTIONS OF TESTIS

Testis performs two functions:

1. Gametogenic function by which gametes are produced in gonads.
2. Endocrine function by which male sex hormones are secreted.

GAMETOGENIC FUNCTIONS OF TESTIS: SPERMATOGENESIS

Spermatogenesis is the process by which male gametes called **spermatozoa** (sperms) are formed from primitive spermatogenic cells (spermatogonia) in the testis **(Fig. 58.4)**. It takes 74 days for the formation of sperm from a primitive germ cell.

STAGES OF SPERMATOGENESIS

Spermatogenesis occurs in four stages:

1. Stage of proliferation.
2. Stage of growth.
3. Stage of maturation.
4. Stage of transformation.

1. Stage of Proliferation

Each spermatogonium contains diploid number (23 pairs) of chromosomes. One member of each pair is derived from mother and the other one from father. The 23 pairs include

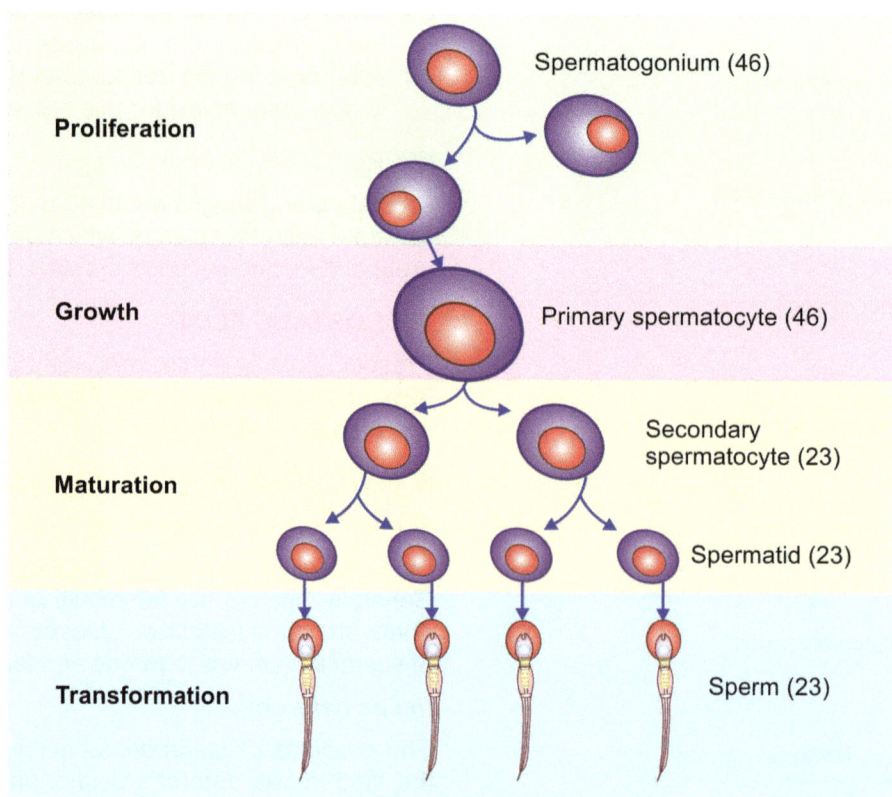

FIGURE 58.4: Spermatogenesis. Number in parenthesis indicates chromosomal number.

22 pairs of autosomal chromosomes and one pair of sex chromosomes. Sex chromosomes are one X chromosome and one Y chromosome.

During the proliferative stage, **spermatogonia** divide by mitosis without any change in chromosomal number. In man, there are usually seven generations of spermatogonia. During this stage, the spermatogonia migrate along with Sertoli cells towards the lumen of seminiferous tubule.

Last generation of spermatogonia enters the stage of growth as **primary spermatocyte**.

2. Stage of Growth

In this stage, the primary spermatocyte grows into a large cell. Apart from growth, there is no other change in spermatocyte during this stage.

3. Stage of Maturation

After reaching the full size, each primary spermatocyte quickly undergoes meiotic or maturation division, which occurs in two phases.

First phase of maturation

In the first phase each primary spermatocyte divides into two **secondary spermatocytes**. Significance of first meiotic division is that each secondary spermatocyte receives only haploid or half the number of chromosomes. Total of 23 chromosomes include 22 autosomes and one X or Y chromosome.

Second phase of maturation

During second phase, each secondary spermatocyte undergoes second meiotic division resulting in two smaller cells called **spermatids**. Each spermatid has haploid number of chromosomes.

4. Stage of Transformation

There is no further division. Spermatids are transformed into **matured spermatozoa** (sperms). Transformation occurs in two stages.

i. Spermiogenesis

Spermiogeneis is the process by which spermatids become matured spermatozoa.

Changes taking place during spermiogenesis stage are:
a. Condensation of nuclear material.
b. Formation of acrosome, mitochondrial spiral filament and tail structures.
c. Removal of unwanted quantity of cytoplasm.

ii. Spermiation

Spermiation is the process by which the matured sperms are released from Sertoli cells into the lumen of seminiferous tubules. Structure of sperm is explained later in this chapter.

ROLE OF SERTOLI CELLS IN SPERMATOGENESIS

Sertoli cells influence spermatogenesis by many ways (see above).

ROLE OF HORMONES IN SPERMATOGENESIS

Spermatogenesis is influenced by many hormones which act either directly or indirectly. Hormones necessary for spermatogenesis are given below **Table 58.1**.

1. Follicle Stimulating Hormone

FSH is responsible for the initiation of spermatogenesis. It binds with Sertoli cells and spermatogonia and induces the proliferation of spermatogonia. It also stimulates formation of estrogen and androgen binding protein from Sertoli cells **(Fig. 58.5)**.

2. Luteinizing Hormone

In males this hormone is called **interstitial cell stimulating hormone**. It is essential for the secretion of testosterone from Leydig cells.

TABLE 58.1: Hormones necessary for spermatogenesis.

Stage of spermatogenesis	Hormones necessary
Stage of proliferation	Follicle-stimulating hormone Growth hormone
Stage of growth	Testosterone Growth hormone
Stage of maturation	Testosterone Growth hormone
Stage of transformation	Testosterone Estrogen

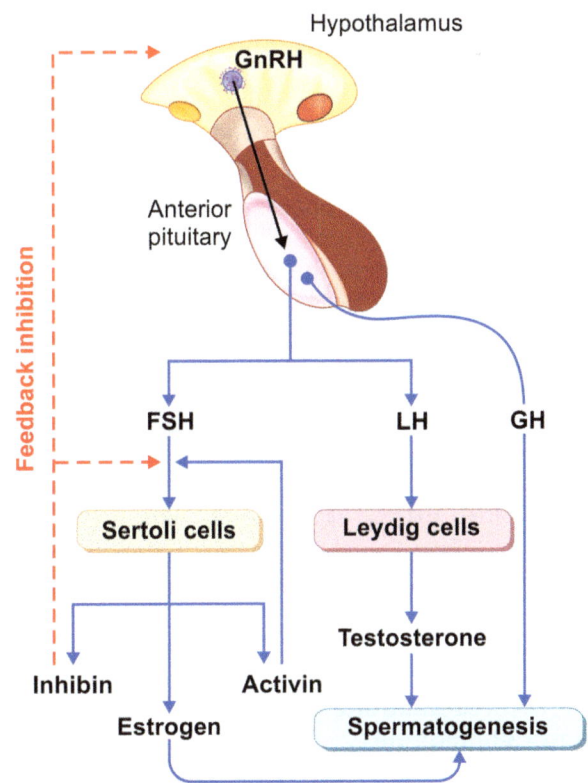

FIGURE 58.5: Role of hormones in spermatogenesis. Blue arrow = Stimulation, Red dotted arrow = Inhibition, GnRH = Gonadotropin-releasing hormone, FSH = Follicle stimulating hormone, LH = Luteinizing hormone, GH = Growth hormone.

3. Growth Hormone

Growth hormone is essential for the general metabolic processes in testis. It is also necessary for proliferation of spermatogonia. In pituitary dwarfs, the spermatogenesis is severely affected.

4. Testosterone

Testosterone is responsible for sequence of later stages in spermatogenesis. It is also responsible for maintenance of spermatogenesis. Testosterone activity is largely influenced by androgen binding protein.

5. Estrogen

Estrogen is formed from testosterone in Sertoli cells. It is necessary for spermiogenesis.

6. Inhibin

Inhibin is a peptide hormone and serves as a transforming growth factor. It is secreted by Sertoli cells. In females, it is secreted by granulosa cells of ovarian follicles. Secretion of inhibin is stimulated by FSH.

In males, inhibin inhibits FSH secretion through feedback mechanism leading to decrease in the pace of spermatogenesis.

7. Activin

It is also a peptide hormone secreted by Sertoli cells and Leydig cells. Activin has opposite actions of inhibin. It increases secretion of FSH and accelerates spermatogenesis.

■ OTHER FACTORS AFFECTING SPERMATOGENESIS

Spermatogenesis is also influenced by some other factors:

1. Increase in the body temperature prevents spermatogenesis. It occurs in cryptorchidism (see below). Normally, temperature in the scrotum is about 2°C less than the body temperature. But in cryptorchidism the testes are in the abdomen where the temperature is always higher than that of scrotum. Increase in temperature stops spermatogenesis.
2. Infectious diseases such as mumps cause degeneration of seminiferous tubules and absence of spermatogenesis.

■ ENDOCRINE FUNCTIONS OF TESTIS

Testis secretes male sex hormones which are collectively called the **androgens**.

Androgens secreted by testis are:

1. **Testosterone**.
2. **Dihydrotestosterone**.
3. **Androstenedione**.

Androgens are secreted in large quantities by interstitial cells of Leydig in testes and in small quantity by zona reticularis in adrenal cortex.

Androgens are steroid hormones synthesized from cholesterol or acetate. Testosterone is a C19 steroid. The plasma level of testosterone in an adult male varies between 300 and 700 ng/dL. In adult female the testosterone level is 30 to 60 mg/dL.

■ TESTOSTERONE SECRETION IN DIFFERENT PERIODS OF LIFE

Testosterone is secreted in fetus by **genital** ridge. In childhood, no testosterone is secreted until 10 to 12 years of age. Afterwards, testosterone secretion starts and, it increases rapidly at the onset of puberty and lasts through most of the remaining part of life. Testosterone secretion starts decreasing after 40 years and becomes almost zero by the age of 90 years.

■ FUNCTIONS OF TESTOSTERONE IN FETAL LIFE

Fetal testes begin to secrete testosterone at about 2nd to 4th month of fetal life.

Testosterone performs three functions in fetus:

1. Sex differentiation in fetus.
2. Development of accessory sex organs.
3. Descent of the testes.

1. Sex Differentiation in Fetus

Testosterone is responsible for the sex differentiation of fetus.

Fetus has two genital ducts:

i. **Müllerian duct** which gives rise to female accessory sex organs such as vagina, uterus and fallopian tube.
ii. **Wolffian duct** which gives rise to male accessory sex organs such as epididymis, vas deferens and seminal vesicles.

If testosterone is secreted from the **genital ridge** of the fetus at about 7th week of intrauterine life, the Müllerian duct system disappears and male sex organs develop from Wolffian duct. In addition to testosterone, **Müllerian regression factor (MRF)** secreted by Sertoli cells is also responsible for regression of Müllerian duct.

In the absence of testosterone, Wolffian duct regresses and female sex organs develop from Müllerian duct.

2. Development of Accessory Sex Organs and External Genitalia

Testosterone is also essential for the growth of the external genitalia viz. penis and scrotum and other accessory sex organs namely genital ducts, seminal vesicles and prostate.

3. Descent of Testes

Testes which are developed in the abdominal cavity are pushed down into the scrotum through inguinal canal just before birth. The process by which testes enter the scrotum is called the descent of testes. Testosterone is necessary for descent of testes.

Cryptorchidism

Cryptorchidism is a congenital disorder characterized by the failure of one or both testes to descent from abdomen into scrotum. In such case, the testes are called

Chapter 58: Male Reproductive System 291

undescended testes. Administration of testosterone or gonadotropic hormones (which stimulate Leydig cells) causes descent of testes. Surgery is required if the inguinal canal is narrow. Males with untreated testes are prone for **testicular cancer**.

■ FUNCTIONS OF TESTOSTERONE IN ADULT LIFE

1. Effect on Sex Organs

Testosterone increases the size of penis, scrotum and the testes after puberty. All these organs are enlarged many folds between the onset of puberty and the age of 20 years, under the influence of testosterone. Testosterone is also necessary for spermatogenesis.

2. Effect on Basal Metabolic Rate

At the time of puberty and earlier part of adult life, testosterone increases the basal metabolic rate to about 5 to 10% by its anabolic effects on protein metabolism.

3. Effect on Electrolyte and Water Balance

Testosterone increases the sodium reabsorption from renal tubules along with water. It leads to increase in ECF volume.

4. Effect on Blood

Testosterone has got **erythropoietic action**. So, after puberty, testosterone causes mild increase in RBC count. It also increases blood volume by increasing the water retention and ECF volume.

5. Effect on Secondary Sexual Characters

Secondary sexual characters are the physical and behavioral characteristics that distinguish the male from female. These characters appear at the time of puberty. Testosterone is responsible for the development of secondary sexual characters in males. Secondary sexual characters in males are given below.

i. Effect on muscular growth

Testosterone increases the muscle mass due to its **anabolic effects** on proteins. It accelerates transport of amino acids into the muscle cells, synthesis of proteins and storage of proteins in the muscles.

ii. Effect on bone growth

After puberty, testosterone increases the thickness of bones by increasing the matrix content and calcium deposition.

In addition to increase in the size and strength of bones, testosterone also causes early **fusion of epiphyses** of long bones with shaft. So, if testes are removed before puberty, the fusion of epiphyses is delayed and the height of the person increases.

iii. Effect on shoulder and rib cage

Testosterone causes broadening of shoulder bones and rib cage.

iv. Effect on pelvic bones

Testosterone has a specific effect on pelvis which results in:

a. Lengthening of pelvis.
b. Funnel-like shape of pelvis.
c. Narrowing of pelvic outlet.

Thus, pelvis in males is different from that of females, which is broad and round or oval in shape.

v. Effect on skin

Testosterone increases the thickness of skin and ruggedness of subcutaneous tissue by increasing the deposition of proteins in skin. It also increases the quantity of **melanin pigment**, which is responsible for deepening of the skin color.

Testosterone enhances the secretory activity of **sebaceous glands**. So, at the time of puberty, when body is exposed to sudden increase in testosterone secretion, the excess secretion of sebum leads to development of **acne** on the face. After few years, the skin gets adapted to testosterone secretion and, the acne disappears.

vi. Effect on hair distribution

Testosterone causes male type of hair distribution on the body, i.e. hair growth over the pubis, along linea alba up to umbilicus, on face, on chest and other parts of the body such as back and limbs. In males, the pubic hair has the base of the triangle downwards whereas in females it is upwards. Testosterone decreases the hair growth on head and may cause baldness if there is genetic background.

vii. Effect on voice

At the time of adolescence, boys have a cracking voice. It is because of testosterone effect which causes:

a. Hypertrophy of laryngeal muscles.
b. Enlargement of larynx and lengthening.
c. Thickening of vocal cords.

Later, the **cracking voice** changes gradually into a typical adult male voice.

■ MODE OF ACTION OF TESTOSTERONE

Testosterone acts via genes.

■ REGULATION OF TESTOSTERONE SECRETION

In Fetus

During fetal life, the testosterone secretion from testis is stimulated by human chorionic gonadotropin, which has the properties similar to those of luteinizing hormone. Human chorionic gonadotropin stimulates the development of Leydig cells in the fetal testes and promotes testosterone secretion.

In Adults

Interstitial cell stimulating hormone (ICSH) or luteinizing hormone (LH) stimulates the Leydig cells and the quantity of testosterone secreted is directly proportional to the amount of LH available.

Secretion of LH from anterior pituitary gland is stimulated by gonadotropin releasing hormone (GnRH) or luteinizing hormone releasing hormone (LHRH) from hypothalamus.

Feedback Control

Testosterone regulates its own secretion by **negative feedback** mechanism. It acts on hypothalamus and inhibits the secretion of LHRH. When LHRH secretion is inhibited, LH is not released from anterior pituitary resulting in stoppage of testosterone secretion from testes. On the other hand, when testosterone production is low, lack of inhibition of hypothalamus leads to secretion of testosterone through LHRH and LH **(Fig. 58.6)**.

■ SEMEN

Semen is a white or gray fluid that contains spermatozoa (sperms). It is the collection of fluids from testes, seminal vesicles, prostate gland and bulbourethral glands. Semen is discharged during sexual act and the process of discharge of semen is called **ejaculation.**

Testes contribute sperms. The prostate secretion gives milky appearance to semen. And, the secretions from seminal vesicles and bulbourethral glands provide mucoid consistency to semen.

At the time of ejaculation, human semen is liquid in nature. Immediately, it coagulates and after some time it becomes liquid again.

The **fibrinogen** secreted from seminal vesicle is converted into a weak **coagulum** by the clotting enzymes secreted from prostate gland. The coagulum is liquefied after about 30 minutes, as it is lysed by **fibrinolysin**. Fibrinolysin is the activated form of **profibrinolysin** produced in prostate gland.

When semen is ejaculated, the sperms are **nonmotile** due to the viscosity of coagulum. When the coagulum dissolves, the sperms become **motile**.

■ PROPERTIES OF SEMEN

Specific gravity : 1.028.
Volume : 2 to 6 mL per ejaculation.
Reaction : It is alkaline with a pH of 7.5. Alkalinity is due to the secretions from prostate gland.

■ COMPOSITION OF SEMEN

Semen contains 10% sperms and 90% of fluid part which is called **seminal plasma**. The seminal plasma contains the products from seminal vesicle and prostate gland **(Fig. 58.7)**. It also has small amount of secretions from the mucus glands, particularly the bulbourethral glands.

■ SPERM

Sperm or spermatozoon (pleural = spermatozoa) is the male reproductive cell, developed in the testis. The matured sperm is 60 μ long.

Sperm Count

Total count of sperm is about 100 million to 150 million/mL of semen. Sterility occurs when the sperm count falls below 20 million/mL.

Survival Time of Sperm

Though the sperms can be stored in male genital tract for longer periods, after ejaculation the survival time is only about 24 to 48 hours at a temperature equivalent to body temperature.

Motility of Sperm

Rate of motility of sperm in female genital tract is about 3 mm/min. Sperms reach the fallopian tube in about 30 to 60 minutes after sexual intercourse. Uterine contractions during sexual act facilitate the movement of sperms.

Structure of Sperm

Each sperm consists four parts:

1. Head.
2. Neck.
3. Body.
4. Tail.

1. Head

Head of sperm is oval in shape (in front view), with a length of 3 to 5 μ and width of up to 3 μ. Anterior portion of head is thin **(Fig. 58.8)**.

Head is formed by thin cytoplasm with a condensed nucleus and it is covered by a thin cell membrane. Anterior two thirds of the head appear like a thick cap and it is called **acrosome**. Acrosome develops from Golgi apparatus and it is made up of mucopolysaccharide and acid phosphatase. It also contains **hyaluronidase** and

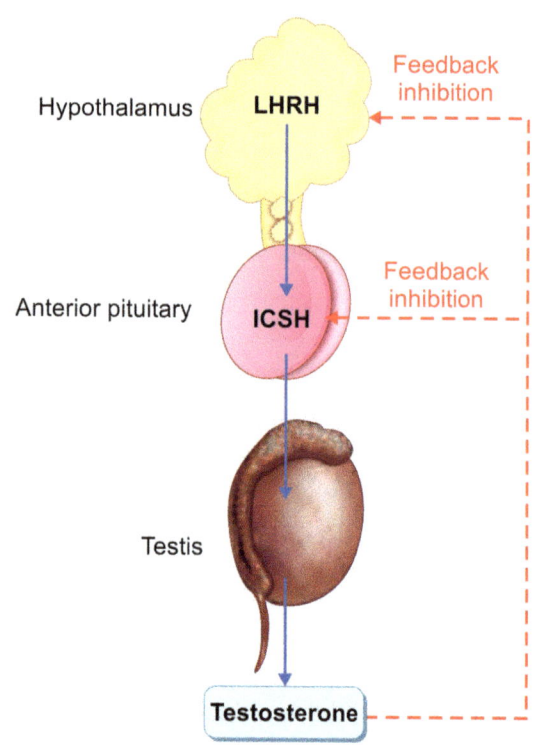

FIGURE 58.6: Regulation of testosterone secretion. LHRH = Luteinizing hormone-releasing hormone, ICSH = Interstitial cell-stimulating hormone.

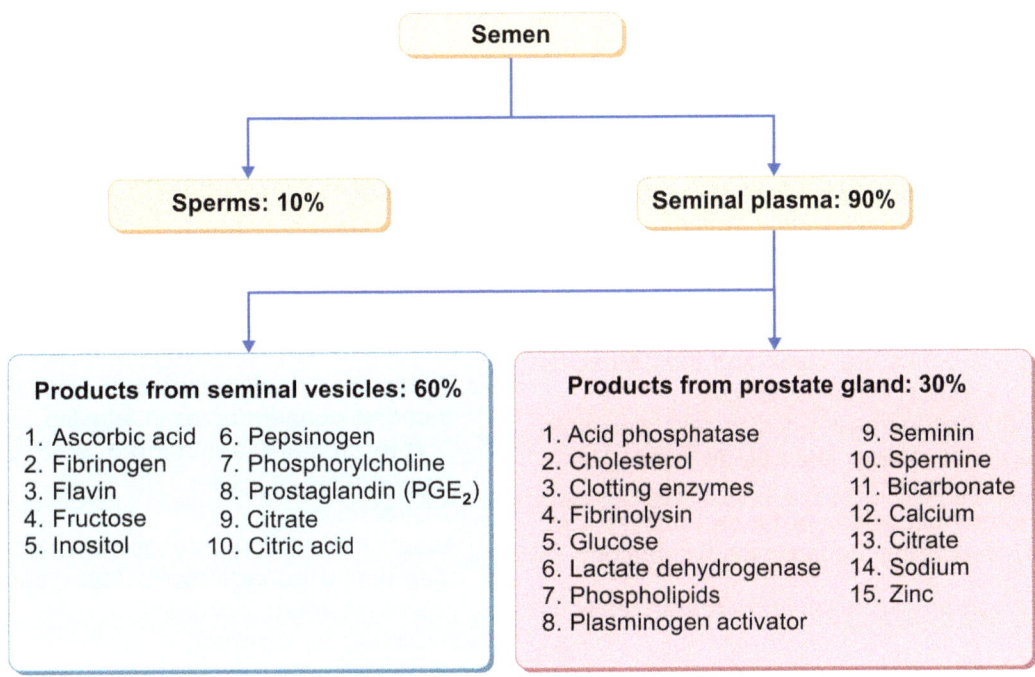

FIGURE 58.7: Composition of semen.

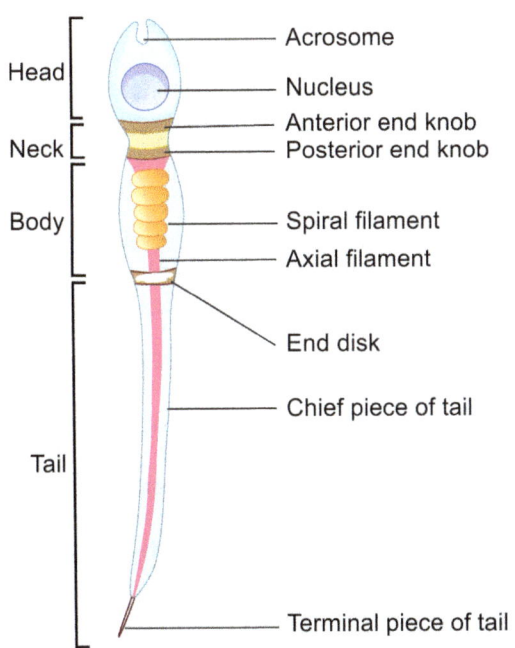

FIGURE 58.8: Human sperm.

proteolytic enzymes which are essential for the sperm to fertilize the ovum.

2. Neck

Head is connected to the body by a short neck. Anterior end of the neck is formed by thick disk-shaped **anterior end knob**, which is also called proximal centriole. Posterior end of neck is formed by another similar structure known as **posterior end knob**. It gives rise to the **axial filament** of body.

Often, the neck and body of sperm are together called **midpiece**.

3. Body

It is cylindrical with a length of 5 to 9 μ and the thickness of 1 μ. Body of the sperm consists of a central core called axial filament covered by thin cytoplasmic capsule.

Axial filament starts from posterior end knob of the neck. It passes through the body and a perforated disk called end disk or end ring centriole. Finally, axial filament reaches the tail as **axial thread**.

In the body, axial filament is surrounded by a closely wound **spiral filament** consisting of mitochondria.

4. Tail

Tail of the sperm consists of two segments:

i. **Chief or main piece** of tail which is enclosed by cytoplasmic capsule and has an axial thread. It is 40 μ to 50 μ long.
ii. **Terminal or end piece** of tail that has only the axial filament.

■ MALE CLIMACTERIC

Male andropause or climacteric is the condition in men characterized by emotional and physical changes in the body due to low androgen level with aging. It is also called **viropause**. After the age of 50, testosterone secretion starts declining because of decrease in number and secretory activity of Leydig cells.

APPLIED PHYSIOLOGY

EFFECTS OF EXTIRPATION OF TESTES

Removal of tests is called **castration**. Effects of castration depend upon the age when testes are removed.

1. Effects of Extirpation of Testes before Puberty: Eunuchism

If a boy loses the testes before puberty, he continues to have **infantile sexual characters** throughout life. This condition is called eunuchism. Height of the person is slightly more but the bones are weak and thin. Muscles become weak and shoulder remains narrow.

Sex organs do not increase in size and the male secondary sexual characters do not develop. Voice remains like that of a child.

There is abnormal deposition of fat on buttocks, hip, pubis and breast, resembling the feminine distribution.

2. Effects of Extirpation of Testes Immediately after Puberty

If testes are removed after puberty, some of the male secondary sexual characters revert to those of a child and other masculine characters are retained.

Functions of sex organs are suppressed. Seminal vesicles and prostate undergo atrophy. Penis remains smaller. Voice remains mostly masculine but other secondary sexual characters like masculine hair distribution, musculature and thickness of bones are lost. There may be loss of sexual desire and sexual activities.

3. Effect of Extirpation of Testes in Adults

Removal of testis in adults does not cause loss of secondary sexual characters. But accessory sex organs start degenerating. Sexual desire is not totally lost. Erection occurs but ejaculation is rare because of degeneration of accessory sex organs and lack of sperms.

HYPERGONADISM IN MALES

Hypergonadism is the condition characterized by hypersecretion of sex hormones from gonads.

Cause of Hypergonadism

Hypergonadism in males is mainly due to the tumor of Leydig cells. It is common in **prepubertal boys** who develop precocious **pseudopuberty**.

Symptoms of Hypergonadism

There is rapid growth of musculature and bones. But, height of the person is less because of early closure of epiphysis. There is excess development of sex organs and secondary sexual characters.

Tumors also secrete estrogenic hormones which cause **gynecomastia** (enlargement of breasts).

HYPOGONADISM IN MALES

Hypogonadism is a condition characterized by reduction in the functional activity of gonads.

Causes of Hypogonadism

Hypogonadism in males is due to various abnormalities of testes:

1. Congenital non-functioning of testes.
2. Under developed testes due to absence of human chorionic gonadotropins in fetal life.
3. Cryptorchidism associated with partial or total degeneration of testes.
4. Castration.
5. Absence of androgen receptors in testes.
6. Disorder of gonadotrophs (cells secreting gonadotropins) in anterior pituitary.
7. Hypothalamic disorder.

Signs and Symptoms of Hypogonadism

Clinical picture of male hypogonadism depends upon whether the testicular deficiency develops before or after puberty.

Before puberty

Features of hypogonadism are similar to those developed due to extirpation of testes before puberty, which are described above.

After puberty

Symptoms are similar to those developed due to the removal of testes after puberty (see above).

In adults

Same symptoms, which develop after extirpation of testis, occur in this condition.

Hypogonadism caused by testicular disorders increases the gonadotropin secretion and the condition is called **hypergonadotropic hypogonadism**. Hypogonadism that occurs due to deficiency of gonadotropins (pituitary or hypothalamic disorder) is called **hypogonadotropic hypogonadism**.

Dystrophia adiposogenitalis

It is the disorder characterized by obesity and hypogonadism in adolescent boys. It is also called **Fröhlich's syndrome** or **hypothalamic eunuchism**. Refer Chapter 50 for details.

Chapter 59: Female Reproductive System

CHAPTER OUTLINE

- FEMALE REPRODUCTIVE ORGANS
- FUNCTIONAL ANATOMY OF OVARY
- ACCESSORY SEX ORGANS IN FEMALES
- UTERUS
- CERVIX
- VAGINA
- FUNCTIONS OF OVARY
- OVARIAN HORMONES
- SEXUAL LIFE IN FEMALES
- CLIMACTERIC AND MENOPAUSE

FEMALE REPRODUCTIVE ORGANS

Female reproductive system comprises primary sex organs and accessory sex organs **(Figs. 59.1 and 59.2)**.

Primary sex organs are a pair of **ovaries**, which produce eggs or **ova** and secrete female sex hormones, the estrogen and progesterone. Accessory sex organs are given below.

FUNCTIONAL ANATOMY OF OVARY

Ovaries are flattened ovoid bodies with dimensions of 4 cm in length, 2 cm in width and 1 cm in thickness. On cross section, each ovary shows two zones:

1. Medulla.
2. Cortex.

MEDULLA

Medulla of ovary or **zona vasculosa** is the inner portion of ovary. It has the stroma of loose connective tissues. It contains blood vessels, lymphatics, nerve fibers and bundles of smooth muscle fibers near the hilum.

CORTEX

Cortex is the outer broader portion of ovary and it has compact cellular layers. Cortex is covered by **germinal**

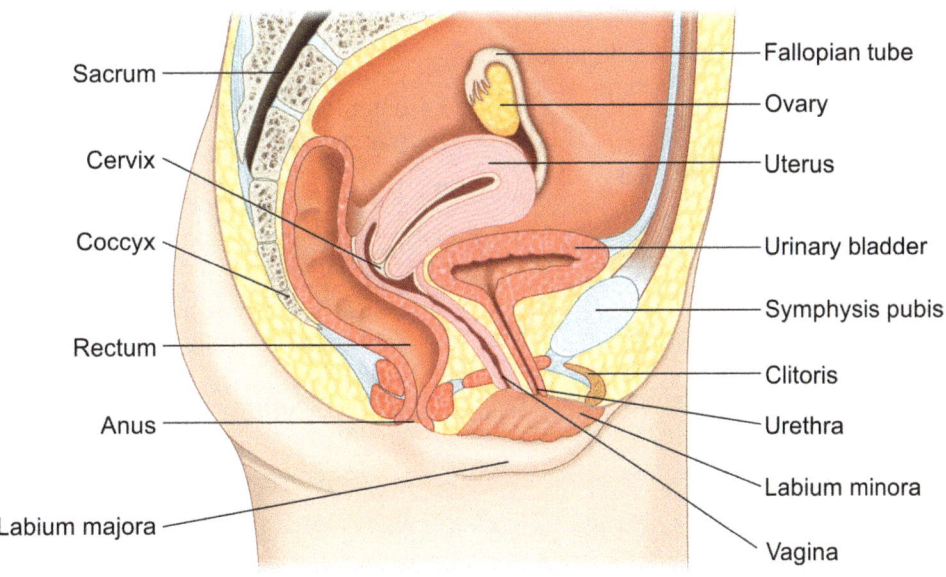

FIGURE 59.1: Female reproductive organs and other organs of pelvis.

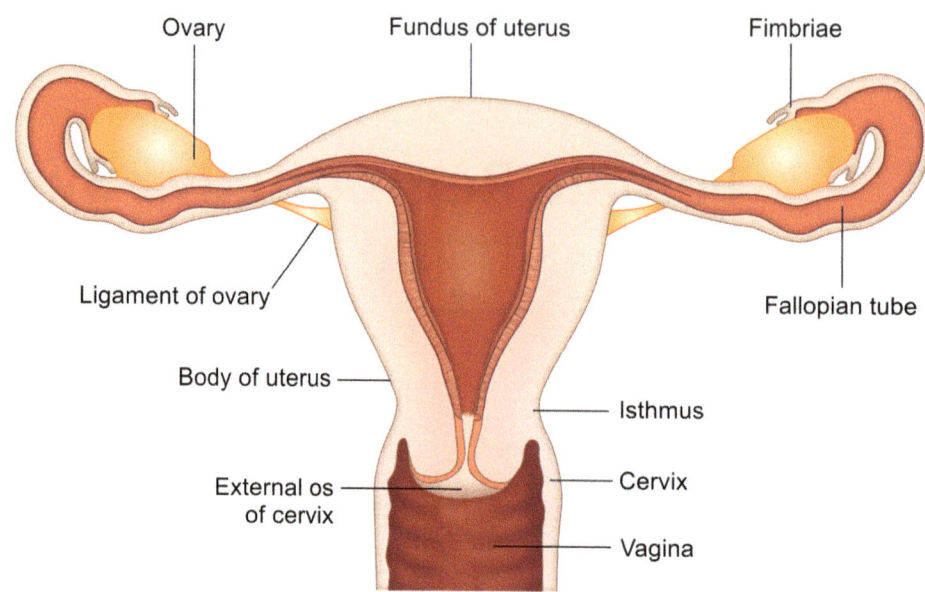

FIGURE 59.2: Female reproductive system.

epithelium underneath a fibrous layer known as **tunica albuginea**. Cortex consists of ovarian follicles at different stages, connective tissue and interstitial cells.

When the fetus develops, **primary germ cells** called **oogonia** develop from germinal epithelium. Oogonia give rise to **immature ova** called **primary oocytes**. Primary oocytes move towards the inner substance of cortex. A layer of **granulose cells** from ovarian stroma surrounds each primary oocyte. Primary oocyte along with granulosa cells is called the **primordial follicle**.

At 7th or 8th month of intrauterine life, about 6 million primordial follicles are found in the ovary. But, at the time of birth, only 1 million primordial follicles are seen in both the ovaries. Remaining follicles degenerate. At the time of puberty, number reduces further to about 3,00,000 to 4,00,000. After menarche, during every menstrual cycle, one of the follicles matures and releases its ovum. Only one ovum is released from any one of the ovaries during each menstrual cycle.

During every cycle, many of the follicles degenerate and become **atretic follicles** which disappear without leaving any scar.

■ ACCESSORY SEX ORGANS IN FEMALES

Accessory sex organs in females are:

1. A system of genital ducts that includes fallopian tubes, uterus, cervix and vagina.
2. External genitalia which are labia majora, labia minora and clitoris.

Mammary glands are not the female genital organs but are the important glands of female reproductive system.

■ UTERUS

Uterus is otherwise known as **womb**. It lies in the pelvic cavity, in between the rectum and urinary bladder. Uterus is a hollow muscular organ with a thick wall. It has a central cavity, which opens into **vagina** through **cervix**. On either side at its upper part, the **fallopian tubes** open. Uterus communicates with peritoneal cavity through fallopian tubes. There is a constriction almost at the middle of uterus called **isthmus**.

Divisions of Uterus

Uterus is divided into three portions:

1. Fundus (above the entrance points of fallopian tubes).
2. Body (between fundus and isthmus).
3. Cervix (below isthmus).

Structure of Uterine Wall

Uterine wall made up of three layers of structures:

1. Outer serous layer or **perimetrium** derived from peritoneum.
2. Middle muscular layer or **myometrium** made up of smooth muscle fibers.
3. Inner mucus layer or **endometrium** made up of ciliated columnar epithelial cells, connective tissue and uterine glands **(Fig. 59.3)**.

■ CERVIX

Cervix is the lower constricted part of uterus. It is divided into two portions:

1. Upper **supravaginal portion** which communicates with body of uterus through **internal os** (orifice) of cervix.
2. Lower **vaginal portion** which communicates with vagina through **external os**.

■ VAGINA

Vagina is a short tubular organ. It is lined by mucous membrane which is formed by stratified epithelial cells.

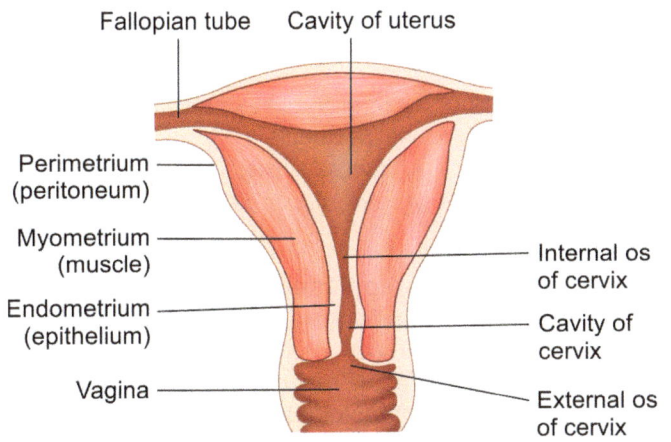

FIGURE 59.3: Section of uterus.

■ FUNCTIONS OF OVARY

Functions of ovaries are:

1. Secretion of female sex hormones.
2. Oogenesis.
3. Menstrual cycle.

Sex hormones and oogenesis are discussed later in this Chapter. Menstrual cycle is explained in the next Chapter.

■ OOGENESIS

Definition

Oogenesis is the process of origin and development of female gamete ovum. Oogenesis is different from spermatogenesis.

Spermatogenesis is continuous process that occurs in testes. Matured sperms are released from testes. Oogenesis that occurs in ovary is not a continuous process. Immature ovum is released from ovary and becomes matured only after fertilization.

Stages of Oogenesis

1. Stage of proliferation

In fetus, cells of germinal epithelium that covers the ovary undergo repeated mitotic division to form diploid **oogonia**. All the oogonia are formed during fetal life itself and not after birth.

2. Stage of growth

Oogonia give rise to **immature ova** called **primary oocytes**. Each primary oocyte is enclosed in primordial ovarian follicle (see above). Primary oocyte has diploid number (23 pairs) of chromosomes.

3. Stage of maturation

Just before ovulation, meiotic division takes place. Primary oocyte divides into a **secondary oocyte** and a **first polar body**. First polar body is expelled out. Secondary oocyte contains only 23 chromosomes (haploid). Remaining 23 chromosomes are lost in the expelled first polar body.

After ovulation the secondary oocyte is released into abdominal cavity because of rupture of Graafian follicle (Chapter 60). Then, the secondary oocyte enters fallopian tube through fimbriated end.

When fertilization occurs, the secondary oocyte divides into a **matured ovum** and a **second polar body**. Second polar body is expelled. Matured ovum has 23 chromosomes.

■ OVARIAN HORMONES

Ovary secretes the female sex hormones estrogen and progesterone. Ovary also secretes few more hormones namely, inhibin, relaxin and small quantities of androgens.

■ ESTROGEN

In a normal non-pregnant female, estrogen is secreted in large quantity by **theca interna** cells of ovarian follicles and in small quantity by **corpus luteum** of the ovaries. A small quantity of estrogen is also secreted by **adrenal cortex**. During pregnancy, a large amount of estrogen is secreted by the **placenta**. Estrogen is a C18 steroid.

Forms of Estrogen

Estrogen is present in three forms in plasma:

1. β-estradiol.
2. Estrone.
3. Estriol.

Quantity and potency of β-estradiol are more than those of estrone and estriol. Plasma level of estrogen in females at normal reproductive age varies during different phases of menstrual cycle. In follicular phase, it is 30 to 200 pg/mL **(Fig. 60.6)**. In normal adult male estrogen level is 12 to 34 pg/mL.

Functions of Estrogen

Major function of the estrogen is to promote cellular proliferation and tissue growth in sex organs and in other tissues related to reproduction.

Effects of estrogen are given below.

1. Effect on ovarian follicles

Estrogen promotes the growth of ovarian follicles by increasing the proliferation of the follicular cells. It also increases the secretory activity of theca cells. Refer Chapter 60 for details.

2. Effect on uterus

Estrogen produces the following changes in uterus:

i. Enlargement of uterus to about double of its childhood size by the proliferation of endometrial cells.
ii. Increase in the blood supply to endometrium.
iii. Deposition of glycogen and fats in endometrium.
iv. Proliferation and dilatation of blood vessels of endometrium.

v. Proliferation and dilatation of the endometrial glands, which become more tortuous with increased blood flow.
vi. Increase in the spontaneous activity of the uterine muscles and their sensitivity to oxytocin.
vii. Increase in the contractility of the uterine muscles due to increase in actomyosin concentration.
All these changes prepare uterus for pregnancy.

3. Effect on fallopian tubes

Estrogen:

i. Acts on mucosal lining of fallopian tubes and increases the number and size of epithelial cells, especially ciliated epithelial cells lining the fallopian tubes.
ii. Increases the activity of cilia, so that the movement of ovum in fallopian tube is facilitated.
iii. Enhances the proliferation of glandular tissues in fallopian tubes.
All these changes are necessary for fertilization of ovum.

4. Effect on vagina

Estrogen:

i. Changes the vaginal epithelium from cuboidal into stratified type. Stratified epithelium is more resistant to trauma and infection.
ii. Increases the layers of vaginal epithelium by proliferation.
iii. Reduces the pH of vagina making it more acidic.

All these changes are necessary for prevention of certain common vaginal infections such as gonorrheal vaginitis. Such infections can be cured by administration of estrogen.

5. Effect on secondary sexual characters

Estrogen is responsible for the development of secondary sexual characters in females.

Secondary sexual characters in female are:

i. *Hair distribution:* Hair develops in the pubic region and axilla. In females, pubic hair has the base of triangle upwards. Body hair growth is less. Scalp hair grows profusely.
ii. *Skin:* Skin becomes soft and smooth. Vascularity also increases in skin.
iii. *Body shape:* Shoulders become narrow, hip broadens, the thighs converge and the arms diverge. Fat deposition increases in the breasts and buttocks.
iv. *Pelvis:* Estrogen has a specific effect on pelvis which results in:
   a. Broadening of pelvis with increased transverse diameter.
   b. Round or oval shaped pelvis
   c. Round or oval shaped pelvic outlet.
   Thus, pelvis in females is different from that of males, which is funnel-like shaped.
v. *Voice:* Larynx remains in prepubertal stage, which produces high-pitch voice.

6. Effect on breast

Estrogen causes:

i. Development of stromal tissues of breasts.
ii. Growth of an extensive ductile system.
iii. Deposition of fat in ductile system.
All these effects prepare the breasts for lactation.

7. Effect on bones

Estrogen increases **osteoblastic activity**. So, at the time of puberty, the growth rate increases enormously. But, at the same time, estrogen causes early **fusion of epiphysis** with the shaft. This effect is much stronger in the females than the similar effect of testosterone in males. As a result, growth of females usually ceases few years earlier than in the males.

In old age, the estrogen is not secreted or it becomes scanty. It leads to **osteoporosis** by which the bones become extremely weak and fragile. And, because of this, the bones are highly susceptible for fractures (Chapter 52).

8. Effect on metabolism

i. *On protein metabolism:* Estrogen induces **anabolism of proteins** by which it increases the total body protein.
ii. *On fat metabolism:* Estrogen causes **deposition of fat** in the subcutaneous tissues, breasts, buttocks and thighs.

9. Effect on electrolyte balance

Estrogen causes sodium and water retention from the renal tubules. This effect is normally insignificant but in pregnancy, it becomes more significant.

Mode of Action of Estrogen

Estrogen acts through genes.

Regulation of Estrogen Secretion

Secretion of estrogen is regulated by **follicle stimulating hormone (FSH)** released from anterior pituitary. Release of FSH is stimulated by the **gonadotropin releasing hormone (GnRH)** secreted from hypothalamus.

FSH stimulates the secretory activities of theca and granulosa cells. Estrogen inhibits secretion of FSH and GnRH by negative feedback. Inhibin secreted by granulosa cells (Chapter 60) also decreases estrogen secretion by inhibiting secretion of FSH and GnRH **(Fig. 59.4)**.

■ PROGESTERONE

A small quantity of progesterone is secreted by **theca interna** cells of ovarian follicles during the first half of menstrual cycle, i.e. during follicular stage. But, a large quantity of progesterone is secreted during the latter half of each menstrual cycle, i.e. during secretory phase by the **corpus luteum**. Small amount of progesterone is secreted from **adrenal cortex** also.

During pregnancy, a large amount of progesterone is secreted by **corpus luteum** in the first trimester. In the second trimester corpus luteum degenerates. **Placenta**

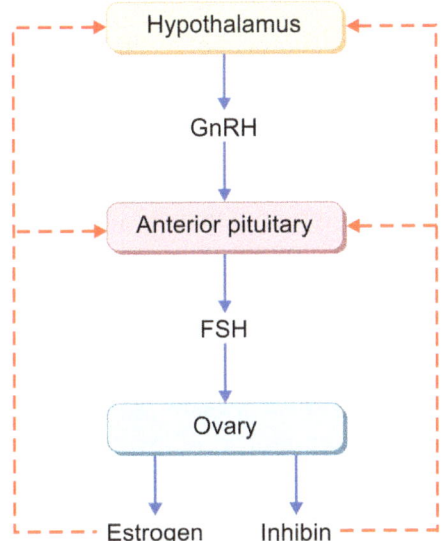

FIGURE 59.4: Regulation of estrogen secretion.
Red dashed lines = Inhibition.

secretes large quantity of progesterone in second and third trimesters.

Progesterone is a C21 steroid. Plasma level of progesterone in females at normal reproductive age varies during different phases of menstrual cycle. In follicular phase, it is about 0.9 ng/mL **(Fig. 60.6)**. In normal adult male progesterone level is 0.3 ng/mL.

Functions of Progesterone

Progesterone is concerned mainly with final preparation of the uterus for pregnancy and the breasts for lactation.

Effects of progesterone are given below.

1. Effect on fallopian tubes

Progesterone promotes secretory activities of mucosal lining of the fallopian tubes. Secretions of fallopian tubes are necessary for nutrition of the fertilized ovum while it is in fallopian tube before implantation.

2. Effect on uterus

Progesterone promotes secretory activities of uterine endometrium during the secretory phase of the menstrual cycle.

Thus, the uterus is prepared for implantation of fertilized ovum by the following actions of progesterone.

Progesterone:

i. Increases thickness of endometrium by increasing the number and size of cells.
ii. Increases size of uterine glands and make them become more tortuous.
iii. Increases secretory activities of epithelial cells of uterine glands.
iv. Increases deposition of lipid and glycogen in the stromal cells of endometrium.
v. Increases the blood supply to endometrium.

vi. Decreases the frequency of uterine contractions during pregnancy. Because of this, expulsion of implanted ovum is prevented.

3. Effect on cervix

Progesterone increases thickness of cervical mucosa and thereby inhibits transport of sperm into uterus. This effect is utilized in the contraceptive actions of mini pills.

4. Effect on mammary glands

Progesterone promotes development of the lobules and alveoli of mammary glands by proliferating and enlarging the alveolar cells. It also makes the breasts secretory in nature. It makes the breasts to swell by increasing the secretory activity and fluid accumulation in subcutaneous tissue.

5. Thermogenic effect

Progesterone increases the body temperature after ovulation. The mechanism of thermogenic action is not known. It is suggested that progesterone increases the body temperature by acting on hypothalamic centers for temperature regulation.

6. Effect on respiration

During luteal phase of menstrual cycle and during pregnancy, progesterone increases the ventilation via respiratory center. This results in decreased partial pressure of carbon dioxide in the alveoli.

Mode of Action of Progesterone

Like estrogen, progesterone also acts through genes.

Regulation of Secretion of Progesterone

Luteinizing hormone (LH) from anterior pituitary activates the corpus luteum to secrete progesterone. Secretion of LH is influenced by the **gonadotropin releasing hormone (GnRH)** secreted in hypothalamus. Progesterone inhibits release of LH from anterior pituitary by negative feedback.

SEXUAL LIFE IN FEMALES

Lifespan of a female is divided into three periods.

FIRST PERIOD

First period extends from birth to puberty. During this period, primary and accessory sex organs do not function. These organs remain quiescent. Puberty occurs at the age of 12 to 15 years.

SECOND PERIOD

Second period extends from onset of puberty to the onset of menopause. First menstrual cycle is known as **menarche**. Permanent stoppage of the menstrual cycle in old age is called **menopause**, which occurs at the age of about 45 to 50 years. During the period between menarche and menopause, women menstruate and reproduce.

THIRD PERIOD

Third period extends after menopause to the rest of the life.

CLIMACTERIC AND MENOPAUSE

Climacteric is the period in old age when reproductive system undergoes changes due to the decreased secretion of sex hormones estrogen and progesterone. It occurs at the age of 45 to 55. In females, climacteric is accompanied by menopause.

Menopause is defined as the period characterized by permanent cessation of menstruation. Normally, it occurs at the age of 45 to 55 years.

In some women, the menstruation stops suddenly. In others, the menstrual flow decreases gradually during every cycle and finally it stops. Sometimes irregular menstruation occurs with lengthening or shortening of the period with less or more flow.

Early menopause may occur because of surgical removal of ovaries (ovariectomy) or uterus (hysterectomy) as a part of treatment for abnormal menstruation. Usually, females with short menstrual cycle attain menopause earlier than the females with longer cycle. Cigarette smoking causes earlier onset of menopause.

CHANGES DURING MENOPAUSE: POSTMENOPAUSAL SYNDROME

Postmenopausal syndrome is the group of symptoms that appear in women immediately after menopause. It is characterized by certain physical, physiological and psychological changes. Symptoms start appearing soon after the ovaries stop functioning.

Cause for symptoms is the lack of estrogen and progesterone. The symptoms may persist till the body gets acclimatized to absence of estrogen and progesterone. Symptoms do not appear in all women. Some women develop mild symptoms and some women develop severe symptoms. Symptoms last for few months to few years.

Most of the women manage it very well. But, about 15% of the women need treatment. In many cases, **psychotherapy** works very well. If it fails, **hormone replacement therapy** is given.

Chapter 60: Menstrual Cycle

CHAPTER OUTLINE

- **DEFINITION, DURATION AND CHANGES**
  - DEFINITION
  - DURATION OF MENSTRUAL CYCLE
  - CHANGES DURING MENSTRUAL CYCLE
- **OVARIAN CHANGES DURING MENSTRUAL CYCLE**
  - FOLLICULAR PHASE
  - OVULATION
  - LUTEAL PHASE
- **UTERINE CHANGES DURING MENSTRUAL CYCLE**
  - MENSTRUAL PHASE
  - PROLIFERATIVE PHASE
  - SECRETORY PHASE
- **CHANGES IN CERVIX DURING MENSTRUAL CYCLE**
  - PROLIFERATIVE PHASE
  - SECRETORY PHASE
- **CHANGES IN VAGINA DURING MENSTRUAL CYCLE**
  - PROLIFERATIVE PHASE
  - SECRETORY PHASE
- **REGULATION OF MENSTRUAL CYCLE**
  - HORMONES INVOLVED IN REGULATION
- **APPLIED PHYSIOLOGY: MENSTRUAL DISORDERS**
  - MENSTRUAL SYMPTOMS
  - PREMENSTRUAL SYNDROME
  - ABNORMAL MENSTRUATION
  - ANOVULATORY CYCLE

DEFINITION, DURATION AND CHANGES

DEFINITION

Menstrual cycle is defined as the cyclic events that take place in a rhythmic fashion during the reproductive period of a woman's life. Menstrual cycle starts at the age of 12 to 15 years, which marks the onset of puberty. Commencement of menstrual cycle is called **menarche**. Menstrual cycle ceases at the age of 45 to 50 years. Permanent cessation of menstrual cycle in old age is called **menopause**.

DURATION OF MENSTRUAL CYCLE

Duration of menstrual cycle is usually 28 days. But, under physiological conditions, it may vary between 20 and 40 days.

CHANGES DURING MENSTRUAL CYCLE

Series of changes occur in ovary and accessory sex organs during each menstrual cycle. All the changes place simultaneously.

Changes taking place during menstrual cycle are:

I. Ovarian changes.
II. Uterine changes.
III. Vaginal changes.
IV. Changes in cervix.

OVARIAN CHANGES DURING MENSTRUAL CYCLE

Changes in ovary during menstrual cycle occur in two phases:

1. Follicular phase.
2. Luteal phase.

FOLLICULAR PHASE

Follicular phase extends from 5th day of cycle until the time of ovulation, which takes place on 14th day. During this phase development of ovarian follicles and maturation of ovum take place.

Ovarian Follicles

Ovarian follicles are glandular structures present in the cortex of ovary. Each follicle consists of an immature ovum surrounded by epithelial cells called **granulosa cells**. The follicles gradually grow into a matured follicle through various stages.

Different follicles are:

1. Primordial follicle.
2. Primary follicle.
3. Vesicular follicle.
4. Matured follicle or Graafian follicle.

1. Primordial Follicle

At the time of puberty, both the ovaries contain about 4,00,000 primordial follicles. Diameter of primordial follicle is about 15 to 20 μ and that of ovum is about 10 μ. Each primordial follicle has an immature ovum which is incompletely surrounded by the **granulosa cells (Fig. 60.1)**. Granulosa cells provide nutrition to ovum during childhood.

Granulosa cells also secrete **oocyte maturation inhibiting factor** which keeps the ovum in the immature stage. All the ova present in ovaries are formed before birth. No new ovum is developed after birth.

During onset of puberty, under the influence of **follicle stimulating hormone (FSH)** and **luteinizing hormone (LH)** the primordial follicles start growing through various stages.

2. Primary Follicle

Primordial follicle becomes the primary follicle, when ovum is completely surrounded by the granulosa cells. During this stage the follicle and ovum inside the follicle increase in size. Diameter of this follicle increases to 30 to 40 μ and that of ovum increases to about 20 μ. Primary follicle is not covered by a definite connective tissue capsule.

Characteristic changes taking place during development of primary follicles are:

i. Proliferation of granulosa cells and increase in size of the follicle.
ii. Increase in size of ovum.
iii. Onset of formation of connective tissue capsule around the follicle.
Primary follicles develop into vesicular follicles.

3. Vesicular Follicle

Under the influence of FSH, about 6 to 12 primary follicles start growing and develop into the vesicular follicles.

During development of vesicular follicles, many changes take place in granulosa cells and ovum. And a covering sheath called theca folliculi is formed around the follicle.

Changes in granulosa cells

i. First, the proliferation of granulosa cells occurs.
ii. A cavity called **follicular cavity** or **antrum** is formed in between the granulosa cells.
iii. Antrum is filled with a serous fluid called the **liquor folliculi**.
iv. Ovum is pushed to one side and it is surrounded by granulosa cells which forms the **germ hill** or **cumulus oophorus**.
v. Granulosa cells which line the antrum form **membrana granulosa**.
vi. Cells of germ hill become columnar and form **corona radiata**.

Changes in ovum

i. First, the ovum increases in size and its diameter increases to 100 to 150 μ.
ii. Nucleus becomes larger and vesicular.
iii. Cytoplasm becomes granular.
iv. Thick membrane is formed around the ovum which is called **zona pellucida**.
v. A narrow cleft called **perivitelline space** appears between ovum and zona pellucida.

Formation of theca folliculi

Spindle cells from the stroma of ovarian cortex are modified and form a covering sheath around the follicle. This covering sheath is known as **follicular sheath** or **theca folliculi**.

Theca folliculi divides into two layers:

i. *Theca interna*

It is the inner vascular layer with loose connective tissue and epithelial cells with lipid granules. Epithelial cells become secretory in nature and start secreting the female

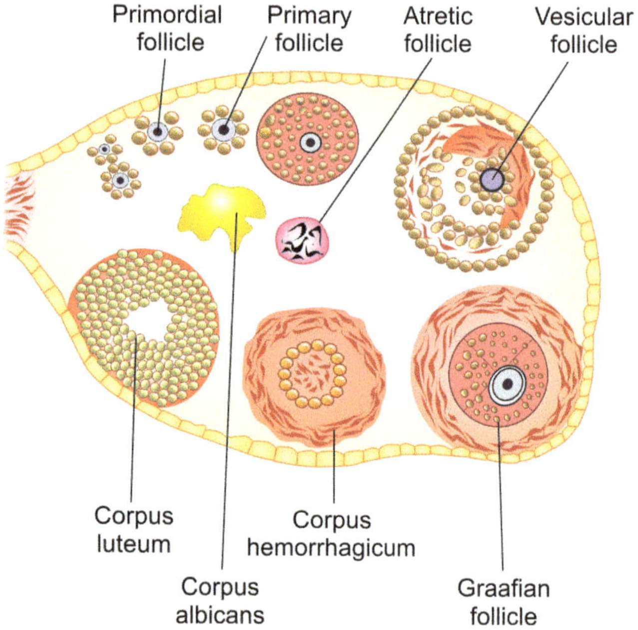

FIGURE 60.1: Ovarian follicles and corpus luteum.

sex hormones, especially estrogen which is released into the fluid of antrum.

ii. Theca externa

It is the outer layer of follicular capsule and consists of thickly packed fibers and spindle shaped cells.

After about 7th day of menstrual cycle, one of the vesicular follicles outgrows the others and becomes **dominant follicle**. It develops further to form graafian follicle. Other vesicular follicles degenerate by means of **apoptosis**.

4. Graafian Follicle

Graafian follicle is the matured ovarian follicle with maturing ovum. It is named after the Dutch physician and anatomist **Regnier De Graaf (Fig. 60.2)**. Many changes take place during the development of graafian follicle:

i. Size of the follicle increases to about 10 to 12 mm.
ii. At one point, follicle encroaches upon tunica albuginea and protrudes upon the surface of ovary. This protrusion is called **stigma**. At the stigma, tunica albuginea becomes thin.
iii. Follicular cavity becomes larger and distended with fluid.
iv. Ovum attains maximum size.
v. Zona pellucida becomes thick.
vi. Corona radiata becomes prominent.
vii. Small spaces filled with fluid appear between the cells of germ hill outside the corona radiata. These spaces weaken the attachment of the ovum to the follicular wall.
viii. Theca interna becomes prominent. Its thickness becomes double with formation of rich capillary network.
ix. On 14th day of menstrual cycle, the graafian follicle is ready for the process of ovulation.

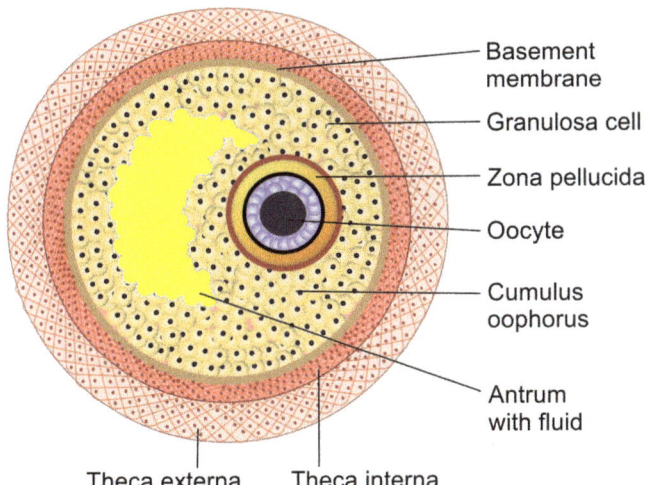

FIGURE 60.2: Graafian follicle.

■ OVULATION

Ovulation is the process by which Graafian follicle is ruptured with consequent discharge of ovum into abdominal cavity. Ovulation occurs usually on 14th day of menstrual cycle in a normal cycle of 28 days.

The ovum, which is released into abdominal cavity, enters the fallopian tube through fimbriated end of tube. Usually, only one ovum is released from any one of the ovaries. LH is responsible for ovulation.

Prior to ovulation, large amount of LH is secreted **(LH surge)** which causes changes in the Graafian follicle leading to ovulation.

LH Surge

LH surge is defined as rapid increase in secretion of luteinizing hormone 24 to 48 hours prior to ovulation.

Stages of Ovulation

1. Graafian follicle moves towards the periphery of ovary.
2. New blood vessels are formed in the ovary by actions of LH and progesterone.
3. The new blood vessels protrude into the wall of the follicle.
4. This increases the blood flow to the follicle.
5. Now, prostaglandin is released from granulosa cells of the follicle.
6. It causes leakage of plasma into the follicle.
7. Just before ovulation, the follicle swells and protrudes against the capsule of the ovary. This protrusion is called stigma.
8. Then, progesterone activates the proteolytic enzymes present in the cells of theca interna.
9. These enzymes weaken the follicular capsule and cause degeneration of the stigma.
10. After about 30 minutes, fluid begins to ooze from the follicle through the stigma.
11. It decreases the size of the follicle causing rupture of stigma.
12. Now, ovum is released from the follicle along with fluid and plenty of small granulosa cells into the abdominal cavity **(Fig. 60.3)**.

Determination of Ovulation Time

Ovulation time can be determined by the following methods:

1. *By determining basal body temperature*: There is a slight fall in the basal temperature just prior to ovulation. And, the temperature increases after ovulation. Alteration in the temperature is very mild and it is about ± 0.3 to 0.5°C.
2. *By determining hormonal excretion in urine*: This test is used determine LH excretion in urine or increased salt content in saliva due to estrogen. Urine test is the most common. During LH surge prior to ovulation, large quantity of hormone is excreted in urine. Detection of LH surge can help determine time of ovulation. This tests is called ovulation predictor test.

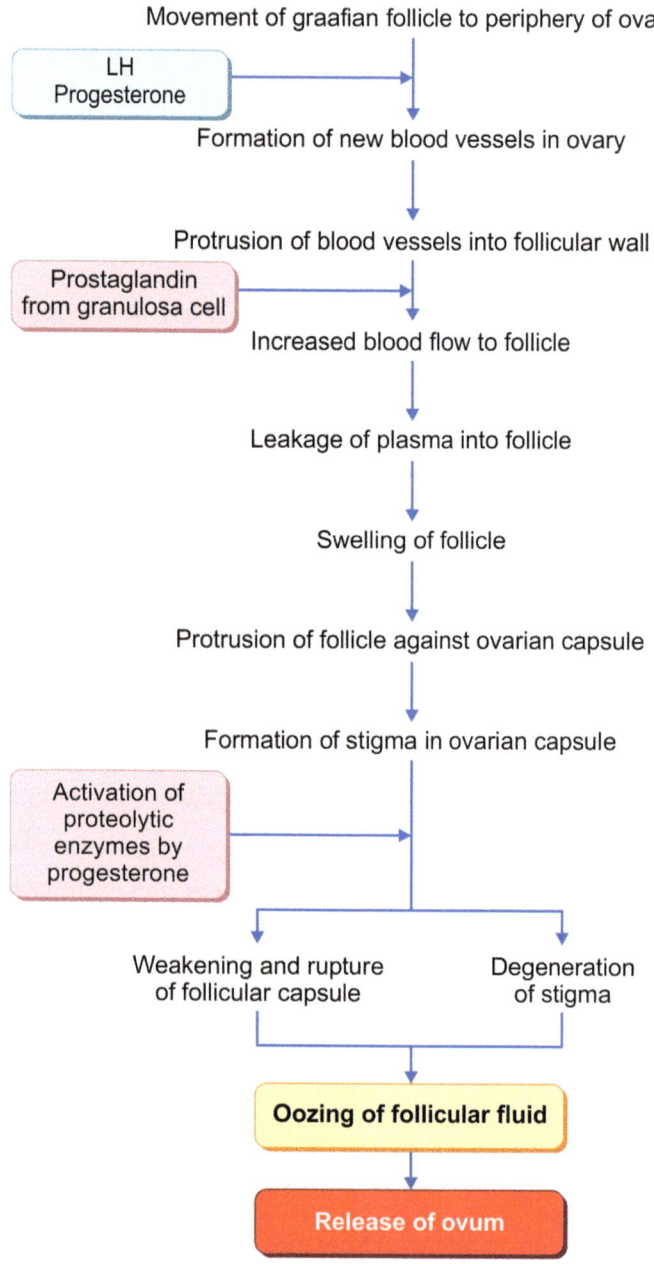

FIGURE 60.3: Process of ovulation.
LH = Luteinizing hormone.

3. *By determination of hormonal level in plasma:* Plasma level of FSH, LH, estrogen and progesterone is altered at the time of ovulation and after ovulation.
4. *Ultrasound scanning:* Process of ovulation is observed by ultrasound scanning.
5. *Cervical mucus pattern:* When the cervical mucus spread on a slide is examined under microscope, it shows a fern pattern. This pattern disappears after ovulation.

Significance of Determining Ovulation Time

Family planning by rhythm method may be well adopted by determination of ovulation time (Chapter 63).

■ LUTEAL PHASE

Luteal phase extends between 15th and 28th day of menstrual cycle. During this phase corpus luteum is developed and hence the name luteal phase **(Fig. 60.4)**.

Corpus Luteum

Corpus luteum is a glandular yellow body developed from the ruptured graafian follicle after the release of ovum. It is also called **yellow body**.

Development of Corpus Luteum

Soon after the rupture of graafian follicle and release of ovum, the follicle is filled with blood. Now the follicle is called **corpus hemorrhagicum**. Blood clots slowly and corpus hemorrhagicum is transformed into a corpus luteum.

In the corpus luteum, the granulosa cells and theca interna cells are transformed into **lutein cells** namely granulosa lutein cells and theca lutein cells by accumulation of fine lipid granules and the yellowish pigment granules. These yellowish pigment granules give the characteristic yellow color to corpus luteum.

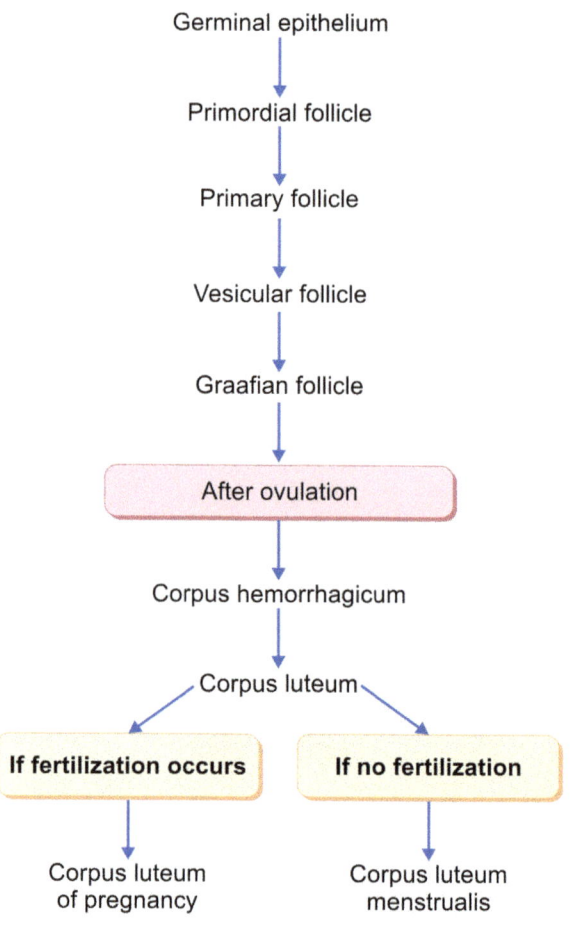

FIGURE 60.4: Schematic diagram showing different ovarian follicles and corpus luteum.

Functions of Corpus Luteum

1. Secretion of hormones

Corpus luteum acts as a **temporary endocrine gland**. It secretes large quantity of progesterone and small amount of estrogen. LH influences the secretion of these two hormones.

2. Maintenance of pregnancy

If pregnancy occurs, corpus luteum maintains the pregnancy for about 3 months of pregnancy till placenta starts secreting estrogen and progesterone. Abortion occurs if corpus luteum becomes inactive or removed before 3rd month of pregnancy, i.e. before placenta starts secreting the hormones.

Fate of Corpus Luteum

Fate of corpus luteum depends upon whether ovum is fertilized or not.

If the ovum is not fertilized

If fertilization does not take place, corpus luteum reaches the maximum size about 1 week after ovulation. During this period, it secretes large quantity of progesterone with small quantity of estrogen. Then, it degenerates into the **corpus luteum menstrualis**. Cells decrease in size and the corpus luteum becomes smaller and involuted. Afterwards, the corpus luteum menstrualis is transformed into a whitish scar called **corpus albicans**. The process by which corpus luteum undergoes regression is called **luteolysis**.

If ovum is fertilized

If ovum is fertilized and pregnancy occurs, the corpus luteum persists and increases in size. It attains a diameter of 20 to 30 mm and it is transformed into **corpus luteum graviditatis (verum)** or **corpus luteum of pregnancy** **(Fig. 60.4)**. It remains in the ovary for 3 to 4 months. During this period, it secretes large amount of progesterone with small quantity of estrogen, which are essential for the maintenance of pregnancy. After 3 to 4 months, placenta starts secreting these hormones and corpus luteum degenerates.

■ UTERINE CHANGES DURING MENSTRUAL CYCLE

During each menstrual cycle, along with ovarian changes, uterine changes also occur simultaneously.

Uterine changes in uterus take place in three phases:

1. Menstrual phase.
2. Proliferative phase.
3. Secretory phase.

■ MENSTRUAL PHASE

After ovulation, if pregnancy does not occur, the thickened endometrium is shed or desquamated. This desquamated endometrium is expelled out through vagina along with some blood and tissue fluid. The process of shedding and exit of uterine lining along with blood and fluid is called **menstruation** or **menstrual bleeding**. It lasts for about 4 to 5 days **(Fig. 60.5)**. This period is called menstrual phase or menstrual period. It is also called **menses**, **emmenia** or **catamenia**.

The day when bleeding starts is considered as the 1st day of the menstrual cycle. Two days before onset of bleeding, that is on 26th or 27th day of the previous cycle, there is sudden reduction in the release of estrogen and progesterone from ovary. Decreased level of these two hormones is responsible for menstruation.

Changes in Endometrium During Menstrual Phase

1. Lack of estrogen and progesterone causes sudden involution of endometrium.
2. It leads to reduction in the thickness of endometrium, up to 65% of original thickness.
3. During the next 24 hours, the tortuous blood vessels in the endometrium undergo severe constriction.

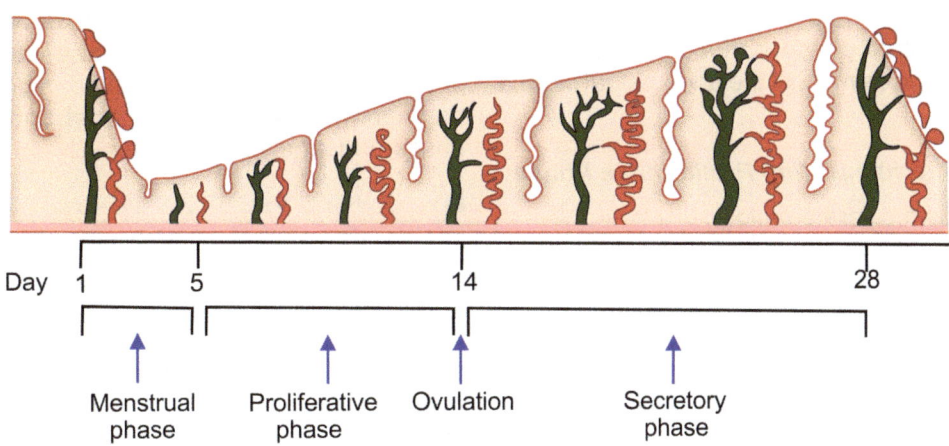

FIGURE 60.5: Uterine changes during menstrual cycle.

Endometrial vasoconstriction is because of three reasons:
   a. Involution of endometrium.
   b. Actions of vasoconstrictor substances like prostaglandin, released from tissues of involuted endometrium.
   c. Sudden lack of estrogen and progesterone (which are vasodilators).
4. Vasoconstriction leads to hypoxia, which results in **necrosis** of the endometrium.
5. Necrosis causes rupture of blood vessels and oozing of blood.
6. Outer layer of the **necrotic endometrium** is separated and passes out along with blood.
7. This process is continued for about 24 to 36 hours.
8. Within 48 hours after the reduction in secretion of estrogen and progesterone, superficial layers of endometrium are completely desquamated.
9. Desquamated tissues and the blood in endometrial cavity initiate the contraction of uterus
10. Uterine contractions expel the blood along with **desquamated uterine tissues** to the exterior through vagina.

During normal menstruation, about 35 mL of blood along with 35 mL of **serous fluid** is expelled. The blood clots as soon as it oozes into the uterine cavity. **Fibrinolysin** causes **lysis of clot** in uterine cavity itself so that, the expelled menstrual fluid does not clot. However, in pathological conditions involving uterus, the lysis of blood clot does not occur. So, the menstrual fluid comes out with blood clot.

Menstruation stops between 3rd and 7th day of menstrual cycle. At the end of menstrual phase, the thickness of endometrium is only about 1 mm. This is followed by proliferative phase.

■ PROLIFERATIVE PHASE

Proliferative phase extends usually from 5th to 14th day of menstruation, i.e. between the day when menstruation stops and the day of ovulation. It corresponds to the follicular phase of ovarian cycle.

At the end of menstrual phase, only a thin layer (1 mm) of endometrium remains as most of the endometrial stroma is desquamated.

Changes in Endometrium During Proliferative Phase

1. Endometrial cells proliferate rapidly.
2. Epithelium reappears on the surface of endometrium within the first 4 to 7 days.
3. Uterine glands start developing within the endometrial stroma.
4. Blood vessels also appear in the stroma.
5. Proliferation of endometrial cells occurs continuously so that the endometrium reaches the thickness of 3 to 4 mm at the end of proliferative phase.

All these uterine changes during proliferative phase occur because of the influence of estrogen released from ovary. On 14th day, **ovulation** occurs under the influence of LH. This is followed by secretory phase.

■ SECRETORY PHASE

Secretory phase extends between 15th and 28th day of the menstrual cycle, i.e. between the day of ovulation and the day when menstruation of next cycle commences.

After ovulation, corpus luteum is developed in the ovary. It secretes a large quantity of progesterone along with a small amount of estrogen. Estrogen causes further proliferation of cells in uterus. Because of this, endometrium becomes very thick. Progesterone causes further enlargement of endometrial stroma and further growth of glands.

Under the influence of progesterone, endometrial glands commence their secretory function. Many changes occur in the endometrium before commencement of secretory function.

Changes in Endometrium During Secretory Phase

1. Endometrial glands become more tortuous. Because of increase in size, the glands become tortuous to get accommodated within the endometrium.
2. Cytoplasm of stromal cells increases because of the deposition of glycogen and lipids.
3. Many new blood vessels appear within endometrial stroma. Blood vessels also become tortuous.
4. Blood supply to endometrium increases.
5. Thickness of endometrium increases up to 6 mm.

Actually, secretory phase is the preparatory period during which, uterus is prepared for **implantation** of ovum. At the end of secretory phase, the thickness of endometrium is 5 to 6 mm. All these uterine changes during secretory phase occur due to the influence of estrogen and progesterone. Estrogen is responsible for repair of damaged endometrium and growth of the glands. Progesterone is responsible for further growth of these structures and secretory activities in the endometrium **(Table 60.1)**.

If a **fertilized ovum** is implanted during this phase and, if the implanted ovum starts developing into a **fetus**, further changes occur in the uterus for the survival of the developing fetus. If the implanted ovum is unfertilized or if pregnancy does not occur, **menstruation** occurs after this phase and a new cycle begins.

■ CHANGES IN CERVIX DURING MENSTRUAL CYCLE

Mucous membrane of cervix also shows cyclic changes during different phases of menstrual cycle.

■ PROLIFERATIVE PHASE

Under the influence of estrogen, during proliferative phase, mucous membrane of cervix becomes thin and **alkaline**. It helps in the survival and motility of spermatozoa.

TABLE 60.1: Menstrual cycle in nutshell.

Organ changes	Phase and hormones involved	Event	Process
Ovarian changes	Follicular phase (5th to 14th day) FSH, LH and E	Maturation of ovum	Ovarian follicle → Primordial follicle → Primary follicle → Vesicular follicle → Graafian follicle
		Release of ovum (ovulation)	Rupture of Graafian follicle → Release of ovum into abdominal cavity
	Luteal phase (15th to 28th day) FSH, LH, E and P	Formation of corpus luteum	Ruptured Graafian follicle → Corpus hemorrhagicum → Corpus luteum
Uterine changes	Menstrual phase (1st to 5th day) Increased E and P Lack of FSH and LH	Desquamation and expulsion of endometrium	Involution of endometrium → Vasoconstriction and hypoxia → Rupture of blood vessels → Necrosis of endometrium → Expulsion of desquamated endometrium → Thinning of endometrium to 1 mm
	Proliferative phase (6th to 14th day) E and P	Increase in the thickness of endometrium	Proliferation of endometrial cells → Development of uterine glands and blood vessels → Increase in the thickness of endometrium to 3 to 4 mm
	Secretory phase (15th to 28th day) E and P	Preparation of uterus to receive fertilized ovum	Increase in number and size of blood vessels and uterine glands → Increase in blood supply → Tortuosity of blood vessels and uterine glands → Deposition of lipid and glycogen in endometrium → Increase in thickness of endometrium to 6 mm
Cervical changes	Proliferative phase	Helps in survival and motility of sperm	Mucous membrane becomes thinner and more alkaline
	Secretory phase	Holding the sperms	Mucous membrane becomes thick and adhesive
Vaginal changes	Proliferative phase	Increase in resistance for infections	Cornification of epithelial cells
	Secretory phase		Proliferation of epithelial cells and infiltration with leukocytes

FSH = Follicle stimulating hormone, LH = Luteinizing hormone, E = Estrogen, P = Progesterone.

■ SECRETORY PHASE

Because of actions of progesterone during secretory phase, the mucous membrane of cervix becomes thick and adhesive.

■ CHANGES IN VAGINA DURING MENSTRUAL CYCLE

■ PROLIFERATIVE PHASE

Epithelial cells of vagina are **cornified**. Estrogen released from ovary is responsible for the cornification of vaginal epithelial cells.

■ SECRETORY PHASE

Vaginal epithelium proliferates due to the actions of progesterone. Vaginal epithelium is **infiltrated with leukocytes**. These two changes increase the resistance for infection.

■ REGULATION OF MENSTRUAL CYCLE

Menstrual cycle is regulated hormones of hypothalamo-pituitary-ovarian axis.

■ HORMONES INVOLVED IN REGULATION

Hormones involved in regulation of menstrual cycle are:
1. Hypothalamic hormone: GnRH.
2. Anterior pituitary hormones: FSH and LH.
3. Ovarian hormones: Estrogen and progesterone.

Hypothalamic Hormone

Gonadotropin releasing hormone (GnRH) from hypothalamus triggers the onset of cyclic changes during menstrual cycle by stimulating secretion of follicle stimulating hormone (FSH) and luteinizing hormone (LH) from anterior pituitary.

Anterior Pituitary Hormones

FSH and LH secreted from anterior pituitary modulate the ovarian and uterine changes by acting directly and/or indirectly via ovarian hormones. FSH stimulates the recruitment and growth of immature ovarian follicles. LH triggers ovulation and sustains corpus luteum.

Secretion of FSH and LH is under the influence of GnRH.

Ovarian Hormones

Estrogen and progesterone which are secreted by follicle and corpus luteum show many activities during menstrual cycle. Ovarian follicle secretes large quantity of estrogen and corpus luteum secretes large quantity of progesterone.

Estrogen secretion reaches the peak twice in each cycle; once during follicular phase just before ovulation and another one during luteal phase (**Fig. 60.6**). On the other hand, progesterone is virtually absent during follicular phase till prior to ovulation. But, it plays a critical role during luteal phase.

Estrogen is responsible for the growth of follicles. Both the steroids act together to produce the changes in uterus, cervix and vagina.

Both the ovarian hormones are under the influence of GnRH which acts via FSH and LH. In addition, the secretion of GnRH, FSH and LH is regulated by ovarian hormones.

■ APPLIED PHYSIOLOGY: MENSTRUAL DISORDERS

■ 1. MENSTRUAL SYMPTOMS

Menstrual symptoms are the unpleasant symptoms with discomfort, which appear in many women during menstruation. These symptoms are due to hormonal withdrawal, leading to cramps in uterine muscle before or during menstruation.

Common menstrual symptoms are abdominal pain, dysmenorrhea (menstrual pain), headache, irritability and depression.

■ 2. PREMENSTRUAL SYNDROME

Premenstrual syndrome (PMS) is the symptom of stress that appears before the onset of menstruation. It is also called premenstrual stress syndrome, premenstrual stress or premenstrual tension. It lasts for about 4 to 5 days prior to menstruation. Symptoms appear due to salt and water retention caused by estrogen.

Common symptoms of this condition are anxiety, emotional instability, headache, depression, constipation, abdominal cramping and bloating (abdominal swelling).

■ 3. ABNORMAL MENSTRUATION

Abnormal types of menstruation are listed in **Table 60.2**.

TABLE 60.2: Abnormal menstruation.

Abnormality	Feature
1. Amenorrhea	Absence of menstrual bleeding
2. Hypomenorrhea or scanty menstruation	Scanty and light menstrual bleeding
3. Menorrhagia or Heavy menstrual bleeding	Heavy and prolonged menstrual bleeding
4. Oligomenorrhea	Less menstrual bleeding with decreased frequency
5. Polymenorrhea	Increased frequency of menstrual bleeding with short menstrual cycle
6. Dysmenorrhea or painful periods or menstrual cramps	Menstruation with pain
7. Metrorrhagia	Abnormal uterine bleeding between menstruations

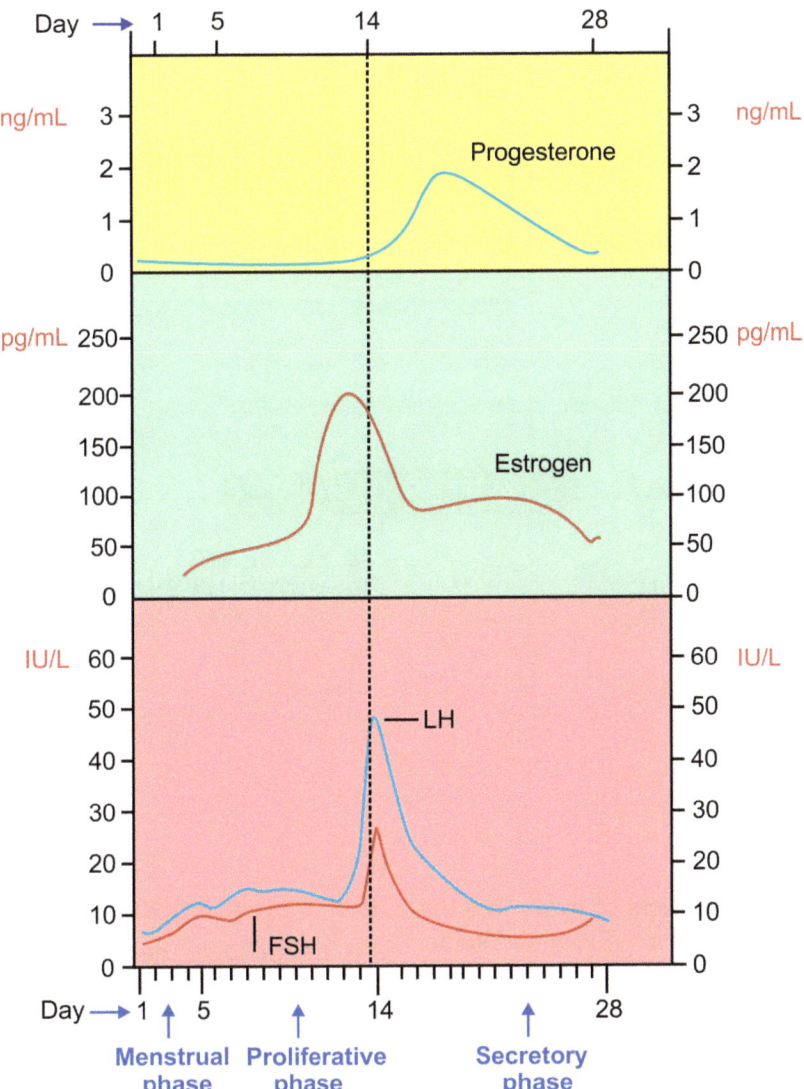

FIGURE 60.6: Hormonal level during menstrual cycle.
LH = Luteinizing hormones, FSH = Follicle-stimulating hormone.

4. ANOVULATORY CYCLE

Anovulatory cycle is the menstrual cycle in which ovulation does not occur. Menstrual bleeding occurs but the release of ovum does not occur. It is common during puberty and few years before menopause.

When it occurs before menopause, it is called **perimenopause**. If it occurs very often during child-bearing years, it leads to infertility.

61 CHAPTER

Pregnancy and Parturition

CHAPTER OUTLINE

- DEVELOPMENT OF OVUM
- FERTILIZATION OF THE OVUM
- SEX CHROMOSOMES AND SEX DETERMINATION
- IMPLANTATION AND DEVELOPMENT OF EMBRYO
- PLACENTA
- MATERNAL CHANGES IN PHYSIOLOGICAL SYSTEMS
- GESTATION PERIOD
- PARTURITION
- PREGNANCY TESTS

■ DEVELOPMENT OF OVUM

Ovum is released from Graafian follicle of ovary into the abdominal cavity at the time of ovulation. From abdominal cavity, ovum enters fallopian tube through the fimbriated end.

Ovum of matured follicle in the ovary is in **primary oocyte** stage with **diploid number** (23 pairs) of chromosomes. Just before ovulation, meiotic division takes place in the ovum. **Primary oocyte** divides into a **secondary oocyte** and a **first polar body**. First polar body is expelled out. Secondary oocyte contains only 23 chromosomes (haploid). Remaining 23 chromosomes are lost in the expelled first polar body.

Thus, when ovum is released into abdominal cavity during ovulation, it is in the **secondary oocyte stage** with haploid number of chromosomes.

■ FERTILIZATION OF THE OVUM

Fertilization is the fusion (union) of male and female gametes (sperm and ovum) to form a new offspring.

Ovum is released into abdominal cavity during ovulation. If sexual intercourse occurs at this time and semen is ejaculated in the vagina, sperms travel through vagina and uterus to reach the fallopian tube. Among 200 to 300 million of sperms entering female genital tract, only one succeeds in fertilizing the ovum.

During fertilization, the sperm enters the ovum by penetrating **granulosa cells** present around the ovum. It is facilitated by **hyaluronidase** and **proteolytic enzymes** present in the acrosome of sperm.

■ SEX CHROMOSOMES AND SEX DETERMINATION

■ SEX CHROMOSOMES

All the dividing cells in the body have 23 pairs of chromosomes. Among the 23 pairs, 22 pairs are called **somatic chromosomes** or **autosomes**. Remaining one pair of chromosomes is called **sex chromosomes**. Sex chromosomes are X and Y chromosomes.

■ SEX DETERMINATION

Sex chromosomes are responsible for sex determination. During fertilization of ovum, 23 chromosomes from ovum and 23 chromosomes from the sperm unite together to form the 23 pairs (46) of chromosomes in the fertilized ovum. Now, sex determination occurs. Ovum contains the X chromosome. Sperm has either X chromosome or Y chromosome. When the ovum is fertilized by a sperm with X chromosome, the child will be female with XX chromosome. And, if the ovum is fertilized by a sperm with Y chromosome, sex of the child will be male with XY chromosome. So, the sex of the child depends upon the male partner.

Role of testosterone in **sex differentiation** is explained in Chapter 58.

Abnormality of Sex Determination

Abnormalities in sex determination leads to following conditions:

1. **Hermaphroditism:** A congenital condition characterized by the presence of both male and female reproductive organs.

2. **Gonadal dysgenesis:** Defective development of gonads.

■ IMPLANTATION AND DEVELOPMENT OF EMBRYO

Implantation is the process by which the fertilized ovum implants (fixes itself or gets attached) in the endometrium of uterus. After fertilization, the ovum is known as **zygote**. Zygote takes 3 to 5 days to reach the uterine cavity from fallopian tube. While travelling through fallopian tube, the zygote receives its nutrition from the secretions of fallopian tube.

After reaching uterus, the developing zygote remains freely in uterine cavity for 2 to 4 days before it is implanted. Just before implantation, the zygote develops into **morula**.

Already uterus is prepared by progesterone secreted from the corpus luteum during secretory phase of menstrual cycle. After implantation, morula develops into **embryo**. Placenta develops between morula and endometrium.

■ PLACENTA

Placenta is a temporary membranous vascular organ that develops during pregnancy. It is expelled after child birth. Placenta forms a link between the fetus and mother. It is considered as an **anchor** for the growing fetus. It is not only the physical attachment between fetus and mother but also forms the **physiological connection** between the two.

Placenta is implanted in the wall of uterus. It is formed from both embryonic and maternal tissues. So, it consists of two parts namely **fetal part** and **mother's part**. It is connected to the fetus by **umbilical cord** which contains blood vessels and connective tissue.

Delivery of fetus is followed by the expulsion of placenta. After expulsion of placenta, the umbilical cord is cut. Site of attachment of placenta in the center of anterior abdomen of fetus is called **naval** or **umbilicus**.

■ FUNCTIONS OF PLACENTA

Nutritive Function

Nutritive substances, electrolytes and hormones necessary for the development of fetus diffuse from the mother's blood into fetal blood through placenta.

Excretory Function

Metabolic end products and other waste products from the fetal body are excreted into the mother's blood through placenta.

Respiratory Function

Fetal lungs are nonfunctioning and placenta forms the **respiratory organ** for fetus. Oxygen necessary for fetus is received by diffusion from maternal blood through placenta. And carbon dioxide from the fetal blood diffuses into mother's blood through placenta.

Endocrine Function

Placenta secretes five hormones:

1. Human chorionic gonadotropin.
2. Estrogen.
3. Progesterone.
4. Human chorionic somatomammotropin.
5. Relaxin.

1. *Human chorionic gonadotropin*

Human chorionic gonadotropin (hCG) is a glycoprotein.

Actions of hCG

i. On corpus luteum: This hormone is responsible for preservation and the secretory activity of corpus luteum. Progesterone and estrogen secreted by corpus luteum are essential for the maintenance of pregnancy. Deficiency or absence of hCG during the first 2 months of pregnancy leads to **termination of pregnancy** (**abortion**), because of involution of corpus luteum.

ii. On fetal testes: Action of hCG on fetal testes is similar to that of LH in adults. It stimulates the interstitial cells of Leydig and causes secretion of testosterone which is necessary for the development of sex organs in male fetus.

2. *Estrogen*

Placental estrogen is similar to ovarian estrogen in structure and function.

Actions of placental estrogen

i. On uterus: Estrogen causes enlargement of uterus, so that the growing fetus can be accommodated.
ii. On breasts: Estrogen is responsible for the enlargement of breasts and growth of duct system in the breasts.
iii. On external genitalia: It causes enlargement of the female external genitalia.
iv. On pelvis: Estrogen relaxes pelvic ligaments. It facilitates the passage of fetus through birth canal at the time of labor.

3. *Progesterone*

Placental progesterone is similar to ovarian progesterone in structure and function.

Actions of placental progesterone

i. On endometrium of uterus: Progesterone accelerates the proliferation and development of decidual cells in the endometrium of uterus. Decidual cells are responsible for the supply of nutrition to embryo in early stage.
ii. On the movements of uterus: Progesterone inhibits the contraction of muscles in pregnant uterus. It is an important function of progesterone, as it prevents expulsion of fetus during pregnancy.
iii. On breasts: Progesterone causes enlargement of breasts and growth of duct system of the breasts.

Progesterone is responsible for further development and preparation of mammary glands for lactation.

4. Human chorionic somatomammotropin

Human chorionic somatomammotropin (HCS) is a protein hormone secreted from placenta. It is often called **placental lactogen**. It acts like prolactin and growth hormone secreted from pituitary. So, it is believed to act on mammary glands and to enhance the growth of fetus by influencing the metabolic activities. It increases the amount of glucose and lipids in the maternal blood which are transferred to fetus.

Actions of human chorionic somatomammotropin

  i. On breasts: In experimental animals, administration of HCS causes enlargement of mammary glands and induces lactation. That is why, it is called mammotropin. However, action of this hormone on the breasts of pregnant women is not clear.
  ii. On protein metabolism: HCS acts like GH on protein metabolism. It causes anabolism of proteins and accumulation of proteins in the fetal tissues. Thus, the growth of fetus is enhanced.
  iii. On carbohydrate metabolism: It reduces the peripheral utilization of glucose in the mother leading to availability of large quantity of glucose to the growing fetus.
  iv. On lipid metabolism: HCS mobilizes fat from adipose tissue of the mother. A large amount of free fatty acid is made available as the source of energy in the mother's body. It compensates the loss of glucose from mother's blood to fetus.

5. Relaxin

Relaxin is a polypeptide which is secreted by corpus luteum. It is also secreted in large quantity by placenta and mammary glands at the time of labor.

FETOPLACENTAL UNIT

Fetoplacental unit is the interaction between fetus and placenta in the formation of steroid hormones. This type of interaction between fetus and placenta occurs, because some of the enzymes involved in steroid synthesis present in fetus are absent in placenta and, those enzymes which are absent in fetus are present in placenta.

Due to this interaction during synthesis of steroid hormones, fetus and placenta are together called fetoplacental unit **(Fig. 61.1)**.

MATERNAL CHANGES IN PHYSIOLOGICAL SYSTEMS DURING PREGNANCY

1. BLOOD

Blood volume increases by about 20% or about 1 L. It is because of increase in plasma volume. This leads to hemodilution. Because of great demand for iron by fetus, the mother usually develops anemia.

2. CARDIOVASCULAR SYSTEM

i. Cardiac Output

Cardiac output increases by about 30% in the first trimester. After the 3rd month, cardiac output starts decreasing and reaches almost the normal level in later stages of pregnancy.

ii. Blood Pressure

Arterial blood pressure remains unchanged during the first trimester. During the second trimester, there is a slight decrease in blood pressure. In third semester blood pressure increases. In some women, hypertension may develop if proper prenatal care is not taken.

Pre-eclampsia or toxemia of pregnancy

Pre-eclampsia or toxemia of pregnancy is the **hypertensive** disorder of pregnancy that occurs in 3 to 4% of the pregnant women. It usually occurs during last trimester of pregnancy.

Eclampsia

Eclampsia is the serious condition of pre-eclampsia characterized by severe **vascular spasm**, dangerous **hypertension** and **convulsions** almost like **seizures**. It occurs just before, during or immediately after delivery. It leads to **death**, if timely treatment is not given.

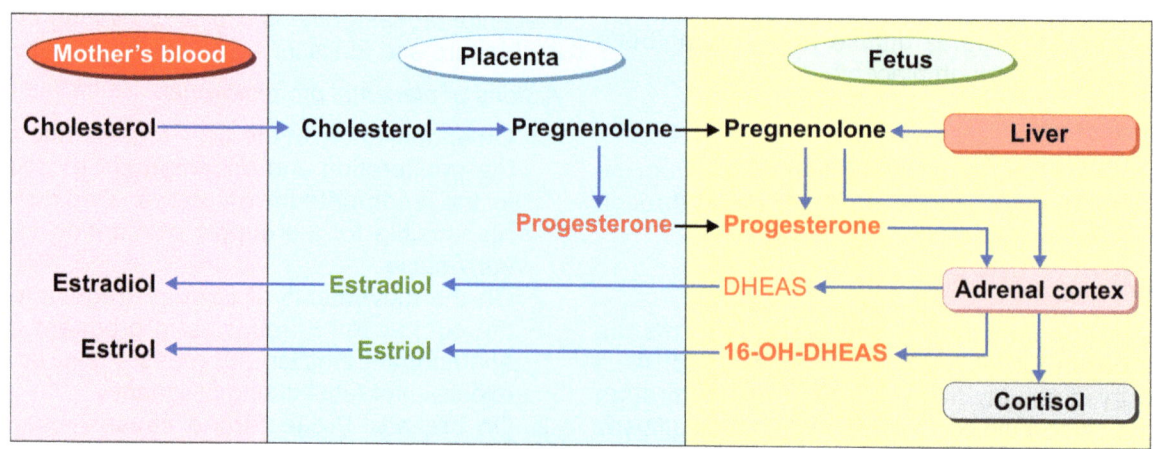

FIGURE 61.1: Fetoplacental unit.
DHEAS = Dehydroepiandrosterone sulfate, 16-OH-DHEAS = 16-hydroxy-dehydroepiandrosterone sulfate.

3. RESPIRATORY SYSTEM

Overall activity of respiratory system increases slightly. Tidal volume, pulmonary ventilation and oxygen utilization are increased.

4. EXCRETORY SYSTEM

Renal blood flow and glomerular filtration rate increase resulting in increase in urine formation. It is because of increase in fluid intake and the increased excretory products from fetus. Urine becomes diluted with the specific gravity of 1,025. In the first trimester, frequency of micturition increases.

5. DIGESTIVE SYSTEM

i. Morning Sickness

Morning sickness is the feeling of sickness during early part of pregnancy. It is characterized by **nausea, vomiting** and tiredness or **giddiness**. Morning sickness starts around 4 to 6 weeks of pregnancy and reaches the peak between 9 and 11 weeks. In most of the women symptoms disappear in 14 to 16 weeks.

Morning sickness is due to high level of **human chorionic gonadotropin (hCG)**.

ii. Other Changes in Digestive System

Indigestion and **hypochlorhydria** (decrease in the amount of hydrochloric acid in gastric juice) and constipation are also common during pregnancy.

6. ENDOCRINE SYSTEM

i. Anterior Pituitary

During pregnancy, size of anterior pituitary increases by about 50%. And secretion of corticotropin, thyrotropin and prolactin increases. However, the secretion of FSH and LH decreases very much. It is because of negative feedback control by estrogen and progesterone which are continuously secreted from corpus luteum initially and placenta later on.

ii. Adrenal Cortex

There is moderate increase in secretion of cortisol and aldosterone. Aldosterone is responsible for the retention of water and sodium.

iii. Thyroid Gland

Size and the secretory activity of thyroid gland increase during pregnancy.

iv. Parathyroid Gland

Parathyroid glands also show an increase in the size and secretory activity.

7. NERVOUS SYSTEM

There is general excitement of nervous system during pregnancy. It leads to the **psychological imbalance**, such as change in the moods, excitement or depression in the early stages of pregnancy. During the later months of pregnancy, the woman becomes very much excited because of anticipation of delivery of the baby, labor pain, etc.

GESTATION PERIOD

Gestation period means the pregnancy period. Average gestation period is about 280 days or 40 weeks from the date of **last menstrual period (LMP)**. Traditionally it is calculated as 10 lunar months. However, in terms of modern calendar, it is calculated as 9 months and 7 days. If the menstrual cycle is normal 28 days cycle, the fertilization of ovum by the sperm occurs on 14th day after last menstrual period.

Thus, the actual duration of human pregnancy is 280 – 14 = 266 days. If the pregnancy ends before 28th week, it is referred as **miscarriage**.

PARTURITION

Parturition is the expulsion or delivery of the fetus from mother's body. It occurs at the end of pregnancy. The process by which **delivery of fetus** occurs is called **labor**. It involves various actions, such as contraction of uterus, dilatation of cervix and opening of vaginal canal.

BRAXTON HICKS CONTRACTIONS

Braxton Hicks contractions are the weak, irregular, short and usually painless uterine contractions which start after 6th week of pregnancy. These contractions are named after the British doctor, who discovered them in 1872. It is suggested that such contractions do not induce cervical dilatation, but may cause softening of cervix. Often called the **practice contractions,** Braxton Hicks contractions help the uterus practice for upcoming labor. Sometimes these contractions cause discomfort.

FALSE LABOR CONTRACTIONS

While nearing the time of delivery, Braxton Hicks contractions become intense and are called **false labor contractions**. False labor contractions are believed to help cervical dilatation.

STAGES OF PARTURITION

Parturition occurs in three stages.

First Stage

First, strong uterine contractions called **labor contractions** commence. These labor contractions arise from the fundus of uterus and move downwards so that the head of fetus is pushed against the cervix. It results in dilatation of cervix and opening of vaginal canal. This stage extends for a variable period of time.

Second Stage

In this stage, the fetus is delivered out from uterus through cervix and vaginal canal. This stage lasts for about one hour.

Third Stage

During this stage, the **placenta** is detached from decidua and is expelled out from uterus. It occurs within 10 to 15 minutes after the delivery of the child.

■ PREGNANCY TESTS

Pregnancy test is the test used to detect or confirm pregnancy. Pregnancy tests are based on presence of **human chorionic gonadotropin (hCG)** in urine of woman suspected for pregnancy. Both biological and immunological tests are available to determine the presence of hCG in the urine of the pregnant woman. However, biological tests for pregnancy are replaced by immunological tests because of several disadvantages.

■ IMMUNOLOGICAL TESTS

Immunological tests are more accurate and the result is obtained quickly within few minutes. These tests are based on **double antigen-antibody reactions**. Most commonly performed immunological test is known as Gravindex test.

Principle

Principle is to determine the agglutination of sheep RBCs coated with hCG. Latex particles could also be used instead of sheep RBCs.

Requisites

Antiserum from rabbit

Urine from a pregnant woman is collected and hCG is isolated. This hCG is injected into a rabbit.

The rabbit develops antibodies against hCG. This antibody is called **hCG antibody** or **anti-hCG**. Rabbit's blood is obtained and serum is separated. Serum containing hCG antibody is called **rabbit antiserum** or **hCG antiserum**. It is readily available in the market.

Red blood cells from sheep

RBCs are obtained from sheep's blood and are coated with pure hCG obtained from urine of the pregnant women. Nowadays, instead of sheep's RBCs, the rubberized synthetic particles called the **latex particles** are used.

Urine

Fresh urine sample of the woman, who needs to confirm pregnancy, is collected.

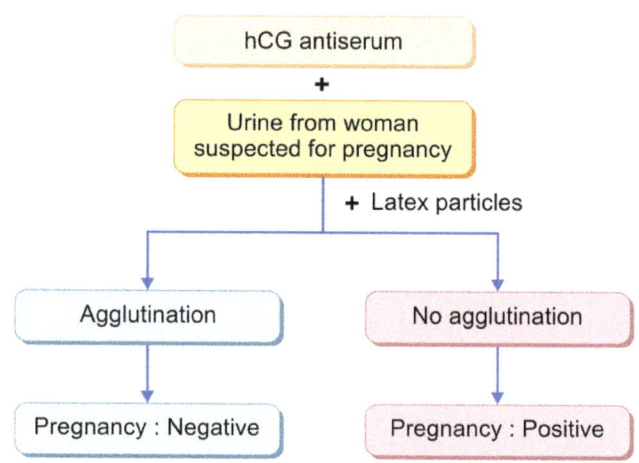

FIGURE 61.2: Immunological test for pregnancy.

Procedure

One drop of hCG antiserum is taken on a glass slide. One drop of urine from the woman who wants to confirm pregnancy is added to this and both are mixed well. If urine contains hCG, all the antibodies of antiserum are used up for agglutination of hCG molecules. The agglutination of hCG molecules by the antiserum is not visible, because it is colorless.

Now, one drop of latex particles is added to this and mixed.

Observation and Result

If the urine contains hCG, it is agglutinated by the antibodies of the antiserum, and all the antibodies are fully used up. No free antibody is available. Later when latex particles are added, these particles are not agglutinated because the free antibody is not available. Thus, the **absence of agglutination** of latex particles indicates that the woman is pregnant.

If the urine without hCG is mixed with antiserum, the antibodies are freely available. When latex particles are added, the antibodies cause agglutination of these latex particles. Agglutination of latex particles can be seen clearly even with naked eye. Thus, the **presence of agglutination** of latex particles indicates that the woman is not pregnant **(Fig. 61.2)**.

Nowadays **pregnancy test strip** is used. Advantage of this test strip is, it can be used even in the first few days of conception. Most sensitive test can detect hCG level as low as 20 mIU/mL.

Chapter 62: Mammary Glands and Lactation

CHAPTER OUTLINE

- DEVELOPMENT OF MAMMARY GLANDS
- ROLE OF HORMONES IN GROWTH OF MAMMARY GLANDS
- APPLIED PHYSIOLOGY: BENIGN BREAST DISEASE
- LACTATION
- BREAST MILK

DEVELOPMENT OF MAMMARY GLANDS

AT BIRTH

At the time of birth, mammary gland is rudimentary and consists of only a tiny nipple and few radiating ducts from it.

AT CHILDHOOD

Till puberty, there is no difference in the structure of mammary gland between male and female.

AT PUBERTY

At the time of puberty and afterwards there is a vast change in the structure of female mammary gland due to hormonal influence. The beginning of changes in the mammary gland is called **thelarche**. It occurs at the time of puberty, just before **menarche** (Chapter 60). At puberty, there is growth of duct system and formation of glandular tissue. Progressive enlargement occurs, which is also due to the deposition of fat.

DURING PREGNANCY

During pregnancy, the mammary glands enlarge to a great extent accompanied by marked changes in structure. During first half of pregnancy, the duct system develops further with appearance of many new alveoli. No milk is secreted by the gland now.

During the second half, there is enormous growth of glandular tissues and the development is completed for the production of milk just before the end of gestation period.

ROLE OF HORMONES IN GROWTH OF MAMMARY GLANDS

Various hormones are involved in the development and growth of breasts at different stages:

1. Estrogen which causes growth and branching of duct system and accumulation of fat in breasts.
2. Progesterone which stimulates the development of glandular tissues and stroma of mammary glands.
3. Prolactin that is necessary for milk secretion. It also accelerates growth of mammary glands during pregnancy by causing proliferation of epithelial cells of alveoli.
4. Placental hormones namely estrogen and progesterone cause further development of mammary glands during pregnancy by stimulating the proliferation of ducts and glandular cells.
5. Other hormones such as growth hormone, thyroxine, cortisol and relaxin enhance the overall growth and development of mammary glands in all stages.

APPLIED PHYSIOLOGY: BENIGN BREAST DISEASE

Benign breast disease is a group of conditions characterized by **noncancerous changes** in tissues of mammary glands. Some type of benign breast conditions may cause pain or discomfort and may need treatment.

Most of the conditions are not life-threatening. But some of the benign breast conditions have the **risk of cancer** development.

TYPES OF BENIGN BREAST DISEASE

1. *Fibroadenoma of breast*: A solid benign tumor formed by tissues of lobules and connective tissues of breast.
2. *Hyperplasia of breast*: Increase in proliferation of epithelial cells in lobules and duct system resulting in overgrowth of mammary glands.
3. *Cysts in breast*: Fluid-filled sacs formed in tissues of breasts.

4. *Intraductal papillomas*: Small tumors in dust system of mammary glands.
5. *Adenosis of breast*: Enragement of lobules due to increase number of glands of breast.
6. *Fat necrosis*: Formation of lumps by fat tissues caused due to injury of breast.

■ LACTATION

Lactation means synthesis, secretion and ejection of milk. It involves two processes:

A. Milk secretion.
B. Milk ejection.

■ A. MILK SECRETION

Milk secretion refers to **synthesis of milk** by alveolar epithelium and its passage through the duct system. This process occurs in two phases:

1. Initiation of milk secretion or lactogenesis.
2. Maintenance of milk secretion or galactopoiesis.

1. Initiation of Milk Secretion or Lactogenesis

Although small amount of milk secretion occurs at later months of pregnancy, a free flow of milk occurs only after the delivery of the child. The milk secreted initially before parturition is called **colostrum**.

Colostrum is lemon yellow in color and it is rich in protein (particularly globulins) and salts. But its sugar content is low. It contains almost all the components of milk except fat.

Role of hormones in lactogenesis

During pregnancy, particularly in later months, large quantity of prolactin is secreted. But the activity of this hormone is suppressed by estrogen and progesterone secreted from placenta. Because of this, lactation is prevented during pregnancy.

Immediately after the delivery of baby and expulsion of placenta, there is sudden lack of estrogen and progesterone. Now, the prolactin is free to exert its action on breasts and to promote lactogenesis.

2. Maintenance of Milk Secretion or Galactopoiesis

Galactopoiesis occurs up to 7 to 9 months after delivery of child provided feeding the baby with mother's milk is continued till then. In fact, the milk production is continued only if feeding the baby is continued.

Role of hormones in galactopoiesis

Galactopoiesis depends upon prolactin secretion. Other hormones like growth hormone, thyroxine and cortisol are essential for continuous supply of glucose, amino acids, fatty acids, calcium and other substances necessary for the milk production **(Fig. 62.1)**.

■ B. MILK EJECTION

Milk ejection is the discharge of milk from mammary gland. It depends upon suckling exerted by the baby and on contractile mechanism in breast, which expels milk from alveoli into the ducts.

Milk ejection is a reflex phenomenon. It is called milk ejection reflex or milk let down reflex. It is a neuroendocrine reflex.

Milk Ejection Reflex

Milk ejection reflex is explained in Chapter 50.

■ BREAST MILK

Breast or human milk forms the primary source of nutrition for infants.

■ COMPOSITION

Breast milk contains about 88.5% of water and 11.5% of solids.

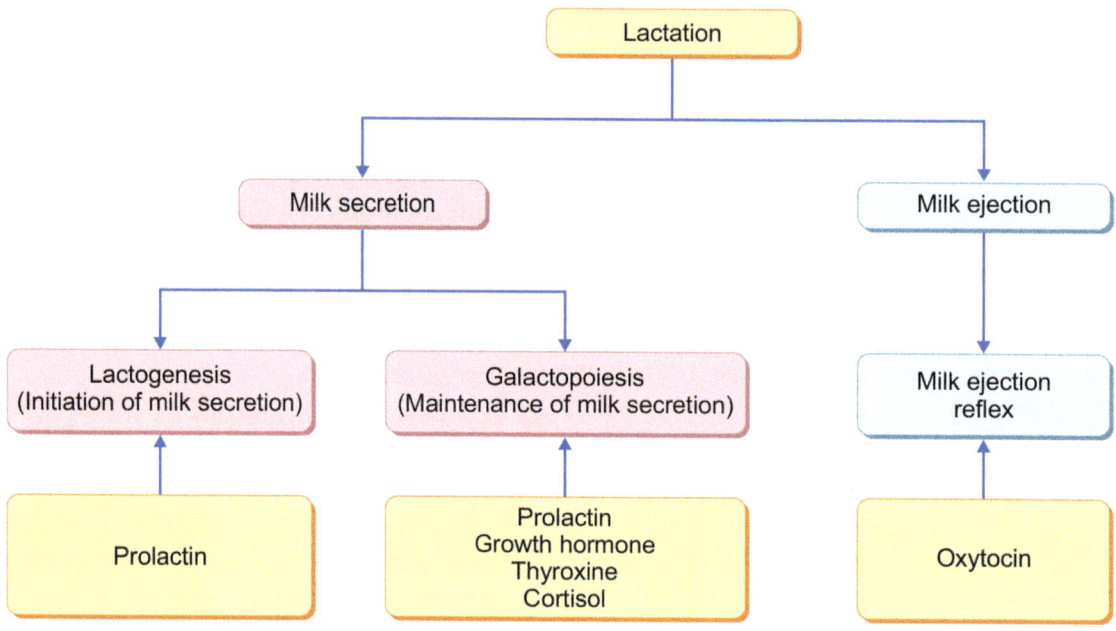

FIGURE 62.1: Process of lactation and role of hormones.

Solids include:

1. Nutrients: Lactose, casein, lactalbumin, lactoglobulin, cholesterol and essential fatty acids
2. Minerals: Sodium, calcium, potassium, magnesium, chloride, phosphorous, negligible quantity of iron and copper
3. Vitamins: A, B, C, D, E and K
4. Immunoglobulins: IgA, IgG and IgM
5. Antibacterial agents: Lysozyme and lactoferrin
6. Cells: Neutrophils and other leukocytes, macrophages and stem cells
7. Other substances: Digestive enzymes, hormones, transforming growth factor-β, interleukin-10 and insulin-like growth factor 1.

■ ADVANTAGES OF BREAST MILK

Breast milk is always considered superior to animal milk (cow milk or goat milk) because it consists of sufficient quantity of all the substances necessary for infants like iron, vitamins and minerals.

Besides nourishment of infant, the breast milk also provides several antibodies which help the infant resist the infection by lethal bacteria. Even some phagocytic cells, such as neutrophils and macrophages are secreted in milk. Phagocytic cells protect the infant by destroying microbes in the infant's body.

Chapter 63: Fertility Control

CHAPTER OUTLINE

- **CONTRACEPTIVE METHODS**
- **RHYTHM METHOD**
  - FERTILE PERIOD
  - INFERTILE PERIOD
  - ADVANTAGES AND DISADVANTAGES
- **BARRIER METHODS**
  - PHYSICAL BARRIERS
  - CHEMICAL BARRIERS
- **INTRAUTERINE CONTRACEPTIVE DEVICE (IUCD)**
  - TYPES OF IUCD
  - DISADVANTAGES
- **HORMONAL CONTRACEPTIVES**
  - ORAL CONTRACEPTIVES
  - HORMONAL IMPLANTS
  - OTHER HORMONAL CONTRACEPTIVES
- **MEDICAL TERMINATION OF PREGNANCY (MTP): ABORTION**
  - DILATATION AND CURETTAGE (D AND C)
  - VACUUM ASPIRATION
  - ADMINISTRATION OF PROSTAGLANDIN
- **SURGICAL METHOD (STERILIZATION): PERMANENT METHOD**
  - TUBECTOMY
  - VASECTOMY

CONTRACEPTIVE METHODS

Contraception means prevention of pregnancy. It is also called birth control, fertility control or family planning.

Contraceptive method or fertility control method is the method or device that is used by a woman to prevent pregnancy. Contraceptive methods may be temporary or permanent. Several methods are available for fertility control. Each method has its own advantages and disadvantages.

RHYTHM METHOD

Rhythm method of fertility control is based on the time of ovulation.

FERTILE PERIOD

After ovulation, i.e. on the 14th day of menstrual cycle, the ovum is fertilized during its passage through fallopian tubes. Its viability is only for 2 days after ovulation, and should be fertilized within this period.

Sperms survive only for about 24 to 48 hours after ejaculation in the female genital tract. If sexual intercourse occurs during this period, i.e. few days before and few days after ovulation, there is chance of pregnancy. This period is called fertile or **dangerous period**. Pregnancy can be avoided if there is no sexual intercourse during this period. Prevention of pregnancy by avoiding sexual mating during this period is called rhythm method.

INFERTILE OR STERILE OR SAFE PERIOD

Periods when pregnancy does not occur are 4 to 5 days after menstrual bleeding and 5 to 6 days before the onset of next cycle. These periods are together called infertile or sterile or **safe period.**

ADVANTAGES AND DISADVANTAGES OF RHYTHM METHOD

It is one of the most successful methods of fertility control, provided the woman knows exact day of ovulation. However, it is not a successful method because of various reasons. Basic knowledge about the menstrual cycle is necessary to determine the day of ovulation. Self restrain is essential to avoid sexual intercourse. Because of these practical difficulties, this method is not popular.

BARRIER METHODS

Barriers are used to prevent the entry of sperm into uterine cavity during sexual intercourse. Barriers are of two types namely, physical barriers and chemical barriers.

■ PHYSICAL BARRIERS

Physical barriers are:
1. Condoms.
2. Cervical cap.
3. Diaphragm.
4. Vaginal sponge.

1. Condom

Condom is one of the barriers used for contraception. It is available for both males and females.

Male condom

Condom is the commonly used barrier by men. Male condom is a thin leak-proof and stretchy pouch made of latex or plastic, polyurethane. It is fitted over erectile penis just before intercourse. It does not permit entrance of semen into the female genital tract during coitus.

Female condom

Female condom, also called **internal condom** is a soft pouch made of polyurethane. It is put inside vagina before intercourse, and it forms a barrier to stop sperm to meet the ovum.

Advantages of condoms

1. If used correctly, condoms are most effective contraceptive devices.
2. Condoms are the only contraceptive devices that protect against **sexually transmitted infections (STI)** including infection by **human immunodeficiency virus (HIV)**.
3. Used only at the time of intercourse.

Disadvantages of condoms

1. If not used correctly, condoms particularly in men may tear or slip off.
2. One or both partners may not feel comfortable with condom and may feel interference of condom with sex sensation.

2. Cervical Cap

Cervical cap is the commonly used barrier device in females. It is a small bowl-shaped cup made from latex or silicon. When inserted into the vagina it fits tightly over cervix. Cervical cap is mostly used with **spermicidal gel** or cream. **Spermicide** is a substance that kills sperms.

Advantages and disadvantages of cervical cap

Cervical cap does not contain hormone, but disadvantages are more. It is not an effective contraceptive device. Also, it does not protect against STI. Cervical cap is not available easily and it is also little difficult to insert.

3. Diaphragm

Diaphragm is a shallow flexible cup shaped device made up of soft silicon. It is inserted into vagina to cover the cervix. It is always used with **spermicidal agent**.

Advantages and disadvantages of diaphragm

For many women diaphragm is a safest device but does not protect from the spread of STI. Repeated use of spermicide along with diaphragm may irritate vagina and increase the risk of infection.

4. Vaginal Sponge

Vaginal sponge is a contraceptive sponge that prevents entry of sperm into uterus. It is a small disk-shaped sponge made up of soft polyurethane foam. It also contains spermicide. After insertion into vagina, it covers cervix tightly.

Advantages and disadvantages of vaginal sponge

Sponge is the most effective device when used correctly. However, it does not protect against STI.

■ CHEMICAL BARRIERS

Chemical barriers are the substances which are applied in female genital tract before coitus to destroy the sperms. Destruction of sperms is called **spermicidal action.** Spermicidal substances are available in the form of foam tablets, jelly, cream and paste which are inserted into vagina deep up to cervix. Common chemical substance present in spermicidal agents is **nonoxynol-9**. Chemical barriers have not become popular because of so many drawbacks.

Advantages and Disadvantages of Chemical Barriers

Any spermicide is cheap and easy to use. But most of the spermicides cause vaginal irritation. Nonoxynal-9 may be allergic to many women. It also increases the risk of getting infected by HIV.

■ INTRAUTERINE CONTRACEPTIVE DEVICE (IUCD): PREVENTION OF FERTILIZATION AND IMPLANTATION OF OVUM

Intrauterine contraceptive device (IUCD) is a contraceptive device that is inserted into uterus. It prevents fertilization and the implantation of ovum. IUCD is a small device made from metal, polyurethane or other polymers.

■ TYPES OF IUCD

Three types of IUCD are available which are given below.

1. Nonmedicated IUCD

Nonmedicated IUCD is the **first generation** IUCD which is made from plastic. It is available in different shapes.

Common one is the **Lippes loop** which is "S" shaped. It is made up of polyethylene. Nonmedicated IUCD works by changing intrauterine environment which becomes spermicidal. This device causes a mild and sterile inflammatory reaction in uterine wall which is enough for spermicidal action.

Lippes loop is outdated now because of availability of new generations of IUCDs.

2. Copper IUCD

Copper IUCD or the **second generation** of IUCD is made from plastic and copper is added to it. Among the different varieties of copper bearing IUCDs, **Copper T** has become more popular. It is a T-shaped device made up of polyethylene frame. Copper-bearing IUCD also works like nonmedicated IUCD. In addition, it releases free copper and copper salts which cause mild changes in endometrial secretions and increase viscosity of cervical mucus to prevent entry of sperm into cervix.

3. Hormone-releasing IUCD

Hormone-releasing IUCD is the **third generation** of IUCD. It releases hormone slowly into uterus after insertion. Most common one is called **progestasert**. It is filled with progesterone and it has a permeable polymer membrane to release the hormone.

Progestasert prevents **implantation of ovum** by maintaining high level of progesterone in endometrium. In addition, it also increases viscosity of cervical mucus to prevent sperm entry. When the hormone is exhausted, the device must be replaced **(Table 63.1)**.

■ DISADVANTAGES OF IUCD

IUCD has some disadvantages. It has the tendency to:

1. Cause heavy bleeding in some women.
2. Promote infection.
3. Come out of uterus accidentally.

TABLE 63.1: Contraceptive methods.

Gender	Name of the method	Devices/Techniques	Mechanism of action
Both genders	Rhythm method	Knowledge and cooperation between the couple	By avoiding coitus during fertile period Fertile Period: Few days before and few days after ovulation Safe period: 5 to 6 days after menstrual bleeding and 5 to 6 days before onset of next cycle
Females	Physical barriers	1. Condom 2. Cervical cap 3. Diaphragm 4. Vaginal sponge	Cover the cervix and prevents entry of sperm into uterus
	Chemical methods	Foam tablets, jelly, cream and paste	Inserted into vagina just before coitus Kills the sperms
	Intrauterine contraceptive devices (IUDC)	1. Non-medicated: Lippe's loop 2. Copper-bearing: Coper T 3. Hormone-releasing: Progestasert	Inserted high in the uterus Prevent fertilization: 1. By reducing chances of sperm survival and entry of sperm into uterus 2. By impeding the movement of ovum into uterus
	Hormonal contraceptives	1. Oral contraceptives: Combination pills, sequential pills and mini pills 2. Hormonal implants 3. Others	Inhibit maturation of ovarian follicles and prevents ovulation
	Medical termination of pregnancy (MTP)	Dilatation and curettage (D and C)	Dilatation of cervix and removal of implanted zygote
		Vacuum aspiration	Removal of implanted zygote by vacuum aspiration
		Prostaglandin administration	Expulsion of implanted zygote by inducing uterine contractions
	Surgical method	Tubectomy	Fallopian tubes are cut and the cut ends are ligated Prevents the entry of fertilized zygote into uterus for implantation
Males	Physical barrier	Male condom	Covers the penis and prevents entry of sperms into vagina
	Surgical method	Vasectomy	Vas deferens are cut and the cut ends are ligated Prevents the entry of sperms into the ejaculatory duct

4. Copper-bearing IUCD cannot be used for long time because release of copper ions is affected after some period due to deposition of materials like minerals. So, the device needs to be replaced periodically.
5. Same with hormone-releasing IUCD also. When the hormone is exhausted, the device must be replaced.

HORMONAL CONTRACEPTIVES

Hormonal contraceptives prevent pregnancy by inhibiting maturation of follicles and ovulation. This leads to alteration of normal menstrual cycle. Menstrual cycle becomes the **anovulatory cycle**. Some chemical contraceptives prevent entry of sperm into cervix by increasing the viscosity of cervical mucus. Some hormonal contraceptives prevent implantation of fertilized ovum.

Hormonal contraceptives are of different types namely, oral contraceptives, hormonal implants, injectable contraceptives, vaginal ring, contraceptive patch and hormonal IUCD.

ORAL CONTRACEPTIVES

Oral contraceptives prevent pregnancy by the mechanism mentioned above.

This method of fertility control is called **pill method** and pills are called **contraceptive pills** or birth control pills. These pills contain **synthetic estrogen** and **synthetic progesterone**.

Contraceptive pills are of four types:

1. Classical or combined pills.
2. Sequential pills.
3. Minipills or micropills.
4. Postcoital or emergency contraceptive pills.

1. Classical or Combined Pills

Classical or combined pills contain a moderate dose of synthetic estrogen like ethinyl estradiol or mestranol and a mild dose of synthetic progesterone like norethindrone or norgestrel.

These pills are taken daily from 5th to 25th day of menstrual cycle. Withdrawal of the pills after 25th day causes menstrual bleeding. Intake of pills is resumed again after 5th day of the next cycle.

Mechanism of action of classical pills

During continuous intake of the pills, there is relatively large amount of estrogen and progesterone in the blood. It suppresses the release of gonadotropins, FSH and LH from pituitary by means of feedback mechanism. Lack of FSH and LH prevents the maturation of follicle, and ovulation. In addition, progesterone increases the thickness of mucosa in cervix, which is not favorable for transport of sperm. When the pills are withdrawn after 21 days, the menstrual flow starts.

2. Sequential Pills

Sequential pills contain a high dose of estrogen along with moderate dose of progesterone. These pills are taken in two courses:

 i. Daily for 15 days from 5th to 20th day of the menstrual cycle.
 ii. Then during the last 5 days, i.e. 23rd to 28th day. Sequential pills also prevent ovulation.

3. Minipills or Micropills

Minipills contain a low dose of only progesterone and are taken throughout the menstrual cycle. It prevents pregnancy without affecting ovulation. Progesterone increases the thickness of cervical mucosa, so that the transport of sperms is inhibited. It also prevents implantation of ovum.

4. Postcoital Pills or Emergency Contraceptive Pills

Postcoital pills or **emergency contraceptive pills** are taken to prevent pregnancy after unprotected sex. These pills contain either **levonorgestrel** (synthetic progesterone) or **ethinyl estradiol** (synthetic estrogen).

Disadvantages of Oral Contraceptives

About 40% of women who use contraceptive pills may have minor transient side effects. However, long-term use of oral contraceptives causes some serious side effects such as hypertension, heart attack, stroke and cancer.

HORMONAL IMPLANTS OR LONG-TERM CONTRACEPTIVES

To avoid taking pills daily, the long-term contraceptives are used. These contraceptives are in the form of implants containing mainly progesterone. The implants which are inserted beneath skin release the drug slowly and prevent fertility for 4 to 5 years. Though it seems to be effective, it may produce amenorrhea.

OTHER HORMONAL CONTRACEPTIVES

Other hormonal contraceptive devices include:

1. Injectables which may be progesterone only injectable or combination injectable.
2. Vaginal ring which contains progesterone.
3. Contraceptive patch containing hormone which is applied to skin over abdomen, buttock, lateral aspect of upper arm and upper torso.
4. Hormone-bearing IUCD which is already described.

MEDICAL TERMINATION OF PREGNANCY (MTP): ABORTION

Abortion is done during first few months of pregnancy. This method is called medical termination of pregnancy (MTP). There are three ways of doing MTP.

1. DILATATION AND CURETTAGE (D AND C)

In this method, the cervix is dilated and the implanted ovum or zygote is removed.

2. VACUUM ASPIRATION

The implanted ovum is removed by vacuum aspiration method. This is done up to 12 weeks of pregnancy.

3. ADMINISTRATION OF PROSTAGLANDIN

Administration of prostaglandin like PGE_2 and PGF_2 intravaginally increases uterine contractions resulting in abortion.

SURGICAL METHOD (STERILIZATION): PERMANENT METHOD

Permanent sterility is obtained by surgical methods. It is also called **sterilization**.

IN FEMALES: TUBECTOMY

In tubectomy, fallopian tubes are cut and both the cut ends are ligated. It prevents entry of ovum into uterus. This operation done through vaginal orifice in the postpartum period. During other periods, it is done by abdominal incision. Tubectomy is done quickly (in few minutes) by using a laparoscope.

Though tubectomy causes permanent sterility, if necessary, **recanalization** of fallopian tube can be done using plastic tube by another surgical procedure.

IN MALES: VASECTOMY

In vasectomy, vas deferens is cut and the cut ends are ligated. So, the sperms cannot enter the ejaculatory duct and semen is devoid of sperms. It is done by surgical procedure with local anesthesia. If necessary, the **recanalization of** vas deferens can be done with plastic tube.

MODEL QUESTIONS IN REPRODUCTIVE SYSTEM

LONG QUESTIONS

1. Describe the functions of testis and regulation of testicular functions.
2. Describe the actions and regulation of secretion of testosterone.
3. What are the female sex hormones? Explain their actions.
4. What is menstrual cycle? Explain the ovarian changes taking place during menstrual cycle.
5. Describe the uterine changes during menstrual cycle.

SHORT QUESTIONS

1. Spermatogenesis.
2. Testosterone.
3. Cryptorchidism.
4. Secondary sexual characters in males.
5. Semen.
6. Effects of removal of testes.
7. Estrogen.
8. Progesterone.
9. Follicle stimulating hormone.
10. Luteinizing hormone.
11. Gonadotropins.
12. Secondary sexual characters in females.
13. Ovarian follicles.
14. Ovulation.
15. Corpus luteum.
16. Functions of placenta.
17. Pregnancy tests.
18. Milk ejection reflex.
19. Safe period/Rhythm method.
20. Oral contraceptives.
21. MTP.
22. Tubectomy.
23. Condoms.
24. IUCD.
25. Vasectomy.

VERY SHORT ANSWER QUESTIONS

1. Prostate gland.
2. Sertoli cells.
3. Sex differentiation in fetus/Müllerian and Wolffian ducts.
4. Descend of testes and cryptorchidism.
5. Secondary sexual characters in males/Puberty in males.
6. Regulation of testosterone secretion.
7. Properties and composition of semen.
8. Structure of sperm.
9. Hypergonadism in males.
10. Hypogonadism in males.
11. Divisions and structure of uterus.
12. Graafian follicle.
13. Corpus luteum.
14. LH surge.
15. Changes in cervix during menstrual cycle.
16. Changes in vagina during menstrual cycle.
17. Abnormal menstruation.
18. Anovulatory cycle.
19. Hormonal regulation of ovulation.
20. Menopause.
21. Fertilization of ovum.
22. Sex chromosome and sex determination.
23. Braxton Hicks contractions.
24. Stages of parturition.
25. Endocrine function of placenta.
26. Fetoplacental unit.
27. Human chorionic gonadotropin.
28. Human chorionic somatomammotropin.
29. Breast milk.
30. Rhythm method of fertility control.
31. Medical termination of pregnancy.
32. Surgical method of fertility control/Sterilization.

SECTION 8: CARDIOVASCULAR SYSTEM

Chapter 64: Overview of Cardiovascular System

CHAPTER OUTLINE

- **CARDIOVASCULAR SYSTEM**
- **HEART**
  - RIGHT SIDE
  - LEFT SIDE
  - SEPTA
  - LAYERS OF WALL
  - PERICARDIUM
  - MYOCARDIUM
  - ENDOCARDIUM
  - VALVES
- **ACTIONS OF HEART**
  - CHRONOTROPIC ACTION
  - INOTROPIC ACTION
  - DROMOTROPIC ACTION
  - BATHMOTROPIC ACTION
  - LUSITROPIC ACTION
- **BLOOD VESSELS**
- **ARTERIAL SYSTEM**
- **VENOUS SYSTEM**
- **DIVISIONS OF CIRCULATION**
  - SYSTEMIC CIRCULATION
  - PULMONARY CIRCULATION

CARDIOVASCULAR SYSTEM

Cardiovascular system is made up of **heart** and **blood vessels**. Heart pumps the blood into blood vessels. Blood vessels circulate the blood throughout body and transport nutrients and oxygen to the tissues and remove carbon dioxide and waste products from the tissues.

HEART

Heart is a muscular organ that pumps blood throughout the circulatory system. It situated in between the two lungs in mediastinum. It is made up of four chambers, viz. two atria and two ventricles. Musculature is more and thick in the ventricles than in the atria. Force of contraction of the heart depends upon the muscles.

RIGHT SIDE OF HEART

Right side of the heart has two chambers, upper **right atrium** and lower **right ventricle**. Right atrium is a thin walled and low-pressure chamber. It has got the **pacemaker** known as **sinoatrial node** that produces cardiac impulses and atrioventricular node that conducts the impulses to the ventricles.

Right atrium receives venous (deoxygenated) blood via two large veins:

1. Superior vena cava that returns venous blood from the head, neck and upper limbs.
2. Inferior vena cava that returns venous blood from lower parts of the body **(Fig. 64.1)**.

Right atrium communicates with right ventricle through **tricuspid valve**. Venous blood from right atrium enters the right ventricle through this valve.

From right ventricle, pulmonary artery arises. This artery carries venous blood from right ventricle to the lungs. In the lungs, deoxygenated blood is oxygenated.

LEFT SIDE OF HEART

Left side of the heart has two chambers, upper **left atrium** and lower **left ventricle**. Left atrium is a thin walled and low-pressure chamber. It receives oxygenated blood from the lungs through pulmonary veins. This is the only exception in the body where an artery carries venous blood and vein carries the arterial blood.

Blood from left atrium enters the left ventricle through the **bicuspid valve** (mitral valve). Wall of the left ventricle

Section 8: Cardiovascular System

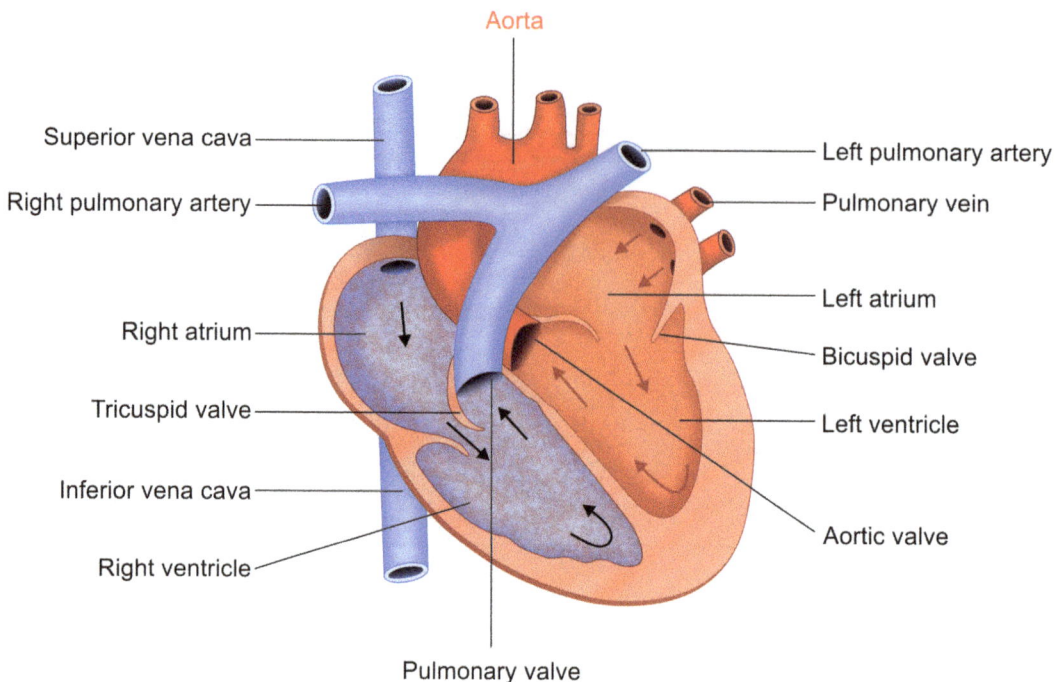

FIGURE 64.1: Section of the heart.

is very thick. Left ventricle pumps the arterial blood to different parts of the body through systemic aorta.

SEPTA OF HEART

Right and left atria of heart are separated from one another by **interatrial septum**. The ventricles are separated from one another by **interventricular septum**.

LAYERS OF WALL OF HEART

Heart is made up of three layers of tissues:

1. Outer pericardium.
2. Middle myocardium.
3. Inner endocardium.

1. PERICARDIUM

Pericardium is the outer covering of heart. It is made up of two layers:

i. Outer **parietal pericardium** which forms a strong protective sac around the heart.
ii. Inner **visceral pericardium** or **epicardium** that covers myocardium.

Layers of pericardium are separated by a space called **pericardial space** or **pericardial cavity** which contains a thin film of fluid.

2. MYOCARDIUM

Myocardium is the middle layer of wall of the heart and it is formed by cardiac muscle fibers. It forms the bulk of heart and it is responsible for pumping action of the heart. Refer Chapter 24 for features of cardiac muscles.

Myocardium is formed by three types of cardiac muscle fibers:

i. Muscle fibers which form contractile unit of heart.
ii. Muscle fibers which form pacemaker.
iii. Muscle fibers which form the conductive system.

i. Muscle Fibers which Form Contractile Unit of Heart

These cardiac muscle fibers are **striated fibers** and are similar to the skeletal muscles in structure. But, unlike the skeletal muscle fibers, cardiac muscle fibers are **involuntary** in nature.

Cardiac muscle fiber is covered by sarcolemma. It has a centrally placed nucleus. Myofibrils are embedded in the sarcoplasm. Sarcomere of the cardiac muscle has all the contractile proteins namely, actin, myosin, troponin and tropomyosin. Cardiac muscles also have sarcotubular system like that of skeletal muscle.

Important difference between skeletal muscle and cardiac muscle is that the cardiac muscle fiber is branched and the skeletal muscle is not branched.

Intercalated disk

Intercalated disk is a tough double membranous structure situated at the junction between branches of neighboring cardiac muscle fibers. It is formed by fusion of the membrane of the cardiac muscle branches **(Fig. 64.2)**.

Intercalated disks form adherens junctions which play an important role in contraction of the muscle as a single unit (Chapter 2).

Syncytium

Structure of the cardiac muscle is considered as a syncytium. The word syncytium refers to tissue in which there is cytoplasmic continuity between the adjacent cells.

However, in cardiac muscle, there is no continuity of the cytoplasm and the muscle fibers are separated

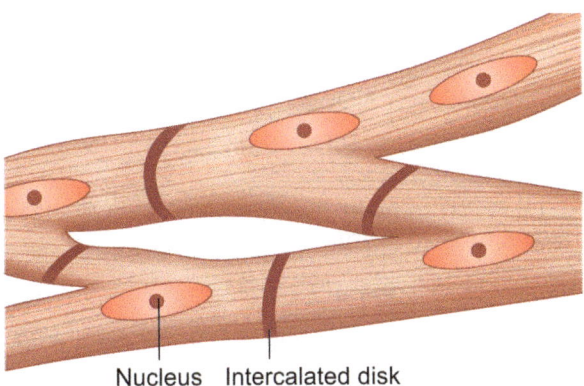

FIGURE 64.2: Cardiac muscle fiber.

from each other by cell membrane. But at the sides, membranes of adjacent muscle fibers fuse together to form gap junctions. Gap junctions facilitate rapid conduction of electrical activity from one fiber to another. This makes the cardiac muscle fibers act like a single unit referred as **physiological syncytium**.

Syncytium in human heart has two portions, atrial syncytium and ventricular syncytium which are connected by atrioventricular ring.

ii. Muscle Fibers which Form Pacemaker

Some of the muscle fibers of heart are modified into a specialized structure known as pacemaker. Muscle fibers forming the pacemaker have less striation.

Pacemaker

Pacemaker is a structure in heart that generates the impulses for heartbeat. It is formed by the **pacemaker cells** called **P cells**. Sinoatrial (SA) node forms the pacemaker in human heart. Details of pacemaker are given in next Chapter.

iii. Muscle Fibers which Form Conductive System

Conductive system of the heart is formed by modified cardiac muscle fibers. Impulses from SA node is transmitted to the atria directly. However, the impulses are transmitted to ventricles, through various components of conducting system which are given in the next Chapter.

3. ENDOCARDIUM

Endocardium is the inner most layer of heart wall. It is a thin, smooth and glistening membrane. It is formed by a single layer of endothelial cells lining the inner surface of the heart. Endocardium continues as endothelium of the blood vessels.

VALVES OF THE HEART

Human heart has four valves. Two of the valves are in between atria and the ventricles called atrioventricular valves. Other two valves are semilunar valves which are placed at the opening of blood vessels arising from the ventricles, i.e. systemic aorta and pulmonary artery. Valves of the heart permit flow of blood through the heart in only one direction.

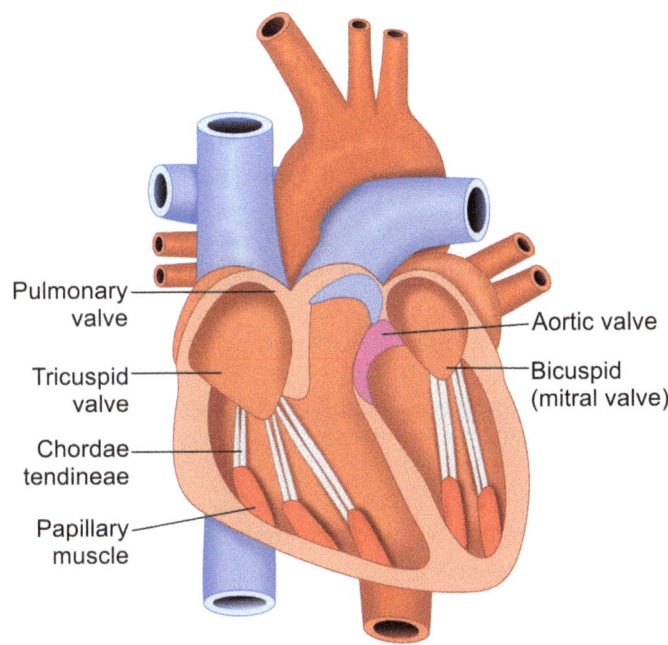

FIGURE 64.3: Valves of the heart.

Atrioventricular Valves

Left atrioventricular valve is otherwise known as **mitral valve** or **bicuspid valve**. It is formed by two valvular cusps or flaps **(Fig. 64.3)**. Right atrioventricular valve is known as **tricuspid valve** and it is formed by three cusps.

Brim of the atrioventricular valves is attached to the **atrioventricular ring**, which is the fibrous connection between the atria and ventricles. **Cusps** of the valves are attached to **papillary muscles** by means of **chordae tendineae**. The papillary muscles arise from the inner surface of ventricles. Papillary muscles play an important role in closure of the cusps and in preventing the back flow of blood from ventricle to atria during ventricular contraction.

Atrioventricular valves open only towards ventricles and prevent the backflow of blood into atria.

Semilunar Valves

Semilunar valves are present at the openings of systemic aorta and pulmonary artery and are known as **aortic valve** and **pulmonary valve** respectively. Because of the half-moon shape, these two valves are called semilunar valves. Semilunar valves are made up of three flaps.

Semilunar valves open only towards the aorta and pulmonary artery, and prevent backflow of blood into the ventricles.

ACTIONS OF HEART

Actions of heart are classified into five types:

1. Chronotropic action.
2. Inotropic action.
3. Dromotropic action.
4. Bathmotropic action.
5. Lusitropic action

1. CHRONOTROPIC ACTION

Chronotropic action is the frequency of heartbeat or heart rate. It is of two types:

i. Tachycardia or increase in heart rate.
ii. Bradycardia or decrease in heart rate.

2. INOTROPIC ACTION

Inotropic action is the force of contraction of heart. It is of two types:

i. Positive inotropic action or increase in force of contraction.
ii. Negative inotropic action or decrease in force of contraction.

3. DROMOTROPIC ACTION

Dromotropic action is the conduction of impulse through heart. It is of two types:

i. Positive dromotropic action or increase in velocity of conduction.
ii. Negative dromotropic action or decrease in velocity of conduction.

4. BATHMOTROPIC ACTION

Bathmotropic action is the excitability of cardiac muscle. It is also of two types:

i. Positive bathmotropic action or increase in excitability of cardiac muscle.
ii. Negative bathmotropic action or the decrease in excitability of cardiac muscle.

5. LUSITROPIC ACTION

Lusitropic action is the ability of cardiac muscle to relax after contraction. It is also of two types:

i. Positive lusitropic action or increase in relaxation of cardiac muscle.
ii. Negative lusitropic action or decrease in relaxation of cardiac muscle (Table 64.1).

Regulation of Actions of Heart

All the actions of heart are continuously regulated. It is essential for the heart to cope up with needs of the body. All the actions are altered by stimulation of nerves supplying the heart, some hormones or hormonal substances secreted in the body and drugs used to treat cardiovascular diseases.

BLOOD VESSELS

Vessels of the circulatory system are divided into arterial system and venous system.

VESSELS OF ARTERIAL AND VENOUS SYSTEMS

Arterial system of circulation includes the aorta, arteries and arterioles. Venous system includes venules, veins and venae cavae. Structural differences between different blood vessels are given in Table 64.2.

CAPILLARIES

Capillaries form the link between arterial system and venous system by connecting arterioles and venules (see below).

END ARTERY OR FUNCTIONAL TERMINAL ARTERY

End artery or functional terminal artery is the artery that does not join with other vessel and it is the only vessel supplying oxygenated blood to an organ or a part of the body. Obstruction of end artery may lead to ischemia and other complications of the organ.

Examples of end artery are arteries in spleen and kidney.

TABLE 64.1: Actions of heart.

Action	Definition
Chronotropic action	Frequency of heartbeat
Inotropic action	Force of contraction of heart
Dromotropic action	Conduction of impulse through heart
Bathmotropic action	Excitability of cardiac muscle
Lusitropic action	Relaxation of cardiac muscle

TABLE 64.2: Structural and dimensional differences between different blood vessel walls.

Blood vessel	Diameter	Thickness of vessel wall	Presence of elastic tissue	Presence of smooth muscle fibers	Presence of fibrous tissue
Aorta	25 mm	2 mm	More	Less	More
Artery	4 mm	1 mm	More	More	Moderate
Bigger arteriole	30 μ	6 μ	Moderate	More	Moderate
Terminal arteriole	10 μ	2 μ	Less	More	Moderate
Capillary	8 μ	0.5 μ	Absent	Absent	Moderate
Venule	20 μ	1 μ	Absent	Absent	Less
Vein	5 mm	0.5 μ	Less	More	Moderate
Vena cava	30 mm	1.5 μ	Less	More	More

ANASTOMOSIS

Anastomosis means connection between two tubular structures. In cardiovascular system, anastomosis refers to connection between two vessels such as one artery and one vein.

COLLATERAL CIRCULATION

Collateral circulation is the alternate circulation of blood maintained to a tissue or an organ through network of minute blood vessels that become enlarged and anastomose with adjacent vessels. This happens when the major blood vessel of that tissue or organ is obstructed.

ARTERIAL SYSTEM

Arterial system comprises the aorta, arteries and arterioles. The walls of aorta and arteries are formed by three layers:

1. Outer **tunica adventitia**, which is made up of connective tissue layer. It is the continuation of parietal pericardium.
2. Middle **tunica media**, which is formed by smooth muscles.
3. Inner **tunica intima**, which is made up of endothelium. It is the continuation of endocardium.

Branches of arteries become narrower and their walls become thinner while reaching the periphery. Aorta has got the maximum diameter of about 25 mm. Diameter of the arteries is gradually decreased and at the end arteries, it is about 4 mm. It further decreases to 30 μ in the arterioles and ends up with 10 μ in terminal arterioles. The resistance (**peripheral resistance**) is offered to the blood flow in the arterioles and so these vessels are called **resistant vessels**.

Arterioles are continued as capillaries which are small, thin walled vessels having a diameter of about 5 to 8 μ. Capillaries are functionally very important, because the exchange of materials between blood and the tissues occurs through these vessels.

VENOUS SYSTEM

From the capillaries, venous system starts and it includes venules, veins and venae cavae. Capillaries end in the venules. The venules are smaller vessels with thin muscular wall than the arterioles. Diameter of the venules is about 20 μ. At a given time, large quantity of blood is held in venules and so the venules are called **capacitance vessels**.

Venules are continued as **veins**, which have the diameter of 5 mm. Veins form **superior** and **inferior venae cavae** which have a diameter of about 30 mm **(Table 64.2)**.

The walls of the veins and venae cavae are made up of inner endothelium, elastic tissues, smooth muscles and outer connective tissue layer. In veins and vena cava, the elastic tissue is less but the smooth muscle fibers are more.

DIVISIONS OF CIRCULATION

Blood flows through two divisions of circulatory system:

1. Systemic circulation.
2. Pulmonary circulation.

SYSTEMIC CIRCULATION

It is otherwise known as **greater circulation (Fig. 64.4)**. Blood which is pumped from left ventricle passes through

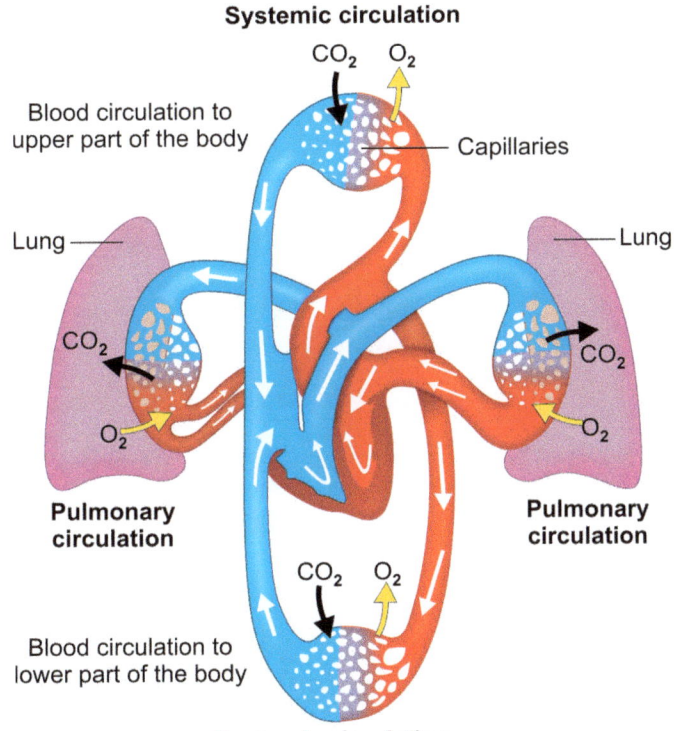

FIGURE 64.4: Systemic and pulmonary circulation.

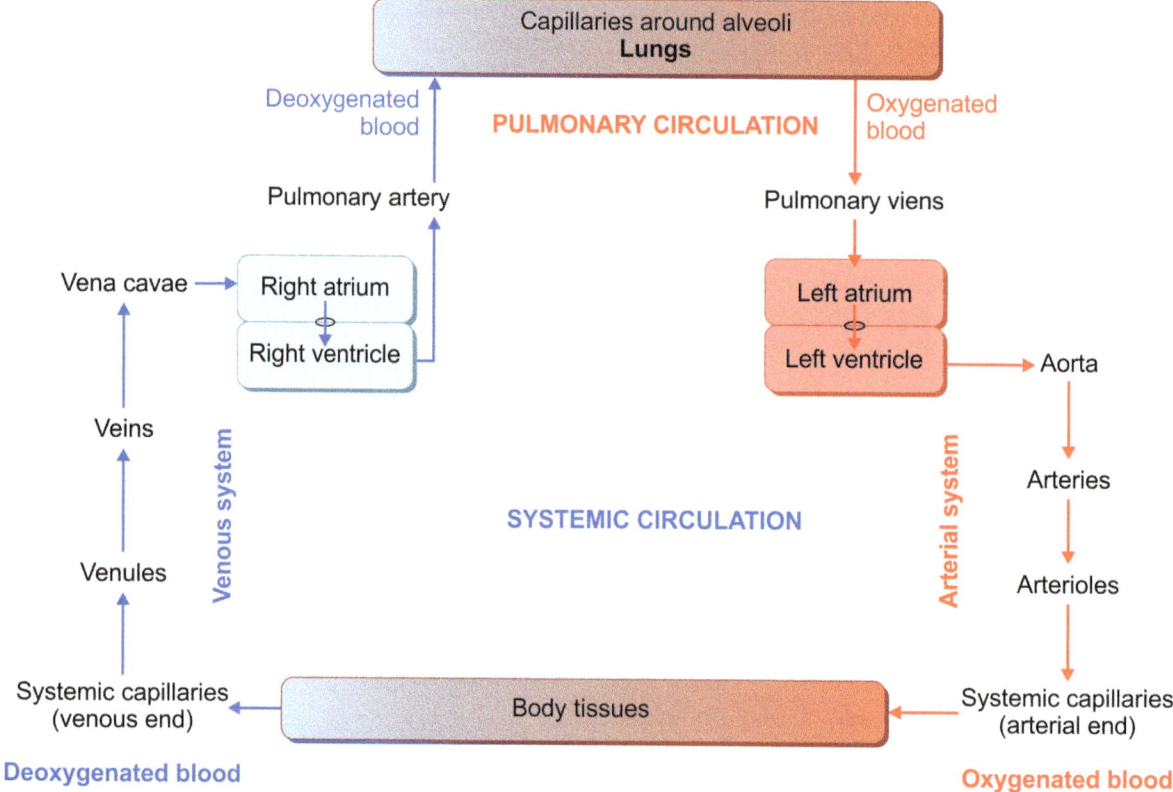

FIGURE 64.5: Schematic diagram showing systemic and pulmonary circulation.

a series of blood vessels of arterial system and reaches the tissues. Exchange of various substances between blood and the tissues takes place in the capillaries. After the exchange of substances in capillaries, blood enters the venous system and returns to right atrium and then the right ventricles.

■ PULMONARY CIRCULATION

It is otherwise called **lesser circulation**. Blood is pumped from right ventricle to lungs through pulmonary artery. The exchange of gases occurs between blood and alveoli of the lungs through pulmonary capillary membrane. Oxygenated blood returns to left atrium through the pulmonary veins **(Fig. 64.5)**.

Thus, the left side of heart contains oxygenated or arterial blood and right side of the heart contains venous blood.

Chapter 65: Properties of Cardiac Muscle

CHAPTER OUTLINE

- **EXCITABILITY**
  - DEFINITION
  - ELECTRICAL POTENTIALS IN CARDIAC MUSCLE
  - IONIC BASIS OF ACTION POTENTIAL
  - SPREAD OF ACTION POTENTIAL THROUGH CARDIAC MUSCLE
- **RHYTHMICITY**
  - DEFINITION
  - PACEMAKER
  - ELECTRICAL POTENTIAL IN SA NODE
- **CONDUCTIVITY**
  - CONDUCTIVE SYSTEM IN HUMAN HEART
  - VELOCITY OF IMPULSES AT CONDUCTIVE SYSTEM
- **CONTRACTILITY**
  - ALL-OR-NONE LAW
  - STAIRCASE PHENOMENON
  - SUMMATION OF SUBLIMINAL STIMULI
  - REFRACTORY PERIOD

■ EXCITABILITY

■ DEFINITION

Excitability is defined as the ability of a living tissue to give response to a stimulus. In all tissues, initial response to a stimulus is the electrical activity in the form of action potential. It is followed by mechanical activity in the form of contraction, secretion, etc.

■ ELECTRICAL POTENTIALS IN CARDIAC MUSCLE

Refer Chapter 27 for basics of electrical potentials in the muscle.

Resting Membrane Potential in Cardiac Muscle

Resting membrane potential in single cardiac muscle fiber is – 85 to – 95 mV.

Action Potential in Cardiac Muscle

Action potential in cardiac muscle is different from that of other tissues such as skeletal muscle, smooth muscle and nervous tissue. Duration of the action potential in cardiac muscle is 250 to 350 msec (0.25 to 0.35 second).

In a single cardiac muscle fiber, action potential occurs in four phases:

1. Initial depolarization.
2. Initial repolarization.
3. A plateau: Final depolarization.
4. Final repolarization.

1. Initial Depolarization

Initial depolarization is very rapid and it lasts for about 2 msec. Amplitude of the depolarization is about + 20 mV **(Fig. 65.1)**.

2. Initial Repolarization

Immediately after depolarization, there is an initial rapid repolarization for a short period of about 2 msec. End of this rapid repolarization is represented by a **notch**.

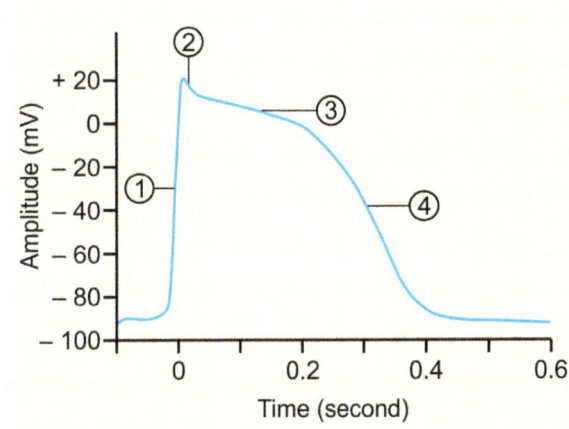

FIGURE 65.1: Action potential in ventricular muscle.
1 = Depolarization, 2 = Initial rapid repolarization, 3 = Plateau, 4 = Final repolarization.

3. Plateau: Final Depolarization

Afterwards, the muscle fiber remains in depolarized state for sometime before further repolarization. It forms the plateau (stable period) in action potential curve. This plateau lasts for about 200 msec (0.2 second) in atrial muscle fibers and for about 300 msec (0.3 second) in ventricular muscle fibers. Due to the long plateau in action potential, the contraction time is longer in cardiac muscle.

4. Final Repolarization

Final repolarization occurs after the plateau. It is a slow process and it lasts for about 50 to 80 msec (0.05 to 0.08 second) before the re-establishment of resting membrane potential.

■ IONIC BASIS OF ACTION POTENTIAL

1. Initial depolarization is due to opening of fast sodium channels and the **rapid influx of sodium ions**
2. Initial repolarization is due to the transient (short duration) opening of potassium channels and **efflux of potassium ions** in a small quantity from the muscle fiber. Simultaneously, the fast sodium channels close suddenly and slow sodium channels open resulting in **slow influx of sodium ions** in a low quantity.
3. Plateau (final depolarization) is because of the opening of calcium channels which are kept opened for a longer period. This causes **influx of calcium ions** in large numbers. Entry of both calcium and sodium ions is responsible for prolonged depolarization, i.e. plateau.
4. Final repolarization is due to increase in **efflux of potassium ions**.

■ SPREAD OF ACTION POTENTIAL THROUGH CARDIAC MUSCLE

Action potential spreads through the cardiac muscle very rapidly. It is because of the presence of gap junctions between cardiac muscle fibers. Gap junctions are permeable junctions and allow free movement of ions. Due to this, the action potential spreads rapidly from one muscle fiber to another fiber.

Action potential is transmitted from atria to ventricles through the fibers of specialized conductive system, which is explained later in this chapter.

■ RHYTHMICITY
■ DEFINITION

Rhythmicity is the ability of a tissue to produce its own impulses regularly. It is more appropriately named as **autorhythmicity**. It is also called **self-excitation**. This property is present in all the tissues of heart.

However, heart has a specialized excitatory structure from which the discharge of impulses is rapid. This specialized structure is called pacemaker. From this, the impulses spread to other parts through the specialized conductive system.

■ PACEMAKER

Pacemaker is defined as the part of heart from which the impulses for heartbeat are produced normally. Pacemaker is formed by **pacemaker cells** called **P cells**. In mammalian heart, the pacemaker is sinoatrial node (SA node).

SA Node

SA node is a small strip of **modified cardiac muscle** situated in the superior part of lateral wall of right atrium, just below the opening of superior vena cava. Fibers of this node do not have contractile elements. These fibers are continuous with fibers of atrial muscle, so that the impulses from SA node spread rapidly through atria.

Other parts of heart like AV node, atria and ventricle also can produce the impulses and function as pacemaker. Still SA node is called the pacemaker because the rate of production of impulse (rhythmicity) is more in SA node than in other parts. It is about 70 to 80/min.

Spread of Impulses from SA Node

Mammalian heart has got a specialized conductive system by which, the impulses from SA node spread to other parts of the heart (see below).

Rate of Generation of Impulses by Different Parts of Human Heart

Rate of generation of impulses by different parts of heart is given in **Table 65.1**.

■ ELECTRICAL POTENTIAL IN SA NODE

Electrical potential in SA node is different from that of other cardiac muscle fibers. In SA node, each impulse triggers the next impulse. It is mainly due to the **unstable resting membrane potential**.

Resting Membrane Potential in SA Node

Resting membrane potential in SA node cells exists only for a very short duration and it has a negativity of -55 to -60 mV. It is different from the negativity of -85 to -95 mV in other cardiac muscle fibers.

Action Potential in SA Node

Action potential in SA node has three phases:

Phase 1: Pacemaker potential
Phase 2: Rapid depolarization
Phase 3: Rapid repolarization

Phase 1: Pacemaker potential

Pacemaker potential is also called spontaneous depolarization or pacemaker current. During this phase the

TABLE 65.1: Rate of generation of impulses by different parts of human heart.

Part of the heart	Rate of generation of impulses (per minute)
1. SA node	70 to 89
2. AV node	40 to 60
3. Atrial muscle	40 to 60
4. Purkinje fibers	35 to 40
5. Ventricular muscle	20 to 40

spontaneous depolarization starts very slowly and reaches the threshold level of – 40 mV very slowly.

Phase 2: Rapid depolarization

Pacemaker potential triggers the rapid depolarization. Depolarization reaches the voltage of + 5 mV.

Phase 3: Rapid repolarization

Rapid depolarization is followed by rapid repolarization. Repolarization reaches a voltage of – 55 to – 60 mV resulting in **hyperpolarization** and ends in resting membrane potential **(Fig. 65.2)**.

Once again, the cycle is repeated with spontaneous depolarization.

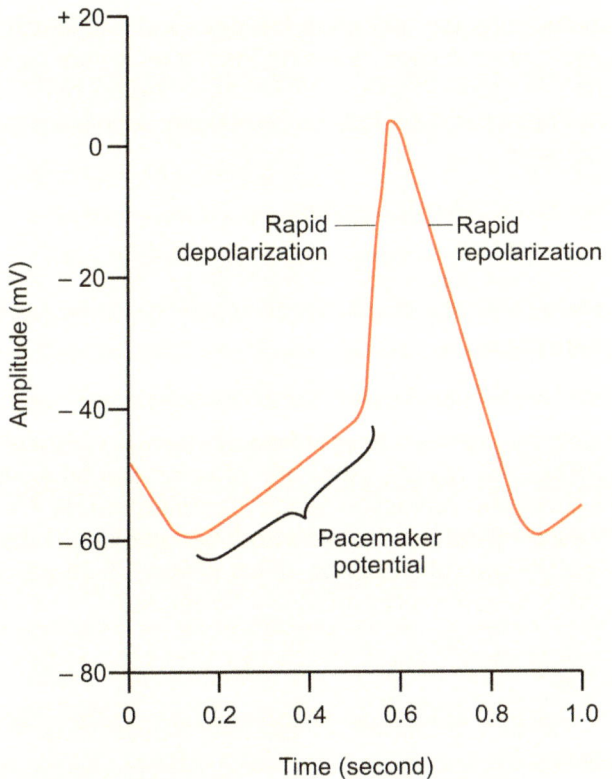

FIGURE 65.2: Action potential in SA node.

Funny Current

Pacemaker current (**pacemaker potential**) is always referred as funny current because of its unusual properties.

■ CONDUCTIVITY

Heart has a specialized conductive system through which the impulses from SA node are transmitted to all other parts of the heart **(Fig. 65.3)**.

■ CONDUCTIVE SYSTEM IN HEART

Conductive system of the heart is formed by the **modified cardiac muscle fibers**. Conductive tissues of the heart are also called the **junctional tissues**.

Components of Conductive System in Heart

1. AV node.
2. Bundle of His.
3. Right and left bundle branches.
4. Purkinje fibers.

SA node is situated in right atrium (see above). AV node is situated in right posterior portion of intra-atrial septum. The impulses from SA node are conducted throughout right and left atria. These impulses also reach the AV node via some specialized fibers called **intermodal fibers**.

From AV node, the **bundle of His** arises. It divides into right and left **bundle branches** which run on either side of the interventricular septum. From each branch of bundle of His, many **Purkinje fibers** arise and spread all over the ventricular myocardium.

■ VELOCITY OF IMPULSES AT DIFFERENT PARTS OF THE CONDUCTIVE SYSTEM

Velocity of electrical impulse through different parts of conductive system is given in **Table 65.2**. Velocity is maximum at Purkinje fibers and minimum at AV node. So, when electrical impulse travels from SA node to AV node it is slowed down for a very short period before traveling down through bundle of His. This delay is called **AV nodal delay.**

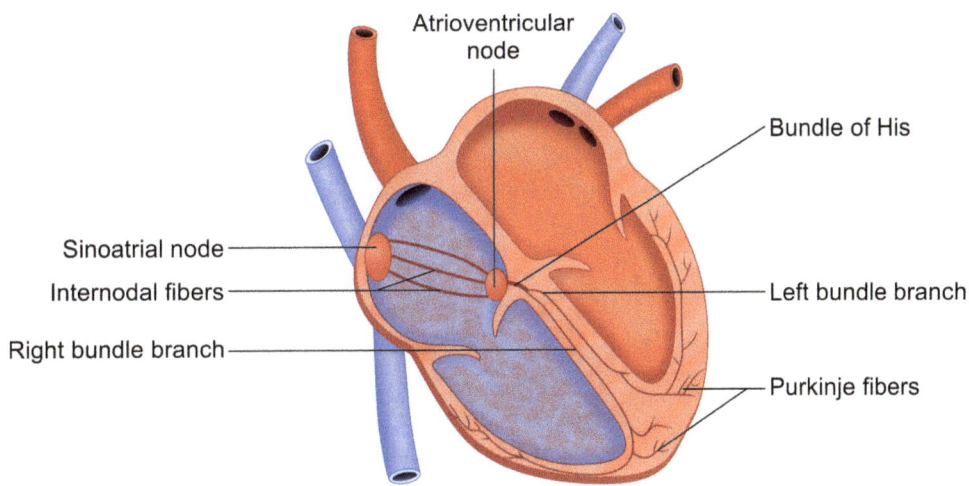

FIGURE 65.3: Sinoatrial node and conductive system of the heart.

CONTRACTILITY

Contractility is ability of the tissue to shorten in length (contraction) when stimulated.

Contractile properties are:

1. ALL-OR-NONE LAW

According to all-or-none law, when a stimulus is applied, whatever may be the strength, the whole cardiac muscle gives maximum response or it does not give any response at all. Below the threshold level, i.e. if strength of stimulus is not adequate, the muscle does not give response.

All-or-none law is applicable to whole cardiac muscle. It is because of **cardiac syncytium**. In skeletal muscle, all-or-none law is applicable only to a single muscle fiber.

2. STAIRCASE PHENOMENON

When the ventricle is stimulated successively (at a short interval of 2 seconds) without changing the strength, the force of contraction increases gradually for the first few contractions, and then it remains same. Gradual increase in the force of contraction is called staircase phenomenon **(Fig. 65.4)**.

Staircase phenomenon occurs because of the beneficial effect which facilitates the force of successive contraction. So, there is a gradual increase in force of contraction.

3. SUMMATION OF SUBLIMINAL STIMULI

When a stimulus with a subliminal strength is applied, the heart does not show any response. When few stimuli with same subliminal strength are applied in succession, the heart shows response by contraction. It is due to summation of the stimuli.

4. REFRACTORY PERIOD

Refractory period is the period in which the muscle does not show any response to a stimulus.

Refractory period is of two types, absolute refractory period and relative refractory period.

Absolute Refractory Period

Absolute refractory period is the period during which the muscle does not show any response at all, whatever may be the strength of stimulus. It is because, the depolarization occurs during this period. So, a second depolarization is not possible.

Relative Refractory Period

Relative refractory period is the period during which the muscle shows response if strength of stimulus is increased to maximum. It is the stage at which the muscle is in repolarizing state.

Refractory Period in Cardiac Muscle

Cardiac muscle has a **long refractory period** compared to that of skeletal muscle. Absolute refractory period extends throughout the contraction period of cardiac muscle. It is for 0.27 second and relative refractory period extends during first half of relaxation period which is about 0.26 second. So, the total refractory period is 0.53 second.

Significance of Long Refractory Period in Cardiac Muscle

Long refractory period in cardiac muscle has three advantages:

1. Summation of contractions does not occur.
2. Fatigue does not occur.
3. Tetanus does not occur.

TABLE 65.2: Velocity of impulse through conductive system of heart.

Part of conductive system	Velocity (M/sec)
1. Atrial muscle	0.3
2. Internodal fibers	1.0
3. AV node	0.05
4. Bundle of His	0.12
5. Purkinje fibers	4.0
6. Ventricular muscle	0.5

Velocity of impulse is maximum at Purkinje fibers and minimum at AV node.

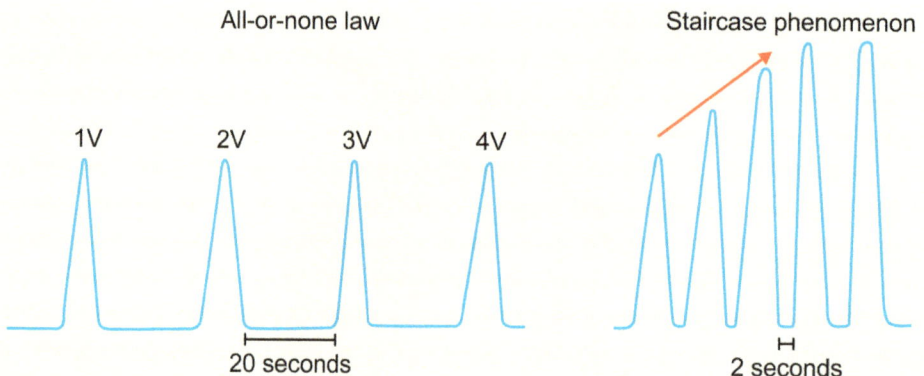

FIGURE 65.4: All-or-none law and staircase phenomenon in cardiac muscle.

Chapter 66: Cardiac Cycle

CHAPTER OUTLINE

- **DEFINITION**
- **EVENTS**
- **DIVISIONS AND DURATION**
  - ATRIAL EVENTS
  - VENTRICULAR EVENTS
- **DESCRIPTION OF ATRIAL EVENTS**
  - ATRIAL SYSTOLE
  - ATRIAL DIASTOLE
- **DESCRIPTION OF VENTRICULAR EVENTS**
  - ISOMETRIC CONTRACTION PERIOD
  - EJECTION PERIOD
  - PROTODIASTOLE
  - ISOMETRIC RELAXATION PERIOD
  - RAPID FILLING PHASE
  - SLOW FILLING PHASE
- **LAST RAPID FILLING PHASE**
- **PRESSURE CHANGES DURING CARDIAC CYCLE**
  - INTRA-ATRIAL PRESSURE CHANGES DURING CARDIAC CYCLE
  - INTRA-VENTRICULAR PRESSURE CHANGES DURING CARDIAC CYCLE
  - AORTIC PRESSURE CHANGES DURING CARDIAC CYCLE
- **VENTRICULAR VOLUME CHANGES DURING CARDIAC CYCLE**
  - SIGNIFICANCE OF VOLUME OF BLOOD IN VENTRICLES
  - VOLUME OF BLOOD IN RIGHT AND LEFT VENTRICLES

DEFINITION

Cardiac cycle is defined as the succession (sequence) of coordinated events in the heart which are repeated during every heartbeat in a cyclic manner.

Each heartbeat consists of two major periods called **systole** and **diastole**. Systole is the contraction of the cardiac muscle and diastole is the relaxation of cardiac muscle.

EVENTS OF CARDIAC CYCLE

Events of cardiac cycle are classified into two divisions:

1. Atrial events which constitute atrial systole and atrial diastole.
2. Ventricular events which constitute ventricular systole and ventricular diastole.

DIVISIONS AND DURATION OF EVENTS OF CARDIAC CYCLE

When the heart beats at the normal rate of 72/minute, the duration of each cardiac cycle is about 0.8 second.

ATRIAL EVENTS

1. Atrial systole : 0.11 (0.1) second.
2. Atrial diastole : 0.69 (0.7) second.

VENTRICULAR EVENTS

Ventricular events are divided into two divisions:

1. Ventricular systole : 0.27 (0.3) second
2. Ventricular diastole : 0.53 (0.5) second

In clinical practice, the term 'systole' refers to ventricular systole and 'diastole' refers to ventricular diastole. Ventricular systole is divided into two subdivisions and ventricular diastole is divided into five subdivisions. Subdivisions of systole and diastole are given in **Box 66.1**.

BOX 66.1: Subdivisions of ventricular events.

Ventricular systole (0.27 sec)	
1. Isometric contraction	0.05 sec
2. Ejection period	0.22 sec
Ventricular diastole (0.53 sec)	
1. Protodiastole	0.04 sec
2. Isometric relaxation	0.08 sec
3. Rapid filling	0.11 sec
4. Slow filling	0.19 sec
5. Last rapid filling (Atrial systole)	0.11 sec

Among the atrial events, atrial systole occurs during last phase of ventricular diastole. So, it is also called **last rapid period**. Atrial diastole is not considered as a separate phase, since it coincides with the whole of ventricular systole and earlier part of ventricular diastole.

■ DESCRIPTION OF ATRIAL EVENTS OF CARDIAC CYCLE

For the sake of better understanding, the description of events of cardiac cycle is commenced with atrial systole.

■ ATRIAL SYSTOLE

Atrial systole is also known as second or **last rapid filling phase** or **presystole**. It is considered as the last phase of ventricular diastole. Its duration is 0.11 second.

During this period, only a small amount, i.e. 10% of blood is forced from atria into ventricles. Atrial systole is not essential for the maintenance of circulation. Many persons with atrial fibrillation survive for years, without suffering from circulatory insufficiency. However, such persons feel difficult to cope up with physical stress like exercise.

Pressure and Volume Changes

During atrial systole, the intra-atrial pressure increases. Intraventricular pressure and ventricular volume also increase, but slightly.

Fourth Heart Sound

Contraction of atrial musculature causes the production of fourth heart sound during this phase.

■ ATRIAL DIASTOLE

After atrial systole, the atrial diastole starts. Atrial diastole lasts for about 0.7 second (accurate duration is 0.69 second). This long atrial diastole is necessary, because this is the period during which atrial filling takes place. Right atrium receives deoxygenated blood from all over the body through superior and inferior venae cavae. Left atrium receives oxygenated blood from lungs through pulmonary veins.

Atrial Events vs Ventricular Events

Out of 0.7 second of atrial diastole, first 0.3 second (0.27 second accurately) coincides with ventricular systole. So, the heart relaxes as a whole for 0.4 second. **Figure 66.1** shows the correlation between atrial and ventricular events of cardiac cycle.

■ DESCRIPTION OF VENTRICULAR EVENTS OF CARDIAC CYCLE

■ ISOMETRIC CONTRACTION PERIOD

Isometric contraction is the type of muscular contraction characterized by increase in tension without any change in the length of muscle fibers. Isometric contraction of ventricular muscle is also called **isovolumetric contraction**.

Isometric contraction period in cardiac cycle is the first phase of ventricular systole. It lasts for 0.05 second

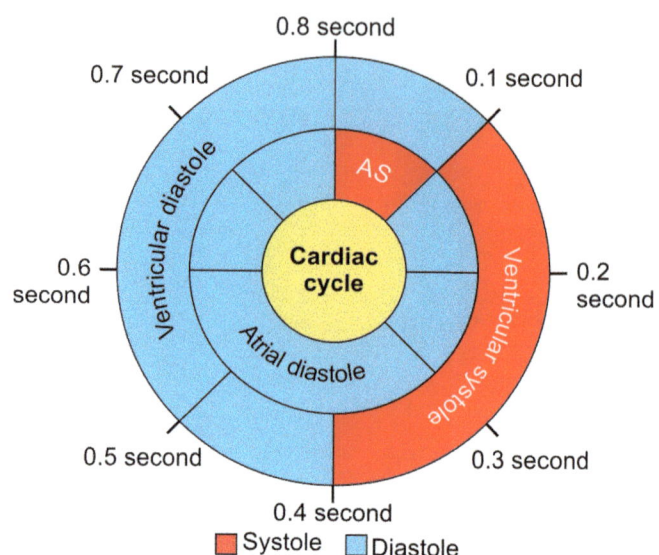

FIGURE 66.1: Atrial and ventricular events of cardiac cycle. AS = Atrial systole.

(Table 66.1). Immediately after atrial systole, the atrioventricular valves are closed due to increase in ventricular pressure. Semilunar valves are already closed. Now, the ventricles contract as **closed cavities** in such a way that, there is no change in the volume of ventricular chambers or in length of muscle fibers. Only, the tension increases in ventricular musculature.

Because of increased tension in ventricular musculature during isometric contraction, the pressure increases sharply inside ventricles.

First Heart Sound

Closure of atrioventricular valves at the beginning of this phase produces first heart sound.

Significance of Isometric Contraction

During isometric contraction period, the ventricular pressure increases greatly **(Table 66.1)**. When this pressure increases above the pressure in aorta and pulmonary artery, semilunar valves open. Thus, the pressure rise in ventricle caused by isometric contraction is responsible for opening of semilunar valves. This leads to ejection of blood from the ventricles into aorta and pulmonary artery.

■ EJECTION PERIOD

Due to the opening of semilunar valves and isotonic contraction of ventricles, the blood is ejected out of both the ventricles. Hence, this period is called ejection period. Duration of this period is 0.22 second.

Ejection period is of two stages:

i. First stage is called **rapid ejection period**. Immediately after the opening of semilunar valves, a large amount of blood is rapidly ejected from both the ventricles. It lasts for 0.13 second.

ii. Second stage is called **slow ejection period**. During this stage, the blood is ejected slowly with much less force. Duration of this period is 0.09 second.

Chapter 66: Cardiac Cycle

TABLE 66.1: Atrial and ventricular events of cardiac cycle.

Events	Duration of events (second)	Divisions	Duration of divisions (second)	Subdivisions	Duration of subdivisions (second)	Primary action
Atrial events	0.8	Atrial systole	0.11	–	–	Ventricular filling
		Atrial diastole	0.69	–	–	Atrial filling
Ventricular events	0.8	Ventricular systole	0.27	Isovolumetric contraction period	0.05	Steep increase in pressure
				Rapid ejection period	0.13	Pumping of blood into systemic and pulmonary blood vessels
				Slow ejection period	0.09	
		Ventricular diastole	0.53	Protodiastole	0.04	Beginning of diastole
				Isovolumetric relaxation period	0.08	Rapid fall in pressure
				First rapid filling phase	0.11	Filling of ventricles
				Slow filling phase	0.19	
				Last rapid filling phase	0.11	

Note: Most of the atrial events and ventricular events overlap.

End-systolic Volume

Ventricles are not emptied at the end of ejection period and some amount of blood remains in each ventricle. Amount of blood remaining in ventricles at the end of ejection period (i.e. at the end of systole) is called end-systolic volume. It is 60 to 80 mL per ventricle.

Ejection Fraction

Ejection fraction means the fraction (or portion) of end-diastolic volume (see below) that is ejected out by each ventricle per beat. From 130 to 150 mL of end-diastolic volume, 70 mL is ejected out by each ventricle (stroke volume). Normal ejection fraction is 60 to 65%.

■ PROTODIASTOLE

This is the first stage of ventricular diastole hence the name protodiastole. Duration of this period is 0.04 second. During this period, the pressure in ventricles drops due to ejection of blood. At the end of this period, intraventricular pressure becomes less than the pressure in aorta and pulmonary artery. This causes closure of semilunar valves. Atrioventricular valves are already closed (see above). No other change occurs in the heart during this period. Thus, protodiastole indicates only the end of systole and beginning of diastole.

Second Heart Sound

Closure of semilunar valves during this phase produces second heart sound.

■ ISOMETRIC RELAXATION PERIOD

Isometric relaxation is the type of muscular relaxation characterized by decrease in tension without any change in the length of muscle fibers. Isometric relaxation of ventricular muscle is also called **isovolumetric relaxation**.

During isometric relaxation period, once again all the valves of the heart are closed. Now, both the ventricles relax as **closed cavities**, without any change in volume or length of the muscle fiber. But intraventricular pressure decreases during this period. Duration of isometric relaxation period is 0.08 second.

Significance of Isometric Relaxation

During isometric relaxation period, the ventricular pressure decreases greatly. When the ventricular pressure becomes less than pressure in atria, the atrioventricular valves open. Thus, the fall in pressure in the ventricles, caused by isometric relaxation is responsible for the opening of atrioventricular valves, resulting in filling of ventricles.

■ RAPID FILLING

When AV valves are opened, there is a sudden rush of blood from atria into ventricles. So, this period is called the **first rapid filling period**. Filling during this period occurs without atrial systole. About 70% of filling takes place during this phase which lasts for 0.11 second.

Third Heart Sound

Rushing of blood into ventricles during this phase produces third heart sound **(Fig. 66.2)**.

■ SLOW FILLING

After a sudden rush of blood, the ventricular filling becomes slow. Now, it is called the slow filling. It is also called **diastasis**. Filling during this phase also occurs without atrial systole. About 20% of filling occurs in this phase. Duration of slow filling phase is 0.19 second.

■ LAST RAPID FILLING

Filling becomes once again rapid because of atrial systole. After slow filling period, the atria contract and push a small amount of blood into the ventricles. About 10% of ventricular filling takes place during this period. Flow of additional amount of blood into ventricle due to atrial systole is called **atrial kick.**

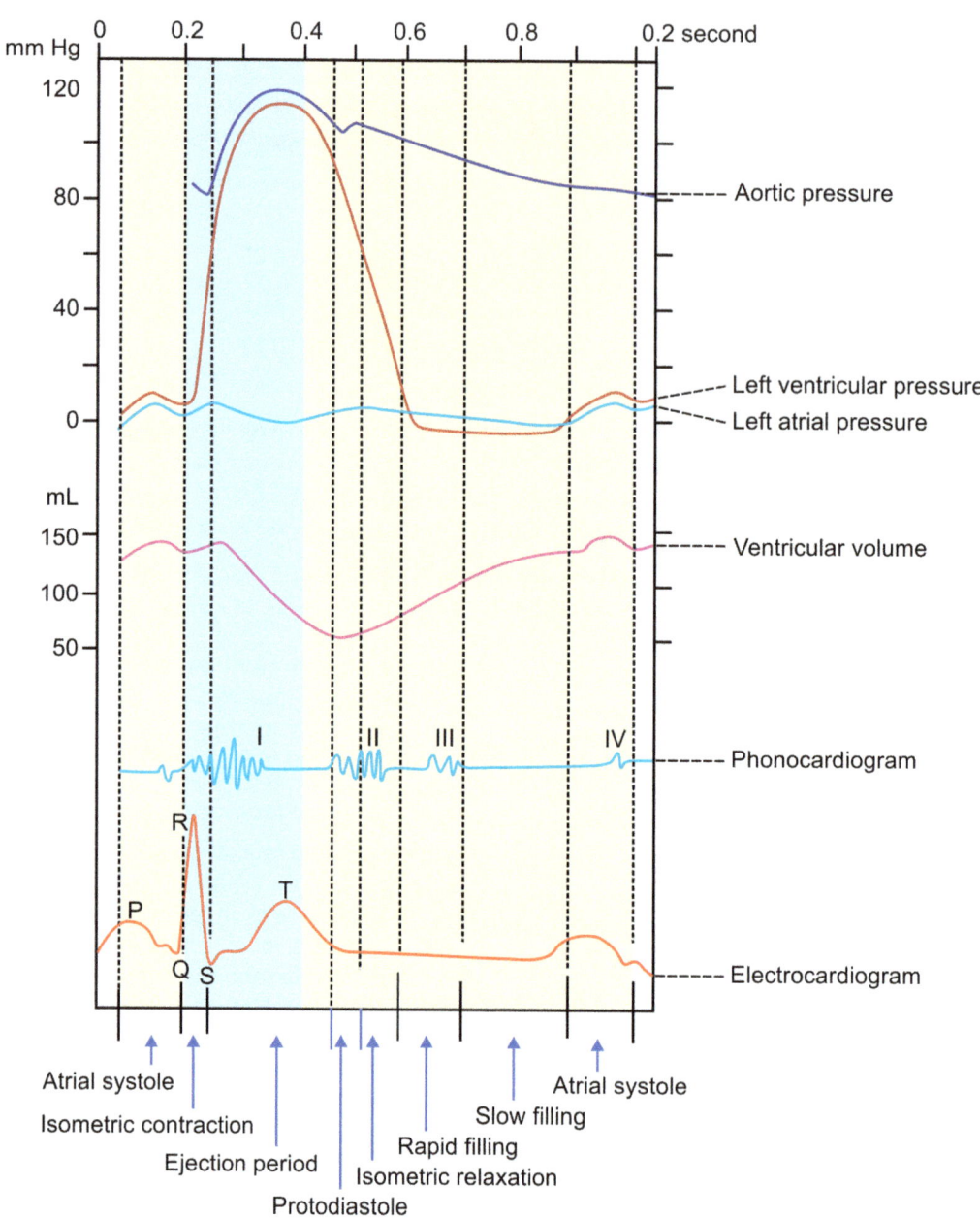

FIGURE 66.2: Comprehensive diagram (Wiggers diagram) ECG, phonocardiogram, pressure changes and volume changes during cardiac cycle.

End-diastolic Volume

End-diastolic volume is the amount of blood remaining in each ventricle at the end of diastole. It is about 130 to 150 mL per ventricle.

PRESSURE CHANGES DURING CARDIAC CYCLE

INTRA-ATRIAL PRESSURE CHANGES DURING CARDIAC CYCLE

Significance of Intra-atrial Pressure

Pressure in the atria is called the intra-atrial pressure. Intra-atrial pressure is responsible for opening of the atrioventricular valves and ventricular filling. It is also the main factor for the development of venous pulse.

Pressure Changes During Cardiac Cycle

During atrial diastole, the pressure in atrial falls down and reaches 0 mm Hg because of relaxation. During atrial systole pressure rises sharply up to 5 mm Hg in right atrium and 7 mm Hg in left atrium.

Maximum and minimum pressures in the left and right atria are given in **Table 66.2**.

INTRA-VENTRICULAR PRESSURE CHANGES DURING CARDIAC CYCLE

Significance of Intra-ventricular Pressure

Intra-ventricular pressure is the pressure developed inside the ventricles of heart. It is essential for the circulation of blood, because the flow of blood through systemic and pulmonary circulation depends upon pressure at which the blood is pumped out of ventricles.

Pressure Changes During Cardiac Cycle

Pressure in ventricles reach maximum during ejection period and reaches minimum during final phase of ventricular diastole.

Maximum and minimum pressures in the left and right ventricles are given in **Table 66.2**.

AORTIC PRESSURE CHANGES DURING CARDIAC CYCLE

Significance Aortic Pressure

Aortic pressure is the pressure developed in the aorta. It is necessary to maintain the blood flow through the circulatory system.

Pressure Changes During Cardiac Cycle

Pressure in systemic aorta is always higher than that of pulmonary artery. It is because of the higher pressure in left ventricle than in the right ventricle. Maximum and minimum pressures in aorta are given in **Table 66.2**.

Minimum pressure in systemic aorta is much greater than the minimum pressure in the left ventricle. It is due to the presence of elastic tissues in the aorta, which enable the aorta to recoil and maintain the minimum pressure at a higher level.

During ejection period of cardiac cycle, the pressure in aorta increases and reaches the peak. During diastole, it reduces gradually and reaches the minimum level. At the time of closure of semilunar valves, an incisura occurs due to back flow of some blood towards the ventricles **(Fig. 66.2)**.

TABLE 66.2: Pressure changes during cardiac cycle.

Area	Maximum Pressure	Minimum pressure
Left atrium	7 to 8 mm Hg	0 to 2 mm Hg
Right atrium	5 to 6 mm Hg	0 to 2 mm Hg
Left ventricle	120 mm Hg	5 mm Hg
Right ventricle	25 mm Hg	2 to 3 mm Hg
Systemic aorta	120 mm Hg	80 mm Hg
Pulmonary artery	25 mm Hg	7 to 8 mm Hg

VENTRICULAR VOLUME CHANGES DURING CARDIAC CYCLE

SIGNIFICANCE OF VOLUME OF BLOOD IN VENTRICLES

Volume of blood in the left ventricle is an important factor to maintain cardiac output and blood circulation. Volume of blood in right ventricle is responsible for flow of blood into pulmonary circulation.

VOLUME OF BLOOD IN RIGHT AND LEFT VENTRICLES

End-diastolic Volume and End-systolic Volume

Amount of blood is the same in both right and left ventricles **(Fig. 66.2)**. Maximum volume of blood in each ventricle after filling (end-diastolic volume) is 130 mL to 150 mL. Minimum volume of blood left in the ventricles at the end of ejection period (end of systolic volume) is 60 mL to 80 mL.

Chapter 67: Heart Sounds and Cardiac Murmur

CHAPTER OUTLINE

- PRODUCTION OF HEART SOUNDS
- DESCRIPTION OF HEART SOUNDS
- TRIPLE AND QUADRUPLE HEART SOUNDS
- METHODS OF STUDY OF HEART SOUNDS
- CARDIAC MURMUR

PRODUCTION OF HEART SOUNDS

Heart sounds are the sounds produced by mechanical activities of the heart during each cardiac cycle. Heart sounds are produced by flow of blood through chambers of the heart contraction of cardiac muscle and closure of valves of the heart.

Heart sounds are heard by placing the ear over the chest or by using a stethoscope or microphone. These sounds are also recorded graphically.

DIFFERENT HEART SOUNDS

Four heart sounds are produced during each cardiac cycle. First and second heart sounds are called **classical heart sounds**. These two sounds are more prominent and resemble the spoken words '**LUB** (or LUBB) and '**DUB**' (or DUP) respectively. These two heart sounds are heard by using the stethoscope.

IMPORTANCE OF HEART SOUNDS

Evaluation of heart sounds has important diagnostic value in clinical practice because alteration in heart sounds indicates the cardiac diseases involving valves of the heart.

DESCRIPTION OF HEART SOUNDS

FIRST HEART SOUND

First heart sound is heard during **isometric contraction** period and earlier part of **ejection period (Table 67.1)**.

TABLE 67.1: Heart sounds.

Features	First heart sound	Second heart sound	Third heart sound	Fourth heart sound
Cause	Closure of atrioventricular valves	Closure of semilunar valves	Rushing of blood into ventricle	Contraction of atrial musculature
Occurs during	Isometric contraction period and part of ejection period	Protodiastole and part of isometric relaxation period	Rapid filling phase	Atrial systole
Characteristics	Long, soft and low pitched. Resembles the word 'LUBB'	Short, sharp and high pitched. Resembles the word 'DUP'	Low pitched	Inaudible sound
Duration (second)	0.10 to 0.17	0.10 to 0.14	0.07 to 0.10	0.02 to 0.04
Frequency (cycles per sec)	25 to 45	50	1 to 6	1 to 4
Relation with ECG	Coincides with peak of 'R' wave	Precedes or appears 0.09 second after peak of 'T' wave	Between 'T' wave and 'P' wave	Between 'P' wave and 'Q' wave
Number of vibrations in phonocardiogram	9 to 13	4 to 6	1 to 4	1 to 2

Causes of First Heart Sound

Major cause for first heart sound is the sudden and synchronous (simultaneous) closure of **atrioventricular valves**. In addition to this, ejection of blood from ventricles into aorta and pulmonary artery and contraction of cardiac muscles also contribute in the production of the first heart sound.

Characteristics of First Heart Sound

First heart sound is a **long, soft and low-pitched** sound. It resembles the spoken word '**LUBB**' (or LUB). Duration of this sound is 0.10 to 0.17 second. Its frequency is 25 to 45 cycles/second.

First Heart Sound and ECG

First heart sound coincides with peak of 'R' wave in ECG.

Applied Physiology

Reduplication of first heart sound

Reduplication means splitting of the heart sound. First heart sound is split when the atrioventricular valves do not close simultaneously (**asynchronous closure**). Splitting of first heart sound in normal conditions (physiological splitting) is rare. Pathological splitting of first heart sound occurs in stenosis of atrioventricular valves and atrial septal defect.

■ SECOND HEART SOUND

Second heart sound is produced at the end of **protodiastolic period**.

Cause for Second Heart Sound

Second heart sound is produced due to the sudden and synchronous closure of **semilunar valves**.

Characteristics for Second Heart Sound

Second heart sound is a **short, sharp and high-pitched** sound. It resembles the spoken word '**DUBB**' (or DUP). Duration of the second heart sound is 0.10 to 0.14 second. Its frequency is 50 cycles/second.

Second Heart Sound and ECG

Second heart sound coincides with the 'T' wave in ECG. Sometimes, it may precede the 'T' wave or it may commence after the peak of 'T' wave.

Applied Physiology

Reduplication of second heart sound

Splitting of second heart sound occurs due to asynchronous closure of **semilunar valves**. It may occur both in physiological and pathological conditions.

Physiological splitting occurs during deep inspiration. Pathological splitting occurs during the conditions such as pulmonary stenosis, right bundle branch block and right ventricular hypertrophy.

■ THIRD HEART SOUND

Third heart sound is a **low-pitched** sound that is produced during **rapid filling period** of the cardiac cycle. Usually, the third heart sound is **inaudible** by stethoscope and it can be heard only by using microphone.

Cause for Third Heart Sound

Third heart sound is produced by the rushing of blood into ventricles during rapid filling phase.

Characteristics of Third Heart Sound

Third heart sound is a **short** and **low-pitched** sound. Duration of this sound is 0.07 to 0.10 second. Its frequency is 1 to 6 cycles/second.

Third Heart Sound and ECG

It appears between 'T' and 'P' waves of ECG.

Applied Physiology

Conditions when third heart sound becomes audible by stethoscope

Third heart sound can be heard by stethoscope in children and athletes. Pathological conditions when third heart sound becomes loud and audible by stethoscope are aortic regurgitation, cardiac failure and cardiomyopathy with dilated ventricles.

When third heart sound is heard by stethoscope the condition is called **triple heart sound** (see below). Third heart sound is usually heard best with the bell of stethoscope placed at the apex beat area when the patient is in left lateral decubitus (lying on left side) position.

■ FOURTH HEART SOUND

Normally, the fourth heart sound is an **inaudible** sound. It becomes audible only in pathological conditions. It is studied only by graphical recording, i.e. by **phonocardiography**. This sound is produced during **atrial systole** (late diastole) and it is considered as the physiologic atrial sound. It is also called **atrial gallop** or **presystolic gallop**.

Cause for Fourth Heart Sound

Fourth heart sound is produced by contraction of atrial musculature during atrial systole.

Characteristics of Fourth Heart Sound

Fourth heart sound is a **short and low-pitched** sound. Duration of this sound is 0.02 to 0.04 second. And its frequency is 1 to 4 cycles/second.

Fourth Heart Sound and ECG

Fourth heart sound coincides with the interval between the end of 'P' wave and the onset of 'Q' wave.

Applied Physiology

Conditions when fourth heart sound becomes audible

Forth heart sound becomes audible by stethoscope when the ventricles become stiff. Ventricular stiffness occurs in conditions like ventricular hypertrophy, longstanding hypertension and aortic stenosis. To overcome the ventricular stiffness, atria contract forcefully producing audible fourth heart sound.

When fourth heart sound is heard by stethoscope the condition is called **triple heart sound** (see below). It is usually heard best with the bell of stethoscope placed at the apex beat area when the patient is in supine or left semilateral position.

TRIPLE AND QUADRUPLE HEART SOUNDS

TRIPLE HEART SOUND OR GALLOP RHYTHM

Triple heart sound or **triple rhythm** is an **abnormal rhythm** of heart, characterized by three clear heart sounds during each heartbeat. It is due to an abnormal third or fourth heart sound that is heard besides first and second heart sounds. It is also called gallop rhythm, since it resembles the sound of a **horse's gallop.** Usually, it is indicative of serious cardiovascular disease.

Triple heart sound is produced in conditions like myocardial infarction and severe hypertension.

QUADRUPLE HEART SOUND

Quadruple heart sound is an abnormal rhythm of heart, characterized by four clear heart sounds during each heartbeat. It is also called **quadruple rhythm.** It is due to third and fourth heart sounds that are heard besides first and second heart sounds. It is also called **quadruple gallop.** Quadruple heart sound is also indicative of serious cardiovascular disease.

Quadruple heart sound is produced in patients with congestive heart failure.

Summation Gallop

Whenever, there is tachycardia in patients with quadruple heart sound, the third and fourth heart sounds merge together and give rise to a single sound. This sound is called summation gallop and it resembles gallop rhythm.

METHODS OF STUDY OF HEART SOUNDS

Heart sounds are studied by three methods:

1. By using stethoscope.
2. By using microphone.
3. By phonocardiogram.

BY USING STETHOSCOPE: AUSCULTATION AREAS

First and second heart sounds are heard on the auscultation areas by using the stethoscope. Chest piece of the stethoscope is placed over 4 areas on the chest, which are called auscultation areas.

Auscultation Areas

1. Mitral area (Bicuspid area)

Mitral area is in the left 5th intercostal space half inch medial to midclavicular line. Sound produced by the closure of mitral valve (first heart sound) is transmitted well into this area. It is also called **apex beat area** because apex beat is felt in this area.

Apex beat is the thrust (pushing forcefully) of the apex of ventricles, against chest wall during systole.

2. Tricuspid area

Tricuspid area is on the left border of lower end of sternum **(Fig. 67.1)**. Sound produced by the closure of tricuspid valve (first heart sound) is transmitted well into this area.

3. Pulmonary area

Pulmonary area is on the left 2nd intercostal space, close to sternum. Sound produced by the closure of pulmonary valve (second heart sound) is heard well on this area.

4. Aortic area

Aortic area is over the right 2nd intercostal space, close to sternum. On this area, the sound produced by closure of aortic valve (second heart sound) is heard well.

First heart sound is best heard in mitral and tricuspid areas. However, it is heard in other areas also but the intensity is less. Similarly, the second heart sound is best heard in pulmonary and aortic areas. It is also heard in other areas with less intensity.

BY MICROPHONE

A highly sensitive microphone is placed over the chest. Heart sounds are amplified by means of an amplifier and heard by using a loudspeaker. First, second and third heart sounds are heard by this method.

BY PHONOCARDIOGRAM

Phonocardiography is the technique used to record the heart sounds. Phonocardiogram is the graphical record of heart sounds. It is done by placing an electronic sound transducer over the chest. This transducer is connected to a recording device like polygraph. All the four heart sounds can be recorded in phonocardiogram. It helps to analyze the frequency of the sound waves **(Fig. 66.2)**.

Appearance of Heart Sounds in Phonocardiogram

First heart sound is recorded as single group of waves which are of small amplitude to start with. Later, the amplitude rapidly rises and falls to form **crescendo** and **diminuendo** series of waves. About 9 to 13 waves appear **(Fig. 66.2)**.

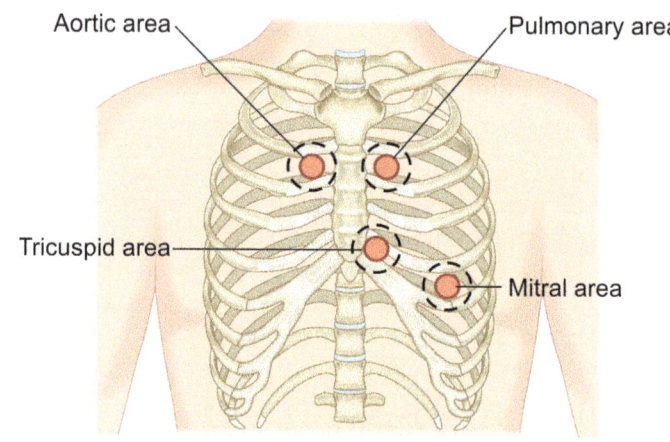

FIGURE 67.1: Auscultatory areas.

Second heart sound appears as single group of waves, which have same amplitude. About 4 to 6 waves are recorded.

Third heart sound is found in phonocardiogram with only 1 to 4 waves grouped together.

Fourth heart sound mostly merges with first heart sound. If it appears as separate form, it has 1 to 2 waves with very low amplitude.

CARDIAC MURMUR

Cardiac murmur is the abnormal or unusual heart sound heard by stethoscope along with normal heart sounds. Cardiac murmur is also called **abnormal heart sound** or **cardiac bruit**. Abnormal sound is produced because of change in the pattern of blood flow. Normally, blood flows in stream line through the heart and the blood vessels. However, during the abnormal conditions like valvular diseases, the blood flow becomes turbulent. This produces the cardiac murmur.

Cardiac murmur is heard by placing the chest piece of the stethoscope over the auscultatory areas. Murmur due to disease of a particular valve is heard well over the auscultatory area of that valve. Sometimes, the murmur is felt by palpation as 'thrills'. In some patients, the murmur is heard without any aid even at a distance of few feet away from the patient.

VALVULAR DISEASES

Valvular diseases are of two types:

1. Stenosis or narrowing of heart valve: Blood flows rapidly with turbulence through narrow orifice of the valve resulting in murmur.
2. Incompetence or weakening of heart valve. When the valve becomes weak, it cannot close properly. It causes back flow of blood resulting in turbulence. This disease is also called regurgitation or valvular insufficiency.

CLASSIFICATION OF MURMUR

Cardiac murmur is classified into three types:

1. **Systolic murmur** produced during systole of the heart.
2. **Diastolic murmur** produced during diastole of the heart.
3. **Continuous murmur** produced continuously heard in conditions such as **patent ductus arteriosus**.

Chapter 68: Electrocardiogram and Arrhythmia

CHAPTER OUTLINE

- DEFINITIONS
- USES OF ECG
- ELECTROCARDIOGRAPHIC GRID
- ECG LEADS
- WAVES OF NORMAL ECG
- INTERVALS AND SEGMENTS OF ECG
- ARRHYTHMIA

■ DEFINITIONS

Electrocardiography

Electrocardiography is a **technique** by which electrical activities of the heart are studied.

Electrocardiograph

Electrocardiograph is the **instrument** (ECG machine) by which the electrical activities of heart are recorded.

Electrocardiogram (ECG)

Electrocardiogram is the record or **graphical registration** of electrical activities of the heart, which occur prior to the onset of mechanical activities. It is the **summed electrical activity** of all the cardiac muscle fibers recorded from the surface of the body.

■ USES OF ECG

ECG is useful in determining heart rate and heart rhythm. ECG is also useful in diagnosing the following conditions:

1. Myocardial ischemia.
2. Heart attack.
3. Coronary artery disease.
4. Hypertrophy of heart chambers.

■ ELECTROCARDIOGRAPHIC (ECG) GRID

Electrocardiograph or ECG machine amplifies the electrical signals produced from the heart and records these signals on a moving strip of paper. Paper that is used for recording ECG is called ECG paper.

ECG grid means to markings (lines) on ECG paper. ECG paper has horizontal and vertical lines at regular intervals of 1 mm. Every 5th line (5 mm) is thickened.

■ DURATION

Time duration of different ECG waves is plotted horizontally on X-axis.

1 mm = 0.04 second
5 mm = 0.20 second.

■ AMPLITUDE

Amplitude of ECG waves is plotted vertically on Y-axis.

1 mm = 0.1 mV
5 mm = 0.5 mV.

■ SPEED OF THE PAPER

Movement of paper through the machine can be adjusted in two speeds, 25 mm/sec and 50 mm/sec. Usually, the speed of the paper during recording is fixed at 25 mm/sec.

If the heart rate is very high, speed of the paper is changed to 50 mm/sec.

■ ECG LEADS

ECG is recorded by placing series of **electrodes** on the surface of the body. These electrodes are called ECG leads and are connected to the ECG machine.

Electrodes are fixed on the limbs. Usually right arm, left arm and left leg are chosen. Heart is said to be in the center of an imaginary equilateral triangle drawn by connecting the roots of these three limbs. This triangle is called **Einthoven's triangle**. Electrical potential generated from the heart appears simultaneously on the roots of these three limbs.

ECG is recorded in 12 leads which are classified into two categories:

I. Bipolar limb leads.
II. Unipolar leads.

1. BIPOLAR LIMB LEADS

Bipolar limb leads are otherwise known as **standard limb leads**. Two limbs are connected to obtain these leads and both the electrodes are **active recording electrodes**, i.e. one electrode is positive and the other one is negative **(Fig. 68.1)**.

Standard limb leads are of three types:

1. Limb lead I.
2. Limb lead II.
3. Limb lead III.

Lead I

Lead I is obtained by connecting **right arm** and **left arm**. Right arm is connected to negative terminal of the instrument and left arm is connected to the positive terminal **(Table 68.1)**.

Lead II

Lead II is obtained by connecting **right arm** and **left leg**. Right arm is connected to negative terminal of the instrument and left leg is connected to the positive terminal.

Lead III

Lead III is obtained by connecting **left arm** and **left leg**. Left arm is connected to negative terminal of the instrument and left leg is connected to the positive terminal.

2. UNIPOLAR LEADS

Here, one electrode is active electrode and the other one is an indifferent electrode. Active electrode is positive and the indifferent electrode is serving as a composite negative electrode.

Unipolar leads are of two types:

A. Unipolar limb leads.
B. Unipolar chest leads.

TABLE 68.1: Twelve leads of ECG.

Bipolar limb leads	Unipolar leads	
	Unipolar limb leads	Unipolar Chest leads
1. Limb lead I 2. Limb lead II 3. Limb lead III	4. aVR lead 5. aVL lead 6. aVF lead	7. V_1 8. V_2 9. V_3 10. V_4 11. V_5 12. V_6

Unipolar Limb Leads

Unipolar limb leads are also called **augmented limb leads**. **Active electrode** is connected to one of the limbs. **Indifferent electrode** is obtained by connecting the other two limbs through a resistance.

Unipolar limb leads are of three types:

1. aVR lead in which active electrode is from **right arm**.
2. aVL lead in which active electrode is from **left arm**.
3. aVF lead in which active electrode is from **left leg** (foot).

Unipolar Chest Leads

Chest leads are also called precardial leads. **Indifferent electrode** is obtained by connecting the three limbs, left arm, left leg and right arm through a resistance of 5,000 ohms. **Active electrode** is placed on six points over the chest **(Fig. 68.2)**. This electrode is known as the **chest electrode** and the six points over the chest are called V_1, V_2, V_3, V_4, V_5 and V_6.

V indicates **vector**, which shows the direction of flow of current.

Position of chest leads

V_1: Over 4th intercostal space near right sternal margin.
V_2: Over 4th intercostal space near left sternal margin.
V_3: In between V_2 and V_4.

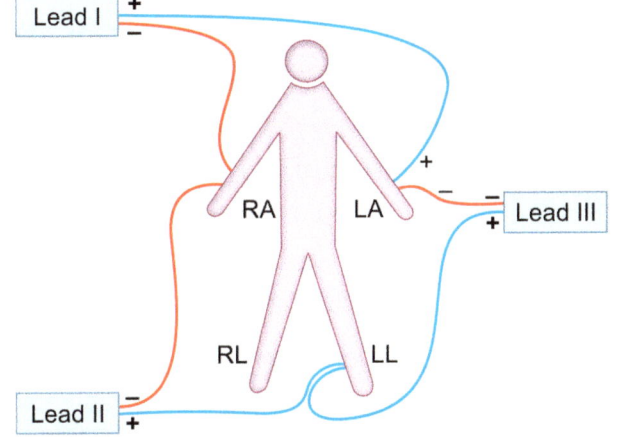

FIGURE 68.1: Position of electrodes for standard limb leads. RA = Right arm, LA = Left arm, LL = Left leg, RL = Right leg (ground electrode).

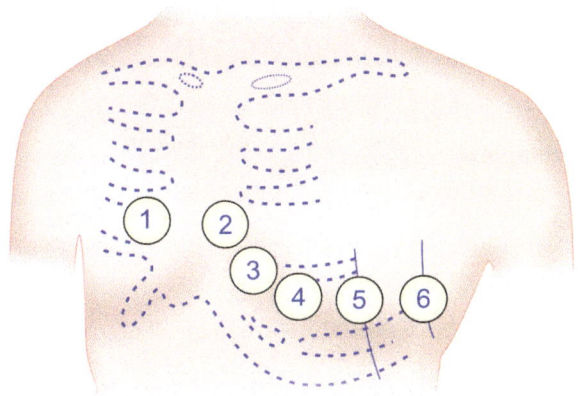

FIGURE 68.2: Position of electrodes for chest leads (V_1 to V_6).

V_4: Over left 5th intercostal space on the midclavicular line.
V_5: Over left 5th intercostal space on the anterior axillary line.
V_6: Over left 5th intercostal space on the mid axillary line.

Ground or Earth Electrode

While recording ECG in each lead, a ground or earth electrode is connected to **right leg** of the subject.

Ground electrode prevents any artifact arising from machine. It also removes noise (produced by electrical power system) that will interfere with low-intensity electrical potential arising from heart.

■ WAVES OF NORMAL ELECTROCARDIOGRAM

A normal ECG consists of waves, complexes, intervals and segments. Waves of ECG recorded by limb lead II are considered as the typical waves.

Normal electrocardiogram has the following waves namely P, Q, R, S and T **(Table 68.2, Figs. 68.3 and 68.4)**. Einthoven had named the waves of ECG starting from the middle of the English alphabets (P) instead of starting from the beginning (A).

Major complexes in ECG are:

1. 'P' wave, the atrial complex.
2. 'QRS' complex, the initial ventricular complex.
3. 'T' wave, the final ventricular complex.
4. 'QRST', the ventricular complex.

■ 'P' WAVE

It is a positive wave and the first wave in ECG. It is also called **atrial complex**.

Cause of 'P' Wave

'P' wave is a positive wave produced due to the **depolarization** of atrial musculature.

Atrial repolarization is not recorded as a separate wave in ECG because it merges with ventricular depolarization (QRS complex).

Duration of 'P' Wave

0.1 second.

Amplitude of 'P' Wave

0.1 to 0.12 mV.

Morphology of 'P' Wave

'P' wave is normally positive (upright) in leads I, II, aVF, V_4, V_5 and V_6. It is normally negative (inverted) in aVR. It is variable in the remaining leads, i.e. it may be positive, negative, biphasic or flat **(Fig. 68.4)**.

■ 'QRS' COMPLEX

It is also called the **initial ventricular complex**. 'Q' wave is a small negative wave. It is continued as the tall 'R' wave, which is a positive wave. 'R' wave is followed by a small negative wave, the 'S' wave.

Cause of 'QRS' Complex

'QRS' complex is due to **depolarization** of ventricular musculature. 'Q' wave is due to the depolarization of basal portion of interventricular septum. 'R' wave is due to the depolarization of apical portion of interventricular septum and apical portion of ventricular muscle. And, 'S' wave is due to the depolarization of basal portion of ventricular muscle near the atrioventricular ring.

Duration of 'QRS' Complex

0.08 to 0.10 second.

Amplitude of 'QRS' Complex

'Q' wave : 0.1 to 0.2 mV.
'R' wave : 1 mV
'S' wave : 0.4 mV

Morphology of 'QRS' Complex

'Q' wave is normally small with amplitude of 4 mm or less. It is less than 25% of amplitude of 'R' wave in leads I, II, aVL, V_5 and V_6. In the remaining leads, its amplitude is less than 0.2 mm.

TABLE 68.2: Waves of normal ECG.

Wave/Segment	From – To	Cause	Duration (second)	Amplitude (mV)
P wave	–	Atrial depolarization	0.1	0.1 to 0.12
QRS complex	Onset of Q wave to the end of S wave	Ventricular depolarization	0.08 to 0.10	Q = 0.1 to 0.2 R = 1 S = 0.4
T wave	–	Ventricular repolarization	0.2	0.3
U wave	–	Repolarization of papillary muscle or Purkinje fibers	0.16 to 0.2	0.1 to 0.2
P-R interval	Onset of P wave to onset of Q wave	Atrial depolarization and conduction through AV node	0.18 (0.12 to 0.2)	–
Q-T interval	Onset of Q wave and end of T wave	Ventricular depolarization and ventricular repolarization	0.4 to 0.42	–
S-T segment	End of S wave and onset of T wave	Isoelectric	0.08	–

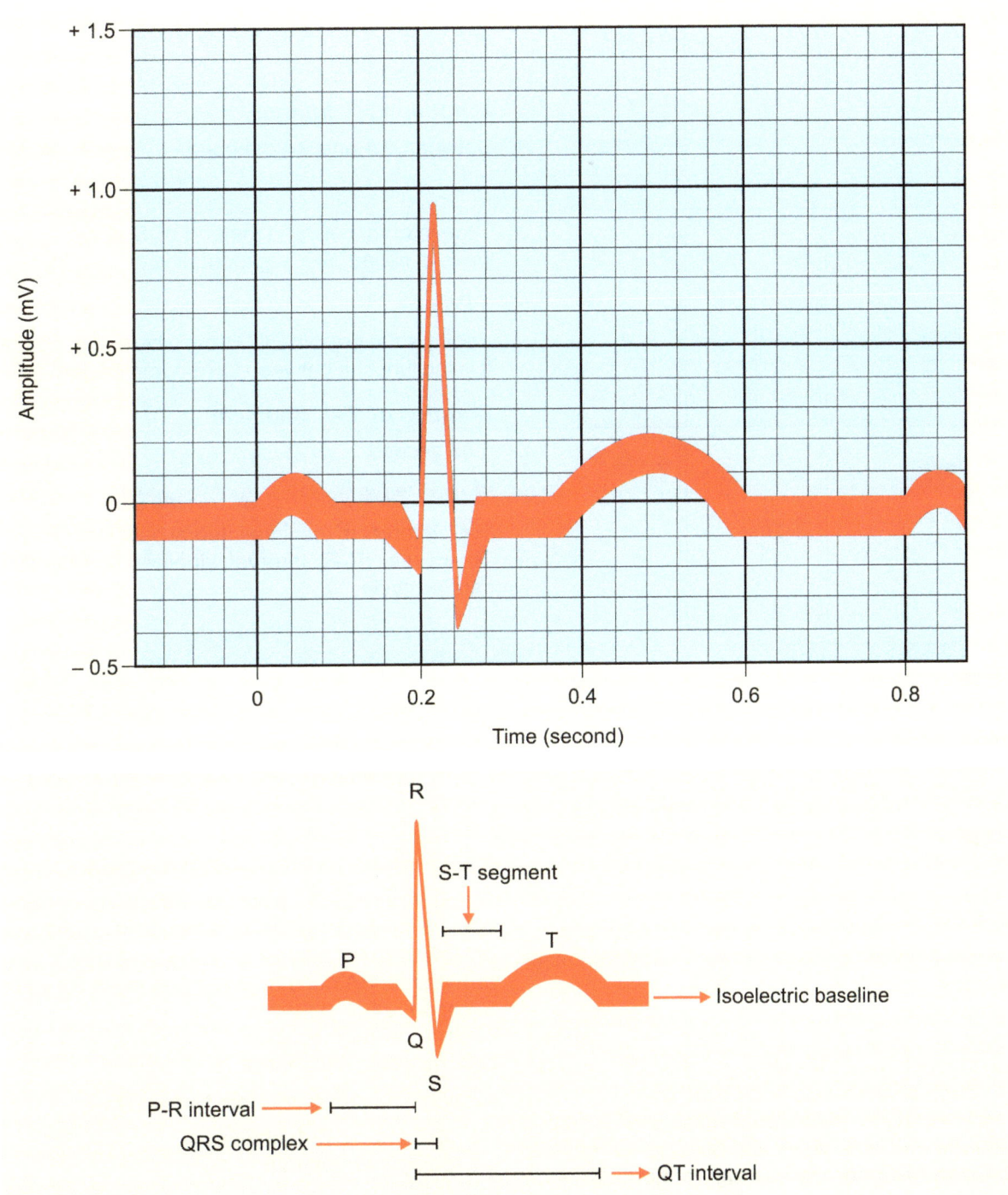

FIGURE 68.3: Waves of normal ECG.

From chest leads V_1 to V_6, 'R' wave becomes gradually larger. It is smaller in V_6 than V_5. 'S' wave is large in V_1 and larger in V_2. It gradually becomes smaller from V_3 to V_6.

■ 'T' WAVE

It is the **final ventricular complex** and is a positive wave.

Cause of 'T' Wave

'T' wave is due to the **repolarization** of ventricular musculature.

Duration of 'T' Wave

0.2 second.

Amplitude of 'T' Wave

0.3 mV.

Morphology of 'T' Wave

'T' wave is normally positive in leads I, II and V_5 and V_6. It is normally inverted in lead aVR. It is variable in the other leads, i.e. it is positive, negative or flat.

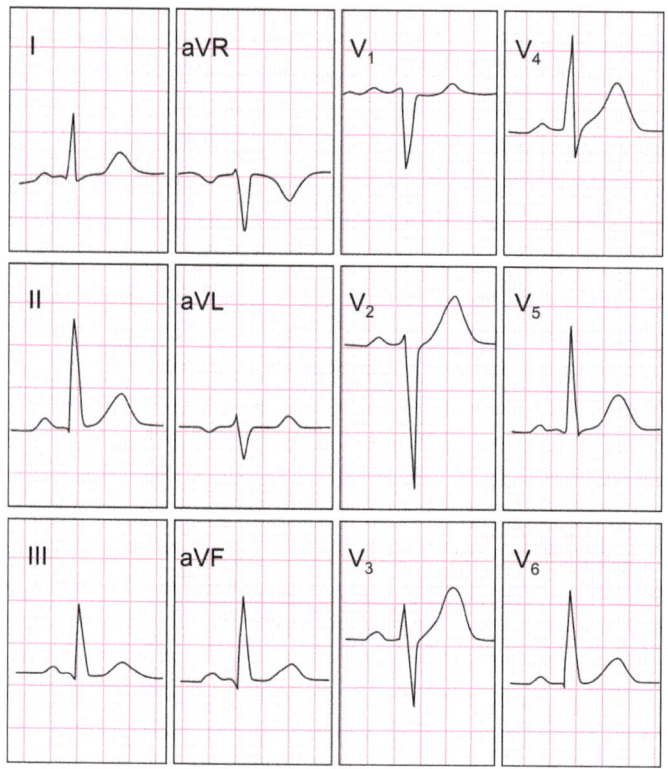

FIGURE 68.4: 12-lead ECG (*Courtesy:* Dr Atul Ruthra).

■ 'U' WAVE

'U' wave is not always seen. It is also an insignificant wave in ECG. It is due to repolarization of papillary muscle and Purkinje fibers.

■ INTERVALS AND SEGMENTS OF ECG

■ 'P-R' INTERVAL

It is the interval between onset of 'P' wave and the onset of 'Q' wave.

'P-R' interval signifies the atrial depolarization and conduction of impulses through AV node. It shows the duration of conduction of the impulses from SA node to ventricles through atrial muscle and AV node.

It is represented by short **isoelectric period** (zero voltage) after the end of 'P' wave and onset of 'Q' wave. It denotes the time taken for the passage of depolarization within AV node.

Duration of 'P-R' Interval

Normal duration is 0.18 second and varies between 0.12 and 0.2 second. If it is more than 0.2 second, that signifies the delay in conduction of impulse from SA node to ventricles. Usually, the delay occurs in AV node. So, it is called the **AV nodal delay**.

■ 'Q-T' INTERVAL

It is the interval between the onset of 'Q' wave and the end of 'T' wave.

'Q-T' interval indicates the ventricular depolarization and ventricular repolarization, i.e. it signifies the electrical activity in ventricles.

Duration 'Q-T' Interval

Between 0.4 and 0.42 second.

■ 'S-T' SEGMENT

Time interval between the end of 'S' wave and onset of 'T' wave is called 'S-T' segment. It is an **isoelectric period.**

J Point

J point is the point in ECG from where 'S-T' segment starts. It is the junction between QRS complex and 'S-T' segment.

Duration of 'S-T' Segment

0.08 second.

■ 'R-R' INTERVAL

'R-R' interval is the time interval between two consecutive 'R' waves. 'R-R' interval signifies the duration of one cardiac cycle.

Significance of 'R-R' Interval

'R-R' interval signifies the duration of one cardiac cycle. Measurement of 'R-R' interval helps to calculate heart rate.

Duration of 'R-R' Interval

Normal duration of 'R-R' interval is 0.8 second.

■ ARRHYTHMIA

■ DEFINITION AND CLASSIFICATION

Arrhythmia refers to **irregular heartbeat** or disturbance in the rhythm of heart. In arrhythmia, heartbeat may be fast or slow or there may be an extra beat or a missed beat. In arrhythmia, SA node may or may not be the pacemaker. If SA node is not the pacemaker, any other part of the heart such as atrial muscle, AV node and ventricular muscle becomes the pacemaker.

Arrhythmia is classified into two types:
  I. Normotopic arrhythmia.
  II. Ectopic arrhythmia.

■ NORMOTOPIC ARRHYTHMIA

Normotopic arrhythmia is the irregular heartbeat, in which SA node is the pacemaker. Normotopic arrhythmia occurs in both physiological and pathological conditions.

Normotopic arrhythmia is of three types:

1. Sinus Arrhythmia

Sinus arrhythmia is a normal rhythmical increase and decrease in heart rate, in relation to respiration. It is also called **respiratory sinus arrhythmia** (RSA). Normal sinus rhythm means the normal heartbeat with SA node as the pacemaker. Normal heart rate is 72 per minute. However, under physiological conditions, in a normal healthy person, heart rate varies according to the phases of respiratory cycle. Heart rate increases during inspiration and decreases during expiration.

2. Sinus Tachycardia

Sinus tachycardia is the increase in discharge of impulses from SA node, resulting in increase in heart rate. Discharge of impulses from SA node is very rapid and the heart rate increases up to 100 per minute and sometimes up to 150 per minute.

3. Sinus Bradycardia

Sinus bradycardia is the reduction in discharge of impulses from SA node resulting in decrease in heart rate. Heart rate is less than 60 per minute.

ECTOPIC ARRHYTHMIA

Ectopic arrhythmia is the abnormal heartbeat, in which one of the structures of heart other than SA node becomes the pacemaker. Impulses produced by these structures are called **ectopic foci**. Ectopic arrhythmia occurs only pathological conditions.

Ectopic arrhythmia is divided into two subtypes:

A. **Homotopic** arrhythmia, in which the impulses for heartbeat arise from any part of conductive system.
B. **Heterotopic** arrhythmia, in which the impulses arise from the musculature of heart other than conductive system.

Different ectopic arrhythmia:

1. Heart block.
2. Extrasystole.
3. Paroxysmal tachycardia.
4. Atrial flutter.
5. Atrial fibrillation.
6. Ventricular fibrillation.

1. Heart Block

Heart block is the blockage of impulses generated by SA node in the conductive system. Because of the blockage, the impulses cannot reach the cardiac musculature, resulting in ectopic arrhythmia. Based on the area affected, the heart block is classified into two types, sinoatrial block and atrioventricular block.

Sinoatrial block

Sinoatrial block is the failure of impulse transmission from SA node to AV node. It is also called **sinus block**.

Atrioventricular block

Atrioventricular block is the heart block in which the impulses are not transmitted from atria (from AV node) to ventricles because of defective conductive system. Atrioventricular block is of two categories, incomplete heart block and complete heart block.

i. *Incomplete heart block*: Incomplete heart block is the condition in which the transmission of impulses from atria to ventricles is slowed down and not blocked completely. Impulses reach ventricles late.
ii. *Complete heart block*: Complete heart block is the condition in which the impulses produced by SA node cannot reach the ventricles. Because of this, the ventricles beat in their own rhythm, independent of atrial beat. It is called **idioventricular rhythm**.

2. Extrasystole

Extrasystole is the premature contraction of the heart before its normal contraction. It is caused by an ectopic focus (discharge of an impulse from any part of the heart other than the SA node). The ectopic focus produces an extra beat of the heart that is always followed by a **compensatory pause**. Compensatory pause is the period during which the heart stops in relaxed state.

3. Paroxysmal Tachycardia

Paroxysmal tachycardia is the sudden attack of increased heart rate due to ectopic foci arising from atria, AV node or ventricle. The attack lasts for a period of few seconds to few hours. It stops suddenly. After the attack, heart functions normally.

4. Atrial Flutter

Atrial flutter is an arrhythmia characterized by rapid ineffective atrial contractions, caused by ectopic foci originating from atrial musculature. It is often associated with atrial paroxysmal tachycardia. Both the atria beat rapidly like the wings of a bird, hence the name atrial flutter. Atrial rate is about 250 to 350 per minute.

5. Atrial Fibrillation

Atrial fibrillation is the type of arrhythmia characterized by rapid and irregular atrial contractions at the rate of 300 to 400 beats per minute.

6. Ventricular Fibrillation

Ventricular fibrillation is the dangerous cardiac arrhythmia, characterized by rapid and irregular twitching of ventricles. Ventricles beat very rapidly and irregularly due to the **circus movement** of impulses within ventricular muscle. The rate reaches 400 to 500 per minute. This is triggered by ventricular extrasystole. This type of arrhythmia is serious as it may lead to death, since the ventricles cannot pump blood.

ABNORMAL PACEMAKER

Abnormal pacemaker is the part of the heart other than SA node that becomes the pacemaker and discharges ectopic foci. Various types of arrhythmia develop when an abnormal pacemaker is activated.

Usual abnormal pacemakers are:

1. Atrioventricular node.
2. Atrial musculature.
3. Ventricular musculature.

■ ARTIFICIAL PACEMAKER

Artificial pacemaker is a small **electronic device** that is surgically implanted to regulate abnormal heartbeat. It contains a battery powered **pulse generator,** which produces electrical impulses capable of stimulating the heart. This pacemaker is implanted under the skin over the chest of the patient. Pulses generated by this device are transmitted to the heart through electrodes. Electrodes connected to the device are inserted and passed through a vein and positioned in the heart chambers. The device has a **lithium battery** that may last for 10 to 15 years. The outer casing of the pacemaker is usually made of titanium, which is rarely rejected by body's immune system.

Pulse generator of the pacemaker has multiple functions. It is programmed to cope up with the needs of the individual patient.

Chapter 69: Cardiac Output

CHAPTER OUTLINE

- **DEFINITIONS AND NORMAL VALUES**
  - STROKE VOLUME
  - MINUTE VOLUME
  - CARDIAC INDEX
- **EJECTION FRACTION**
- **CARDIAC RESERVE**
- **VARIATIONS IN CARDIAC OUTPUT**
  - PHYSIOLOGICAL VARIATIONS
  - PATHOLOGICAL VARIATIONS
- **DISTRIBUTION OF CARDIAC OUTPUT**
- **FACTORS MAINTAINING CARDIAC OUTPUT**
  - VENOUS RETURN
- **FORCE OF CONTRACTION**
- **HEART RATE**
- **PERIPHERAL RESISTANCE**
- **MEASUREMENT OF CARDIAC OUTPUT**
  - BY USING FICK'S PRINCIPLE
  - INDICATOR DILUTION METHOD
  - THERMODILUTION TECHNIQUE
  - ESOPHAGEAL DOPPLER ECHOCARDIOGRAPHY
  - DOPPLER ECHOCARDIOGRAPHY
  - BALLISTOCARDIOGRAPHIC METHOD

DEFINITIONS AND NORMAL VALUES

Cardiac output is the amount of blood pumped from each ventricle. Usually, it refers to the left ventricular output through aorta.

Cardiac output is expressed in three ways namely, stroke volume, minute volume and cardiac index. However, in routine clinical practice cardiac output refers to minute volume.

1. STROKE VOLUME

It is the amount of blood pumped out by each ventricle during each beat.

Stroke volume =
    End-diastolic volume – End-systolic volume.

Normal Value of Stroke Volume

70 mL (60 to 80 mL) when the heart rate is normal (72/min).

2. MINUTE VOLUME

Minute volume is the amount of blood pumped out by each ventricle in one minute. It is the product of stroke volume and heart rate.

Minute volume = Stroke volume × Heart rate

Normal Value of Minute Volume

5 liters/ventricle/minute.

3. CARDIAC INDEX

Cardiac index is the minute volume expressed in relation to square meter of body surface area. It is defined as the amount of blood pumped out per ventricle/minute/square meter of the body surface area.

Normal Value of Cardiac Index

Cardiac index = 2.8 ± 0.3 L/ sq. M of body surface area/minute.

Average **body surface area** in an adult is 1.734 sq. M and normal minute volume is 5 L/min.

EJECTION FRACTION

Ejection fraction is the fraction of end-diastolic volume that is ejected out by each ventricle. Normal ejection fraction is 60 to 65%. Refer Chapter 68 for details.

CARDIAC RESERVE

Cardiac reserve is the maximum amount of blood that can be pumped out by heart above the normal value. Cardiac reserve plays an important role in increasing the cardiac output during the conditions such as exercise. It is essential to withstand the stress of exercise. Cardiac reserve in normal healthy adult is 300 to 400%.

■ VARIATIONS IN CARDIAC OUTPUT

● PHYSIOLOGICAL VARIATIONS

1. *Age:* In children, cardiac output is less because of less blood volume. Cardiac index is more than in adults because of less body surface area.
2. *Sex:* In females, cardiac output is less. Cardiac index is more than in males, because of less body surface area.
3. *Body build:* Greater the body build, more is the cardiac output.
4. *Diurnal variation:* Cardiac output is low in early morning and increases in day time.
5. *Environmental temperature:* Moderate change in temperature does not affect cardiac output. Increase in temperature above 30°C raises cardiac output.
6. *Emotional conditions:* Anxiety, apprehension and excitement increase cardiac output about 50% to 100%.
7. *After meals:* During the first 1 hour after taking meals, cardiac output increases.
8. *Exercise:* Cardiac output increases during exercise.
9. *High altitude:* In high altitude, the cardiac output increases.
10. *Posture:* While changing from recumbent to upright position, the cardiac output decreases.
11. *Pregnancy:* During the later months of pregnancy, cardiac output increases by 40%.
12. *Sleep:* Cardiac output is slightly decreased or unaltered during sleep.

● PATHOLOGICAL VARIATIONS

Conditions When Cardiac Output Increases

1. Fever.
2. Anemia.
3. Hyperthyroidism.

Conditions When Cardiac Output Decreases

1. Hypothyroidism.
2. Atrial fibrillation.
3. Heart block.
4. Congestive cardiac failure.
5. Shock.
6. Hemorrhage.

■ DISTRIBUTION OF CARDIAC OUTPUT

Whole amount of blood pumped out by right ventricle goes to lungs. But the blood pumped by left ventricle is distributed to different parts of the body. Fraction of cardiac output distributed to a particular region or organ depends upon the metabolic activities of that region or organ.

Distribution of Blood Pumped Out of Left Ventricle

Distribution of blood pumped out of left ventricle to different organs and the percentage of cardiac output are given in **Table 69.1**.

TABLE 69.1: Distribution of blood pumped out of left ventricle.

Organ	Amount of blood (mL/min)	Percentage
Liver	1,500	30
Kidney	1,300	26
Skeletal muscles	900	18
Brain	800	16
Skin, bone and GI tract	300	6
Heart	200	4
Total	5,000	100

Liver receives maximum amount of blood. Heart, which pumps the blood to all the other organs, receives the least amount of blood.

■ FACTORS MAINTAINING CARDIAC OUTPUT

Cardiac output is maintained (determined) by four factors:

1. Venous return.
2. Force of contraction.
3. Heart rate.
4. Peripheral resistance.

■ 1. VENOUS RETURN

Venus return is amount of blood, which is returned to the heart from different parts of the body. When venous return increases, the ventricular filling and cardiac output are increased. Thus, cardiac output is **directly proportional** to venous return provided the other three factors (force of contraction, heart rate and peripheral resistance) remain constant.

Venous return in turn depends upon respiratory pump and muscle pump.

i. Respiratory Pump

Respiratory pump is the respiratory activity that helps return of blood back to heart during inspiration. It is also called **abdominothoracic pump**. During inspiration, thoracic cavity expands and makes the intrathoracic pressure more negative. It increases the diameter of inferior vena cava resulting in increased venous return. At the same time, descent of diaphragm increases the intra-abdominal pressure. This compresses abdominal veins and pushes the blood upward towards heart and thereby the venous return is increased.

Respiratory pump is much stronger in forced respiration and in severe muscular exercise.

ii. Muscle Pump

Muscle pump is the muscular activity that helps return of the blood back to heart. When muscular activity increases the venous return is more.

When skeletal muscles contract the vein located in between the muscles is compressed. Valve of the vein proximal to contracting muscles **(Fig. 69.1A)** is opened and blood is propelled towards the heart. Valve of the vein distal to the muscles is closed by the back flow of blood.

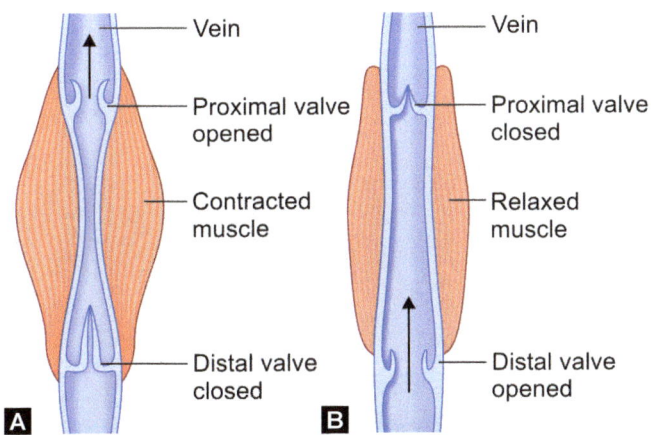

FIGURE 69.1: Mechanism of muscle pump. **A.** During contraction of muscle. **B.** During relaxation of muscle.

During relaxation of the muscles **(Fig. 69.1B)**, the valve proximal to muscles closes and prevents the back flow of blood. And the valve distal to muscles opens and allows the blood to flow upwards.

2. FORCE OF CONTRACTION

Cardiac output is **directly proportional** to the force of contraction provided other three factors remain constant. Force of contraction depends upon diastolic period and ventricular filling. Frank-Starling law of heart is applicable to this.

According to **Frank-Starling law**, the force of contraction of heart is directly proportional to initial length of muscle fibers before the onset of contraction.

Force of contraction also depends upon preload and after load.

Preload

Preload is the stretching of the cardiac muscle fibers at the end of diastole just before contraction. Preload depends upon venous return and ventricular filling. During diastolic period due to the ventricular filling, ventricular pressure increases. This causes stretching of muscle fibers resulting in increase in their length. Increase in length of the muscle fibers increases the force of contraction and cardiac output.

Thus, force of contraction of heart and cardiac output are **directly proportional** to preload.

Afterload

Afterload is the force against which the ventricles must contract and eject the blood. This force is determined by the arterial pressure. At the end of isometric contraction period, semilunar valves are opened and blood is ejected into the aorta and pulmonary artery. So, the pressure increases in these two vessels. Now, the ventricles have to work against this pressure for further ejection. Thus, the afterload for left ventricle is determined by aortic pressure and afterload for right ventricular pressure is determined by pressure in pulmonary artery.

Force of contraction of heart and cardiac output are **inversely proportional** to afterload.

3. HEART RATE

Cardiac output is **directly proportional** to heart rate provided the other three factors remain constant. Moderate change in heart rate does not alter the cardiac output. If there is a marked increase in heart rate, cardiac output is increased.

If there is marked decrease in heart rate, cardiac output is decreased.

4. PERIPHERAL RESISTANCE

Peripheral resistance is the resistance offered to blood flow at the peripheral blood vessels. It is the resistance or load against which the heart has to pump the blood. So, the cardiac output is **inversely proportional** to peripheral resistance.

Resistance is offered at arterioles. So, the arterioles are called **resistant vessels**. In the body, the maximum peripheral resistance is offered at the **splanchnic region**.

MEASUREMENT OF CARDIAC OUTPUT

Cardiac output is measured by direct methods and indirect methods. Direct methods are used only in animals. Indirect methods are used both in animals and human beings.

Several indirect methods are available to measure cardiac output in human beings. Each method has got its own advantages and disadvantages. Generally, the safe and accurate method is preferred. In view of safety, always non-invasive methods are preferred to measure cardiac output.

Invasive method is a procedure which involves invasion or penetration of healthy tissues, organs or parts of the body by means of perforation, puncture, incision, injection or catheterization.

Non-invasive method is the procedure that does not involve invasion or penetration of tissues, organs or parts of the body.

Methods used to measure cardiac output in human beings are:

1. By using Fick's principle.
2. Indicator (dye) dilution technique.
3. Thermodilution technique.
4. Ultrasonic Doppler transducer technique.
5. Doppler echocardiography.
6. Ballistocardiography.

1. BY USING FICK'S PRINCIPLE

According to Fick's principle, amount of a substance taken up by an organ (or by the whole body) or given out in a unit of time is the product of amount of blood flowing through the organ and arteriovenous difference of that substance across the organ.

| Amount of substance taken or given | = | Amount of blood flow/minute | × | Arteriovenous difference |

For Example

Amount of blood flowing through lungs is 5,000 mL/min/O_2 content in arterial blood = 20 mL/100 mL of blood.
O_2 content in venous blood = 15 mL/100 mL of blood.
So, amount of O_2 moved from lungs to blood =

$$= 5,000 \times \frac{20-15}{100}$$

$$= 5,000 \times \frac{5}{100} = 250$$

Thus, amount of O_2 moved from lungs to blood = 250 mL/min.

Modification of Fick Principle to Measure Cardiac Output

Fick's principle is modified to measure the cardiac output or a part of cardiac output (amount of blood to an organ). Thus, cardiac output or amount of blood flowing through an organ in a given unit of time is determined by the formula given below.

$$\text{Cardiac output} = \frac{\text{Amount of substance taken or given by the organ/minute}}{\text{Arteriovenous difference of the substance across the organ}}$$

By using Fick's principle, cardiac output is measured in two ways:

i. By using oxygen consumption.
ii. By using carbon dioxide given out.

Measurement of Cardiac Output by Using Oxygen Consumption

Fick's principle is used to measure cardiac output by determining the amount of oxygen consumed in body in a given period of time and dividing this value by arteriovenous difference across the lungs.

Oxygen consumption

Amount of oxygen consumed is measured by using a **respirometer** or **BMR apparatus (Benedict-Roth apparatus)**.

Oxygen content in arterial blood

Blood is collected from any artery to determine the oxygen content in arterial blood. Oxygen content is determined by **blood gas analysis**.

Oxygen content in venous blood

Only mixed venous blood is used to determine the oxygen content of venous blood, since oxygen content is different in different veins. **Mixed venous blood** is collected from right atrium. From this blood oxygen content is measured by blood gas analysis **(Fig. 69.2)**.

Calculation

For example, in a subject the following data are obtained:
O_2 consumed (by lungs) = 250 mL/min
O_2 content in arterial blood = 20 mL/100 mL of blood

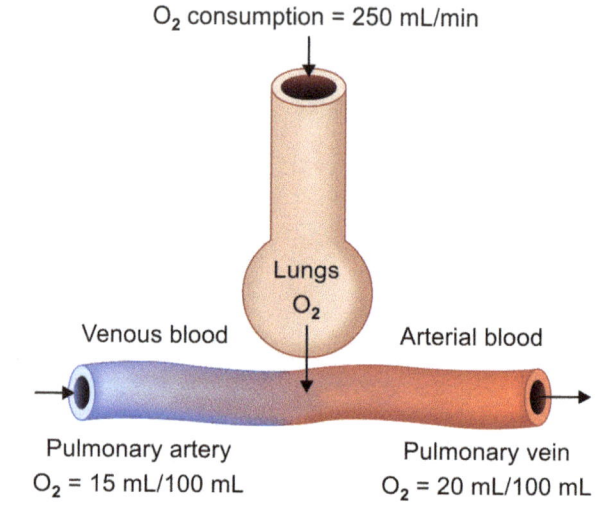

FIGURE 69.2: Oxygen consumption.

O_2 content in venous blood = 15 mL/100 mL of blood

$$\text{Cardiac output} = \frac{O_2 \text{ consumed (in mL/min)}}{\text{Arteriovenous } O_2 \text{ difference}}$$

$$= \frac{250}{5/100} = \frac{250 \times 100}{5}$$

$$= 5,000 \text{ mL/min}$$

5 mL of oxygen is taken by 100 mL of blood while passing through the lungs. Thus, 250 mL of oxygen is taken by 5,000 mL of blood. Since, cardiac output is equivalent to the amount of blood passing through pulmonary circulation, the cardiac output = 5 L/min.

Measurement of Cardiac Output by Using Carbon Dioxide

Cardiac output is also measured by knowing the arteriovenous difference of carbon dioxide and amount of carbon dioxide given out from lungs **(Fig. 69.3)**.

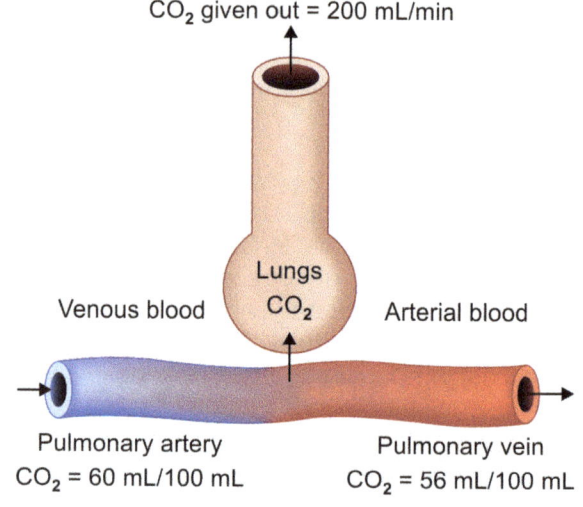

FIGURE 69.3: Carbon dioxide given.

Calculation

For example, in a subject:
CO_2 removed by lungs = 200 mL/min
CO_2 content in arterial blood = 56 mL/100 mL of blood
CO_2 content in venous blood = 60 mL/100 ml of blood

$$\text{Cardiac output} = \frac{CO_2 \text{ given out (in mL/min)}}{\text{Arteriovenous } CO_2 \text{ difference}}$$

$$= \frac{200}{60 - 56 \text{ mL} / 100 \text{ mL}}$$

$$= \frac{200 \times 100}{6}$$

$$= 5,000 \text{ mL} / \text{min} = 5 \text{ L} / \text{min}$$

Since, cardiac output is equal to amount of blood passing through lungs (pulmonary circulation), the cardiac output = 5 L/min.

■ 2. INDICATOR (DYE) DILUTION METHOD

Indicator dilution technique is described in detail in Chapter 5. Marker substance used to measure cardiac output is lithium chloride.

■ 3. THERMODILUTION TECHNIQUE

Cardiac output can also be measured by thermodilution technique or **thermal indicator method**. This method is the modified indicator dilution method. It is the popular method to measure cardiac output.

In this method, a known volume of cold sterile solution is injected into the right atrium by using a catheter. Cardiac output is measured by determining the resultant change in the blood temperature in pulmonary artery. For this purpose, **two thermistors** (temperature transducers) are used. One of them is placed in the inferior vena cava and the second one is placed in pulmonary artery.

■ 4. ESOPHAGEAL DOPPLER TRANSDUCER TECHNIQUE

This technique involves insertion of a flexible probe into midthoracic part of esophagus. A pulse wave **ultrasonic Doppler transducer** is fixed at the tip of the probe. This transducer calculates the velocity of blood flow in descending aorta. Diameter of aorta is determined by echocardiography. Cardiac output is calculated by using the values of velocity of blood flow and diameter of aorta.

■ 5. DOPPLER ECHOCARDIOGRAPHY

Doppler echocardiography is a method for detecting the direction and velocity of moving blood within the heart. This is also a popular method to measure cardiac output.

■ 6. BALLISTOCARDIOGRAPHIC METHOD

Ballistocardiography is the technique to record the movements of the body caused by ballistic recoil associated with contraction of heart and ejection of blood. It is based on **Newton's third law of motion** (for every action there is an equal and opposite reaction).

When heart pumps blood into aorta and pulmonary artery, a recoiling force is exerted against heart and the body. It is similar to that of ballistic recoil when a bullet is fired from a riffle.

Pulsations due to this ballistic recoil can be recorded graphically by making the subject to lie on a suspended bed movable in the long axis of the body. Cardiac output is determined by analyzing the graph obtained.

Chapter 70: Heart Rate

CHAPTER OUTLINE

- **HEART RATE**
  - NORMAL HEART RATE
  - TACHYCARDIA
  - BRADYCARDIA
- **REGULATION OF HEART RATE**
- **VASOMOTOR CENTER: CARDIAC CENTER**
  - VASOCONSTRICTOR AREA
  - VASODILATOR AREA
  - SENSORY AREA
- **MOTOR (EFFERENT) NERVE FIBERS TO HEART**
  - PARASYMPATHETIC NERVE FIBERS
  - SYMPATHETIC NERVE FIBERS
- **SENSORY (AFFERENT) NERVE FIBERS FROM HEART**
- **FACTORS AFFECTING VASOMOTOR CENTER: REGULATION OF VAGAL TONE**
  - IMPULSES FROM HIGHER CENTERS
  - IMPULSES FROM RESPIRATORY CENTERS
  - IMPULSES FROM BARORECEPTORS
  - IMPULSES FROM CHEMORECEPTORS
  - IMPULSES FROM RIGHT ATRIUM: BAINBRIDGE REFLEX
  - IMPULSES FROM OTHER AFFERENT NERVES
  - BEZOLD-JARISCH REFLEX

HEART RATE

NORMAL HEART RATE

Normal heart rate is 72/minute. It ranges between 60 and 80 per minute.

TACHYCARDIA

Tachycardia is the increase in heart rate above 100 per minute.

Physiological Conditions when Tachycardia Occurs

1. Childhood.
2. Exercise.
3. Pregnancy.
4. Emotional conditions such as anxiety.

Pathological Conditions when Tachycardia Occurs

1. Fever.
2. Anemia.
3. Hypoxia.
4. Hyperthyroidism.
5. Hypersecretion of catecholamines.
6. Cardiomyopathy.
7. Valvular heart diseases.

Drugs which Induce Bradycardia

1. Beta blockers.
2. Channel blockers.
3. Digitalis and other antiarrhythmic drugs.

BRADYCARDIA

Bradycardia is the decrease in heart rate below 60 per minute.

Physiological Conditions when Bradycardia Occurs

1. During sleep.
2. In athletes.

Pathological Conditions when Bradycardia Occurs

1. Hypothermia.
2. Hypothyroidism.
3. Heart attack.
4. Congenital heart disease.

5. Degenerative process of aging.
6. Obstructive jaundice.
7. Increased intracranial pressure.

REGULATION OF HEART RATE

Heart rate is maintained within normal range constantly. It is subjected for variation during conditions such as exercise, emotion, etc. However, under physiological conditions, the altered heart rate is quickly brought back to normal. Heart rate is regulated by the nervous mechanism which consists of three components.

Components of Nervous Mechanism Regulating Heart Rate

I. Vasomotor center.
II. Motor (efferent) nerve fibers to the heart.
III. Sensory (afferent) nerve fibers from the heart.

VASOMOTOR CENTER: CARDIAC CENTER

Vasomotor center is the nervous center that regulates the heart rate. It also regulates the blood pressure. Earlier it was called the **cardiac center**.

Vasomotor center is bilaterally situated in the **reticular formation** of medulla oblongata and lower part of pons. It has three areas.

Areas of Vasomotor Center

1. Vasoconstrictor area.
2. Vasodilator area.
3. Sensory area.

VASOCONSTRICTOR AREA: CARDIOACCELERATOR CENTER

Situation

It is situated in the **reticular formation of medulla** in the floor of IV ventricle and it forms the lateral portion of vasomotor center. Vasoconstrictor area is otherwise known as **pressor area** or cardioaccelerator center.

Functions of Vasoconstrictor Area

This area increases the heart rate by sending accelerator impulses to heart through sympathetic nerves. It also causes constriction of blood vessels.

Control of Vasoconstrictor Area

Vasoconstrictor area is under the control of **cerebral cortex** and **hypothalamus**.

VASODILATOR AREA: CARDIOINHIBITORY CENTER

Situation

It is also situated in the **reticular formation of medulla** oblongata in the floor of IV ventricle. It forms the medial portion of vasomotor center. It is also called **depressor area** or cardioinhibitory center.

Functions of Vasodilator Area

Vasodilator area decreases the heart rate by sending inhibitory impulses to the heart through vagus nerve. It also causes dilatation of blood vessels.

Control of Vasodilator Area

Vasodilator area is under the control of **cerebral cortex** and **hypothalamus**. It is also controlled by the impulses from baroreceptors, chemoreceptors and other sensory impulses via afferent nerves.

SENSORY AREA

Situation

Sensory area is in **nucleus of tractus solitarius** in medulla. It forms posterior part of vasomotor center.

Functions of Sensory Area

Sensory area receives sensory impulse via glossopharyngeal nerve and **vagus nerve** from periphery, particularly, from the baroreceptors. In turn, this area controls the vasoconstrictor and vasodilator areas.

MOTOR (EFFERENT) NERVE FIBERS TO HEART

Heart receives efferent nerves from both the divisions of autonomic nervous system. Parasympathetic fibers arise from the medulla oblongata and pass through vagus nerve. Sympathetic fibers arise from upper thoracic (T1 to T4) segments of spinal cord **(Fig. 70.1)**.

PARASYMPATHETIC NERVE FIBERS

Origin

Parasympathetic nerve fibers supplying heart arise from **dorsal nucleus of vagus** situated in the floor of fourth ventricle in medulla oblongata.

Distribution of Parasympathetic Nerve Fibers

Preganglionic parasympathetic nerve fibers from dorsal nucleus of vagus reach the heart and terminate on postganglionic neurons. Postganglionic fibers from these neurons innervate heart muscle.

Most of the fibers from right vagus terminate in SA node. Remaining fibers supply the atrial muscles and AV node. Most of the fibers from left vagus supply AV node and some fibers supply the atrial muscle and SA node.

Ventricles do not receive the vagus nerve supply.

Functions of Parasympathetic Nerve

Vagus nerve is **cardioinhibitory** in function and carries inhibitory impulses from vasodilator area to heart. These impulses decrease the rate and force contraction of heart.

Vagal Tone

Vagal tone is the continuous stream of **inhibitory impulses** from vasodilator area to heart via vagus nerve. Heart rate is kept under control because of vagal tone.

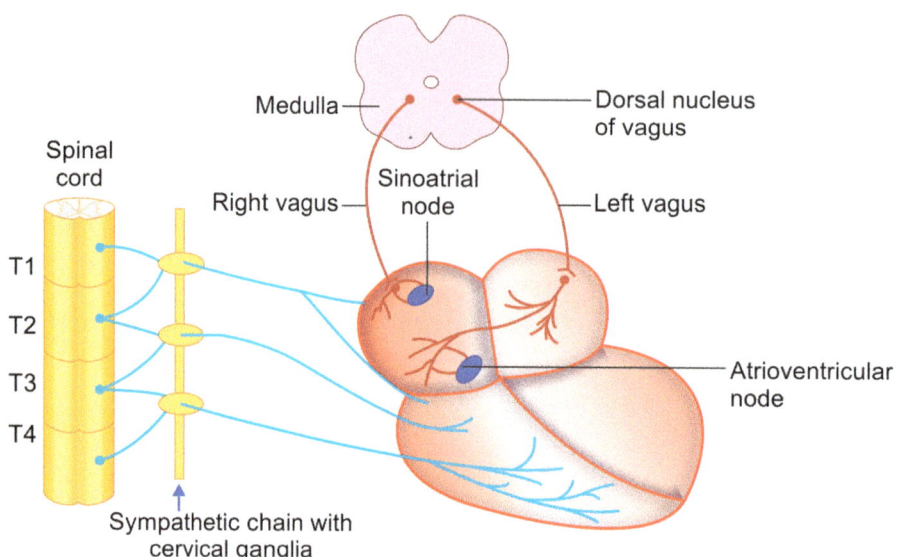

FIGURE 70.1: Nerve supply to heart.

These impulses reach the heart and exert inhibitory effect on heart. Heart rate is **inversely proportional** to vagal tone. In experimental animals (dog), removal of vagal input (by sectioning vagus) increases the heart rate. This proves the existence of vagal tone. Under resting conditions, vagal tone dominates sympathetic tone (see below).

Impulses from different parts of the body regulate the heart rate through vasomotor center, by altering the vagal tone. Vagal tone is also called **cardioinhibitory tone** or **parasympathetic tone.**

Effects of Stimulation of Vagus Nerve

Effects of stimulation of right vagus nerve: Vagal escape

Right vagus supplies mainly SA node. Stimulation of right vagus in experimental animals such as dog, with a weak stimulus causes reduction in heart rate and force of contraction. Stimulation with strong stimulus causes stoppage of heart due to inhibition of SA node. If the stimulus is continued for some time, the ventricle starts beating; but the rate of contraction is slower than before. This is because of vagal escape.

Vagal escape is the escape of ventricle from inhibitory effect of vagal stimulation. If stimulation of vagus nerve is stopped, heart starts beating normally.

Causes for vagal escape

Stimulation of right vagus stops the heartbeat due to inhibition of SA node and atria. However, ventricles are not supplied by vagus. So, the ventricles are not inhibited by vagal stimulation. Because of this, when stoppage of heartbeat is continued for some time (by vagal stimulation), a part of ventricular musculature becomes pacemaker and starts producing impulses. It results in contraction of ventricles, which is called vagal escape.

Thus, vagal escape includes only ventricular contractions. Rhythmicity of ventricular muscle is less and it is about 20 per minute.

Effects of stimulation of left vagus nerve: Heart block

Left vagus supplies mainly the AV node. Stimulation of left vagus in dog with a weak stimulus causes inhibition of AV node. Because of inhibition of AV node, some of the impulses from SA node are not conducted to ventricles. This is called the **partial heart block.** Ratio between atrial contraction and ventricular contraction is 2:1, 3:1 or 4:1, depending upon the strength of stimulus.

Stimulation of left vagus with strong stimulus causes stoppage of ventricular contraction, which is called **complete heart block.** This is because of the complete inhibition of AV node. The prolongation of stimulation **causes idioventricular rhythm**, which is different from the rhythm of atrial contraction.

Mode of Action of Vagus Nerve

Vagus nerve inhibits the heart by secreting the neurotransmitter called **acetylcholine.**

■ SYMPATHETIC NERVE FIBERS

Origin

Preganglionic fibers of the sympathetic nerves to heart arise from lateral gray horns of the first 4 thoracic segments (T1 to T4) of the spinal cord.

Course and Distribution of Sympathetic Nerve Fibers

Preganglionic fibers reach the superior, middle and inferior **cervical sympathetic ganglia** situated in the sympathetic chain. Inferior cervical sympathetic ganglion fuses with first thoracic sympathetic ganglion forming **stellate ganglion**. From these ganglia, the postganglionic fibers arise.

Postganglionic fibers form superior, middle and inferior **cervical sympathetic nerves**.

Nerves Formed by Sympathetic Postganglionic Fibers

1. Superior cervical sympathetic nerve, which innervates larger arteries and base of the heart.
2. Middle cervical sympathetic nerve, which supplies the rest of the heart.
3. Inferior cervical sympathetic nerve, which serves as **sensory (afferent) nerve** from the heart.

Functions of Sympathetic Nerves

Sympathetic nerves are **cardioaccelerator** in function and carry cardioaccelerator impulses from vasoconstrictor area to the heart. These impulses increase the rate and force of contraction of heart.

Sympathetic Tone

Sympathetic tone or **cardioaccelerator tone** is the continuous stream of impulses produced by the vasoconstrictor area. These impulses pass through sympathetic nerves and accelerate the heart rate.

Under normal conditions, vagal tone is dominant over sympathetic tone. Whenever vagal tone is reduced or abolished, the sympathetic tone becomes powerful.

Effects of Stimulation of Sympathetic Nerves

Stimulation of sympathetic nerves increases the rate and force of contraction of heart. Effect depends upon the strength of stimulus.

Mode of Action of Sympathetic Nerves

Sympathetic nerves increase heart rate by secreting the neurotransmitter called **noradrenaline.**

SENSORY (AFFERENT) NERVE FIBERS FROM HEART

Afferent (sensory) nerve fibers from the heart pass through the **inferior cervical sympathetic nerve**. These nerve fibers carry sensations of **stretch** and **pain** from the heart to the brain via spinal cord.

FACTORS AFFECTING VASOMOTOR CENTER: REGULATION OF VAGAL TONE

Vasomotor center regulates the cardiac activity by receiving impulses from different sources in the body. After receiving the impulses from different sources, the vasodilator area alters the vagal tone and modulates the activities of the heart. Various sources from which the impulses reach the vasomotor center are detailed below.

1. IMPULSES FROM HIGHER CENTERS

Vasomotor center is mainly controlled by the impulses from following higher centers in the brain.

Cerebral Cortex

Area 13 in cerebral cortex is concerned with emotional reactions of the body. During emotional conditions, this area sends inhibitory impulses to the vasodilator area. This causes reduction in vagal tone leading to cardioacceleration.

Hypothalamus

Hypothalamus influences the heart rate via vasomotor center. Stimulation of posterior and lateral hypothalamic nuclei causes tachycardia. Stimulation of preoptic and anterior nuclei causes bradycardia.

2. IMPULSES FROM RESPIRATORY CENTERS

In forced breathing, heart rate increases during inspiration and decreases during expiration. This variation is called **respiratory sinus arrhythmia**. This is common in some children and in some adults even during quiet breathing.

3. IMPULSES FROM BARORECEPTORS: MAREY'S REFLEX

Baroreceptors or **pressoreceptors** are the receptors, which give response to change in blood pressure.

Situation of Baroreceptors

Baroreceptors are of two types, **carotid baroreceptors** and **aortic baroreceptors**. Carotid baroreceptors are situated in the carotid sinus, which is present in the wall of internal carotid artery near the bifurcation of common carotid artery. Aortic baroreceptors are situated in the wall of arch of aorta.

Nerve Supply to Baroreceptors

Carotid baroreceptors are supplied by **Hering's nerve**, a branch of glossopharyngeal (IX cranial) nerve. Aortic baroreceptors are supplied by **aortic nerve**, a branch of vagus (X cranial) nerve **(Fig. 70.2)**. Nerve fibers from the baroreceptors reach the nucleus of tractus solitarius situated adjacent to vasomotor center.

Functions of Baroreceptors: Marey's Reflex

Baroreceptors regulate the heart rate through a reflex called Marey's reflex. Stimulus for this reflex is increase in blood pressure.

Marey's reflex is a **cardioinhibitory reflex** that decreases heart rate when blood pressure increases.

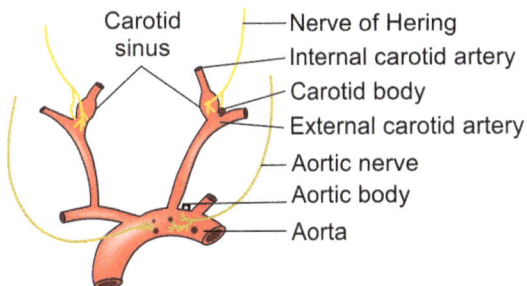

FIGURE 70.2: Nerve supply to baroreceptors and chemoreceptors.

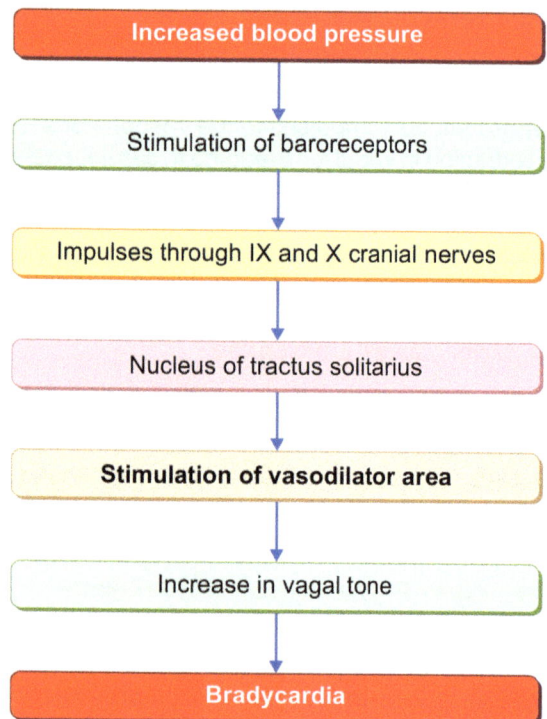

FIGURE 70.3: Marey's (cardioinhibitory) reflex.

Whenever blood pressure increases, the aortic and carotid baroreceptors are stimulated and stimulatory impulses are sent to nucleus of tractus solitarius via Hering's nerve and aortic nerve (afferent nerves). Now, the nucleus of tractus solitarius stimulates the vasodilator area, which in turn increases vagal tone leading to decrease in heart rate **(Fig. 70.3)**.

When pressure is less, the baroreceptors are not stimulated. So, no impulses go to the nucleus of tractus solitaries and heart rate is not decreased.

Thus, the heart rate is **inversely proportional** to blood pressure.

Marey's Law

According to Marey's law, the pulse rate (which represents heart rate) is inversely proportional to blood pressure.

Baroreceptors produce the Marey's reflex only during resting conditions. So, in many conditions such as exercise, there is an increase in both blood pressure and heart rate.

4. IMPULSES FROM CHEMORECEPTORS

Chemoreceptors are the receptors giving response to change in chemical constituents of blood, particularly oxygen, carbon dioxide and hydrogen ion concentration.

Situation of Chemoreceptors

Peripheral chemoreceptors are situated in the **carotid body** and **aortic body** adjacent to baroreceptors.

Nerve Supply to Chemoreceptors

Chemoreceptors in carotid body are supplied by **Hering's nerve**. Chemoreceptors in aortic body are supplied by the **aortic nerve (Fig. 70.2)**.

Functions of Chemoreceptors

Whenever there is hypoxia, hypercapnia, and increased hydrogen ions concentration in the blood, the chemoreceptors are stimulated and inhibitory impulses are sent to vasodilator area. Vagal tone decreases and heart rate increases. Chemoreceptors play a major role in maintaining respiration than the heart rate.

Sinoaortic Mechanism and Buffer Nerves

Sinoaortic mechanism is the mechanism of baroreceptors and chemoreceptors in carotid and aortic regions which regulates heart rate, blood pressure and respiration. The nerves from these receptors are called buffer nerves.

5. IMPULSES FROM RIGHT ATRIUM: BAINBRIDGE REFLEX

Bainbridge reflex is a **cardioaccelerator reflex** that increases the heart rate when venous return is increased. Since this reflex arises from right atrium, it is also called **right atrial reflex**.

There are some **stretch receptors** in the wall of right atrium. When venous return increases, the right atrium is distended. Right atrial distention stimulates the stretch receptors. Stretch receptors, in turn, send inhibitory impulses through inferior cervical sympathetic nerve to vasodilator area of vasomotor center. Vasodilator area is inhibited resulting in decrease in vagal tone and increase in heart rate **(Fig. 70.4)**.

6. IMPULSES FROM OTHER AFFERENT NERVES

Stimulation of sensory nerves produces varying effects.

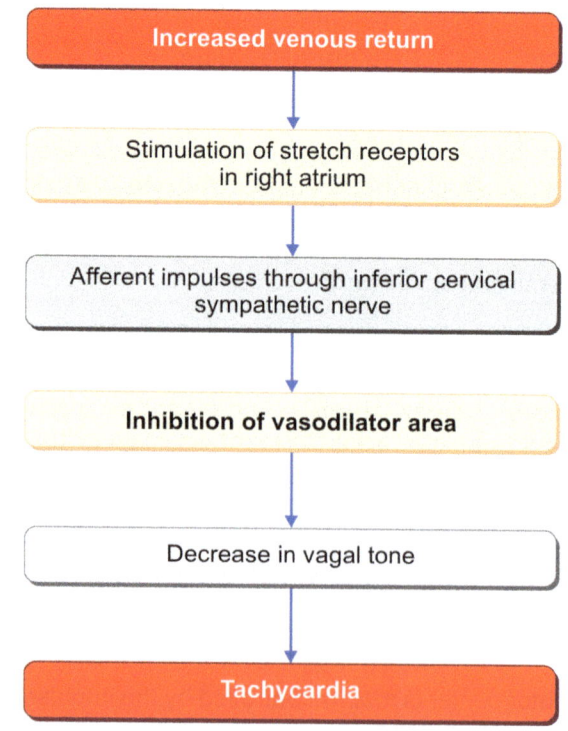

FIGURE 70.4: Bainbridge (cardioaccelerator) reflex.

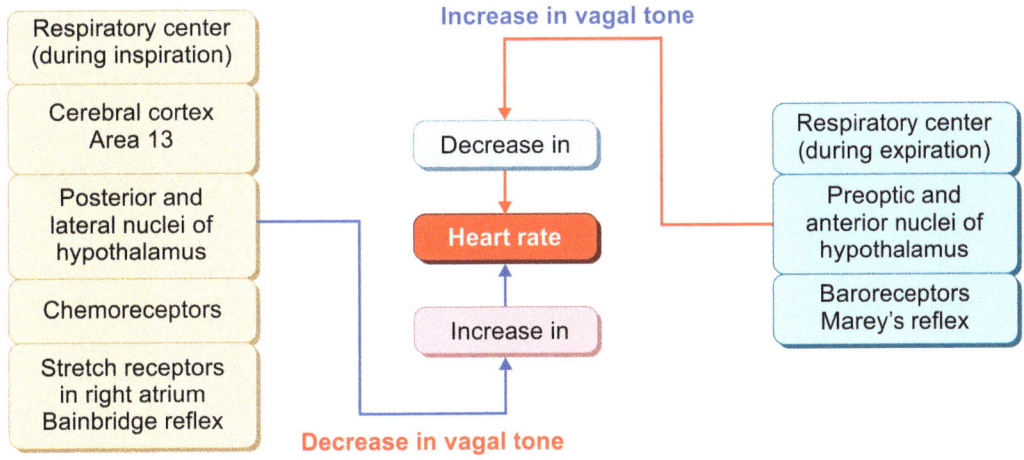

FIGURE 70.5: Factors regulating vagal tone and heart rate.

Examples

i. Stimulation of receptors in nasal mucous membrane causes bradycardia. The impulses from nasal mucous membrane pass via the branches of V cranial nerve and decrease the heart rate.

ii. Most of the **painful stimuli** cause tachycardia and some cause **bradycardia**. The impulses are transmitted via pain nerve fibers **(Fig. 70.5)**.

■ BEZOLD-JARISCH REFLEX

Bezold-Jarisch reflex is the reflex characterized by **bradycardia** and **hypotension**, caused by stimulation of **chemoreceptors** present in the wall of left ventricle by substances such as alkaloids. It is also called **coronary chemoreflex.** Vagal fibers form the afferent and efferent pathways of this reflex.

Conditions when Bezold-Jarisch Reflex Occurs:

1. Myocardial infarction.
2. Administration of thrombolytic agents.
3. Hemorrhage.
4. Aortic stenosis.
5. Syncope.

Chapter 71: Arterial Blood Pressure

CHAPTER OUTLINE

- **DEFINITIONS AND NORMAL VALUES**
  - SYSTOLIC BLOOD PRESSURE
  - DIASTOLIC BLOOD PRESSURE
  - PULSE PRESSURE
  - MEAN ARTERIAL BLOOD PRESSURE
- **VARIATIONS**
  - PHYSIOLOGICAL VARIATIONS
  - PATHOLOGICAL VARIATIONS
- **DETERMINANTS OF ARTERIAL BLOOD PRESSURE**
  - CENTRAL FACTORS
  - PERIPHERAL FACTORS
- **REGULATION OF ARTERIAL BLOOD PRESSURE**
- **NERVOUS MECHANISM: SHORT-TERM REGULATION**
  - VASOMOTOR CENTER
  - VASOCONSTRICTOR FIBERS
  - VASODILATOR FIBERS
  - MECHANISM OF ACTION OF VASOMOTOR CENTER
- **RENAL MECHANISM: LONG-TERM REGULATION**
  - BY REGULATION OF EXTRACELLULAR FLUID VOLUME
  - THROUGH RENIN-ANGIOTENSIN MECHANISM
- **HORMONAL MECHANISM**
- **LOCAL MECHANISM**
  - LOCAL VASOCONSTRICTORS
  - LOCAL VASODILATORS
- **MEASUREMENT OF ARTERIAL BLOOD PRESSURE**
- **APPLIED PHYSIOLOGY**
  - HYPERTENSION
  - HYPOTENSION

■ DEFINITIONS AND NORMAL VALUES

Arterial blood pressure is defined as the **lateral pressure** exerted by the column of blood on the wall of arteries. This pressure is exerted when blood flows through the arteries. Generally, the term 'blood pressure' refers to arterial blood pressure.

Arterial blood pressure is expressed in four different terms:

1. Systolic blood pressure.
2. Diastolic blood pressure.
3. Pulse pressure.
4. Mean arterial blood pressure.

■ 1. SYSTOLIC BLOOD PRESSURE

Systolic blood pressure or systolic pressure is defined as the **maximum pressure** exerted in the arteries during systole of heart.

Normal systolic pressure:

120 mm Hg (110 to 140 mm Hg).

■ 2. DIASTOLIC BLOOD PRESSURE

Diastolic blood pressure or diastolic pressure is defined as the **minimum pressure** in the arteries during diastole of heart.

Normal diastolic pressure:

80 mm Hg (60 to 80 mm Hg).

■ 3. PULSE PRESSURE

Pulse pressure is the **difference** between systolic pressure and diastolic pressure.

Normal pulse pressure:

40 mm Hg (120 – 80).

■ 4. MEAN ARTERIAL BLOOD PRESSURE

It is the average pressure existing in the arteries. It is not the **arithmetic mean** of systolic and diastolic pressures. It is the diastolic pressure plus one third of pulse pressure. To determine the mean pressure, diastolic pressure is considered than the systolic pressure. It is because diastolic period of cardiac cycle is longer (0.53 second) than the systolic period (0.27 second).

Normal mean arterial pressure:

93 mm Hg (80 + 13 = 93).

■ VARIATIONS OF ARTERIAL BLOOD PRESSURE
■ PHYSIOLOGICAL VARIATIONS

1. Age

Arterial blood pressure increases as age advances. **Table 71.1** shows systolic and diastolic pressures at different age.

2. Sex

In females, up to the period of menopause, arterial pressure is about 5 mm Hg less than in males of same age. After menopause, the pressure in females becomes equal to that in males of same age.

3. Body Built

Pressure is more in obese persons than in lean persons.

4. Diurnal Variation

In early morning, the pressure is slightly low. It gradually increases and reaches the maximum at noon. It becomes low in evening.

5. After Meals

Arterial blood pressure is increased for few hours after meals due to increase in cardiac output.

6. During Sleep

Usually, the pressure is reduced up to 15 to 20 mm Hg during deep sleep. However, it increases slightly during sleep associated with dreams.

7. Emotional Conditions

During excitement or anxiety, the blood pressure is increased due to release of adrenaline.

8. After Exercise

After moderate exercise, systolic pressure increases by 20 to 30 mm Hg above the basal level due to increase in force of contraction and stroke volume. Normally, diastolic pressure is not affected by moderate exercise. It is because the diastolic pressure depends upon peripheral resistance, which is not altered by moderate exercise.

After severe muscular exercise, the systolic pressure rises by 40 to 50 mm Hg above the basal level. But the diastolic pressure reduces because the peripheral resistance decreases in severe muscular exercise. More details are given in Chapter 77.

■ PATHOLOGICAL VARIATIONS

Pathological variations of arterial blood pressure are hypertension and hypotension. Refer applied physiology of this chapter for details.

■ DETERMINANTS OF ARTERIAL BLOOD PRESSURE: FACTORS MAINTAINING ARTERIAL BLOOD PRESSURE

Some factors are necessary for the maintenance of normal arterial blood pressure, which are called **local factors**, **mechanical factors** or **determinants** of arterial blood pressure.

Types of Local Factors

Local factors are divided into two types:

I. Central factors which are pertaining to the heart:
 1. Cardiac output.
 2. Heart rate.
II. Peripheral factors which are pertaining to blood and blood vessels:
 3. Peripheral resistance.
 4. Blood volume.
 5. Venous return.
 6. Elasticity of blood vessels.
 7. Velocity of blood flow.
 8. Diameter of blood vessels.
 9. Viscosity of blood.

■ CENTRAL FACTORS

1. Cardiac Output

Systolic pressure is **directly proportional** to cardiac output **(Table 71.2)**. Whenever the cardiac output increases, the systolic pressure is increased and, when cardiac output is less, the systolic pressure is reduced. Cardiac output increases in muscular exercise, emotional

TABLE 71.1: Arterial blood pressure in different age.

Age	Systolic pressure (mm Hg)	Diastolic pressure (mm Hg)
Newborn	70	40
After 1 month	85	45
After 6 months	90	50
After 1 year	95	55
After puberty	120	80
After 50 years	140	85
After 70 years	160	90
After 80 years	180	95

TABLE 71.2: Local factors determining arterial blood pressure.

Arterial blood pressure	Factors
Directly proportional to	1. Cardiac output 2. Heart rate 3. Peripheral resistance 4. Blood volume 5. Venous return 6. Velocity of blood flow 7. Viscosity of blood
Inversely proportional to	1. Elasticity of blood vessel 2. Diameter of blood vessel

conditions, etc. So, in these conditions the systolic pressure is increased. In conditions like myocardial infarction, the cardiac output decreases resulting in fall in systolic pressure.

2. Heart Rate

Moderate changes in heart rate do not affect arterial blood pressure much. However, marked alteration in the heart rate affects the blood pressure by altering cardiac output (Chapter 69).

■ PERIPHERAL FACTORS

3. Peripheral Resistance

Peripheral resistance is the resistance offered to blood flow at the periphery. Resistance is offered at arterioles, which are called the **resistant vessels**. This is the important factor, which maintains diastolic pressure. Diastolic pressure is **directly proportional** to peripheral resistance. When peripheral resistance increases, diastolic pressure increases and when peripheral resistance decreases, the diastolic pressure decreases.

4. Blood Volume

Blood pressure is **directly proportional** to blood volume. Blood volume maintains the blood pressure through venous return and cardiac output. If the blood volume increases, there is increase in venous return and cardiac output resulting in elevation of blood pressure.

5. Venous Return

Blood pressure is **directly proportional** to venous return. When venous return increases, there is increase in ventricular filling and cardiac output resulting in elevation of arterial blood pressure **(Fig. 71.1)**.

6. Elasticity of Blood Vessels

Blood pressure is **inversely proportional** to the elasticity of blood vessels. Due to the elastic property, blood vessels are distensible and are able to maintain the pressure. When the elastic property is lost, blood vessels become rigid (**arteriosclerosis**) and pressure increases as in old age. Deposition of cholesterol, fatty acids and calcium ions cause rigidity of blood vessels (**atherosclerosis**) leading to increased blood pressure.

7. Velocity of Blood Flow

Pressure in a blood vessel is **directly proportional** to the velocity of blood flow. If the velocity of the blood flow increases, the resistance increases. So, the pressure is increased.

8. Diameter of Blood Vessels

Arterial blood pressure is **inversely proportional** to diameter of the blood vessel. If the diameter decreases, the peripheral resistance increases leading to increase in the pressure.

9. Viscosity of Blood

Arterial blood pressure is **directly proportional** to the viscosity of blood. When viscosity of blood increases, the frictional resistance is increased and this increases the pressure.

■ REGULATION OF ARTERIAL BLOOD PRESSURE

Arterial blood pressure varies even under physiological conditions. However, immediately it is brought back to normal level because of the presence of well-organized regulatory mechanisms in the body.

Regulatory mechanisms which maintain the blood pressure within normal limits are:

 I. Nervous mechanism or short-term regulatory mechanism.
 II. Renal mechanism or long-term regulatory mechanism.
 III. Hormonal mechanism.
 IV. Local mechanism.

■ NERVOUS MECHANISM FOR REGULATION OF BLOOD PRESSURE: SHORT-TERM REGULATION

Nervous regulation is rapid among all the mechanisms involved in regulation of arterial blood pressure. When blood pressure is altered, nervous system brings the pressure back to normal within few minutes. Although nervous mechanism is **quick in action**, it operates only for a short period and then it adapts to the new pressure. Hence, it is called **short-term regulation**. Nervous mechanism regulating the arterial blood pressure operates through vasomotor system.

Components of Vasomotor System

Vasomotor system includes three components:

 1. Vasomotor center.
 2. Vasoconstrictor fibers.
 3. Vasodilator fibers.

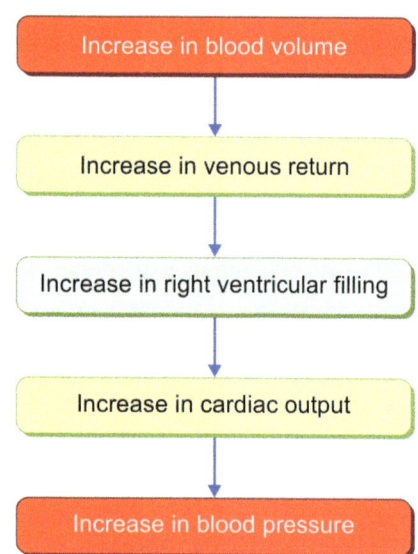

FIGURE 71.1: Effect of blood volume and venous return on arterial blood pressure.

Chapter 71: Arterial Blood Pressure

■ 1. VASOMOTOR CENTER

Vasomotor center is bilaterally situated in the reticular formation of medulla oblongata and lower part of the pons.

Vasomotor center consists of three areas:
  i. Vasoconstrictor area.
  ii. Vasodilator area.
  iii. Sensory area.

i. *Vasoconstrictor Area*

Vasoconstrictor area is also called the **pressor area**. It forms the lateral portion of vasomotor center. Vasoconstrictor area sends impulses to blood vessels through sympathetic vasoconstrictor fibers. This area is also concerned with **acceleration of heart rate** (Chapter 70).

ii. *Vasodilator Area*

Vasodilator area is also called **depressor area**. It forms the medial portion of vasomotor center. This area suppresses the vasoconstrictor area and causes vasodilatation. It is also concerned with **inhibition of heart rate** (Chapter 70).

iii. *Sensory Area*

Sensory area is in the nucleus of tractus solitarius, which is situated in the posterolateral part of medulla and pons. This area receives sensory impulses via glossopharyngeal and vagal nerves from the periphery, particularly, from the baroreceptors. Sensory area in turn, controls the vasoconstrictor and vasodilator areas.

■ 2. VASOCONSTRICTOR FIBERS

Vasoconstrictor fibers belong to the sympathetic division of autonomic nervous system. These fibers cause vasoconstriction by the release of the neurotransmitter substance, noradrenaline.

Vasomotor Tone or Sympathetic Tone

Vasomotor tone or sympathetic tone is the continuous discharge of impulses from vasoconstrictor center through the vasoconstrictor fibers. Vasomotor tone plays an important role in regulating the pressure by producing a constant partial state of constriction of the blood vessels. Thus, the arterial blood pressure is **directly proportional** to vasomotor tone. Vasomotor tone is also called **sympathetic vasoconstrictor tone** or **sympathetic tone**.

■ 3. VASODILATOR FIBERS

Vasodilator fibers are of three types:
  i. Parasympathetic vasodilator fibers.
  ii. Sympathetic vasodilator fibers.
  iii. Antidromic vasodilator fibers.

i. *Parasympathetic Vasodilator Fibers*

Parasympathetic vasodilator fibers cause dilatation of blood vessels by releasing the chemical mediator, **acetylcholine**.

ii. *Sympathetic Vasodilator Fibers*

Some of the sympathetic fibers cause vasodilatation in certain areas by secreting **acetylcholine**. Such fibers are called sympathetic vasodilator or sympathetic cholinergic fibers. Sympathetic cholinergic fibers, which supply the blood vessels of skeletal muscles are important in increasing the blood flow to muscles by vasodilatation during conditions like exercise.

iii. *Antidromic Vasodilator Fibers*

Normally, the impulses produced by a cutaneous receptor (like pain receptor) pass through sensory nerve fibers. But, some of these impulses pass through the other branches of the axon in opposite direction and reach the blood vessels supplied by these branches. Now, these impulses dilate the blood vessels. It is called the antidromic or **axon reflex**. And, the nerve fibers are called **antidromic vasodilator fibers**.

■ MECHANISM OF ACTION OF VASOMOTOR CENTER IN REGULATION OF BLOOD PRESSURE

Vasomotor center regulates the arterial blood pressure by causing vasoconstriction or vasodilatation. However, its actions depend upon the impulses it receives from other structures such as baroreceptors, chemoreceptors, higher centers and respiratory centers. Among these structures, baroreceptors and chemoreceptors play a major role in short-term regulation of blood pressure.

1. *Baroreceptor Mechanism*

Baroreceptors are the receptors, which give response to **change in blood pressure**. Baroreceptors are situated in carotid sinus and wall of aorta. Refer Chapter 70 for details of baroreceptors.

Functions of Baroreceptors

Role of baroreceptors when pressure increases

When arterial blood pressure rises rapidly, the baroreceptors are activated and send stimulatory impulses to nucleus of tractus solitarius through glossopharyngeal and vagus nerves. Now, the nucleus of tractus solitarius acts on both vasoconstrictor area and vasodilator areas of vasomotor center. It inhibits the vasoconstrictor area and excites the vasodilator area.

Inhibition of vasoconstrictor area reduces vasomotor tone. Reduction in vasomotor tone causes vasodilatation resulting in decreased peripheral resistance. Simultaneous excitation of vasodilator center increases vagal tone (Chapter 70). This decreases the rate and force of contraction of heart leading to reduction in cardiac output. These two factors, i.e. decreased peripheral resistance and reduced cardiac output bring the arterial blood pressure back to normal level **(Fig. 71.2)**.

Role of baroreceptors when pressure decreases

Fall in arterial blood pressure or the occlusion of common carotid arteries decreases the pressure in carotid sinus. This causes inactivation of baroreceptors. Now, there is no inhibition of vasoconstrictor center or excitation of vasodilator center. Therefore, the blood pressure rises.

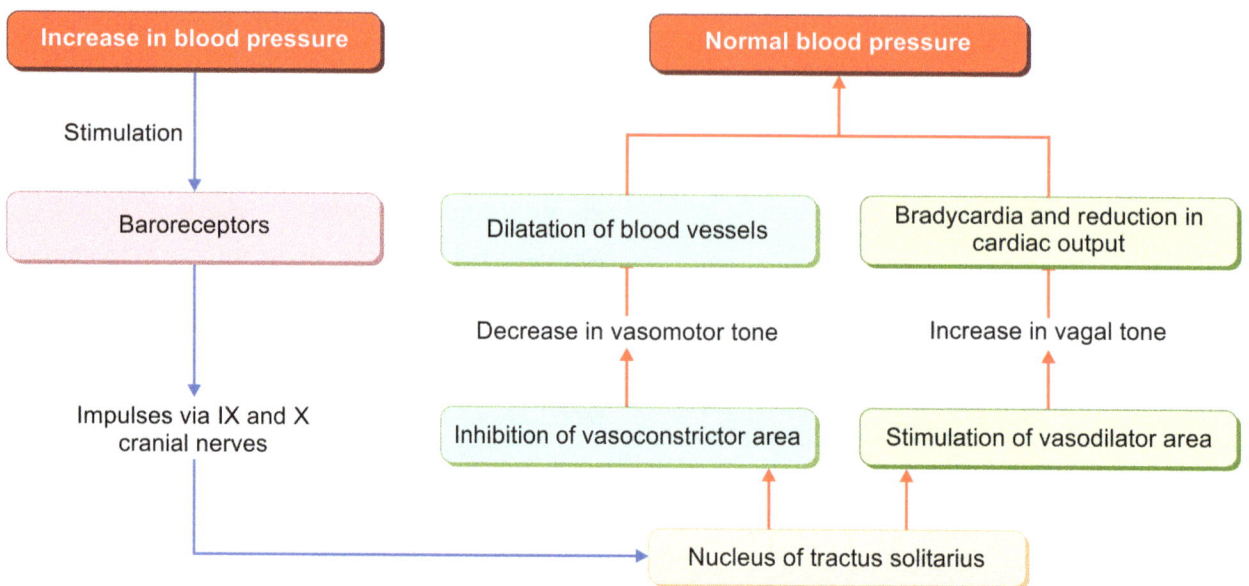

FIGURE 71.2: Regulation of blood pressure by baroreceptor mechanism.

2. Chemoreceptor Mechanism

Chemoreceptors are the receptors giving response to change in chemical constituents of blood. Peripheral chemoreceptors. are situated in the carotid body and aortic body.

Peripheral chemoreceptors influence the vasomotor center. Refer Chapter 70 for details of peripheral chemoreceptors.

Function of chemoreceptors

Peripheral chemoreceptors are sensitive to lack of oxygen and excess of carbon dioxide and hydrogen ion concentration in blood. But lack of oxygen is the most potent stimulant for peripheral chemoreceptors. Whenever blood pressure decreases, the blood flow decreases resulting in decreased oxygen content and excess of carbon dioxide and hydrogen ion. These factors stimulate the chemoreceptors, which send impulses to stimulate the vasoconstrictor center. Blood pressure rises and blood flow increases.

Chemoreceptors play a major role in maintaining respiration (Chapter 83) rather than blood pressure.

Sinoaortic mechanism and buffer nerves

Mechanism of action of baroreceptors and chemoreceptors in carotid and aortic region constitute sinoaortic mechanism. Nerves from the baroreceptors and chemoreceptors are called buffer nerves because these nerves regulate the heart rate (Chapter 70), blood pressure and respiration (Chapter 83).

3. Higher Centers

Vasomotor center is also controlled by the impulses from two higher centers in brain.

i. Cerebral cortex

Area 13 in cerebral cortex is concerned with emotional reactions. During emotional conditions, this area sends impulses to vasomotor center. Now, vasomotor center is activated, the vasomotor tone is increased and blood pressure rises.

ii. Hypothalamus

Stimulation of posterior and lateral nuclei of hypothalamus causes vasoconstriction and increase in blood pressure. Stimulation of preoptic area causes vasodilatation and decrease in blood pressure. Impulses from hypothalamus are mediated via vasomotor center.

4. Respiratory Centers

During the beginning of expiration, arterial blood pressure increases slightly, i.e. by 4 to 6 mm Hg. And it decreases during later part of expiration and during inspiration. It is because of two factors:

i. Radiation of impulses from respiratory centers towards vasomotor center at different phases of respiratory cycle.
ii. Pressure changes in thoracic cavity leading to alteration of venous return and cardiac output.

■ RENAL MECHANISM FOR REGULATION OF BLOOD PRESSURE: LONG-TERM REGULATION

Kidneys play an important role in the long-term regulation of arterial blood pressure. When blood pressure alters slowly in several days/months/years, nervous mechanism adapts to the altered pressure and loses the sensitivity for changes. It cannot regulate the pressure any more. In such conditions, the renal mechanism operates efficiently to regulate the blood pressure. Therefore, it is called long-term regulation.

Kidneys regulate arterial blood pressure by two ways:

1. By regulation of ECF volume.
2. Through renin-angiotensin mechanism.

Chapter 71: Arterial Blood Pressure

1. BY REGULATION OF EXTRACELLULAR FLUID VOLUME

When the blood pressure increases, kidneys excrete large amounts of water and salt, particularly sodium by means of pressure diuresis and pressure natriuresis. **Pressure diuresis** is the excretion of large quantity of water in urine because of increased blood pressure. Even a slight increase in blood pressure doubles the water excretion. **Pressure natriuresis** is the excretion of large quantity of sodium in urine because of increased blood pressure.

Because of diuresis and natriuresis, there is decrease in the ECF volume and blood volume, which in turn brings the arterial blood pressure back to normal level.

When blood pressure decreases, the reabsorption of water from renal tubules is increased. This in turn, increases ECF volume, blood volume and cardiac output resulting in restoration of blood pressure.

2. THROUGH RENIN-ANGIOTENSIN MECHANISM

Details about source of renin secretion, formation of angiotensin and conditions when renin is secreted are described in Chapter 40.

Actions of Angiotensin II

When blood pressure and ECF volume decrease, renin secretion from kidneys is increased. It converts angiotensinogen into angiotensin I. This is converted into angiotensin II by **angiotensin-converting enzyme** (ACE). Angiotensin II acts in two ways to restore the blood pressure:

i. It causes constriction of arterioles in the body so that the peripheral resistance is increased, and blood pressure rises. In addition, angiotensin II causes constriction of afferent arterioles in kidneys so that the glomerulali filtration reduces. This results in retention of water and salts. This increases ECF volume to normal level. This in turn increases the blood pressure to normal level.

ii. Simultaneously, angiotensin II stimulates the adrenal cortex to secrete aldosterone. This hormone increases reabsorption of sodium from renal tubules. Sodium reabsorption is followed by water reabsorption resulting in increased ECF volume and blood volume. It increases the blood pressure to normal level **(Fig. 71.3)**.

Actions of Angiotensin III and Angiotensin IV

Like angiotensin II, the angiotensins III and IV also increase the blood pressure and stimulate adrenal cortex to secrete aldosterone (Chapter 40).

HORMONAL MECHANISM FOR REGULATION OF BLOOD PRESSURE

Many hormones are involved in the regulation of blood pressure. Hormones, which increase or decrease the arterial blood pressure are listed in **Table 71.3**.

LOCAL MECHANISM FOR REGULATION OF BLOOD PRESSURE

In addition to nervous, renal and hormonal mechanisms, some local substances also regulate the blood pressure. The local substances regulate the blood pressure by vasoconstriction or vasodilatation **(Fig. 71.4)**.

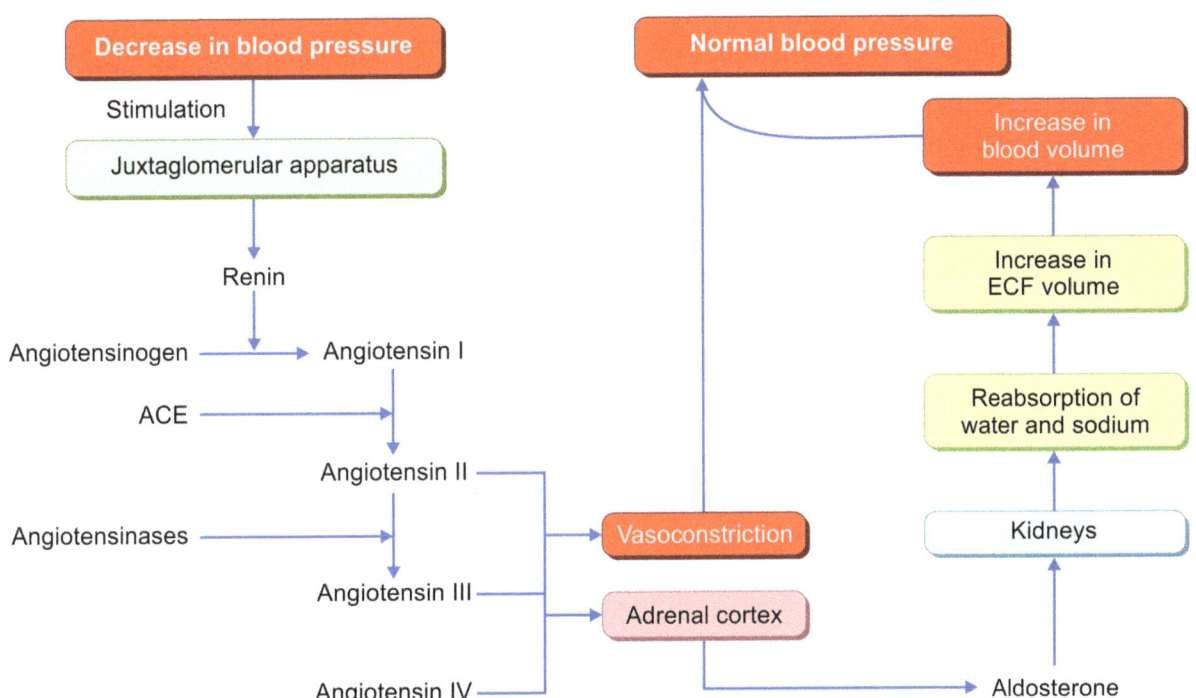

FIGURE 71.3: Regulation of blood pressure by renin-angiotensin mechanism.
ACE = Angiotensin-converting enzyme.

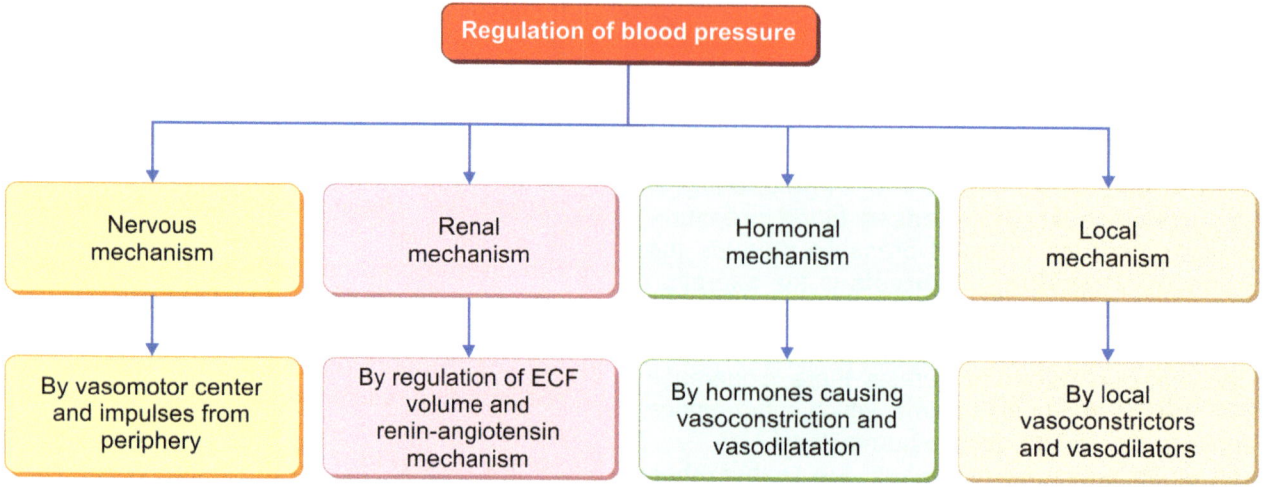

FIGURE 71.4: Regulation of blood pressure.
ECF = Extracellular fluid.

TABLE 71.3: Hormones regulating of arterial blood pressure.

Hormones which increase arterial blood pressure	Hormones which decrease arterial blood pressure
1. Adrenaline* 2. Noradrenaline 3. Thyroxine* 4. Aldosterone 5. Vasopressin 6. Angiotensin 7. Serotonin	1. Vasoactive intestinal polypeptide (VIP) 2. Bradykinin 3. Prostaglandin 4. Histamine 5. Acetylcholine 6. Atrial natriuretic peptide 7. Brain natriuretic peptide 8. C-type natriuretic peptide

*Adrenaline and thyroxine increase systolic pressure but decrease diastolic pressure.

TABLE 71.4: Local substances regulating arterial blood pressure.

Local vasoconstrictors (endothelins)	Local vasodilators	
	Metabolic products	Endothelins (ET)
EDCF: 1. ET1 2. ET2 3. ET3	1. Carbon dioxide 2. Lactate 3. Hydrogen 4. Adenosine	EDRF: 1. Nitric oxide

EDCF = Endothelium-derived constricting factor. EDRF = Endothelium-derived relaxing factor.

■ LOCAL VASOCONSTRICTORS

Local vasoconstrictor substances are of vascular endothelial origin and are known as **endothelins (ET)**. Endothelins are peptides with 21 amino acids. Endothelins are produced by stretching of blood vessels. These peptides act by activating phospholipase, which in turn activates **prostacyclin** and **thromboxane A$_2$**. These two substances cause constriction of blood vessels and increase in blood pressure.

■ LOCAL VASODILATORS

Local vasodilators are of two types:

1. Vasodilators of metabolic origin such as carbon dioxide, lactate, hydrogen ions and **adenosine (Table 71.4)**.
2. Vasodilators of endothelial origin such as **nitric oxide (NO)**.

■ MEASUREMENT OF ARTERIAL BLOOD PRESSURE

Blood pressure is measured by direct and indirect methods. Direct method which is used in animals only. Indirect method which is used in human beings as well animals.

■ INDIRECT METHOD

Apparatus

Apparatus used to measure blood pressure in human beings is called **sphygmomanometer**. Along with sphygmomanometer, **stethoscope** is also necessary to measure blood pressure.

Principle

When an external pressure is applied over the artery, the blood flow through that artery is obstructed. And the pressure required to cause occlusion of blood flow indicates pressure inside the vessel.

Procedure

Brachial artery is usually chosen because of convenience. The arm cuff of sphygmomanometer is tied around upper arm, above the cubital fossa. Cuff should not be too tight or too loose. It is connected to sphygmomanometer.

Pressure can be measured by three methods:

1. Palpatory method.
2. Auscultatory method.
3. Oscillatory method.

1. Palpatory method

First, the **radial pulse** is felt. While feeling the pulse, pressure is increased in the cuff by inflating air into it, with the help of a hand pump. While doing this, mercury column in the sphygmomanometer shows the pressure in the cuff.

When pressure is increased in the arm cuff, brachial artery is compressed and blood flow is obstructed. So, radial pulse disappears. When radial pulse disappears, the pressure is further increased by about 20 mm Hg. Then, the pressure in the cuff is slowly reduced by releasing the valve of the hand pump, i.e. the cuff is deflated slowly. This is done by feeling the pulse and simultaneously watching the mercury column in the apparatus. Pressure is noted when the pulse reappears. Pressure at which pulse reappears indicates the **systolic pressure**.

Disadvantage of palpatory method is that the diastolic pressure cannot be measured.

2. Auscultatory method

Auscultatory method is the most accurate method to determine arterial blood pressure. After determining systolic pressure in palpatory method, the pressure in the cuff is raised by about 20 mm Hg above that level, so that the brachial artery is occluded due to compression. Now, the chest piece of stethoscope is placed over antecubital fossa and the arm cuff is slowly deflated. While doing so, series of sounds are heard through the stethoscope. These sounds are known as Korotkoff sounds, named after the discoverer **Korotkoff** (1905). While reducing the pressure, Korotkoff sounds have five phases.

First phase: Tapping sound

While decreasing the pressure from arm cuff, occlusion of the artery is relieved and when blood starts flowing through the artery, first sound appears suddenly. In a normal person, it appears, when the pressure is reduced to 120 mm Hg. It is a clear tapping sound.

Appearance of tapping sound indicates **systolic pressure**. When the pressure is reduced further by 10 mm Hg from the initial level, this sound slowly becomes louder.

Second phase: Murmuring sound

Following the clear taping sound, a soft murmuring sound is heard when the pressure is reduced further by about 15 mm Hg.

Third phase: Gong sound

After the murmuring sound, a very clear and louder sound is heard. It is of gong type. It is heard while reducing the pressure by another 15 mm Hg **(Table 71.5)**.

TABLE 71.5: Phases of Korotkoff sounds.

Phase	Sound
First phase	Tapping sound **Indicates systolic pressure**
Second phase	Murmuring sound
Third phase	Gong sound
Fourth phase	Muffled sound
Fifth phase	Disappearance of sound **Indicates diastolic pressure**

Fourth phase: Muffled sound

Next to the gong type sound, a mild and muffled sound is heard when the pressure is decreased further by 5 mm Hg.

Fifth phase: Disappearance of sound

Muffling sound disappears. **Disappearance of the sound** indicates **diastolic pressure.**

Thus, in auscultatory method, appearance of clear tapping sound during first phase indicates the systolic pressure and disappearance of the muffling sound in fifth phase indicates diastolic pressure.

3. Oscillatory method

When pressure in arm cuff is increased above the level of systolic pressure, the artery is occluded due to compression. At this stage, mercury column in the manometer remains static. When the pressure is gradually reduced, some oscillations occur at the top of the mercury column. While deflating the cuff further, the amplitude and duration of oscillations increase suddenly. It denotes systolic pressure. When the cuff pressure is reduced further, the amplitude and duration of oscillations is reduced. It reflects the diastolic pressure.

Because of its inaccuracy, this method is not followed in routine clinical practice. By connecting the manometer to an appropriate recording device, the oscillations of mercury column can be recorded graphically.

Aneroid Sphygmomanometer

Aneroid sphygmomanometer consists of an **aneroid device** instead of mercury column. It is commonly used in hospitals and clinics because of the concerns about environmental **toxicity of mercury**. However, it is less accurate compared to mercury sphygmomanometer.

Automatic Blood Pressure Instrument

Nowadays automatic blood pressure instrument is widely used. This instrument has a **microprocessor driven air** pump, which automatically inflates the arm cuff at a fixed pressure value. Then, it records the pressure oscillation pattern during a stepwise deflation. This instrument determines the pulse rate also. The results are shown on digital screen.

Automatic instrument does not need expert personnel to measure the blood pressure since it has the self-measuring facilities. However, accuracy of this instrument is controversial.

■ APPLIED PHYSIOLOGY

Pathological variations of arterial blood pressure are:
I. Hypertension.
II. Hypotension.

■ HYPERTENSION

Definition

Hypertension is defined as the persistent high arterial blood pressure. Clinically, when the systolic pressure remains elevated above 150 mm Hg and diastolic pressure remains elevated above 90 mm Hg, it is considered as hypertension. If there is increase only in systolic pressure, it is called **systolic hypertension.**

Types of Hypertension

Hypertension is divided into two types:

1. Primary hypertension.
2. Secondary hypertension.

1. *Primary hypertension or essential hypertension*

Primary hypertension is the elevated blood pressure in the absence of any underlying disease. It is also called essential hypertension. Arterial blood pressure is increased because of increased peripheral resistance, which occurs due to some unknown cause.

2. *Secondary hypertension*

Secondary hypertension is the high blood pressure due to some underlying disorders.

Different forms of secondary hypertension are:

  i. **Cardiovascular hypertension** that is produced due to cardiovascular disorders **(Table 71.6)**.
 ii. **Endocrine hypertension** which is due to hyperactivity of some endocrine glands.
iii. **Renal hypertension** that is caused by renal diseases.
 iv. **Neurogenic hypertension** which is developed by nervous disorders.
  v. **Hypertension during pregnancy** which is due to toxemia of pregnancy (Chapter 61).

■ HYPOTENSION

Definition

Hypotension is the low blood pressure. When the systolic pressure is less than 90 mm Hg, it is considered as hypotension.

Types of Hypotension

1. Primary hypotension.
2. Secondary hypotension.

1. *Primary hypotension*

Primary hypotension is the low blood pressure that develops in the absence of any underlying disease and develops due to some unknown cause. It is also called **essential hypotension**. Frequent fatigue and weakness are the common symptoms of this condition. However, the persons with primary hypotension are not easily susceptible to heart or renal disorders.

2. *Secondary hypotension*

Secondary hypotension occurs due to some underlying diseases such as:

  i. Myocardial infarction.
 ii. Hypoactivity of pituitary gland.
iii. Hypoactivity of adrenal glands.
 iv. Tuberculosis.
  v. Nervous disorders.

Orthostatic hypotension

Orthostatic hypotension is the sudden fall in blood pressure while standing for some time. It is due to the effect of gravity. Gravity causes pooling of blood in lower limbs and decrease in blood pressure. It develops in persons affected by **myasthenia gravis** or some nervous disorders like tabes dorsalis, syringomyelia and diabetic neuropathy. Common symptom of this condition is **orthostatic syncope**. Syncope is described in detail in Chapter 76.

TABLE 71.6: Types of secondary hypertension.

Type	Cause
Cardiovascular hypertension	1. Atherosclerosis: Hardening of blood vessels by fat deposition 2. Coarctation (narrowing) of aorta
Endocrine hypertension	1. Pheochromocytoma: Hypersecretion of adrenaline 2. Hyperaldosteronism: Hypersecretion of aldosterone 3. Cushing' syndrome: Hypersecretion of glucocorticoids
Renal hypertension	1. Stenosis of renal arteries 2. Hypersecretion of angiotensin II 3. Glomerulonephritis
Neurogenic hypertension	1. Increased intracranial pressure 2. Lesion in tractus solitarius 3. Sectioning of nerve fibers in carotid sinus
Hypertension in pregnancy	1. Toxemia of pregnancy

Chapter 72: Venous Blood Pressure and Capillary Blood Pressure

CHAPTER OUTLINE

- **VENOUS BLOOD PRESSURE**
  - DEFINITION
  - NORMAL VALUES
  - EFFECT OF RESPIRATION ON VENOUS BLOOD PRESSURE
- **CAPILLARY BLOOD PRESSURE**
  - DEFINITION AND NORMAL VALUES
  - REGIONAL VARIATIONS
  - CAPILLARY ONCOTIC PRESSURE

VENOUS BLOOD PRESSURE

DEFINITION

Venous blood pressure is the pressure exerted by the contained blood in veins. Pressure in vena cava and right atrium is called **central venous pressure**. And the pressure in peripheral veins is called **peripheral venous pressure**.

Pressure is not same in all the veins. It varies in different veins in the extremities of the body and also varies from central veins to peripheral veins.

NORMAL VALUES

Venous Blood Pressure in Extremities of the Body

Venous pressure is less in parts of the body above the level of heart and it is more in parts below the level of heart. Refer **Box 72.1** for values.

Venous Pressure in Central and Peripheral Veins

Pressure is greater in peripheral veins than in central veins. Refer **Box 72.1** for values.

BOX 72.1: Normal values of venous blood pressure.

In extremities of the body	
Dorsal venous arch of foot	: 13.2 mm Hg (17.9 cm H_2O)
Jugular vein	: 5.1 mm Hg (6.9 cm H_2O)
In peripheral and central veins	
Antecubital vein	: 7.1 mm Hg (9.6 cm H_2O).
Superior vena cava	: 4.6 mm Hg (6.2 cm H_2O)

(1 mm Hg pressure = 1.359 cm H_2O pressure.)

EFFECT OF RESPIRATION ON VENOUS BLOOD PRESSURE

Effect of respiration on venous blood pressure is demonstrated by two procedures:

1. Valsalva maneuver or Valsalva experiment.
2. Müller maneuver or Müller experiment.

Valsalva Maneuver: Valsalva Experiment

Valsalva maneuver is the **forced expiratory effort** with closed glottis. It is performed by attempting to exhale forcibly while closing the mouth and nose.

Effects of Valsalva maneuver

During this maneuver, the intrathoracic pressure increases greatly and becomes positive. It may reach + 50 mm Hg **(Table 72.1)**.

High intrathoracic pressure produces following effects:

1. Compression of central vein in thorax.
2. Decrease in venous return to right atrium.
3. Decrease in central venous pressure.
4. Increase in peripheral venous blood pressure to about 30 cm H_2O, due to accumulation of blood in peripheral veins such as veins of neck, face and limbs.

Uses of Valsalva maneuver

1. Valsalva maneuver is used as a diagnostic tool to evaluate the cardiovascular disorders. Best example is the 30 minutes endurance test.
2. Valsalva maneuver is practiced to relieve chest pain.
3. It is used to correct the abnormal heart rhythms.

TABLE 72.1: Valsalva maneuver vs Müller maneuver.

Features	Valsalva maneuver	Müller maneuver
1. Performance	Forced expiratory effort with closed glottis	Forced inspiratory effort with closed glottis
2. Intrathoracic pressure	Increases up to + 50 mm Hg	Decreases up to – 70 mm Hg
3. Central veins in thorax	Compressed	Dilated and blood rushes
4. Venous return to right atrium	Decreases	Increases
5. Peripheral venous blood pressure	Increases to 30 cm H_2O	Decreases to 3 cm H_2O
6. Central venous blood pressure	Decreases	Increases
7. Uses	To evaluate cardiovascular disorders To relieve chest pain To correct abnormal heart rhythms	To evaluate upper respiratory problems To evaluate sleep apnea syndrome

30 Seconds endurance test

The subject is asked to blow against **sphygmomanometer**, in which the pressure is maintained at 40 mm Hg for 30 seconds. Then the changes in heart rate, blood pressure or murmurs are observed to evaluate the cardiovascular disorders.

Müller Maneuver: Müller Experiment

Müller maneuver or **reverse Valsalva maneuver** is the **forced inspiratory effort** with closed glottis. It is performed by attempting to inhale forcibly, while closing the mouth and nose.

Effects of Müller maneuver

During this maneuver, the intrathoracic pressure decreases greatly and becomes more negative. It is about – 70 mm Hg **(Table 72.1)**.

More negative intrathoracic pressure produces following effects:

1. Dilatation of right atrium and central vein because of increase in negative intrathoracic pressure.
2. Rapid emptying of blood from peripheral veins into the central veins and increase in venous return to right atrium.
3. Decrease in peripheral venous blood pressure to less than 3 to 4 cm H_2O.
4. Increase in central venous blood pressure.

Uses of Müller maneuver

Müller maneuver is used to evaluate:

1. Upper respiratory tract problems.
2. **Sleep apnea syndrome** (temporary stoppage of breathing repeatedly during sleep).

CAPILLARY BLOOD PRESSURE
DEFINITION AND NORMAL VALUES

Definition

Capillary blood pressure is the pressure exerted by the blood contained in capillary. It is also called **capillary hydrostatic pressure**.

Significance

Capillary blood pressure is responsible for the exchange of various substances between blood and interstitial fluid through capillary wall.

Normal Values

Arterial end of capillary : 30 to 32 mm Hg.
Venous end of capillary : 15 mm Hg **(Fig. 72.1)**.

However, capillary pressure varies depending upon the function of the organ or region of the body.

REGIONAL VARIATIONS OF CAPILLARY BLOOD PESSURE

Capillary blood pressure varies in different organs particularly in kidneys and lungs. Regional variation in capillary pressure is in relation to the physiological activities of the particular region. So, it has some functional significance.

Capillary Blood Pressure in Kidney

In kidney, the glomerular capillaries form **high pressure bed** with a pressure of 60 to 70 mm Hg. This high capillary pressure is responsible for glomerular filtration.

Peritubular capillaries form **low pressure bed** with a pressure of 8 to 10 mm Hg. This low pressure helps tubular reabsorption.

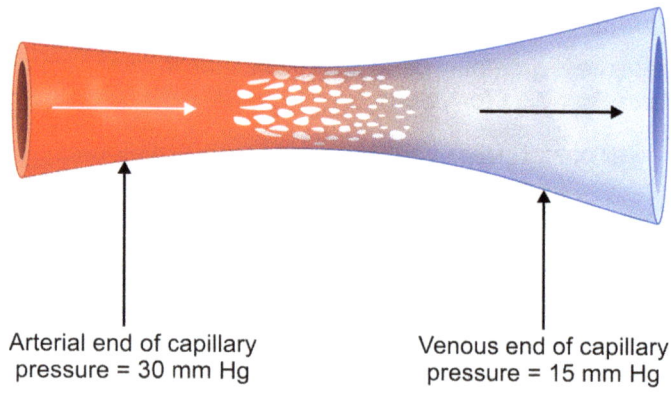

Arterial end of capillary pressure = 30 mm Hg
Venous end of capillary pressure = 15 mm Hg

FIGURE 72.1: Capillary blood pressure.

Capillary Blood Pressure in Lungs

In lungs, the pulmonary capillaries form **low pressure bed**. Capillary pressure of about 7 mm Hg favors exchange of gases between blood and alveoli.

■ CAPILLARY ONCOTIC PRESSURE

Capillary oncotic pressure or **colloidal pressure** is the pressure exerted by plasma protein which stay within capillaries because of impermeability of capillary membrane to plasma proteins. Normal oncotic pressure is about 25 mm Hg. Among the plasma proteins, albumin exerts 70% of oncotic pressure.

Oncotic pressure plays an important role in regulating filtration across capillary membrane, particularly in renal glomerular capillaries.

Chapter 73: Arterial Pulse and Venous Pulse

CHAPTER OUTLINE

- **ARTERIAL PULSE**
  - DEFINITION AND FORMATION
  - TRANSMISSION
  - ARTERIAL PULSE TRACING
  - PULSE POINTS
  - EXAMINATION OF RADIAL PULSE
  - APPLIED PHYSIOLOGY: ABNORMAL ARTERIAL PULSE
- **VENOUS PULSE**
  - DEFINITION AND IMPORTANCE
  - EXAMINATION OF VENOUS PULSE
  - JUGULAR VENOUS PULSE TRACING
  - APPLIED PHYSIOLOGY: ABNORMAL VENOUS PULSE

ARTERIAL PULSE

DEFINITION AND FORMATION OF ARTERIAL PULSE

Arterial pulse is defined as the pressure changes transmitted in the form of waves through arterial wall and blood column from heart to periphery.

During contraction of left ventricle, the blood ejected forcefully into aorta. It causes distension of aorta and rise in pressure. So, a pressure wave is produced on the elastic wall of aorta. It travels rapidly from the heart towards periphery. And, it can be felt after a brief interval, at any superficial peripheral artery like radial artery at wrist.

Pulse rate is the accurate measure of heart rate except in conditions such as **pulses deficit**.

TRANSMISSION OF ARTERIAL PULSE

Central arterial pulse is transmitted to the peripheral arteries as **peripheral arterial pulse.** Formation and transmission of pulse wave depends upon the elasticity of blood vessels. Thus, when the walls of arteries are more distensible, the pressure rise is less and so transmission of pulse is less. When the arterial wall loses its elastic property and becomes rigid as in old age, the pressure rise is more and the transmission of pulse is also more.

Pulse is not transmitted to capillaries because capillaries do not have elastic tissues.

Velocity of Transmission of Pulse

Average velocity at which the pulse wave is transmitted varies between 7 and 9 m/sec. Pulse wave travels faster than blood flow. Maximum velocity of blood flow in the body (in larger arteries) is only 50 cm/sec.

ARTERIAL PULSE TRACING

Arterial pulse is recorded by using **polygraph**. Pulse recorded in radial artery or femoral artery is the typical peripheral pulse (**Fig. 73.1**). Peripheral pulse tracing has three main features.

1. *Anacrotic Limb*

Anacrotic limb or ascending limb is due to the rise in pressure during systole.

2. *Catacrotic Limb*

Catacrotic limb or descending limb is due to the fall in pressure during diastole.

3. *Catacrotic Notch*

In the upper part of catacrotic limb of pulse tracing, a small notch appears. It is known as catacrotic notch or **incisura**.

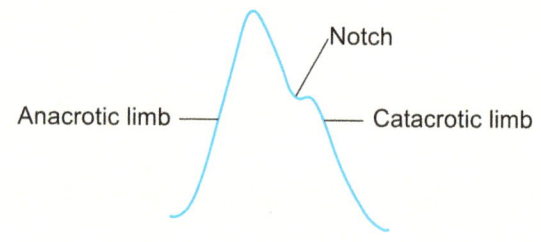

FIGURE 73.1: Radial pulse tracing.

This notch is produced by the backflow of blood during the closure of semilunar valves at the beginning of diastolic period, which produces slight increase in the pressure.

4. Pre- and Post-catacrotic Waves

The wave appearing before the notch is called **precatacrotic wave**. The wave appearing after the notch is called **postcatacrotic wave**.

PULSE POINTS

Usually, pulse is palpated on the radial artery because it is easily approachable and placed superficially. However, arterial pulse can be felt in different areas on the body. These areas are called pulse points. Pulse points and the area of palpation are given in **Table 73.1**.

EXAMINATION OF RADIAL PULSE

Examination of pulse is a valuable clinical procedure. Pulse represents the heartbeat. By examining pulse, important information regarding cardiac function such as rate of contraction, rhythmicity, etc. can be obtained. In addition, an experienced physician can determine the mean arterial pressure by hardness of pulse and its amplitude.

Method of Examining Radial Pulse

Subject is made to sit comfortably with forearm placed in mid- or semi-prone position, with wrist slightly flexed. The observer must stand by the right side of subject. Tips of the middle three fingers (index finger, middle finger and ring finger) of the observer are placed over the radial artery of the subject at wrist below the base of thumb. Light pressure is applied by the fingers until the pulse is felt. If necessary, fingers are moved around till the pulse is felt.

Index finger is used to occlude blood flow from radial artery. **Ring finger** is used to occlude retrograde flow of blood from ulnar artery through palmar arch. **Middle finger** is used to assess the pulse.

Observations During Examination of Pulse

1. Rate.
2. Rhythm.
3. Character.
4. Volume.
5. Condition of blood vessel wall.
6. Delayed pulse.

1. Rate

Pulse rate is the number of pulses per minute. It has to be counted at least for 30 seconds. Pulse rate in adults is 72/min. Pulse rate at different age is given in **Table 73.2**.

2. Rhythm

Rhythm is the regularity of pulse. Under normal conditions, the pulse appears at regular intervals. Rhythm of the pulse becomes irregular in some pathological conditions such as atrial fibrillation. Irregular rhythm of pulse is of two types, regularly irregular and irregularly irregular.

3. Character

Character of pulse is observed while examining the pulse. It denotes the tension on vessel wall produced by the waves of pulse.

4. Volume

Volume is the determination of movement of the vessel wall produced by transmission of pulse wave. It is also a measure of pulse pressure. It depends upon condition of the blood vessel.

5. Condition of Wall of the Blood Vessel

Condition of wall of the blood vessel is assessed by feeling and rolling the radial artery against the underlying bones. Normally, wall of the vessel is not palpable in children

TABLE 73.2: Pulse rate at different age.

Age	Pulse rate (per min)
In fetus	150 to 180
At birth	130 to 140
At 10 years of age	90
After puberty	72

TABLE 73.1: Pulse points.

Pulse point	Area of palpation
1. Temporal pulse	Over the temple, in front of ear on superficial temporal artery
2. Facial pulse	On facial artery at the angle of jaw
3. Carotid pulse	In the neck along anterior border of sternocleidomastoid muscle on common carotid artery
4. Axillary pulse	In axilla on axillary artery
5. Brachial pulse	In cubital fossa along medial border of biceps muscle on brachial artery
6. Radial pulse	Over the thumb side of wrist between tendons of brachioradialis and flexor carpi radialis muscles on radial artery
7. Ulnar pulse	Over the little finger side of wrist on ulnar artery
8. Femoral pulse	In the groin on femoral artery
9. Popliteal pulse	Behind knee, in the popliteal fossa on popliteal artery
10. Dorsalis pedis pulse	Over the dorsum of foot on dorsalis pedis artery
11. Tibialis pulse	Over the back of the ankle behind medial malleolus on posterior tibial artery.

and young adults. However, in old age wall of the vessel becomes rigid and palpable. In abnormal conditions like arteriosclerosis, it is felt as a hard rope.

6. Delayed Pulse

Sometimes the arrival of pulse in certain peripheral arteries is delayed. It is an important feature to be noted because it is useful in diagnosis of certain diseases. For example, while palpating radial pulse and femoral pulse simultaneously, there is a short delay in the arrival of femoral pulse wave. It is called **femoral delay**, radial femoral delay or radiofemoral delay.

■ APPLIED PHYSIOLOGY: ABNORMAL ARTERIAL PULSE

1. Pulsus Deficit

Pulsus deficit is the abnormal condition in which the pulse rate is less than the heart rate. Pulsus deficit is the only condition in which pulse rate is less than the heart rate. It occurs during atrial fibrillation. **Atrial fibrillation** is the type of arrhythmia (irregular heart beat) characterized by rapid and irregular atrial contractions at the rate of 300 to 400 beats per minute.

2. Pulsus Alternans

Pulsus alternans is the abnormal condition characterized by alternation of strong and weak pulse. It is common in severe myocardial diseases.

3. Anacrotic Pulse

Anacrotic pulse is the abnormal pulse, characterized by a slow ascending limb which has a notch called anacrotic notch. It is produced in aortic stenosis (narrowing).

4. Thready Pulse

Thready or weak pulse is the abnormally weak and very feeble pulse because of its low volume. And it is hardly felt at the arteries. It usually occurs during severe hemorrhage or severe chills.

5. Pulsus Paradoxus

Pulsus paradoxus is the condition characterized by a weak pulse with marked decrease in volume during inspiration caused by fall in systolic blood pressure by 10 mm Hg. The pulse becomes normal or stronger with increase in volume during expiration. It occurs in many cardiac and respiratory diseases.

6. Water Hammer Pulse

Water hammer pulse or **collapsing pulse** is the abnormal pulse, characterized by a rapid upstroke and an equally rapid downstroke. In other words, it is a bounding and forceful pulse that quickly increases in volume and subsequently and decreases in volume resulting in collapse. It is seen in patent ductus arteriosus, aortic regurgitation (see below).

7. Abnormal Pulse in Patent Ductus Arteriosus

Pulse during patent ductus arteriosus is a strong water hammer pulse. Patent ductus arteriosus is the permanent existence of ductus arteriosus.

8. Abnormal Pulse in Aortic Regurgitation

Pulse during aortic regurgitation also is a strong water hammer pulse. Aortic regurgitation is the backflow of blood from aorta into left ventricle. It is common during **incompetence** of **semilunar valve** in aorta.

■ VENOUS PULSE

■ DEFINITION AND IMPORTANCE OF VENOUS PULSE

Venous pulse is defined as the pressure changes transmitted in the form of waves from right atrium to the veins near the heart. Venous pulse is observed only in larger veins near the heart such as jugular vein.

Evaluation of the venous pulse is an integral part of the physical examination because it reflects right atrial pressure and **hemodynamic events** in **right atrium**. Venous pulse recording is used to determine rate of atrial contraction, just as the record of arterial pulse is used to determine rate of ventricular contraction.

In addition, many phases of cardiac cycle can be recognized by means of venous pulse tracing. It is the simple and accurate method to measure duration of different phases in diastole. It also represents the atrial pressure changes taking place during cardiac cycle.

■ EXAMINATION OF VENOUS PULSE

Inspection of jugular vein pulsations is routinely done by bedside examination of neck veins. It provides valuable information about the cardiac function.

To observe the pulsation of internal jugular vein, head of the subject is tilted upwards at 45°. However, in patients with increased venous pressure, the head should be tilted as much as 90°. Pulsations of jugular vein can be noticed when light is passed across the skin overlying internal jugular vein with relaxed neck muscles. Simultaneous palpation of the left carotid artery helps the examiner confirm the venous pulsations.

■ JUGULAR VENOUS PULSE TRACING

Recording of jugular venous pulse is also called **phlebogram**. It is similar to intra-atrial pressure curve **(Fig. 73.2)**.

Phlebogram has three positive waves and three negative waves:

Positive waves: a, c, and v.
Negative waves: x, x_1 and y.

'a' Wave

It is the first wave and is a positive wave. It is due to rise in atrial pressure during atrial systole.

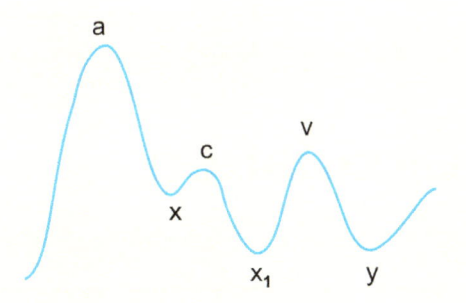

FIGURE 73.2: Phlebogram.

'x' Wave

This negative wave is due to fall of pressure in atrium and coincides with atrial diastole and beginning of ventricular systole.

'c' Wave

This positive wave occurs due to rise in atrial pressure during isometric contraction period. During this period the atrioventricular valves bulge into the atria and increase the pressure in the atria slightly.

'x_1' Wave

It is a negative wave and it is due to fall in pressure during ejection period. During ejection period, the atrioventricular ring is pulled towards ventricles causing fall in atrial pressure.

'v' Wave

This positive wave is due to rise in atrial pressure. The pressure increases because of atrial filling (venous return). It is obtained during isometric relaxation period or during atrial diastole.

'y' Wave

This negative wave denotes fall in pressure in atria. It is due to the opening of atrioventricular valve and emptying of blood into the ventricle. It appears during rapid and slow filling periods. 'y' wave is followed by 'a' wave and the cycle is repeated.

■ APPLIED PHYSIOLOGY: ABNORMAL VENOUS PULSE

1. Elevated Jugular Venous Pulse

Elevated jugular venous pulse indicates the rise in right ventricular pressure. It occurs in diseases of heart.

2. Kussmaul's Sign

Kussmaul's sign is the increase in venous distention and venous pressure. Normally, it occurs during inspiration.

It also occurs in pathological conditions of the heart.

Chapter 74: Regional Circulation

CHAPTER OUTLINE

- REGIONAL CIRCULATION
- CORONARY CIRCULATION
- CEREBRAL CIRCULATION
- SPLANCHNIC CIRCULATION
- CAPILLARY CIRCULATION
- SKELETAL MUSCLE CIRCULATION
- CUTANEOUS CIRCULATION

REGIONAL CIRCULATION

Circulation of blood through a particular organ or a region of the body is called regional circulation. Blood flow through a region is proportional to the local activity.

Various regional circulations are:

1. Coronary circulation.
2. Cerebral circulation.
3. Splanchnic circulation.
4. Capillary circulation.
5. Skeletal muscle circulation.
6. Cutaneous circulation.
7. Pulmonary circulation.
8. Renal circulation.

Pulmonary circulation is explained in Chapter 78. Renal circulation is explained in Chapter 41. Other regional circulations are given below.

CORONARY CIRCULATION

DISTRIBUTION OF CORONARY BLOOD VESSELS

Coronary Arteries

Heart muscle is supplied by two coronary arteries, the right and left coronary arteries, which are the first branches of aorta. Coronary arteries encircle the heart in the manner of a **crown** hence the name coronary arteries (Latin word corona = crown).

Branches of coronary arteries

Coronary arteries divide and subdivide into smaller branches, which run all along the surface of the heart. Smaller arterial branches are called **epicardiac arteries**. Epicardiac arteries give rise to further smaller branches known as **intramural vessels** or **final arteries**. Final arteries run at right angles through heart muscle near the inner aspect of wall of the heart.

Venous Drainage

Venous drainage from the heart muscle is by three types of vessels:

1. Coronary sinus

Coronary sinus is the larger vein draining 75% of total coronary flow. It drains blood from left side of the heart and opens into right atrium near tricuspid valve.

2. Anterior coronary veins

Anterior coronary veins drain blood from right side of the heart and open directly into right atrium.

3. Thebesian veins

Thebesian veins drain deoxygenated blood from myocardium directly into the concerned chamber of heart.

Physiological Shunt

Physiological shunt is a **diverted route** (diversion) through which the venous blood is mixed with arterial blood. Deoxygenated blood flowing from thebesian veins into cardiac chambers makes up part of normal physiological shunt. Other component of physiological shunt is the drainage of deoxygenated blood from bronchial circulation into pulmonary vein without being oxygenated (Chapter 78).

NORMAL CORONARY BLOOD FLOW

Normal blood flow through coronary circulation is about 200 mL/min. It forms 4% of cardiac output. It is about 65 to 70 mL/min/100 g of cardiac muscle.

PHASIC CHANGES IN CORONARY BLOOD FLOW

Blood flow through coronary arteries is not constant. It decreases during systole and increases during diastole **(Fig. 74.1)**.

During systole, the coronary blood vessels are compressed and blood flow is reduced. During diastole, the compression is released and the blood vessels are distended. So, the blood flow is increased.

REGULATION OF CORONARY BLOOD FLOW

Like any other organ, heart also has the capacity to regulate its own blood flow by **autoregulation** (Chapter 41). Coronary blood flow is not affected when mean arterial pressure varies between 60 mm Hg and 150 mm Hg.

Factors regulating coronary blood flow are:

1. Need for oxygen.
2. Metabolic factors.
3. Coronary perfusion pressure.
4. Nervous factors.

1. Need for Oxygen

Amount of blood passing through coronary circulation is directly proportional to the consumption of oxygen by cardiac muscle. Even in resting condition, a large amount of oxygen, i.e. 70 to 80% is consumed from the blood by heart muscle than by any other tissues. In conditions associated with increased cardiac activity, the need for oxygen increases enormously. This leads to **coronary vasodilatation** and increase in blood flow to heart.

2. Metabolic Factors

Metabolic products increase coronary blood flow by **coronary vasodilatation** during hypoxic conditions. Increase in blood flow due to vasodilator effects of metabolites is called **reactive hyperemia**.

Metabolic products which increase the coronary blood flow by vasodilation are:

i. Adenosine.
ii. Potassium.
iii. Hydrogen.
iv. Carbon dioxide.
v. Adenosine phosphate compounds.

3. Coronary Perfusion Pressure

Coronary perfusion pressure is the balance between mean arterial pressure in aorta and the right atrial pressure. Since right atrial pressure is low, the mean arterial pressure becomes the major factor that maintains coronary blood flow.

4. Nervous Factors

Coronary blood vessels are innervated both by parasympathetic and sympathetic divisions of autonomic nervous system. These nerves influence the coronary blood flow only indirectly by acting on the musculature of heart.

During sympathetic stimulation, the rate and force of contraction of heart are increased resulting in liberation of metabolites. The metabolites dilate the blood vessels and increase the coronary blood flow. During parasympathetic stimulation, cardiac functions are inhibited and the liberation of metabolites is less. And coronary blood flow decreases.

APPLIED PHYSIOLOGY: CORONARY ARTERY DISEASE

Coronary artery disease (CAD) is a heart disease caused by inadequate blood supply to cardiac muscle that is due to occlusion of coronary artery. It is also called **coronary heart disease**.

Coronary Occlusion

Coronary occlusion means the partial or complete obstruction of the coronary artery. Occlusion occurs because of **atherosclerosis**, a condition associated with deposition of cholesterol on the walls of the artery. In due course, this part of the arterial wall becomes **fibrotic** and it is called **atherosclerotic plague**. The plaque is made up of cholesterol, calcium and other substances from blood.

Because of the atherosclerotic plague the lumen of the coronary artery becomes narrow. In severe conditions, the artery is completely occluded.

Smaller blood vessels are occluded by the **thrombus** or part of atherosclerotic plague detached from coronary artery. This thrombus or part of the plague is called **embolus**.

Myocardial Ischemia

Myocardial ischemia is the reaction of a part of myocardium in response to hypoxia. Hypoxia develops when blood flow to a part of myocardium decreases severely due to occlusion of a coronary artery.

When the ischemia is mild due to obstruction of smaller blood vessel, the blood flow can be restored by rapid development of **coronary collateral arteries**.

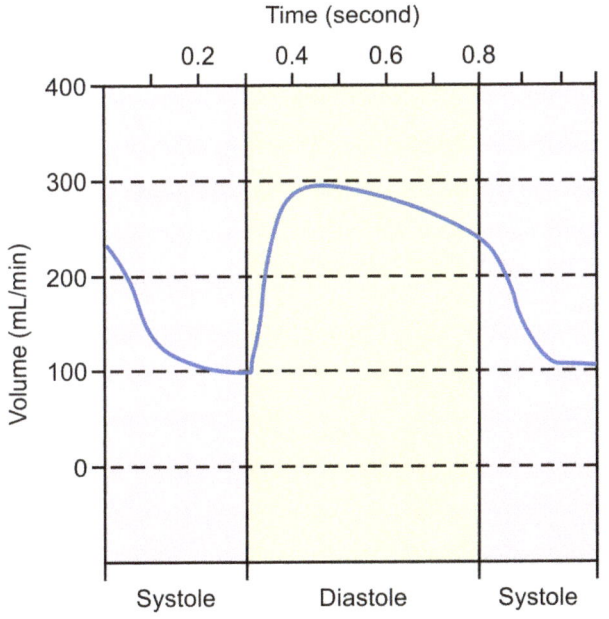

FIGURE 74.1: Phasic changes in coronary blood flow.

Necrosis

Necrosis is the death of cells or tissues by injury or disease in a localized area. When coronary occlusion is severe involving larger blood vessels, severe ischemia develops and it leads to **necrosis of myocardium**. Necrosis is irreversible.

Myocardial Infarction: Heart Attack

Myocardial infarction is the necrosis of myocardium caused by insufficient blood flow due to embolus, thrombus or vascular spasm. It is also called heart attack. In myocardial infarction, death occurs rapidly due to ventricular fibrillation.

Common symptoms of myocardial infarction are:

1. Cardiac pain.
2. Nausea.
3. Vomiting.
4. Palpitations.
5. Difficulty in breathing.
6. Extreme weakness.
7. Sweating.
8. Anxiety.

Cardiac Pain: Angina Pectoris

Cardiac pain is the **chest pain** caused by **myocardial ischemia**. It is also called angina pectoris. It is the common manifestation of coronary artery disease. Pain starts beneath the sternum and radiates to the surface of left arm and left shoulder. Cardiac pain is a **referred pain** (Chapter 96) since it is felt over the body away from the heart. It is because, heart and left arm develop from the same dermatomal segment in embryo.

■ CEREBRAL CIRCULATION

Cerebral circulation means flow of blood through the blood vessels of brain.

■ IMPORTANCE OF CEREBRAL CIRCULATION

Brain tissues need adequate blood supply continuously. Stoppage of blood flow for 5 seconds leads to **unconsciousness** and for 5 minutes leads to **irreparable damage** to the brain cells.

■ CEREBRAL BLOOD VESSELS

Brain receives blood from the **basilar artery** and **internal carotid artery**. Branches from these arteries form **circle of Willis**. The venous drainage is by sinuses, which open into internal jugular vein.

■ NORMAL CEREBRAL BLOOD FLOW

Normally, brain receives 750 to 800 mL of blood per minute. It is about 15 to 16% of total cardiac output and about 50 to 55 mL/100 g of brain tissue per minute.

■ REGULATION OF CEREBRAL BLOOD FLOW

Cerebral circulation is regulated by three factors:

1. Autoregulation.
2. Chemical factors.
3. Neural factors.

1. Autoregulation

Like any other vital organ, brain also regulates its own blood flow by means of autoregulation (Chapter 41). However, the autoregulation in brain has got its own limitations.

2. Chemical Factors

Chemical factors which increase the cerebral blood flow:

i. Decreased oxygen tension.
ii. Increased carbon dioxide tension.
iii. Increased hydrogen ion concentration.

3. Nervous Factors

Cerebral blood vessels are supplied by sympathetic vasoconstrictor fibers. But these fibers do not regulate cerebral blood flow under normal conditions. In pathological conditions like hypertension, the sympathetic nerves cause constriction of cerebral blood vessels, leading to reduction in blood flow. It prevents cerebral vascular hemorrhage and cerebral stroke.

■ APPLIED PHYSIOLOGY: STROKE

Definition

Stroke is the sudden death of neurons in localized area of brain due to inadequate blood supply. It is characterized by reversible or irreversible paralysis with other symptoms. Stroke is also called **cardiovascular accident** (CVA) or **brain attack**.

Causes of Stroke

1. Heart disease.
2. Hypertension.
3. High cholesterol in blood.
4. High blood sugar (diabetes mellitus).
5. Heavy smoking.
6. Heavy alcohol consumption.

Symptoms of Stroke

Symptoms of stroke depend upon the area of brain that is damaged.

Common symptoms of stroke are:

1. Weakness.
2. Numbness or paralysis particularly on one side of the body.
3. Impairment of speech.
4. Emotional disturbances.
5. Loss of coordination.
6. Loss of memory.
7. Dizziness.
8. Loss of consciousness.
9. Coma or death.

SPLANCHNIC CIRCULATION

INTRODUCTION

Splanchnic or visceral circulation constitutes three portions:

1. Mesenteric circulation supplying blood to GI tract.
2. Splenic circulation supplying blood to spleen.
3. Hepatic circulation supplying blood to liver.

Unique feature of splanchnic circulation is that, the blood from mesenteric bed and spleen forms a major amount of blood flowing to liver. Blood flows to liver from GI tract and spleen through portal system.

MESENTERIC CIRCULATION

Distribution of Blood Flow in Mesenteric Circulation

Stomach : 35 mL/100 g/min
Intestine : 50 mL/100 g/min
Pancreas : 80 mL/100 g/min

SPLENIC CIRCULATION

Importance of Splenic Circulation

Spleen is the main **reservoir for blood**. Due to the dilatation of blood vessels, a large amount of blood is stored in spleen. And the constriction of blood vessels by sympathetic stimulation releases blood into circulation.

Storage of Blood in Spleen

Two structures are involved in spleen in storage of blood namely, splenic venous sinuses and splenic pulp.

Small arteries and arterioles open directly into the venous sinuses. When spleen expands, the sinuses swell and large quantity of blood is stored. The capillaries of splenic pulp are highly permeable. So, most of the blood cells pass through capillary membrane and are stored in the pulp.

HEPATIC CIRCULATION

Hepatic Blood Vessels

Liver receives blood from two sources:

1. Hepatic artery from aorta.
2. Portal vein from mesenteric and splenic vascular bed. More details are given in Chapter 34.

Normal Blood Flow to Liver

Liver receives maximum amount of blood as compared to any other organ in the body since, most of the metabolic activities are carried out in the liver. Blood flow to liver is 1,500 mL/min, which forms 30% of cardiac output. It is about 100 mL/100 g of tissue per minute.

Normally, about 1,100 mL of blood flows through portal vein and remaining 400 mL of blood flows through hepatic artery. However, portal vein carries only about 25% of oxygen to liver. It is because it carries the blood, which has already passed through the blood vessels of GI tract where oxygen might have been used. Hepatic artery transports 75% of oxygen to the liver.

CAPILLARY CIRCULATION

MICROCIRCULATION

Microcirculation is the flow of blood through the minute blood vessels such as arterioles, capillaries and venules. Capillary circulation forms the major part of microcirculation. Capillaries are formed by single layer of endothelial cells which are wrapped around by pericytes.

SALIENT FEATURES OF CAPILLARIES

1. Capillaries arise from arterioles and form the area for exchange of materials between blood and tissues.
2. Capillaries outnumber the other blood vessels. About **10 billion capillaries** are present in the body.
3. Each capillary lies in a very close proximity to the cells of the tissues at a distance of about 20 to 30 mm. This enables easy and rapid exchange of substances between blood and the tissues through interstitial fluid.

PATTERN OF CAPILLARY SYSTEM

Capillaries are disposed between arterioles and venules. From the arterioles, the meta-arterioles take origin **(Fig. 74.2)**.

From meta-arterioles, two types of capillaries arise:

1. Preferential channels.
2. True capillaries.

1. Preferential Channels or Continuous Capillaries

After arising from the meta-arterioles, the preferential channels form a network and finally join the venules.

2. True Capillaries

After arising from meta-arterioles, the true capillaries also form a network and join the venules. Smooth muscle fibers encircle the beginning of true capillaries forming a sphincter called **precapillary sphincter**. This sphincter controls the blood flow through true capillaries.

ANATOMICAL AND PHYSIOLOGICAL SHUNTS

Anatomical Shunt: Arteriovenous Shunt

Anatomical shunt is the direct link between arterioles and venules. It is also called arteriovenous shunt. Flow of blood through the capillaries where exchange of nutrients, gases and other substances takes place is called **nutritional flow**. Flow of blood through anatomical shunt is called **non-nutritional flow**. Non-nutritional blood flow occurs in many tissues of the body particularly during resting conditions when metabolic activities are low.

Physiological Shunt

Physiological shunt is the link between arterial and venous side of circulation provided by meta-arteriole. Many tissues of the body such as muscles do not have anatomical shunts. However, the meta-arteriole in these tissues acts as the physiological shunt between arterial and venous sides of the circulation. Non-nutritional blood flow occurs through physiological shunt under resting conditions.

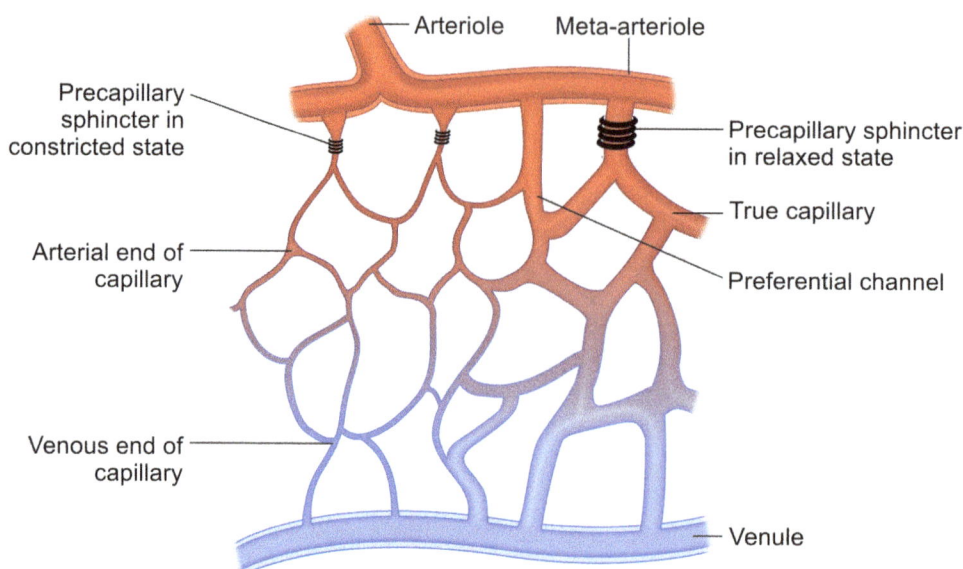

FIGURE 74.2: Capillary bed.

Shunt in Capillaries vs Shunt in Heart

Physiological shunt in capillaries is different from physiological shunt in heart. In capillaries the oxygenated blood flows towards deoxygenated blood. But in heart, the deoxygenated blood flows towards the oxygenated blood (see above).

■ PECULIARITIES OF CAPILLARY BLOOD FLOW

1. Blood does not pass through the capillary system continuously. It is because of the alternate constriction and dilatation of meta-arterioles and alternate opening and closure of precapillary sphincters.
2. Direction of blood flow through the capillaries is not fixed as in the case of other blood vessels. Blood may flow in opposite direction in two adjacent capillaries.
3. In capillaries, blood flows as a single pile or single row of blood cells. In other blood vessels, the blood flows in either axial stream containing mainly blood cells or peripheral stream containing plasma.
4. Under resting conditions, most of the capillaries lie in collapsed state. Only during activity, all the capillaries open up and increase the vascularity.
5. Amount of blood flowing through the capillary system throughout the body is very low. It is only about 150 mL/min.
6. Velocity of blood flow is least in capillaries. It is only about 0.5 to 1 mm/sec. It facilitates exchange of substances between the capillaries and tissues.

■ FUNCTIONS OF CAPILLARIES

Most important function of capillaries is the exchange of substances between blood and tissues. Oxygen, nutrients and other essential substances enter the tissues from capillary blood; carbon dioxide, metabolites and other unwanted substances are removed from the tissues by capillary blood.

Exchange of materials across the capillary endothelium occurs primarily by **diffusion**. It also occurs by means of filtration and **pinocytosis**.

■ SKELETAL MUSCLE CIRCULATION
■ BLOOD FLOW TO SKELETAL MUSCLES

During resting condition, blood flow to skeletal muscle is 4 to 7 mL/100 g/min. During exercise, it increases to about 100 mL/100 g/min.

■ MUSCULAR CONTRACTION AND BLOOD FLOW

During contraction of muscle, the blood vessels are compressed and the blood flow decreases. And during relaxation of muscle, the compression of blood vessels is relieved and the blood flow increases.

In severe muscular exercise, blood flow increases in between the muscular contractions.

■ APPLIED PHYSIOLOGY: VARICOSE VEINS

Varicose vein is the vein that becomes irregularly swollen (twisted or tortuous) and enlarged. Superficial veins of the leg are mostly affected.

Causes for Varicose Vein

1. Permanent dilatation of veins due to **incompetence** of the valves of the veins or absence of muscular activity for long periods. So, varicose veins are common in the individuals with occupations, which require standing for long periods.
2. **Thrombophlebitis:** Inflammation of vein associated with formation of thrombus.

■ CUTANEOUS CIRCULATION
■ ARCHITECTURE OF CUTANEOUS BLOOD VESSELS

1. **Arterioles** arising from the smaller arteries reach the dermis.

2. After taking origin, the arterioles turn horizontally and give rise to **meta-arterioles**.
3. From meta-arterioles, hairpin-shaped **capillary loops** arise. Arterial limb of the loop ascends vertically and turns to form a venous limb, which descends down. After reaching the base of dermis, few venous limbs of neighboring papillae unite to form the **collecting venule**.
4. Collecting venules anastomose with one another to form the **subpapillary venous plexus**.
5. Subpapillary plexus runs horizontally and drain into the **deeper veins**.

FUNCTIONS OF CUTANEOUS CIRCULATION

Cutaneous blood flow performs two functions:

1. Supply of nutrition to skin.
2. Loss of heat from the body and regulation of body temperature.

NORMAL BLOOD FLOW TO SKIN

Under normal conditions, the blood flow to skin is about 250 mL/sq.m/min. When the body temperature increases, cutaneous blood flow increases up to 2,800 mL/sq.m/min because of cutaneous vasodilatation.

Chapter 75: Fetal Circulation and Respiration

CHAPTER OUTLINE

- FETAL HEART AND PLACENTA
- BLOOD VESSELS IN FETUS
- FETAL LUNGS
- CHANGES IN CIRCULATION AND RESPIRATION AFTER BIRTH: NEONATAL CIRCULATION AND RESPIRATION
  - FIRST BREATH OF THE CHILD
- FLOW OF BLOOD TO LUNGS
- CLOSURE OF FORAMEN OVALE
- REVERSAL OF BLOOD FLOW IN DUCTUS ARTERIOSUS
- CLOSURE OF DUCTUS VENOSUS
- CLOSURE OF DUCTUS ARTERIOSUS

FETAL HEART AND PLACENTA

Development of heart is completed at fourth week of intrauterine life and, it starts beating at the rate of 65 per minute. Along with heart, the blood vessels also develop. Heart rate gradually increases and reaches the maximum rate of about 140 beats per minute just before birth.

Fetal circulation is different from that of adults because of the presence of **placenta**. Since **fetal lungs** are **nonfunctioning**, placenta is responsible for exchange of gases between fetal blood and mother's blood. So, the blood from right ventricle is diverted to placenta.

Fetus is connected with the mother through placenta. Fetal blood passes to placenta through **umbilical vessels** and the maternal blood runs through **uterine vessels**. These two sets of blood vessels lie in close proximity in the placenta through which the exchange of substances takes place between mother's blood and fetal blood. However, there is **no direct admixture** of maternal and fetal blood (Fig. 75.1).

BLOOD VESSELS IN FETUS

Due to nonfunctioning of fetal lungs, fetal heart pumps large quantity of blood into the placenta for exchange of substances. From placenta, the umbilical veins collect the blood, which has more oxygen and nutrients. **Umbilical vein** passes through liver. Some amount of blood is supplied to liver from umbilical vein. However, a large quantity of blood is diverted from umbilical vein into the inferior vena cava through **ductus venosus**. Liver receives blood from **portal vein** also.

In liver, the oxygenated blood mixes slightly with deoxygenated blood and enters the right atrium via inferior vena cava. From right atrium, major portion of blood is diverted into left atrium via **foramen ovale**. Foramen ovale is an opening in intra-atrial septum.

Blood from upper part of the body enters the right atrium through superior vena cava. From right atrium, blood enters right ventricle. From here, blood is pumped into pulmonary artery. From pulmonary artery, blood enters the systemic aorta through **ductus arteriosus**. Only a small quantity of blood is supplied to fetal lungs. Blood from left ventricle is pumped into aorta. 50% of blood from aorta reaches the placenta through umbilical arteries.

FETAL LUNGS

Pulmonary vascular resistance is the resistance offered to blood flow through pulmonary vascular bed. This resistance is very high in fetus because of the **nonfunctioning of fetal lungs**. High resistance in fetal lungs increases the pressure in the blood vessels of lungs. Because of the high pressure, the blood is diverted from pulmonary artery into aorta via **ductus arteriosus**.

CHANGES IN CIRCULATION AND RESPIRATION AFTER BIRTH: NEONATAL CIRCULATION AND RESPIRATION

1. FIRST BREATH OF THE CHILD

When fetus is delivered and umbilical cord is cut and tied, the lungs start functioning. When placental blood flow is

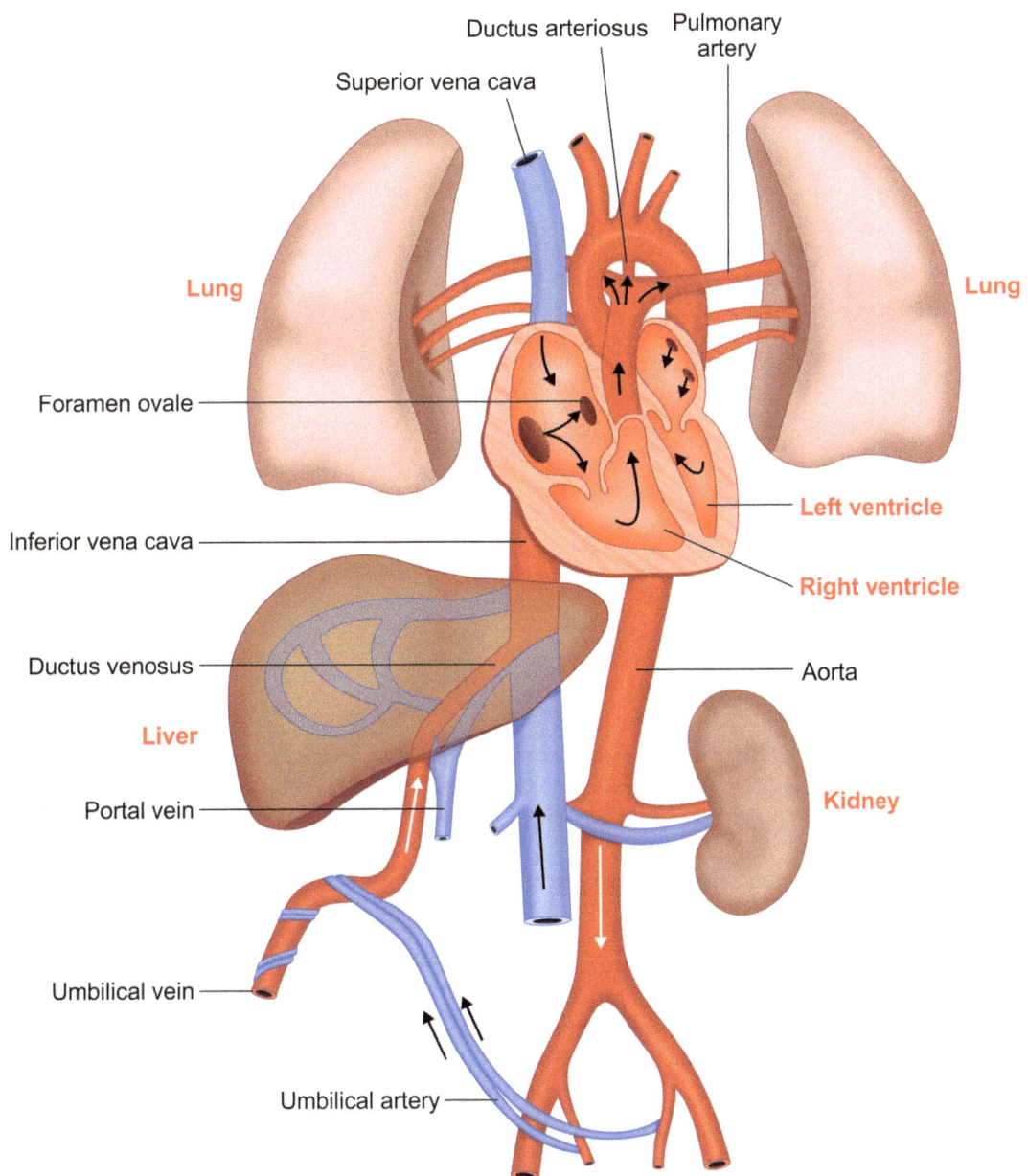

FIGURE 75.1: Fetal circulation.

cut off, there is sudden hypoxia and hypercapnia. Now, the respiratory center is strongly stimulated by these two factors and, the respiration starts. Initially, there is gasping, which is followed by normal respiration.

■ 2. FLOW OF BLOOD TO LUNGS

Lungs expand during the first breath of the infant. Expansion of lungs causes immediate reduction in the pulmonary vascular resistance and a sudden fall in pressure in the blood vessels of lungs. Therefore, the blood flow from pulmonary artery to lungs increases.

■ 3. CLOSURE OF FORAMEN OVALE

When blood starts flowing through the pulmonary circulation, the oxygenated blood from lungs returns to left atrium. It causes increase in the left atrial pressure. Simultaneously, due to stoppage of blood from placenta, pressure in inferior vena cava is decreased. It leads to fall in right atrial pressure. Thus, the pressure in right atrium is less and the pressure in left atrium is already high. This causes the closure of foramen ovale. Within few days after birth, the foramen ovale closes completely and fuses with the atrial wall.

■ 4. REVERSAL OF BLOOD FLOW IN DUCTUS ARTERIOSUS

In fetus, since pulmonary arterial pressure is very high, the blood passes from pulmonary artery into aorta via ductus arteriosus. However, in neonatal life, since the systemic arterial pressure is more than pulmonary arterial pressure, the blood passes in opposite direction in ductus arteriosus, i.e. from systemic aorta into pulmonary aorta

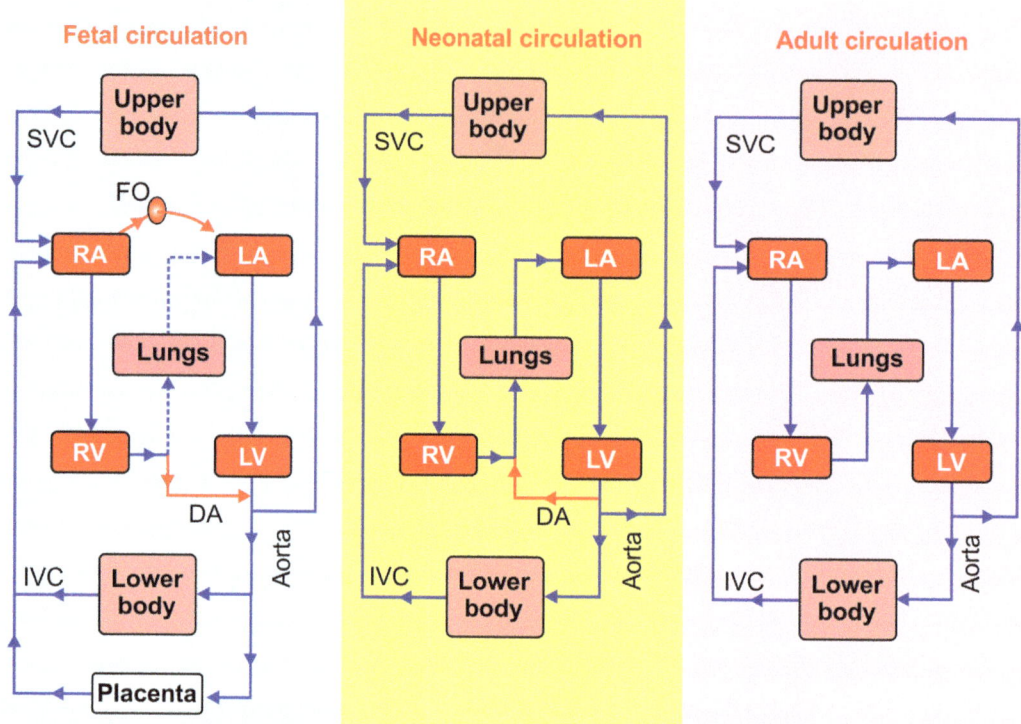

FIGURE 75.2: Fetal, neonatal and adult circulation.
RA = Right atrium, LA = Left atrium, RV = Right ventricle, LV = Left ventricle, FO = Foramen ovale, DA = Ductus arteriosus, SVC = Superior vena cava, IVC = Inferior vena cava. Dashed blue line in fetal circulation = Flow of very less quantity of blood.

(Fig. 75.2). The reversed flow in ductus arteriosus is heard as **continuous murmur** in infants.

■ 5. CLOSURE OF DUCTUS VENOSUS

Due to the contraction of smooth muscle near junction between umbilical vein and ductus venosus, the constriction and closure of ductus venosus occurs. Later, the ductus venosus becomes **fibrous band**.

■ 6. CLOSURE OF DUCTUS ARTERIOSUS

Ductus arteriosus starts closing due to narrowing. It closes completely after 2 days and the adult type of circulation starts. In some rare cases, the ductus arteriosus does not close. It remains intact producing a continuous murmur. The condition with intact ductus arteriosus is known as **patent ductus arteriosus**.

Chapter 76: Hemorrhage, Circulatory Shock and Heart Failure

CHAPTER OUTLINE

- **HEMORRHAGE**
  - DEFINITION
  - TYPES AND CAUSES
  - EFFECTS OF HEMORRHAGE
- **CIRCULATORY SHOCK**
  - DEFINITION
  - MANIFESTATIONS OF CIRCULATORY SHOCK
- **TYPES OF CIRCULATORY SHOCK**
- **SYNCOPE: FAINTING**
- **HEART FAILURE**
  - DEFINITION AND TYPES
  - CAUSES
  - SIGNS AND SYMPTOMS

HEMORRHAGE

DEFINITION

Hemorrhage is defined as excess loss of blood due to rupture of the blood vessels.

TYPES AND CAUSES OF HEMORRHAGE

Hemorrhage occurs because of various reasons. Based on the cause, hemorrhage is classified into five categories:

1. *Accidental Hemorrhage*

It occurs in road accidents and industrial accidents.

2. *Capillary Hemorrhage*

Capillary hemorrhage is the bleeding due to rupture of capillaries. It is very common in brain and heart during cardiovascular diseases.

3. *Internal Hemorrhage*

Internal hemorrhage is the bleeding in viscera. It is caused by rupture of blood vessels in the viscera.

4. *Postpartum Hemorrhage*

Postpartum hemorrhage is the excess bleeding that occurs immediately after labor.

5. *Hemorrhage due to Premature Detachment of Placenta*

In some cases, the placenta is detached from uterus of mother before the due date of delivery causing severe hemorrhage.

EFFECTS OF HEMORRHAGE

Many effects are observed during and after hemorrhage. Effects are different in acute hemorrhage and chronic hemorrhage.

Acute Hemorrhage

Acute hemorrhage is the sudden loss of large quantity of blood. It occurs in conditions like accidents. Decreased blood volume in acute hemorrhage causes hypovolemic shock.

Chronic Hemorrhage

Chronic hemorrhage is the loss of blood either by internal or by external bleeding over a long period of time. Internal bleeding occurs in conditions such as ulcer. External bleeding occurs in conditions like hemophilia and excess vaginal bleeding (menorrhagia). Chronic hemorrhage produces different types of effects such as anemia.

Compensatory Effects

After hemorrhage, series of compensatory reactions develop in the body to cope up with the blood loss. Some of the compensatory reactions take place immediately after hemorrhage and others at a later period.

CIRCULATORY SHOCK

DEFINITION

Shock is a general term that refers to depression or suppression of body functions produced by any disorder. Circulatory shock is the shock developed by inadequate blood flow throughout the body. It is a life-threatening condition and if the affected person is not treated immediately, it may result in death.

■ MANIFESTATIONS OF SHOCK

1. Cardiovascular System

Common feature of circulatory shock is fall in arterial blood pressure which results decreased blood flow to all organs.

2. Respiratory System

Breathing becomes rapid and shallow resulting in hypoventilation. Some persons may develop **respiratory distress syndrome**.

3. Kidneys

Initially, urinary output is reduced. Later **tubular necrosis** develops resulting in **acute renal failure**.

4. Skin

Because of stagnant hypoxia skin becomes **pale** and cold. **Cyanosis** develops in many parts of the body, particularly in earlobes and fingertips. There is excess sweating.

5. Vital Organs

Vital organs such as **liver** and endocrine glands fail to function due to necrosis.

6. Brain

Lack of blood flow to brain tissues produces **ischemia** resulting in **fainting** and irreparable damage of brain tissues.

Finally, the **brain damage** and **cardiac arrest** cause death of the victim.

■ TYPES OF CIRCULATORY SHOCK

Circulatory shock is primarily classified into four types:
I. Shock due to decreased blood volume.
II. Shock due to increased vascular capacity.
III. Shock due to cardiac disease.
IV. Shock due to obstruction to blood flow.

I. Shock due to Decreased Blood Volume: Hypovolemic Shock

Shock due to decreased blood volume is called hypovolemic shock. It occurs when there is acute loss of at least 10 to 15% of blood. Important manifestations of hypovolemic shock are decrease in cardiac output, low blood pressure, increase in respiratory rate, and restlessness or lethargy.

Common types of hypovolemic shock are:

1. Hemorrhagic shock

Hemorrhagic shock is the shock that occurs due to hemorrhage. Acute hemorrhage as in the case of accident causes shock.

2. Traumatic shock

Traumatic shock is developed due to **trauma** (serious injury or wound caused by some external force).

3. Surgical shock

It is caused by internal **hemorrhage**, external hemorrhage or **dehydration** that occur during or after surgical procedures.

4. Burn shock

Burn shock is produced by the effects of burn.

5. Dehydration shock

Shock which is developed during severe dehydration is called dehydration shock.

II. Shock due to Increased Vascular Capacity: Vasogenic Shock

Shock occurs because of inadequate blood supply to the tissues due to increased vascular capacity. Capacity of the vascular system increases by the extensive dilatation of blood vessels. It is also known as vasogenic shock **(Fig. 76.1)**.

Common types of vasogenic shock are:

1. Neurogenic shock

Neurogenic shock is the type of shock characterized by sudden depression of nervous system due to extensive

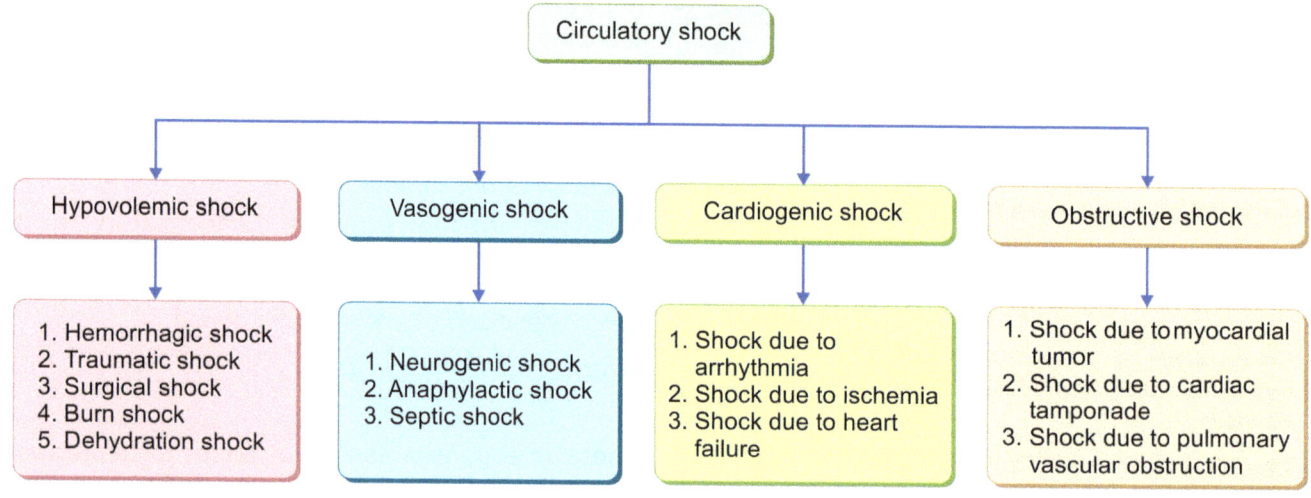

FIGURE 76.1: Different types of circulatory shock.

vasodilatation caused by loss of vasomotor tone. Common feature of neurogenic shock is syncope (see below).

2. Anaphylactic shock

Anaphylaxis means exaggerated allergic reaction to a foreign protein or antigen or any other substance to which the person has been previously sensitized. Shock that develops during anaphylactic reactions is called anaphylactic shock.

3. Septic shock

Sepsis is the condition characterized by the presence of pathogenic organisms or their toxins in blood or tissues. Shock developed during sepsis is known as septic shock or **blood poisoning**.

III. Shock due to Cardiac Diseases: Cardiogenic Shock

Shock due to cardiac disease is also called cardiogenic shock.

Types of cardiogenic shock
1. Shock due to arrhythmia (abnormal heart beat)
2. Shock due to myocardial ischemia.
3. Shock due to congestive heart failure.

IV. Shock due to Obstruction of Blood Flow: Obstructive Shock

Shock developed due to the obstruction to blood flow through circulatory system is called obstructive shock.

Causes of obstructive shock
1. Tumor in myocardium.
2. **Cardiac tamponade** (compression of heart due to accumulation of fluid in pericardial space).
3. Obstruction of blood vessels in lungs due to embolism.

SYNCOPE: FAINTING

Syncope or fainting is the sudden and transient (short-time) loss of consciousness and postural tone with spontaneous recovery. It occurs due to temporary inadequate cerebral blood flow.

Types of Syncope

1. Vasovagal syncope or emotional fainting

Fainting is caused by sudden stimulation of **vagus nerve**. It is also called **neurocardiogenic syncope**. Vasovagal syncope is common in conditions such as severe emotional distress and exertion.

2. Postural syncope

Postural syncope is the loss of consciousness caused by **prolonged standing**. It occurs due to pooling of blood in lower limbs during prolonged standing resulting in decreased blood supply to the brain.

3. Micturition syncope

It is the fainting during micturition. It is common in patients who suffer from **orthostatic hypotension** (Chapter 71).

4. Effort syncope

Fainting caused **during exercise** or any other **strain** is called effort syncope. It is the common symptom in patients with stenosis of semilunar valves.

5. Cough syncope

This is the fainting while coughing. Severe cough increases intrathoracic pressure, which reduces the venous return and cardiac output leading to fainting.

6. Carotid sinus syncope

Fainting in persons wearing **tight collar dress**. Tight collar of the dress exerts pressure over the region of carotid sinus. This leads to reduction in heart rate, vasodilatation and fainting.

HEART FAILURE

DEFINITION AND TYPES

Definition of Heart Failure

Heart failure or **cardiac failure** is defined as the condition in which the heart loses the ability to pump sufficient amount of blood to all parts of the body. Heart failure may involve left ventricle or right ventricle or both.

Types of Heart Failure

Heart failure may be acute or chronic.

Acute heart failure

Acute heart failure is the sudden and rapid onset of signs and symptoms of abnormal heart functions. The symptoms last for a very short time and the condition improves rapidly.

Chronic heart failure

Chronic heart failure is the heart failure that is characterized by the symptoms that appear slowly over a period of time and become worst gradually.

Congestive Heart Failure

It is the heart failure resulting in **accumulation of fluid** in lungs and other tissues. When heart is not able to pump blood through aorta, the blood remains in heart. It results in dilatation of the chambers and accumulation of blood in veins (**vascular congestion**). This condition is also manifested by **fluid retention** and **pulmonary edema**.

CAUSES OF HEART FAILURE

Common causes of heart failure are:
1. Coronary artery disease.
2. Defective heart valves.
3. Arrhythmia.
4. Cardiac muscle disease such as cardiomyopathy.
5. Hypertension.
6. Congenital heart disease.
7. Diabetes.
8. Hyperthyroidism.
9. Anemia.
10. Lung disorders.

11. Myocarditis (inflammation of cardiac muscle due to viral infection, drugs, alcohol, etc.).

■ SIGNS AND SYMPTOMS OF HEART FAILURE

Signs and Symptoms of Chronic Heart Failure

1. Fatigue and weakness.
2. Rapid and irregular heartbeat.
3. Shortness of breathing.
4. Fluid retention and weight gain.
5. Loss of appetite, nausea and vomiting.
6. Cough.
7. Chest pain, if developed by myocardial infarction.

Signs and Symptoms of Acute Heart Failure

Signs and symptoms of acute heart failure may be same as chronic heart failure. But the signs and symptoms appear suddenly and severely. When heart starts to fail suddenly, the fluid accumulates in lungs causing pulmonary edema. It results in sudden and severe shortness of breath, cough with pink, foamy mucus and heart palpitations. It may lead to sudden death, if not attended immediately.

Chapter 77: Cardiovascular Adjustments During Exercise

CHAPTER OUTLINE

- ADJUSTMENTS DURING EXERCISE
- TYPES OF EXERCISE
  - DYNAMIC EXERCISE
  - STATIC EXERCISE
- AEROBIC AND ANAEROBIC EXERCISES
  - AEROBIC EXERCISE
  - ANAEROBIC EXERCISE
  - METABOLISM IN AEROBIC AND ANAEROBIC EXERCISES
- SEVERITY OF EXERCISE
  - MILD EXERCISE
  - MODERATE EXERCISE
- SEVERE EXERCISE
- EFFECTS OF EXERCISE ON CARDIOVASCULAR SYSTEM
  - ON BLOOD
  - ON BODY FLUID
  - ON HEART RATE
  - ON CARDIAC OUTPUT
  - ON VENOUS RETURN
  - ON BLOOD FLOW TO SKELETAL MUSCLES
  - ON BLOOD PRESSURE

ADJUSTMENTS DURING EXERCISE

During exercise, there is an increase in metabolic needs of body tissues, particularly the muscles.

Various adjustments, which take place in the body, are aimed at:

1. Supply of nutrients and oxygen to muscles and other tissues involved in exercise.
2. Prevention of increase in body temperature.

TYPES OF EXERCISE

Exercise is generally classified into two types depending upon the type of muscular contraction:
1. Dynamic exercise.
2. Static exercise.

DYNAMIC EXERCISE

Dynamic exercise involves **isotonic contraction** of muscles. It keeps the joints and muscles moving. Examples are swimming, bicycling, walking, etc. External work is involved in this type of exercise. External work is the shortening of muscle fibers against load.

In this type of exercise, the heart rate, force of contraction, cardiac output and systolic blood pressure increases. However, the diastolic blood pressure is unaltered or decreased. It is because, during dynamic exercise, the peripheral resistance is unaltered or decreased.

STATIC EXERCISE

Static exercise involves **isometric contraction** of muscles without movement of joints. Example is pushing heavy object. This is a type of exercise without the performance of external work. While doing this exercise, apart from increase in heart rate, force of contraction, cardiac output and systolic blood pressure, the diastolic blood pressure also increases. It is because of increase in peripheral resistance during static exercise.

AEROBIC AND ANAEROBIC EXERCISES

Based on the type of metabolism (energy producing process) involved, the exercise is classified into two types:

1. Aerobic exercise.
2. Anaerobic exercise.

AEROBIC EXERCISE

Aerobic means 'with air' or 'with oxygen'. The energy is obtained by utilizing nutrients in the presence of oxygen. Aerobic exercise involves activities with **lower intensity**, which is performed for **longer period** (see below). Aerobic exercise requires large amount of oxygen to obtain the energy needed for prolonged performance.

Examples of Aerobic Exercise

1. Fast walking.
2. Jogging.
3. Running.
4. Bicycling.
5. Skiing.
6. Skating.
7. Hockey.
8. Soccer.
9. Tennis.
10. Badminton.
11. Swimming.
12. Rowing.

ANAEROBIC EXERCISE

Anaerobic means 'without air' or 'without oxygen'. Body obtains energy by burning glycogen stored in the muscles without oxygen. Anaerobic exercise involves **exertion** for **short periods** followed by periods of rest. It uses the muscles at high intensity and a high rate of work for a short period.

Burning glycogen without oxygen liberates lactic acid. Accumulation of lactic acid leads to fatigue. Therefore, this type of exercise cannot be performed for longer period. And a recovery period is essential before going for another burst of anaerobic exercise. Anaerobic exercise helps to increase the muscle strength.

Examples of Anaerobic Exercise

1. Pull ups.
2. Push ups.
3. Weightlifting.
4. Sprinting.
5. Any other rapid burst of strenuous exercise.

METABOLISM IN AEROBIC AND ANAEROBIC EXERCISES

When a person starts doing some exercise like jogging, bicycling or swimming, the muscles start utilizing energy. In order to have quick energy during the first few minutes, the muscles burn glycogen stored in them. During this period, fat is not burnt. Only glycogen is burnt and it is burnt without using oxygen. This is called **anaerobic metabolism.** Lactic acid is produced during this period. Presence of lactic acid causes some sort of **burning sensation** in the muscles particularly the muscles of arms, legs and back.

Muscles burn all the muscle glycogen within 3 to 5 minutes. If the person continues the exercise beyond this, glycogen stored in liver is converted into glucose, which is transported to muscles through blood. Now the body moves into **aerobic metabolism**. Glucose obtained from liver is burnt in the presence of oxygen. No more lactic acid is produced. So, the burning sensation in the muscles disappears. Proper breathing is essential during this period so that adequate oxygen is supplied to the muscles to extract the energy from glucose. Supply of glucose from liver in combination with adequate availability of oxygen allows the person to continue the exercise.

Utilization of all the glycogen stored in liver is completed by about 20 minutes. If the exercise is continued beyond this, the body starts utilizing the fat. The stored fat called body fat is converted into carbohydrate, which is utilized by the muscles. This allows the person to do the exercise for a longer period.

SEVERITY OF EXERCISE

Cardiovascular and other changes in the body depend upon the severity of exercise also.

Based on severity, the exercise is classified into three types:

1. Mild exercise.
2. Moderate exercise
3. Severe exercise.

1. MILD EXERCISE

It is the very simple form of exercise like slow walking. Little or no change occurs in cardiovascular system during mild exercise.

2. MODERATE EXERCISE

Moderate exercise does not involve strenuous muscular activity and it can be performed for a longer period. Exhaustion does not occur at the end of moderate exercise. The examples of this type of exercise are fast walking and slow running.

3. SEVERE EXERCISE

Severe exercise involves strenuous muscular activity and it can be performed only for short duration. Fast running for a distance of 100 or 400 meters is the best example of this type of exercise. Complete exhaustion occurs at the end of severe exercise.

EFFECTS OF EXERCISE ON CARDIOVASCULAR SYSTEM

1. ON BLOOD

Red blood cell count increases because of release of **erythropoietin** from kidney due to hypoxia. The pH of blood decreases due to increased carbon dioxide content.

2. ON BODY FLUIDS

More heat is produced during exercise and the **thermoregulatory system** is activated. This in turn, causes secretion of large amount of **sweat** leading to:

i. Fluid loss.
ii. Reduced blood volume.
iii. Hemoconcentration.
iv. Sometimes, severe exercise leads to dehydration.

3. ON HEART RATE

Heart rate increases during exercise. Even the thought of exercise or preparation for exercise increases the heart rate. It is because of impulses from cerebral cortex to medullary centers, which reduces vagal tone.

In moderate exercise, the heart rate increases to 180 beats/minute. In severe muscular exercise it reaches 240 to 260 beats/minute. Increased heart rate during exercise is mainly due to **vagal withdrawal** and **increase in sympathetic tone**.

4. ON CARDIAC OUTPUT

Cardiac output increases up to 20 L/minute in moderate exercise and up to 35 L/minute during severe exercise. Increase in cardiac output is directly proportional to the increase in amount of oxygen consumed during exercise.

5. ON VENOUS RETURN

Venous return increases during exercise because of muscle pump, respiratory pump and splanchnic vasoconstriction.

6. ON BLOOD FLOW TO SKELETAL MUSCLES

There is increase in the amount of blood flowing to skeletal muscles during exercise. In resting condition, the blood supply to the skeletal muscles is 3 to 4 mL/100 gram of the muscle/minute. It increases up to 60 to 80 mL in moderate exercise and up to 90 to 120 mL in severe exercise.

During the muscular activity, stoppage of blood flow occurs when the muscles contract. It is because of compression of blood vessels during contraction. And in between the contractions, the blood flow increases.

7. ON BLOOD PRESSURE

During moderate **isotonic exercise**, the systolic pressure is increased. It is due to increase in heart rate and stroke volume. Diastolic pressure is not altered because peripheral resistance is not affected during moderate isotonic exercise.

In severe exercise involving isotonic muscular contraction, the systolic pressure enormously increases, but the diastolic pressure decreases. Decrease in diastolic pressure is because of the decrease in peripheral resistance. Decrease in peripheral resistance is due to vasodilatation caused by metabolites.

During exercise involving **isometric contraction**, the peripheral resistance increases. So, the diastolic pressure also increases along with systolic pressure.

Blood Pressure After Exercise

After exercise, the blood pressure falls below the resting level. It is because of vasodilatation caused by metabolic end products accumulated in muscles during exercise. However, the pressure returns to resting level quickly as soon as the metabolic end products are removed from muscles.

MODEL QUESTIONS IN CARDIOVASCULAR SYSTEM

■ LONG QUESTIONS

1. Define cardiac cycle. Describe various events of cardiac cycle.
2. Define electrocardiogram. Describe the waves, segments and intervals of normal ECG. Add a note on ECG leads.
3. Give the definitions, normal values and variations of cardiac output. Explain the factors regulating cardiac output.
4. What is cardiac output? Enumerate the various methods to measure cardiac output and, explain the measurement of cardiac output by applying Fick's principle.
5. Describe the innervation of heart and the regulation of heart rate.
6. Define arterial blood pressure. Describe the nervous regulation (short term) of arterial blood pressure.
7. Describe renal mechanism of (long term) regulation of arterial blood pressure.
8. Describe the cardiovascular and respiratory changes during exercise.

■ SHORT QUESTIONS

1. Action potential in cardiac muscle.
2. Pacemaker.
3. Conductive system in heart.
4. Isometric contraction period.
5. Heart sounds.
6. Waves of normal ECG.
7. ECG leads.
8. Nerve supply to heart.
9. Vagal tone.
10. Baroreceptors.
11. Chemoreceptors.
12. Determinants of arterial blood pressure.
13. Renal regulation of blood pressure.
14. Hypertension.
15. Venous pressure.
16. Capillary pressure.
17. Arterial pulse.
18. Phlebogram/Venous pulse.
19. Coronary artery disease.
20. Stroke.
21. Capillary circulation (microcirculation).
22. Syncope.
23. Heart failure.
24. Effect of exercise on blood pressure.

■ VERY SHORT ANSWER QUESTIONS

1. Pericardium.
2. Syncytium in cardiac muscle.
3. Valves of the heart.
4. Actions of heart.
5. Divisions of circulation.
6. Velocity of impulse at different parts of conductive system.
7. All-or-none law and staircase phenomenon.
8. Refractory period in cardiac muscle.
9. End systolic volume, end diastolic volume and ejection fraction.
10. Reduplication of first and second heart sounds.
11. Triple and quadruple heart sounds.
12. Auscultation areas.
13. Cardiac murmurs.
14. P wave/QRS complex/T wave of ECG.
15. Definitions and normal values of cardiac output.
16. Respiratory pump.
17. Muscle pump.
18. Preload and afterload.
19. Peripheral resistance.
20. Fick's principle and its application.
21. Pathological conditions when tachycardia or bradycardia occurs.
22. Vagal tone.
23. Vagal escape.
24. Sympathetic tone.
25. Role of baroreceptors in regulating heart rate.
26. Marey's reflex/Marey's law.
27. Sinoaortic mechanism and buffer nerves.
28. Bainbridge reflex.
29. Bezold-Jarisch reflex/Coronary chemoreflex.
30. Role of baroreceptors in regulation of arterial blood pressure.
31. Renin-angiotensin mechanism.
32. List the hormones which increase, and hormones which decrease the arterial blood pressure.
33. Korotkoff sounds.
34. Hypotension.
35. Valsalva maneuver.
36. Müller maneuver.
37. Physiological shunt in heart.
38. Myocardial infarction.
39. Angina pectoris/cardiac pain.
40. Importance of cerebral circulation.
41. Mesenteric circulation.
42. Splenic circulation.
43. Hepatic circulation.
44. Physiological shunt in capillaries.
45. Peculiarities of capillary circulation.
46. Circulation through skeletal muscles.
47. Definition, types and causes of hemorrhage.
48. Dynamic exercise.
49. Static exercise.
50. Aerobic and anaerobic exercise.

Chapter 78: Respiratory Tract and Pulmonary Circulation

SECTION 9: RESPIRATORY SYSTEM AND ENVIRONMENTAL PHYSIOLOGY

CHAPTER OUTLINE

- **RESPIRATION**
  - NORMAL RATE OF RESPIRATION
  - TYPES OF RESPIRATION
  - PHASES OF RESPIRATION
- **FUNCTIONAL ANATOMY OF RESPIRATORY TRACT**
- **RESPIRATORY UNIT**
  - STRUCTURE OF RESPIRATORY UNIT
  - RESPIRATORY MEMBRANE
- **NON-RESPIRATORY FUNCTIONS OF RESPIRATORY TRACT**
- **RESPIRATORY PROTECTIVE REFLEXES**
  - COUGH REFLEX
  - SNEEZING REFLEX
  - SWALLOWING REFLEX
- **PULMONARY CIRCULATION**
  - PULMONARY BLOOD VESSELS
  - PHYSIOLOGICAL SHUNT
  - SALIENT FEATURES OF PULMONARY BLOOD VESSELS
  - PULMONARY BLOOD FLOW
  - PULMONARY BLOOD PRESSURE
  - MEASUREMENT OF PULMONARY BLOOD FLOW
  - REGULATION OF PULMONARY BLOOD FLOW

RESPIRATION

Respiration is the process by which oxygen is taken in and carbon dioxide is given out. The first breath takes place only after birth. **Fetal lungs** are **nonfunctional.** So, during intrauterine life the exchange of gases between fetal blood and mother's blood occurs through **placenta**.

After the first breath, the respiratory process continues throughout the life. Permanent stoppage of respiration occurs only at death.

NORMAL RATE OF RESPIRATION

Newborn	: 30 to 60/min
Early childhood	: 20 to 40/min
Late childhood	: 15 to 25/min
Adult	: 12 to 16/min

TYPES OF RESPIRATION

Respiration is often classified into two types:

1. **External respiration** that involves exchange of respiratory gases, i.e. oxygen and carbon dioxide between lungs and blood.
2. **Internal respiration** which involves exchange of gases between blood and tissues.

PHASES OF RESPIRATION

Respiration occurs in two phases:

1. **Inspiration** during which the air enters the lungs from atmosphere.
2. **Expiration** during which the air leaves the lungs.

FUNCTIONAL ANATOMY OF RESPIRATORY TRACT

Respiratory tract is the anatomical structure through which air moves in and out. It consists of nose, pharynx, larynx, trachea, bronchi and lungs **(Fig. 78.1)**.

Covering of Lungs: Pleura

Each lung is covered by a bilayered serous membrane called pleura or **pleural sac**. Pleura is formed by two layers namely, **visceral layer** and **parietal layer**. Visceral (inner) layer lines the surface of the lungs. At hilum, it is continuous with parietal (outer) layer, which is attached to the wall of the thoracic cavity.

Intrapleural Space or Pleural Cavity

Intrapleural space or pleural cavity is the narrow space in between the two layers of pleura.

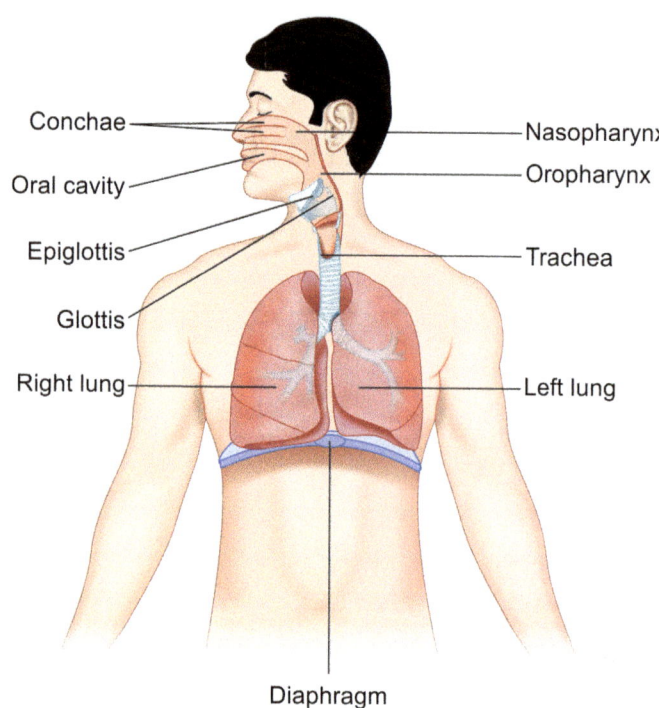

FIGURE 78.1: Respiratory tract.

Intrapleural Fluid

Intrapleural fluid is a thin film of serous fluid that occupies intrapleural space. This fluid is secreted by visceral layer of pleura.

Functions of intrapleural fluid

1. It functions as the lubricant and prevents friction between two layers of pleura.
2. It is involved in creating the negative pressure called **intrapleural pressure** within intrapleural space.

Tracheobronchial Tree

Tracheobronchial tree is a part of air passage formed by trachea and bronchi.

Components of tracheobronchial tree

1. Trachea bifurcates into two main or **primary bronchi** called right and left primary bronchi **(Fig. 78.2)**.
2. Each primary bronchus enters the lungs and divides into **secondary bronchi**.
3. Secondary bronchi divide into **tertiary bronchi**. In right lung, there are 10 tertiary bronchi and, in left lung, there are 8 tertiary bronchi.
4. Tertiary bronchi divide several times with reduction in length and diameter into many generations of **bronchioles**.
5. When the diameter of bronchioles becomes 1 mm or less, it is called **terminal bronchiole**.
6. Terminal bronchiole continues or divides into **respiratory bronchiole**, which has a diameter of 0.5 mm.

Upper and Lower Respiratory Tracts

Generally, respiratory tract is divided into two parts:

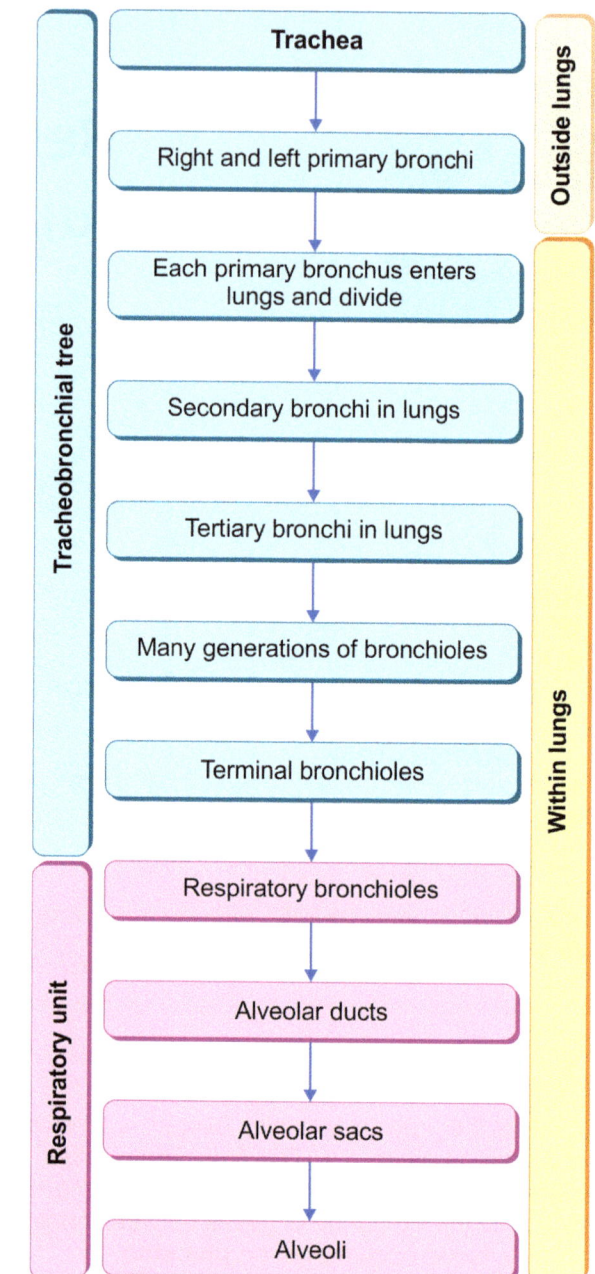

FIGURE 78.2: Schematic representation of tracheobronchial tree and respiratory unit.

1. **Upper respiratory tract** which includes all the structures from nose up to vocal cords.
2. **Lower respiratory tract** that includes trachea, bronchi and lungs.

■ RESPIRATORY UNIT

Lung parenchyma is formed by respiratory unit that forms the **terminal portion** of respiratory tract. Respiratory unit is defined as the structural and functional unit of lung. Exchange of gases occurs only in this part of the respiratory tract.

■ STRUCTURE OF RESPIRATORY UNIT

Respiratory unit starts from the **respiratory bronchioles (Fig. 78.3)**. Each respiratory bronchiole divides into **alveolar ducts**. Each alveolar duct enters an enlarged structure

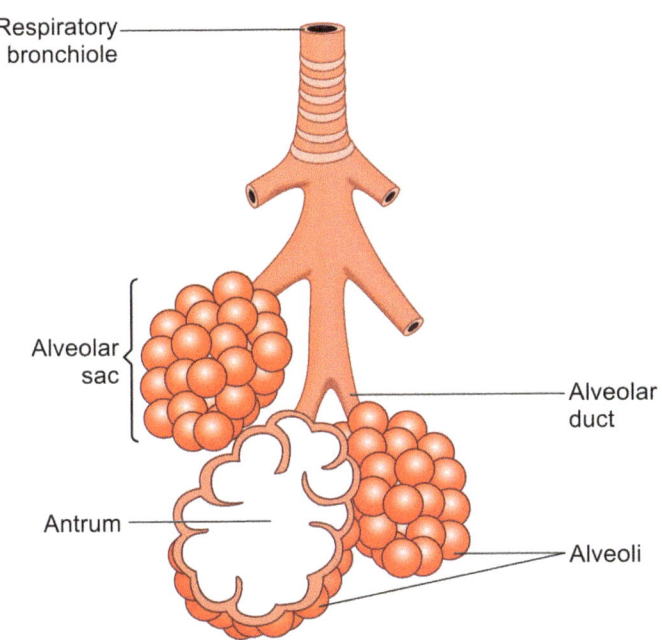

FIGURE 78.3: Structure of respiratory unit.

called the **alveolar sac**. Space inside the alveolar sac is called **antrum**. Alveolar sac consists of a cluster of **alveoli**. Few alveoli are present in the wall of alveolar duct also.

Thus, respiratory unit includes:

1. Respiratory bronchioles.
2. Alveolar ducts.
3. Alveolar sacs.
4. Alveoli.

Each alveolus is like a pouch with the diameter of about 0.2 to 0.5 mm. It is lined by epithelial cells.

Alveolar Cells or Pneumocytes

Alveolar epithelium consists of alveolar cells or pneumocytes.

Alveolar cells are of two types:

i. Type I alveolar cells which form the site of gaseous exchange between alveolus and blood.
ii. Type II alveolar cells which secrete the alveolar fluid and surfactant.

■ RESPIRATORY MEMBRANE

Respiratory membrane is the membranous structure through which exchange of gases occurs in lungs.

Respiratory membrane separates air in the alveoli from blood in capillary. It is formed by **the alveolar membrane** and **capillary membrane**. Respiratory membrane has a surface area of 70 sq. M and thickness of 0.6 μ. Structure of respiratory membrane is explained in Chapter 82 **(Fig. 82.1)**.

■ NON-RESPIRATORY FUNCTIONS OF RESPIRATORY TRACT

Besides the primary function of gaseous exchange, the respiratory tract is involved in several non-respiratory functions of the body.

■ 1. OLFACTION

Olfactory receptors present in the mucous membrane of nostril are involved in **olfactory sensation**.

■ 2. VOCALIZATION

Along with other structures, larynx forms the **speech apparatus**. However, larynx alone plays major role in the process of vocalization. Therefore, it is called **sound box**.

■ 3. PREVENTION OF DUST PARTICLES

Dust particles, which enter the nostrils from air, are prevented from reaching the lungs by filtration action of **hairs** in nasal mucous membrane. The small particles, which escape the hairs, are held by the **mucus** secreted by nasal mucous membrane. Those dust particles, which escape the nasal hairs and nasal mucous membrane, are removed by the phagocytic action of **macrophages** in alveoli.

Particles which escape the protective mechanisms in nose and alveoli are thrown out by **cough reflex** and **sneezing reflex**.

■ 4. DEFENSE MECHANISM

Defense functions of the lungs are performed by their own defenses and by the presence of various types of cells in mucous membrane lining the alveoli of lungs. These cells are leukocytes, macrophages, mast cells, natural killer cells and dendritic cells.

Lung's Own Defenses

Epithelial cells lining the air passage secrete some innate immune factors called **defensins** and **cathelicidins**. These two substances are **antimicrobial peptides** and help in lung's natural defenses.

Defense Through Leukocytes

Leukocytes, particularly the neutrophils and lymphocytes present in alveoli of lungs provide defense mechanism against bacteria and virus. **Neutrophils** kill the bacteria by phagocytosis. **Lymphocytes** develop immunity against bacteria.

Defense Through Macrophages

Macrophages engulf dust particles and pathogens, which enter the alveoli and thereby act as **scavengers** in lungs. Macrophages are also involved in the development of immunity by functioning as **antigen presenting cells**.

Defense Through Mast Cells

Mast cells are responsible for allergic reactions.

Defense Through Natural Killer Cell

Natural killer (NK) cell destroys the **microorganisms** such as viruses and the viral infected or damaged cells, which may form the tumors. It also destroys the **malignant cells** and prevents development of cancer.

Defense Through Dendritic Cells

Dendritic cells in the lungs function as **antigen presenting cells**.

5. MAINTENANCE OF WATER BALANCE

Respiratory tract plays a role in **water loss mechanism**. During expiration, water evaporates through the expired air and some amount of body water is lost by this process.

6. REGULATION OF BODY TEMPERATURE

During expiration, along with water, heat is also lost from the body. Thus, respiratory tract help **heat loss** mechanism.

7. REGULATION OF ACID-BASE BALANCE

Lungs play a role in maintenance of acid base balance of the body by regulating the carbon dioxide content in blood. Carbon dioxide is produced during various metabolic reactions in the tissues of the body. When it enters the blood, **carbon dioxide** combines with water to form **carbonic acid**. Since carbonic acid is unstable, it splits into hydrogen and bicarbonate ions.

$$CO_2 + H_2O \longrightarrow H_2CO_3 \longrightarrow H^+ + HCO_3^-$$

The entire reaction is reversed in lungs when carbon dioxide is removed from blood into the alveoli of lungs.

$$H^+ + HCO_3^- \longrightarrow H_2CO_3 \longrightarrow CO_2 + H_2O$$

As carbon dioxide is a volatile gas, it is practically blown out by ventilation.

8. ANTICOAGULANT FUNCTION

Mast cells in lungs secrete **heparin**. Heparin is an anticoagulant and it prevents the intravascular clotting.

9. SECRETION OF ANGIOTENSIN CONVERTING ENZYME

Endothelial cells of the pulmonary capillaries secrete the angiotensin-converting enzyme (ACE). It converts the angiotensin I into active angiotensin II which plays an important role in the regulation of ECF volume and blood pressure (Chapter 40).

10. SYNTHESIS OF HORMONAL SUBSTANCES

Lung tissues are also known to synthesize the hormonal substances, prostaglandins, acetylcholine and serotonin which have many physiological actions in the body including regulation of blood pressure (Chapter 57).

RESPIRATORY PROTECTIVE REFLEXES

Respiratory protective reflexes are the reflexes that protect the lungs and air passage from foreign particles. Respiratory protective reflexes are explained below.

COUGH REFLEX

Cough is a modified respiratory process characterized by forced expiration. It is the protective reflex that occurs because of irritation of respiratory tract and some other areas such as external auditory meatus.

Causes of Cough Reflex

Cough is produced mainly by irritant agents. It is also produced by cardiac disorders such as congestive heart failure, pulmonary disorders such as chronic obstructive pulmonary disease (COPD) and tumor in thorax, which may exert pressure on larynx, trachea, bronchi or lungs.

Mechanism of Cough Reflex

Cough begins with deep inspiration followed by forced expiration with closed glottis. This increases the intrapleural pressure above 100 mm Hg. Then, glottis opens suddenly with explosive outflow of air at a high velocity. The velocity of the airflow may reach 960 km/h. It causes expulsion of irritants out of the respiratory tract.

SNEEZING REFLEX

Sneezing is also a modified respiratory process characterized by forced expiration. It is the protective reflex caused by irritation of nasal mucous membrane.

Causes of Sneezing Reflex

Irritation of the nasal mucous membrane occurs because of dust particles, debris, mechanical obstruction of the airway, and excess fluid accumulation in the nasal passages.

Mechanism Sneezing Reflex

Sneezing starts with deep inspiration, followed by forceful expiration with opened glottis resulting in expulsion of irritant agents out of respiratory tract.

SWALLOWING (DEGLUTITION) REFLEX

Swallowing is a respiratory protective reflex that prevents entrance of food particles into the air passage during swallowing.

While swallowing of the food, the respiration is arrested for a while. The temporary arrest of respiration is called **apnea**. The arrest of breathing during swallowing is called swallowing apnea or **deglutition apnea**. It takes place during pharyngeal stage, i.e. II stage of deglutition and prevents entry of food particles into the respiratory tract (Chapter 37).

PULMONARY CIRCULATION
PULMONARY BLOOD VESSELS

Pulmonary blood vessels include **pulmonary artery** which carries **deoxygenated blood** to alveoli of lungs and **bronchial artery** which supply **oxygenated blood** to other structures of lungs (see below).

Pulmonary Artery

Pulmonary artery supplies deoxygenated blood pumped from right ventricle to alveoli of lungs (pulmonary circulation). After leaving the right ventricle, it divides into right and left branches. Each branch enters the corresponding lung along with primary bronchus. After entering the lung, the branch of the pulmonary artery divides into small vessels and finally forms the **capillary plexus** that is in intimate relationship to alveoli. Capillary plexus is solely concerned with alveolar gas exchange.

Oxygenated blood from the alveoli is carried to left atrium by one pulmonary vein from each side.

Bronchial Artery

Bronchial artery arises from descending thoracic aorta. It supplies arterial blood to bronchi, connective tissue and other structures of lung stroma, visceral pleura and pulmonary lymph nodes.

Venous blood from these structures is drained by two **bronchial veins** from each side. However, the blood from distal portion of bronchial circulation is drained directly into the tributaries of pulmonary veins.

■ PHYSIOLOGICAL SHUNT

Physiological shunt is defined as a connection between arterial and venous side of circulation (Chapter 74). In lungs, the physiological shut provides a diversion through which the venous blood is mixed with arterial blood.

Components of Physiological Shunt

Physiological shunt has two components:

1. Flow of deoxygenated blood from **bronchial circulation** into **pulmonary veins** without being oxygenated makes up part of normal physiological shunt.
2. Flow of deoxygenated blood from **thebesian veins** into **cardiac chambers** directly (Chapter 74).

Venous Admixture and Wasted Blood

Venous admixture is the mixing of deoxygenated blood with oxygenated blood. It is caused by physiological shunt.

Fraction of venous blood, which is not fully oxygenated, is generally considered as wasted blood.

■ SALIENT (CHARACTERISTIC) FEATURES OF PULMONARY CIRCULATION

1. Pulmonary artery has a thin wall and it has only about one-third of thickness of the systemic aortic wall. Wall of other pulmonary blood vessels is also thin.
2. Pulmonary blood vessels are highly elastic and more distensible.
3. Smooth muscle coat is not well developed in the pulmonary blood vessels.
4. True arterioles have less smooth muscle fibers.
5. Pulmonary capillaries are larger than systemic capillaries.
6. Vascular resistance in pulmonary circulation is very less; it is only one tenth of systemic circulation.
7. Pulmonary vascular system is a low-pressure system (see below).
8. Pulmonary artery carries deoxygenated blood from heart to lungs and pulmonary veins carry oxygenated blood from lungs to heart.
9. Physiological shunt is present.

■ PULMONARY BLOOD FLOW

Both the lungs receive whole amount of blood that is pumped out from right ventricle. Output of blood per minute is same in both the right and left ventricle. It is about 5 liters.

■ PULMONARY BLOOD PRESSURE

Pulmonary blood pressure is less than systemic blood pressure because the pulmonary blood vessels are more distensible than systemic blood vessels. Thus, the entire pulmonary vascular system is a low-pressure bed.

Pulmonary Arterial Pressure

Systolic pressure : 25 mm Hg
Diastolic pressure : 10 mm Hg
Mean arterial pressure : 15 mm Hg

Mean pulmonary arterial pressure is not calculated by using the same formula for mean systemic arterial pressure.

$$\text{Mean pulmonary arterial pressure} = \frac{2}{3} \text{ of pulmonary diastolic pressure} + \frac{1}{3} \text{ of pulmonary systolic pressure}$$

Pulmonary Capillary Pressure

Pulmonary capillary pressure is about 7 mm Hg.

■ MEASUREMENT OF PULMONARY BLOOD FLOW

Pulmonary blood flow is measured by applying **Fick principle**. Details are given in Chapter 69.

■ REGULATION OF PULMONARY CIRCULATION

Under normal conditions, pulmonary blood flow is regulated by the following factors:

1. Cardiac Output

Pulmonary blood flow is **directly proportional** to cardiac output.

Cardiac output is in turn is regulated by four other factors:

1. Venous return.
2. Force of contraction.
3. Heart rate.
4. Peripheral resistance.

Refer Chapter 69 for details of factors affecting cardiac output.

2. Vascular Resistance

Pulmonary blood flow is **inversely proportional** to the pulmonary vascular resistance. Pulmonary vascular resistance is low compared to systemic vascular resistance.

3. Nervous Factors

Sympathetic stimulation increases the pulmonary vascular resistance by vasoconstriction. Parasympathetic stimulation decreases the vascular resistance by vasodilatation. However, under physiological conditions, it is doubtful whether autonomic nerves play any role in regulating the blood flow to lungs.

Chapter 79: Mechanics of Respiration

CHAPTER OUTLINE

- **RESPIRATORY MOVEMENTS**
  - MUSCLES OF RESPIRATION
  - MOVEMENTS OF THORACIC CAGE
  - MOVEMENTS OF LUNGS
- **RESPIRATORY PRESSURES**
  - INTRAPLEURAL PRESSURE
  - INTRA-ALVEOLAR PRESSURE
- **TRANSPULMONARY PRESSURE**
- **COMPLIANCE**
  - DEFINITION
  - NORMAL VALUES
  - VARIATIONS: APPLIED PHYSIOLOGY
- **WORK OF BREATHING**
  - WORK DONE BY RESPIRATORY MUSCLES

RESPIRATORY MOVEMENTS

During normal quiet breathing, inspiration is the **active process** and expiration is the **passive process**. During inspiration, thoracic cage enlarges and lungs expand so that air enters the lungs easily. During expiration, the thoracic cage and lungs decrease in size and attain the **preinspiratory position** so that air leaves the lungs easily.

MUSCLES OF RESPIRATION

Muscles involved in respiratory movements are inspiratory muscles and expiratory muscles. However, the respiratory muscles are generally classified into two types:

1. Primary or major respiratory muscles which are responsible for change in size of thoracic cage during normal quiet breathing.
2. Accessory respiratory muscles that help primary respiratory muscles during forced respiration.

Inspiratory Muscles

Muscles involved in inspiratory movements are known as inspiratory muscles which are primary or accessory muscles.

1. Primary inspiratory muscles are the diaphragm, which is supplied by **phrenic nerve** (C3 to C5) and external intercostal muscles, supplied by **intercostal nerves** (T1 to T11).
2. Accessory inspiratory muscles are sternocleidomastoid, scalene, anterior serrati, elevators of scapulae and pectorals.

Expiratory Muscles

Muscles involved in expiratory movements are known as expiratory muscles which are primary or accessory muscles.

1. Primary expiratory muscles are the internal intercostal muscles, which are innervated by **intercostal nerves**.
2. Accessory expiratory muscles are the abdominal muscles.

MOVEMENTS OF THORACIC CAGE

During inspiration thoracic cage enlarges in all axis, viz. anteroposterior, transverse and vertical axis. Increase in anteroposterior and transverse diameters occurs due to the elevation of ribs. Vertical diameter of thoracic cage is increased by the descent of diaphragm.

Change in the size of thoracic cavity occurs because of the movements of four units of structures:

1. Thoracic lid.
2. Upper costal series.
3. Lower costal series.
4. Diaphragm.

1. Thoracic Lid

Thoracic lid is formed by **manubrium sterni** and the first pairs of ribs. Movement of thoracic lid increases the **anteroposterior diameter** of thoracic cage.

2. Upper Costal Series

Upper costal series is constituted by second to sixth pairs of ribs. Upper costal series increases the **anteroposterior** diameter and **transverse diameter** of the thoracic cage by pump handle movement and bucket handle movements.

Pump handle movement

During inspiration, there is elevation of upper costal series of ribs and upward and forward movement of sternum. This movement is called pump handle movement. It increases **anteroposterior diameter** of the thoracic cage.

Bucket handle movement

Simultaneously, central portions of these ribs (arches of ribs) move upwards and outwards to a more horizontal position. This movement is called bucket handle movement and it increases the **transverse diameter** of thoracic cage.

3. Lower Costal Series

It is formed by the seventh to tenth pairs of ribs. Movement of lower costal series increases the **transverse diameter** of the thoracic cage. These ribs also show bucket handle movement by swinging outward and upward.

Eleventh and twelfth pairs of ribs are the **floating ribs**, which are not involved in changing the size of thoracic cage.

4. Diaphragm

Movement of diaphragm increases the **vertical diameter** of thoracic cage. Normally, before inspiration diaphragm is dome shaped with convexity facing upwards. During inspiration, due to the contraction of muscle fibers the central tendinous portion is drawn downwards so the diaphragm is flattened and increases the vertical diameter of the thoracic cage.

MOVEMENTS OF LUNGS

During inspiration, due to the enlargement of **thoracic cage**, negative pressure is increased in the thoracic cavity. It causes expansion of the **lungs**. During expiration, the thoracic cavity decreases in size to the preinspiratory position. Pressure in the thoracic cage also comes back to the preinspiratory level. It compresses the lung tissues so that, the air is expelled out of lungs.

Collapsing Tendency of Lungs

Lungs are under constant threat to collapse even under resting conditions because of certain factors.

Factors causing collapsing tendency of lungs

Two factors are responsible for the collapsing tendency of lungs:
1. Elastic property of lung tissues.
2. Surface tension exerted on the surface of alveolar membrane by the fluid secreted from alveolar epithelium.

Fortunately, there are some factors which save the lungs from collapsing.

Factors Preventing Collapsing Tendency of Lungs

In spite of elastic property of the lungs and surface tension in the alveoli of lungs, collapsing tendency of lungs is prevented by two factors:

1. Intrapleural pressure

Intrapleural pressure which is always negative (see below) keeps the lungs expanded and prevents the collapsing tendency of lungs.

2. Surfactant

Surfactant is a surface acting material or agent that is responsible for lowering the surface tension of a fluid and thereby prevents collapsing tendency of lungs. Surfactant that lines the epithelium of alveoli in lungs is known as **pulmonary surfactant** and it decreases the **surface tension** on the alveolar membrane.

Source of secretion of pulmonary surfactant

Pulmonary surfactant is secreted by two types of cells:
i. **Type II alveolar epithelial cells** in lungs.
ii. **Clara cells** in bronchioles.

Chemistry of surfactant

Surfactant is a lipoprotein complex formed by lipids especially phospholipids, proteins and ions. The phospholipid called **dipalmitoylphosphatidylcholine** (DPPC) is the major component of surfactant.

Functions of surfactant

1. Surfactant reduces the surface tension in the alveoli of lungs and prevents the collapsing tendency of lungs. The phospholipid molecule in the surfactant is responsible for this.
2. Surfactant is responsible for stabilization of the alveoli, which is necessary to withstand the collapsing tendency.
3. It plays an important role in the inflation of lungs after birth. In fetus, lungs are solid and not expanded. First breath starts soon after birth. Although the respiratory movements are attempted by the infant, the lungs tend to collapse repeatedly. And, the presence of surfactant in the alveoli prevents the lungs from collapsing.
4. The hydrophilic proteins in surfactant play a role in defense in the lungs by destroying the bacteria and viruses.

Effect of deficiency of surfactant:
Respiratory distress syndrome

Deficiency or absence of surfactant in infants causes collapse of lungs. This condition is called respiratory distress syndrome or hyaline membrane disease.

Deficiency of surfactant occurs in adults also and it is called **adult respiratory distress syndrome** (**ARDS**).

RESPIRATORY PRESSURES

Two types of pressures are exerted in thoracic cavity and lungs during the process of respiration:

1. Intrapleural pressure.
2. Intra-alveolar pressure.

INTRAPLEURAL PRESSURE: INTRATHORACIC PRESSURE

Definition

Intrapleural pressure is the pressure existing in pleural cavity, that is, in between the visceral and parietal layers of pleura. It is exerted by the suction of the fluid that lines the pleural cavity **(Fig. 79.1)**. It is also called **intrathoracic pressure** since it is exerted in the whole of thoracic cavity.

Normal Values of Intrapleural Pressure

Respiratory pressures are always expressed in relation to atmospheric pressure, which is 760 mm Hg. Under physiological conditions, the intrapleural pressure is always negative.

Normal values of intrapleural pressure are given in **Table 79.1**.

Cause for Negativity of Intrapleural Pressure

Pleural cavity is always lined by a thin layer of fluid that is secreted by the visceral layer of pleura. This fluid is constantly pumped from the pleural cavity into the lymphatic vessels. The pumping of fluid creates the negative pressure in the pleural cavity.

Measurement of Intrapleural Pressure

Intrapleural pressure is measured by direct method and indirect method. In the direct method, intrapleural pressure is determined by introducing a needle into the pleural cavity and connecting the needle to a **mercury manometer**. In indirect method, intrapleural pressure is measured by introducing the **esophageal balloon**, which is connected to a **manometer**. Intrapleural pressure is considered as equivalent to the pressure existing in the esophagus.

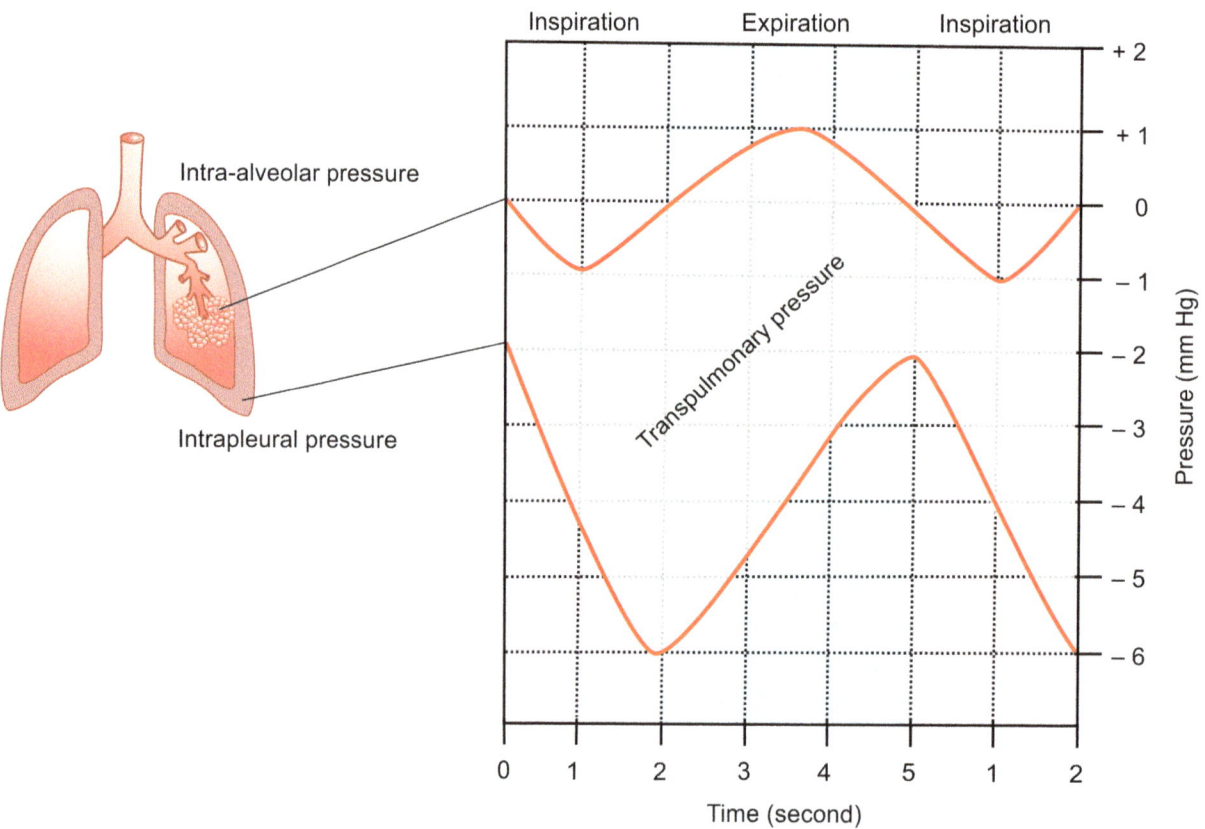

FIGURE 79.1: Changes in respiratory pressures during inspiration and expiration. '0' = Normal atmospheric pressure (760 mm Hg).

TABLE 79.1: Normal values of intrapleural pressure.

Condition	Intrapleural pressure
At the end of normal inspiration	− 6 mm Hg (760 − 6 = 754 mm Hg)
At the end of normal expiration	− 2 mm Hg (760 − 2 = 758 mm Hg)
At the end of forced inspiration	− 30 mm Hg
During forced inspiration with closed glottis: Müller maneuver	− 70 mm Hg
During forced expiration with closed glottis: Valsalva maneuver	+ 50 mm Hg

Chapter 79: Mechanics of Respiration

Significance of Intrapleural Pressure

i. Throughout the respiratory cycle intrapleural pressure remains lower than intra-alveolar pressure. This keeps the lungs always inflated.
ii. It prevents the collapsing tendency of lungs.
iii. It causes dilatation of vena cava and larger veins in thorax. Also, the negative pressure acts like suction pump and pulls the venous blood from lower part of body towards the heart against gravity. Thus, the intrapleural pressure is responsible for the venous return. So, it is called the **respiratory pump** for venous return (Chapter 69).

INTRA-ALVEOLAR PRESSURE: INTRAPULMONARY PRESSURE

Definition

Intra-alveolar pressure is the pressure existing in the alveoli of the lungs. It is also known as **intrapulmonary pressure**.

Normal Values of Intra-alveolar Pressure

Normally, intra-alveolar pressure is equal to the atmospheric pressure, which is 760 mm Hg. It becomes negative during inspiration and positive during expiration.

Normal values of intra-alveolar pressure are given in **Table 79.2**.

Measurement of Intra-alveolar Pressure

Intra-alveolar pressure is measured by using **plethysmograph**.

Significance of Intra-alveolar Pressure

Intra-alveolar pressure has two important functions:

i. It causes flow of air in and out of alveoli. During inspiration, the intraalveolar pressure becomes negative, so the atmospheric air enters the alveoli. And, during expiration, the air is expelled out of alveoli.
ii. It also helps in the exchange of gases between the alveolar air and the blood.

TRANSPULMONARY PRESSURE

Transpulmonary pressure is the difference between intraalveolar pressure and intrapleural pressure. It is the measure of elastic forces in lungs, which is responsible for collapsing tendency of lungs.

COMPLIANCE

DEFINITION AND SIGNIFICANCE

Compliance is the ability of lungs and thorax to expand or it is the **expansibility** of lungs and thorax. It is defined as the change in volume that occurs per unit change in the pressure.

Determination of compliance is useful as it is the measure of stiffness of lungs. Stiffer the lungs, less is the compliance.

NORMAL VALUES

Compliance is expressed in relation to respiratory pressures.

Compliance in Relation to Intra-alveolar Pressure

Compliance is the volume increase in lungs per unit increase in the intra-alveolar pressure:

1. Compliance of lungs and thorax together:
   130 mL/1 cm H_2O pressure.
2. Compliance of lungs alone:
   220 mL/1 cm H_2O pressure.

Compliance in Relation to Intrapleural Pressure

Compliance is the volume increase in lungs per unit decrease in the intrapleural pressure:

1. Compliance of lungs and thorax together:
   100 mL/1 cm H_2O pressure.
2. Compliance of lungs alone:
   200 mL/1 cm H_2O pressure.

Thus, if lungs are removed from thorax, the expansibility (compliance) of lungs alone is doubled. It is because of absence of the inertia and the restriction exerted by structures of thoracic cage, which interfere with expansion of lungs.

APPLIED PHYSIOLOGY: VARIATIONS IN COMPLIANCE

Increase in Compliance

Compliance increases in physiological and pathological conditions:

1. In old age, lung compliance increases due to loss of elastic property of lung tissues.

TABLE 79.2: Normal values of intra-alveolar pressure.

Condition	Intra-alveolar pressure
During normal inspiration	– 1 mm Hg (760 – 1 = 759 mm Hg)
During normal expiration	+ 1 mm Hg (760 + 1 = 761 mm Hg).
At the end of inspiration and expiration	Equal to atmospheric pressure: 760 mm Hg
During forced inspiration with closed glottis: Müller maneuver	– 80 mm Hg
During forced expiration with closed glottis: Valsalva maneuver	+ 100 mm Hg

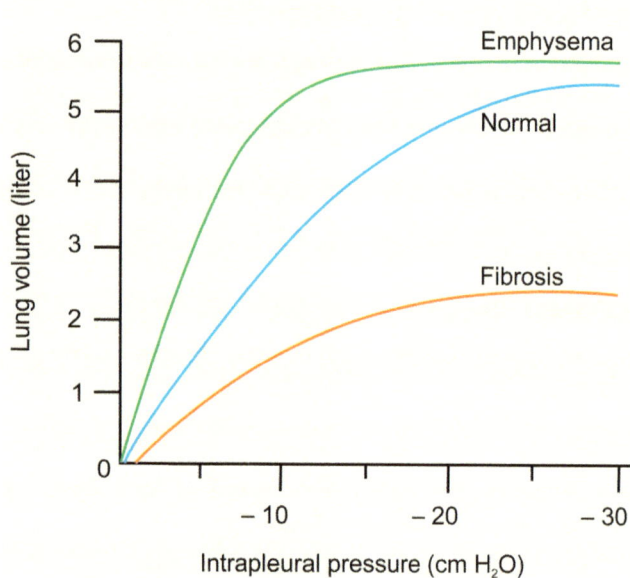

FIGURE 79.2: Variations in lung compliance.

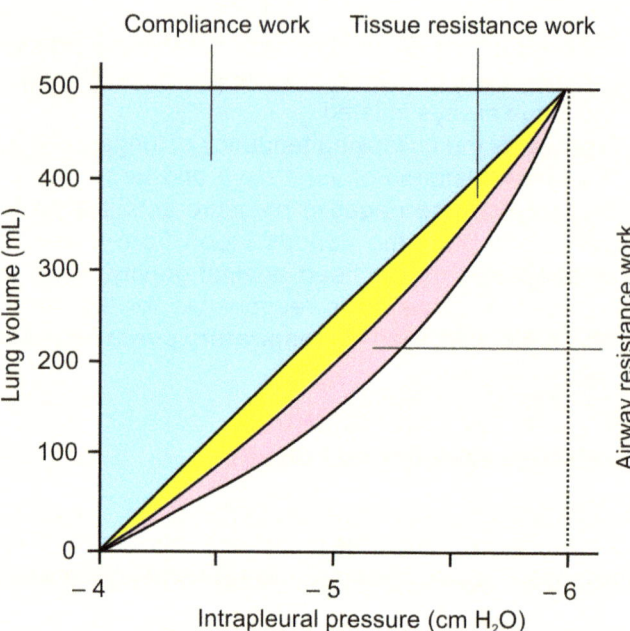

FIGURE 79.3: Work of breathing.

2. In **emphysema** (obstructive respiratory disease), lung compliance increases because of damage of alveolar membrane **(Fig. 79.2)**.

Decrease in Compliance

Compliance decreases in pathological conditions such as:

1. Deformities of thorax like **kyphosis** and **scoliosis** (Chapter 52).
2. Paralysis of respiratory muscles.
3. **Pleural effusion** (accumulation of fluid in pleural cavity).
4. **Fibrotic pleurisy** (inflammation of pleura resulting in fibrosis).
5. **Abnormal thorax** due to presence of air (**pneumothorax**), fluid (**hydrothorax**), blood (**hemothorax**) and pus (**pyothorax**) in pleural space.

■ WORK OF BREATHING

Work done by respiratory muscles during breathing to overcome the resistance in the thorax and respiratory tract is known as work of breathing.

■ WORK DONE BY RESPIRATORY MUSCLES

During the respiratory processes, inspiration is active process and the expiration is a passive process. So, during quiet breathing, the respiratory muscles perform the work only during inspiration and not during expiration.

Energy obtained during the work of breathing is utilized to overcome three types of resistance:

1. Airway resistance.
2. Elastic resistance of lungs and thorax.
3. Nonelastic viscous resistance.

1. Airway Resistance

Airway resistance is the resistance offered to the passage of air through respiratory tract. Work done to overcome this is called airway **resistance work**.

2. Elastic Resistance of Lungs and Thorax

Work done to overcome this elastic resistance is called **compliance work**.

3. Nonelastic Viscous Resistance

Work done to overcome this viscous resistance is called the **tissue resistance work**.

Above factors are explained by a curve that shows the relation between lung volume and pleural pressure **(Fig. 79.3)**.

Chapter 80: Pulmonary Function Tests

CHAPTER OUTLINE

- **TYPES OF LUNG FUNCTION TESTS**
- **LUNG VOLUMES**
  - TIDAL VOLUME (TV)
  - INSPIRATORY RESERVE VOLUME (IRV)
  - EXPIRATORY RESERVE VOLUME (ERV)
  - RESIDUAL VOLUME (RV)
- **LUNG CAPACITIES**
  - INSPIRATORY CAPACITY (IC)
  - VITAL CAPACITY (VC)
  - FUNCTIONAL RESIDUAL CAPACITY (FRC)
  - TOTAL LUNG CAPACITY (TLC)
- **MEASURMENT OF LUNG VOLUMES AND CAPACITIES**
- **MEASUREMENT OF FUNCTIONAL RESIDUAL CAPACITY AND RESIDUAL VOLUME**
- **VITAL CAPACITY**
- **FORCED EXPIRATORY VOLUME (FEV) OR TIMED VITAL CAPACITY**
- **RESPIRATORY MINUTE VOLUME**
- **MAXIMUM BREATHING CAPACITY OR MAXIMUM VENTILATION VOLUME (MVV)**
- **PEAK EXPIRATORY FLOW RATE**
- **RESTRICTIVE AND OBSTRUCTIVE RESPIRATORY DISEASES**

■ TYPES OF LUNG FUNCTION TESTS

Pulmonary function tests or **lung function tests** are useful in assessing the functional status of respiratory system. Pulmonary function tests are carried out mostly by using spirometer.

Lung function tests are of two types:
  I. Static lung function tests.
  II. Dynamic lung function tests.

Static Lung Function Tests

Static lung function tests are based on **volume of air that flows** into or out of lungs. These tests do not depend upon the rate at which air flows.

Static lung function tests are:
  A. Static lung volumes.
  B. Static lung capacities.

Dynamic Lung Function Tests

Dynamic lung function tests are based on time, i.e. the **rate at which air flows** into or out of lungs. These tests are useful in determining the severity of obstructive and restrictive lung diseases.

Dynamic lung function tests are:
  A. Forced vital capacity.
  B. Forced expiratory volume.
  C. Maximum ventilation volume.
  D. Peak expiratory flow.

■ LUNG VOLUMES

Lung volumes are the static volumes of air breathed by an individual. Lung volumes are of four types.

■ 1. TIDAL VOLUME (TV)

Tidal volume is the volume of air breathed in and out of lungs in a single normal quiet respiration. Tidal volume signifies the normal depth of breathing.

Normal value = 500 mL (0.5 L)

■ 2. INSPIRATORY RESERVE VOLUME (IRV)

Inspiratory reserve volume is an additional volume of air that can be inspired forcefully after the end of normal inspiration.

Normal value = 3,300 mL (3.3 L)

3. EXPIRATORY RESERVE VOLUME (ERV)

Expiratory reserve volume is the additional volume of air that can be expired out forcefully, after normal expiration.

Normal value = 1,000 mL (1 L)

4. RESIDUAL VOLUME (RV)

Residual volume is the volume of air remaining in the lungs even after forced expiration. Normally, lungs cannot be emptied completely even by forceful expiration. Some quantity of air always remains in the lungs even after the forced expiration. Residual volume helps to aerate the blood in between breathing and during expiration.

Normal value = 1,200 mL (1.2 L)

LUNG CAPACITIES

Lung capacities are the combination of two or more lung volumes. Lung capacities are of four types **(Figs 80.1 to 80.3)**.

1. INSPIRATORY CAPACITY (IC)

Inspiratory capacity is the maximum volume of air that is inspired after normal expiration (end expiratory position). It includes tidal volume and inspiratory reserve volume.

IC = TV + IRV
= 500 + 3,300 = 3,800 mL

2. VITAL CAPACITY (VC)

It is the maximum volume of air that can be expelled out forcefully after a maximal or deep inspiration. Vital capacity includes inspiratory reserve volume, tidal volume and expiratory reserve volume.

VC = IRV + TV + ERV
= 3,300 + 500 + 1,000 = 4,800 mL

3. FUNCTIONAL RESIDUAL CAPACITY (FRC)

It is the volume of air remaining in the lungs after normal expiration (after normal tidal expiration). Functional residual capacity includes expiratory reserve volume and residual volume.

FRC = ERV + RV
= 1,000 + 1,200 = 2,200 mL

4. TOTAL LUNG CAPACITY (TLC)

Total lung capacity is the volume of air present in the lungs after a deep (maximal) inspiration. It includes all the volumes.

TLC = IRV + TV + ERV + RV
= 3,300 + 500 + 1,000 + 1,200
= 6,000 mL

MEASUREMENT OF LUNG VOLUMES AND CAPACITIES

Spirometry is the method to measure lung volumes and capacities. Simple instrument used for this purpose is called **spirometer**. Modified spirometer is known as **respirometer**. Nowadays **plethysmograph** is also used to measure lung volumes and capacities.

SPIROMETER

Spirometer contains two chambers, namely outer chamber and inner chamber **(Fig. 80.2)**. Outer chamber is filled with water. A **floating drum** is immersed in the water in an inverted position. Drum is counter balanced by a **weight.** Weight is attached to the top of the inverted drum by means of string or chain. A **pen with ink** is attached to the counter weight. Pen is made to write on a **calibrated paper,** which is fixed to a recording device.

Inner chamber is inverted and has a small hole at the top. A **rubber tube** is connected to bottom of inner chamber via a metal tube. At the other end of this rubber tube, a mouthpiece is attached. Subject respires through this mouthpiece by closing the nose with a **nose clip.**

When the subject breathes with spirometer, during expiration, drum moves up and the counter weight comes down. Reverse of this occurs when the subject breathes the air from the spirometer, i.e. during inspiration. Upward and downward movements of the counter weight are recorded in the form of a graph. Upward deflection of the curve in the graph shows **inspiration** and the downward deflection denotes **expiration**.

Spirogram

Spirogram is the graphical record of lung volumes and capacities using spirometer. In spirogram upward curve indicates inspiration and the downward curve indicates

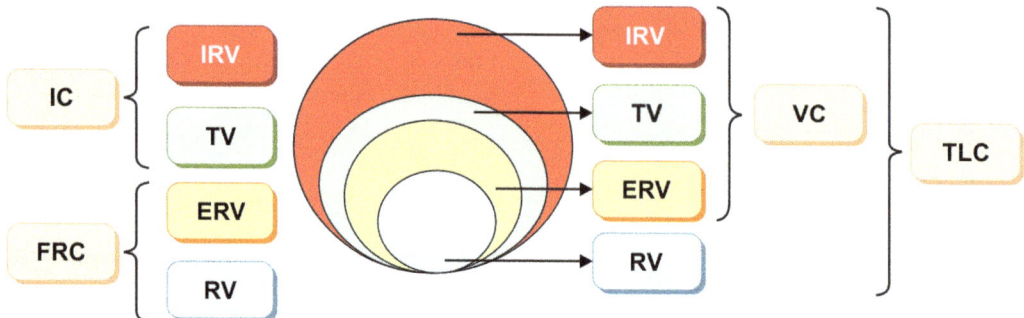

FIGURE 80.1: Lung volumes and capacities.
TV = Tidal volume. IRV = Inspiratory reserve volume. ERV = Expiratory reserve volume. RV = Residual volume.
IC = Inspiratory capacity. FRC = Functional residual capacity. VC = Vital capacity. TLC = Total lung capacity.

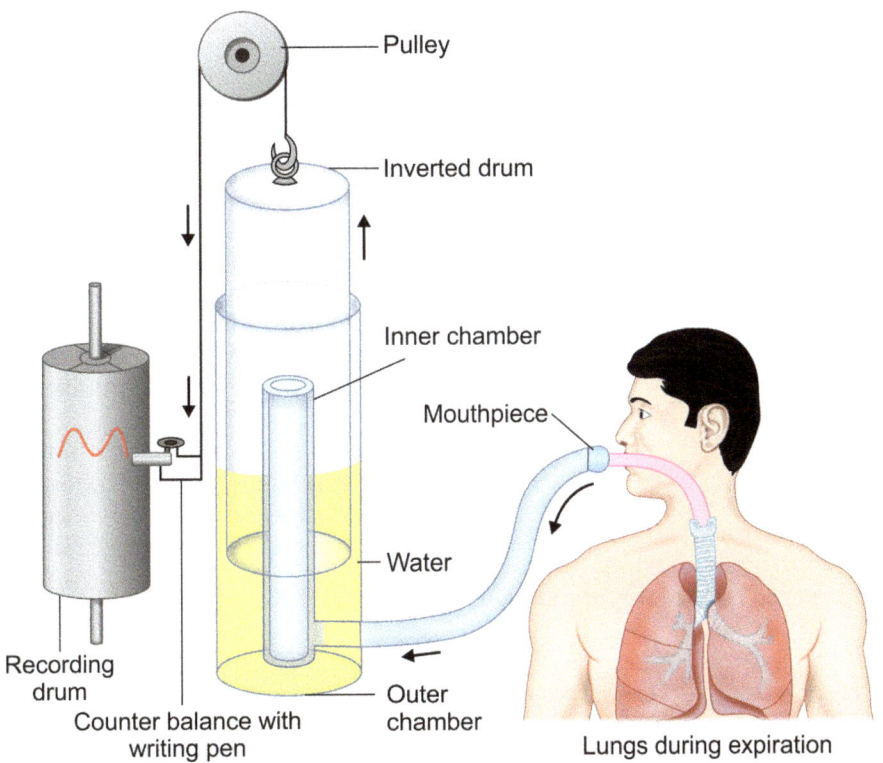

FIGURE 80.2: Spirometer. During expiration, the air enters the spirometer from lungs. Inverted drum moves up and the pen draws a downward curve on the recording drum.

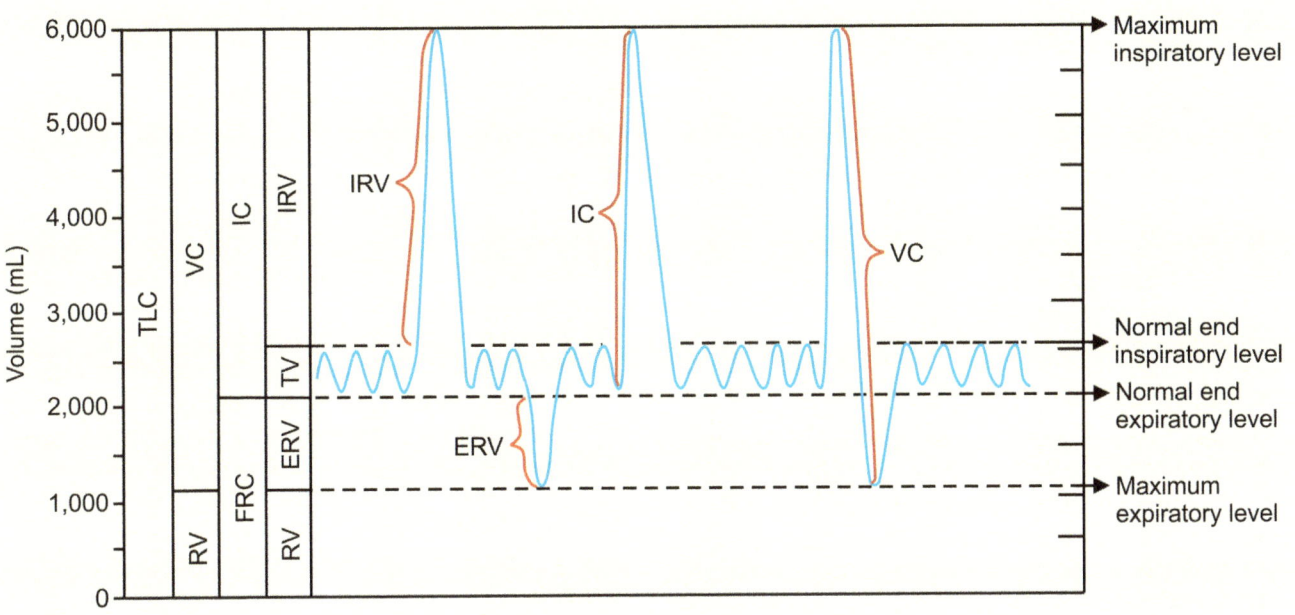

FIGURE 80.3: Spirogram.
TV = Tidal volume. IRV = Inspiratory reserve volume. ERV = Expiratory reserve volume. RV = Residual volume.
IC = Inspiratory capacity. FRC = Functional residual capacity. VC = Vital capacity. TLC = Total lung capacity.

expiration **(Fig. 80.3)**. In order to determine the lung volumes and capacities, following four levels are to be noted in spirogram:

1. Normal end expiratory level.
2. Normal end inspiratory level.
3. Maximum expiratory level.
4. Maximum inspiratory level.

Computerized Spirometer

Computerized spirometer is the solid-state electronic equipment. It does not contain a drum or water chamber.

Subject has to respire into a sophisticated transducer, which is connected to the instrument by means of a cable.

Disadvantages of Spirometry

Spirometer is used only for a **single breath.** Repeated cycles of respiration cannot be recorded by using this instrument because carbon dioxide accumulates in the spirometer and oxygen or fresh air cannot be provided to the subject.

So, all the lung volumes and lung capacities can not be measured by using simple or computerized spirometer.

Volume, which cannot be measured by spirometry, is the **residual volume.** Capacities, which include residual volume, also cannot be measured. Capacities that include residual volume are **functional residual capacity** and **total lung capacity.**

Volume and capacities, which cannot be measured by spirometry, are measured by **nitrogen washout** technique or **helium dilution technique** or by body **plethysmograph.**

■ RESPIROMETER

Respirometer is the modified spirometer. It has provision for removal of carbon dioxide and supply of oxygen.

Carbon dioxide is removed by placing soda lime inside the instrument. Oxygen is supplied to the instrument from the oxygen cylinder, by a suitable valve system.

■ PLETHYSMOGRAPHY

Plethysmography is another technique used to measure all the lung volumes and capacities (see below).

■ MEASUREMENT OF FUNCTIONAL RESIDUAL CAPACITY AND RESIDUAL VOLUME

Residual volume and the functional residual capacity cannot be measured by spirometer and can be determined by three methods:

1. Helium dilution technique.
2. Nitrogen washout method.
3. Plethysmography.

■ 1. HELIUM DILUTION TECHNIQUE

A respirometer is filled with air containing a known quantity of **helium.** Initially, the subject breathes normally. Then, after the end of expiration, subject breathes from respirometer. Helium from respirometer enters the lungs and starts mixing with air in lungs. After few minutes of breathing, concentration of helium in the respirometer becomes equal to concentration of helium in the lungs of subject. It is called the equilibration of helium. After **equilibration of helium** between respirometer and lungs, concentration of helium in respirometer is determined. Functional residual capacity is calculated by using the data such as initial volume of air in respirometer, initial concentration of helium in respirometer and final concentration of helium in respirometer.

To determine functional residual capacity, the subject starts breathing with respirometer after normal expiration. To measure residual volume, the subject should start breathing from the respirometer after forced expiration.

■ 2. NITROGEN WASHOUT METHOD

Normally, concentration of nitrogen in air is 80%. So, if total quantity of nitrogen in the lungs is measured, the volume of air present in lungs can be calculated.

Subject is asked to breathe normally. At the end of normal expiration, the subject inspires **pure oxygen** through a valve and expires into a Douglas bag. This procedure is repeated for 6 to 7 minutes, until the **nitrogen** in lungs is displaced by oxygen. Nitrogen comes to the **Douglas bag.** Afterwards, functional residual capacity is calculated from the data such as volume of air collected in Douglas bag and concentration of nitrogen in Douglas bag.

To measure the functional residual capacity, the subject starts inhaling pure oxygen after normal expiration and to determine the residual volume, the subject starts breathing pure oxygen after forceful expiration.

■ 3. PLETHYSMOGRAPHY

Plethysmography is a technique to study the variations in the size or volume of a part of the body such as limb. **Plethysmograph** is the instrument used for this purpose. Whole body plethysmograph is the instrument used to measure the lung volumes including residual volume.

■ VITAL CAPACITY

■ DEFINITION AND NORMAL VALUE

Definition and normal value of vital capacity are given on page 406.

■ VARIATIONS OF VITAL CAPACITY

Pathological Variations

1. *Sex:* In females, vital capacity is less than in males.
2. *Body built:* Vital capacity is slightly more in heavily built persons.
3. *Posture:* Vital capacity is more in standing position and less in lying position.
4. *Athletes:* Vital capacity is more in athletes.
5. *Occupation:* Vital capacity is decreased in people with sedentary jobs. It is increased in persons who play musical wind instruments such as bugle and flute.

Pathological Variations

Vital capacity is reduced in the following respiratory diseases:

1. Asthma.
2. Emphysema.
3. Weakness or paralysis of respiratory muscle.
4. Pulmonary congestion.
5. Pneumonia.
6. Pneumothorax.
7. Hemothorax.
8. Pyothorax.
9. Hydrothorax.
10. Pulmonary edema.
11. Pulmonary tuberculosis.

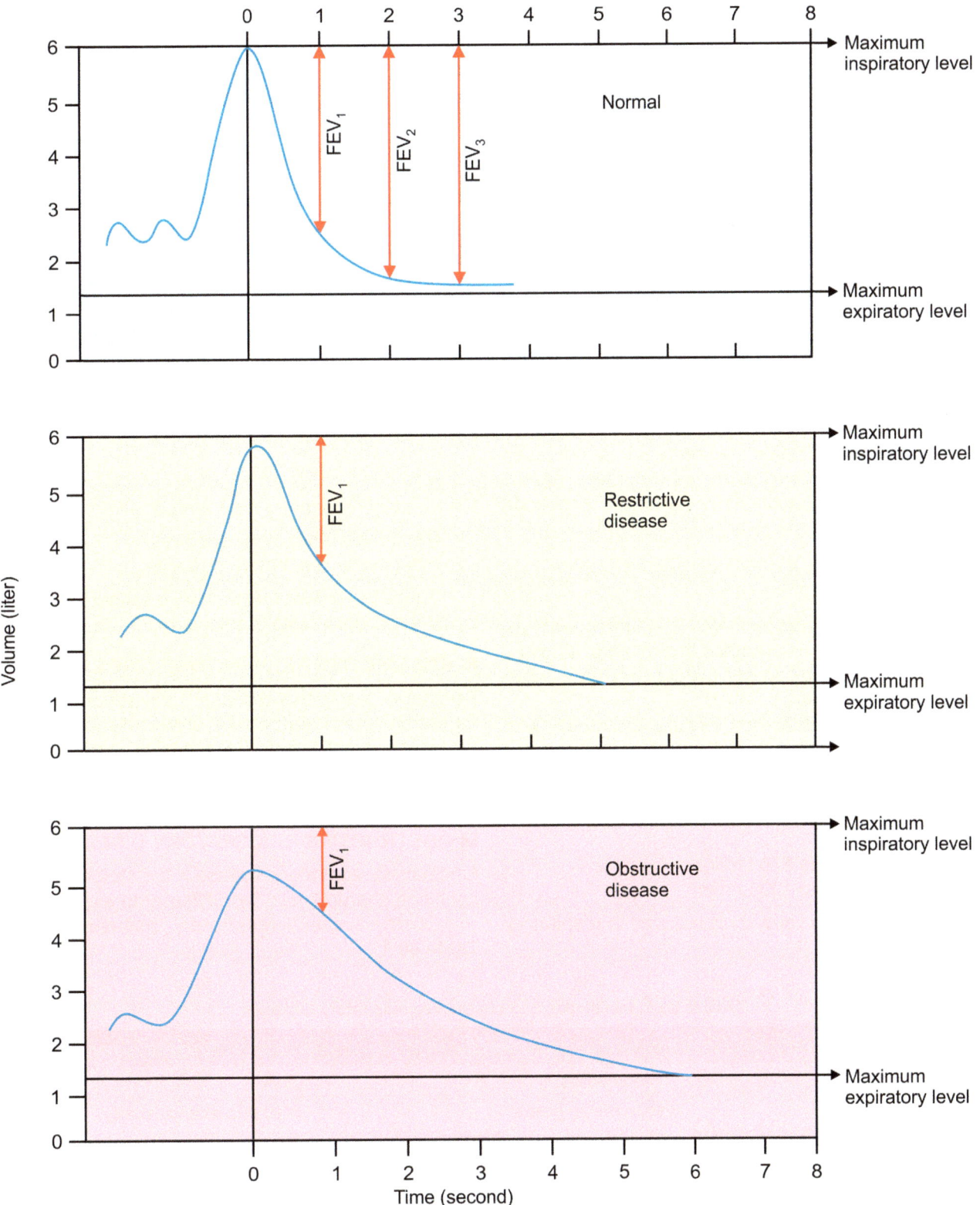

FIGURE 80.4: Forced expiratory volume (FEV).

■ FORCED EXPIRATORY VOLUME (FEV) OR TIMED VITAL CAPACITY

■ DEFINITION

Forced expiratory volume (FEV) is the volume of air, which can be expired forcefully in a given unit of time after a deep inspiration. It is also called timed vital capacity.

FEV_1 = Volume of air expired forcefully in 1 second
FEV_2 = Volume of air expired forcefully in 2 seconds
FEV_3 = Volume of air expired forcefully in 3 seconds.

■ NORMAL VALUES

Forced expiratory volume in persons with normal respiratory functions is as follows:

FEV_1 = 83% of total vital capacity
FEV_2 = 94% of total vital capacity

FEV_3 = 97% of total vital capacity
After 3rd second = 100% of total vital capacity.

■ SIGNIFICANCE OF DETERMINING FEV

Vital capacity may be almost normal in some of the respiratory diseases. However, the FEV has great diagnostic value, as it is decreased significantly in some respiratory diseases. For example, it is very much decreased in the obstructive diseases like asthma and emphysema. It is slightly reduced in some of the restrictive respiratory diseases like fibrosis **(Fig. 80.4)**.

■ RESPIRATORY MINUTE VOLUME (RMV)

Respiratory minute volume is the volume of air breathed in and out of lungs every minute. It is the product of tidal volume (TV) and respiratory rate (RR).

RMV = TV × RR = 500 × 12 = 6,000 mL

Normal respiratory minute volume is 6 L. It increases in physiological conditions, such as voluntary hyperventilation, exercise and emotional conditions. It is reduced in respiratory diseases.

■ MAXIMUM BREATHING CAPACITY (MBC) OR MAXIMUM VENTILATION VOLUME (MVV)

Maximum breathing capacity (MBC) is the maximum volume of air which can be breathed in and out of lungs by rapid and forceful respiration per minute. It is also called maximum ventilation volume (MVV).

Subject is asked to breathe forcefully and rapidly with a respirometer for 15 seconds. Volume of air inspired and expired is measured from the spirogram. From this value, the MBC is calculated for 1 minute.

Normal value:

In adult male : 150 to 170 L/min.
In adult female: 80 to 100 L/ min.

Maximum breathing capacity is reduced in respiratory diseases.

■ PEAK EXPIRATORY FLOW RATE (PEFR)

Peak expiratory flow rate (PEFR) is the maximum rate at which the air can be expired after deep inspiration. It is measured by **Wright's peak flowmeter** or a **mini peak flowmeter**.

Normal value: 400 L/min

■ SIGNIFICANCE OF DETERMINING PEFR

Determination of peak expiratory flow rate is useful to diagnose respiratory diseases especially the obstructive respiratory diseases. Generally, PEFR is reduced in all type of respiratory diseases. However, reduction is more significant in the obstructive diseases than in restrictive diseases.

Thus, in restrictive diseases, the PEFR is 200 L/min and in obstructive diseases, it is only 100 L/min.

■ RESTRICTIVE AND OBSTRUCTIVE RESPIRATORY DISEASES

Diseases of respiratory tract are classified into two types:

1. Restrictive respiratory diseases.
2. Obstructive respiratory diseases.

These two types of respiratory diseases are determined by lung functions tests, particularly FEV.

■ RESTRICTIVE RESPIRATORY DISEASE

Restrictive respiratory disease is the abnormal respiratory condition characterized by **difficulty in inspiration**. Expiration is not affected. Restrictive respiratory disease may be because of abnormality of lungs, thoracic cavity or/and nervous system.

■ OBSTRUCTIVE RESPIRATORY DISEASE

Obstructive respiratory disease is the abnormal respiratory condition characterized by **difficulty in expiration**. Obstructive and respiratory diseases are listed in **Table 80.1**.

TABLE 80.1: Restrictive and obstructive respiratory diseases.

Type	Disease	Structures involved
Restrictive respiratory diseases	Poliomyelitis	CNS
	Myasthenia gravis	CNS and thoracic cavity
	Flail chest (broken ribs)	Thoracic cavity
	Paralysis of diaphragm	CNS
	Spinal cord diseases	CNS
	Pleural effusion	Thoracic cavity
Obstructive respiratory diseases	Asthma Chronic bronchitis Emphysema Cystic fibrosis	Lower respiratory tract
	Laryngotracheobronchitis Epiglottis Tumors Severe cough and cold with phlegm	Upper respiratory tract

Chapter 81: Ventilation and Dead Space

CHAPTER OUTLINE

- **PULMONARY VENTILATION**
  - DEFINITION
  - NORMAL VALUE AND CALCULATION
- **ALVEOLAR VENTILATION**
  - DEFINITION
  - NORMAL VALUE AND CALCULATION
- **DEAD SPACE**
  - DEFINITION
  - TYPES
  - NORMAL VALUE
- **MEASUREMENT**
- **VENTILATION-PERFUSION RATIO**
  - DEFINITION
  - NORMAL VALUE AND CALCULATION
  - SIGNIFICANCE
  - VARIATIONS
- **INSPIRED AIR**
- **ALVEOLAR AIR**
- **EXPIRED AIR**

PULMONARY VENTILATION

DEFINITION

Pulmonary ventilation is the volume of air moving in and out of lungs per minute in quiet breathing. It is also called **respiratory minute volume** (RMV).

NORMAL VALUE AND CALCULATION

Normal value of pulmonary ventilation is 6 L/minute. It is the product of tidal volume (TV) and the rate of respiration (RR).

Pulmonary ventilation is calculated by the following formula.

Pulmonary ventilation
= Tidal volume × Respiratory rate
= 500 mL × 12/minute
= 6,000 mL = 6 L/minute

ALVEOLAR VENTILATION

DEFINITION

Alveolar ventilation is the amount of **air utilized for gaseous exchange** every minute. Alveolar ventilation is different from pulmonary ventilation. In pulmonary ventilation, 6 L of air moves in and out of lungs in every minute. But the whole volume of air is not utilized for exchange of gases. Volume of air subjected for exchange of gases is the alveolar ventilation. Air that is trapped in the respiratory passage (dead space) does not take part in gaseous exchange.

NORMAL VALUE AND CALCULATION

Normal value of alveolar ventilation is 4,200 mL (4.2 L)/minute.

Alveolar ventilation is calculated by the following formula.

Alveolar ventilation
= (Tidal volume − Dead space) × Respiratory rate
= (500 − 150) mL × 12/min
= 4,200 mL (4.2 L)/min

DEAD SPACE

DEFINITION

Dead space is defined as the part of respiratory tract, where gaseous exchange does not take place. Air present in the dead space is called **dead space air**.

TYPES OF DEAD SPACE

Dead space is of two types:
I. Anatomical dead space.
II. Physiological dead space.

Anatomical Dead Space

Anatomical dead space includes nose, pharynx, trachea, bronchi and branches of bronchi up to terminal bronchioles.

Physiological Dead Space

Physiological dead space includes the anatomical dead space plus two additional volumes:

  i. *Air in the alveoli, which are nonfunctioning:* In some respiratory diseases, alveoli do not function due to destruction of alveolar membrane.
  ii. *Air in the alveoli, which do not receive adequate blood flow:* Gaseous exchange does not take place during inadequate blood supply.

Wasted ventilation and wasted air

Wasted ventilation is the volume of air that occupies physiological dead space. Wasted air is the air that is not utilized for gaseous exchange. Dead space air is generally considered as wasted air.

■ NORMAL VALUE OF DEAD SPACE

Under normal conditions, physiological dead space is equal to anatomical dead space. It is because, all the alveoli are functioning and all alveoli receive adequate blood flow in normal conditions. Volume of normal dead space is 150 mL.

In respiratory disorders, which affect the pulmonary blood flow or the alveoli, the dead space increases. It is associated with reduction in alveolar ventilation.

■ MEASUREMENT OF DEAD SPACE

Dead space is measured by single breath **nitrogen wash-out method**. Subject respires normally for few minutes. Then, he takes a sudden inhalation of pure oxygen. Oxygen replaces the air in dead space (air passage), i.e. the dead space air contains only oxygen and it pushes the other gases into alveoli.

Now, the subject exhales through a **nitrogen meter**. Nitrogen meter determines the concentration of nitrogen in expired air continuously.

First portion of expired air comes from upper part of respiratory tract or air passage, which contains only **oxygen**. Next portion of expired air comes from the alveoli, which contains **nitrogen**. Now, the nitrogen meter shows the nitrogen concentration, which rises sharply and reaches the plateau soon. By using data obtained from nitrogen meter, a graph is plotted. From this graph, the dead space is calculated (**Fig. 81.1**).

The graph has two areas, area without nitrogen and area with nitrogen. Area of the graph is measured by planimeter or by computer. Area without nitrogen indicates dead space air.

It is calculated by the formula:

$$\text{Dead space} = \frac{\text{Area without } N_2}{\text{Area with } N_2 + \text{Area without } N_2} \times \text{Volume of expired air}$$

For example, in a subject:

Area with nitrogen = 70 sq. cm

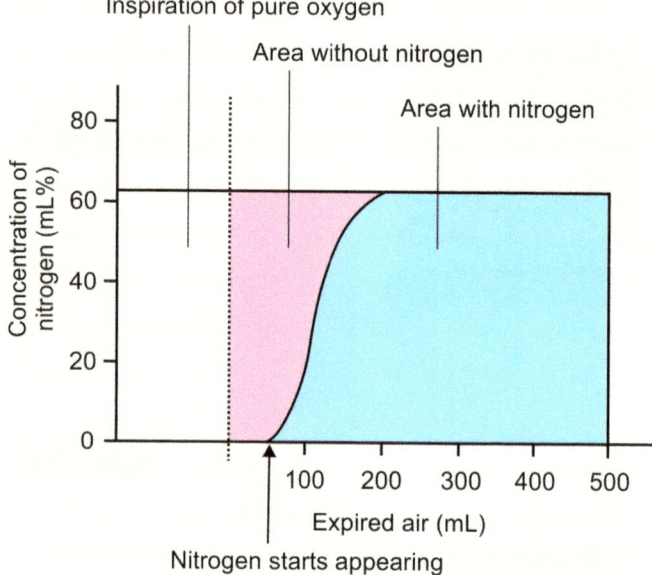

FIGURE 81.1: Measurement of dead space.

Area without nitrogen = 30 sq. cm
Volume of air expired = 500 mL

$$\text{Dead space} = \frac{30}{70 + 30} \times 500$$

$$= \frac{30}{100} \times 500$$

$$= 150 \text{ mL}$$

■ VENTILATION-PERFUSION RATIO

■ DEFINITION

Ventilation-perfusion ratio is the ratio of alveolar ventilation and amount of blood that perfuse the alveoli.

It is expressed as V_A/Q. V_A is alveolar ventilation and Q is the blood flow (perfusion).

■ NORMAL VALUE AND CALCULATION OF VENTILATION-PERFUSION RATIO

Normal value of ventilation-perfusion ratio is about 0.84.

Ventilation-perfusion ratio is calculated by the formula:

$$\text{Ventilation-perfusion ratio} = \frac{\text{Alveolar ventilation}}{\text{Pulmonary blood flow}}$$

Alveolar ventilation = (Tidal volume − Dead space) × Respiratory rate
= (500 − 150 mL) × 12/min
= 4,200 mL/min

Blood flow through alveoli (pulmonary blood flow) = 5,000 mL/min

Therefore,

$$\text{Ventilation-perfusion ratio} = \frac{4,200}{5,000}$$

$$= 0.84$$

TABLE 81.1: Composition of alveolar air, inspired air and expired air.

Components	Inspired (atmospheric) air		Alveolar air		Expired air	
	Volume (mL%)	Partial pressure (mm Hg)	Volume (mL%)	Partial pressure (mm Hg)	Volume (mL%)	Partial pressure (mm Hg)
Oxygen	20.84	159.00	13.60	104.00	15.70	120.00
Carbon dioxide	0.04	0.30	5.30	40.00	3.60	27.00
Nitrogen	78.62	596.90	74.90	569.00	74.50	566.00
Water vapor, etc.	0.50	3.80	6.20	47.00	6.20	47.00
Total	100.00	760.00	100.00	760.00	100.00	760.00

■ SIGNIFICANCE OF VENTILATION-PERFUSION RATIO

Ventilation-perfusion ratio signifies the gaseous exchange. It is affected if there is any change in alveolar ventilation or in blood flow.

■ VARIATIONS IN VENTILATION-PERFUSION RATIO

Physiological Variation

1. Ratio increases, if ventilation increases without any change in blood flow.
2. Ratio decreases, if blood flow increases without any change in ventilation.

Pathological Variation

In **chronic obstructive pulmonary diseases (COPD)**, ventilation is affected because of destruction of alveolar membrane. So, the ventilation-perfusion ratio reduces greatly.

■ INSPIRED AIR

Inspired air is the atmospheric air, which is inhaled during inspiration. Composition of inspired air is given in **Table 81.1**.

■ ALVEOLAR AIR

Alveolar air is the air present in the alveoli of lungs. It is collected by **Haldane-Priestly tube**.

Importance of Alveolar Air

1. Alveolar air is different from the inspired air or atmospheric air. Alveolar air is partially replaced by atmospheric air during each breath.
2. Oxygen diffuses from alveolar air into pulmonary capillaries constantly.
3. Carbon dioxide diffuses from pulmonary blood into alveolar air constantly.
4. Dry atmospheric air is humidified, while passing through respiratory passage just before entering the alveoli **(Table 81.1)**.

■ RENEWAL ALVEOLAR AIR

Alveolar air is constantly renewed. Rate of renewal is slow during normal breathing. During each breath, out of 500 mL of tidal volume, only 350 mL of air enters the alveoli and the remaining quantity of 150 mL (30%) becomes dead space air.

Hence, the amount of alveolar air replaced by new atmospheric air with each breath is only about 70% of total alveolar air.

Thus,

$$\text{Alveolar air} = \frac{350}{500} \times 100 = 70\%$$

■ EXPIRED AIR

Expired air is the amount of air that is exhaled during expiration. It is a combination of dead space air and alveolar air. Expired air is collected by using **Douglas bag**.

Concentration of gases in expired air is somewhere between inspired air and alveolar air. Composition of expired air is given in **Table 81.1**.

Chapter 82: Exchange and Transport of Respiratory Gases

CHAPTER OUTLINE

- **EXCHANGE OF GASES**
- **EXCHANGE OF RESPIRATORY GASES IN LUNGS**
  - RESPIRATORY MEMBRANE
  - DIFFUSING CAPACITY
  - DIFFUSION OF OXYGEN
  - DIFFUSION OF CARBON DIOXIDE
- **EXCHANGE OF RESPIRATORY GASES AT TISSUE LEVEL**
  - DIFFUSION OF OXYGEN FROM BLOOD INTO TISSUES
  - DIFFUSION OF CARBON DIOXIDE FROM TISSUES INTO BLOOD
- **RESPIRATORY EXCHANGE RATIO**
  - DEFINITION
  - NORMAL VALUES
- **RESPIRATORY QUOTIENT**
  - DEFINITION
  - NORMAL VALUE
- **TRANSPORT OF GASES**
- **TRANSPORT OF OXYGEN**
  - AS SIMPLE SOLUTION
  - IN COMBINATION WITH HEMOGLOBIN
  - OXYGEN-HEMOGLOBIN DISSOCIATION CURVE
- **TRANSPORT OF CARBON DIOXIDE**
  - AS DISSOLVED FORM
  - AS CARBONIC ACID
  - AS BICARBONATE
  - AS CARBAMINO COMPOUNDS
  - CARBON DIOXIDE DISSOCIATION CURVE

■ EXCHANGE OF GASES

Oxygen is essential for the cells. Carbon dioxide, which is produced as waste product in the cells must be expelled from cells and body. Lungs serve to exchange these two gases with blood.

■ EXCHANGE OF RESPIRATORY GASES IN LUNGS

In the lungs, exchange of respiratory gases takes place between the alveoli and the blood. Exchange of gases occurs through **bulk flow** diffusion (Chapter 3).

Respiratory unit is the structure through which the exchange of gases between blood and alveoli takes place. Refer Chapter 78 for details.

■ RESPIRATORY MEMBRANE

Exchange of respiratory gases takes place through respiratory membrane. It is formed by **epithelium** of the respiratory unit and **endothelium** of pulmonary capillary. Epithelium of the respiratory unit is a very thin layer (Chapter 78). Since the capillaries are in close contact with this membrane, the alveolar air is in close proximity to capillary blood. This facilitates the gaseous exchange between air and blood **(Fig. 82.1)**.

Respiratory membrane is formed by different layers of structures belonging to the alveoli and capillaries.

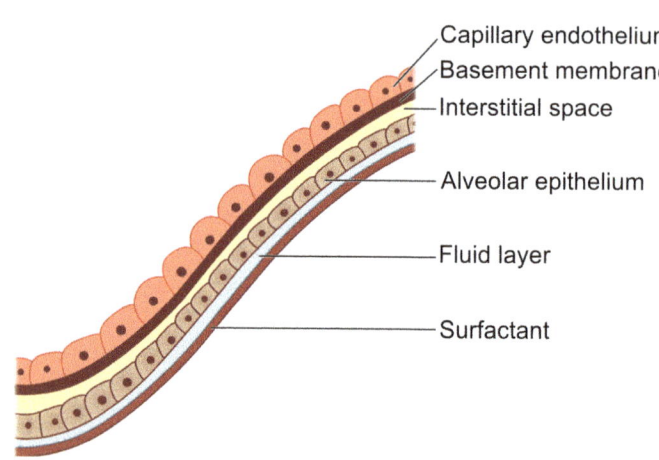

FIGURE 82.1: Structure of respiratory membrane.

Layers of Respiratory Membrane

Different layers of respiratory membrane from inside out are given in **Table 82.1**.

Average thickness of respiratory membrane is 0.6 μ in spite of having many layers. Total surface area of the respiratory membrane in both the lungs is about 70 sq. m.

Average diameter of pulmonary capillary is only 8 μ, which means that the RBCs with a diameter of 7.4 μ actually squeeze through the capillaries. Therefore, the membrane of RBCs is in close contact with capillary wall. This facilitates quick exchange of oxygen and carbon dioxide between the blood and alveoli.

■ DIFFUSING CAPACITY

Diffusing capacity is defined as the volume of gas that diffuses through the respiratory membrane each minute for a pressure gradient of 1 mm Hg.

Diffusing Capacity for Oxygen and Carbon Dioxide

Diffusing capacity for oxygen is 21 mL/min/1 mm Hg. Diffusing capacity for carbon dioxide is 400 mL/min/1 mm Hg. Thus, the diffusing capacity for carbon dioxide is about 20 times more than that of oxygen.

Factors Affecting Diffusing Capacity

1. Pressure gradient

Diffusing capacity is **directly proportional** to the pressure gradient. Pressure gradient is the difference between partial pressure of a gas in the alveoli and pulmonary capillary blood (see below). It is the major factor which affects the diffusing capacity.

2. Solubility of gas in fluid medium

Diffusing capacity is **directly proportional** to solubility of the gas. If the solubility of a gas is more in the fluid medium, a large number of molecules dissolve in it and diffuse easily.

3. Total surface area of respiratory membrane

Diffusing capacity is **directly proportional** to surface area of respiratory membrane. Surface area of respiratory membrane in each lung is about 70 sq. m. If the total surface area of respiratory membrane decreases, the diffusing capacity for the gases is decreased.

4. Molecular weight of the gas

Diffusing capacity is **inversely proportional** to molecular weight of the gas. If the molecular weight is more, the density is more and rate of diffusion is less.

5. Thickness of respiratory membrane

Diffusing capacity is **inversely proportional** to the thickness of respiratory membrane. More the thickness of respiratory membrane less is the diffusion. It is because the distance through which the diffusion takes place is long.

■ DIFFUSION OF OXYGEN

Entrance of Oxygen from Atmospheric Air into Alveoli

Partial pressure of oxygen in the atmospheric air is 159 mm Hg and, in the alveoli, it is 104 mm Hg. Because of the pressure gradient of 55 mm Hg, oxygen easily enters from atmospheric air into the alveoli **(Table 82.2)**.

Diffusion of Oxygen from Alveoli into Blood

When the blood is flowing through the pulmonary capillary, RBC is exposed to oxygen only for 0.75 sec at rest and only for 0.25 sec during severe exercise. So, the diffusion of oxygen must be quicker and effective. Fortunately, this is possible because of pressure gradient.

Partial pressure of oxygen in the pulmonary capillary is 40 mm Hg and, in the alveoli, it is 104 mm Hg. The pressure gradient is 64 mm Hg. It facilitates the diffusion of oxygen from alveoli into the blood **(Fig. 82.2)**.

■ DIFFUSION OF CARBON DIOXIDE

Diffusion of Carbon Dioxide from Blood into Alveoli

Partial pressure of carbon dioxide in alveoli is 40 mm Hg, whereas in the blood it is 46 mm Hg. Pressure gradient of

TABLE 82.1: Layers of respiratory membrane.

Parts of respiratory membrane	Different layers
Alveolar part	1. Layer of surfactant 2. Thin layer of alveolar fluid 3. Layer of alveolar epithelium 4. Basement membrane of alveolar epithelial
Between alveolar and capillary parts	5. Interstitial space
Capillary part	6. Basement membrane of capillary endothelium 7. Capillary endothelium

TABLE 82.2: Partial pressure, and content of oxygen and carbon dioxide in alveoli, capillaries and tissue.

Gas	Arterial end of pulmonary capillary	Alveoli	Venous end of pulmonary capillary	Arterial end of systemic capillary	Tissue	Venous end of systemic capillary
pO_2 (mm Hg)	40	104	104	95	40	40
Oxygen content (mL%)	14	–	19	19	–	14
pCO_2 (mm Hg)	46	40	40	40	46	46
Carbon dioxide content (mL%)	52	–	48	48	–	52

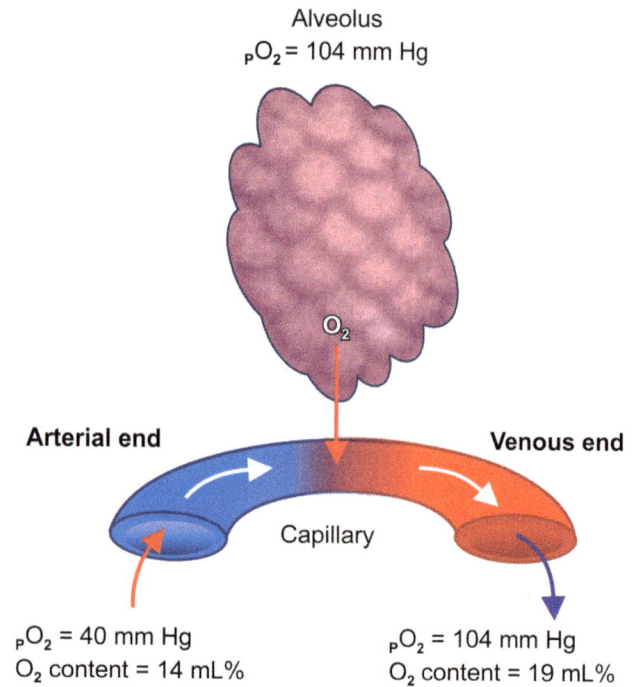

FIGURE 82.2: Diffusion of oxygen from alveolus to pulmonary capillary.

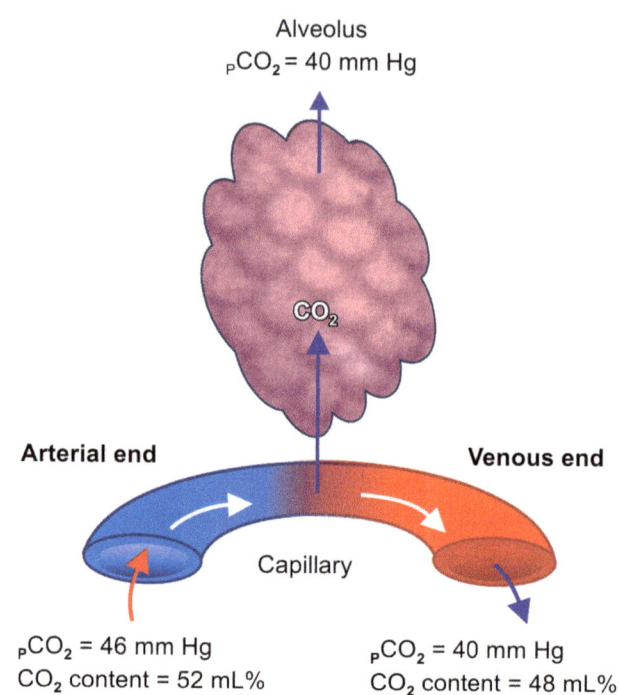

FIGURE 82.3: Diffusion of carbon dioxide from pulmonary capillary to alveolus.

6 mm Hg is responsible for the diffusion of carbon dioxide from blood into the alveoli **(Fig. 82.3)**.

Diffusion of Carbon Dioxide from Alveoli into Atmospheric Air

In the atmospheric air, partial pressure of carbon dioxide is very insignificant and is only about 0.3 mm Hg, whereas in the alveoli, it is 40 mm Hg. So, carbon dioxide enters the atmosphere from alveoli easily.

■ EXCHANGE OF RESPIRATORY GASES AT TISSUE LEVEL

■ DIFFUSION OF OXYGEN FROM BLOOD INTO TISSUES

Partial pressure of oxygen in arterial end of systemic capillary is 95 mm Hg. Average oxygen tension in the tissues is 40 mm Hg. It is because of continuous metabolic activity and constant utilization of oxygen. Thus, a pressure gradient of about 55 mm Hg exists between capillary blood and the tissues, so that oxygen can easily diffuse into the tissues **(Fig. 82.4)**.

Oxygen content in arterial blood is 19 mL%, and in the venous blood, it is 14 mL%. Thus, the diffusion of oxygen from blood to the tissues is 5 mL/100 mL of blood.

■ DIFFUSION OF CARBON DIOXIDE FROM TISSUES INTO BLOOD

Due to continuous metabolic activity, carbon dioxide is produced constantly in the cells of the tissues. So, the partial pressure of carbon dioxide is high in the cells and is about 46 mm Hg. The partial pressure of carbon dioxide in arterial blood is 40 mm Hg. Pressure gradient of 6 mm Hg is responsible for the diffusion of carbon dioxide from tissues to the blood **(Figs. 82.5 and 82.6)**.

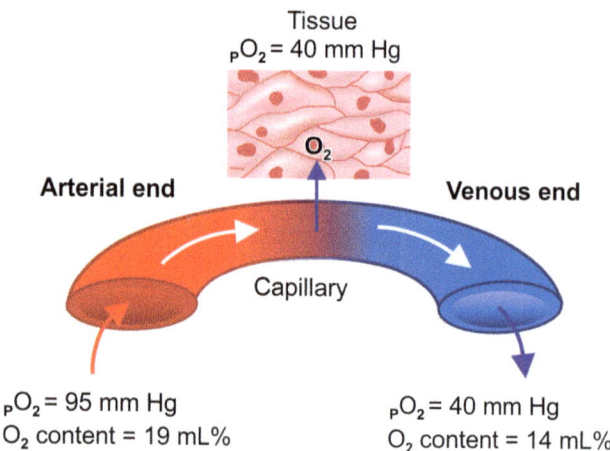

FIGURE 82.4: Diffusion of oxygen from capillary to tissue.

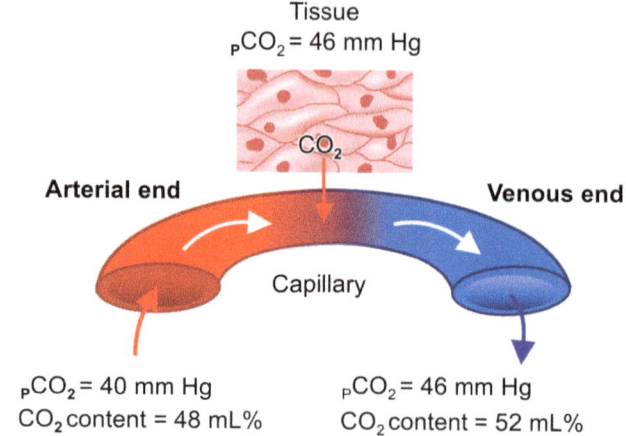

FIGURE 82.5: Diffusion of carbon dioxide from tissue to capillary.

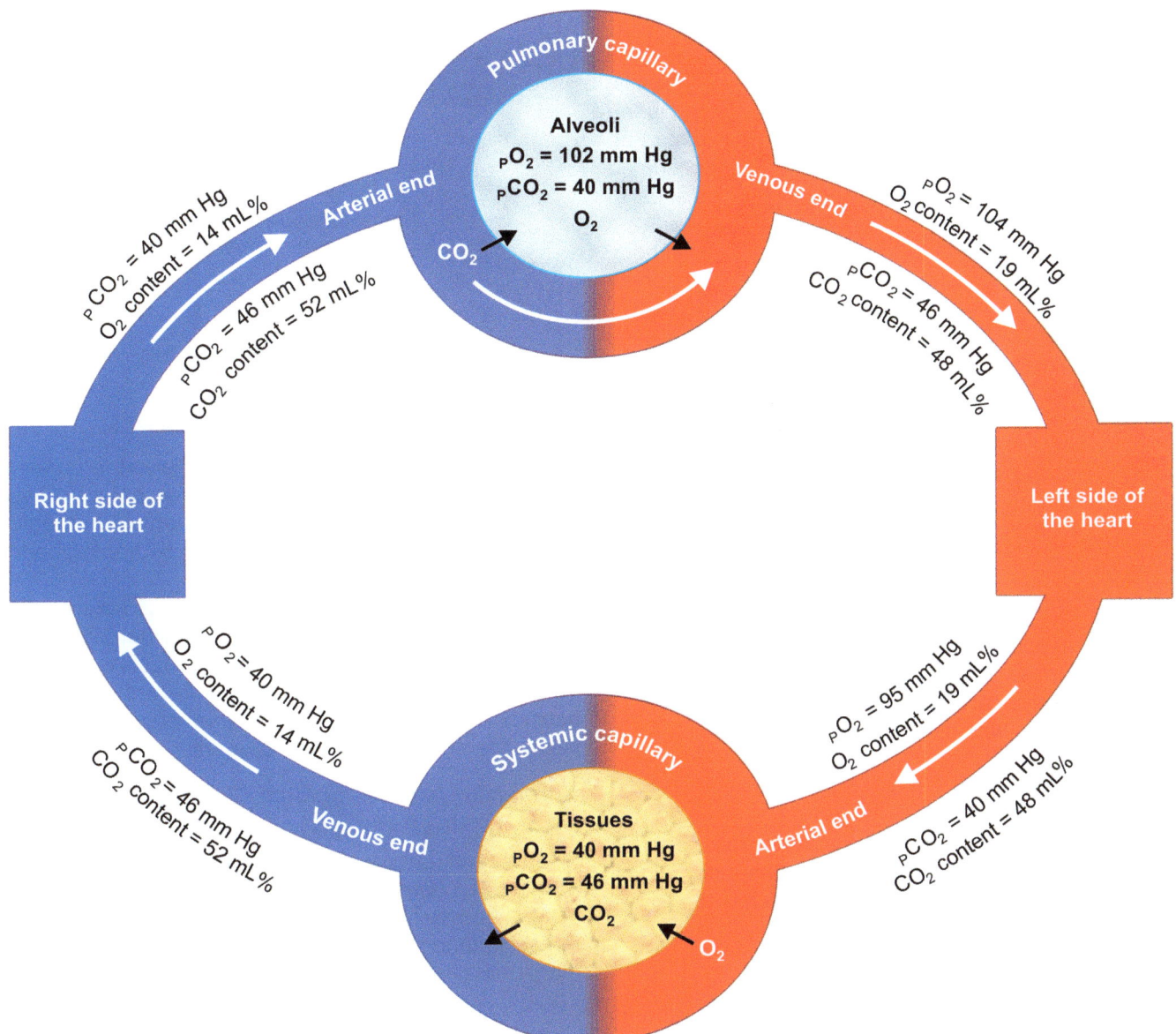

FIGURE 82.6: Partial pressure and content of oxygen and carbon dioxide in blood, alveoli and tissues.

Carbon dioxide content in arterial blood is 48 mL%, and, in the venous blood, it is 52 mL%. So, the diffusion of carbon dioxide from tissues to the blood is 4 mL/100 mL of blood.

■ RESPIRATORY EXCHANGE RATIO

■ DEFINITION

Respiratory exchange ratio (R) is the ratio between net output of carbon dioxide from tissues to simultaneous net uptake of oxygen by the tissues.

$$R = \frac{CO_2 \text{ output}}{O_2 \text{ uptake}}$$

■ NORMAL VALUES OF RESPIRATORY EXCHANGE RATIO

Normal value of respiratory exchange ratio depends upon the type of food substance that is metabolized. However, when a balanced diet containing average quantity of proteins, carbohydrates and lipids is utilized, the R is about 0.825. In steady conditions, respiratory exchange ratio is equal to respiratory quotient.

Respiratory exchange ratio during utilization of different food substances for metabolism is given in **Table 82.3**.

■ RESPIRATORY QUOTIENT

■ DEFINITION

Respiratory quotient is the molar ratio of carbon dioxide production to oxygen consumption. It is used to determine the utilization of different foodstuffs.

TABLE 82.3: Values of respiratory exchange ratio (R).

Food substances utilized for metabolism	R
Only carbohydrate	1.0
Only fat	0.7
Only protein	0.803
Balanced diet	0.825

NORMAL VALUE

For about 1 hour after meals, the respiratory quotient is 1.0. It is because usually, immediately after taking meals, only the carbohydrates are utilized by the tissues. During the metabolism of carbohydrates, one molecule of carbon dioxide is produced for every molecule of oxygen consumed by the tissues. Respiratory quotient is 1.0, which is equal to respiratory exchange ratio.

After utilization of all the carbohydrates available, body starts utilizing fats. Now the respiratory quotient becomes 0.7. When the proteins are metabolized, it becomes 0.8.

During exercise, the respiratory quotient increases (Chapter 88).

■ TRANSPORT OF GASES

Blood serves to transport the respiratory gases. Oxygen, which is essential for the cells of the body, is transported from alveoli of lungs to tissues. Carbon dioxide, which is the waste product in cells, is transported from tissues to alveoli of lungs.

■ TRANSPORT OF OXYGEN

Oxygen is transported from alveoli to the tissue by the blood in two forms:
1. As simple physical solution.
2. In combination with hemoglobin.

■ TRANSPORT OF OXYGEN AS SIMPLE SOLUTION

Oxygen dissolves in water of plasma and is transported in this **physical form**. Amount of oxygen transported in this way is very negligible. It is only 0.3 mL/100 mL of plasma. It is about 3% of total oxygen in blood.

■ IN COMBINATION WITH HEMOGLOBIN

Oxygen combines with hemoglobin in blood and is transported as **oxyhemoglobin**. Transport of oxygen in this form is important, because maximum amount (97%) of oxygen is transported by this method.

Oxygen combines with hemoglobin only as a physical combination. It is only **oxygenation** and not oxidation. This type of combination of oxygen with hemoglobin has got some advantages. Oxygen can be readily released from hemoglobin when it is needed.

Oxygen combines with the iron in heme part of hemoglobin.

Oxygen Carrying Capacity of Blood

Oxygen carrying capacity of blood is the amount of oxygen transported by blood. One gram of hemoglobin carries 1.34 mL of oxygen. It is called oxygen carrying capacity of hemoglobin.

Normal hemoglobin content in blood is 15 g%. So, the blood with 15 g% of hemoglobin should carry 20.1 mL% of oxygen, i.e. 20.1 mL of oxygen in 100 mL of blood. But, the blood with 15 g% of hemoglobin carries only 19 mL% of oxygen, i.e. 19 mL of oxygen is carried by 100 mL of blood **(Table 82.4)**. Oxygen carrying capacity of blood is only 19 mL% because the hemoglobin is not fully saturated with oxygen. It is saturated only for about 95%.

TABLE 82.4: Gases in arterial and venous blood.

Gas		Arterial blood	Venous blood
Oxygen	Partial pressure (mm Hg)	95	40
	Content (mL%)	19	14
Carbon dioxide	Partial pressure (mm Hg)	40	46
	Content (mL%)	48	52

■ OXYGEN-HEMOGLOBIN DISSOCIATION CURVE

Oxygen-hemoglobin dissociation curve is the curve that demonstrates the relationship between partial pressure of oxygen and percentage saturation of hemoglobin with oxygen. It explains the affinity of hemoglobin for oxygen.

Normally in the blood, hemoglobin is saturated with oxygen only up to 95%. Saturation of hemoglobin with oxygen depends upon the partial pressure of oxygen. When the partial pressure of oxygen is more, hemoglobin accepts oxygen and when the partial pressure of oxygen is less, hemoglobin releases oxygen.

Normal Oxygen-Hemoglobin Dissociation Curve

Under normal conditions, the oxygen-hemoglobin dissociation curve is 'S' shaped or sigmoid shaped **(Fig. 82.7)**. Lower part of the curve indicates dissociation of oxygen from hemoglobin. Upper part of the curve indicates the acceptance of oxygen by hemoglobin depending upon the partial pressure of oxygen.

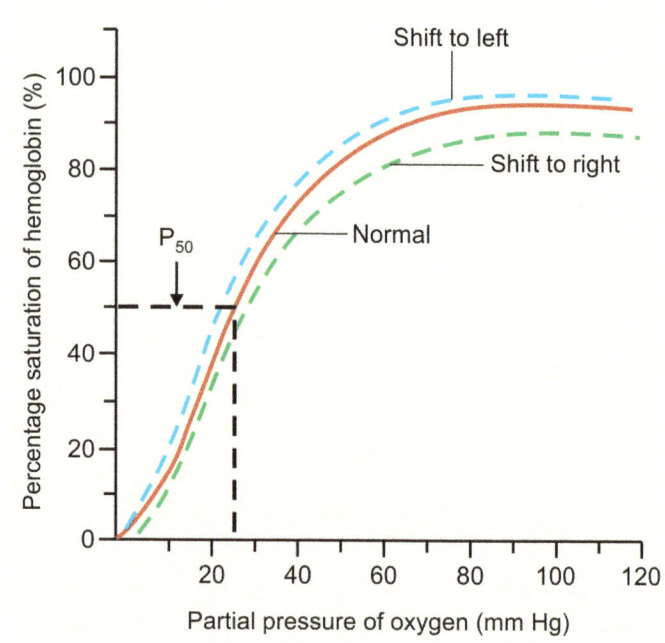

FIGURE 82.7: Oxygen-hemoglobin dissociation curve.

P_{50}

P_{50} is the partial pressure of oxygen at which hemoglobin saturation with oxygen is 50%. When the partial pressure of oxygen is 25 to 27 mm Hg, the hemoglobin is saturated to about 50%. That is, the blood contains 50% of oxygen. At 40 mm Hg of partial pressure of oxygen, the saturation is 75%. It becomes 95% when the partial pressure of oxygen is 100 mm Hg.

Factors Affecting Oxygen-Hemoglobin Dissociation Curve

Oxygen-hemoglobin dissociation curve is shifted to left or right by various factors:

I. Shift to left indicates acceptance (association) of oxygen by hemoglobin.
II. Shift to right indicates dissociation of oxygen from hemoglobin.

I. Shift to left

Oxygen-hemoglobin dissociation curve is shifted to left in the following conditions:

1. In fetal blood, because fetal hemoglobin has got more affinity for oxygen than the adult hemoglobin.
2. Decrease in hydrogen ion concentration and increase in pH (alkalinity).

II. Shift to right

Oxygen-hemoglobin dissociation curve is shifted to right in the following conditions:

1. Decrease in partial pressure of oxygen.
2. Increase in partial pressure of carbon dioxide (Bohr effect).
3. Increase in hydrogen ion concentration and decrease in pH (acidity).
4. Increased body temperature.
5. Excess of 2,3-diphosphoglycerate (DPG) which is a byproduct of carbohydrate metabolism present in red blood corpuscles.

Bohr Effect

Bohr effect is the effect by which presence of carbon dioxide decreases the affinity of hemoglobin for oxygen. In the tissues, due to continuous metabolic activities, the partial pressure of carbon dioxide is very high. Because of this, carbon dioxide enters the blood. Presence of carbon dioxide in blood decreases the affinity of hemoglobin for oxygen, so that oxygen is released from the blood to the tissues and, oxygen dissociation curve is shifted to right.

■ TRANSPORT OF CARBON DIOXIDE

Carbon dioxide is transported in the blood from tissues to the alveoli. Partial pressure and content of carbon dioxide in arterial blood and venous blood are given in **Table 82.2**.

Carbon dioxide is transported in the blood in four ways:

1. As dissolved form   : 7%
2. As carbonic acid   : Negligible
3. As bicarbonates   : 63%
4. As carbamino compounds   : 30%.

■ TRANSPORT OF CARBON DIOXIDE AS DISSOLVED FORM

Carbon dioxide diffuses into blood and dissolves in the fluid of plasma forming a **simple solution**. Only about 3 mL/100 mL of plasma of carbon dioxide is transported as dissolved state. It is about 7% of total carbon dioxide in the blood.

■ TRANSPORT OF CARBON DIOXIDE AS CARBONIC ACID

Part of dissolved carbon dioxide in plasma combines with the water to form carbonic acid. This reaction is very slow and the transport of carbon dioxide in this form is negligible.

■ TRANSPORT OF CARBON DIOXIDE AS BICARBONATE

About 63% of carbon dioxide is transported as bicarbonate. From plasma, the carbon dioxide enters the RBCs. In the RBCs, carbon dioxide combines with water to form carbonic acid. This reaction inside RBCs is very rapid. Rapid formation of carbonic acid inside RBCs is due to the presence of an enzyme called **carbonic anhydrase**. This enzyme accelerates the reaction. Carbonic anhydrase is present only inside the RBCs and not in the plasma. That is why the carbonic acid formation is at least 200 to 300 times more in the RBCs than in plasma.

Carbonic acid is very unstable. Almost all carbonic acid (99.9%) formed in RBCs, dissociates into bicarbonate and hydrogen ions. Concentration of bicarbonate ions in RBC increases more and more. Due to concentration gradient, bicarbonate ions diffuse through the cell membrane into the plasma.

Chloride Shift or Hamburger Phenomenon

Chloride shift or Hamburger phenomenon is the exchange of a chloride ion for a bicarbonate ion across the erythrocyte membrane.

Chloride shift occurs when carbon dioxide enters the blood from tissues. In plasma, plenty of sodium chloride is present. It dissociates into sodium and chloride ions **(Fig. 82.8)**. When the negatively charged bicarbonate, ions move out of RBC into the plasma, the negatively charged chloride ions move into the RBC in order to maintain the **electrolyte equilibrium** (ionic balance).

Reverse Chloride Shift

Reverse chloride shift is the process by which the chloride ions are moved back into plasma from RBC. This occurs in lungs.

When the blood reaches the alveoli, sodium bicarbonate in the plasma dissociates into the sodium and bicarbonate ions. Bicarbonate ion moves into the RBC. It makes chloride ion to move out of the RBC into the plasma, where it combines with sodium and forms sodium chloride.

Bicarbonate ion inside the RBC combines with hydrogen ion, forms carbonic acid, which dissociates into water and carbon dioxide. Carbon dioxide is then expelled into alveoli.

Thus, **chloride shift** occurs in **tissues** and **reverse chloride shift** occurs in **lungs**.

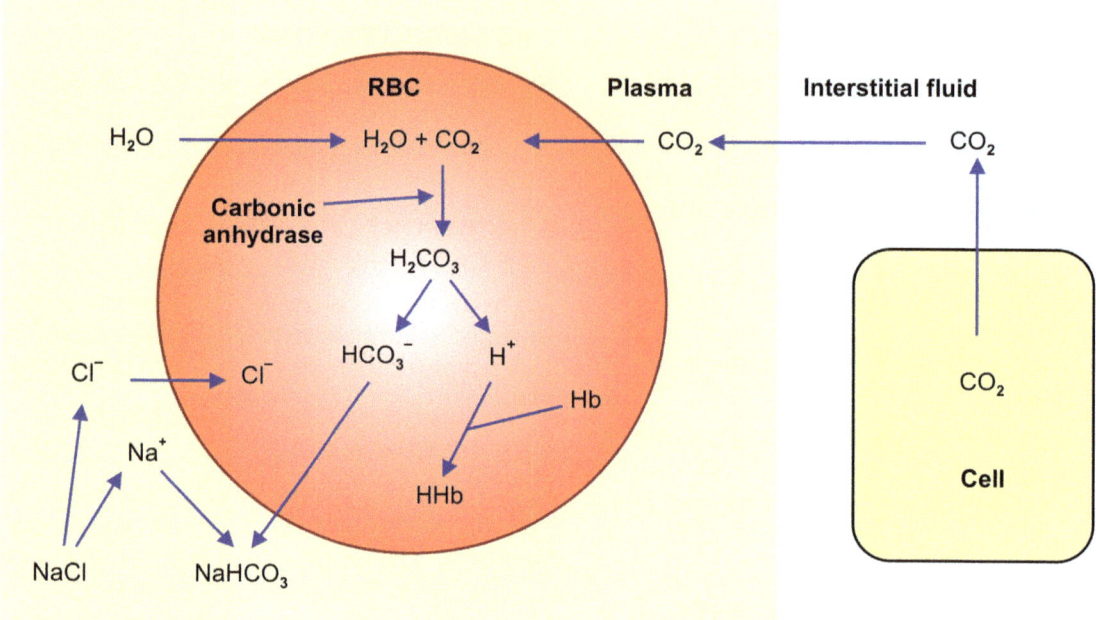

FIGURE 82.8: Transport of carbon dioxide in blood in the form of bicarbonate and chloride shift.

TRANSPORT OF CARBON DIOXIDE AS CARBAMINO COMPOUNDS

About 30% of carbon dioxide is transported as carbamino compounds. Carbon dioxide is transported in blood in combination with hemoglobin and plasma proteins. Carbon dioxide combines with hemoglobin to form carbamino hemoglobin or **carbhemoglobin**. And, it combines with plasma proteins to form carbamino proteins. Carbamino hemoglobin and **carbamino proteins** are together called carbamino compounds.

Carbon dioxide combines with proteins or hemoglobin with a loose bond, so that carbon dioxide is easily released into alveoli, where the partial pressure of carbon dioxide is low. Thus, the combination of carbon dioxide with proteins and hemoglobin is a reversible one. Amount of carbon dioxide transported in combination with plasma proteins is very less compared to the amount transported in combination with hemoglobin. It is because, the quantity of proteins in plasma is only half of the quantity of hemoglobin.

CARBON DIOXIDE DISSOCIATION CURVE

Carbon dioxide is transported in blood as physical solution and in combination with water, plasma proteins and hemoglobin. Amount of carbon dioxide combining with blood depends upon the partial pressure of carbon dioxide.

Carbon dioxide dissociation curve is the curve that demonstrates the relationship between partial pressure of carbon dioxide and quantity of carbon dioxide that combines with blood.

Normal Carbon Dioxide Dissociation Curve

Normal carbon dioxide dissociation curve shows that the carbon dioxide content in the blood is 48 mL% when the partial pressure of carbon dioxide is 40 mm Hg. It becomes 52 mL% when the partial pressure of carbon dioxide is 48 mm Hg. Carbon dioxide content becomes 70 mL% when the partial pressure is about 100 mm Hg **(Fig. 82.9)**.

Haldane Effect

Haldane effect is the effect by which combination of oxygen with hemoglobin displaces carbon dioxide from hemoglobin. Excess of oxygen content in blood causes shift of the carbon dioxide dissociation curve to the right.

Significance of Haldane effect

Haldane's effect is essential for release of carbon dioxide from blood into the alveoli of lungs and uptake of oxygen by the blood.

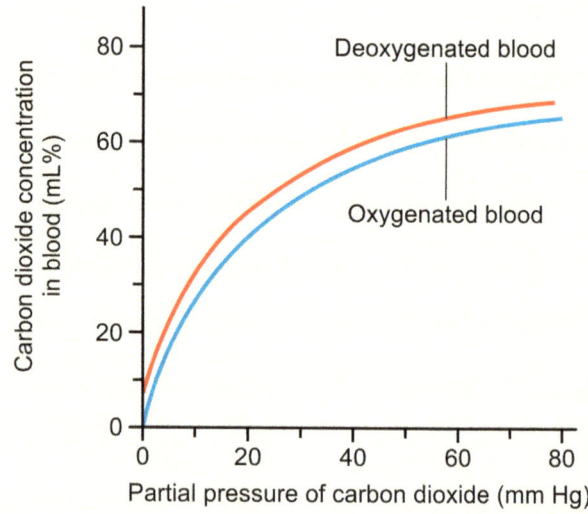

FIGURE 82.9: Carbon dioxide dissociation curve.

Chapter 83: Regulation of Respiration

CHAPTER OUTLINE

- **REGULATORY MECHANISMS**
- **NERVOUS MECHANISM**
  - RESPIRATORY CENTERS
  - MEDULLARY CENTERS
  - PONTINE CENTERS
  - CONNECTIONS OF RESPIRATORY CENTERS
- **INTEGRATION OF RESPIRATORY CENTERS**
  - FACTORS AFFECTING RESPIRATORY CENTERS
- **CHEMICAL MECHANISM**
  - CENTRAL CHEMORECEPTORS
  - PERIPHERAL CHEMORECEPTORS

REGULATORY MECHANISMS

Respiration is a reflex process. But it can be controlled voluntarily (voluntary breath holding) for a short period. **Breath holding time** in a normal healthy adult is 45 to 55 seconds. However, by practice, breathing can be withheld for a long period.

Respiration is subjected to variation, even under normal physiological conditions. For example, emotion and exercise increase the rate and force of respiration. But the altered pattern of respiration is brought back to normal within a short time by some regulatory mechanisms in the body.

Regulatory mechanisms responsible for quiet regular breathing are:

1. Nervous or neural mechanism.
2. Chemical mechanism.

NERVOUS MECHANISM

Nervous mechanism that regulates respiration includes:

1. Respiratory centers
2. Afferent nerves
3. Efferent nerves.

RESPIRATORY CENTERS

Respiratory centers are group of neurons, which control the rate, rhythm and force of respiration. These centers are bilaterally situated in reticular formation of brainstem **(Fig. 83.1)**. Depending upon the situation in brainstem, respiratory centers are classified into two groups:

I. Medullary centers:
   1. Dorsal respiratory group of neurons.
   2. Ventral respiratory group of neurons.
II. Pontine centers:
   1. Pneumotaxic center.
   2. Apneustic center.

MEDULLARY CENTERS

1. Dorsal Respiratory Group of Neurons

Situation

Dorsal respiratory group of neurons are diffusely situated in nucleus of tractus solitarius which is present in upper medulla oblongata **(Fig. 83.1)**. Usually, these neurons are collectively called **inspiratory center**.

All the neurons of dorsal respiratory group are **inspiratory neurons** and generate **inspiratory ramp** by the virtue of their **autorhythmic property (Table 83.1)**.

Function

Dorsal group of neurons are responsible for basic rhythm of respiration (see below for details).

Experimental evidence

Electrical stimulation of these neurons in animals by using needle electrode causes contraction of inspiratory muscles and prolonged inspiration.

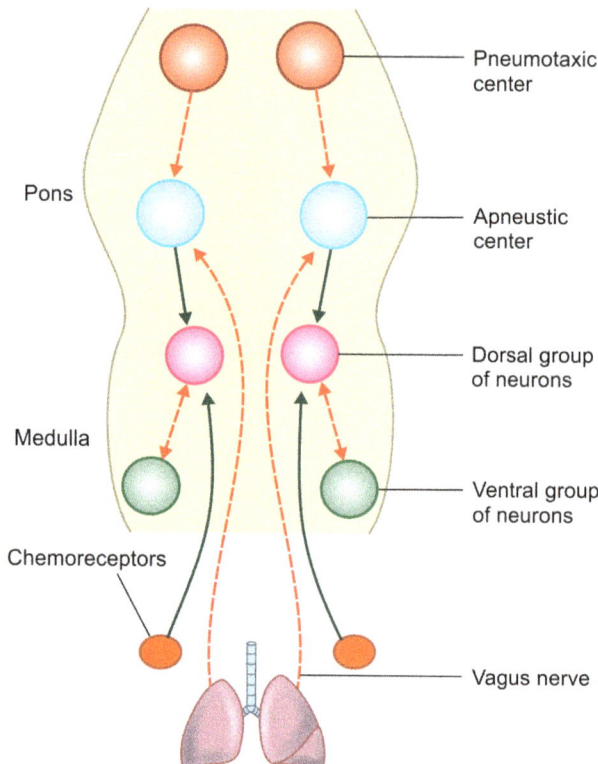

FIGURE 83.1: Nervous regulation of respiration.
Solid blue line = Stimulation, Dotted red line = Inhibition.

2. Ventral Respiratory Group of Neurons Situation

Situation

Ventral respiratory group of neurons are present in nucleus ambiguus and nucleus retroambiguus. These two nuclei are situated in the medulla oblongata, anterior and lateral to the nucleus of tractus solitarius. Earlier, ventral group neurons were collectively called **expiratory center**.

Ventral respiratory group has both **inspiratory** and **expiratory neurons.** Inspiratory neurons are found in central area of the group. Expiratory neurons are in caudal and rostral areas of the group.

Function

Normally, ventral group neurons are inactive during quiet breathing and become active during forced breathing. During forced breathing, these neurons stimulate both inspiratory muscles and expiratory muscles.

Experimental evidence

Electrical stimulation of the inspiratory neurons in ventral group causes contraction of inspiratory muscles and prolonged inspiration. Stimulation of expiratory neurons causes contraction of expiratory muscles and prolonged expiration.

■ PONTINE CENTERS

1. Apneustic Center

Situation

Apneustic center is situated in the nuclei of reticular formation of **lower pons**.

Function

Apneustic center increases depth of inspiration by acting directly on dorsal respiratory group of neurons.

Experimental evidence

Stimulation of apneustic center causes **apneusis.** Apneusis is an abnormal pattern of respiration, characterized by prolonged inspiration followed by inefficient short expiration.

2. Pneumotaxic Center

Situation

Pneumotaxic center is situated in the dorsolateral part of reticular formation **in upper pons**. It is formed by neurons of medial parabrachial and subparabrachial nuclei. Subparabrachial nucleus is also called ventral parabrachial or Kölliker-Fuse nucleus.

Function

Primary function of pneumotaxic center is to control the medullary respiratory centers, particularly the dorsal group neurons. It acts through apneustic center. Pneumotaxic center inhibits the apneustic center so that the dorsal group neurons are inhibited. Because of this, inspiration stops and expiration starts. Thus, pneumotaxic center influences the switching between inspiration and expiration.

Pneumotaxic center **increases respiratory rate** by reducing the duration of inspiration.

TABLE 83.1: Respiratory centers.

Features	Medullary centers		Pontine centers	
	Dorsal respiratory group of neurons	Ventral respiratory group of neurons	Apneustic center	Pneumotaxic center
Situation	Nucleus of tractus solitarius	Nucleus ambiguus and Nucleus retroambiguus	Nuclei of reticular formation of lower pons	Nuclei of reticular formation of upper pons
Type of neurons	Inspiratory neurons	Inspiratory neurons and Expiratory neurons	Inspiratory neurons	Neurons of medial parabrachial and subparabrachial nuclei
Function	Generate inspiratory ramp Has autorhythmicity Always active	Inactive during quiet breathing Active during forced breathing	Prolonged inspiration and Short expiration	Switching between inspiration and expiration by inhibiting inspiration through apneustic center

Experimental evidence

Stimulation of pneumotaxic center does not produce any typical effect, except slight **prolongation of expiration,** by inhibiting the dorsal respiratory group of neurons through apneustic center. Destruction or inactivation of pneumotaxic center results in apneusis.

■ CONNECTIONS OF RESPIRATORY CENTERS

Efferent Pathway

Nerve fibers from respiratory centers leave brainstem and descend in spinal cord and terminate on the motor neurons in the anterior horn cells of cervical and thoracic segments of spinal cord.

From the motor neurons of spinal cord two sets of nerve fibers arise:

1. **Phrenic nerve fibers** (C3 to C5) which supply the diaphragm.
2. **Intercostal nerve fibers** (T1 to T11) which supply the external intercostal muscles.

Afferent Pathway

Impulses from peripheral chemoreceptors and baroreceptors are carried to respiratory centers by the branches of glossopharyngeal and vagus nerves. Vagal nerve fibers also carry impulses from stretch receptors of lungs to the respiratory centers.

Thus, the respiratory centers receive afferent impulses from different parts of the body and modulate the movements of thoracic cage and lungs accordingly through efferent nerve fibers.

■ INTEGRATION OF RESPIRATORY CENTERS

Role of Medullary Centers

Rhythmic discharge of inspiratory impulses

Dorsal respiratory group neurons maintain the **normal rhythm of respiration** by discharge of impulses (action potentials) **rhythmically**. These impulses are transmitted to the respiratory muscles by phrenic and intercostal nerves.

Inspiratory ramp

Inspiratory ramp is the pattern of discharge from dorsal respiratory group neurons characterized by steady increase in amplitude of the action potential. To start with, the amplitude of action potential is low due to the activation of only few neurons. Later, more and more neurons are activated leading to gradual increase in the amplitude of the action potential in a **ramp fashion**. Impulses of this type of firing from dorsal group neurons are called **inspiratory ramp signals**.

Impulses from dorsal group of neurons are produced only for a period of **2 seconds** during which inspiration occurs. After 2 seconds, the ramp signals stop abruptly and do not appear for another **3 seconds**. Switching off ramp signals causes expiration. At the end of 3 seconds, the inspiratory ramp signals reappear in same pattern, and the cycle is repeated.

Normally, during inspiration, dorsal respiratory group neurons inhibit expiratory neurons of ventral group. During expiration, the expiratory neurons inhibit the dorsal group neurons. Thus, the medullary respiratory centers control each other.

Significance of inspiratory ramp signals

Significance of inspiratory ramp signals is that there is a slow and steady inspiration so that, the filling of lungs with air is also steady.

Role of Pontine Centers

Pontine respiratory centers regulate the medullary centers. Apneustic center accelerates the activity of dorsal group of neurons and the stimulation of this center causes prolonged inspiration.

Pneumotaxic center inhibits the apneustic center and restricts the duration of inspiration.

Pre-Bötzinger Complex

Pre-Bötzinger complex **(pre-BötC)** is an **additional respiratory center** found in animals. It is formed by a group of neurons called **pacemaker neurons,** which generate the rhythmic respiratory impulses. Exact functioning mechanism of this complex is not known.

■ FACTORS AFFECTING RESPIRATORY CENTERS

Respiratory centers regulate the respiratory movements, by receiving impulses from various sources in the body.

1. Impulses from Higher Centers

Higher centers alter the respiration by sending impulses directly to dorsal group neurons. Impulses from various parts of **cerebral cortex** such as anterior cingulate gyrus, olfactory tubercle and posterior orbital gyrus inhibit the respiration. Impulses from motor area and Sylvian area of cerebral cortex produce forced breathing.

2. Impulses from Stretch Receptors of Lungs: Hering-Breuer Reflex

Hering-Breuer reflex is a **protective reflex** that restricts the inspiration and prevents overstretching of lung tissues. It is initiated by the stimulation of stretch receptors of bronchi and bronchioles.

Stretch receptors give response to stretch of the tissues. During inspiration, there is stretching of lungs due to entrance of air resulting in stimulation of stretch receptors. Impulses from stretch receptors pass through vagal afferent fibers to respiratory centers and inhibit the dorsal group neurons. So, **inspiration stops** and **expiration starts (Fig. 83.2)**. Thus, overstretching of lung tissues is prevented.

However, Hering-Breuer reflex does not operate during quiet breathing. It operates, only when the tidal volume increases beyond 1,000 mL.

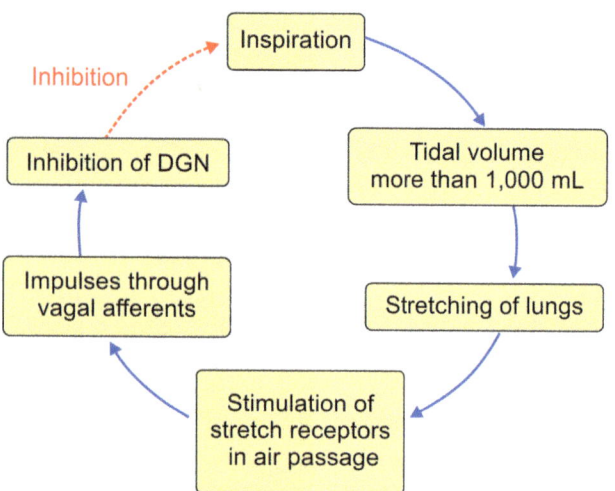

FIGURE 83.2: Hering-Breuer inflation reflex.
DGN = Dorsal respiratory group of neurons.

This reflex is also called **Hering-Breuer inflation reflex** since occurs due to inflation of lungs during inspiration. The reverse of this reflex is called **Hering-Breuer deflation reflex** and it takes place during expiration. During expiration as the stretching of lungs is abolished, the deflation of lungs occurs.

3. Impulses from 'J' Receptors of Lungs

'J' receptors are **juxtacapillary receptors** which are present on the wall of alveoli and having close contact with pulmonary capillaries.

Stimulation of the 'J' receptors produces a reflex response, which is characterized by apnea followed by hyperventilation, bradycardia, hypotension and weakness of skeletal muscles.

Role of 'J' receptors in physiological conditions is not clear. However, these receptors are responsible for hyperventilation in the patients affected by pulmonary congestion and left heart failure.

4. Impulses from Irritant Receptors of Lungs

Besides stretch receptors, there is another type of receptors in the bronchi and bronchioles, called irritant receptors. The irritant receptors are stimulated by irritant chemical agents such as ammonia and sulfurdioxide.

Stimulation of **irritant receptors** produces reflex **hyperventilation** along with **bronchospasm**. Hyperventilation along with bronchospasm prevents further entry of harmful agents into the alveoli.

5. Impulses from Baroreceptors

Baroreceptors are the receptors which give response to change in blood pressure. Refer Chapter 70 for details of baroreceptors.

Whenever arterial blood pressure increases, baroreceptors are activated and send inhibitory impulses to vasomotor center in medulla oblongata. This causes decrease in blood pressure and inhibition of respiration. However, in physiological conditions, the role of baroreceptors in regulation of respiration is insignificant.

6. Impulses from Chemoreceptors

Chemoreceptors play an important role in the chemical regulation of respiration. Details of the chemoreceptors and chemical regulation of respiration are explained later in this chapter.

7. Impulses from Proprioceptors

Proprioceptors are the receptors, which give response to the change in the position of body. These receptors are situated in joints, tendons and muscles.

Proprioceptors are stimulated during the muscular exercise and, send impulses to brain particularly, the cerebral cortex through somatic afferent nerves. Cerebral cortex in turn causes **hyperventilation** by sending impulses to the medullary respiratory centers.

8. Impulses from Thermoreceptors

Thermoreceptors are the cutaneous receptors, which give response to change in the environmental temperature. There are two types of temperature receptors, namely, the receptors for cold and the receptors for warmth.

When the body is **exposed to cold** or when cold water is applied over the body, cold receptors are stimulated and, send impulses to cerebral cortex via somatic afferent nerves. Cerebral cortex in turn stimulates the respiratory centers and causes **hyperventilation**.

9. Impulses from Pain Receptors

Pain receptors are the receptors which give response to pain stimulus. Whenever pain receptors are stimulated, the impulses are sent to cerebral cortex via somatic afferent nerves. Cerebral cortex in turn stimulates the respiratory centers and causes **hyperventilation (Fig. 83.3)**.

■ CHEMICAL MECHANISM

Chemical mechanism of regulation of respiration is operated through the **chemoreceptors** which give response to changes in chemical constituents of blood such as:

1. Hypoxia (decreased partial pressure of oxygen).
2. Hypercapnia (increased partial pressure of carbon dioxide).
3. Increased hydrogen ion concentration.

Types of Chemoreceptors

Chemoreceptors are classified into two groups:

1. Central chemoreceptors.
2. Peripheral chemoreceptors.

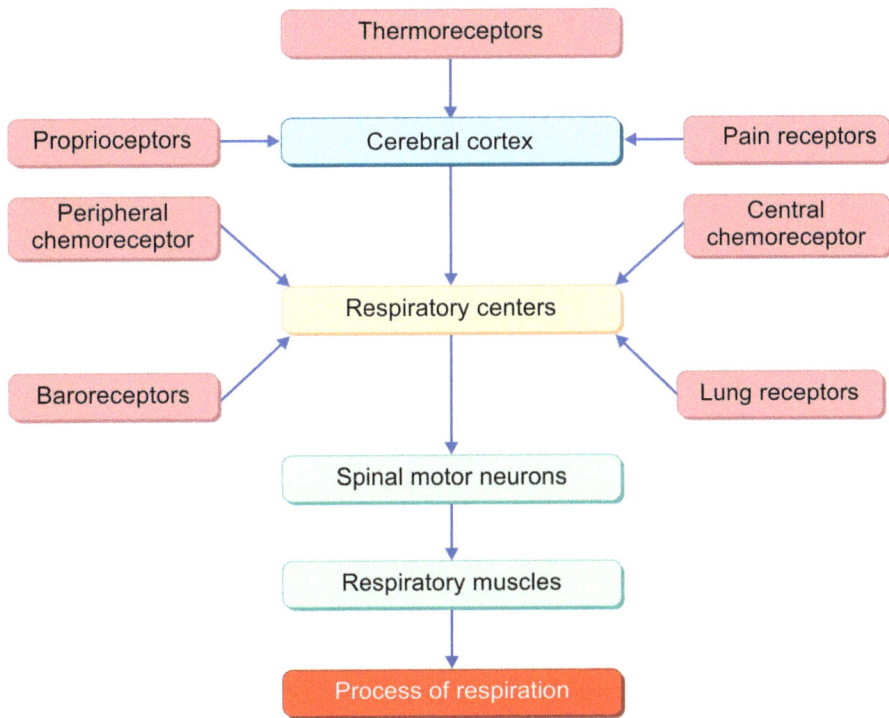

FIGURE 83.3: Factors affecting respiratory centers.

■ CENTRAL CHEMORECEPTORS

Chemoreceptors present in the brain are called the central chemoreceptors. These chemoreceptors are situated in **medulla oblongata**, close to dorsal respiratory group of neurons. This area with chemoreceptors is known as **chemosensitive area**.

Mechanism of Action

Main stimulant for the central chemoreceptors is the **increased hydrogen ion** concentration.

However, hydrogen ions from blood cannot cross the blood-brain barrier and blood cerebrospinal fluid barrier. On the other hand, carbon dioxide can easily cross these barriers and enter the interstitial fluid of brain or the cerebrospinal fluid. There, the carbon dioxide combines with water to form carbonic acid. Since carbonic acid is unstable, it immediately dissociates into hydrogen ion and bicarbonate ion **(Fig. 83.4)**.

$$CO_2 + H_2O \longrightarrow H_2CO_3 \longrightarrow H^+ + HCO_3^-$$

Hydrogen ions stimulate the central chemoreceptors. Chemoreceptors in turn send stimulatory impulses to dorsal respiratory group of neurons causing increased ventilation (increased rate and force of breathing). Because of this, the excess carbon dioxide is washed out and the respiration is brought back to normal.

■ PERIPHERAL CHEMORECEPTORS

Chemoreceptors present in the carotid and aortic region are called peripheral chemoreceptors. Refer Chapter 70 for details.

Mechanism of Action

Reduction in partial pressure of oxygen is the most potent stimulant for peripheral chemoreceptors. Whenever, partial pressure of oxygen decreases, the chemoreceptors are stimulated and send impulses through aortic and Hering's nerves. These impulses reach the respiratory centers, particularly the dorsal group of neurons and stimulate them. Dorsal group of neurons send stimulatory impulses to respiratory muscles resulting in increased ventilation.

This provides enough oxygen and rectifies the lack of oxygen.

Peripheral chemoreceptors are mildly sensitive to the increased partial pressure of carbon dioxide and increased hydrogen ion concentration.

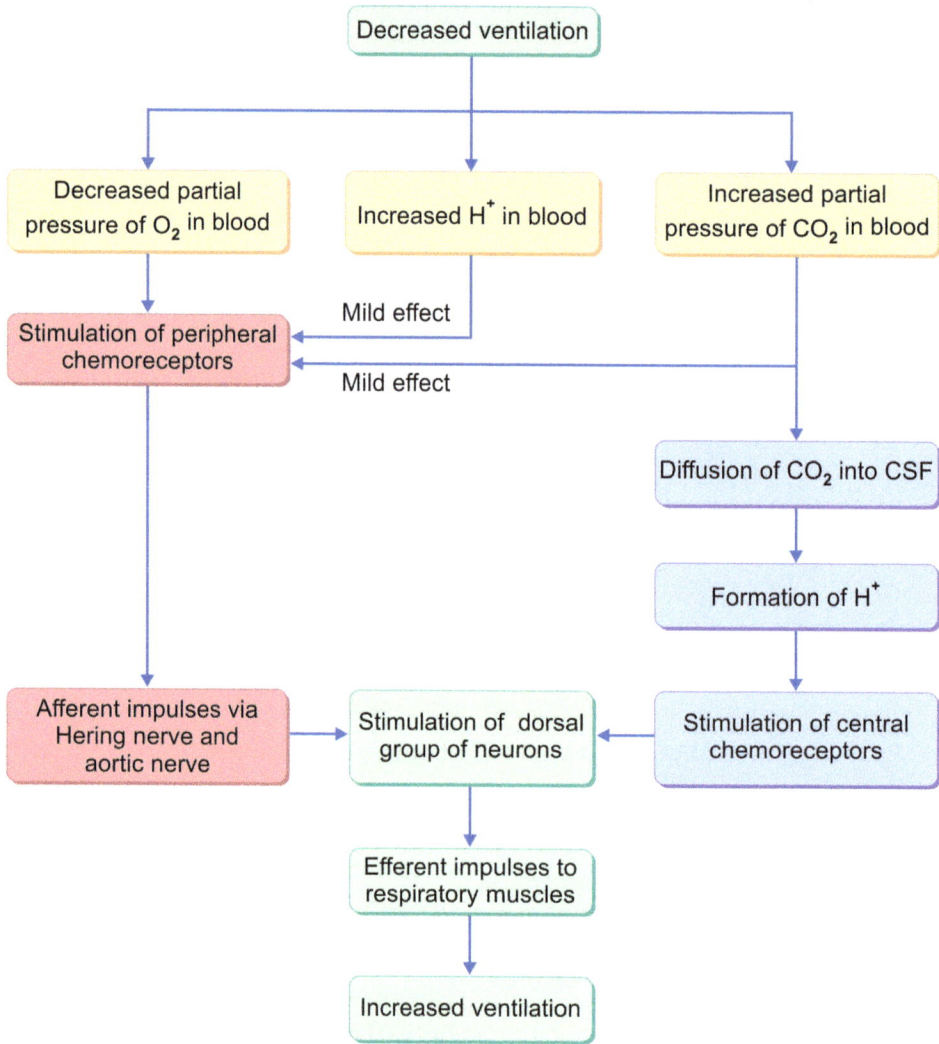

FIGURE 83.4: Chemical regulation of respiration.
CSF = Cerebrospinal fluid.

Chapter 84: Diseases and Disorders of Respiration

CHAPTER OUTLINE

- RESPIRATORY PATTERNS
- APNEA
- HYPERVENTILATION
- HYPOVENTILATION
- HYPOXIA
- OXYGEN TOXICITY (POISONING)
- HYPERCAPNIA
- HYPOCAPNIA
- ASPHYXIA
- DYSPNEA
- PERIODIC BREATHING
- CYANOSIS
- CARBON MONOXIDE POISONING
- BRONCHIAL ASTHMA
- OTHER RESPIRATORY DISORDERS

RESPIRATORY PATTERNS

Normal respiratory pattern is called **eupnea**. Respiratory pattern is altered by many ways.

ALTERED PATTERNS OF RESPIRATION

1. *Tachypnea:* Increase in rate of respiration.
2. *Bradypnea:* Decrease in rate of respiration.
3. *Polypnea:* Rapid, shallow breathing resembling panting in dogs. In this type of breathing, only the rate of respiration increases but the force does not increase significantly.
4. *Apnea:* Temporary arrest of breathing.
5. *Hyperpnea:* Increase in pulmonary ventilation due to increase in force of breathing with or without increase in rate of respiration. Partial pressure of respiratory gases particularly of carbon dioxide is not altered. It occurs after exercise. It also occurs in abnormal conditions like fever or other disorders.
6. *Hyperventilation:* Abnormal increase in rate and force of respiration. It is also called over breathing and it results in excess removal of carbon dioxide (see below for details).
7. *Hypoventilation:* Decrease in rate and force of respiration.
8. *Dyspnea:* Difficulty in breathing.
9. *Periodic breathing:* Abnormal respiratory rhythm.
10. *Apneusis:* Abnormal breathing pattern with deep and prolonged inspiration followed by short insufficient expiration.

APNEA

Apnea is defined as **temporary arrest of breathing**. Apnea can also be produced voluntarily which is called **breath holding** or **voluntary apnea**. The breath holding time is known as **apnea time**. It is about 45 to 55 seconds in a normal adult, after a deep inspiration.

Apnea occurs in the following conditions:

1. Voluntary effort (voluntary breath holding or apnea).
2. After hyperventilation.
3. During deglutition (deglutition apnea: Chapter 37).
4. During stimulation of vagus nerve in animals (**vagal apnea**).
5. After injection of adrenaline (**adrenaline apnea**).
6. Sleep apnea (**apnea during sleep**).

HYPERVENTILATION

DEFINITION

Hyperventilation or **over breathing** or **over ventilation** is increased pulmonary ventilation due to rapid and forced breathing. Both rate and force of breathing are increased.

CAUSES OF HYPERVENTILATION

Hyperventilation mostly occurs in conditions like exercise when partial pressure of carbon dioxide (pCO_2) is increased. Excess of carbon dioxide stimulates the respiratory centers. Voluntarily also, hyperventilation can be produced. It is called **voluntary hyperventilation**.

EFFECTS OF HYPERVENTILATION

During hyperventilation, excessive carbon dioxide is washed out. In blood, the partial pressure of carbon dioxide is reduced. It causes suppression of respiratory centers, resulting in **apnea.** Apnea is followed by Cheyne-Stokes type of periodic breathing. After a period of **Cheyne-Stokes breathing,** normal respiration is restored.

Common symptoms of hyperventilation are headache, weakness, dizziness, numbness or tingling on fingers and arms. Severe hyperventilation leads to loss of consciousness.

HYPOVENTILATION

DEFINITION

Hypoventilation is the decrease in pulmonary ventilation caused by decrease in rate or force of breathing. Thus, the amount of air moving in and out of lungs is reduced.

CAUSES OF HYPOVENTILATION

Hypoventilation occurs when respiratory centers are suppressed or by administration of some drugs. It also occurs during partial **paralysis of respiratory muscles.**

EFFECTS OF HYPOVENTILATION

Hypoventilation results in development of **hypoxia** along with **hypercapnia**. It increases the rate and force of respiration, leading to **dyspnea**. Severe conditions result in lethargy, coma and death.

HYPOXIA

DEFINITION

Hypoxia is defined as the reduced availability of oxygen to the tissues.

CAUSES OF HYPOXIA

Four important causes of hypoxia are:

1. Decreased oxygen tension in arterial blood.
2. Decreased oxygen carrying capacity of blood.
3. Decreased velocity of blood flow.
4. Decreased utilization of oxygen by the cells.

CLASSIFICATION OF HYPOXIA

On the basis of these factors, hypoxia is classified into four types **(Table 84.1)**:

I. Hypoxic hypoxia.
II. Anemic hypoxia.
III. Stagnant hypoxia.
IV. Histotoxic hypoxia.

Each type of hypoxia may be acute or chronic. Simultaneously, two or more types of hypoxia may be present.

I. Hypoxic Hypoxia

Hypoxic hypoxia means the decreased oxygen content in the blood. It is also called **arterial hypoxia.**

Causes for hypoxic hypoxia

1. Low oxygen tension in inspired (atmospheric).
2. Respiratory disorders.
3. Cardiac disorders.

Characteristic features of hypoxic hypoxia

Hypoxic hypoxia is characterized by **decreased oxygen tension** in arterial blood. All other features remain normal **(Table 84.1)**.

II. Anemic Hypoxia

Anemic hypoxia is the condition characterized by the inability of blood to carry enough amount of oxygen. The oxygen availability is normal. But the blood is not able to take up sufficient amount of oxygen due to anemic condition.

Causes of anemic hypoxia

Any condition that causes anemia can cause anemic hypoxia.

Anemic hypoxia occurs because of the following conditions:

1. Decreased number of RBCs.
2. Decreased hemoglobin content in the blood.
3. Formation of altered hemoglobin.
4. Combination of hemoglobin with gases other than oxygen and carbon dioxide.

Characteristic features of anemic hypoxia

Anemic hypoxia is characterized by the **decreased oxygen carrying capacity** of blood. All other features remain normal **(Table 84.1)**.

III. Stagnant Hypoxia

It is the hypoxia caused by decreased velocity of blood flow. It is otherwise called **hypokinetic hypoxia.**

Causes of stagnant hypoxia

Stagnant hypoxia occurs mainly due to reduction in velocity of blood flow.

Velocity of blood flow decreases in the following conditions:

1. Congestive cardiac failure.
2. Hemorrhage.
3. Surgical shock.
4. Vasospasm.
5. Thrombosis.
6. Embolism.

Characteristic features of stagnant hypoxia

Characteristic feature of stagnant hypoxia is the **decreased velocity of blood flow**. All other features remain normal **(Table 84.1)**.

IV. Histotoxic Hypoxia

Histotoxic hypoxia is the type of hypoxia produced by the inability of tissues to utilize oxygen.

Causes for histotoxic hypoxia

Histotoxic hypoxia occurs due to cyanide or sulfide poisoning. These substances destroy the cellular oxidative

TABLE 84.1: Characteristic features of different types of hypoxia.

Features	Hypoxic hypoxia	Anemic hypoxia	Stagnant hypoxia	Histotoxic hypoxia
1. PO_2 in arterial blood	Reduced	Normal	Normal	Normal
2. Oxygen carrying capacity of blood	Normal	Reduced	Normal	Normal
3. Velocity of blood flow	Normal	Normal	Reduced	Normal
4. Utilization of oxygen by tissues	Normal	Normal	Normal	Reduced
5. Efficacy of oxygen therapy	100%	75%	< 50%	Not useful

enzymes. So, even if oxygen is supplied, the tissues are not able to utilize it.

Characteristic features of histotoxic hypoxia

Histotoxic hypoxia is characterized by **inability of tissues to utilize oxygen** even if it is delivered. All other features remain normal **(Table 84.1)**.

■ EFFECTS OF HYPOXIA

Acute and severe hypoxia leads to unconsciousness. If not treated immediately, brain death occurs.

Chronic hypoxia produces various symptoms in the body.

Effects of hypoxia are of two types:

A. Immediate effects.
B. Delayed effects.

A. Immediate Effects of Hypoxia

1. Effects on blood

Hypoxia stimulates the secretion of erythropoietin from kidney. Erythropoietin increases production of RBCs. Thus, the oxygen carrying capacity of blood is improved by increase in RBC count and hemoglobin content.

2. Effects on cardiovascular system

Initially, due to the reflex stimulation of cardiac and vasomotor centers, there is increase in rate and force of contraction of heart, cardiac output and blood pressure. Later, there is reduction in the rate and force of contraction of heart. Cardiac output and blood pressure are also decreased.

3. Effects on respiration

Initially, the respiratory rate is increased due to chemoreceptor reflex. Because of this large amount of carbon dioxide is washed out leading to alkalemia. Later, the respiration tends to be shallow and periodic. Finally, the rate and force of breathing are reduced to a great extent due to the failure of respiratory centers.

4. Effects on digestive system

Hypoxia is associated with loss of appetite, nausea and vomiting. Mouth becomes dry and there is a feeling of thirst.

5. Effects on kidney

Juxtaglomerular apparatus of kidney secretes erythropoietin. Alkaline urine is excreted.

6. Effects on central nervous system

In mild hypoxia, the symptoms are similar to those of **alcoholic intoxication**.

The individual is depressed, apathic with general loss of self-control. Person becomes talkative, quarrelsome, ill-tempered and rude. The subject starts shouting, singing or crying.

There is disorientation, and loss of discriminative ability and loss of power of judgment. Memory is impaired. Weakness, lack of coordination and fatigue of muscles are common in hypoxia.

If hypoxia is acute and severe, there is sudden loss of consciousness. If not treated immediately, coma occurs which leads to death.

■ TREATMENT FOR HYPOXIA: OXYGEN THERAPY

Best treatment for hypoxia is oxygen therapy, i.e. treating the affected person with oxygen. Pure oxygen or oxygen combined with another gas is administered.

Depending upon the situation, oxygen therapy can be given either under normal atmospheric pressure or under high pressure (**hyperbaric oxygen**).

In Normal Atmospheric Pressure

With normal atmospheric pressure, i.e. at one atmosphere (760 mm Hg), administration of pure oxygen is well tolerated by the patient for long hours.

In High Atmospheric Pressure: Hyperbaric Oxygen

Hyperbaric oxygen is the pure oxygen with high atmospheric pressure of 2 or more than 2 atmospheres. Hyperbaric oxygen therapy with 2 to 3 atmospheres is tolerated by the patient for about 5 hours. But oxygen toxicity develops when pure oxygen is administered for long periods. Refer oxygen toxicity below.

Efficacy of Oxygen Therapy in Different Types of Hypoxia

Oxygen therapy is the best treatment for hypoxia. Value of oxygen therapy depends upon the type of hypoxia.

In hypoxic hypoxia, the oxygen therapy is 100% useful. In anemic hypoxia, oxygen therapy is moderately effective to about 70%. In stagnant hypoxia, the effectiveness of oxygen therapy is less than 50%. In histotoxic hypoxia, the oxygen therapy is not useful at all. It is because, even if oxygen is delivered, the cells cannot utilize oxygen.

OXYGEN TOXICITY

DEFINITION

Oxygen toxicity or **oxygen poisoning** is the increased oxygen content in tissues beyond certain critical level. It is also called oxygen poisoning.

CAUSE OF OXYGEN TOXICITY

Oxygen toxicity is caused by breathing **hyperbaric oxygen** (see above). In this condition, an excess amount of oxygen is transported in plasma as dissolved form because oxygen carrying capacity of hemoglobin is decreased.

EFFECTS OF OXYGEN TOXICITY

1. Lung tissues are affected first with tracheobronchial irritation and pulmonary edema.
2. Metabolic rate increases in all the body tissues and tissues are burnt out by excess heat. The heat also destroys cytochrome system leading to damage of tissues.
3. When brain is affected, first hyperirritability occurs. Later, it is followed by increased muscular twitching, ringing in ears and dizziness.
4. Finally, the toxicity results in convulsions, coma and death.

HYPERCAPNIA

DEFINITION

Hypercapnia is the increased carbon dioxide content of blood.

CAUSES OF HYPERCAPNIA

It occurs in conditions, which leads to blockage of respiratory pathway as in case of asphyxia. It also occurs while breathing air containing excess carbon dioxide content.

EFFECTS OF HYPERCAPNIA

1. Excess stimulation of respiratory centers leading to dyspnea.
2. Reduction in pH of blood.
3. Increase in heart rate and blood pressure.
4. Headache, depression and laziness.
5. Muscular rigidity, tremors and convulsions.
6. Giddiness and loss of consciousness.

HYPOCAPNIA

DEFINITION

Hypocapnia is the decreased carbon dioxide content in blood.

CONDITIONS WHEN HYPOCAPNIA OCCURS

It occurs in conditions associated with hypoventilation. It also occurs after prolonged hyperventilation, because of washing out of excess carbon dioxide.

EFFECTS OF HYPOCAPNIA

1. Rate and force of respiration decrease.
2. The pH of blood increases leading to respiratory alkalosis.
3. Tetany develops because of decreased calcium concentration.
4. Dizziness, mental confusion, muscular twitching and loss of consciousness.

ASPHYXIA

Asphyxia is the condition characterized by combination of hypoxia and hypercapnia due to obstruction of air passage.

CONDITIONS WHEN ASPHYXIA OCCURS

Asphyxia develops in conditions characterized by acute obstruction of air passage such as, hanging, strangulation and drowning.

EFFECTS OF ASPHYXIA

Effects of asphyxia develop in three stages:

1. Stage of Hyperpnea

Hyperpnea is the first stage of asphyxia. It extends for about 1 minute. In this stage, breathing becomes deep and rapid. It is due to the powerful stimulation of respiratory centers by carbon dioxide accumulated. Hyperpnea is followed by **dyspnea** and **cyanosis**. The eyes become more prominent.

2. Stage of Convulsions

This stage is characterized by **convulsions** (uncontrolled involuntary muscular contractions). Duration of this stage is less than one minute. Following effects develop in this stage due to the effect of hypercapnia on brain and spinal cord:

i. Expiratory efforts become more violent.
ii. Generalized convulsions appear.
iii. Heart rate increases.
iv. Arterial blood pressure increases.
v. Consciousness is lost.

3. Stage of Collapse

This stage lasts for about three minutes. Effects developed in this stage are:

i. Depression of brain centers due to lack of oxygen. So, convulsions disappear.
ii. Respiratory gasping occurs with stretching of the body and opening of mouth as if gasping for breath.
iii. Dilatation of pupils.
iv. Reduction in heart rate.
v. Loss of all reflexes.
vi. Gradual increase in the duration between the gasps.
vii. Finally, the death.

All together asphyxia extends only for 5 minutes. The person can be saved by timely help such as relieving the respiratory obstruction, good aeration, etc. Otherwise, death occurs.

DYSPNEA

DEFINITION

Dyspnea means **difficulty in breathing**. It is otherwise called the **air hunger**. Normally, breathing goes on without our consciousness. When breathing enters the consciousness and produces discomfort, it is called dyspnea. Dyspnea is also defined as "a consciousness of necessity for increased respiratory effort".

■ DYSPNEA POINT

Dyspnea point is the level at which there is increased ventilation with severe breathing discomfort. A normal person is not aware of any increase in breathing until the pulmonary ventilation is doubled. Real discomfort develops when ventilation increases by 4 or 5 times.

■ CONDITIONS WHEN DYSPNEA OCCURS

Physiologically, dyspnea occurs during severe muscular exercise.

Pathological conditions when dyspnea occurs are the following:

1. Respiratory disorders which involve obstruction in any part of respiratory tract.
2. Cardiac disorders such as left ventricular failure and mitral stenosis.
3. Metabolic disorders such as diabetic acidosis.

■ PERIODIC BREATHING

Periodic breathing is the abnormal or uneven respiratory rhythm.

It is of two types:

A. Cheyne-Stokes breathing.
B. Biot breathing.

■ CHEYNE-STOKES BREATHING

Definition

Cheyne-Stokes breathing is the periodic breathing characterized by rhythmic hyperpnea and apnea. It is the most common type of periodic breathing.

Features of Cheyne-Stokes Breathing

Cheyne-Stokes breathing is marked by two alternate patterns of respiration:

1. Hyperpneic period.
2. Apneic period.

1. Hyperpneic Period: Waxing and Waning of Breathing

To begin with the breathing is shallow. Force of respiration increases gradually and reaches the maximum (hyperpnea). Then, it decreases gradually and reaches minimum. Now it is followed by apnea. The gradual increase followed by gradual decrease in force of respiration is called waxing and waning of breathing **(Fig. 84.1)**.

2. Apneic Period

When, the force of breathing is reduced to minimum, cessation of breathing occurs for a short period. It is again followed by hyperpneic period and the cycle is repeated.

Causes for waxing and waning

Initially, during forced breathing, large quantity of carbon dioxide is washed out from blood leading to inactivation of respiratory centers. It causes apnea. During apnea, there is accumulation of carbon dioxide with reduction in oxygen tension resulting in activation of respiratory centers. This causes gradual increase in the force of breathing to the maximum. And the cycle is repeated.

Conditions when Cheyne-Stokes Breathing Occurs

Cheyne-Stokes breathing occurs in both physiological and pathological conditions.

Physiological conditions when Cheyne-Stokes breathing occurs

1. During deep sleep.
2. In high altitude.
3. After prolonged voluntary hyperventilation.
4. In newborn babies.
5. After severe muscular exercise.

Pathological conditions when Cheyne-Stokes breathing occurs

1. During increased intracranial pressure.
2. During cardiac failure.
3. During renal diseases.
4. Poisoning by narcotics.
5. In premature infants.

■ BIOT BREATHING

Definition

Biot breathing is another form of periodic breathing characterized by period of apnea and hyperpnea.

Features of Biot Breathing

There is no waxing and waning of breathing **(Fig. 84.1)**. After apneic period, hyperpnea occurs abruptly.

Causes of Abrupt Apnea and Hyperpnea

Due to apnea, carbon dioxide accumulates and it stimulates the respiratory centers leading to hyperpnea. During hyperpnea, lot of carbon dioxide is washed out. So, the respiratory centers are not stimulated and apnea occurs.

Conditions when Biot's Breathing Occurs

Biot's breathing occurs only in pathological conditions such as nervous disorders involving lesions in respiratory centers.

■ CYANOSIS

■ DEFINITION

Cyanosis is defined as diffused bluish coloration of skin and mucous membrane.

■ CAUSE FOR CYANOSIS

Cyanosis is caused by due to the presence of large amount of reduced hemoglobin in the blood. Quantity of reduced hemoglobin should be at least 5 to 7 g/dL in the blood to cause cyanosis.

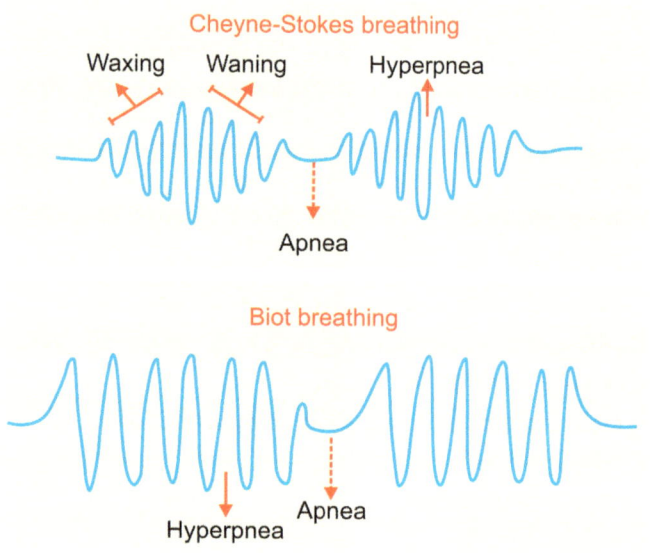

FIGURE 84.1: Periodic breathing.

DISTRIBUTION OF CYANOSIS

Cyanosis is distributed all over the body. But it is more marked in certain regions such as lips, cheeks, ear lobes, nose and fingertips above the base of the nail.

CONDITIONS WHEN CYANOSIS OCCURS

1. Any condition which leads to arterial hypoxia and stagnant hypoxia.
2. Conditions when altered hemoglobin like methemoglobin or sulfhemoglobin is formed.
3. Conditions like polycythemia when blood flow is slow.

CARBON MONOXIDE POISONING

SOURCE

Common sources for carbon monoxide are exhaust of gasoline engines, coal mines, gases from guns, deep wells and underground drainage system.

EFFECTS OF CARBON MONOXIDE

Carbon monoxide is a dangerous gas because it **displaces oxygen from hemoglobin** by binding with same site in hemoglobin for oxygen. So, oxygen transport and oxygen carrying capacity of the blood are decreased.

SYMPTOMS OF CARBON MONOXIDE POISONING

Symptoms of carbon monoxide poisoning depend upon its concentration in air:

1. While breathing air with 1% of carbon monoxide, mild symptoms like headache and nausea appear.
2. While breathing air containing carbon monoxide above 1% causes convulsions, cardiorespiratory arrest, loss of consciousness and coma occur.
3. High carbon monoxide content in air causes death.

BRONCHIAL ASTHMA

DEFINITION

Bronchial asthma is the inflammatory disease of respiratory tract characterized by recurrent attacks of difficult breathing with **wheezing.**

Wheezing

Wheezing is a high-pitched **whistling** sound produced while breathing. It is associated with difficult breathing.

Wheezing occurs due to obstruction of air passage because bronchiolar constriction.

CAUSES OF BRONCHIAL ASTHMA

1. Leukotrienes released from eosinophils and mast cells during inflammation cause bronchoconstriction (bronchospasm).
2. Allergic substances such as foreign proteins produce hypersensitivity of nerve fibers to larynx and nose resulting in asthma.
3. Pulmonary edema with congestion of lungs caused by left ventricular failure leads to asthma. Asthma developed in this condition is called **cardiac asthma**.

FEATURES OF BRONCHIAL ASTHMA

1. Asthma is a **paroxysmal** (sudden) **disorder** because the attack commences and ends abruptly. During the attack, the difficulty is felt both during inspiration and expiration. More difficulty is experienced during expiration.
2. Because of difficulty during expiration, the lungs are not deflated completely, so that the residual volume and functional residual capacity are increased.
3. Tidal volume, vital capacity, FEV1 and alveolar ventilation are decreased.
4. Carbon dioxide accumulates, resulting in acidosis, dyspnea and cyanosis.

OTHER RESPIRATORY DISORDERS

ATELECTASIS

Atelectasis is the partial or complete **collapse of lungs.** When a large portion of lung is collapsed, the partial pressure of oxygen is reduced in blood, leading to dyspnea and death.

Atelectasis is caused by deficiency of surfactant, obstruction of bronchus or bronchiole. It is also caused by presence of air **(pneumothorax),** fluid **(hydrothorax),** blood **(hemothorax)** or pus **(pyothorax)** in the pleural cavity.

PNEUMOTHORAX

Pneumothorax is the presence of air in pleural space resulting in collapse of lungs.

Air enters the pleural cavity because of damage of chest wall or lungs during accident, bullet injury or stab injury.

PNEUMONIA

Pneumonia is the **inflammation** of lung tissues, followed by the accumulation of blood cells, fibrin and exudates in the alveoli. Affected part of the lungs becomes **consolidated**.

Inflammation of lung is caused by bacterial or viral infection and inhaling noxious chemical substance.

Features of pneumonia include fever, chest compression, chest pain, shallow breathing, cyanosis, insomnia (sleeplessness) and delirium (disturbed mental state).

PULMONARY EDEMA

Pulmonary edema is the accumulation of serous fluid in the alveoli and the interstitial tissue of lungs.

It is caused by increased pulmonary capillary pressure (due to left ventricular failure or mitral valve disease), pneumonia, and breathing harmful chemicals.

Features of pulmonary edema are severe dyspnea and cough. Death occurs in severe conditions.

PLEURAL EFFUSION

Pleural effusion is the accumulation of large amount of fluid in pleural cavity.

Pleural effusion occurs because of blockage of lymphatic drainage, flow of fluid from pulmonary capillaries and inflammation of pleural membrane.

Pleural effusion causes atelectasis, leading to dyspnea and other respiratory disturbances.

PULMONARY TUBERCULOSIS

Tuberculosis is the disease caused by **tubercle bacilli**. This disease can affect any organ in the body. However, the lungs are affected more commonly. Infected tissue is invaded by macrophages and later it becomes fibrous. Affected tissue is called **tubercle.**

Initially, alveoli in the affected part become non-functioning. In severe conditions, the destruction of the lung tissue is followed by formation of large **abscess cavities**.

EMPHYSEMA

Emphysema is an **obstructive respiratory disease** characterized by extensive **damage of lung tissues**. Damage of lung tissues results in loss of alveolar walls. Because of this, the elastic recoil of lungs is also lost.

Emphysema is caused by cigarette smoking, exposure to oxidant gases and untreated bronchitis.

Chronic emphysema could lead to hypoxia, hypercapnia, severe dyspnea and death.

Chapter 85: High Altitude and Deep Sea Physiology

CHAPTER OUTLINE

- **HIGH ALTITUDE PHYSIOLOGY**
  - BAROMETRIC PRESSURE AND PARTIAL PRESSURE OF OXYGEN AT DIFFERENT ALTITUDES
  - CHANGES IN THE BODY AT HIGH ALTITUDE
  - MOUNTAIN SICKNESS
  - ACCLIMATIZATION
- AVIATION PHYSIOLOGY
- SPACE PHYSIOLOGY
- **DEEP SEA PHYSIOLOGY**
  - BAROMETRIC PRESSURE AT DIFFERENT DEPTHS
  - EFFECT OF HIGH BAROMETRIC PRESSURE: NITROGEN NARCOSIS
  - DECOMPRESSION SICKNESS

■ HIGH ALTITUDE PHYSIOLOGY

Any altitude above 8,000 ft from mean sea level is called high altitude. People can ascend up to this level without any adverse effect.

At high altitudes, the barometric pressure is low. However, amount of oxygen available in the atmosphere is same as it is at the sea level. Due to **low barometric pressure**, the partial pressure of gases, particularly oxygen decreases leading to hypoxia.

Carbon dioxide at high altitude is very much negligible and it does not create any problem.

■ BAROMETRIC PRESSURE AND PARTIAL PRESSURE OF OXYGEN AT DIFFERENT ALTITUDES

Barometric pressure decreases at different altitudes, and accordingly the partial pressure of oxygen also decreases leading to various effects on the body. Barometric pressure and partial pressure of oxygen at different altitudes and their common effects on the body are given in **Table 85.1**.

■ CHANGES IN THE BODY AT HIGH ALTITUDE

When a person is exposed to high altitude particularly by rapid ascent, various systems in the body cannot cope with lowered oxygen tension, and the effects of hypoxia start. Besides hypoxia, some other factors are also responsible for changes in the functions of the body at high altitude.

Factors Affecting Physiological Functions at High Altitude

1. Hypoxia.
2. Expansion of gases.
3. Fall in atmospheric temperature.
4. Light rays.

1. Effect of Hypoxia

Refer Chapter 84 for effects of hypoxia on physiological functions.

2. Effects of Expansion of Gases

Volume of gases increases when the barometric pressure is reduced. So, at high altitude, volume of all gases increases in atmospheric air, as well as in the body due to the decreased barometric pressure.

Expansion of gases in GI tract causes painful distention of stomach and intestine. It is minimized by supporting the abdomen with a belt or by evacuation of the gases. Expansion of gases also destroys the alveoli.

During very rapid ascent from sea level to over 30,000 feet height, the gases evolve as bubbles, particularly nitrogen, resulting in decompression sickness (see below).

3. Effects of Reduced Atmospheric Temperature

Environmental temperature falls gradually at high altitudes. Temperature decreases to about 0°C at the height of 10,000 feet. It becomes – 22°C at the height of 20,000 feet. At the altitude of 40,000 feet, the temperature falls to – 44°C.

TABLE 85.1: Barometric pressure, partial pressure of oxygen and common effects at different altitudes.

Altitude (feet)	Barometric pressure (mm Hg)	Partial pressure of oxygen (mm Hg)	Common effects
Sea level	760	159	–
5,000	600	132	No hypoxia
10,000	523	110	Mild symptoms of hypoxia start appearing
15,000	400	90	Moderate hypoxia develops with following symptoms: 1. Reduction in visual acuity 2. Effects on mental functions 3. Improper judgment 4. Feeling of overconfidence
20,000	349	73	Severe hypoxia appears with cardiorespiratory symptoms such as: 1. Increase in heart rate and cardiac output 2. Increase in respiratory rate and respiratory minute volume This is the highest level for permanent inhabitants
25,000	250	62	This is the critical altitude for survival: 1. Hypoxia becomes severe 2. Breathing oxygen becomes essential
29,628	235	49	This is the height of Mount Everest
30,000	226	47	Symptoms become severe even with oxygen
50,000	87	18	Hypoxia becomes more severe even with pure oxygen

Injury or **frostbite** occurs if the body is not adequately protected by warm clothing.

4. Effects of Light Rays

Skin becomes susceptible for injury due to many harmful rays such as **ultraviolet rays** of sunlight. Moreover, the sunrays reflected by the snow might injure the retina of the eye, if it is not protected with suitable tinted glasses.

■ MOUNTAIN SICKNESS

Definition

Mountain sickness is the condition characterized by adverse effects of **hypoxia** at high altitude. It commonly develops in persons going to high altitude for the first time. It occurs within a day in these persons before they get acclimatized to high altitude.

Symptoms

In mountain sickness, the symptoms occur mostly in digestive system, cardiovascular system, respiratory system and nervous system. Symptoms of mountain sickness are detailed below.

1. Digestive system

Loss of appetite, nausea and vomiting occur because of expansion of gases in the gastrointestinal tract.

2. Cardiovascular system

Heart rate increases.

3. Respiratory system

Pulmonary blood pressure increases due to increased blood flow. Blood flow increases because of vasodilatation induced by hypoxia. Increased pulmonary blood pressure results in pulmonary edema which causes breathlessness.

4. Nervous system

Symptoms of nervous system are headache, depression, disorientation, irritability, lack of sleep, weakness and fatigue.

Treatment

Treatment depends upon severity of sickness. Symptoms can be reverted by returning to lower altitude or by breathing oxygen. Medical attention is required if symptoms are very severe.

■ ACCLIMATIZATION

Definition

Acclimatization is defined as adaptations or the adjustments by the body in high altitude. While staying at high altitudes for several days to several weeks, a person slowly gets adapted or adjusted to low oxygen tension, so that hypoxic effects are reduced. It enables the person to ascent further.

Changes During Acclimatization

Various changes during acclimatization help the body to cope with the adverse effects of hypoxia at high altitude. Following changes occur in the body during acclimatization.

1. Changes in blood

During acclimatization, the RBC count increases and packed cell volume rises from the normal value of 45% to about 59%. Hemoglobin content in the blood rises from 15 to 20 g%. So, the oxygen carrying capacity of the blood is increased. Thus, more oxygen can be carried to tissues in spite of hypoxia.

Increase in RBC count, packed cell volume and hemoglobin content is due to erythropoietin that is released from juxtaglomerular apparatus of kidney.

2. Changes in cardiovascular system

Overall activity of cardiovascular system is increased in high altitude. There is increase in rate and force of contraction of heart, cardiac output and blood pressure. Hypoxia-induced vasodilatation increases the vascularity in the body. So, blood flow to the vital organs such as heart, brain and muscles increases.

3. Respiratory system

i. Pulmonary ventilation increases up to 65% due to the stimulation of chemoreceptors. This helps the person to ascend several thousand feet.
ii. **Pulmonary hypertension** develops due to increased cardiac output and pulmonary blood flow.
iii. Diffusing capacity of gases increases in the alveoli due to the increase in pulmonary blood flow and pulmonary ventilation. It enables more diffusion of oxygen into blood.

4. Changes in tissues

Both in human beings and animals residing at high altitudes permanently, the cellular oxidative enzymes involved in metabolic reactions are more than in the inhabitants at sea level.

Even when a sea level inhabitant stays at high altitude for certain period, quantity of the oxidative enzymes is not increased. So, the elevation in quantity of oxidative enzymes occurs only in fully acclimatized persons. An increase in the number of mitochondria is observed in these persons.

■ AVIATION PHYSIOLOGY

Aviation physiology is the study of physiological responses of the body in **aviation environment.**

Flying affects the body through **accelerative forces** and **gravitational forces,** which are developed during the **flight maneuvering.** Pilots and other crew members of aircraft are trained to overcome the effects of these forces.

Accelerative Force

Acceleration means **change in velocity**. Flying straight in horizontal plane with constant velocity has minimum effects on the body. However, changes in velocity produce severe physiological effects. Accelerative forces are developed in the flight during linear, radial or centripetal and angular acceleration.

Gravitational Force: G Unit

Gravitational force (G force) is the major factor that develops accelerative force. Force or pull of gravity upon the body is expressed in **G unit**. On the earth, this pull is responsible for body weight. Force of gravity while sitting, standing or lying position is considered to be equal to body weight and it is referred as 1 G. G unit increases in acceleration.

While traveling in an airplane, elevator or a car, if there is a sudden change in speed or direction, the passengers are thrown or centrifuged in opposite direction. It is because of change in the G unit.

G unit is of two types namely G positive and G negative. Increase in G unit is called **positive G** and it occurs while increasing the speed (acceleration). Decrease in G unit is called **negative G** and it occurs while decreasing the speed (slowing down; deceleration). G unit is altered during the change in direction also.

While flying, both positive G and negative G cause physiological changes in the body.

Body can be protected from the effects of G forces, particularly positive G by using abdominal belt and anti-G suit.

■ SPACE PHYSIOLOGY

Space physiology is the study of physiological responses of the body in space and space crafts.

Major differences between the environments of earth and space are atmospheric factors, radiation and gravity. These three factors challenge the human survival in space. Atmospheric factors are atmospheric pressure, temperature, humidity and gas composition.

Spacecraft or **spacelab** is provided with stable and sophisticated environmental control system, which maintains all the atmospheric factors close to earth's environment. **Astronauts** also wear **launch and entry suit (LES)** which is a pressurized suit that protects the body from space environment.

Another factor which affects the body in the space is **weightlessness.** Weightlessness is because of absence of gravity (microgravity).

■ DEEP SEA PHYSIOLOGY

In high altitude, the problem is with low atmospheric (barometric) pressure. In deep sea or mines, the problem is with high barometric pressure. Increased barometric pressure in deep sea produce two major problems:

1. Compression effect on the body and internal organs.
2. Decrease in volume of gases.

■ BAROMETRIC PRESSURE AT DIFFERENT DEPTHS

At sea level, the barometric pressure is 760 mm Hg, which is referred as 1 atmosphere. At the depth of every 33 feet (about 10 m), the pressure increases by 1 atmosphere.

Thus, at the depth of 33 feet, the pressure is 2 atmospheres. It is due to the air above water and the weight of water itself. Pressure at different depths is given in **Table 85.2.**

■ EFFECT OF HIGH BAROMETRIC PRESSURE: NITROGEN NARCOSIS

Narcosis means unconsciousness or **stupor** (lethargy with suppression of sensations and feelings) produced by drugs. **Nitrogen narcosis** means narcotic effect produced by nitrogen at high pressure.

Nitrogen narcosis is common in deep sea divers who breathe **compressed air** (air under high pressure). Breathing compressed air is essential for a deep sea diver or an underwater tunnel worker in order to equalize the surrounding high pressure acting on thoracic wall and abdomen.

TABLE 85.2: Barometric pressure and the effects at different depth.

Depth (feet)	Atmospheric pressure (atmosphere)	Effects on the subject
Sea level	1	–
33	2	–
66	3	–
100	4	Symptoms of nitrogen narcosis appear
133	5	Lack of concentration Becomes jovial and careless
166	6	Starts feeling drowsy
200	7	Feels fatigued and weak Becomes very careless
233	8	Loses power of judgment Unable to do skilled work
266	9	Becomes unconscious

Symptoms of Nitrogen Narcosis

1. First symptom starts appearing at a depth of 120 feet. The person becomes very jovial, careless and does not understand the seriousness of the conditions.
2. At the depth of 150 to 200 feet, the person becomes drowsy.
3. At 200 to 250 feet depth, the person becomes extremely fatigued and weak. There is lack of concentration and judgment. Ability to perform skilled work or movements is also lost.
4. Beyond the depth of 250 feet, the person becomes unconscious **(Table 85.2)**.

Mechanism of Nitrogen Narcosis

Nitrogen is soluble in fat. During compression by high barometric pressure in deep sea, nitrogen escapes from blood vessels and gets dissolved in the fat present in various parts of the body, especially the neuronal membranes. The dissolved nitrogen acts like an anesthetic agent suppressing the neuronal excitability. Nitrogen remains in dissolved form in the fat till the person remains in the deep sea. When the person ascends up, decompression sickness develops.

■ DECOMPRESSION SICKNESS

Definition

Decompression sickness is the disorder that occurs when a person returns rapidly to normal surroundings (atmospheric pressure) from the area of high atmospheric pressure such as deep sea. It is also known as dysbarism, compressed air sickness, caisson disease, bends or diver's palsy.

Causes of Decompression Sickness

High barometric pressure at deep sea leads to compression of gases in the body. Compression reduces the volume of gases.

Among the respiratory gases, oxygen is utilized by tissues. Carbon dioxide can be expired out. But, nitrogen, which is present in high concentration, i.e. 80% is an inert gas. So, it is neither utilized nor expired. When nitrogen is compressed by high atmospheric pressure in deep sea, it escapes from blood vessels and enters the organs. As it is fat soluble, it gets dissolved in the fat of the tissues and tissue fluids. It is very common in the brain tissues.

As long as the person remains in deep sea, nitrogen remains in solution and does not cause any problem. But, if the person ascends rapidly and returns to atmospheric pressure, decompression sickness occurs.

Due to sudden return to atmospheric pressure, the nitrogen is decompressed and escapes from the tissues at a faster rate. Being a gas, it forms **bubbles** while escaping rapidly. The bubbles travel through blood vessels and ducts. In many places, the bubbles obstruct the blood flow and produce air **embolism,** leading to decompression sickness.

Underground tunnel workers who use the **caissons** (pressurized chambers) also develop decompression sickness (**caisson disease**). Pressure in the chamber is increased to prevent the entry of water inside. Decompression sickness also occurs in a person who ascends up rapidly from sea level in an airplane without any precaution.

Symptoms of Decompression Sickness

Symptoms of decompression sickness are

1. Severe pain in tissues, particularly the joints, produced by nitrogen bubbles in the myelin sheath of sensory nerve fibers.
2. Sensation of numbness, tingling or pricking (paresthesia) and itching.
3. Temporary paralysis due to nitrogen bubbles in the myelin sheath of motor nerve fibers.
4. Muscle cramps associated with severe pain.
5. Occlusion of coronary arteries followed by coronary ischemia, caused by bubbles in the blood.
6. Occlusion of blood vessels in brain and spinal cord also.
7. Damage of tissues of brain and spinal cord because of obstruction of blood vessels by the bubbles.
8. Dizziness, paralysis of muscle, shortness of breath and choking.
9. Finally, fatigue, unconsciousness and death.

Prevention of Decompression Sickness

Decompression sickness is prevented by taking proper precautionary measures. While returning to mean sea level, the ascent should be very slow with short stay at regular intervals. Stepwise ascent allows nitrogen to come back to the blood without forming bubbles. It prevents the decompression sickness.

Treatment

If a person is affected by decompression sickness, first **recompression** should be done. It is done by keeping the person in a **recompression chamber**. Then, he is brought back to atmospheric pressure by reducing the pressure slowly. Oxygen therapy may be useful.

Chapter 86: Effects of Exposure to Cold and Heat

CHAPTER OUTLINE

- EFFECTS OF EXPOSURE TO COLD
  - HEAT PRODUCTION
  - PREVENTION OF HEAT LOSS
- EFFECTS OF EXPOSURE TO SEVERE COLD
  - LOSS OF TEMPERATURE REGULATING CAPACITY
- FROSTBITE
- EFFECTS OF EXPOSURE TO HEAT
  - HEAT EXHAUSTION
  - DEHYDRATION EXHAUSTION
  - HEAT CRAMPS
  - HEATSTROKE: SUNSTROKE

EFFECTS OF EXPOSURE TO COLD

During exposure to cold, the body temperature is maintained by two mechanisms:

A. Heat production.
B. Prevention of heat loss.

HEAT PRODUCTION

When the body is exposed to cold, the heat is produced by the following activities.

1. By Accelerating Metabolic Activities

During exposure to cold **heat gain center** in hypothalamus is stimulated. It causes secretion of adrenaline and noradrenaline by activating sympathetic centers. These hormones, especially adrenaline increase heat production by accelerating cellular metabolic activities (Chapter 48).

2. By Shivering

Shivering is the increased **involuntary muscular activity** with slight vibration of the body in response to fear, onset of fever or exposure to cold. Shivering occurs when the body temperature falls to about 25°C (77°F).

During exposure to cold, the heat gain center activates the motor center for shivering situated in posterior hypothalamus leading to shivering. Enormous heat is produced during shivering due to severe muscular activities.

PREVENTION OF HEAT LOSS

When the body is exposed to cold, the heat gain center in hypothalamus is stimulated and it activates the sympathetic centers in posterior hypothalamus resulting in **cutaneous vasoconstriction** and decrease in blood flow. Due to decrease in cutaneous blood flow, sweat secretion is decreased and heat loss is prevented.

EFFECTS OF EXPOSURE TO SEVERE COLD

Exposure of body to severe cold leads to death if quick remedy is not provided. Survival time depends upon the temperature of the environment.

If a person is exposed to ice cold water, i.e. 0°C for 20 to 30 minutes, the body temperature falls below 25°C (77°F) and the person can survive if he is placed immediately in hot water tub with a temperature of 43°C (110°F). The survival time at 9°C (28°F) is about 1 hour and the survival time at 15.5°C (60°F) is about 5 hours.

Effects of exposure of body to extreme cold are:

1. Loss of temperature regulating capacity.
2. Frostbite.

LOSS OF TEMPERATURE REGULATING CAPACITY

Temperature regulating capacity of hypothalamus is affected when the body temperature reduces to about 34.4°C (94°F). Hypothalamus totally loses the power of temperature regulation when body temperature falls below 25°C (77°F). Shivering does not occur.

In addition to loss of hypothalamic function, the metabolic activities are also suppressed. Sleep or coma develops due to depression of the central nervous system.

FROSTBITE

Frostbite is the **freezing** of the surface of the body when it is exposed to cold. It occurs due to sluggishness of blood flow. It mainly affects the exposed areas such as ear lobes and digits of hands and feet. Frostbite is common in mountaineers. Prolonged exposure will lead to permanent damage of the cells followed by thawing and **gangrene** (death and decay of tissues) formation.

■ EFFECTS OF EXPOSURE TO HEAT

Effects of exposure to heat are:

1. Heat exhaustion.
2. Dehydration exhaustion.
3. Heat cramps.
4. Heatstroke: Sunstroke.

■ HEAT EXHAUSTION

Heat exhaustion is the body's response to excess loss of water and salt through sweat caused by exposure to hot environmental conditions. In fact, it is the warning that body is getting too hot. Heat exhaustion results in loss of consciousness and collapse.

■ DEHYDRATION EXHAUSTION

Prolonged exposure to heat results in dehydration. It is due to excess sweating. Dehydration leads to fall in cardiac output, and blood pressure. Collapse occurs if treatment is not given immediately.

■ HEAT CRAMPS

Severe **muscle cramps** (sudden painful involuntary spasmodic contractions of muscles) involving chest, abdomen and legs occur. Cramps are due to reduction in the quantity of salts and water as a result of increased sweating during the continuous exposure to heat.

■ HEATSTROKE: SUNSTROKE

Heatstroke is an abnormal increase in body temperature that occurs during exposure to extreme heat. It is characterized by increase in body temperature above 41°C (106°F) accompanied by some physical and neurological symptoms. Heatstroke is a very severe condition and often becomes fatal if not treated immediately. Hypothalamus loses the power of regulating body temperature.

Sunstroke is the heatstroke that is caused by prolonged exposure to sun during summer in desert or tropical areas.

Features

Common features of heatstroke or sunstroke are:

1. Nausea and vomiting.
2. Dizziness.
3. Headache.
4. Abdominal pain.
5. Difficulty in breathing.
6. Vertigo.
7. Confusion.
8. Muscle cramps and convulsions.
9. Paralysis.
10. Unconsciousness.

If immediate and vigorous treatment is not given, the damage of brain tissues occurs, resulting in coma and death.

Treatment

Person affected by heatstroke or sunstroke must be treated before the damage of organs. The subject should be immediately moved from hot environment and **hospitalized** as soon as possible. Immediate cooling of the body is the usual treatment. The person must be immersed in **cold water** or cold water may be sprayed on the skin. If water supply is not sufficient, cooling the head and neck of the subject should be done first. Ice cubes can be rubbed on head and neck. Ice packs must be kept under armpits and groin. Cooling efforts should be continued till the body temperature falls to about 35°C.

Chapter 87: Artificial Respiration

CHAPTER OUTLINE

- CONDITIONS WHEN ARTIFICIAL RESPIRATION IS REQUIRED
- METHODS OF ARTIFICIAL RESPIRATION
- MANUAL METHODS
- MECHANICAL METHODS

CONDITIONS WHEN ARTIFICIAL RESPIRATION IS REQUIRED

Artificial respiration is required whenever there is arrest of breathing without cardiac failure.

Arrest of breathing occurs in the following conditions:

1. Accidents.
2. Drowning.
3. Gas poisoning.
4. Electric shock.
5. Anesthesia.

Stoppage of oxygen supply for 5 minutes causes **irreversible changes** in tissues of brain, particularly tissues of cerebral cortex. So, the artificial respiration (resuscitation) must be started quickly without any delay, before the development of cardiac failure.

Purpose of artificial respiration is to ventilate the alveoli and to stimulate the respiratory centers.

METHODS OF ARTIFICIAL RESPIRATION

Methods of artificial respiration are of two types:

I. Manual methods.
II. Mechanical methods.

MANUAL METHODS

Manual methods of **resuscitation** (process carried out to revive someone from unconsciousness or apparent death) can be applied quickly without waiting for the availability of any mechanical aids.

Affected person must be provided with clear air. The clothes around neck and chest regions must be loosened. Mouth, face and throat should be cleared off mucus, saliva, foreign particles, etc. Tongue must be drawn forward and, it must be prevented from falling posteriorly which may cause airway obstruction.

Manual methods are of two types:

1. Mouth-to-mouth method.
2. Holger-Nielsen method.

1. Mouth-to-Mouth Method

1. Subject is kept in supine position and the **resuscitator** (person who give resuscitation) kneels at the side of the subject.
2. By keeping the thumb on subject's mouth, the lower jaw is pulled downwards. Nostrils of the subject are closed with thumb and index finger of the other hand.
3. Resuscitator then takes a deep inspiration and exhales into the subject's mouth forcefully. Volume of exhaled air must be twice the normal tidal volume. This expands the subject's lungs **(Fig. 87.1)**.
4. Then, the resuscitator removes his mouth from that of the subject. Now, a passive expiration occurs in the subject due to elastic recoil of the lungs.

This procedure is repeated at a rate of 12 to 14 times a minute, till normal respiration is restored.

Mouth-to-mouth method is the most effective manual method because carbon dioxide in expired air of the resuscitator directly stimulates the respiratory centers and facilitates onset of respiration.

Only disadvantage is that the close contact between the mouths of resuscitator and subject may not be acceptable for various reasons.

Holger-Nielsen Method or Back Pressure Arm Lift Method

1. Subject is placed in prone position with head turned to one side. Hands are placed under the cheeks with flexion at elbow joint and abduction of arms at the

Chapter 87: Artificial Respiration

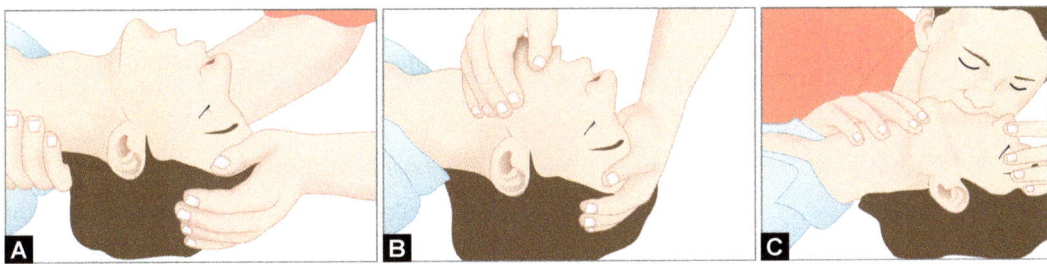

FIGURE 87.1: Mouth-to-mouth method of artificial respiration. **A.** Resuscitator kneels by the side of subject. **B.** Subject's lower jaw is pulled down and nostrils are closed. **C.** Resuscitator takes a deep inspiration and exhales into subject's mouth.
(*Courtesy:* Dr CL Ghai).

shoulders. Resuscitator kneels beside the head of the subject and places the palm of hands over back of the subject.

2. Now, the resuscitator bends forward with straight arms (without flexion at elbow) and applies pressure on the back of the subject. Weight of the resuscitator and pressure on back of the subject compresses his chest and expels air from the lungs.
3. Later, the resuscitator leans back. At the same time, he draws the subject's arm forward by holding it just above elbow **(Fig. 87.2)**.

This procedure causes expansion of thoracic cage and flow of air into the lungs. The movements are repeated at the rate of 12 per minute, till the normal respiration is restored.

■ MECHANICAL METHODS

Mechanical methods of artificial respiration become necessary when the subject needs artificial respiration for long periods. It is essential during the respiratory failure due to paralysis of respiratory muscles or any other cause.

Mechanical methods are of two types:
1. Drinker method.
2. Ventilation method.

1. *Drinker Method*

Drinker respirator is the machine used in this method. It is also called **iron lung chamber** or **tank respirator**. This equipment has an airtight chamber made of iron or steel. The subject is placed inside this chamber with head outside the chamber.

By means of some pumps, the pressure inside the chamber is made positive and negative alternately. During the negative pressure in chamber, the subject's thoracic cage expands and inspiration occurs. And, during positive pressure the expiration occurs.

By using the tank respirator, the patient can survive for a longer time, even up to the period of 1 year till the natural respiratory functions are restored.

2. *Ventilation Method*

A rubber tube is introduced into the trachea of the patient through the mouth. By using a pump, air or oxygen is

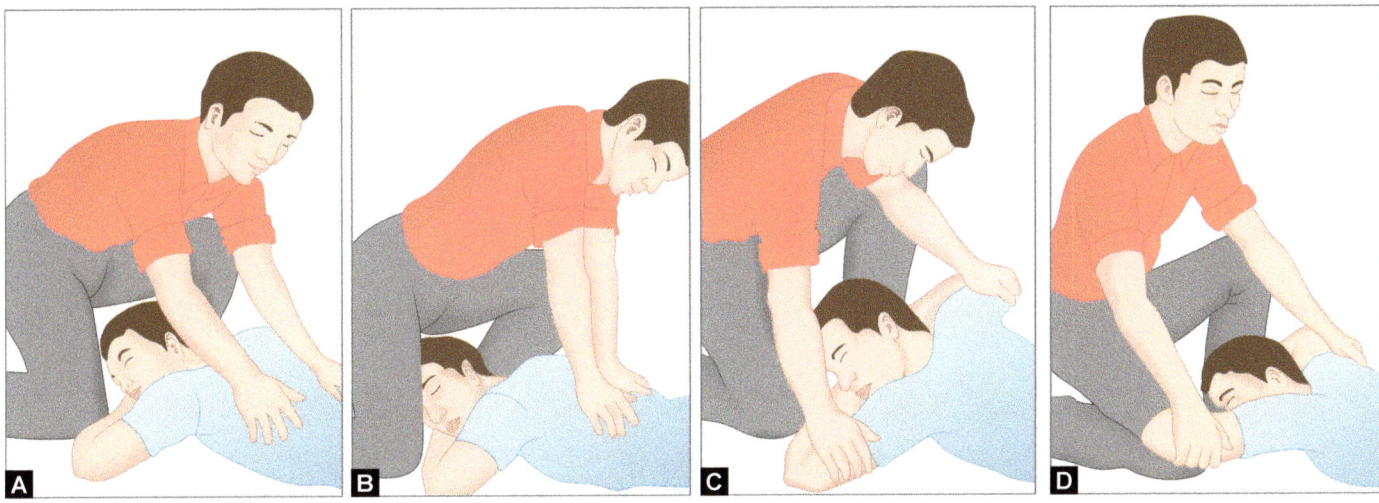

FIGURE 87.2: Holger-Nelsen method of artificial respiration. **A.** Resuscitator places his palms over back of subject. **B.** Applying pressure on back of subject for expiration. **C.** Resuscitator leans back and holds subject's arms. **D.** He draws subject's arms forward for inspiration.
(*Courtesy:* Dr CL Ghai).

pumped into the lungs with pressure intermittently. When air is pumped, inflation of lungs occurs. When it is stopped, expiration occurs and the cycle is repeated.

The apparatus used for ventilation is called ventilator.

Ventilator is of two types:

i. Volume ventilator.
ii. Pressure ventilator.

i. *Volume ventilator*

By volume ventilator, a constant volume of air is pumped into the lungs of patient intermittently with minimum pressure.

ii. *Pressure ventilator*

By pressure ventilator, air is pumped into the lungs of subject with constant high pressure.

Chapter 88: Effects of Exercise on Respiration

CHAPTER OUTLINE

- **EFFECTS OF EXERCISE ON RESPIRATION**
  - **PULMONARY VENTILATION**
  - **DIFFUSING CAPACITY FOR OXYGEN**
  - **CONSUMPTION OF OXYGEN**
- **OXYGEN DEBT**
- **VO$_2$ MAX**
- **RESPIRATORY QUOTIENT**

EFFECTS OF EXERCISE ON RESPIRATION

Muscular exercise brings about many changes on various systems of the body. The degree of changes depends upon the severity of exercise. Refer Chapter 77 for types and severity of exercise.

EFFECT ON PULMONARY VENTILATION

During exercise, **hyperventilation** occurs. In moderate exercise, respiratory rate increases to about 30 per minute and tidal volume increases to about 2,000 mL. Thus, the pulmonary ventilation increases to about 60 L/min during moderate exercise. In severe muscular exercise, it rises further up to 100 L/min.

EFFECT ON DIFFUSING CAPACITY FOR OXYGEN

Diffusing capacity for oxygen is about 21 mL/min/1 mmHg at resting condition. It rises to 45 to 50 mL/min/1 mmHg during moderate exercise due to increase in blood flow through the pulmonary capillaries.

EFFECT ON CONSUMPTION OF OXYGEN

Oxygen consumed by the tissues, particularly the skeletal muscles is greatly enhanced during exercise. Because of vasodilatation in muscles during exercise, more amount of blood flows through the muscles and more amount of oxygen diffuses into the muscles from blood. The amount of oxygen utilized by the muscles is directly proportional to the amount of oxygen available.

OXYGEN DEBT

Oxygen debt is the **extra amount of oxygen** required by the muscles during recovery from severe muscular exercise. After a period of severe muscular exercise, amount of oxygen consumed is greatly increased. Oxygen required is more than the quantity available to the muscle. This much of oxygen is required not only for the activity of the muscle but also for reversal of some metabolic processes such as:

1. Reformation of glucose from lactic acid, accumulated during exercise.
2. Resynthesis of ATP and creatine phosphate.
3. Restoration of amount of oxygen dissociated from hemoglobin and myoglobin.

Thus, for the above reversal phenomena, an extra amount of oxygen must be made available in the body after severe muscular exercise. Oxygen debt is about six times more than the amount of oxygen consumed under resting conditions.

VO$_2$ MAX

VO$_2$ max is the amount of oxygen consumed under maximal aerobic metabolism. It is the product of maximal cardiac output and maximal amount of oxygen consumed by the muscle.

In a normal active and healthy male, the VO$_2$ max is 35 to 40 mL/kg body weight/minute. In females, it is 30 to 35 mL/kg/min.

There is an increase of VO$_2$ max by 50% during exercise.

RESPIRATORY QUOTIENT

Respiratory quotient is the molar ratio of carbon dioxide production to oxygen consumption. Refer Chapter 82 for details.

Respiratory quotient in resting condition is 1.0 and during exercise it increases to 1.5 to 2. However, at the end of exercise, respiratory quotient reduces to 0.5.

MODEL QUESTIONS IN RESPIRATORY SYSTEM AND ENVIRONMENTAL PHYSIOLOGY

■ LONG QUESTIONS

1. Describe lung volumes and capacities. Add a note on their measurement.
2. Give an account of exchange of respiratory gases.
3. Explain the transport of oxygen in blood.
4. Explain the transport of carbon dioxide in blood.
5. Describe the nervous regulation of respiration.
6. Describe the chemical regulation of respiration.
7. What is hypoxia? Describe the types, causes and effects of hypoxia. Add a note on oxygen therapy.
8. Describe changes in the body at high altitude and explain the acclimatization.
9. Describe in detail the respiratory and cardiovascular changes during exercise.

■ SHORT QUESTIONS

1. Respiratory unit.
2. Nonrespiratory functions of respiratory tract.
3. Salient features of pulmonary circulation.
4. Respiratory pressures.
5. Compliance.
6. Work of breathing.
7. Lung volumes/capacities.
8. Dead space.
9. Oxygen hemoglobin dissociation curve.
10. Carbon dioxide dissociation curve.
11. Exchange of gases between alveoli and blood.
12. Exchange of gases between blood and tissues.
13. Respiratory centers.
14. Chemoreceptors.
15. Hypoxia.
16. Asphyxia.
17. Periodic breathing.
18. Mountain sickness.
19. Acclimatization.
20. Decompression sickness.
21. Effects of sudden exposure to cold.
22. Effects of sudden exposure to heat.
23. Heatstroke or sunstroke.
24. Artificial respiration.
25. Respiratory changes during exercise.

■ VERY SHORT ANSWER QUESTIONS

1. Types and phases of respiration.
2. Upper and lower respiratory tract.
3. Intrapleural cavity and intrapleural fluid.
4. Tracheobronchial tree.
5. Role of lungs in defense mechanism.
6. Role of lungs in acid-base balance.
7. Cough reflex.
8. Sneezing reflex.
9. Pulmonary blood vessels.
10. Physiological shunt and physiological dead space.
11. Pulmonary blood pressure.
12. Respiratory muscles.
13. Pump handle and bucket handle movements.
14. Surfactant.
15. Respiratory distress syndrome.
16. intrapleural and intra-alveolar pressure.
17. Any one lung volume/lung capacity.
18. Vital capacity.
19. Forced expiratory volume or timed vital capacity.
20. Respiratory minute volume.
21. Maximum breathing capacity or maximum ventilation volume.
22. Peak expiratory flow meter.
23. Define ventilation and describe pulmonary ventilation and alveolar ventilation.
24. Ventilation-perfusion ratio.
25. Composition of inspired air, alveolar air and expired air.
26. Differences between inspired air and alveolar air.
27. Respiratory membrane.
28. Diffusion capacity and factors affecting it.
29. P_{50}.
30. Oxygen carrying capacity of hemoglobin and blood.
31. What is indicated by shift to the right of oxygen hemoglobin dissociation curve? Name some of the factors causing it.
32. What is indicated by shift to the left of oxygen hemoglobin dissociation curve? Name some of the factors causing it.
33. Chloride shift or Hamburger phenomenon.
34. Reverse chloride shift.
35. Bohr effect.
36. Haldane effect.
37. Any one respiratory center.
38. Inspiratory ramp.
39. Hering-Breuer reflex.
40. Different types of receptors in lungs which alter the respiration.
41. Apnea.
42. Characteristic features of different types of hypoxia.
43. Oxygen toxicity.
44. Dyspnea.
45. Cheyne-Stokes breathing/Biot breathing.
46. Pneumothorax/Hydrothorax/Hemothorax/Pyothorax.
47. Pneumonia.
48. Pulmonary edema.
49. Pleural effusion.
50. Nitrogen narcosis.
51. Frostbite.
52. Ventilator.
53. VO_2 max.
54. Fetal respiration and first breath.

SECTION 10: NERVOUS SYSTEM

CHAPTER 89: Overview of Nervous System

CHAPTER OUTLINE
- DIVISIONS OF NERVOUS SYSTEM
- CENTRAL NERVOUS SYSTEM
- PERIPHERAL NERVOUS SYSTEM

DIVISIONS OF NERVOUS SYSTEM

Nervous system controls all the activities of the body. It is quicker than the other control system in the body namely, endocrine system.

Nervous system is divided into two parts:

I. Central nervous system.
II. Peripheral nervous system.

CENTRAL NERVOUS SYSTEM

Central nervous system (CNS) includes **brain** and **spinal cord**. It is formed by **neurons** and the supporting cells called **neuroglia**. Structures of brain and spinal cord are arranged in two layers namely, the gray matter and white matter. **Gray matter** is formed by nerve cell bodies and proximal parts of nerve fibers arising from the nerve cell body. **White matter** is formed by nerve fibers.

In brain, white matter is in inner part and gray matter is placed in the outer part. In spinal cord, white matter is placed in the outer part and gray matter is in inner part.

Brain is situated in the skull. It is continued as spinal cord in the vertebral canal through the **foramen magnum** of the skull bone. Brain and spinal cord are surrounded by three layers of meninges called the outer **dura mater**, middle **arachnoid mater** and inner **pia mater**. The space between the arachnoid mater and pia mater is known as **subarachnoid space**. This space is filled with a fluid called **cerebrospinal fluid (CSF)**. Both, the brain and spinal cord are actually suspended in CSF. Important parts of brain and segments of the spinal cord are shown in **Figure 89.1**.

Parts of Brain

Brain consists of three major divisions:

1. Prosencephalon.
2. Mesencephalon.
3. Rhombencephalon.

1. **Prosencephalon**

Prosencephalon or **forebrain** is subdivided into two parts:

i. **Telencephalon** which includes cerebral hemispheres, basal ganglia, hippocampus and amygdaloid nucleus.
ii. **Diencephalon** which consists of thalamus, hypothalamus, metathalamus and subthalamus.

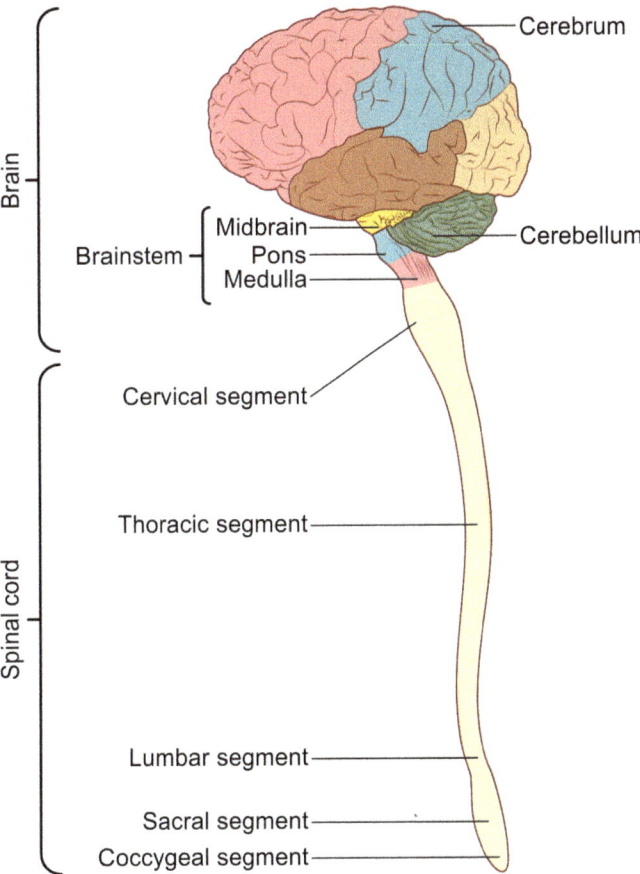

FIGURE 89.1: Parts of central nervous system.

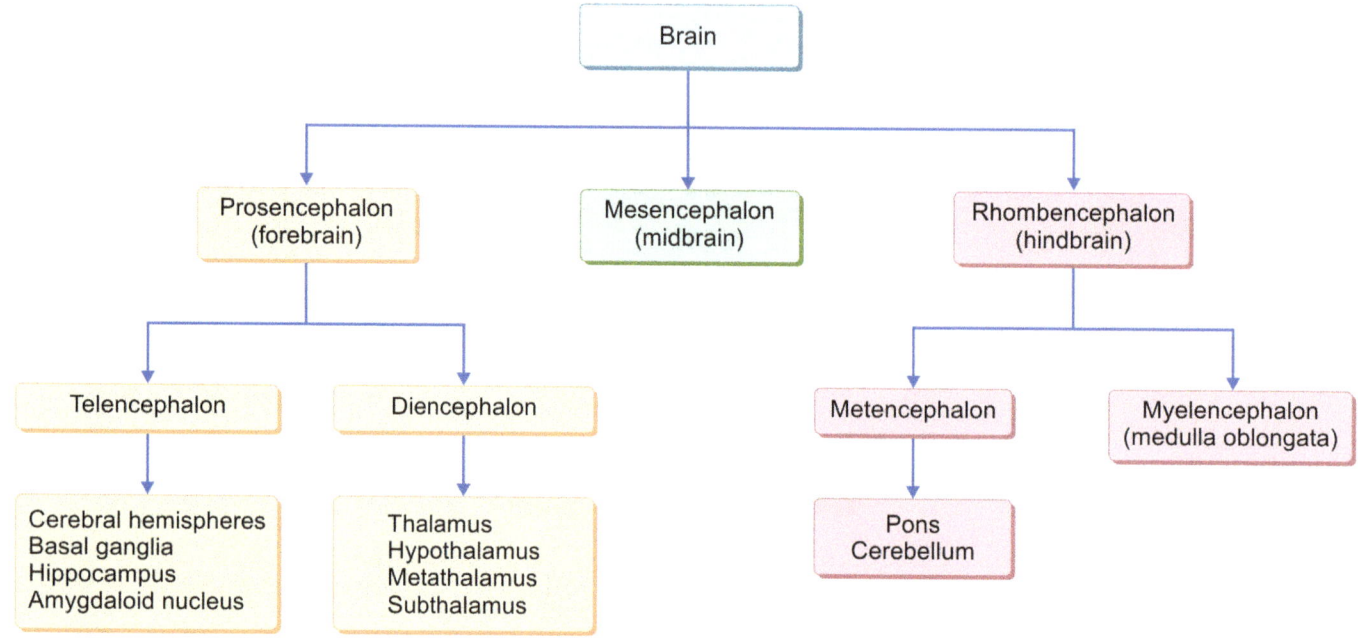

FIGURE 89.2: Parts of brain.

2. Mesencephalon

Mesencephalon is also known as **midbrain**.

3. Rhombencephalon

Rhombencephalon or **hindbrain** is subdivided into two portions:

i. **Metencephalon** formed by pons and cerebellum.
ii. **Myelencephalon** or medulla oblongata **(Fig. 89.2)**.

Midbrain, pons and medulla oblongata are together called the **brainstem**.

■ PERIPHERAL NERVOUS SYSTEM

Peripheral nervous system (PNS) is formed by the neurons and their processes present in all regions of the body. It consists of cranial nerves arising from brain and spinal nerves arising from the spinal cord. It is again divided into two subdivisions:

1. Somatic nervous system.
2. Autonomic nervous system.

1. Somatic Nervous System

Somatic nervous system is concerned with **somatic functions**. It includes the nerves supplying the skeletal muscles. Somatic nervous system controls the movements of the body by acting on skeletal muscles **(Fig. 89.3)**.

2. Autonomic Nervous System

Autonomic nervous system is concerned with regulation of visceral or vegetative functions. So, it is otherwise called **visceral** or **vegetative** or **involuntary** nervous system.

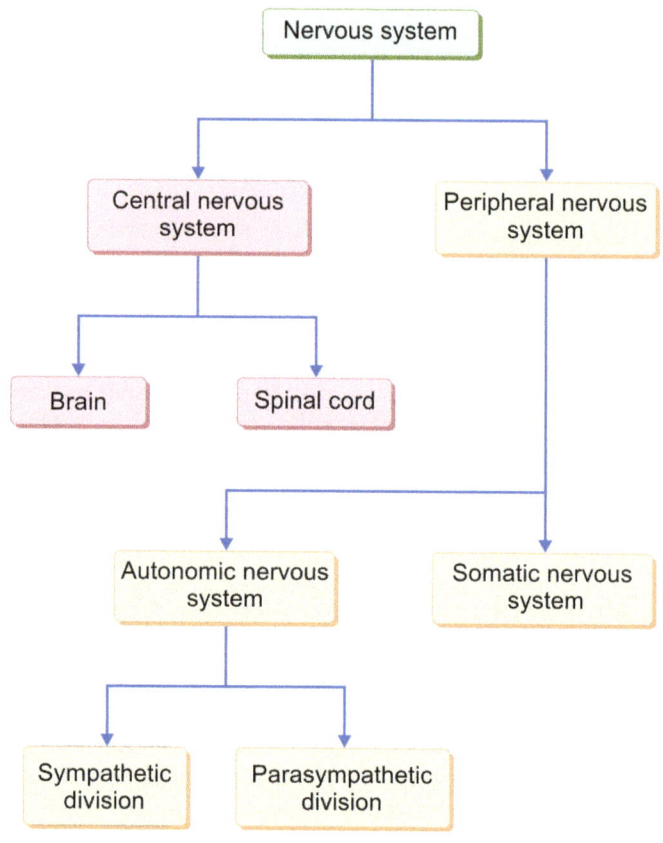

FIGURE 89.3: Organization of nervous system.

Autonomic nervous system consists of two divisions:

i. Sympathetic division.
ii. Parasympathetic division.

Chapter 90

Neuron and Neuroglia

CHAPTER OUTLINE

- **NEURON**
  - CLASSIFICATION
  - STRUCTURE
  - NEUROTROPHINS: NEUROTROPHIC FACTORS
- **CLASSIFICATION OF NERVE FIBERS**
  - DEPENDING UPON STRUCTURE
  - DEPENDING UPON DISTRIBUTION
  - DEPENDING UPON ORIGIN
  - DEPENDING UPON FUNCTION
  - DEPENDING UPON SECRETION OF NEUROTRANSMITTER
  - DEPENDING UPON DIAMETER AND CONDUCTION OF IMPULSE
- **PROPERTIES OF NERVE FIBERS**
  - EXCITABILITY
  - CONDUCTIVITY
  - REFRACTORY PERIOD
- **SUMMATION**
- **ADAPTATION**
- **INFATIGABILITY**
- **ALL-OR-NONE LAW**
- **DEGENERATION OF NERVE FIBERS**
  - DEGREES OF INJURY
  - DEGENERATIVE CHANGES
  - WALLERIAN DEGENERATION
  - RETROGRADE DEGENERATION
  - TRANSNEURONAL DEGENERATION
- **REGENERATION OF NERVE FIBER**
  - CRITERIA FOR REGENERATION
  - STAGES OF REGENERATION
- **NEUROGLIA**
  - DEFINITION
  - CLASSIFICATION
  - FUNCTIONS

■ NEURON

Neuron or nerve cell is defined as the structural and functional unit of the nervous system. Like any other cell in the body, neuron has nucleus and all the organelles in the cytoplasm. However, it is different from other cells by two ways:

1. Neuron has branches or processes called **axon** and **dendrites**.
2. Neuron has **no centrosome**. So, it cannot undergo division.

■ CLASSIFICATION OF NEURON

Neurons are classified by three different methods:

I. Depending upon number of poles.
II. Depending upon function.
III. Depending upon length of the axon.

I. Classification Depending upon Number of Poles

Based on the number of poles from which the nerve fibers arise, neurons are divided into three types:

1. **Unipolar neurons** that have only **one pole** from which, both the axon and dendrite arise **(Fig. 90.1)**.

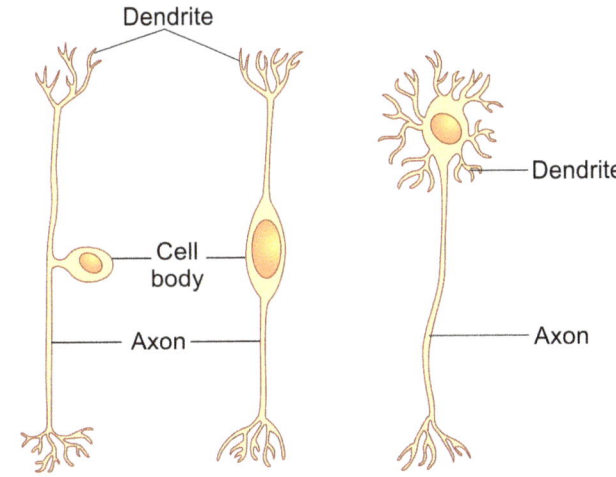

FIGURE 90.1: Types of neuron.

2. **Bipolar neurons** which have **two poles**. Axon arises from one pole and dendrites arise from the other pole.
3. **Multipolar neurons** which have **many poles**. One of the poles gives rise to axon and, all other poles give rise to dendrites.

II. *Classification Depending upon Function*

On the basis of function, the nerve cells are classified into two types:

1. **Motor** or **efferent neurons** which carry the **motor impulses** from central nervous system to the peripheral effector organs such as muscles, glands, blood vessels, etc.
2. **Sensory** or **afferent neurons** which carry the **sensory impulses** from periphery to the central nervous system.

III. *Classification Depending upon Length of Axon*

Depending upon the length of axon, neurons are divided into two types:

1. **Golgi type I neurons** that have **long axons**. Cell body of these neurons is in central nervous system and their axons leave the central nervous system and reach the remote peripheral organs.
2. **Golgi type II neurons** that have **short axons**. These neurons are present in large numbers in cerebral cortex and cerebellar cortex.

■ STRUCTURE OF NEURON

Each neuron is made up of three parts:

1. Nerve cell body.
2. Dendrite.
3. Axon.

Dendrite and axon together form the **processes of neuron (Fig. 90.2)**. In general, the dendrites are short processes and the axons are long processes. The dendrites and axons are usually called **nerve fibers**.

1. *Nerve Cell Body*

Nerve cell body is also known as **soma** or **perikaryon**. It is irregular in shape and, it is constituted by a mass of cytoplasm called **neuroplasm** which is covered by a cell membrane. Neuroplasm contains a large nucleus, Nissl bodies, neurofibrils, mitochondria and Golgi apparatus. Nissl bodies and neurofibrils are found only in nerve cell and not in other cells.

Centrioles are absent in nerve cell. So, the nerve cell cannot multiply with other cells of the body.

Nucleus

Each neuron has one nucleus which is centrally placed in the nerve cell body. Nucleus has one or two prominent nucleoli.

Nissl bodies or Nissl granules

Nissl bodies are small basophilic granules found in neuroplasm of neurons and are named after the discoverer. These bodies are present in the soma **except axon hillock**. Nissl bodies are called **tigroid substances** since these bodies are responsible for the spotted or **tigroid appearance** of soma after suitable staining. Nissl granules flow into the dendrites from soma, but not into axon. So, the dendrites are distinguished from axons by the presence of Nissl granules under microscope.

Nissl bodies are membranous organelles containing ribosomes. So, these bodies are concerned with synthesis of proteins in the soma of neurons. The proteins formed in soma are transported to the axon by **axonal flow**.

Neurofibrils

Neurofibrils are thread-like structures present in the form of network in the soma and the nerve processes. Presence of neurofibrils is another characteristic feature of the neurons.

Mitochondria

Mitochondria are present in the soma and in axon. As in other cells, mitochondria form the **powerhouse** of nerve cell, where ATP is produced (Chapter 1).

Golgi apparatus

Golgi apparatus of the nerve cell body is similar to that of other cells. It is concerned with processing and packaging of proteins into granules (Chapter 1).

2. *Dendrite of Neuron*

Dendrite is the **branched process** of the neuron and it is branched repeatedly. Dendrite may be present or absent. If present, it may be one or many in number. Dendrite has Nissl granules and neurofibrils.

Dendrite is conductive in nature. It transmits impulses towards the nerve cell body.

3. *Axon of Neuron*

Axon is longer than dendrite. Each neuron has only one axon. Axon arises from **axon hillock** of the nerve cell body. Axon extends for a long distance away from the nerve cell body. Length of the longest axon is about 1 meter.

Organization of nerve

Many axons together form a bundle called **fasciculus**. Many fasciculi together form a **nerve**.

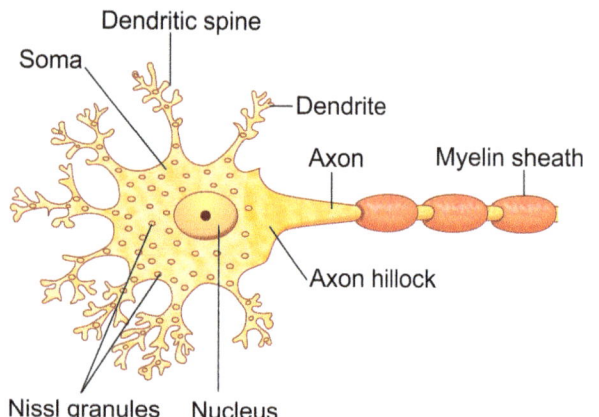

FIGURE 90.2: Structure of a neuron.

Coverings of nerve

Whole nerve is covered by tubular sheath, called **epineurium**. Each fasciculus is covered by **perineurium** and each nerve fiber (axon) is covered by **endoneurium** (Fig. 90.3).

Internal structure of axon: Axis cylinder

Axon has a long central core of cytoplasm called **axoplasm**. Axoplasm is covered by the tubular sheath like membrane called **axolemma** which is the continuation of the cell membrane of nerve cell body. The axoplasm along with axolemma is called the **axis cylinder** of the nerve fiber (Fig. 90.4).

Axoplasm contains mitochondria, neurofibrils and axoplasmic vesicles. But Nissl bodies are absent in the axon. Axis cylinder of the nerve fiber is covered by a membrane called **neurilemma** (see below).

Non-myelinated nerve fiber

Nerve fiber described above is the non-myelinated nerve fiber which is not covered by myelin sheath.

Myelinated nerve fiber

Nerve fibers which are insulated by myelin sheath are called myelinated nerve fibers.

Myelin Sheath

Myelin sheath is a thick **lipoprotein** sheath that insulates the myelinated nerve fiber. Myelin sheath is not a continuous sheath. It is absent at regular intervals. The area where the myelin sheath is absent is called **node of Ranvier**. The segment of the nerve fiber between two nodes is called **internode**. Myelin sheath is responsible for white color of the nerve fibers.

Chemistry of myelin sheath

Myelin sheath is formed by concentric layers of proteins alternating with lipids. The lipids are cholesterol, lecithin and cerebroside (sphingomyelin).

Formation of myelin sheath: Myelinogenesis

Formation of myelin sheath around the axon is called the myelinogenesis. It is formed by **Schwann cells** in neurilemma.

Functions of myelin sheath

1. *Faster conduction:* Myelin sheath is responsible for **faster conduction** of impulse through the nerve fibers. In the myelinated nerve fibers, the impulses jump from one node to another node by **saltatory conduction** (see below).
2. *Insulating capacity:* Myelin sheath has a high insulating capacity. Because of this quality, the myelin sheath restricts the nerve impulse within the single nerve fiber, and prevents the stimulation of neighboring nerve fibers.

Neurilemma or Sheath of Schwann

Neurilemma is a thin membrane which surrounds the axis cylinder. It is also called **neurilemmal sheath** or **sheath of Schwann**. It contains **Schwann cells**, which have flattened and elongated nuclei. The cytoplasm is thin and modified to form the thin sheath of neurilemma.

One nucleus is present in each internode of the axon. Nucleus is situated between myelin sheath and neurilemma.

In non-myelinated nerve fiber, the neurilemma continuously surrounds axolemma. In myelinated nerve fiber, it covers the myelin sheath. At the node of Ranvier (where myelin sheath is absent), the neurilemma invaginates and runs up to axolemma in the form of a finger like process.

Functions of neurilemma

In non-myelinated nerve fiber, the neurilemma serves as a covering membrane. In myelinated nerve fiber, it

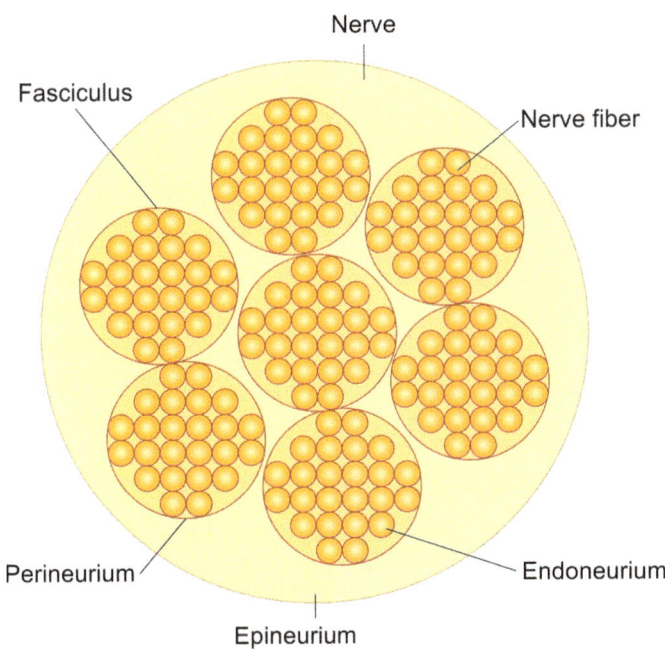

FIGURE 90.3: Cross-section of a nerve.

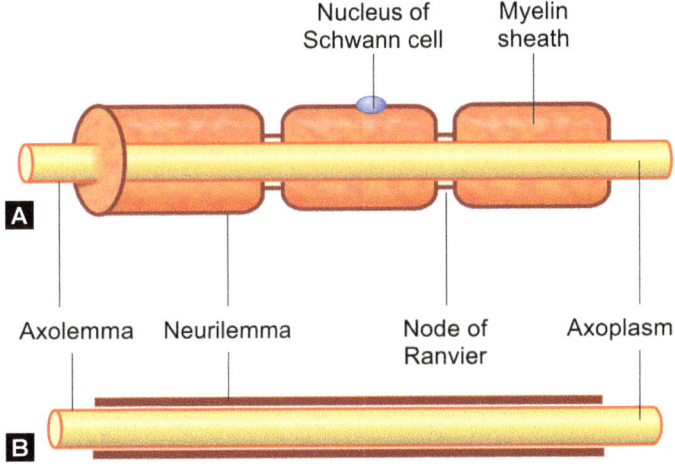

FIGURE 90.4: A. Myelinated nerve fiber. B. Non-myelinated nerve fiber.

is necessary for **myelinogenesis** (formation of myelin sheath).

NEUROTROPHINS: NEUROTROPHIC FACTORS

Neurotrophins or neurotrophic factors are the protein substances, which play important role in growth and functioning of nervous tissue.

Source of Secretion of Neurotrophins

Neurotrophins are secreted by many tissues in the body, particularly **muscles**, **neurons** and neuroglial cells called **astrocytes.**

Functions of Neurotrophins

Neurotrophins:

1. Facilitate initial growth and development of nerve cells in central and peripheral nervous system.
2. Promote survival and repair of the nerve cells.
3. Play an important role in the maintenance of nervous tissue and neural transmission.

Commercial preparations of neurotrophins are used for the treatment of neural diseases.

Types of Neurotrophins

Many types of neurotophic factors are identified.

Nerve growth factor

Nerve growth factor (NGF) is the first neurotrophin protein substance identified as neurotrophin. It is found in many tissues. It promotes early growth and development of neurons.

Commercial preparation of NGF extracted from animals is used to treat many nervous disorders such as Alzheimer's disease, neuron degeneration in aging and neuron regeneration in spinal cord injury.

Other neurotrophins

1. Brain-derived neurotrophic factor (BDNF) found in brain and human sperm.
2. Ciliary neurotrophic factor (CNTF).
3. Glial cell line-derived neurotrophic factor (GDNF).
4. Fibroblast growth factor (FGF).
5. Neurotrophin-3, 4 and 5 (NT-3, NT-4 and NT-5).

CLASSIFICATION OF NERVE FIBERS

Nerve fibers are classified by different methods. The basis of classification differs in each method. Nerve fibers are classified by six methods.

1. CLASSIFICATION DEPENDING UPON STRUCTURE

Based on the structure, the nerve fibers are classified into two types:

i. **Myelinated nerve fibers** that are covered by myelin sheath.
ii. **Non-myelinated nerve fibers** which are not covered by myelin sheath.

2. CLASSIFICATION DEPENDING UPON DISTRIBUTION

Nerve fibers are classified into two types on the basis of the distribution:

i. **Somatic nerve fibers** which supply the skeletal muscles of the body.
ii. **Visceral** or **autonomic nerve fibers** which supply internal organs of the body.

3. CLASSIFICATION DEPENDING UPON ORIGIN

On the basis of origin, the nerve fibers are divided into two types:

i. **Cranial nerves** arising from **brain**.
ii. **Spinal nerves** arising from **spinal cord**.

4. CLASSIFICATION DEPENDING UPON FUNCTION

On the basis of functions, the nerve fibers are of two types:

i. **Sensory** or **afferent nerve fibers** which carry **sensory impulses** from different parts of the body to the central nervous system.
ii. **Motor** or **efferent nerve fibers** which carry **motor impulses** from central nervous system to different parts of the body **(Box 90.1)**.

5. CLASSIFICATION DEPENDING UPON SECRETION OF NEUROTRANSMITTER

Depending upon the neurotransmitter substance secreted the nerve fibers are divided into two types:

i. Adrenergic nerve fibers that secrete **noradrenaline**.
ii. Cholinergic nerve fibers that secrete **acetylcholine**.

6. CLASSIFICATION DEPENDING UPON DIAMETER AND CONDUCTION OF IMPULSE: ERLANGER-GASSER CLASSIFICATION

Erlanger and Gasser classified the nerve fibers into three major types on the basis of diameter of the fibers and the rate of conduction of impulses:

i. Type A nerve fibers.
ii. Type B nerve fibers.
iii. Type C nerve fibers.

Among these fibers, type A nerve fibers are the **thickest fibers** and type C nerve fibers are the **thinnest fibers**. Type A nerve fibers are divided into four subtypes. Except 'C' type of fibers, all the nerve fibers are myelinated.

BOX 90.1: Efferent and afferent nerve fibers.

Efferent nerve fiber
Carry motor information from central nervous system to different parts of the body
Afferent nerve fiber
Carry sensory information from different parts of the body to central nervous system

Velocity of impulse through a nerve fiber is directly proportional to the **thickness** of the fibers.

Different types of nerve fibers along with diameter and velocity of conduction are given in the **Table 90.1**.

■ PROPERTIES OF NERVE FIBERS
■ EXCITABILITY

Excitability is defined as the **physiochemical change** that occurs in a tissue when a stimulus is applied.

Stimulus is defined as an external agent, which produces excitability in the tissues. When the nerve fiber is stimulated action potential develops.

Response to Stimulus

When a nerve fiber is stimulated, based on the strength of stimulus, two types of response develop.

1. Action potential or nerve impulse.
2. Electrotonic potential or local potential

Action Potential or Nerve Impulse

Action potential or nerve impulse develops in a nerve fiber when it is stimulated by a stimulus with adequate strength. Adequate strength of stimulus, necessary for producing the action potential in a nerve fiber is known as **threshold** or **minimal stimulus**. Action potential is **propagated**.

Action potential in a nerve fiber is similar to that in a muscle, except for some minor differences **(Table 90.2)**. The action potential in a skeletal muscle fiber is described in Chapter 27.

Resting membrane potential in the nerve fiber is – 70 mV. The firing level is at – 55 mV. Depolarization ends at + 35 mV **(Fig. 90.5)**. Usually, the action potential starts in the initial segment of nerve fiber.

Electrotonic Potential or Local Potential

When the stimulus with **subliminal strength** is applied, only electrotonic potential develops and the action potential does not develop. Electrotonic potential is **non-propagated**.

TABLE 90.2: Differences in electrical potentials between nerve fiber and skeletal muscle fiber.

Event	Nerve fiber	Skeletal muscle fiber
Resting membrane potential	– 70 mV	– 90 mV
Firing level	– 55 mV	– 75 mV
End of depolarization	+ 35 mV	+ 55 mV

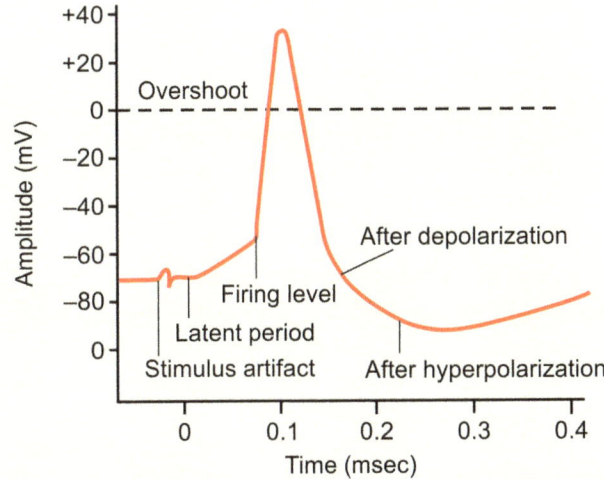

FIGURE 90.5: Action potential in nerve fiber.

Cathelectrotonic and anelectrotonic potentials

While recording electrical potential in a nerve fiber, two electrodes, namely **cathode** and **anode** are used. Potential change that is produced at cathode is called cathelectrotonic potential. Potential that is developed at anode is known as anelectrotonic potential.

Only the cathelectrotonic potential can be transformed into action potential or electrotonic potential.

■ CONDUCTIVITY

Conductivity is the ability of nerve fibers to transmit the impulse from area of stimulation to the other areas. Action potential is transmitted through the nerve fiber as

TABLE 90.1: Types of nerve fibers.

Type	Structure	Diameter (μ)	Velocity of conduction (m/sec)	Functions
A alpha	Large with thick myelin sheath	12 to 24	70 to 120	Sensory fibers from proprioceptors and touch receptors Motor fibers to skeletal muscle
A beta	Medium with thick myelin sheath	6 to 12	30 to 70	Sensory fibers from proprioceptors, touch receptors and pressure receptors
A gamma	Medium with thick myelin sheath	5 to 6	15 to 30	Motor to muscle spindle
A delta	Medium with thin myelin sheath	2 to 5	12 to 15	Sensory fibers from pain (fast) receptors and temperature receptors
B	Small with thin myelin sheath	1 to 2	3 to 10	Preganglionic autonomic fibers
C	Small without myelin sheath	<1.5	0.5 to 2	Sensory from pain (slow) and temperature receptors Postganglionic autonomic fibers

nerve impulse. Normally in the body, action potential is transmitted through the nerve fiber in only **one direction**.

Mechanism of Conduction of Action Potential

Depolarization occurs first at the site of stimulation in the nerve fiber. It causes depolarization of the neighboring areas. Like this, depolarization travels throughout the nerve fiber. Depolarization is followed by **repolarization**.

Conduction Through Myelinated Nerve Fiber: Saltatory Conduction

Saltatory conduction is a form of conduction of nerve impulse in which the impulse jumps from one node to another. Conduction of impulse through a myelinated nerve fiber is about 50 times faster than through a nonmyelinated fiber. It is because the action potential jumps from one node to another **node of Ranvier** instead of travelling through the entire nerve fiber **(Fig. 90.6)**.

Mechanism of saltatory conduction

Myelin sheath is not permeable to ions. So, the entry of sodium from extracellular fluid into nerve fiber occurs only in the node of Ranvier, where the myelin sheath is absent. It causes depolarization in the node, and not in the internode. Thus, the depolarization occurs at **successive nodes**. So, the action potential jumps from one node to another. Hence, it is called saltatory conduction (saltare = jumping).

■ REFRACTORY PERIOD

Refractory period is the period at which the nerve does not give any response to a stimulus. Refractory period is of two types.

1. Absolute Refractory Period

Absolute refractory period is the period during which the nerve does not show any response at all, whatever may be the strength of stimulus.

2. Relative Refractory Period

It is the period, during which the nerve fiber shows response, if the strength of stimulus is increased to maximum.

Absolute refractory period corresponds to the period from the time when firing level is reached till the time when 1/3 of repolarization is completed. Relative refractory period extends through rest of the repolarization period.

■ SUMMATION

One **subliminal stimulus** does not produce any response in the nerve fiber because the subliminal stimulus is very weak. However, if two or more subliminal stimuli are applied within a short interval of about 0.5 msec, the response is produced. It is because the subliminal stimuli are summed up together to become strong enough to produce the response. This phenomenon is known as summation.

■ ADAPTATION

While stimulating a nerve fiber continuously, excitability of the nerve fiber is greater in the beginning. Later the response decreases slowly and finally the nerve fiber does not show any response at all. This phenomenon is known as adaptation or **accommodation**.

Causes for adaptation are:

1. When a nerve fiber is stimulated continuously, depolarization occurs continuously.
2. Continuous depolarization inactivates the sodium pump and increases the efflux of potassium ions.

■ INFATIGABILITY

A nerve fiber cannot be fatigued, even if it is stimulated continuously for a long time. Reason for this is the nerve fiber can conduct only **one action potential** at a time. At that time, it is completely **refractory** and does not conduct another action potential.

■ ALL-OR-NONE LAW

All-or-none law states that when a nerve is stimulated by a stimulus it gives maximum response or does not give response at all. Refer Chapter 65 for more details of all-or-none law.

■ DEGENERATION OF NERVE FIBERS

When a nerve fiber is injured, various changes occur in the nerve fiber and nerve cell body. All these changes are together called the **degenerative changes**.

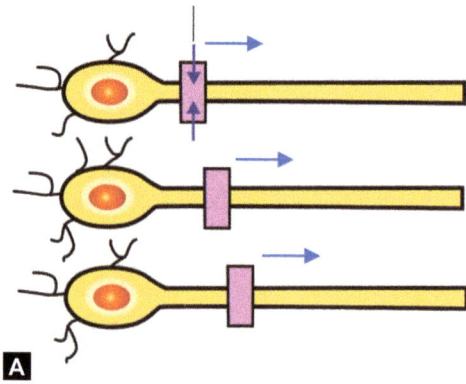

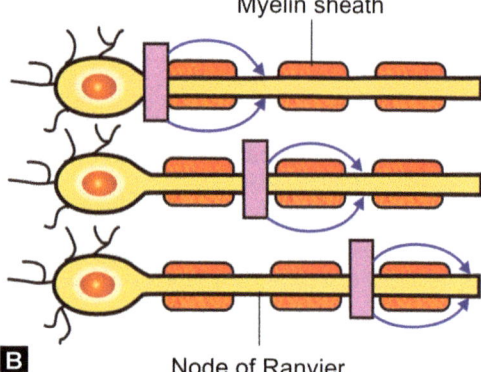

FIGURE 90.6: Mode of conduction through nerve fibers. **A.** Non-myelinated nerve fiber: Continuous conduction. **B.** Myelinated nerve fiber: Saltatory conduction (impulse jumps from node to node).

AP = Action potential.

Causes for Injury

Injury to a nerve fiber occurs due to following causes:

1. Obstruction of blood flow.
2. Local injection of toxic substances.
3. Crushing of nerve fiber.
4. Transection of nerve fiber.

■ DEGREES OF INJURY

According to **Sunderland**, injury to nerve fibers is classified into five types depending upon the order of **severity**.

First Degree Injury

First degree injury is very common type of injury. It is caused by pressure applied over a nerve for a short period leading to occlusion of blood flow and hypoxia. Axon loses the function temporarily for a short time, which is called **conduction block**. The function returns within few hours to few weeks. First degree of injury is called **Seddon neuropraxia**.

Second Degree Injury

Second degree is due to the prolonged severe pressure, which causes **Wallerian degeneration** (see below). However, the endoneurium is intact. Repair and restoration of function take about 18 months. Second degree of injury is called **axonotmesis**.

Third Degree Injury

In this case, the **endoneurium** is interrupted. Epineurium and perineurium are intact. After degeneration, the recovery is slow and poor or incomplete. Third, fourth and fifth degrees of injury are called **neurotmesis**.

Fourth Degree Injury

This type of injury is more severe. Epineurium and perineurium are also interrupted. Fasciculi of nerve fibers are disturbed and disorganized. Regeneration is poor or incomplete.

Fifth Degree Injury

Fifth degree of injury involves **complete transaction** of the nerve trunk with loss of continuity. Useful regeneration is not possible unless the cut ends are rearranged and approximated quickly by surgery.

■ DEGENERATIVE CHANGES IN NEURON

Degeneration means deterioration or impairment or pathological changes of an injured tissue. When a peripheral nerve fiber is injured, the degenerative changes occur in the nerve cell body and the nerve fiber of same neuron and the adjoining neuron.

Accordingly, the degenerative changes are classified into three types:

1. Wallerian degeneration.
2. Retrograde degeneration.
3. Transneural degeneration.

■ 1. WALLERIAN OR ORTHOGRADE DEGENERATION

Wallerian or orthograde degeneration is the pathological change that occurs in the distal cut end of nerve fiber (axon). It is named after the discoverer **Waller**. Wallerian degeneration starts within 24 hours of injury. The change occurs throughout the length of distal part of nerve fiber simultaneously.

Changes in nerve

i. Axis cylinder swells and breaks up into small pieces. After few days, the broken pieces appear as debris in the space occupied by axis cylinder (**Fig. 90.7**).
ii. Myelin sheath is slowly disintegrated into fat droplets. The changes in myelin sheath occur from 8th to 35th day.
iii. Neurilemmal sheath is unaffected, but the Schwann cells multiply rapidly. The macrophages invade from outside. Macrophages remove the debris of axis

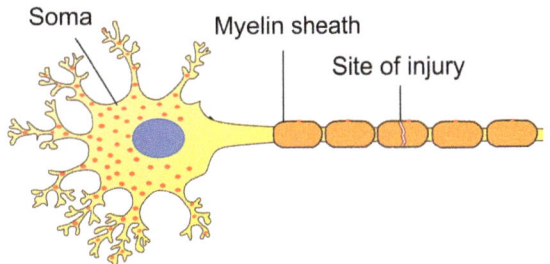

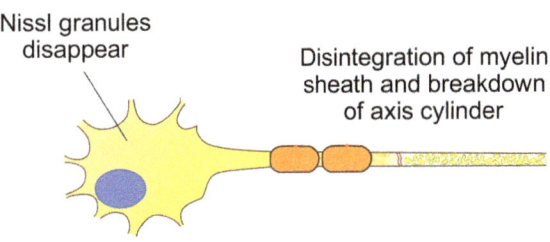

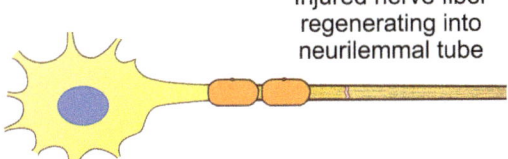

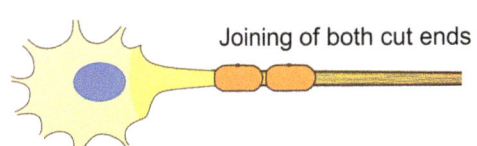

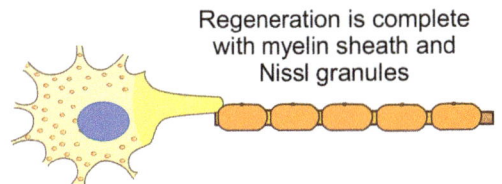

FIGURE 90.7: Degeneration and regeneration of nerve fiber.

cylinder and the fat droplets of disintegrated myelin sheath.

iv. So, the neurilemmal tube becomes empty. Later it is filled by the cytoplasm of Schwann cell. All these changes take place for about 2 months from the day of injury.

■ 2. RETROGRADE DEGENERATION

Retrograde degeneration is the pathological changes which occur in the nerve cell body and axon proximal to the cut end.

Changes in nerve cell body

Changes in the nerve cell body commence within 48 hours after the section of nerve.

Changes in nerve cell body are:

i. First, Nissl granules disintegrate into fragments by **chromatolysis**.
ii. Golgi apparatus is disintegrated.
iii. Nerve cell body swells due to accumulation of fluid and becomes round.
iv. Neurofibrils disappear followed by displacement of the nucleus towards the periphery.
v. Sometimes, the nucleus is extruded out of the cell. In this case, death of the neuron occurs and regeneration of the injured nerve is not possible.

Changes in axon proximal to cut end

In the axon, changes occur only up to first node of Ranvier from the site of injury. Degenerative changes that occur in proximal cut end of axon are similar to those changes occurring in distal cut end of the nerve fiber.

■ 3. TRANSNEURONAL DEGENERATION

If an afferent nerve fiber is cut, the degenerative changes occur in another neuron with which the afferent nerve fiber synapses. It is called transneuronal degeneration.

REGENERATION OF NERVE FIBER

Regeneration is the **regrowth** of lost or destroyed part of a tissue. The injured and degenerated nerve fiber can regenerate. It starts as early as 4th day after injury, but, becomes more effective only after 30 days and is completed in about 80 days.

■ CRITERIA FOR REGENERATION

Regeneration is possible only if certain criteria are fulfilled by the degenerated nerve fiber:

1. Gap between the cut ends of the nerve should not exceed 3 mm.
2. Neurilemma should be present.
3. Nucleus must be intact.
4. Two cut ends should remain in the same line.

■ STAGES OF REGENERATION

1. First, some pseudopodia-like extensions grow from the proximal cut end of the nerve. These extensions are called **fibrils** or **regenerative sprouts**. Number of fibrils is up to 100.
2. Fibrils move towards the distal cut end of the nerve fiber.
3. Some of the fibrils enter the neurilemmal tube of distal end and form axis cylinder.
4. Schwann cells line up in the neurilemmal tube and actually guide the fibrils into the tube. Schwann cells also synthesize nerve growth factors, which attract the fibrils from proximal segment.
5. Axis cylinder is fully established inside the neurilemmal tube. These processes are completed in about 3 months after injury.
6. Myelin sheath is formed by Schwann cells slowly. Myelination is completed in 1 year.
7. Diameter of the nerve fiber gradually increases. However, the degenerated nerve fiber has only 80% of original diameter. Newly formed internodes are also shorter than the original ones.
8. In the nerve cell body, first the Nissl granules appear followed by Golgi apparatus.
9. Cell loses the excess fluid and nucleus occupies the central portion.

Though anatomical regeneration occurs in the nerve, functional recovery occurs after a long period.

NEUROGLIA

■ DEFINITION

Neuroglia or **glial cell** or glia (glia = glue) is the **supporting cell** of the nervous system. Neuroglial cells are **non-excitable** and do not transmit nerve impulse (action potential). So, these cells are also called **non-neural cells.**

■ CLASSIFICATION OF NEUROGLIAL CELLS

Neuroglial cells are distributed in central nervous system (CNS) as well as peripheral nervous system (PNS). Refer **Table 90.3** for functions of different types of neuroglia.

Central Neuroglial Cells

Neuroglial cells in CNS are of three types:

1. Astrocytes.
2. Microglia.
3. Oligodendrocytes.

1. Astrocytes

Astrocytes are star-shaped neuroglial cells present in brain **(Fig. 90.8)**. Astrocytes are of two types namely fibrous astrocytes and protoplasmic astrocytes.

TABLE 90.3: Situation, types and functions of neuroglia.

Classification	Situation	Types	Functions
Central neuroglia	Central nervous system	Astrocytes	1. Form blood-brain barrier 2. Provide supporting network 3. Maintain the ECF status around neurons 4. Regulate calcium and potassium level in ECF 5. Regulate the level and recycling of neurotransmitters at synaptic level 6. Secrete neurotrophins
		Microglia	1. Function as macrophages 2. Protect brain from microorganisms by phagocytic action 3. Provide immune and inflammatory response in brain damage
		Oligodendrocytes	1. Provide myelination 2. Form supporting network
Peripheral neuroglia	Peripheral nervous system	Schwann cells	1. Provide myelination 2. Help in regeneration of injured nerve fibers 3. Scavenge cellular debris by phagocytosis
		Satellite cells	1. Provide supporting network 2. Maintain the ECF status around neurons

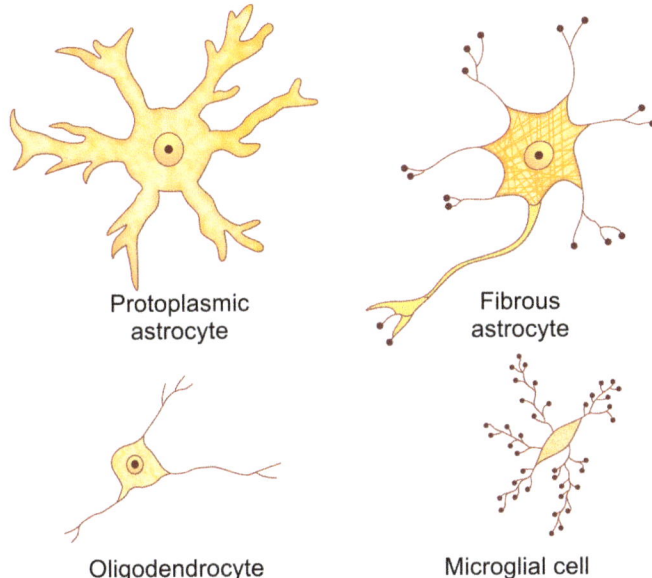

FIGURE 90.8: Neuroglial cells in CNS.

2. Microglia

Microglia are the smallest neuroglial cells. These cells are derived from monocytes. These phagocytic cells often called the macrophages of CNS.

3. Oligodendrocytes

Oligodendrocytes or **oligodendroglia** are the neuroglial cells, which produce myelin sheath around the nerve fibers in CNS.

Peripheral Neuroglial Cells

Neuroglial cells in PNS are of two types:

1. **Schwann cells** which are the major glial cells in PNS.
2. **Satellite cells** which are the glial cells present on the exterior surface of neurons in peripheral nervous system.

FUNCTIONS OF NEUROGLIAL CELLS

Refer **Table 90.3** for functions of different types of neuroglia.

Chapter 91: Receptors

CHAPTER OUTLINE

- DEFINITION
- CLASSIFICATION
  - EXTEROCEPTORS
  - INTEROCEPTORS
- PROPERTIES
  - SPECIFICITY OF RESPONSE: MÜLLER LAW
- ADAPTATION: SENSORY ADAPTATION
- RESPONSE TO INCREASE IN THE STRENGTH OF STIMULUS
- SENSORY TRANSDUCTION
- RECEPTOR POTENTIAL
- LAW OF PROJECTION

DEFINITION

Receptors are the sensory nerve endings which give response to sensory stimuli. These sensory nerve endings terminate in periphery as bare **unmyelinated endings** or in the form of specialized **capsulated structures**. When stimulated, receptors produce a series of impulses which are transmitted through the afferent nerves.

Biological Transducers

Actually receptors function like a transducer. **Transducer** is a device, which converts one form of energy into another.

So, receptors are often defined as the **biological transducers** which convert various forms of energy (stimuli) in the environment into **action potentials** in nerve fiber.

CLASSIFICATION OF RECEPTORS

Generally, the receptors are classified into two types:

I. Exteroceptors.
II. Interoceptors.

EXTEROCEPTORS

Exteroceptors are the receptors which give response to stimuli arising **from outside** the body. Exteroceptors are divided into three groups.

1. Cutaneous Receptors

Receptors situated in the **skin** are called the cutaneous receptors. Cutaneous receptors are also called **mechanoreceptors** because of their response to mechanical stimuli such as touch, pressure and pain (**Figs. 91.1 and 91.2.**). Touch and pressure receptors give response to vibration also. Different types of cutaneous receptors are given in **Table 91.1**.

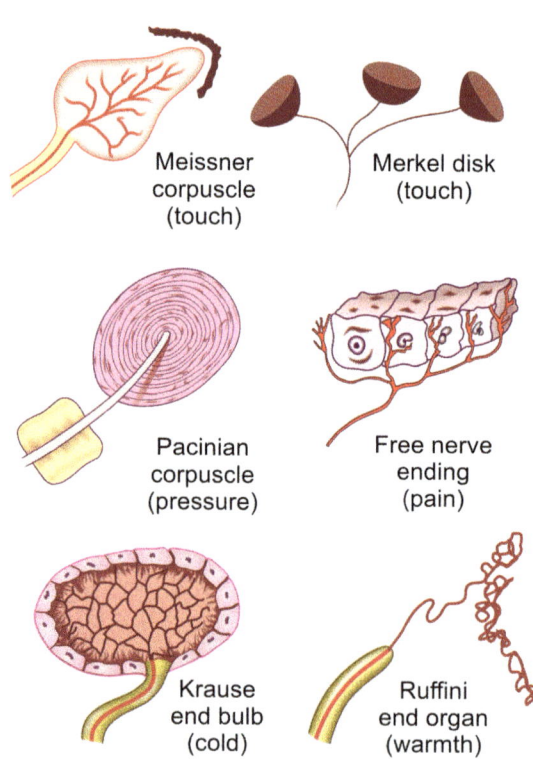

FIGURE 91.1: Cutaneous receptors.

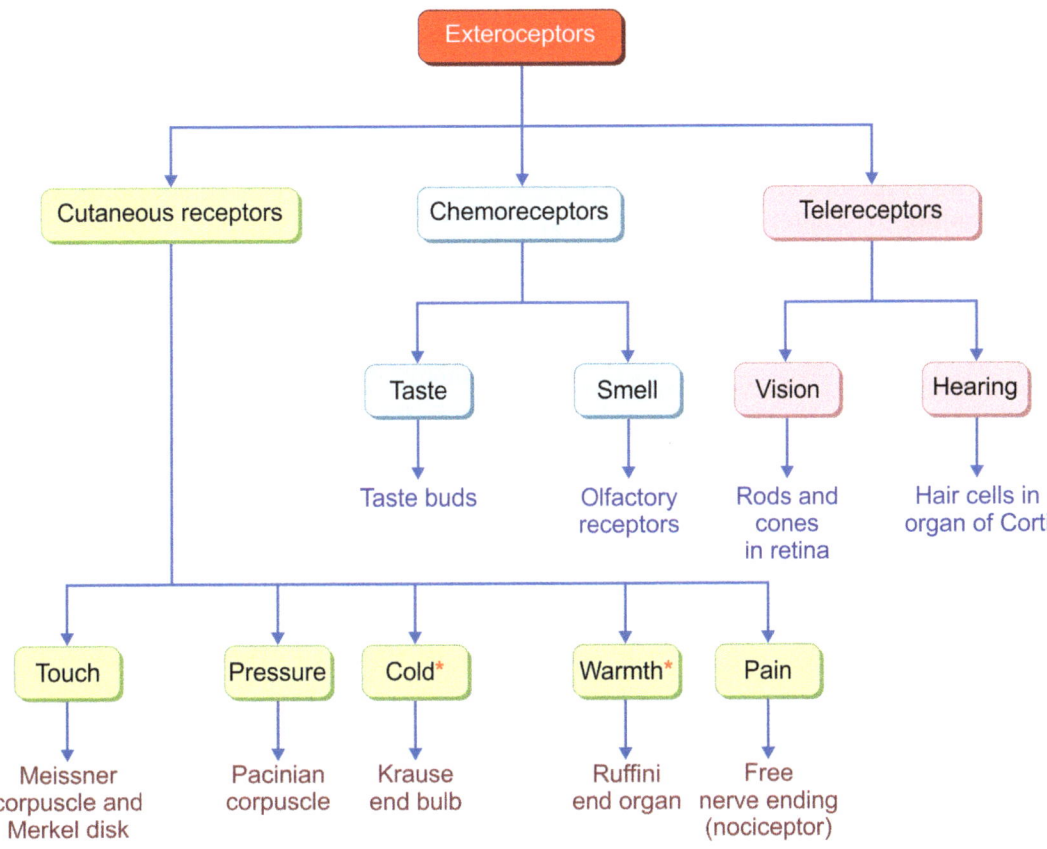

FIGURE 91.2: Exteroceptors.

TABLE 91.1: Cutaneous receptors.

Receptor	Situation	Structure	Type of nerve fiber	Sensation
Meissner corpuscle	Upper dermis between papillae	Encapsulated with collagen fiber network	Aβ	Touch
Merkel disk	Base of epidermis	Branched dendrite. Each branch is expanded like a disk and not encapsulated	Aβ	Touch
Pacinian corpuscle	Onion like concentric laminae encapsulated with connective tissue	Deeper layer of dermis Fascia over muscles Tendons Tissues around joint capsule	C	Pressure and vibration
Krause end bulb	Dermis	Encapsulated with collagen fiber network	Aδ	Cold temperature
Ruffini end organ	Covered by elongated cylindrical capsule	Deeper layer of dermis	C	Warm temperature
Free nerve ending	Uncapsulated ramified nerve fibers	Skin, muscle, tendon, fascia, joints	Aδ C	Pain, temperature and crude touch

2. Chemoreceptors

Receptors, which give response to **chemical stimuli**, are called the chemoreceptors (**Fig. 91.2**).

3. Telereceptors

Telereceptors are the receptors that give response to stimuli arising **away from body**. These receptors are also called the **distance receptors**. Examples are given in **Figure 91.2**.

■ INTEROCEPTORS

Interoceptors are the receptors which give response to stimuli arising **from within** the body. Interoceptors are of two types.

1. *Visceroceptors*

Receptors situated in the viscera are called visceroceptors. Visceroceptors are listed in **Figure 91.3**.

2. *Proprioceptors*

Proprioceptors are the receptors which give response to **change in the position** of different parts of the body (Chapter 103). Proprioceptors are listed in **Figure 91.3**.

■ PROPERTIES OF RECEPTORS

■ 1. SPECIFICITY OF RESPONSE: MÜLLER LAW

According to Müller law, each type of receptor gives response only to one **specific sensation**. This phenomenon is called specificity of response. For example, pain receptors give response only to pain sensation. Similarly, temperature receptors give response only to temperature sensation.

Specificity of response is also called **doctrine of specific nerve energies**.

■ 2. ADAPTATION: SENSORY ADAPTATION

Adaptation is the decrease in discharge of sensory impulses from a receptor when it is stimulated continuously with constant strength. It is also called sensory adaptation or **desensitization**. Depending upon adaptation time, the receptors are divided into two types:

  i. **Phasic receptors**, which get adapted rapidly. Touch and pressure receptors are the phasic receptors.
  ii. **Tonic receptors**, which get adapted slowly. Muscle spindle, pain receptors and cold receptors are the tonic receptors.

■ 3. RESPONSE TO INCREASE IN STRENGTH OF STIMULUS

During the stimulation of a receptor, if the response given by the receptor is to be doubled, strength of stimulus must be increased 100 times. This phenomenon is called **Weber-Fechner law**, which states that the change in response of a receptor is directly proportional to the logarithmic increase in the intensity of stimulus.

■ 4. SENSORY TRANSDUCTION

Sensory transduction in a receptor is a process by which the energy (stimulus) in the environment is converted into electrical impulses (action potentials) in nerve fiber. **Transduction** means conversion of one form of energy into another.

When a receptor is stimulated, it gives response by sending information about the stimulus to CNS. Series of events occur to carry out this function such as the development of receptor potential in the receptor cell and development of action potential in the sensory nerve.

Sensory transduction varies depending upon the type of receptor. For example, the **chemoreceptor** converts **chemical energy** into action potential in the sensory nerve fiber. The **touch receptor** converts **mechanical energy** into action potential in the sensory nerve fiber.

■ 5. RECEPTOR POTENTIAL

Receptor potential is a non-propagated transmembrane potential difference that develops when a receptor is stimulated. It is also called **generator potential**. The receptor potential is short lived and hence, it is called **transient receptor potential**.

Receptor potential is not action potential. It is a **graded potential** (Chapter 27). It is similar to excitatory postsynaptic potential (EPSP) in synapse, endplate potential in neuromuscular junction and electrotonic potential in the nerve fiber.

Properties of Receptor Potential

Receptor potential has two important properties:
  i. Receptor potential is nonpropagated. It is confined within the receptor itself.
  ii. It does not obey all-or-none law.

Interoceptors

Visceroceptors

Receptors	Situation
1. Stretch receptors	Heart
2. Baroreceptors	Blood vessels
3. Chemoreceptors	GI tract
4. Osmoreceptors	Urinary tract
	Brain

Proprioceptors

Receptors	Situation
1. Muscle spindle	Muscle
2. Golgi tendon organ	Tendon
3. Pacinian corpuscle	Ligament
4. Free nerve ending	Fascia
	Joint
5. Hair cells	Vestibular apparatus

FIGURE 91.3: Interoceptors.

Significance of Receptor Potential

When the receptor potential is sufficiently strong (when the magnitude is about 10 mV), it causes development of action potential in the sensory nerve.

Mechanism of Development of Receptor Potential

Pacinian corpuscles are generally used to study the receptor potential because of their large size and anatomical configuration.

Pacinian corpuscles give response to **pressure** stimulus. When pressure stimulus is applied, Pacinian corpuscle is compressed. This compression causes elongation or change in shape of the corpuscle. Change in shape of the corpuscle leads to deformation of central fiber of the corpuscle. This results in the opening of mechanically gated sodium channels (Chapter 3). So, the positively charged sodium ions enter the interior of fiber. This produces a **mild depolarization**, i.e. receptor potential.

Generation of Action Potential in the Nerve Fiber

Receptor potential causes development of a **local circuit of current**, which spreads along the unmyelinated part of nerve fiber within the corpuscle.

When this local circuit of current reaches the first node of Ranvier within the corpuscle, it causes opening of voltage-gated sodium channels and entrance of sodium ions into the nerve fiber. This leads to the development of action potential in the nerve fiber (**Figs. 91.4 and 91.5**).

■ LAW OF PROJECTION

When a sensory pathway from receptor to cerebral cortex is stimulated on any particular site along its course, the

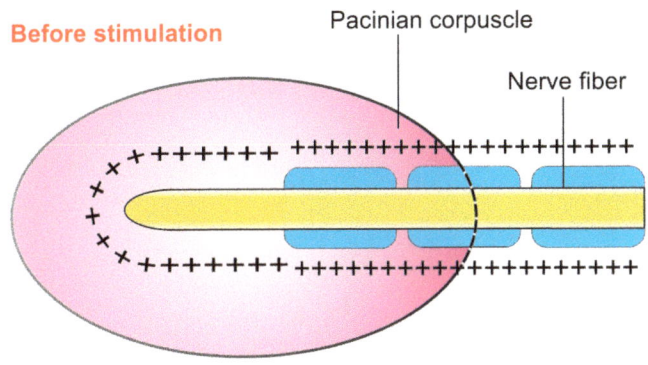
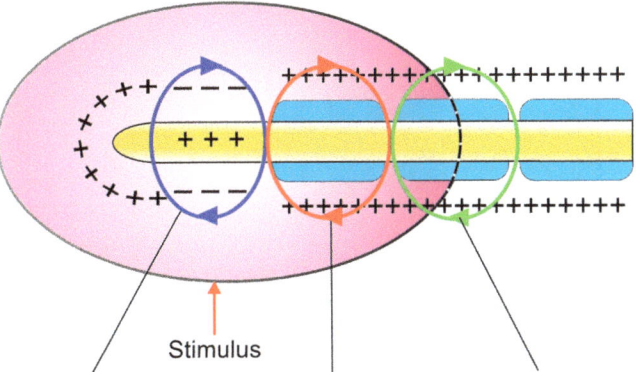

FIGURE 91.4: Receptor potential in Pacinian corpuscle. Receptor potential leads to development of local circuit current which spreads up to first node within the capsule. Local circuit current causes development of action potential in the first node of nerve fiber.

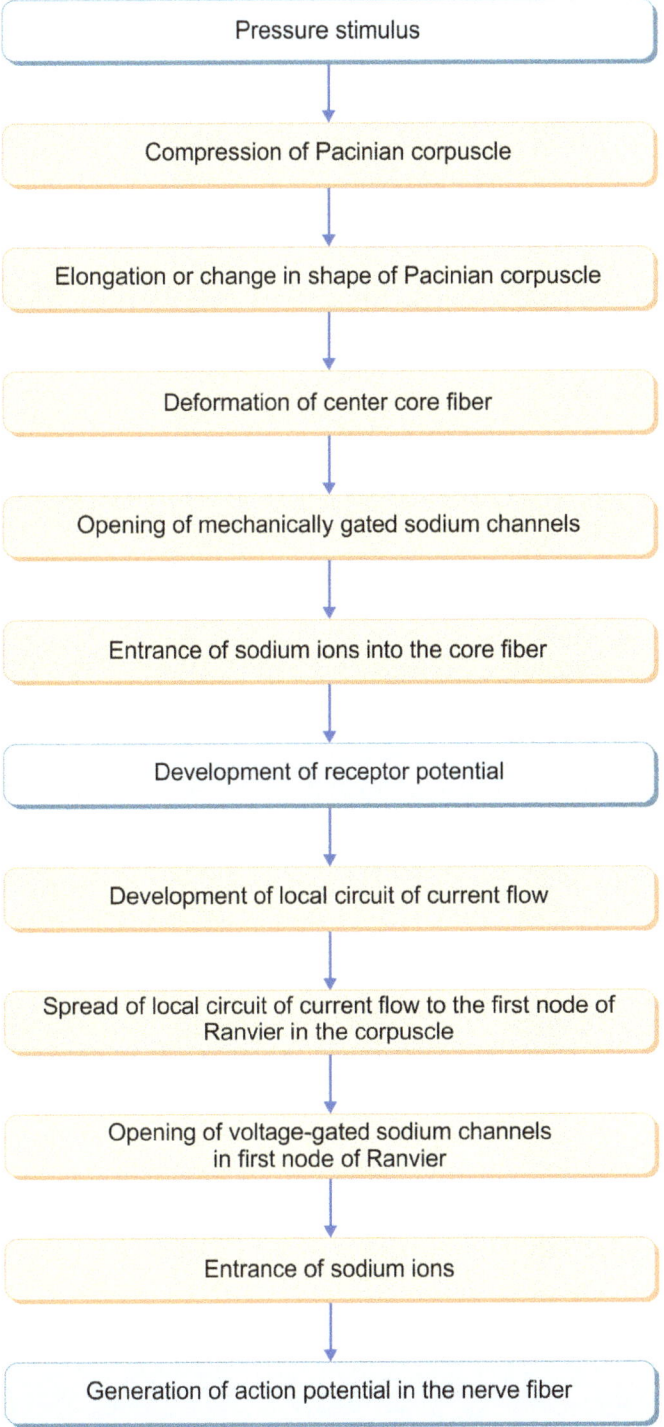

FIGURE 91.5: Schematic diagram showing development of receptor potential and generation of action potential in the nerve fiber.

sensation caused by stimulus is always felt (**referred**) at the location of receptor, irrespective of site stimulated. This phenomenon is known as law of projection.

Examples of Law of Projection

1. If somesthetic area in right cerebral cortex, which receives sensation from left hand, is stimulated, sensations are felt in left hand and not in head.
2. Sensation complained by amputated patients in the missing limb (**phantom limb**) is the best example of law of projection. For example, if a leg has been amputated, the cut end heals with scar formation. The cut ends of nerve fibers are merged within the scar.

If the cut ends of sensory fibers are stimulated during movement of thigh, the patient feels as if the sensation is originating from **non-existent leg**. Sometimes, the patient feels pain in non-existent limb. This type of pain is called **phantom limb pain**.

Chapter 92: Synapse and Neurotransmitters

CHAPTER OUTLINE

- DEFINITION
- CLASSIFICATION
  - ANATOMICAL CLASSIFICATION
  - FUNCTIONAL CLASSIFICATION
- FUNCTIONAL ANATOMY
- FUNCTIONS
  - EXCITATORY SYNAPSE
  - INHIBITORY SYNAPSE
- PROPERTIES
  - ONE WAY CONDUCTION: BELL-MAGENDIE LAW
- SYNAPTIC DELAY
- FATIGUE
- SUMMATION
- ELECTRICAL PROPERTY
- CONVERGENCE AND DIVERGENCE
- NEUROTRANSMITTERS
  - DEFINITION
  - CLASSIFICATION
  - TRANSPORT AND RELEASE
- NEUROMODULATORS
  - CHEMISTRY AND TYPES

DEFINITION

Synapse is the **junction** between the two neurons. It is not an anatomical continuation. It is only a **physiological** continuity between two nerve cells.

CLASSIFICATION OF SYNAPSE

Synapse is classified by two methods, anatomical classification and functional classification.

ANATOMICAL CLASSIFICATION

Synapse is formed by axon of one neuron ending on the cell body, dendrite or axon of the next neuron. First neuron from which the axon arises is called the **presynaptic neuron.**

Second neuron on which the axon of first neuron ends is called **postsynaptic neuron**.

Depending upon ending of axon, synapse is classified into three types:

1. Axoaxonic Synapse

In this type of synapse, axon of presynaptic neuron terminates on **axon** of postsynaptic neuron.

2. Axodendritic Synapse

Here, axon of presynaptic neuron terminates on **dendrite** of postsynaptic neuron.

3. Axosomatic Synapse

In this, presynaptic neuron ends on soma (cell body) of postsynaptic neuron (Fig. 92.1).

FUNCTIONAL CLASSIFICATION

Functional classification depends upon mode of **impulse transmission**.

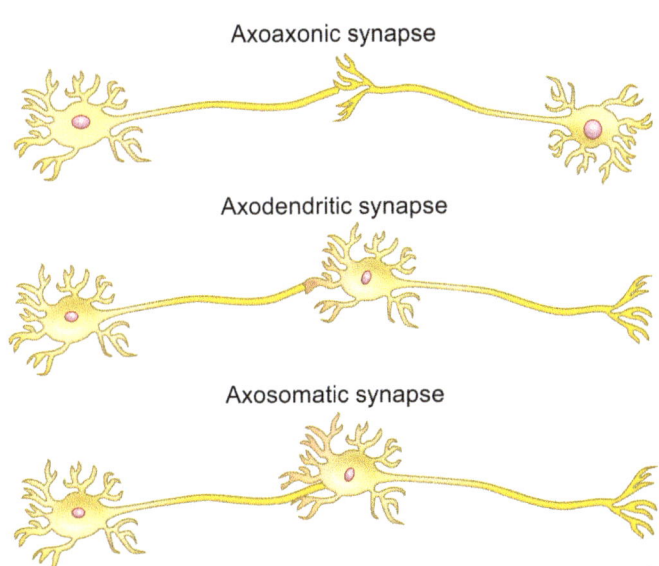

FIGURE 92.1: Anatomical synapses.

On the basis of function, synapse is classified into two types:

1. Electrical Synapse

Electrical synapse is a type of synapse in which the **physiological continuity** between presynaptic and postsynaptic neurons is provided by **gap junction** between these two neurons (Fig. 92.2). There is **direct exchange** of ions between the two neurons through the gap junction. So, the action potential reaching the terminal portion of presynaptic neuron directly enters the postsynaptic neuron.

2. Chemical Synapse

Chemical synapse is the junction between a nerve fiber and a muscle fiber or between two nerve fibers, through which the signals are transmitted by the release of chemical transmitter. In the chemical synapse, there is no continuity between the presynaptic and postsynaptic neurons. These two neurons are separated by a space called **synaptic cleft** between the two neurons.

FUNCTIONAL ANATOMY OF CHEMICAL SYNAPSE

Functional anatomy of a chemical synapse is shown in **Figure 92.3**. Axon of the presynaptic neuron divides into many small branches before forming the synapse. These branches are known as presynaptic **axon terminals**.

Membrane of presynaptic axon terminal is called **presynaptic membrane**.

Presynaptic terminal has two important structures:

1. **Mitochondria**, which help in the synthesis of neurotransmitter substances.
2. **Synaptic vesicles**, which store neurotransmitter substance.

Membrane of the postsynaptic neuron is called **postsynaptic membrane**. It contains some **receptor proteins**. The small space in between the presynaptic membrane and the postsynaptic membrane is called **synaptic cleft**. **Basal lamina** of this cleft contains cholinesterase, which destroys acetylcholine.

FUNCTIONS OF SYNAPSE

Function of the synapse is to transmit the impulses from one neuron to another. However, some synapses inhibit the impulses.

Accordingly, synapse is divided into two types:

1. Excitatory synapses, which transmit the impulses (excitatory function).
2. Inhibitory synapses, which inhibit the transmission of impulses (inhibitory function).

EXCITATORY SYNAPSE

Excitatory synapse transmits the impulses from presynaptic neuron to postsynaptic neuron by the development of excitatory postsynaptic potential.

Excitatory Postsynaptic Potential: EPSP

Excitatory postsynaptic potential (EPSP) is a **non-propagated** electrical potential that develops during the process of synaptic transmission.

When action potential reaches the presynaptic axon terminal, the voltage-gated **calcium channels** at the presynaptic membrane are opened and **calcium ions** enter the axon terminal from ECF. Calcium ions cause bursting of synaptic vesicles and release of **neurotransmitter**. Now, the neurotransmitter diffuses through presynaptic membrane and enters the synaptic cleft by means of **exocytosis (Fig. 92.4)**. Common neurotransmitter in synapse is **acetylcholine**.

The neurotransmitter binds with receptor protein present in the postsynaptic membrane to form the **neurotransmitter-receptor complex**.

Neurotransmitter-receptor complex causes opening of ligand-gated **sodium channels**. Now, **sodium ions** from ECF enter the cell body of postsynaptic neuron. As the sodium ions are positively charged, resting membrane

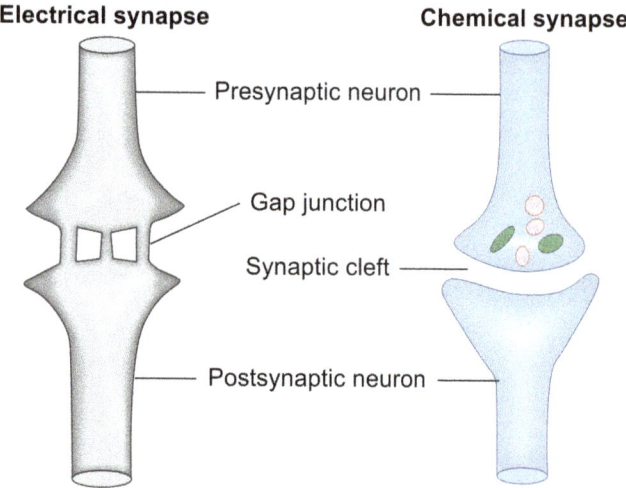

FIGURE 92.2: Electrical and chemical synapse.

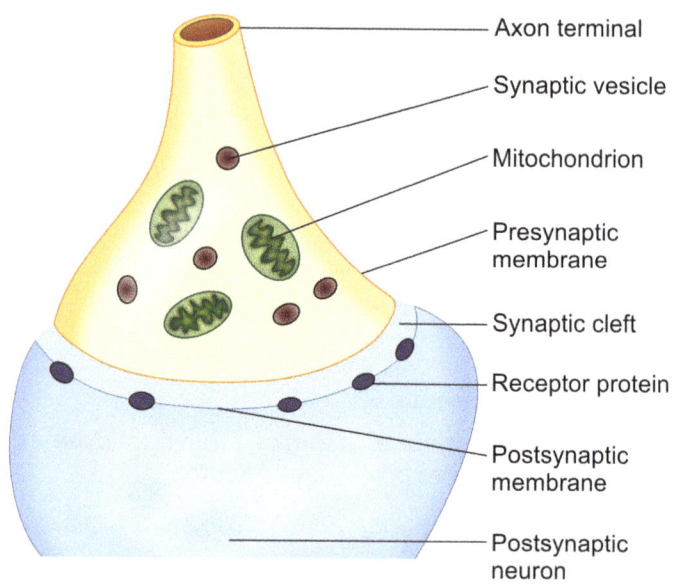

FIGURE 92.3: Structure of chemical synapse.

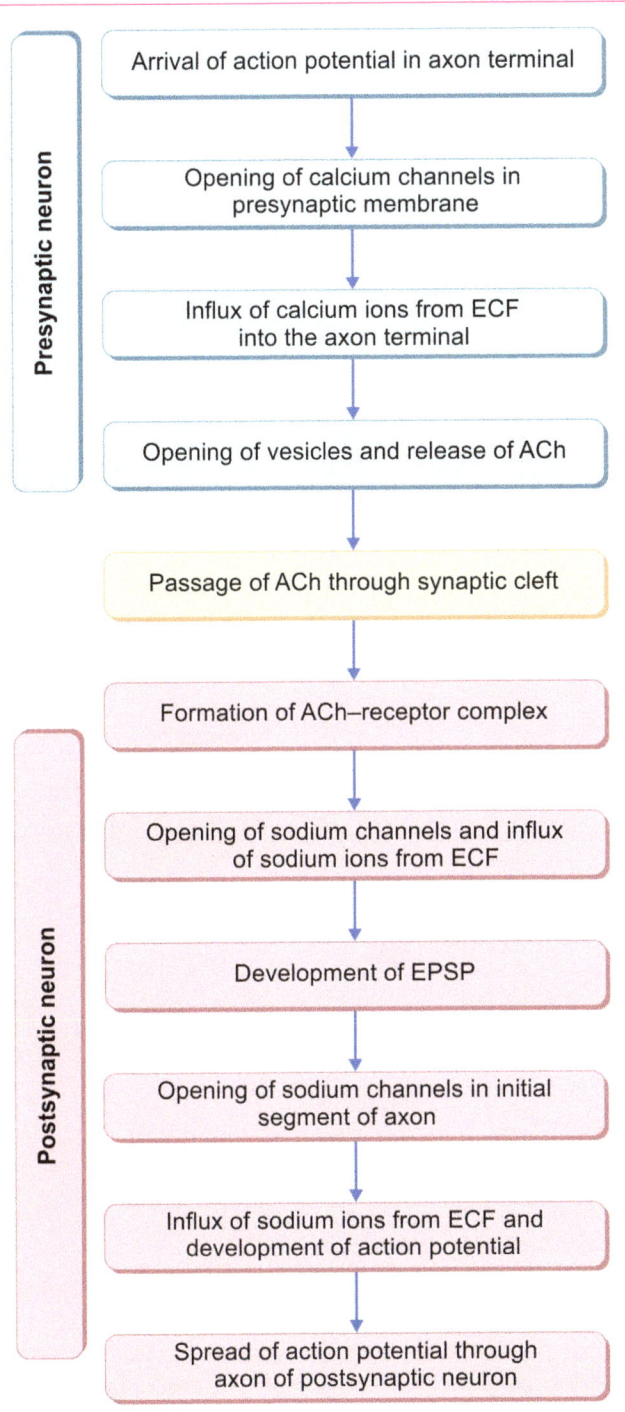

FIGURE 92.4: Sequence of events during synaptic transmission. ACh = Acetylcholine, ECF = Extracellular fluid, EPSP = Excitatory postsynaptic potential.

potential inside the cell body becomes slightly positive and a **mild depolarization** develops. This type of mild depolarization is called **excitatory postsynaptic potential (EPSP)**.

EPSP is confined only to the synapse. It is a **graded potential** (Chapter 27). It is similar to receptor potential and endplate potential.

Properties of EPSP

1. EPSP is nonpropagated.
2. It does not obey all-or-none law.

Significance of EPSP

EPSP is not transmitted into the axon of postsynaptic neuron. However, it causes development of action potential in the axon.

When EPSP is strong enough, it causes the opening of voltage-gated sodium channels in the initial segment of axon. Now, due to the entrance of sodium ions, depolarization occurs in the initial segment of axon and thus, the action potential develops. From here, the action potential spreads to other segments of the axon.

■ INHIBITORY SYNAPSE

Inhibitory synapse does not transmit the impulses from presynaptic neuron to postsynaptic neuron.

Inhibition of synaptic transmission is classified into three types:

1. Postsynaptic inhibition.
2. Presynaptic inhibition.
3. Renshaw cell inhibition.

1. Postsynaptic Inhibition

Postsynaptic inhibition or **direct inhibition** is the type of synaptic inhibition that occurs due to the release of an **inhibitory neurotransmitter** from presynaptic terminal instead of an excitatory neurotransmitter substance. The inhibitory neurotransmitter develops **inhibitory postsynaptic potential (IPSP)** instead of EPSP. Inhibitory neurotransmitters are **gamma-aminobutyric acid** (GABA), dopamine and glycine.

Action of GABA: Development of IPSP

IPSP is the electrical potential in the form of **hyperpolarization** that develops during postsynaptic inhibition. The inhibitory neurotransmitter substance acts on postsynaptic membrane by binding with receptor. Neurotransmitter-receptor complex opens the ligand-gated **potassium channels** instead of sodium channels. Now, the **potassium ions** which are available in plenty in the cell body of postsynaptic neuron move to ECF. Simultaneously, chloride channels also open and chloride ions move from ECF into the cell body of postsynaptic neuron. Exit of potassium ions and influx of chloride ions cause more negativity inside, leading to **hyperpolarization**. The hyperpolarized state of the synapse inhibits synaptic transmission (Fig. 92.5).

2. Presynaptic Inhibition

Presynaptic or **indirect inhibition** is a type of synaptic inhibition that occurs due to failure of presynaptic axon terminal to release sufficient quantity of **excitatory neurotransmitter** substance.

Presynaptic inhibition is mediated by axoaxonic synapses. It is prominent in **spinal cord** and regulates the propagation of information to higher centers in brain.

Normally, during synaptic transmission, action potential reaching the **presynaptic neuron** produces development of EPSP in the postsynaptic neuron. But, in spinal cord,

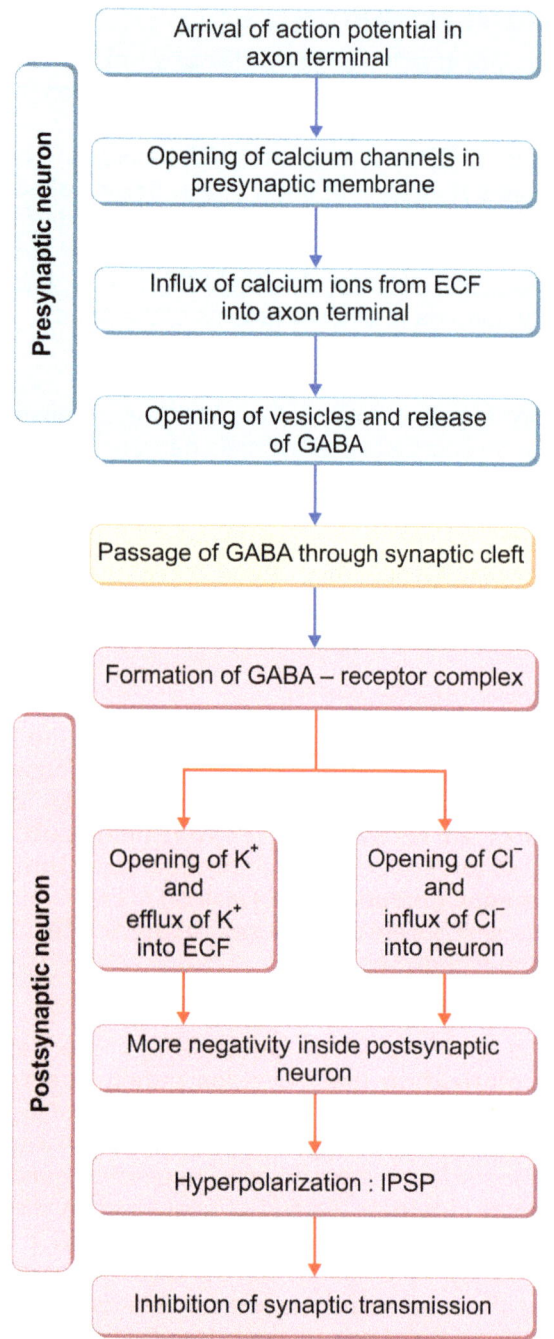

FIGURE 92.5: Sequence of events during postsynaptic inhibition.
GABA = Gamma-aminobutyric acid, ECF = Extracellular fluid, IPSP = Inhibitory postsynaptic potential.

a modulatory neuron called **presynaptic inhibitory neuron** forms an **axoaxonic synapse** with the presynaptic neuron **(Fig. 92.6)**.

This inhibitory neuron inhibits the presynaptic neuron and decreases the magnitude of action potential in presynaptic neuron. This **smaller action potential** reduces **calcium influx.** This in turn decreases the quantity of neurotransmitter released by presynaptic neuron. So, the magnitude of EPSP in postsynaptic neuron is decreased resulting in synaptic inhibition.

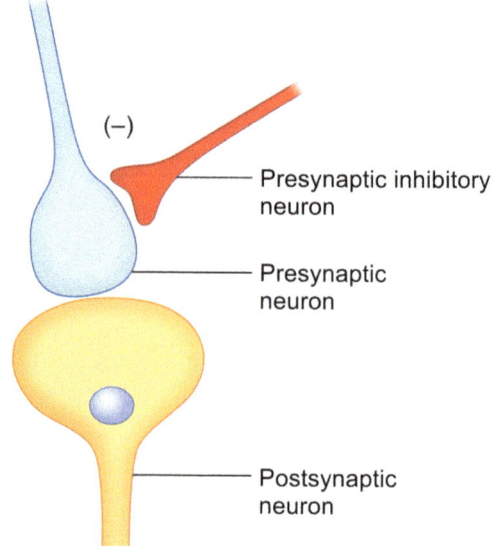

FIGURE 92.6: Presynaptic inhibition.

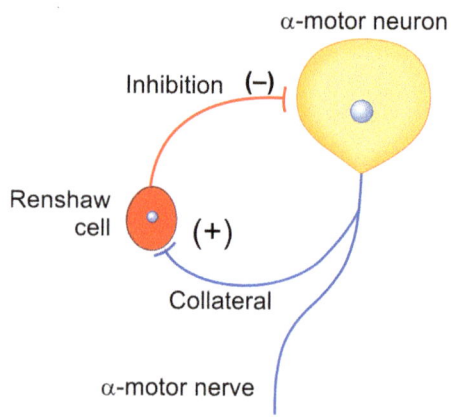

FIGURE 92.7: Renshaw cell inhibition.

3. Renshaw Cell Inhibition

This is a type of synaptic inhibition caused by **Renshaw cells** in spinal cord. Renshaw cells are small motor neurons scattered among the large **α-motor neurons** in anterior gray horn of spinal cord (Chapter 94). The motor nerve fibers to effector organs arise from α-motor neurons. Some of these fibers send **collateral fibers** to Renshaw cells.

When the motor neurons send motor impulses to effector organs, some of the impulses reach Renshaw cell by passing through collaterals. Now, Renshaw cell is stimulated. This in turn, sends inhibitory impulses to α-**motor neurons,** so that the discharge from α-motor neurons is reduced **(Fig. 92.7)**.

Significance of Synaptic Inhibition

Synaptic inhibition in CNS limits the number of impulses going to muscles and enables the muscles to act **properly and appropriately.**

PROPERTIES OF SYNAPSE

1. ONE WAY CONDUCTION: BELL-MAGENDIE LAW

According to Bell-Magendie law, the impulses are transmitted only in one direction in synapse, i.e. from presynaptic neuron to postsynaptic neuron.

2. SYNAPTIC DELAY

Synaptic delay is a short delay that occurs during the transmission of impulses through the synapse.

It is due to the time taken for:

i. Release of neurotransmitter.
ii. Passage of neurotransmitter from axon terminal to postsynaptic membrane.
iii. Action of the neurotransmitter to open the ionic channels in postsynaptic membrane.

Normal duration of synaptic delay is 0.3 to 0.5 msec. Synaptic delay is one of the causes for **reaction time** of the reflex activity.

Significance of Determining Synaptic Delay

Determination of synaptic delay helps to find out whether the pathway for a reflex is monosynaptic or polysynaptic.

3. FATIGUE

During continuous muscular activity, synapse forms the seat of fatigue along with Betz cells present in the motor area of frontal lobe of cerebral cortex. Refer Chapter 26 for details of fatigue. Fatigue at the synapse is due to the **depletion of acetylcholine** (neurotransmitter).

Depletion of acetylcholine occurs by two factors:

i. Soon after the action, acetylcholine is destroyed by acetylcholinesterase.
ii. Due to continuous action, new acetylcholine is not synthesized.

These two factors lead to depletion of acetylcholine resulting in fatigue.

4. SUMMATION

Summation is the **fusion of effects** or progressive increase in the excitatory postsynaptic potential (EPSP) in postsynaptic neuron when many presynaptic excitatory terminals are stimulated simultaneously or when single presynaptic terminal is stimulated repeatedly. Increased EPSP triggers the action potential in the initial segment of the axon of postsynaptic neuron **(Fig. 92.8)**.

Summation is of two types:

i. **Spatial summation** which occurs when many presynaptic terminals are stimulated simultaneously.
ii. **Temporal summation** which occurs when one presynaptic terminal is stimulated repeatedly.

5. ELECTRICAL PROPERTY

Electrical properties of the synapse are the EPSP and IPSP, which are already described in this Chapter.

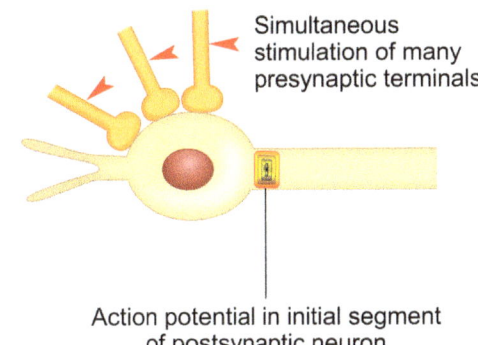

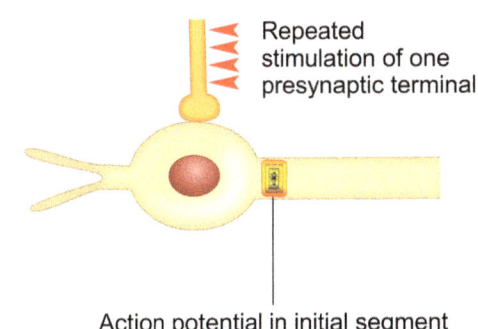

FIGURE 92.8: Spatial and temporal summation.

CONVERGENCE AND DIVERGENCE

Convergence is the process by which many presynaptic neurons terminate on a single postsynaptic neuron **(Fig. 92.9)**.

Divergence is the process by which one presynaptic neuron terminates on many postsynaptic neurons.

NEUROTRANSMITTERS

DEFINITION

Neurotransmitter is a chemical substance that acts as a mediator for the transmission of nerve impulse from one neuron to another neuron through a synapse.

CLASSIFICATION OF NEUROTRANSMITTERS

Depending upon Chemical Nature

Depending upon chemical nature, neurotransmitters are classified into three groups **(Table 92.1)**:

1. Amino acids.
2. Amines.
3. Others.

Depending upon Function

Depending upon function, neurotransmitters are classified into two types:

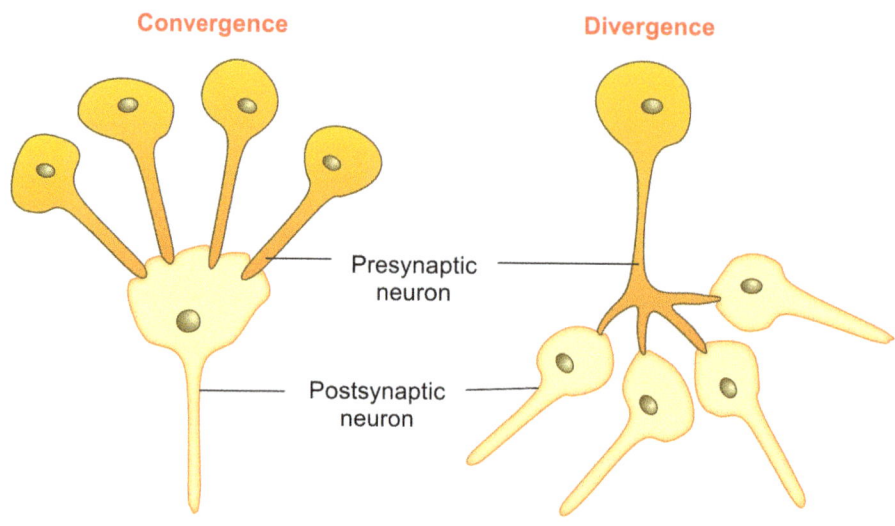

FIGURE 92.9: Convergence and divergence.

TABLE 92.1: Neurotransmitters.

Group	Name	Site of secretion	Action
Amino acids	GABA	Cerebral cortex, cerebellum, basal ganglia, retina and spinal cord	Inhibitory
	Glycine	Forebrain, brainstem, spinal cord and retina	Inhibitory
	Glutamate	Cerebral cortex, brainstem and cerebellum	Excitatory
	Aspartate	Cerebellum, spinal cord and retina	Excitatory
Amines	Noradrenaline	Postganglionic adrenergic sympathetic nerve endings, cerebral cortex, hypothalamus, basal ganglia, brainstem, locus ceruleus and spinal cord	Excitatory and Inhibitory
	Adrenaline	Hypothalamus, thalamus and spinal cord	Excitatory and Inhibitory
	Dopamine	Basal ganglia, hypothalamus, limbic system, neocortex, retina and sympathetic ganglia	Inhibitory
	Serotonin	Hypothalamus, limbic system, cerebellum, spinal cord, retina, gastrointestinal (GI) tract, lungs and platelets	Inhibitory
	Histamine	Hypothalamus, cerebral cortex, GI tract and mast cells	Excitatory
Others	Nitric oxide	Many parts of CNS, neuromuscular junction and GI tract	Excitatory
	Acetylcholine	Neuromuscular junction Synapse Preganglionic parasympathetic nerve and postganglionic parasympathetic nerve Preganglionic sympathetic nerve, postganglionic sympathetic cholinergic nerve Amacrine cells of retina and Many regions of brain	Excitatory

GABA = Gamma-aminobutyric acid

1. **Excitatory neurotransmitters** which are responsible for the conduction of impulse.
2. **Inhibitory neurotransmitters** which inhibit the conduction of impulse **(Tables 92.2)**.

TRANSPORT AND RELEASE OF NEUROTRANSMITTER

Neurotransmitter is produced in the cell body of the neuron and is transported through axon. At the axon terminal, the neurotransmitter is stored in small packets called **vesicles**. Under the influence of a stimulus, these vesicles get ruptured and release the neurotransmitter into synaptic cleft. It binds to specific receptors on the surface of the postsynaptic cell.

NEUROMODULATORS

Neuromodulator is a chemical messenger, which **modifies and regulates** the activities which take place during synaptic transmission. Neuromodulator does not propagate nerve impulses like neurotransmitter.

TABLE 92.2: Excitatory and inhibitory neurotransmitters.

Excitatory neurotransmitters	Inhibitory neurotransmitters	Neurotransmitters with excitatory and inhibitory actions
1. Acetylcholine 2. Nitric oxide 3. Histamine 4. Glutamate 5. Aspartate	1. Gamma-aminobutyric acid 2. Glycine 3. Dopamine 4. Serotonin	1. Noradrenaline 2. Adrenaline

■ CHEMISTRY AND TYPES OF NEUROMODULATORS

Generally, the neuromodulators are **peptides.** So, neuromodulators are often called **neuropeptides**. Almost all the peptides found in nervous tissues are neuromodulators.

Neuromodulators are classified into two types:

1. **Non-opioid neuromodulators** which act by binding with G-protein-coupled receptors.
2. **Opioid neuromodulators** which act by binding with opioid receptors located in nerve endings in brain and GI tract.

Chapter 93: Reflex Activity

CHAPTER OUTLINE

- DEFINITION AND SIGNIFICANCE OF REFLEXES
- REFLEX ARC
- CLASSIFICATION OF REFLEXES
- SUPERFICIAL REFLEXES
- DEEP REFLEXES OR TENDON REFLEXES
- VISCERAL REFLEXES
- PATHOLOGICAL REFLEXES
- PROPERTIES OF REFLEXES
- RECIPROCAL INHIBITION AND RECIPROCAL INNERVATION
- APPLIED PHYSIOLOGY: REFLEXES IN MOTOR NEURON LESION

DEFINITION AND SIGNIFICANCE OF REFLEXES

Reflex activity is the **involuntary** response to a stimulus. It is a type of **protective mechanism** and it protects the body from irreparable damages.

For example, when hand is placed on a hot object, it is withdrawn immediately. When a bright light is thrown into the eyes, eyelids are closed and **pupil** is constricted to prevent the damage of retina by entrance of excess light into the eyes.

REFLEX ARC

Reflex arc is the anatomical nervous pathway for a reflex action.

Simple reflex arc includes five components:

1. Receptor

Receptor is the **end organ**, which receives the stimulus. When the receptor is stimulated, impulses are generated in afferent nerve.

2. Afferent Nerve

Afferent or **sensory nerve** transmits sensory impulses from the receptor to the center.

3. Center

Center receives the sensory impulses via afferent nerve fibers and in turn, it generates appropriate motor impulses. Center is located in the brain or spinal cord.

In simple reflex arc, the **synapse** between afferent nerve and efferent nerve forms the center.

4. Efferent Nerve

Efferent or **motor nerve** transmits motor impulses from the center to the effector organ (Fig. 93.1).

5. Effector Organ

Effector organ is the structure such as muscle or gland where the activity occurs in response to the stimulus.

Afferent and efferent nerve fibers may be connected directly to the center. In some places, one or more neurons are interposed between these nerve fibers and the center. Such neurons are called **connector neurons** or **internuncial neurons** or **interneurons**.

CLASSIFICATION OF REFLEXES

Reflexes are classified by six different methods depending upon various factors as given below:

I. Depending upon whether inborn or acquired reflexes.
II. Depending upon situation: **Anatomical classification**.
III. Depending upon purpose: **Physiological classification**.

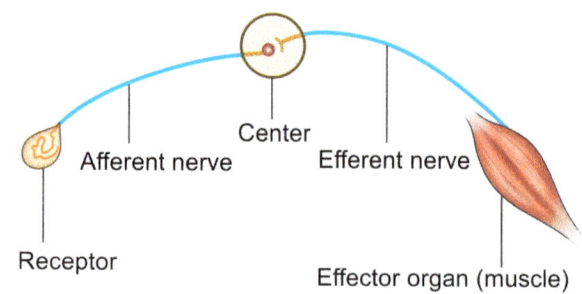

FIGURE 93.1: Simple reflex arc.

Chapter 93: Reflex Activity

IV. Depending upon number of synapses.
V. Depending upon whether visceral or somatic.
VI. Depending upon clinical basis.

■ I. CLASSIFICATION DEPENDING UPON WHETHER INBORN OR ACQUIRED

1. Inborn Reflexes or Unconditioned Reflexes

Inborn reflexes or unconditioned reflexes are the natural reflexes which are present since the time of birth. Such reflexes do not require previous learning, training or conditioning.

Example is the secretion of saliva when a drop of honey is kept in the mouth of a newborn baby for the first time. The baby does not know the taste of the honey but still saliva is secreted.

2. Acquired Reflexes or Conditioned Reflexes

Acquired reflexes or conditioned reflexes are the reflexes that are developed after conditioning or training. These reflexes are not inborn but acquired after birth. Such reflexes require previous learning, training or conditioning.

Example is the secretion of saliva by the sight, smell, thought or hearing of a known edible substance.

■ II. CLASSIFICATION DEPENDING UPON SITUATION OF CENTER: ANATOMICAL CLASSIFICATION

1. Cerebellar Reflexes.
2. Cortical Reflexes.
3. Midbrain Reflexes.
4. Bulbar or Medullary Reflexes.
5. Spinal Reflexes.

■ III. CLASSIFICATION DEPENDING UPON THE PURPOSE: PHYSIOLOGICAL CLASSIFICATION

1. Protective Reflexes or Flexor Reflexes

Protective reflexes are the reflexes which protect the body from **nociceptive** (harmful) **stimuli**. These reflexes are also called **withdrawal reflexes** or flexor reflexes. Protective reflexes involve flexion at different joints hence the name flexor reflexes.

2. Antigravity Reflexes or Extensor Reflexes

Antigravity reflexes are the reflexes which protect the body against **gravitational force**. These reflexes are also called extensor reflexes because, the extensor muscles contract during these reflexes resulting in extension at joints.

■ IV. CLASSIFICATION DEPENDING UPON NUMBER OF SYNAPSE

1. Monosynaptic Reflexes

Reflexes having only **one synapse** in the reflex arc are called monosynaptic reflexes. **Stretch reflex** is the best example for monosynaptic reflex and it is elicited by the stimulation of muscle spindle.

2. Polysynaptic Reflexes

Reflexes having **more than** one synapse in the reflex arc are called polysynaptic reflexes. Examples are **flexor reflexes** (withdrawal reflexes).

■ V. CLASSIFICATION DEPENDING UPON WHETHER SOMATIC OR VISCERAL REFLEXES

1. Somatic Reflexes

Somatic reflexes are the reflexes, for which the reflex arc is formed by **somatic nerve fibers.** These reflexes involve the participation of skeletal muscles. And there may be flexion or extension at different joints during these reflexes.

2. Visceral or Autonomic Reflexes

Visceral or autonomic reflexes are the reflexes, for which at least a part of reflex arc is formed by **autonomic nerve fibers.** These reflexes involve participation of smooth muscle or cardiac muscle. Visceral reflexes include pupillary reflexes, gastrointestinal reflexes, cardiovascular reflexes, respiratory reflexes, etc.

Some reflexes like swallowing, coughing or vomiting are considered as visceral reflexes. However, these reflexes involve participation of skeletal muscles also.

■ VI. CLASSIFICATION DEPENDING UPON CLINICAL BASIS

Depending upon clinical basis reflexes are classified into four types:

A. Superficial reflexes.
B. Deep reflexes.
C. Visceral reflexes.
D. Pathological reflexes.

■ SUPERFICIAL REFLEXES

Superficial reflexes are the reflexes, which are elicited from the **surface of the body**.

Superficial reflexes are elicited from:

1. Cornea (**corneal reflex**) and conjunctiva (**conjunctival reflex**) of eyeball.
2. Mucous membrane (**mucous membrane reflexes**).
3. Skin (**cutaneous reflexes**).

Details of superficial reflexes are given in **Tables 93.1 and 93.2**.

■ DEEP REFLEXES OR TENDON REFLEXES

Deep reflexes or tendon reflexes are elicited from **deeper structures** beneath the skin such as tendon.

Details of deep reflexes are given in **Table 93.3**.

■ VISCERAL REFLEXES

Visceral reflexes are the reflexes arising from the **pupil** and the **visceral organs**.

TABLE 93.1: Superficial reflexes elicited from the eye and the mucous membrane.

Reflex	Method of eliciting reflex	Response	Afferent nerve	Center	Efferent nerve
1. Corneal reflex	Touching cornea with a wisp of cotton	Closing of eyelids (blinking)	Ophthalmic branch of V cranial nerve	Pons: Trigeminal nucleus	VII cranial nerve
2. Conjunctival reflex	Touching conjunctiva with wisp of cotton				
3. Nasal reflex (sneezing reflex)	Stimulating the nasal mucosa with a wisp of cotton	Sneezing	V cranial nerve	Medulla: Nucleus tractus solitarius	V, VII, IX and X cranial nerves
4. Pharyngeal reflex (gag reflex)	Touching roof of mouth, back of tongue, uvula, tonsils or back of throat pharynx with a wisp of cotton or any other object.	Elevation of soft palate and retching (strong involuntary effort to vomit) or gagging (opening of mouth)	IX cranial nerve	Medulla: Nucleus tractus solitarius	X cranial nerve

TABLE 93.2: Superficial reflexes elicited from the skin (cutaneous reflexes).

Reflex	Method of eliciting reflex	Response	Afferent nerve	Center (spinal segments)	Efferent nerve
1. Scapular reflex	Stroking the skin at interscapular space	Contraction of scapular muscles and Drawing in of scapula	Suprascapular nerve	C5 and C6	Suprascapular nerve
2. Upper abdominal reflex	Stroking the abdominal wall below the costal margin (supraumbilical level)	Ipsilateral contraction of abdominal muscle and Movement of umbilicus towards site of stroke	T7 and T8 spinal nerves	T7 and T8	T7 and T8 spinal nerves
3. Middle abdominal reflex	Scratching the abdominal wall near umbilicus (umbilical level)		T9 and T10 spinal nerves	T9 and T10	T9 and T10 spinal nerves
4. Lower abdominal reflex	Stroking the abdominal wall at umbilical and iliac level (infraumbilical level)		T11 and T12 spinal nerves	T11 and T12	T11 and T12 spinal nerves
5. Cremasteric reflex	Scratching the skin at upper and inner aspect of thigh	Elevation of testicles	L1 and L2 spinal nerves	L1 and L2	L1 and L2 spinal nerves
6. Gluteal reflex	Stroking the skin over buttock	Contraction of gluteus muscles	Posterior femoral cutaneous nerve	S1 to S3	Inferior gluteal nerve
7. Plantar reflex	Stroking the sole	Plantar flexion and adduction of toes	Sciatic nerve	L5 to S1	Sciatic nerve
8. Bulbocavernosus reflex	Stroking the dorsum of glans penis	Contraction of bulbocavernosus	Perineal nerve	S3 and S4	Perineal nerve
9. Anal reflex	Stroking the perianal region	Contraction of anal sphincter	Inferior rectal nerve	S3 and S4	Inferior rectal nerve

C = Cervical. T = Thoracic. L = Lumbar. S = Sacral.

Visceral reflexes are:
1. **Pupillary reflexes** in which the size of pupil is altered. Details are given in Chapter 113.
2. **Oculocardiac reflex** in which heart rate decreases by the pressure applied over eyeball.
3. **Carotid sinus reflex** in which the pressure over carotid sinus in neck by **tight collar dress** decreases heart rate and blood pressure.

PATHOLOGICAL REFLEXES

Pathological reflexes are the reflexes that are elicited only in pathological conditions. Three pathological reflexes are well known.

1. BABINSKI REFLEX

Babinski reflex is the **abnormal plantar reflex**. It is also called **Babinski sign** or **phenomenon**. In normal plantar

TABLE 93.3: Deep (tendon) reflexes.

Reflex	Method of eliciting reflex	Response	Afferent nerve	Center	Efferent nerve
1. Jaw jerk	Tapping the middle of the chin with slightly opened mouth	Closure of mouth	V cranial nerve	Pons: V cranial nerve nuclei	V cranial nerve
2. Biceps jerk	Tapping the biceps tendon	Flexion of forearm	Musculocutaneous nerve	V and VI cervical spinal segments	Musculocutaneous nerve
3. Triceps jerk	Tapping the triceps tendon	Extension of forearm	Radial nerve	VI and VII cervical spinal segments	Radial nerve
4. Supinator jerk or brachioradialis jerk or radial periosteal reflex	Tapping the tendon over distal end (styloid process) of radius	Supination and flexion of forearm	Radial nerve	V and VI cervical spinal segments	Radial nerve
5. Knee jerk or patellar tendon reflex	Tapping the patellar tendon	Extension of knee due to contraction of quadriceps muscle	Femoral nerve	II, III and IV lumbar spinal segments	Femoral nerve
6. Ankle jerk or Achilles tendon reflex	Tapping the Achilles tendon	Plantar flexion of foot	Tibial nerve	I and II sacral spinal segments	Tibial nerve

reflex, a gentle scratch over the outer edge of the sole of the foot causes plantar flexion and adduction of all toes.

But in Babinski reflex, there is dorsiflexion of great toe and fanning of other toes.

Babinski reflex is present in **upper motor neuron lesion** particularly in lesion of corticospinal (pyramidal) tracts. It is noticed in some physiological conditions also.

It is present in infants up to 2 years because of incomplete myelination of pyramidal tracts. In adults this reflex may be elicited in deep sleep and in old age.

2. CLONUS

Clonus is a series of rapid and repeated involuntary jerky movements, which occur while eliciting a deep reflex. It occurs in **upper motor neuron lesion** (Chapter 95).

When a deep reflex is elicited in a normal person, the contractions of a muscle or group of muscles are smooth and continuous. But in upper motor neuron lesion clonus occurs. It is because of hypertonicity of muscles and exaggeration of deep reflexes.

Clonus is well seen in calf muscles producing **ankle clonus** and quadriceps producing **patella clonus**. Clonus is also seen in wrists, fingers, jaw and elbow.

3. PENDULAR MOVEMENTS

Pendular movements are the slow **oscillatory movements** (instead of brisk movements) which are developed while eliciting a tendon jerk. The pendular movements are very common while eliciting the knee jerk in patients affected by **cerebellar lesion**. Such movements are similar to movements of **clock's pendulum** hence the name pendular movements.

PROPERTIES OF REFLEXES

ONE WAY CONDUCTION: BELL-MAGENDIE LAW

During any reflex activity, the impulses are transmitted in only one direction through the reflex arc as per Bell-Magendie law. Impulses pass from receptors to the center and then from center to effector organ.

REACTION TIME

Reaction time is the **time interval** between application of stimulus and the onset of reflex. It depends upon the length of afferent and efferent nerve fibers, velocity of impulse through these fibers and central delay. **Central delay** is the delay at the synapse. It is also called **synaptic delay** (Chapter 92).

SUMMATION

Refer Chapter 92 for details of summation. Summation (fusion of effects) in reflex action is of two types:

1. Spatial Summation

When two afferent nerve fibers supplying a muscle are stimulated separately with subliminal stimulus, there is no response. But the muscle contracts when both the nerve fibers are stimulated together with same strength of stimulus. It is called spatial summation.

2. Temporal Summation

When one nerve fiber is stimulated repeatedly with subliminal stimuli, these stimuli are summed up to give response in the muscle. It is called temporal summation.

Thus, both spatial summation and temporal summation play an important role in the facilitation of responses during the reflex activity.

RECRUITMENT

Recruitment is defined as the successive activation of additional motor units (Chapter 28) with progressive increase in force of muscular contraction.

When an excitatory nerve is stimulated for a long time, there is a gradual increase in the response of reflex activities. It is due to the activation of more and more motor units. Recruitment is similar to the effect of temporal summation.

AFTER DISCHARGE

After discharge is the persistence or continuation of response for some time even after cessation of stimulus. When a reflex action is elicited continuously for some time and then the stimulation is stopped, the reflex activity (contraction) will be continued for some time even after the stoppage of the stimulus. It is because of the discharge of impulses from the center even after stoppage of stimulus. The internuncial neurons are responsible for after discharge.

REBOUND PHENOMENON

Reflex activities can be inhibited forcefully for some time. But, when the inhibition is suddenly removed, the reflex activity becomes more forceful than before inhibition. It is called rebound phenomenon. The reason for this state of over excitation is not known.

FATIGUE

When a reflex activity is continuously elicited for a long time, the response is reduced slowly and at one stage, the response does not occur. This type of failure to give response to the stimulus is called fatigue. The center or the synapse of the reflex arc is the first seat of fatigue.

RECIPROCAL INHIBITION AND RECIPROCAL INNERVATION

RECIPROCAL INHIBITION

Reciprocal inhibition is the process during reflex activity, by which there is relaxation of a group of muscles during contraction of their antagonistic muscles.

When a **flexor reflex** is elicited, the **flexor muscles** are excited (contracted) and the **extensor muscles** are inhibited (relaxed) in that side. This phenomenon is called the reciprocal inhibition.

Reciprocal inhibition occurs because of reciprocal innervation.

RECIPROCAL INNERVATION

Reciprocal innervation is a type of innervation of muscles, because of which contraction of a group of muscles is accompanied by relaxation of their **antagonistic muscles**.

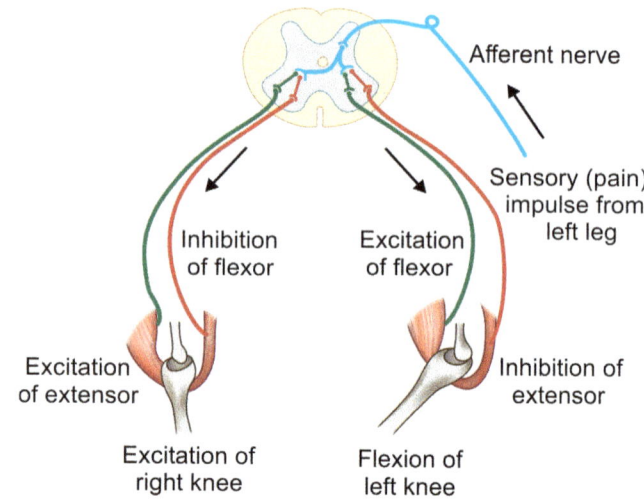

FIGURE 93.2: Crossed extensor reflex.
Green lines = Excitation. Red lines = Inhibition.

Afferent nerve fibers, which produce flexor reflex in a limb, have connections with motor neurons supplying flexor muscles and the motor neurons supplying the extensor muscles of same side.

Afferent nerve **excites** the motor neurons, which supply the **flexor muscles**. Simultaneously, it **inhibits** the motor neurons supplying **extensor muscles** through an interneuron. Accordingly, the flexor muscles contract and extensor muscles relax resulting in flexion of the limb.

CROSSED EXTENSOR REFLEX

Crossed extensor reflex is the **withdrawal reflex** in which the flexors of the withdrawing limb are excited (contracting) and extensors are inhibited (relaxed), while the opposite occurs in the other limb. For example, while eliciting a flexor reflex activity in a limb, that limb is flexed. Simultaneously the opposite limb is extended **(Fig. 93.2)**.

Flexors are excited and extensors are inhibited in this limb, but in the opposite limb, the flexors are inhibited and extensors are excited. This type of crossed extensor reflex is because of reciprocal inhibition.

SIGNIFICANCE OF RECIPROCAL INHIBITION

Reciprocal inhibition and reciprocal innervation are very important in spinal reflexes, which are involved in **locomotion.** It helps in the forward movement of one limb while causing the backward movement of the opposite limb.

APPLIED PHYSIOLOGY: REFLEXES IN MOTOR NEURON LESION

UPPER MOTOR NEURON LESION

During upper motor neuron lesion, all the superficial reflexes are lost. The deep reflexes are exaggerated and Babinski's sign is present (Chapter 95).

LOWER MOTOR NEURON LESION

During lower motor lesion, all the superficial and deep reflexes are lost. Refer Chapter 95 for details.

Chapter 94: Spinal Cord

CHAPTER OUTLINE

- FEATURES OF SPINAL CORD
- INTERNAL STRUCTURE OF SPINAL CORD
- GRAY MATTER
- WHITE MATTER
- TRACTS IN SPINAL CORD
- ASCENDING TRACTS
- DESCENDING TRACTS
- APPLIED PHYSIOLOGY

■ FEATURES OF SPINAL CORD

Spinal cord is a part of central nervous system, the other part being the brain.

Situation and Extent of Spinal Cord

Spinal cord is situated loosely in the **vertebral canal**. It extends between **foramen magnum** where it is continuous with medulla oblongata of brain, and lower border of **first lumbar vertebra**.

Coverings of Spinal Cord

Spinal cord is covered by membranous sheaths called **meninges** which continue as coverings of brain. Meninges are **dura mater, pia mater** and **arachnoid mater**. Meninges are responsible for **protection and nourishment** of the nervous tissues.

Shape and Length of Spinal Cord

Spinal cord is cylindrical in shape. It has a length of about 45 cm in males and about 43 cm in females.

Enlargements of Spinal Cord

Spinal cord has two spindle-shaped swellings, called **cervical enlargement** and **lumbar enlargement**. These two portions of spinal cord innervate upper and lower extremities respectively.

Conus Medullaris and Filum Terminale of Spinal Cord

Spinal cord becomes narrow rapidly below the lumbar enlargement and forms a cone-shaped termination called **conus medullaris**. A slender non-nervous filament called **filum terminale** extends from conus medullaris downward at the level of second sacral vertebra.

Fissure and Sulci in Spinal Cord

A deep furrow called **anterior median fissure** is present on the anterior surface of spinal cord. Depth of this fissure is about 3 mm. Lateral to the anterior median fissure on either side, there is a slight depression called the **anterolateral sulcus**. It denotes the exit of anterior nerve root **(Fig. 94.1)**.

A depression called **posterior median sulcus** is present on the posterior surface of spinal cord. This sulcus is continuous with a thin glial partition called the **posterior median septum**. It extends inside the spinal cord for about 5 mm and reaches the gray matter.

On either side, lateral to posterior median sulcus, there is **posterior intermediate sulcus**. It is continuous with **posterior intermediate septum,** which extends for about 3 mm into the spinal cord. Lateral to the posterior intermediate sulcus, is the **posterolateral sulcus**. This denotes the entry of posterior nerve root.

■ SEGMENTS OF SPINAL CORD

Spinal cord is made up of 31 segments, which are listed in **Table 94.1**. Spinal cord is a continuous structure. The appearance of segments is because of spinal nerves arising from spinal cord.

■ SPINAL NERVES

Spinal nerve is a **mixed nerve** consisting of both motor and sensory fibers which carry the information between spinal cord and specific regions of the body. Spinal nerves form a part of **peripheral nervous system**.

In humans there are 31 pairs of spinal nerves corresponding to the segments of spinal cord in a symmetrical manner. Spinal nerves are listed in **Table 94.1**.

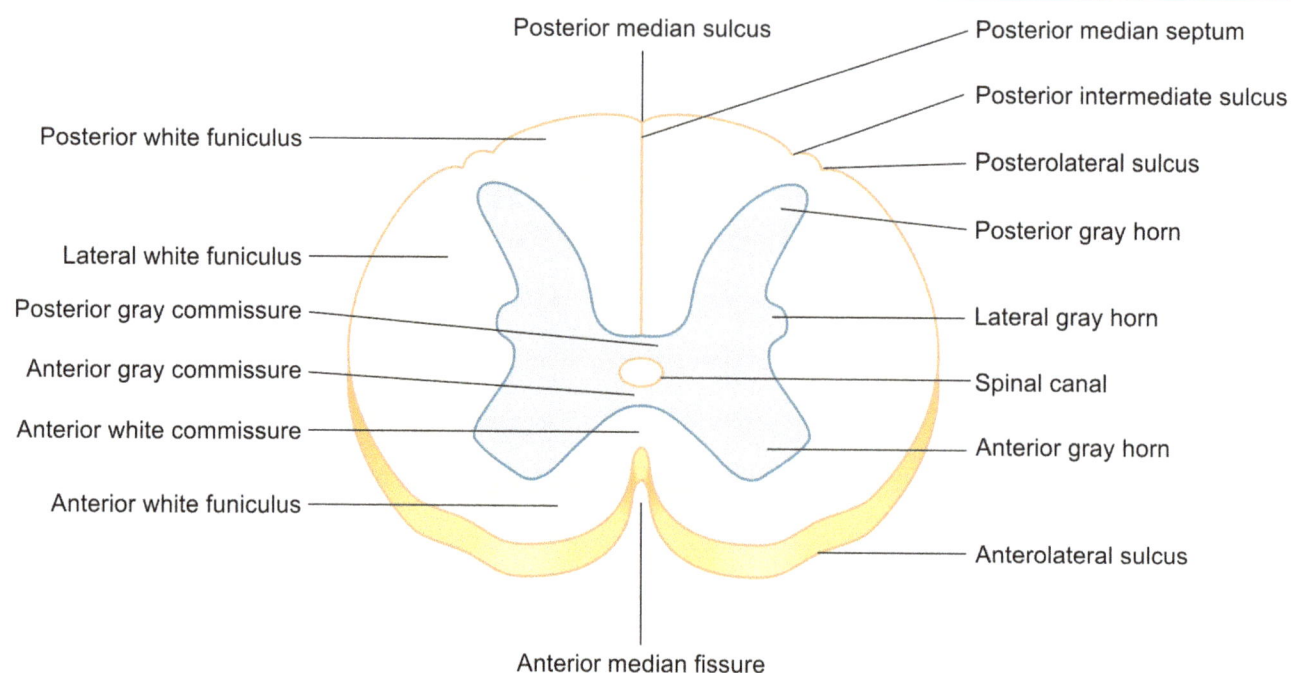

FIGURE 94.1: Section of spinal cord: Thoracic segment.

TABLE 94.1: Segments of spinal cord and spinal nerve.

Spinal segments/Spinal nerves	Number
Cervical segments/Cervical spinal nerves	8
Thoracic segments/Thoracic spinal nerves	12
Lumbar segments/Lumbar spinal nerves	5
Sacral segments/Sacral spinal nerves	5
Coccygeal segment/Coccygeal spinal nerves	1
Total segments/Spinal nerves	**31**

■ SPINAL NERVE ROOTS

Each spinal nerve is formed by a posterior (dorsal) root and an anterior (ventral) root.

1. Posterior or Dorsal Root

It is formed by afferent (sensory) nerve fibers. Posterior root has a small bulging called **posterior root ganglion** which is formed by the soma of neurons. Dendrites of these neurons form sensory nerve fibers and their axons reach the spinal cord.

2. Anterior or Ventral Root

This root is formed by efferent (motor) nerve fibers. Both the nerve roots on either side leave the spinal cord and pass through the corresponding **intervertebral foramina**.

Cervical and thoracic roots are shorter whereas, the lumbar and sacral roots are longer. Long nerves descend down to reach their respective **intervertebral foramina**. This bundle of descending roots surrounding the **filum terminale** resembles the tail of horse. Hence, it is called **cauda equina**.

■ INTERNAL STRUCTURE OF SPINAL CORD

Neural substance of the spinal cord is divided into inner gray matter and outer white matter **(Fig. 94.1)**.

■ GRAY MATTER OF SPINAL CORD

Gray matter of the spinal cord has nerve cell bodies, dendrites and parts of axons. It is placed centrally in the form of wings of butterfly and it resembles the letter 'H'. In the center of gray matter, there is a canal called the **spinal canal**.

Ventral and the dorsal portions of each lateral half of gray matter are called ventral or **anterior gray horn** and dorsal or **posterior gray horn** respectively. In addition, the gray matter forms a small projection in between the anterior and posterior horns in all thoracic and first two lumbar segments. This projection is called the **lateral gray horn**.

Part of the gray matter anterior to central canal is called the **anterior gray commissure.** And, part of gray matter posterior to the central canal is called the **posterior gray commissure**.

Neurons in Gray Matter of Spinal Cord

Gray matter contains two types of multipolar neurons.

1. **Golgi type I neurons** which have long axons.
2. **Golgi type II neurons** which have short axons.

Organization of Neurons in Gray Matter

Organization of neurons in the gray matter of spinal cord is described in two methods:

 I. Nuclei or columns.
 II. Laminae or layers.

I. Nuclei in Spinal Cord

Clusters of neurons are present in the form of nuclei or cell column in gray matter **(Fig. 94.2)**.

1. Nuclei in anterior gray horn

Anterior gray horn contains the **nuclei of lower motor neurons** which are involved in motor function.

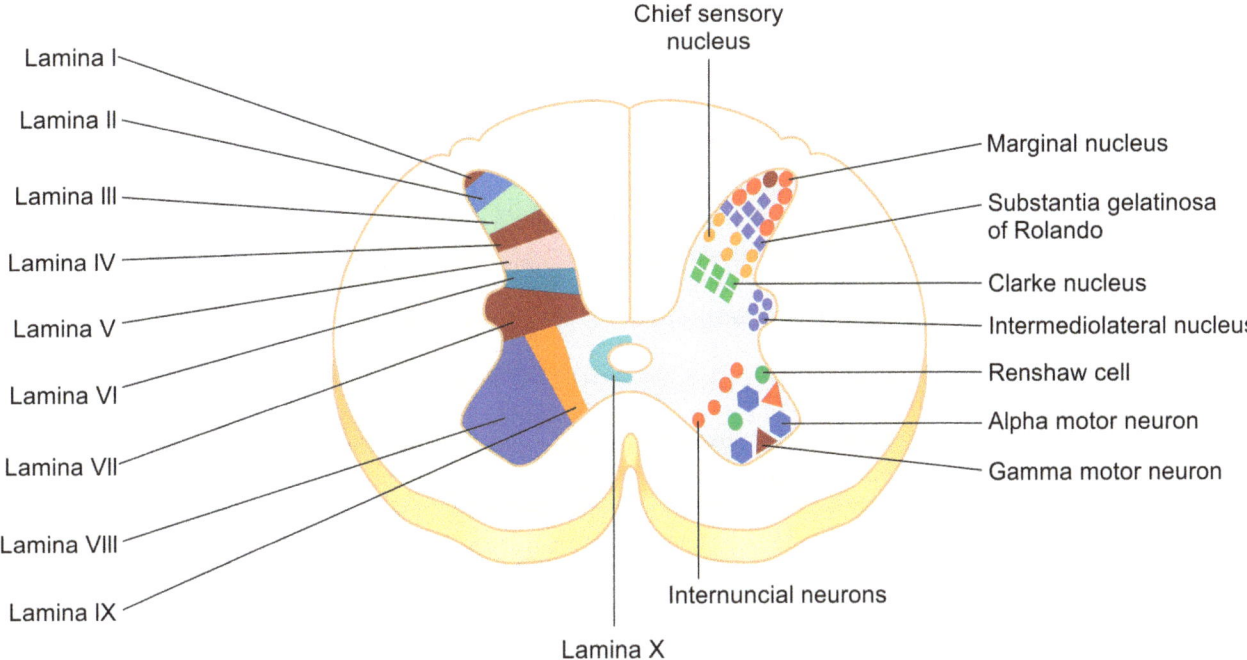

FIGURE 94.2: Nuclei and laminae in gray horn of spinal cord: Thoracic segment.

Lower motor neurons are of three types:

i. Alpha motor neurons.
ii. Gamma motor neurons.
iii. Renshaw cells.

2. Nuclei in lateral gray horn

Lateral gray horn has **intermediolateral nucleus**. Neurons of this nucleus give rise to **sympathetic preganglionic fibers**, which leave the spinal cord through the anterior nerve root **(Table 94.2)**. Intermediolateral nucleus extends between T1 and L2 segments of spinal cord.

3. Nuclei in posterior gray horn

Posterior gray horn contains the **nuclei of sensory neurons**, which receive impulses from various receptors of the body through posterior nerve root fibers.

Nuclei of sensory neurons are of four types:

i. Marginal nucleus.
ii. Substantia gelatinosa of Rolando.
iii. Chief sensory nucleus (nucleus proprius).
iv. Clarke's nucleus.

TABLE 94.2: Neurons and nuclei in gray horns of spinal cord.

Gray horn	Nuclei/Neurons
Anterior gray horn	1. Alpha motor neurons 2. Gamma motor neurons 3. Renshaw cells
Lateral gray horn	1. Intermediolateral nucleus
Posterior gray horn	1. Marginal cells 2. Substantia gelatinosa of Rolando 3. Chief sensory nucleus (nucleus proprius) 4. Clarke nucleus

II. Laminae of Spinal Cord: Rexed Laminae

Neurons of gray matter are distributed in laminae or layers. Each lamina consists of neurons of different size and shape. **Bror Rexed** classified the neurons in 10 laminae. Hence, the laminae are called **Rexed laminae (Table 94.3)**.

1. Laminae in posterior gray horn

Laminae I to VI constitute the posterior gray horn. These laminae contain **nuclei of sensory neurons**.

2. Lamina in lateral gray horn

Lateral gray horn contains only one lamina, the lamina VII. It contains **intermediolateral nucleus**.

3. Laminae in anterior gray horn

Laminae VIII and IX form the anterior gray horn. These laminae contain **nuclei of motor neurons**.

TABLE 94.3: Neurons and nuclei present in laminae of spinal cord.

Gray horn/area	Lamina	Neuron/Nucleus
Posterior gray horn	Lamina I	Marginal nucleus
	Lamina II and III	Substantia gelatinosa of Rolando
	Lamina III, IV and V	Chief sensory nucleus
	Lamina VI	Dorsal nucleus of Clarke
Lateral gray horn	Lamina VII	Intermediolateral nucleus
Anterior gray horn	Lamina VIII	Motor interneurons
	Lamina IX	Motor neurons
Around central canal	Lamina X	Neuroglia

4. Lamina around central canal

Lamina X is present around the spinal canal. It contains **neuroglia**, which form the supporting tissue.

■ WHITE MATTER OF SPINAL CORD

White matter of spinal cord surrounds the gray matter. It is formed by the bundles of nerve fibers. **Anterior median fissure** and the **posterior median septum** divide the entire mass of white matter into two lateral halves. The band of white matter lying in front of anterior gray commissure is called the **anterior white commissure**.

■ DIVISIONS OF WHITE MATTER

Each half of the white matter is divided by the fibers of anterior and posterior nerve roots into three **white columns** or **white funiculi**.

1. Anterior or Ventral White Column

Anterior white column lies between the anterior median fissure on one side and anterior nerve root and anterior gray horn on the other side. It is also called **anterior or ventral funiculus.**

2. Lateral White Column

Lateral white column is present between the anterior nerve root and anterior gray horn on one side and posterior nerve root and posterior gray horn on the other side. It is also called **lateral funiculus.**

3. Posterior or Dorsal White Column

Posterior white column is situated between the posterior nerve root and posterior gray horn on one side and posterior median septum on the other side. It is also called **posterior or dorsal funiculus.**

■ TRACTS IN SPINAL CORD

Tract means collection of nerve fibers. Tracts of the spinal cord are collections of nerve fibers passing through the spinal cord. **Spinal tracts** are divided into two main groups namely short tracts and long tracts.

Short Tracts of Spinal Cord

Fibers of the short tracts connect different parts of spinal cord itself.

Short tracts are of two types:

1. **Association or intrinsic tracts,** which connect adjacent segments of spinal cord on the same half.
2. **Commissural tracts,** which connect opposite halves of same segment of spinal cord.

Long Tracts of Spinal Cord

Long tracts or **projection tracts** of spinal cord connect the spinal cord with other parts of central nervous system.

Long tracts are of two types:

1. **Ascending tracts**, which carry sensory impulses from the spinal cord to brain.
2. **Descending tracts**, which carry motor impulses from brain to the spinal cord.

■ ASCENDING TRACTS OF SPINAL CORD

Ascending tracts of spinal cord carry the impulses of various sensations to the brain. Pathway for each sensation is formed by two or three groups of neurons:

1. First order neurons.
2. Second order neurons.
3. Third order neurons.

First Order Neurons

First order neurons receive sensory impulses from the **receptors** and send them to sensory neurons present in the posterior gray horn of spinal cord through their fibers. Nerve cell bodies of these neurons are located in the **posterior nerve root ganglion** that lies outside the spinal cord.

Second Order Neurons

Second order neurons are the sensory neurons present in **posterior gray horn**. Fibers from these neurons form the **ascending tracts** of spinal cord. These fibers carry sensory impulses from spinal cord to different **subcortical areas** brain areas below cerebral cortex such as thalamus, cerebellum, etc.

All the ascending tracts are formed by fibers of second order neurons of the sensory pathways except the ascending tracts in the posterior white column which are formed by the fibers of first order neurons.

Third Order Neurons

Third order neurons are in the **subcortical areas**. The fibers of these neurons carry the sensory impulses from subcortical areas to **cerebral cortex.**

Ascending tracts situated in different white columns are listed in **Table 94.4**. Features of the ascending tracts are given in **Table 94.5**.

■ 1. ANTERIOR SPINOTHALAMIC TRACT

Anterior spinothalamic tract is formed by the fibers of second order neurons of the pathway for **crude touch**

TABLE 94.4: List of ascending tracts of spinal cord.

White column	Tract
Anterior white column	1. Anterior spinothalamic tract
Lateral white column	1. Lateral spinothalamic tract 2. Ventral spinocerebellar tract 3. Dorsal spinocerebellar tract 4. Spinotectal tract 5. Fasciculus dorsolateralis 6. Spinoreticular tract 7. Spino-olivary tract 8. Spinovestibular tract
Posterior white column	1. Fasciculus gracilis 2. Fasciculus cuneatus 3. Comma tract of Schultze

Chapter 94: Spinal Cord 477

TABLE 94.5: Ascending tracts of spinal cord.

Situation	Tract	Origin	Course	Termination	Function
Anterior white column	1. Anterior spinothalamic tract	Chief sensory nucleus	Crossing in spinal cord Forms spinal lemniscus	Ventral posterolateral nucleus of thalamus	Crude touch sensation
	2. Lateral spinothalamic tract	Substantia gelatinosa	Crossing in spinal cord Forms spinal lemniscus	Ventral posterolateral nucleus of thalamus	Pain sensation Temperature sensations
	3. Ventral spinocerebellar tract	Marginal nucleus	Crossing in spinal cord	Anterior lobe of cerebellum	Subconscious kinesthetic sensations
	4. Dorsal spinocerebellar tract	Clarke nucleus	Uncrossed fibers	Anterior lobe of cerebellum	Subconscious kinesthetic sensations
Lateral white column	5. Spinotectal tract	Chief sensory nucleus	Crossing in spinal cord	Superior colliculus	Spinovisual reflex
	6. Fasciculus dorsolateralis	Posterior nerve root ganglion	Component of lateral spinothalamic tract	Substantia gelatinosa	Pain sensation Temperature sensations
	7. Spinoreticular tract	Intermediolateral cells	Crossed and uncrossed fibers	Reticular formation of brainstem	Consciousness Awareness
	8. Spino-olivary tract	Non-specific	Uncrossed fibers	Olivary nucleus	Proprioception
	9. Spinovestibular tract	Non-specific	Crossed and uncrossed fibers	Lateral vestibular nucleus	Proprioception
	10. Fasciculus gracilis	Posterior nerve root ganglia	Uncrossed fibers No synapse in spinal cord	Nucleus gracilis in medulla	Tactile sensation Tactile localization Tactile discrimination Vibratory sensation
Posterior white column	11. Fasciculus cuneatus	Posterior nerve root ganglia	Uncrossed fibers No synapse in spinal cord	Nucleus cuneatus in medulla	Conscious kinesthetic sensation Stereognosis
	12. Comma tract of Shultze	Posterior nerve root ganglia	Short descending branches of fasciculus gracilis and fasciculus gracilis	Cervical and thoracic segments of spinal cord	Establishment of intersegmental communications Formation short reflex arc

sensation. This tract is situated in anterior white column (**Figs. 94.3 and 94.4**).

Origin

Fibers of anterior spinothalamic tract arise from cells of **chief sensory nucleus (nucleus proprius)** of posterior gray horn which form the **second order neurons**.

(First order neurons are situated in the posterior nerve root ganglia. These neurons receive the impulses from the **pressure receptors**. Axons of the first order neurons reach the chief sensory nucleus through the posterior nerve root).

Course

This tract contains **crossed fibers**. After taking origin from chief sensory nucleus, these fibers cross obliquely in the anterior white commissure and enter the anterior white column of opposite side. Here, the fibers ascend through other segments of spinal cord and brainstem (medulla, pons and midbrain) and reach thalamus.

Termination

Fibers of anterior spinothalamic tract terminate in the **ventral posterolateral nucleus** of thalamus. The fibers from thalamic nucleus carry the impulses to somesthetic area (sensory cortex) of cerebral cortex.

Function

Anterior spinothalamic tract carries impulses of **crude touch** (protopathic) sensation.

Effect of Lesion

Bilateral lesion of this tract leads to **loss of crude touch** sensation and loss of sensations like **itching and tickling** below the level of lesion on both sides.

Unilateral lesion of this tract causes loss of crude touch sensation below the level of lesion in **opposite side** (because fibers of this tract cross to the opposite side in spinal cord).

2. LATERAL SPINOTHALAMIC TRACT

Lateral spinothalamic tract is formed by the fibers from the second order neurons of the pathway for **pain and temperature sensations**. This tract is situated in the lateral white column (**Figs. 94.3 and 94.4**).

Origin

Fibers of lateral spinothalamic tract take origin from **marginal nucleus** and **substantia gelatinosa of Rolando**.

Course

This tract has **crossed fibers**. After origin, the fibers cross the midline, reach the lateral column of opposite side and ascend and reach thalamus.

Termination

Fibers of lateral spinothalamic tract terminate in the **ventral posterolateral nucleus** of thalamus. From here, third order neuron fibers relay to the somesthetic area (sensory cortex) of cerebral cortex.

Function

Fibers of this tract carry impulses of **pain** and **thermal sensations**.

Effect of Lesion

Bilateral lesion of this tract leads to total loss of pain and temperature sensations on both sides below the level of lesion. Unilateral lesion of the lateral spinothalamic tract causes loss of pain and temperature below the level of lesion in the opposite side.

3. VENTRAL SPINOCEREBELLAR TRACT

Ventral spinocerebellar tract or **Gower's tract**, is formed by fibers of second order neurons of the pathway for **subconscious kinesthetic sensation**. This tract is situated in lateral white column (**Figs. 94.3 and 94.5**).

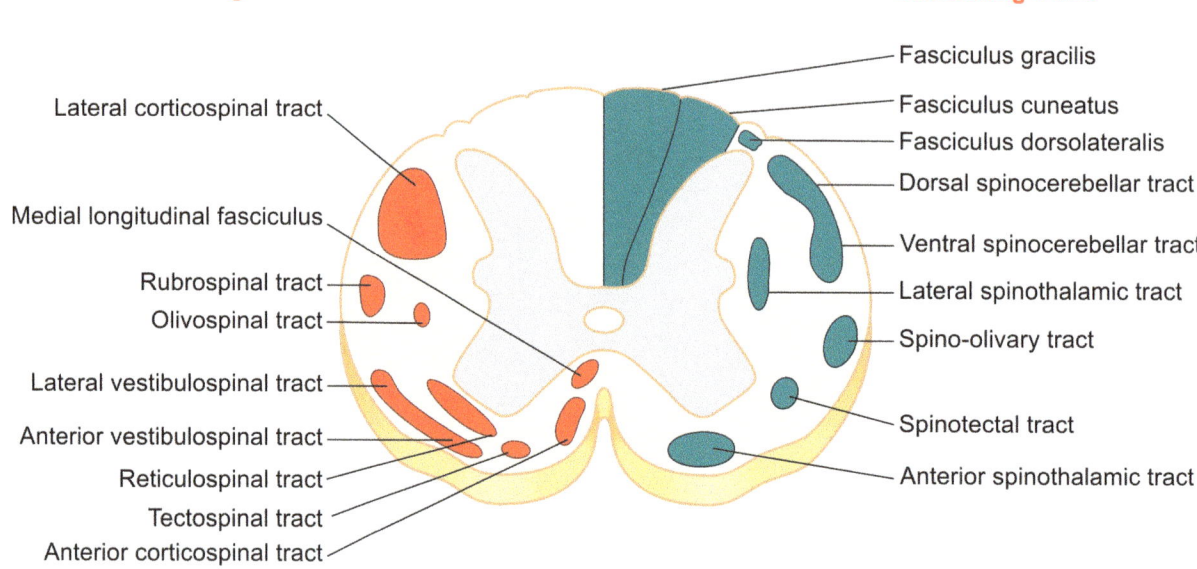

FIGURE 94.3: Tracts of spinal cord.

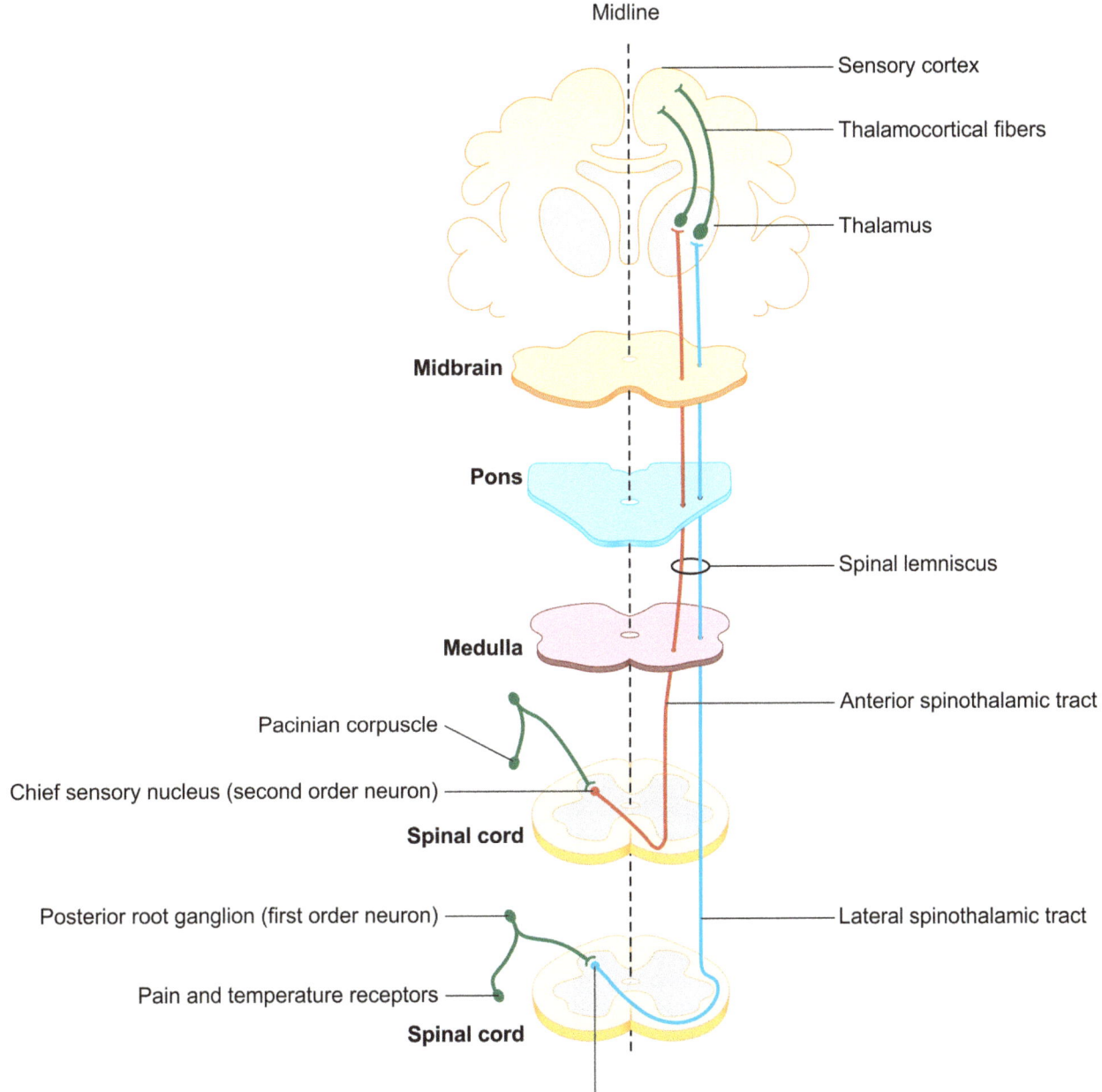

FIGURE 94.4: Spinothalamic tracts and pathways for crude touch, pain and temperature sensations. Anterior spinothalamic tract (red) carries crude touch sensation. Lateral spinothalamic tract (blue) carries pain and temperature sensations.

Origin

Fibers of this tract arise from the **marginal nucleus**. Fibers from these neurons make their first appearance in **lower lumbar** segments of spinal cord.

Course

Majority of the fibers from the marginal nucleus **cross** the midline and ascend in lateral white column of opposite side. Few fibers ascend in the lateral white column of the same side. All the fibers ascend and reach the cerebellum via superior cerebellar peduncle.

Termination

These fibers terminate in the **anterior lobe** of cerebellum.

Function

This tract carries the impulses of subconscious kinesthetic sensation (proprioceptive impulses) from muscles, tendons and joints. The impulses of **subconscious kinesthetic sensation** are also called **non-sensory impulses**.

Effect of Lesion

Lesion of this tract leads to loss of subconscious kinesthetic sensation in the opposite side.

■ 4. DORSAL SPINOCEREBELLAR TRACT

It is otherwise called **Flechsig's tract**, formed by the fibers of second order neurons of the pathway for **subconscious kinesthetic sensation** (Figs. 94.3 and 94.4).

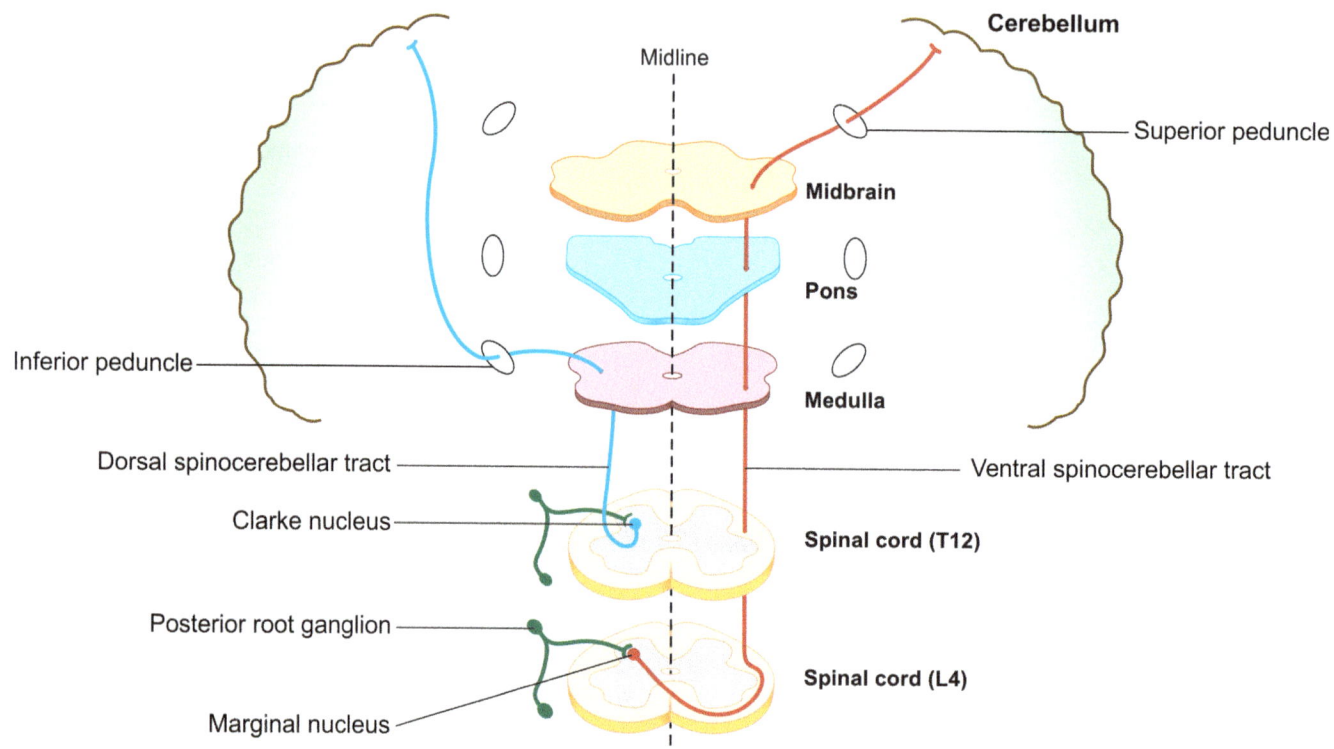

FIGURE 94.5: Spinocerebellar tracts and pathway for subconscious kinesthetic sensation.

Origin

Fibers of this tract arise from the **Clarke's nucleus** in posterior gray matter. First appearance is in **upper lumbar segments**. From lower lumbar and sacral segments, the impulses are carried upwards by the dorsal nerve roots to the upper lumbar segments.

Course

This tract is formed by **uncrossed fibers**. The axons from Clarke's nucleus run to lateral column of same side ascend and reach medulla oblongata. From here, the fibers reach the cerebellum through inferior cerebellar peduncle.

Termination

Fibers of this tract end in the cortex of anterior lobe of cerebellum along with ventral spinocerebellar tract fibers.

Function

Along with ventral spinocerebellar tract, the dorsal spinocerebellar tract carries the impulses of subconscious kinesthetic sensation (non-sensory impulses).

Effect of Lesion

Unilateral loss of the subconscious kinesthetic sensation occurs in lesion of this tract on the **same side.**

■ 5. SPINOTECTAL TRACT

Spinotectal tract is considered as a component of **anterior spinothalamic tract**. It is constituted by the fibers of second order neurons **(Fig. 94.3)**. Fibers of this tract originate from the **chief sensory nucleus**. This tract contains **crossed fibers**. After taking origin, the fibers cross to opposite lateral column. Then, the fibers ascend to the midbrain **along with** anterior spinothalamic tract.

Fibers of spinotectal tract end in the **superior colliculus** in midbrain. This tract is concerned with **spinovisual reflex**.

■ 6. FASCICULUS DORSOLATERALIS

It is otherwise called **tract of Lissauer**. It is considered as a component of **lateral spinothalamic tract**. And, it is constituted by the fibers of first order neurons. This tract is situated in the lateral white column **(Fig. 94.3)**.

Fibers of the dorsolateral fasciculus carry impulses of **pain and temperature sensations**.

■ 7. SPINORETICULAR TRACT

Spinoreticular tract is formed by the fibers of second order neurons. It is situated in anterolateral white column. Fibers of this tract arise from **intermediolateral nucleus**. This tract consists of **crossed** and **uncrossed fibers**. After taking origin, some of the fibers cross the midline and then ascend upwards. Remaining fibers ascend up in the same side without crossing. All the fibers terminate in the **reticular formation** of brainstem.

Fibers of the spinoreticular tract are the components of ascending reticular activating system and are concerned with **consciousness and awareness**.

■ 8. SPINO-OLIVARY TRACT

This tract is situated in anterolateral part of white column. Origin of the fibers of this tract is not specific. However, the fibers terminate in the **olivary nucleus** of medulla oblongata at the same side. From here, the neurons project into cerebellum. This tract is concerned with **proprioception**.

■ 9. SPINOVESTIBULAR TRACT

Spinovestibular tract is situated in the lateral white column of the spinal cord. The fibers of this tract arise from all the segments of spinal cord and terminate on the **lateral vestibular nucleus**. This tract is also concerned with **proprioception**.

■ 10. FASCICULUS GRACILIS (TRACT OF GOLL) AND
■ 11. FASCICULUS CUNEATUS (TRACT OF BURDACH)

These two tracts are together called **ascending posterior column tracts**. These tracts are formed by the fibers from posterior root ganglia. Thus, both the tracts are constituted by the fibers of **first order neurons** of the sensory pathway (Fig. 94.6).

These two tracts are situated in posterior white column of spinal cord hence the name posterior column tracts (Fig. 94.3). In the cervical and upper thoracic segments of spinal cord, the posterior white column is divided into medial **fasciculus gracilis** and lateral **fasciculus cuneatus**.

Origin

Fibers of these two tracts are the axons of **first order neurons**. The cell body of these neurons is in the posterior root ganglia and, the fibers form the medial division (bundle) of the posterior nerve root.

Course

After entering the spinal cord, the fibers ascend through the posterior white column. These fibers do not synapse in the spinal cord.

Fasciculus gracilis contains the fibers from lower parts of the body, i.e. from lower thoracic, lumbar and sacral ganglia of posterior nerve root. **Fasciculus cuneatus** contains fibers from upper part of the body, i.e. from cervical and upper thoracic ganglia of posterior nerve root.

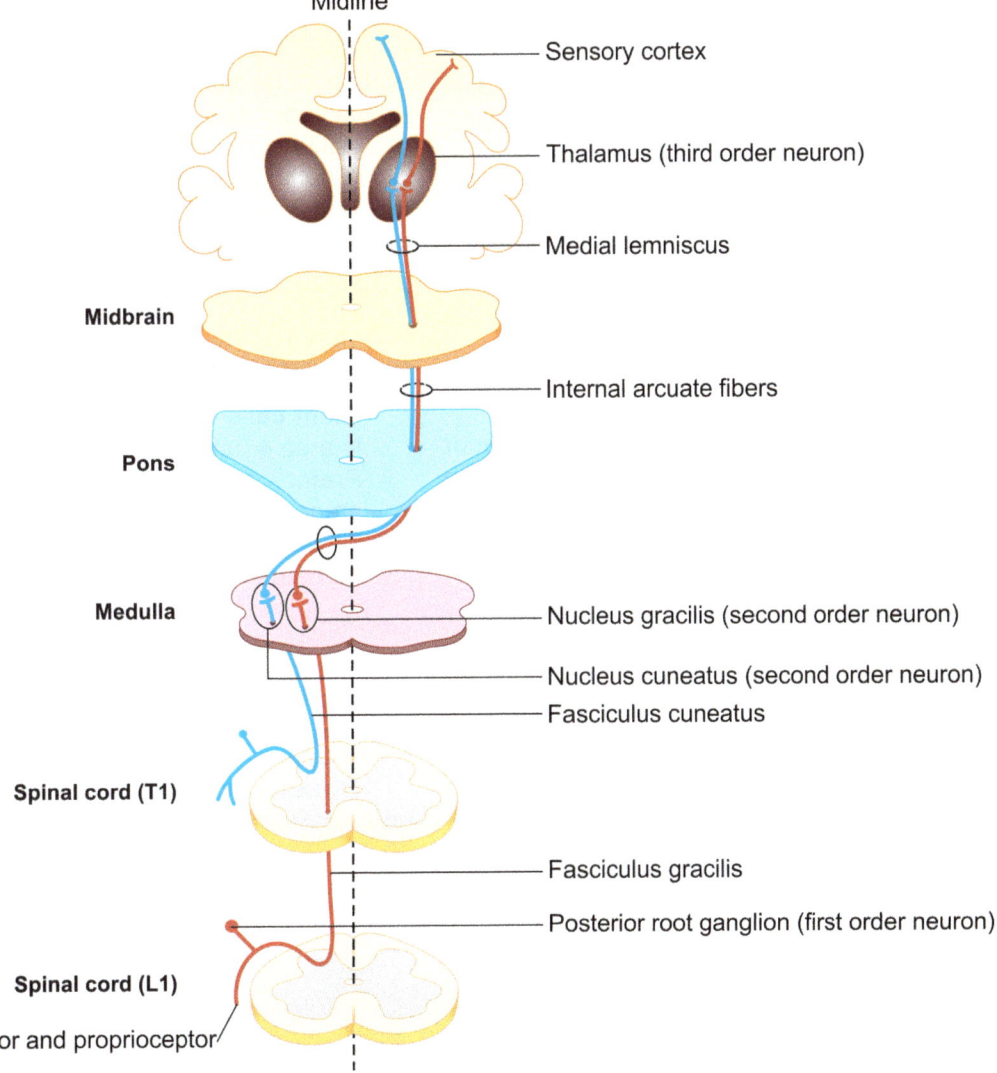

FIGURE 94.6: Ascending tracts in posterior white column of spinal cord and pathway for: 1. Fine touch sensation. 2. Tactile localization. 3. Tactile discrimination. 4. Vibratory sensation. 5. Conscious kinesthetic sensation. 6. Stereognosis.

Termination

These two tracts terminate in the **medulla oblongata** of same side. The fibers of fasciculus gracilis terminate in the **nucleus gracilis** and the fibers of fasciculus cuneatus terminate in the **nucleus cuneatus**. The cells of these medullary nuclei form the **second order neurons**.

Axons of the second order neurons form **internal arcuate fibers**. The internal arcuate fibers from both the sides cross the midline forming **sensory decussation** and then ascend through pons and midbrain as **medial lemniscus**. The fibers of medial lemniscus terminate in **ventral posterolateral nucleus** of thalamus. From here, fibers of the third order neurons relay to **sensory area** of cerebral cortex.

Functions

Tracts of the posterior white column convey impulses of following sensations:

i. **Fine** (epicritic) **tactile** (touch) **sensation**.
ii. **Tactile localization**: It is the ability to locate the area of skin where tactile stimulus is applied with closed eyes.
iii. **Tactile discrimination** (two-point discrimination): It is the ability to recognize the two stimuli applied over the skin simultaneously with closed eyes.
iv. **Sensation of vibration**: It is the ability to perceive the vibrations (from a vibrating tuning fork placed over bony prominence) conducted to deep tissues through skin.
v. **Conscious kinesthetic sensation**: It is the sensation or awareness of various muscular activities in different parts of the body.
vi. **Stereognosis**: It is the ability to recognize the known objects by touch with closed eyes.

Effect of Lesion

Lesion in the fibers of these tracts or lesion in the posterior white column leads to the following symptoms on the same side below the lesion:

i. Loss of fine tactile sensation. However, crude touch sensation is normal.
ii. Loss of tactile localization.
iii. Loss of two-point discrimination.
iv. Loss of sensation of vibration.
v. **Astereognosis**: It is the inability to recognize known objects by touch while closing the eyes.
vi. Lack of ability to differentiate the weight of different objects.
vii. Loss of proprioception: It is inability to appreciate the position and movement of different parts of the body.
viii. **Sensory ataxia** or **posterior column ataxia**: It is the condition characterized by uncoordinated, slow and clumsy voluntary movements because of the loss of proprioception.

■ COMMA TRACT OF SCHULTZE

Comma tract of Schultze is also called **interfascicular fasciculus.** It is situated in between tracts of Goll and Burdach and looks like a comma in transection. This tract is formed by the short descending fibers, arising from the medial division of posterior nerve root. These fibers are also considered as the descending branches of the tracts of Goll and Burdach. This tract establishes **intersegmental communications** and forms short reflex arc.

■ DESCENDING TRACTS OF SPINAL CORD

Descending tracts of the spinal cord are formed by motor nerve fibers arising from brain and descend into the spinal cord. These tracts carry motor impulses from brain to spinal cord. Descending tracts of the spinal cord are of two types:

I. Pyramidal tracts which are concerned with voluntary movements.
II. Extrapyramidal tracts which are concerned with regulation of muscle tone, posture and equilibrium.

Descending tracts are listed in **Table 94.3**. Features of the descending tract are given in **Table 94.6**.

■ PYRAMIDAL TRACTS

Pyramidal tracts were the first tracts to be found in man. These tracts of the spinal cord are concerned with voluntary motor activities of the body. These tracts are otherwise known as **corticospinal tracts**. There are two corticospinal tracts, the anterior corticospinal tract and lateral corticospinal tract.

While running from cerebral cortex towards spinal cord, the fibers of these two tracts give the appearance of a pyramid on the upper part of anterior surface of medulla oblongata **(Fig. 94.7)** and hence the name pyramidal tracts.

Origin

Fibers of pyramidal tracts arise from the following nerve cells in the cerebral cortex:

i. **Giant cells** or **Betz cells** or **pyramidal cells** situated in area 4 (primary motor area) of frontal lobe.
ii. Premotor area (area 6) and supplementary motor areas.
iii. Other parts of frontal lobe.
iv. Somatosensory areas of parietal lobe.

Course

After taking origin, the nerve fibers run downwards through cerebral hemisphere and converge in the form of a fan-like structure called **corona radiata**.

TABLE 94.6: List of descending tracts of spinal cord.

Type	Tract
Pyramidal tracts	1. Anterior corticospinal tract 2. Lateral corticospinal tract
Extrapyramidal tracts	1. Medial longitudinal fasciculus 2. Anterior vestibulospinal tract 3. Lateral vestibulospinal tract 4. Reticulospinal tract 5. Tectospinal tract 6. Rubrospinal tract 7. Olivospinal tract

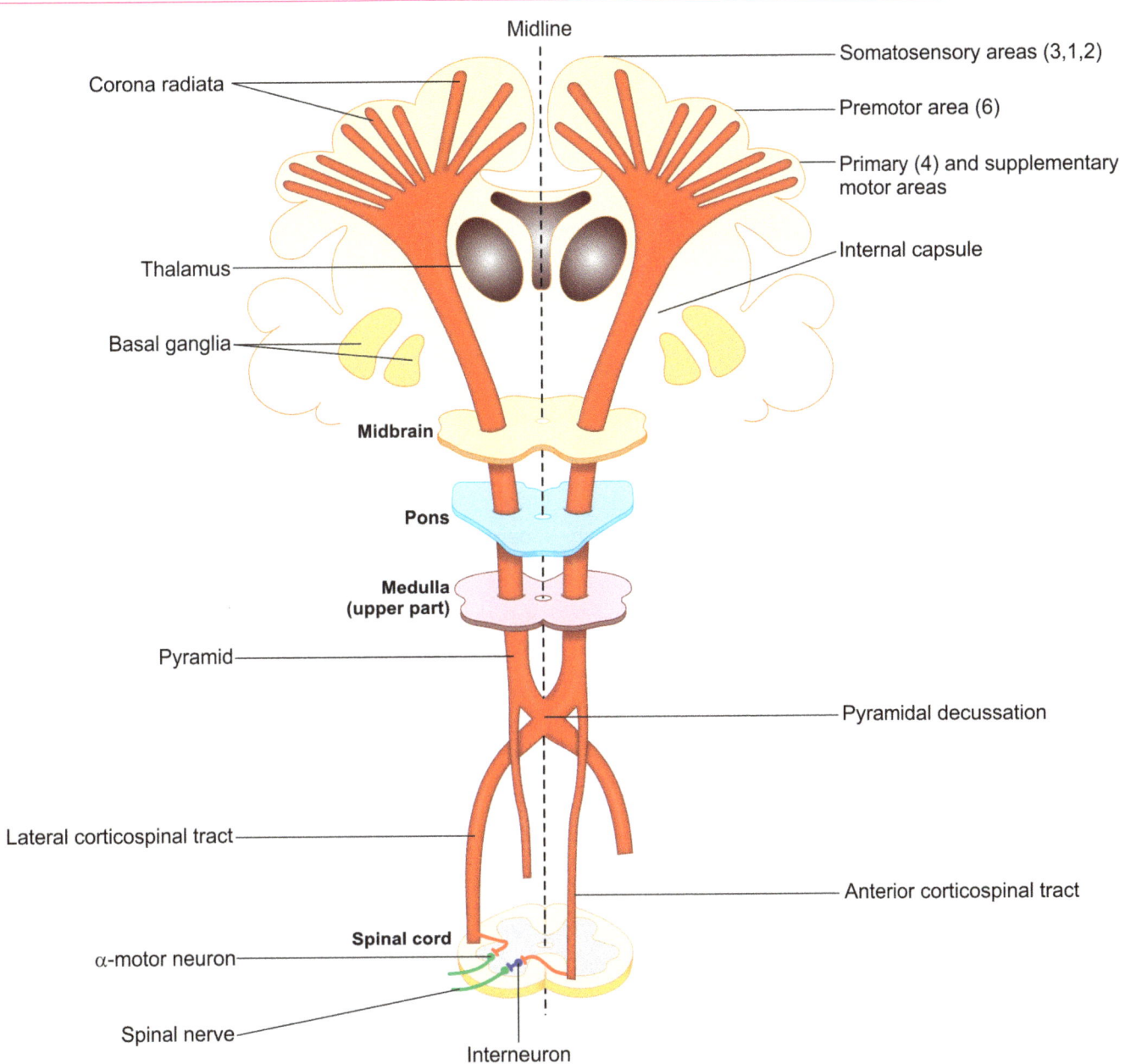

FIGURE 94.7: Pyramidal tracts.

Then the fibers descend down through internal capsule, midbrain and pons. In the upper part of medulla these fibers give the appearance of a **pyramid**.

In the lower part of medulla, 80% of fibers from each side cross to the opposite side. While crossing the midline, the fibers of both sides form the **pyramidal decussation**. After crossing and forming pyramidal decussation, these fibers descend through the posterior part of lateral white column of the spinal cord as **crossed pyramidal tract** or **lateral corticospinal tract** or indirect corticospinal tract.

Remaining 20% of fibers do not cross to the opposite side but descend down through the anterior white column of the spinal cord as **uncrossed pyramidal tract** or **anterior corticospinal tract** or direct corticospinal tract.

Termination

All the fibers of pyramidal tracts terminate in the **motor neurons** of anterior gray horn. Axons of the motor neurons leave the spinal cord as spinal nerves through anterior nerve roots and supply the skeletal muscles.

Neurons giving origin to the fibers of pyramidal tract are called the **upper motor neurons**. The motor neurons in the spinal cord are called the **lower motor neurons**.

Function

Pyramidal tracts are concerned with **voluntary movements** of the body. Fibers of the pyramidal tracts transmit motor impulses from motor area of cerebral cortex to the anterior motor neurons of the spinal cord. These two tracts are responsible for fine, skilled movements.

Effect of Lesion

Lesion in the neurons of motor cortex and the fibers of pyramidal tracts is called the **upper motor neuron lesion**. Effects of upper motor lesion are given in the next Chapter.

■ EXTRAPYRAMIDAL TRACTS

Descending tracts of spinal cord other than pyramidal tracts are called extrapyramidal tracts. Extrapyramidal tracts are listed in **Table 94.7**.

■ 1. MEDIAL LONGITUDINAL FASCICULUS

Origin

Fibers of this tract take origin from **brainstem**. It is situated in anterior white column of the spinal cord.

Course

After entering the spinal cord from the brainstem, the fibers descend through anterior white column of the **same side**. In the spinal cord, this tract runs along with anterior vestibulospinal tract.

Termination

Fibers of this tract terminate in anterior motor neurons of the spinal cord along with fibers of anterior vestibulospinal tract.

Function

This tract helps in the coordination of **reflex ocular movements** and the integration of **ocular and neck movements**.

Effect of Lesion

Reflex ocular movements and reflex neck movements are affected in the lesion of this tract.

■ 2. ANTERIOR VESTIBULOSPINAL TRACT

Origin

Fibers of this tract arise from the **medial vestibular nucleus** in medulla oblongata. This tract is situated in the anterior white column.

Course

Fibers of this tract run down from medulla into the anterior column of spinal cord. All the fibers are **uncrossed**.

Termination

Along with fibers of lateral vestibulospinal tract, the fibers of this tract terminate in anterior motor neurons directly or through internuncial neurons.

Function and Effect of Lesion

Function and effect of lesion of this tract is explained along with the function of lateral vestibulospinal tract.

■ 3. LATERAL VESTIBULOSPINAL TRACT

Origin

Fibers of this tract take origin from the **lateral vestibular nucleus** or **Deiter nucleus** in medulla. This tract occupies the lateral white column of spinal cord.

Course

From medulla, most of the fibers descend directly through lateral column.

Termination

Fibers of this tract terminate in the anterior motor neurons.

Functions

Vestibulospinal tracts are concerned with adjustment of **position of head** and **body** during angular and linear acceleration.

Effect of Lesion

During lesion of vestibulospinal tracts, the adjustment of head and body becomes difficult during acceleration.

■ 4. RETICULOSPINAL TRACT

Origin

Fibers of this tract arise from the **reticular formation** of pons and medulla. These fibers descend in anterior column and to some extend in the anterior part of lateral column. The reticulospinal tract is situated in the anterior white column.

Termination

Fibers of reticulospinal tract terminate in the **gamma motor neurons** of anterior gray horn.

Functions

Reticulospinal tract is concerned with control of **movements** and maintenance of **muscle tone**, respiration and diameter of blood vessels.

Effect of Lesion

Lesion of this tract causes disturbances in respiration, blood pressure, movements of body and muscle tone.

■ 5. TECTOSPINAL TRACT

Origin

Nerve fibers of this tract arise from **superior colliculus** of midbrain. This tract is situated in the anterior white column of the spinal cord.

Course

After taking origin from the superior colliculus, the fibers **cross the midline** in the dorsal tegmental decussation and descend in anterior column.

Termination

Fibers of this tract terminate in the anterior motor neurons of the spinal cord.

Function

This tract is responsible for the **movement of head** in response to visual and auditory stimuli.

TABLE 94.7: Descending tracts of spinal cord.

	Tract	Situation	Origin	Course	Function
Pyramidal tracts	1. Anterior corticospinal tract	Anterior white column	Primary motor area Premotor area	Uncrossed fibers	Control of voluntary movements Form upper motor neurons
	2. Lateral corticospinal tract	Lateral white column	Supplementary motor areas Somatosensory areas	Crossed fibers	
Extrapyramidal tracts	1. Medial longitudinal fasciculus	Anterior white column	Vestibular nucleus Reticular formation Superior colliculus Cells of Cajal	Uncrossed fibers Extend up to upper cervical segments	Coordination of reflex ocular movements Integration of movements of eyes and neck
	2. Anterior vestibulospinal tract	Anterior white column	Medial vestibular nucleus	Uncrossed fibers Extend up to upper thoracic segments	Maintenance of muscle tone and posture Maintenance of position of head and body during acceleration
	3. Lateral vestibulospinal tract	Lateral white column	Lateral vestibular nucleus	Mostly uncrossed Extend to all segments	Coordination of voluntary and reflex movements
	4. Reticulospinal tract	Lateral white fasciculus	Reticular formation of pons and medulla	Mostly uncrossed Extend up to thoracic segments	Control of muscle tone Control of respiration Control of diameter of blood vessels
	5. Tectospinal tract	Anterior white column	Superior colliculus	Crossed fibers Extend up to lower cervical segments	Control of movement of head in response to visual and auditory impulses
	6. Rubrospinal tract	Lateral white column	Red nucleus	Crossed fibers Extend up to thoracic segments	Facilitatory influence on flexor muscle tone
	7. Olivospinal tract	Lateral white column	Inferior olivary nucleus	Mostly crossed Extent: Not clear	Control of movements due to proprioception

Termination: Fibers of all the tracts terminate on motor neurons situated in the anterior gray horn of spinal cord.

6. RUBROSPINAL TRACT

Origin

Fibers of this tract arise from **red nucleus** in midbrain. The rubrospinal tract is situated in the lateral white column.

Course

After arising from the red nucleus, the fibers **cross the midline** and descend into spinal cord through the reticular formation of pons and medulla.

Termination

Fibers of rubrospinal tract end in the anterior motor neurons of the spinal cord.

Function

This tract exhibits facilitatory influence upon the **flexor muscle tone**.

7. OLIVOSPINAL TRACT

Origin

Nerve fibers of this tract take origin from the **inferior olivary nucleus** present in the medulla oblongata. Olivospinal tract is present in the lateral white column.

Termination

Fibers of this tract terminate in the anterior motor neurons of the spinal cord.

Function

This tract is involved in **reflex movements** arising from the proprioceptors.

APPLIED PHYSIOLOGY

Injury to spinal cord or any disease of spinal cord leads to either temporary or permanent dysfunction. Dysfunction of spinal cord occurs because of:

I. Complete transection.
II. Incomplete transection.
III. Hemisection.
IV. Diseases of spinal cord.

I. COMPLETE TRANSECTION OF SPINAL CORD

Complete transection of spinal cord occurs due to:

1. Bullet injury, which causes dislocation of spinal cord.
2. Accidents, which cause dislocation of spinal cord or occlusion of blood vessels.

Complete transection causes immediate **loss of sensation** and **voluntary movement** below the level of lesion. In quick transection of spinal cord, the patient feels himself cut into two. Then the effects (symptoms) of complete transection of spinal cord start appearing.

Effects occur in three stages:

1. Stage of spinal shock.
2. Stage of reflex activity.
3. Stage of reflex failure.

1. *Stage of Spinal Shock*

Stage of spinal shock is the first stage of effects that occurs immediately after injury. Common symptoms during this stage are **paralysis of limbs**, **loss of reflexes**, and **loss of sensations**. There is decreased venous return resulting in accumulation of blood in lower limbs. When lesion is at or above T1 segment, the blood pressure falls drastically.

Severity of complete transection depends upon the level of lesion. Complete transection at the level of cervical region can be very fatal. Because, the diaphragm and other respiratory muscles are cut off from respiratory centers. It causes paralysis of respiratory muscles leading to sudden arrest of breathing.

2. *Stage of Reflex Activity*

Stage of reflex activity is also called **stage of recovery.** After 3 weeks period, depending largely upon the general health of the patient, the reflex activity begins to return to the isolated segments of spinal cord below the level of lesion.

After three months, tone returns in skeletal muscle. Tone returns to **flexor muscles** first. Limbs in this condition tend to adopt a position of slight flexion and the paralysis is therefore called **paraplegia in flexion.** Limbs cannot support weight of the body.

After few weeks, when tone returns to more muscles, reflex movements can occur. In some cases, a widespread reaction can be elicited by scratching the skin over the lower limbs or the anterior abdominal wall. This reaction includes the spasm in flexor muscles of both the lower limbs, evacuation of urinary bladder and profuse sweating. This is known as the **mass reflex.**

3. *Stage of Reflex Failure*

Though the reflex movements return, muscles below the level of injury have less power and less resistance. Usually, general condition of the patient starts **deteriorating**. General infection or **toxemia** becomes common. Due to this, the failure of reflex function develops. The reflexes become more difficult to elicit. Muscles become extremely **flaccid** and undergo **wasting**.

II. INCOMPLETE TRANSECTION OF SPINAL CORD

If spinal cord is gravely injured, but does not suffer complete division, the condition is called as incomplete transection.

After incomplete transection of the spinal cord, all the three stages of complete transection occur:

1. Stage of spinal shock.
2. Stage of reflex activity.
3. Stage of reflex failure.

1. *Stage of Spinal Shock*

Features are similar to those of complete transection.

2. *Stage of Reflex Activity*

During this stage, tone returns to **extensor muscles** first and not to the flexor muscles. So, there is **extensor**

hypertonia and so, the lower limbs are extended at hip and knee with toes pointing slightly downwards. This condition is known as **paraplegia in extension.**

Stretch reflex reappears first. Flexor reflexes return later.

3. Stage of Reflex Failure

Features are similar to those of complete transection.

III. HEMISECTION OF SPINAL CORD: BROWN-SÉQUARD SYNDROME

Lesion involving one lateral half of the spinal cord is called hemisection **(Fig. 94.8)**. It can occur due to injury during accidents. It can also be produced experimentally in animals.

Symptoms of Hemisection of Spinal Cord

Signs and symptoms, which occur after hemisection of the spinal cord, constitute Brown-Séquard syndrome.

If the hemisection is due to injury, spinal shock occurs immediately. Muscles lose the tone and become flaccid. The reflexes are abolished. In case the patient survives, this stage gradually passes off and certain signs and symptoms develop.

Effects occur below the level of lesion and at the level of lesion. Effects in these areas differ on the same side and opposite side. There are changes in sensory and motor functions **(Fig. 94.8)**.

IV. DISEASES OF SPINAL CORD

1. Syringomyelia

Syringomyelia is a spinal cord disorder characterized by the presence of **fluid-filled cavities** in the spinal cord.

Syringomyelia occurs due to the over growth of **neuroglial cells** in spinal cord accompanied by cavity formation and accumulation of fluid. Characteristic features of this disease are the loss of pain and temperature sensations and muscular weakness. Severity of the loss of sensations depends upon the extent of disease in spinal cord.

2. Tabes Dorsalis

Tabes dorsalis is a slowly progressive nervous disorder affecting both the motor and sensory functions of spinal cord.

It occurs due to the degeneration of posterior (sensory) nerve roots. It usually occurs in **syphilis.** In tabes dorsalis, both sensory and motor functions are affected.

3. Multiple Sclerosis

Multiple sclerosis (MS) is a chronic and **progressive inflammatory disease** characterized by **demyelination** in brain and spinal cord. It affects the myelinated nerve fibers of brain, spinal cord and optic nerve and causes gradual destruction of myelin sheath (**demyelination**). When the disease progresses, there is transection of axons in patches throughout brain and spinal cord. The term **sclerosis** refers to **scars** in the myelin sheath.

Initial symptoms include loss of sensations on face, arms and legs, weakness and disturbances in maintenance of posture and double vision followed by partial blindness. Symptoms when the disease progresses include tremor, fatigue and muscle spasms, speech difficulty, difficulty in performing day-to-day activities, complete blindness and suicidal tendency.

4. Disk Prolapse

Intervertebral or **spinal disk** is the cartilaginous structure of vertebral column that separates each vertebra. It is made up of a tough outer fibrous layer and a soft inner part.

Disk prolapse is the rupture of spinal disk. During disk prolapse, the soft inner material bulges out. The bulged disk material may irritate or compress or damage the nerve root that passes through the gap between the vertebrae. Severity of the condition depends upon the degree of bulging.

Symptoms of disk prolapse include pain and weakness in the area of prolapse. Most common areas of disk prolapse are neck and lower part of vertebral column.

488 Section 10: Nervous System

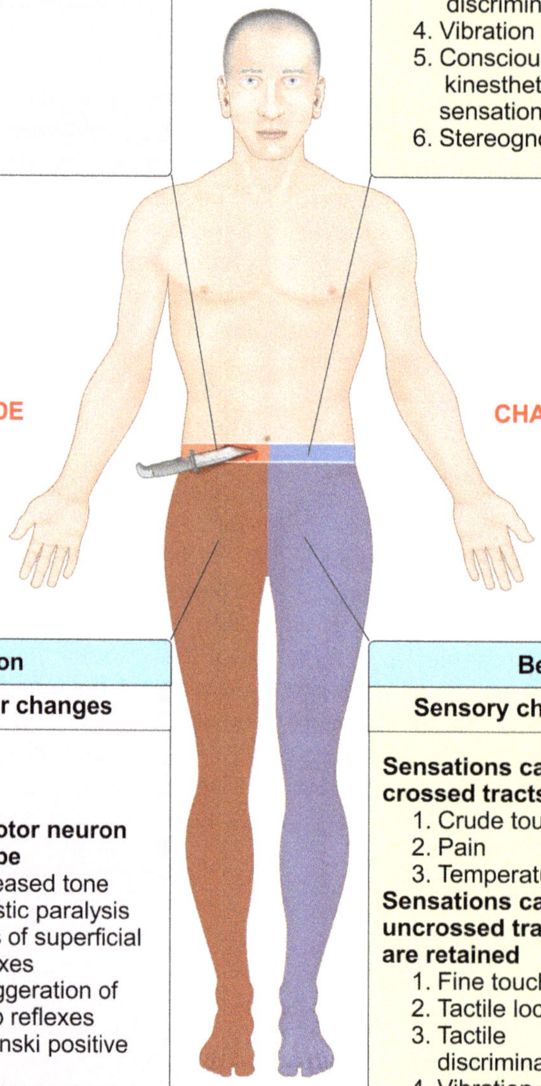

CHANGES ON THE SAME SIDE OF LESION

At the level of lesion

Sensory changes	Motor changes
Complete anesthesia	**Lower motor neuron lesion type** 1. Loss of muscle tone 2. Flaccid paralysis 3. Loss of all reflexes 4. Wastage of muscle 5. Loss of vasomotor tone

Below the level of lesion

Sensory changes	Motor changes
Sensations carried by uncrossed tracts are lost 1. Fine touch 2. Tactile localization 3. Tactile discrimination 4. Vibration sense 5. Conscious kinesthetic sensation 6. Stereognosis **Sensations carried by crossed tracts are retained** 1. Crude touch 2. Pain 3. Temperature	**Upper motor neuron lesion type** 1. Increased tone 2. Spastic paralysis 3. Loss of superficial reflexes 4. Exaggeration of deep reflexes 5. Babinski positive sign 6. Rigidity in the limbs 7. No muscular wastage

CHANGES ON THE OPPOSITE SIDE OF LESION

At the level of lesion

Sensory changes	Motor changes
Sensations carried by crossed tracts are lost 1. Crude touch 2. Pain 3. Temperature **Sensations carried by uncrossed tracts are retained** 1. Fine touch 2. Tactile localization 3. Tactile discrimination 4. Vibration sense 5. Conscious kinesthetic sensation 6. Stereognosis	**No paralysis** *If it occurs:* 1. Very mild 2. Resembles lower motor neuron lesion type

Below the level of lesion

Sensory changes	Motor changes
Sensations carried by crossed tracts are lost 1. Crude touch 2. Pain 3. Temperature **Sensations carried by uncrossed tracts are retained** 1. Fine touch 2. Tactile localization 3. Tactile discrimination 4. Vibration sense 5. Conscious kinesthetic sensation 6. Stereognosis	**No paralysis** *If it occurs:* 1. Very mild 2. Resembles upper motor neuron lesion type

FIGURE 94.8: Effect of hemisection of spinal cord at the same level and below the level of lesion.

Chapter 95: Somatosensory System and Somatomotor System

CHAPTER OUTLINE

- **SENSATIONS**
- **SOMATOSENSORY SYSTEM**
  - **DEFINITION**
  - **TYPES OF SOMATIC SENSATIONS**
  - **SENSORY PATHWAYS**
  - **SENSORY FIBERS PASSING THROUGH SPINAL CORD**
  - **SENSORY FIBERS PASSING THROUGH TRIGEMINAL NERVE**
  - **APPLIED PHYSIOLOGY**
- **MOTOR ACTIVITIES OF THE BODY**
- **SOMATOMOTOR SYSTEM**
  - **ACTIVITIES OF SKELETAL MUSCLES**
  - **STRUCTURE OF MOTOR SYSTEM**
  - **MOTOR NEURONS IN SPINAL CORD AND CRANIAL NERVE NUCLEI**
  - **CLASSIFICATION OF MOTOR PATHWAYS**
  - **UPPER MOTOR NEURON AND LOWER MOTOR NEURON**
  - **APPLIED PHYSIOLOGY**

SENSATIONS

Sensation is a process of detecting and sensing external or internal stimuli received by sensory receptors. It is different from **perception** which means identification and interpretation of sensations.

Sensations are of two types:

1. Somatic Sensations

Somatic sensations are the sensations arising from skin, muscles, tendons, joints and visceral organs. These sensations have **specific receptors**, which respond to a particular type of stimulus.

2. Special Sensations

Special sensations are the **complex sensations** for which the body has some **specialized sense organs**. Such sensations are usually called **special senses**. Special senses are vision, hearing, taste and smell.

Special senses are described in Section 11. This chapter deals only with somatic sensations.

SOMATOSENSORY SYSTEM

DEFINITION

Somatosensory system is defined as the sensory system associated with different parts of the body. It is a wide neural system that spreads in all major areas of the body. It includes specific receptors, sensory or afferent neurons and the centers.

TYPES OF SOMATIC SENSATIONS

Generally, somatic sensations are classified into three types:

1. Epicritic sensations.
2. Protopathic sensations.
3. Deep sensations.

1. Epicritic Sensations

Epicritic sensations are the mild or **light sensations** which are perceived and localized more accurately.

Epicritic sensations are:

i. Fine touch or tactile sensation.
ii. Tactile localization.
iii. Tactile discrimination.
iv. Temperature sensation with finer range between 25°C and 40°C.

2. Protopathic Sensations

Protopathic sensations are the **crude sensations** which are primitive type of sensations.

Protopathic sensations are:

i. Pressure sensation.
ii. Pain sensation.

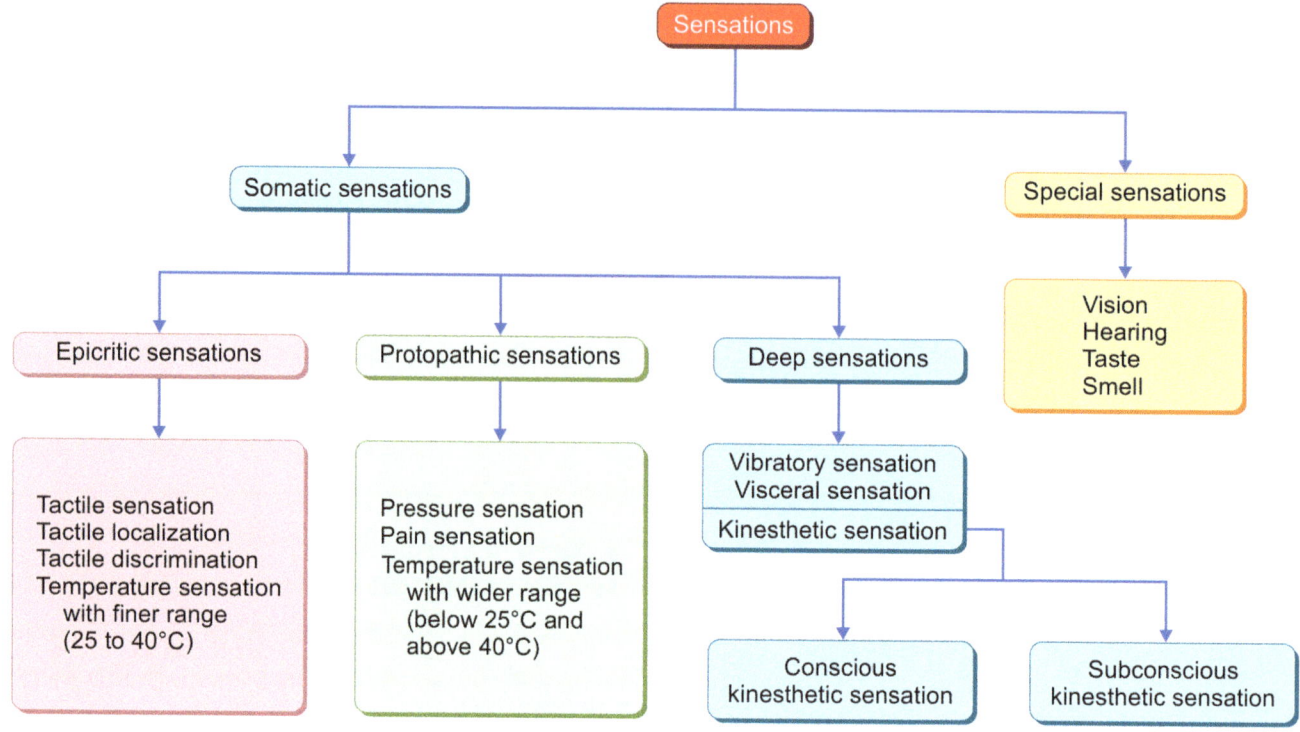

FIGURE 95.1: Classification of sensations.

iii. Temperature sensation with a wider range, i.e. below 25°C and above 40°C.

3. Deep Sensations

Deep sensations are sensations arising from **deeper structures** beneath the skin and visceral organs.

Deep sensations are:

i. Sensation of vibration or **pallesthesia**, which is the combination of touch and pressure sensation.
ii. Kinesthetic sensation or **kinesthesia** which is the sensation of position and movements of different parts of the body. This sensation arises from the proprioceptors present in muscles, tendons, joints and ligaments. Proprioceptors are the receptors, which give response during various movements of a joint. Kinesthetic sensation is of two types:
   a. Conscious kinesthetic sensation (Chapter 94).
   b. Subconscious kinesthetic sensation. Impulses of this sensation are called nonsensory impulses.
iii. **Visceral sensations** arising from viscera **(Fig. 95.1)**.

Combined or Synthetic Sensations

Combined or synthetic sensations are the sensations synthesized at cortical level by integration of impulses of basic sensations. Two or more basic sensations are combined in some of the synthetic senses.

Examples of synthetic senses are **vibratory sensation**, and **stereognosis (Box 95.1)**.

Paresthesia or Abnormal Sensations

Paresthesia or abnormal sensations are the unusual feelings on skin without any specific stimulus.

BOX 95.1: Combined sensations.

Vibratory sensation
Ability to perceive vibrations from a vibrating tuning fork placed over bony prominence conducted to deep tissues through skin
Produced by combination of touch and pressure sensations
Stereognosis
Ability to recognize the known objects by touch with closed eyes
Produced by combination of touch and pressure sensations

BOX 95.2: Abnormal sensations.

Numbness
Lack of sensation in a part of the body
Prickling
Sensation of being pierced or pricked
Tingling
Sensation of slight prickling or sensation of tapping by several needle-like objects
Burning
Sensation of a type of pain that is different from aching or stabbing pain

Examples of abnormal sensations are numbness, prickling, tingling and burning **(Box 95.2)**.

■ SENSORY PATHWAYS

Sensory pathways are the nervous pathways of sensations. These pathways carry the impulses from receptors in different parts of the body to centers in brain.

Sensory pathways are of two types:

1. Pathways of somatosensory system.
2. Pathways of viscerosensory system.

Pathways of somatosensory system convey the information from sensory receptors in skin, skeletal muscles and joints. Pathways of this system are constituted by somatic nerve fibers called **somatic afferent nerve fibers**.

Pathways of viscerosensory system convey the information from receptors of the viscera. Pathways of this system are constituted by **visceral or autonomic fibers**. This chapter deals mainly with the somatosensory system. Somatosensory fibers from different parts of the body run through:

i. Spinal tracts
ii. Trigeminal nerve

■ SENSORY FIBERS PASSING THROUGH SPINAL CORD

Sensory fibers from different parts of the body except face and scalp form the sensory pathways which pass through spinal cord. These sensory pathways are constituted by two or three groups of neurons:

i. First order or primary neurons.
ii. Second order or secondary neurons.
iii. Third order or tertiary neurons.

These three groups of neurons are described along with ascending tracts of spinal cord in Chapter 94. Pathways of some sensations such as kinesthetic sensation have only first and second order neurons.

Details of pathways are given in **Table 95.1**. Diagrams of pathways are given in Chapter 94, along with ascending tracts of spinal cord.

■ SENSORY FIBERS PASSING THROUGH TRIGEMINAL NERVE

Trigeminal nerve carries somatosensory information from face, teeth, periodontal tissues (tissues around teeth), oral cavity, nasal cavity, cranial dura mater and major part of scalp to sensory cortex. It also conveys proprioceptive impulses from the extrinsic muscles of the eyeball **(Table 95.2)**.

TABLE 95.1: Sensory pathways.

Sensation	Receptor	First order neuron in	Second order neuron in	Third order neuron in	Center
Fine touch Tactile localization Tactile discrimination Vibratory sensation Stereognosis	Meissner corpuscle and Merkel disk	Posterior nerve root ganglion fibers form Fasciculus gracilis and Fasciculus cuneatus	Nucleus gracilis and Nucleus cuneatus: Fibers form internal arcuate fibers	Ventral posterolateral nucleus of thalamus	Sensory cortex
Pressure Crude touch	Pacinian corpuscle	Posterior nerve root ganglion	Chief sensory nucleus Fibers form anterior spinothalamic tract	Ventral posterolateral nucleus of thalamus	Sensory cortex
Temperature	Warmth: Ruffini end bulb Cold: Krause end bulb	Posterior nerve root ganglion	Substantia gelatinosa Fibers form lateral spinothalamic tract	Ventral posterolateral nucleus of thalamus	Sensory cortex
Conscious kinaesthetic sensation	Proprioceptors: Muscle spindle Golgi tendon apparatus	Posterior nerve root ganglion Fibers form: Fasciculus gracilis and Fasciculus cuneatus	Nucleus gracilis and Nucleus cuneatus: Fibers form internal arcuate fibers	Ventral posterolateral nucleus of thalamus	Sensory cortex
Subconscious kinaesthetic sensation	Proprioceptors: Muscle spindle Golgi tendon apparatus	Posterior nerve root ganglion	Nucleus of Clarke and Marginal nucleus Fibers form dorsal and ventral spinocerebellar tracts	– – –	Anterior lobe of cerebellum
Pain	Free nerve endings	Posterior nerve root ganglion Fast pain: Aδ-fibers Slow pain: C fibers	Fast pain: Marginal nucleus in spinal cord Slow pain: Substantia gelatinosa of Rolando Fibers form lateral spinothalamic tract	Ventral posterolateral nucleus of thalamus Reticular formation and Midbrain	Sensory cortex

TABLE 95.2: Functions of three divisions of trigeminal nerve.

Division	Areas supplied	Function
Ophthalmic	Forehead Eye Front portion of nose	Sensory
Maxillary	Upper teeth, gums and lip Lower eyelid Sides of nose	Sensory
Mandibular	Lower teeth, gums and lip	Sensory
	Jaw	Motor

Origin

Sensory fibers of trigeminal nerve arise from the **trigeminal ganglion** situated near temporal bone. Peripheral processes of neurons in this ganglion form three divisions of trigeminal nerve, namely **ophthalmic, mandibular** and **maxillary** divisions. Cutaneous distribution of the three divisions of trigeminal nerve is shown in **Figure 95.2**.

Central processes from neurons of trigeminal ganglion enter pons in the form of sensory root.

Termination

After reaching the pons, fibers of sensory root divide into two groups, namely descending fibers and ascending fibers.

Descending fibers

Descending fibers terminate on primary sensory nucleus and spinal nucleus of trigeminal nerve. Primary sensory nucleus is situated in pons. Spinal nucleus of trigeminal nerve is situated below the primary sensory nucleus and extends up to the upper segments of spinal cord.

Ascending fibers

Ascending fibers of sensory root terminate in the mesencephalic nucleus of trigeminal nerve, situated in brainstem above the level of primary sensory nucleus **(Fig. 95.3)**.

Central Connections

Majority of fibers from the primary sensory nucleus and spinal nucleus of trigeminal nerve ascend and form

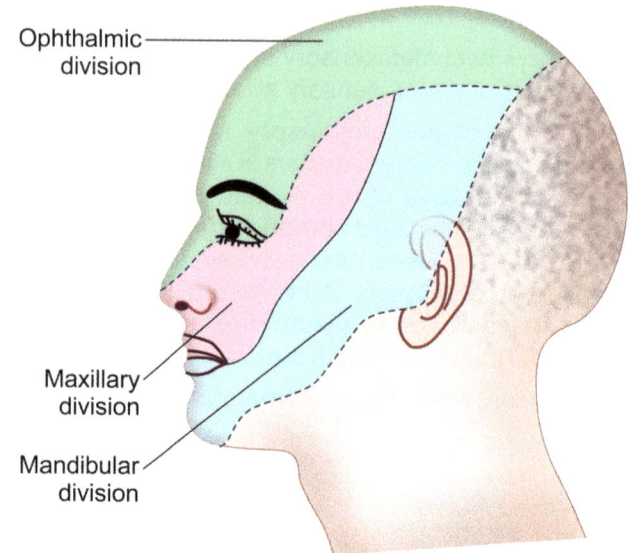

FIGURE 95.2: Cutaneous distribution (sensory) of the three divisions of trigeminal nerve.

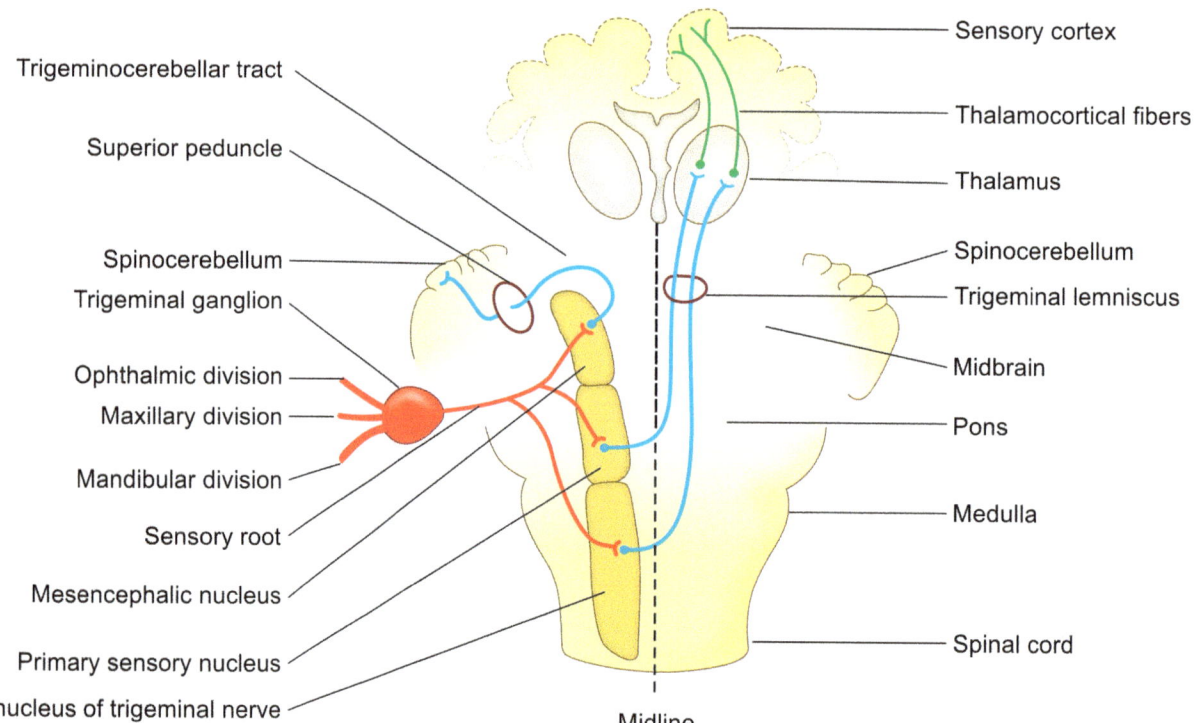

FIGURE 95.3: Diagrammatic representation of trigeminal pathway. Trigeminal lemniscus carries impulses of touch, pressure, pain and temperature sensations to somatosensory cortex. Trigeminocerebellar tract carries proprioceptive impulses to spinocerebellum.

Chapter 95: Somatosensory System and Somatomotor System

trigeminal lemniscus and terminate in ventral posteromedial nucleus of thalamus in the opposite side. Remaining fibers from these two nuclei terminate on the thalamic nucleus of same side. From thalamus, the fibers pass via superior thalamic radiation and reach the somatosensory areas of cerebral cortex.

Primary sensory nucleus and spinal nucleus of trigeminal nerve relay the sensations of touch, pressure, pain and temperature from the regions mentioned above.

Fibers from mesencephalic nucleus form the trigeminocerebellar tract that enters spinocerebellum via the superior cerebellar peduncle of the same side. This nucleus conveys proprioceptive impulses from facial muscles, muscles of mastication and ocular muscles.

■ APPLIED PHYSIOLOGY

Lesions or other nervous disorders in sensory pathway affect the sensory functions of the body. Effects are given in **Table 95.3**.

■ MOTOR ACTIVITIES OF THE BODY

Motor activities of the body are divided into two types:

1. Activities of skeletal muscles which are involved in the posture and movement.
2. Activities of smooth muscles, cardiac muscles and other tissues, which are involved in the functions of various visceral organs.

Activities of the skeletal muscles (voluntary functions) are controlled by the somatomotor system. Activities of other tissues or the visceral organs (involuntary functions) are controlled by the visceral or autonomic nervous system, which is constituted by the sympathetic and parasympathetic systems. Autonomic nervous system is described in Chapter 109.

This chapter deals with somatomotor system.

■ SOMATOMOTOR SYSTEM

Somatomotor system is the part of nervous system that controls the activities of the skeletal muscles (voluntary functions). It is constituted by somatic motor nerve fibers.

■ ACTIVITIES OF SKELETAL MUSCLES

Movements of the body depend upon the different groups of skeletal muscles. Various types of movements or the motor activities brought about by these muscles are:

1. Execution of smooth, precise and accurate voluntary movements.
2. Coordination of movements responsible for skilled activities.
3. Coordination of movements responsible for maintenance of posture and equilibrium.

All these motor activities are controlled by different parts of the nervous system, which are together called the motor system.

TABLE 95.3: Effects of disorders of sensory pathways.

Condition	Definition
1. Anesthesia	Loss of all sensations
2. Hyperesthesia	Increased sensitivity to sensory stimuli
3. Hypoesthesia	Reduction in sensitivity to stimuli
4. Hemianesthesia	Loss of all sensations in one side of body
5. Paresthesia	Abnormal sensations such as tingling, burning, prickling and numbness
6. Hemiparesthesia	Abnormal sensations in one side of body
7. Dissociated anesthesia	Loss of some sensations while other sensations are intact
8. General anesthesia	Loss of all sensations with loss of consciousness produced by anesthetic agents
9. Local anesthesia	Loss of sensations in a restricted area of the body
10. Spinal anesthesia	Loss of sensations without loss of consciousness due to spinal cord lesion or anesthetic agents injected beneath the coverings of spinal cord
11. Tactile anesthesia	Loss of tactile sensations
12. Tactile hyperesthesia	Increased sensitivity to tactile stimulus
13. Analgesia	Loss of pain sensation
14. Hyperalgesia	Increased sensitivity to pain
15. Paralgesia	Abnormal pain sensation
16. Thermoanesthesia or thermanesthesia or thermanalgesia	Loss of thermal sensation
17. Pallanesthesia	Loss of sensation of vibration
18. Astereognosis	Loss of ability to recognize known object with closed eyes due to loss of cutaneous sensations
19. Illusion	Mental depression due to misinterpretation of a sensory stimulus
20. Hallucination	Feeling of a sensation without any stimulus

■ STRUCTURE OF MOTOR SYSTEM

Motor system includes spinal cord and its nerves, cranial nerves, brainstem, cerebral cortex, cerebellum and basal ganglia. The neuronal circuits between these parts of the nervous system which are responsible for the motor activities are called the **motor pathways**.

■ MOTOR NEURONS IN SPINAL CORD AND CRANIAL NERVE NUCLEI

Activities of skeletal muscles are executed by the impulses discharged from alpha motor neurons situated in ventral (anterior) gray horn of spinal cord and nuclei of many of the cranial nerves present in brainstem.

Alpha motor neurons in the spinal cord which innervate the **extrafusal fibers** of skeletal muscles are responsible for the **contraction of muscles** in upper limbs, trunk and lower part of the body. The **gamma motor neurons** which innervate the **intrafusal fibers** of muscle are responsible for the maintenance of **muscle tone**. Motor neurons of the cranial nerve nuclei situated in brainstem send their signals to the muscles of neck and upper part of trunk via cranial nerves.

Final Common Pathway

Alpha motor neurons in spinal cord or cranial nerve nuclei are called **'final common pathway'** of motor system because the motor impulses from different parts of nervous system reach the muscles only through them.

CLASSIFICATION OF MOTOR PATHWAYS

Motor pathways are divided into pyramidal and extrapyramidal tracts.

Pyramidal Tracts

Pyramidal tracts are those fibers, which form the pyramids in the upper part of medulla. Pyramidal tracts are the anterior and lateral corticospinal tracts. These tracts control the voluntary movements of the body (Chapter 94).

Extrapyramidal Tracts

Motor pathways other than pyramidal tracts are known as extrapyramidal tracts. Details of theses tracts are given in Chapter 94. Extrapyramidal tracts which are concerned with coordination muscle tone, posture, equilibrium and integration and the regulation of motor activities.

UPPER MOTOR NEURON AND LOWER MOTOR NEURON

Neurons of the motor system are divided into upper motor neurons and lower motor neurons depending upon their location and termination.

Upper Motor Neuron

Upper motor neurons are the neurons in the higher centers of brain, which control the lower motor neurons.

Upper motor neurons are of three types:

1. Motor neurons in the **cerebral cortex**. Fibers of these neurons form corticospinal (pyramidal) and corticobulbar tracts.
2. Neurons in the **basal ganglia** and **brainstem nuclei**.
3. Neurons in the **cerebellum**.

Motor neurons in the cerebral cortex, which give origin to pyramidal tracts, belong to the pyramidal system and the remaining motor neurons belong to extrapyramidal system.

Lower Motor Neuron

Lower motor neurons are the anterior gray horn cells in the **spinal cord** and the motor neurons of the **cranial nerve nuclei** situated in brainstem, which innervate the muscles directly.

Lower motor neurons constitute the **'final common pathway'** of motor system. The lower motor neurons are under the influence of the upper motor neurons.

APPLIED PHYSIOLOGY

Effects of Lesion of Motor Neurons

Effects of lesions of upper motor neurons and lower motor neurons are given in **Table 95.4**. The effects of lower motor neuron lesion are the loss of muscle tone and flaccid paralysis.

TABLE 95.4: Effects of upper motor neuron lesion and lower motor neuron lesion.

	Effects	Upper motor neuron lesion	Lower motor neuron lesion
Clinical observation	1. Muscle tone	Hypertonia	Hypotonia
	2. Paralysis	Spastic type of paralysis	Flaccid type of paralysis
	3. Wastage of muscle	Wastage of muscle occurs	Wastage of muscle occurs
	4. Superficial reflexes	Lost	Lost
	5. Plantar reflex	Abnormal plantar reflex: Babinski sign	Absent
	6. Deep reflexes	Exaggerated	Lost
	7. Clonus	Present	Absent
Clinical confirmation	8. Electrical activity	Normal	Absent
	9. Muscles affected	Groups of muscles are affected	Individual muscles are affected
	10. Fascicular twitch in EMG	Absent	Present

Effects of upper motor neuron lesion depend upon the site:

1. Lesion in pyramidal system causes hypertonia and spastic paralysis.
2. Lesion in basal ganglia produces hypertonia and rigidity involving both flexor and extensor muscles.
3. Lesion in cerebellum causes hypotonia, muscular weakness and incoordination of movements.

Paralysis

Paralysis is defined as the complete loss of strength and functions of muscle group or a limb.

Causes for paralysis

Common causes for paralysis are:

1. Trauma.
2. Tumor.
3. Stroke.
4. Cerebral palsy (condition caused by brain injury immediately after birth)
5. Neurodegenerative diseases.

Types of paralysis

Paralysis of the muscles in the body depends upon the type and location of motor neurons affected by lesion. Different types of paralysis are given in **Table 95.5**.

TABLE 95.5: Types of paralysis

Paralysis	Parts of the body affected	Causes
Monoplegia	Paralysis of one limb	Isolated damage of central nervous system or peripheral nervous system
Diplegia	Paralysis of both the upper limbs or both the lower limbs	Isolated damage of brain
Hemiplegia	Paralysis of upper limb and lower limb on one side of the body	Lesion in motor cortex and corticospinal tracts in posterior limb of internal capsule on the side opposite to the paralysis
Paraplegia	Paralysis of lower half of the body	Injury to lower part of spinal cord
Quadriplegia or tetraplegia	Paralysis of all the four limbs	Injury to upper part of spinal cord (shoulder level or above, at which the motor nerves of upper limbs leave the spinal cord)

Chapter 96: Physiology of Pain

CHAPTER OUTLINE

- PAIN SENSATION
- BENEFITS OF PAIN SENSATION
- COMPONENTS OF PAIN SENSATION
- PATHWAYS OF PAIN SENSATION
- VISCERAL PAIN
- NEUROTRANSMITTERS INVOLVED IN PAIN SENSATION
- REFERRED PAIN
- ANALGESIA SYSTEM
- GATE CONTROL THEORY
- APPLIED PHYSIOLOGY

■ PAIN SENSATION

Pain sensation is defined as an unpleasant and emotional experience associated with or without actual tissue damage. Pain sensation is described in many ways like sharp, prickling, electric, dull ache, shooting, cutting, stabbing, etc. Often it induces crying and fainting.

Pain is produced by real or potential injury to the body. Often it is expressed in terms of injury. For example, pain produced by fire is expressed as **burning sensation**. Pain produced by severe sustained contraction of skeletal muscles is expressed as **cramps**.

■ BENEFITS OF PAIN SENSATION

Pain is an important sensory symptom. Though it is an unpleasant sensation, it has protective or survival benefits.

Protective or survival benefits of pain.

1. Pain gives warning signal about the existence of a problem or threat. It also creates the awareness of injury.
2. Pain prevents further damage by causing reflex withdrawal of the body from the source of injury.
3. Pain forces the person to rest or to minimize the activities thus enabling the rapid healing of the injured part.
4. Pain urges the person to take required treatment to prevent major damage.

■ COMPONENTS OF PAIN SENSATION

Pain has two components:
1. Fast pain.
2. Slow pain.

Fast pain is the first sensation whenever a pain stimulus is applied. It is experienced as a bright, sharp and localized pain sensation. Fast pain is followed by the **slow pain** which is experienced as a dull, diffused and unpleasant pain.

Receptors for both the components of pain are the same, i.e. the **free nerve endings**. But the afferent nerve fibers are different. Fast pain sensation is carried by **Aδ fibers** and the slow pain sensation is carried by **C type fibers**.

■ PATHWAYS OF PAIN SENSATION

Pain sensation from various parts of body is carried to brain by different pathways which are:
1. Pathway from skin and the deeper structures.
2. Pathway from face.
3. Pathway from viscera.
4. Pathway from pelvic region.

■ 1. PATHWAY OF PAIN SENSATION FROM SKIN AND DEEPER STRUCTURES

Receptors

Receptors of pain sensation are the free nerve endings which are distributed throughout the body.

First Order Neurons

First order neurons are the cells in the posterior nerve root ganglia which receive the impulses of pain sensation from the pain receptors through their dendrites. These impulses are transmitted to spinal cord through the axons of these neurons.

Fast pain fibers

Fast pain sensation is carried by Aδ type afferent fibers which synapse with neurons of **marginal nucleus** in the posterior gray horn.

Slow pain fibers

Slow pain sensation is carried by C type afferent fibers which synapse with neurons of **substantia gelatinosa of Rolando** in the posterior gray horn **(Fig. 94.4)**.

Second Order Neurons

Neurons of marginal nucleus and substantia gelatinosa of Rolando form the second order neurons. Fibers from these neurons ascend in the form of the **lateral spinothalamic tract**.

Third Order Neurons

Third order neurons are **ventral posterolateral nucleus** of thalamus and **reticular formation**. Axons from these neurons reach the sensory area of **cerebral cortex**. Some fibers from reticular formation reach **hypothalamus**.

Center for Pain Sensation

Center for pain sensation is in the postcentral gyrus of **parietal cortex**. Fibers reaching **hypothalamus** are concerned with arousal mechanism due to pain stimulus.

2. PATHWAY OF PAIN SENSATION FROM FACE

Pain sensation from face is carried by **trigeminal nerve**. Refer Chapter 95 for details.

3. PATHWAY OF PAIN SENSATION FROM VISCERA

Pain sensation from thoracic and abdominal viscera is transmitted by **thoracolumbar** (sympathetic) **nerves**. Pain from esophagus, trachea and pharynx is carried by **vagus nerve** and **glossopharyngeal nerve**.

4. PATHWAY OF PAIN SENSATION FROM PELVIC REGION

Pain sensation from deeper structures of pelvic region is conveyed by **sacral parasympathetic nerves**.

VISCERAL PAIN

Pain from viscera is unpleasant. It is poorly localized.

CAUSES OF VISCERAL PAIN

1. Ischemia

Substances released during ischemic reactions such as **bradykinin** and **proteolytic enzymes** stimulate the pain receptors of viscera.

2. Chemical Stimuli

Chemical substances such as **acidic gastric juice** leaks from ruptured ulcers into peritoneal cavity and produce pain.

3. Spasm of Hollow Organs

Spastic contraction of smooth muscles in gastrointestinal tract and other hollow organs of viscera cause pain by stimulating the free nerve endings.

4. Overdistension of Hollow Organs

Overdistention of hollow organs also causes pain.

NEUROTRANSMITTERS INVOLVED IN PAIN SENSATION

Glutamate and **substance P** are the neurotransmitters secreted by pain nerve endings.

Glutamate is secreted by Aδ afferent fibers, which transmit impulses of fast pain. Substance P is secreted by C type fibers, which transmit impulses of slow pain.

REFERRED PAIN

Referred pain is the pain that is perceived at a site adjacent to or away from the site of origin. The deep pain and some visceral pain are referred to other areas. But the superficial pain is not referred.

EXAMPLES OF REFERRED PAIN

1. Cardiac pain is felt at the inner part of left arm and left shoulder.
2. Pain in ovary is referred to umbilicus.
3. Pain from testis is felt in abdomen.
4. Pain in diaphragm is referred to right shoulder.
5. Pain in gallbladder is referred to epigastric region.
6. Renal pain is referred to loin **(Fig. 96.1)**.

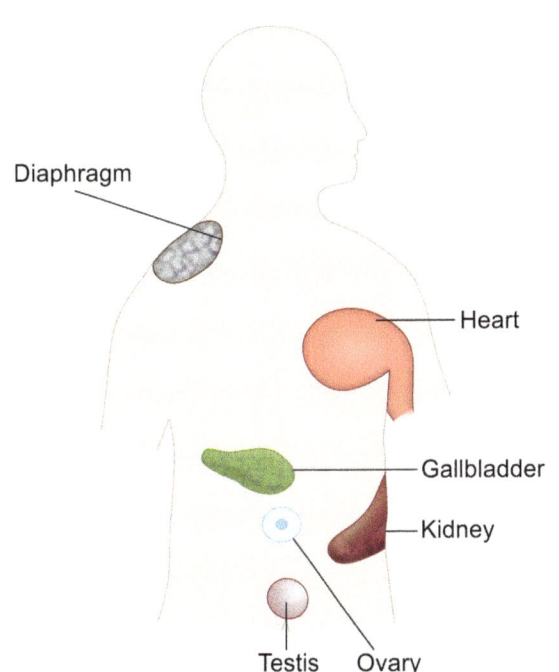

FIGURE 96.1: Sites of referred pain.

MECHANISM OF REFERRED PAIN

Dermatomal Rule

According to dermatomal rule, pain is referred to a structure, which is developed from the same dermatome from which the pain producing structure is developed.

A **dermatome** includes all the structures or parts of the body, which are innervated by afferent nerve fibers of one dorsal root. For example, the heart and inner aspect of left arm originate from the same dermatome. So, the pain in heart is referred to left arm.

ANALGESIA SYSTEM

Analgesia system means the **pain control system**. Body has its own analgesia system in brain which provides a short-term relief from pain. It is also called **endogenous analgesia system**. It includes gray matter surrounding the III ventricle and aqueduct of Sylvius and reticular formation of brainstem.

Analgesia system has got its own pathway through which it blocks the synaptic transmission of pain sensation in spinal cord and suppresses pain. In fact, analgesic drugs such as **opioids** act through this system and provide a controlled pain relief.

ANALGESIC PATHWAY

Analgesic pathway is considered as **descending pain pathway**, the ascending pain pathway being the afferent fibers that transmit pain sensation to the brain. Analgesic pathway commences from brainstem **(Fig. 96.2)**.

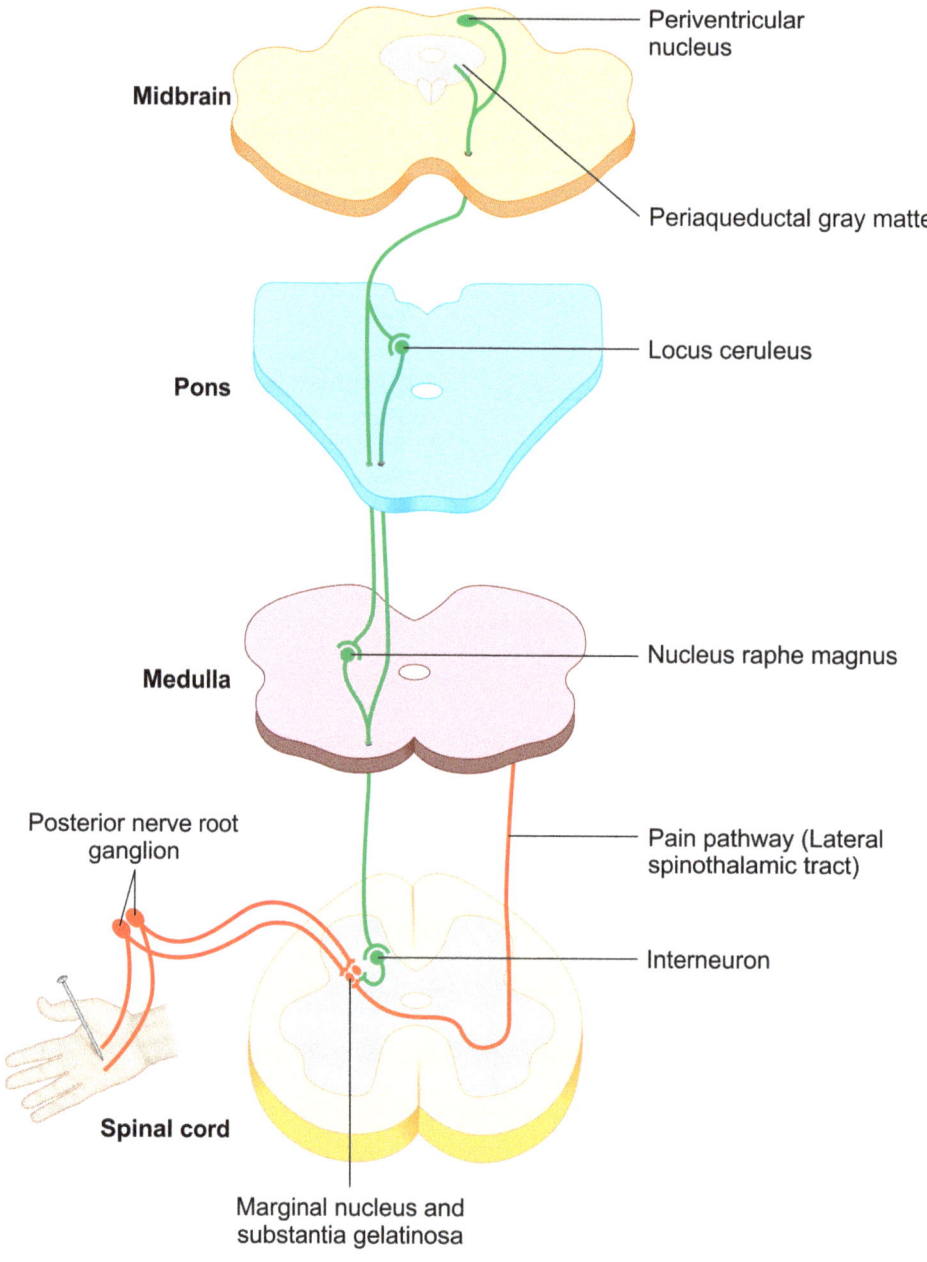

FIGURE 96.2: Analgesic pathway.

Nerve Fibers Forming Analgesic Pathway

1. Nerve fibers of analgesic pathway arise from two sources namely, **periventricular nucleus** and **periaqueductal gray matter** (PAG) situated in midbrain.
2. Nerve fibers from above areas terminate in two areas called **nucleus raphe** magnus and **nucleus locus ceruleus** situated in reticular formation of midbrain.
3. Fibers from the above nuclei descend through dorsal horn of spinal cord and synapse with interneurons.
4. Interneurons form synapses with the neurons of **marginal nucleus** and **substantia gelatinosa** of Rolando. Neurons of these nuclei form second order neurons of afferent (ascending) pathway for pain.

Mechanism of Analgesic Pathway in Inhibiting Pain Transmission

1. Whenever sensory cortex receives impulses of pain sensation via afferent pain pathway, it activates the periventricular nucleus and periaqueductal gray matter.
2. These two areas in turn activate nucleus raphe magnus and nucleus locus ceruleus of reticular formation.
3. Now, impulses from these two nuclei are transmitted to interneurons present in lateral horn of spinal cord.
4. Interneurons of spinal cord now, inhibit pain transmission at the synaptic level before being relayed to brain.

GATE CONTROL THEORY

Gate control theory explains the **pain suppression**. According to this theory, the pain stimuli transmitted by afferent pain fibers are blocked by gate mechanism located at the posterior gray horn of spinal cord. If the gate is opened, pain is felt. If the gate is closed, pain is suppressed. Brain also plays some important role in the gate control system of the spinal cord.

Significance of Gate Control

Thus, the gating of pain at spinal level is similar to **presynaptic inhibition**. Gate control forms the basis for pain relief through rubbing, massage techniques, application of ice packs, acupuncture and electrical analgesia. All these techniques relieve pain by stimulating the release of endogenous pain relievers such as **opioid peptides** which close the gate and block the pain signals.

APPLIED PHYSIOLOGY

Analgesia

Analgesia means loss of pain sensation.

Hyperalgesia

Hyperalgesia is defined as the increased sensitivity to pain sensation.

Paralgesia

Abnormal pain sensation is called paralgesia.

Chapter 97: Thalamus

CHAPTER OUTLINE

- SITUATION
- THALAMIC NUCLEI
- FUNCTIONS OF THALAMUS
  - RELAY CENTER FOR SENSATIONS
  - CENTER FOR PROCESSING OF SENSORY INFORMATION
  - CENTER FOR DETERMINING QUALITY OF SENSATIONS
  - CENTER FOR SEXUAL SENSATIONS
- ROLE IN AROUSAL AND ALERTNESS REACTIONS
- CENTER FOR REFLEX ACTIVITY
- CENTER FOR INTEGRATION OF MOTOR ACTIVITY
- APPLIED PHYSIOLOGY
  - THALAMIC LESION
  - THALAMIC SYNDROME

■ SITUATION OF THALAMUS

Thalamus is a large ovoid mass of gray matter, situated bilaterally in **diencephalon**. Both thalami form 80% of diencephalon **(Fig. 97.1)**.

■ THALAMIC NUCLEI

Thalamus on each side is divided into five main nuclear groups by means of "Y" shaped internal medullary septum.

■ 1. MIDLINE NUCLEI

It is a group of small nuclei, situated on the medial surface of thalamus **near midline**.

■ 2. INTRALAMINAR NUCLEI

Intralaminar nuclei are smaller nuclei present in the **medullary septum** of the thalamus.

■ 3. MEDIAL MASS OF NUCLEI

Medial mass of nuclei is situated **medial to septum** and it comprises two nuclei:
1. Anterior nucleus.
2. Dorsomedial nucleus.

■ 4. LATERAL MASS OF NUCLEI

This group of nuclei is situated **lateral to septum**.

Lateral mass of nuclei is again divided into two subgroups:

a. Dorsal group of lateral mass with two nuclei:
   1. Dorsolateral nucleus.
   2. Posterolateral nucleus.

b. Ventral group of lateral mass with three nuclei:
   1. Ventral anterior nucleus.
   2. Ventral lateral nucleus.
   3. Posteroventral nucleus. It consists of two parts:
      i. Ventral posterolateral nucleus.
      ii. Ventral posteromedial nucleus.

■ 5. POSTERIOR GROUP OF NUCLEI

It is the continuation of lateral mass of nuclei. It has two subgroups:

a. Pulvinar.
b. Metathalamus which consists of two structures:
   1. Medial geniculate body.
   2. Lateral geniculate body.

Thalamic Reticular Nucleus

Thalamus also includes thalamic reticular nucleus, which is a thin layer of neurons covering the lateral aspect of thalamus.

■ FUNCTIONS OF THALAMUS

Thalamus is primarily concerned with somatic functions. Various functions of thalamus are given below.

■ 1. RELAY CENTER FOR SENSATIONS

Thalamus forms the relay center for the sensations. Impulses of almost all the sensations reach the thalamic nuclei, particularly in the **ventral posterolateral nucleus**.

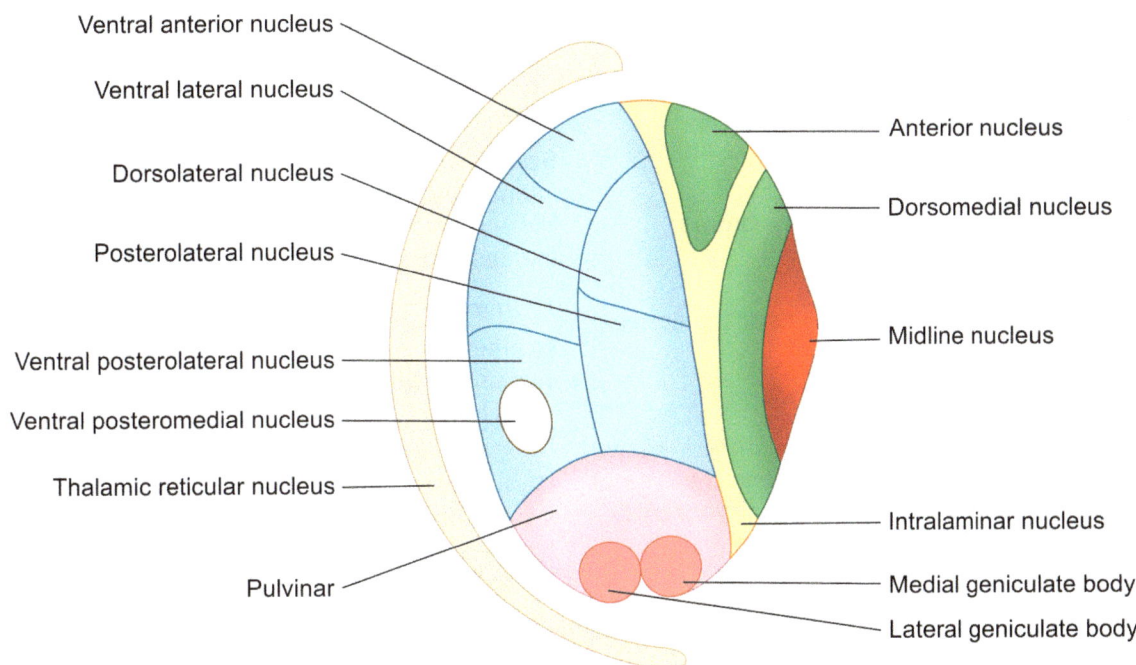

FIGURE 97.1: Thalamic nuclei. Red = Midline nuclei. Yellow = Intralaminar nuclei. Green = Medial mass of nuclei. Blue = Lateral mass of nuclei. Pink = Posterior group of nuclei.

After being processed in the thalamus, the impulses are carried to cerebral cortex.

2. CENTER FOR PROCESSING OF SENSORY INFORMATION

Thalamus forms the major center for processing the sensory information. All the peripheral sensory impulses reaching thalamus are **integrated and modified** before being sent to specific areas of cerebral cortex. This function of thalamus is usually called the processing of sensory information.

Functional Gateway for Cerebral Cortex

Almost all the sensations are processed in thalamus before reaching cerebral cortex. Very little information of somatosensory function is sent directly to cerebral cortex without being processed by the thalamic nuclei. Because of this function, thalamus is usually called a 'Functional gateway' for cerebral cortex.

3. CENTER FOR DETERMINING QUALITY OF SENSATIONS

Thalamus is also the center for determining the quality of sensations, that is, to determine the affective nature of sensations.

Usually the sensations have two qualities:

i. Discriminative nature.
ii. Affective nature.

i. Discriminative Nature of Sensation

Discriminative nature is the ability to recognize the type, location and other details of the sensations. It is the function of cerebral cortex.

ii. Affective Nature of Sensation

Affective nature is the capacity to determine whether a sensation is pleasant or unpleasant and agreeable or disagreeable. Determining the affective nature of sensations is the function of thalamus.

4. CENTER FOR SEXUAL SENSATIONS

Thalamus forms the center for perception of sexual sensations.

5. ROLE IN AROUSAL AND ALERTNESS REACTIONS

Because of its connections with nuclei of reticular formation, thalamus plays an important role in arousal and alertness reactions.

6. CENTER FOR REFLEX ACTIVITY

Since the sensory fibers relay here, thalamus forms the center for many reflex activities.

7. CENTER FOR INTEGRATION OF MOTOR ACTIVITY

Through the connections with cerebellum and basal ganglia, thalamus serves as a center for integration of motor functions.

APPLIED PHYSIOLOGY

THALAMIC LESION

Thalamic lesion occurs mainly because of blockage (due to thrombosis) in blood vessels supplying thalamus. Mostly, posteroventral nuclei of thalamus are affected because the thalamogeniculate branch of posterior cerebral artery supplies this part of thalamus. Lesion of thalamus leads to a condition called thalamic syndrome.

THALAMIC SYNDROME

Thalamic syndrome is the neurological disease caused by infarction of posteroventral part of thalamus.

Following are the symptoms of thalamic syndrome:

1. Loss of Sensations

Loss of all sensations (**anesthesia**) occurs as the sensory relay system in thalamus is affected.

2. Astereognosis

Astereognosis is the loss of ability to recognize a known object by touch with closed eyes. It is due to the loss of tactile and kinesthetic sensations in thalamic syndrome.

3. Ataxia

Ataxia is the **incoordination** of voluntary movements.

4. Thalamic Phantom Limb

Persons with amputated limb, sometimes feel sensations in the missing limb. This is called phantom limb. It is because of response by thalamus to inputs from cut ends of sensory nerves. Refer Chapter 91 for **phantom limb pain.**

5. Amelognosia

It is the **illusion** felt by the patient that his limb is absent.

6. Pain Sensation

Spontaneous pain occurs often. The pain may be so intense, that it even resists the action of powerful sedatives like morphine. Sometimes, the patient feels pain even in the absence of pain stimulus.

7. Involuntary Movements

Thalamic syndrome is always associated with some involuntary motor movements:

  i. **Athetosis** (slow writhing and twisting movements).
  ii. **Chorea** (quick jerky involuntary movements).
  iii. Intention tremor: **Tremor** is defined as rapid alternate rhythmic and involuntary movement of flexion and extension in the joints of fingers and wrist or elbow. **Intention tremor** is the tremor that develops while attempting to do any voluntary act. Intention tremor is the common feature of thalamic syndrome.

8. Thalamic Hand or Athetoid Hand

It is the abnormal attitude of the hand in thalamic lesion. It is characterized by moderate flexion at wrist and hyperextension of all fingers.

Chapter 98: Hypothalamus

CHAPTER OUTLINE

- SITUATION AND FORMATION
- NUCLEI
- FUNCTIONS
  - SECRETION OF POSTERIOR PITUITARY HORMONES
  - CONTROL OF ANTERIOR PITUITARY
  - REGULATION OF ADRENAL CORTEX
  - REGULATION OF ADRENAL MEDULLA
  - REGULATION OF AUTONOMIC NERVOUS SYSTEM
  - REGULATION OF HEART RATE
  - REGULATION OF BLOOD PRESSURE
  - REGULATION OF BODY TEMPERATURE
  - REGULATION OF HUNGER AND FOOD INTAKE
  - REGULATION OF WATER BALANCE
- REGULATION OF SLEEP AND WAKEFULNESS
- ROLE IN BEHAVIOR AND EMOTIONAL CHANGES
- REGULATION OF SEXUAL FUNCTION
- ROLE IN RESPONSE TO SMELL
- ROLE IN CIRCADIAN RHYTHM
- APPLIED PHYSIOLOGY: DISORDERS OF HYPOTHALAMUS
  - DIABETES INSIPIDUS
  - DYSTROPHIA ADIPOSOGENITALIS
  - KALLMANN SYNDROME
  - LAURENCE-MOON-BIEDL SYNDROME
  - NARCOLEPSY
  - CATAPLEXY

SITUATION AND FORMATION OF HYPOTHALAMUS

Hypothalamus is a diencephalic structure. It is situated just below thalamus in the ventral part of **diencephalon**. It is formed by groups of nuclei scattered in the walls and floor of third ventricle. It extends from optic chiasma to mammillary body.

NUCLEI OF HYPOTHALAMUS

Nuclei of hypothalamus are divided into three groups:

1. Anterior or preoptic group.
2. Middle or tuberal group.
3. Posterior or mammillary group.

Nuclei of each group are listed in **Table 98.1** and represented diagrammatically in **Figure 98.1**.

FUNCTIONS OF HYPOTHALAMUS

Hypothalamus is the important part of the brain concerned with **homeostasis** of the body. It regulates many vital functions of the body such as endocrine functions, visceral functions, metabolic activities, hunger, thirst, sleep, wakefulness, emotion, sexual functions, etc. **(Table 98.2)**.

1. SECRETION OF POSTERIOR PITUITARY HORMONES

Posterior pituitary hormones namely, antidiuretic hormone (ADH) and oxytocin are secreted by supraoptic

TABLE 98.1: Nuclei of hypothalamus.

Anterior or preoptic group	Middle or tuberal group	Posterior or mammillary group
1. Preoptic nucleus 2. Paraventricular nucleus 3. Anterior nucleus 4. Supraoptic nucleus 5. Suprachiasmatic nucleus	1. Dorsomedial nucleus 2. Ventromedial nucleus 3. Lateral nucleus 4. Arcuate (tuberal) nucleus	1. Posterior nucleus 2. Mammillary body

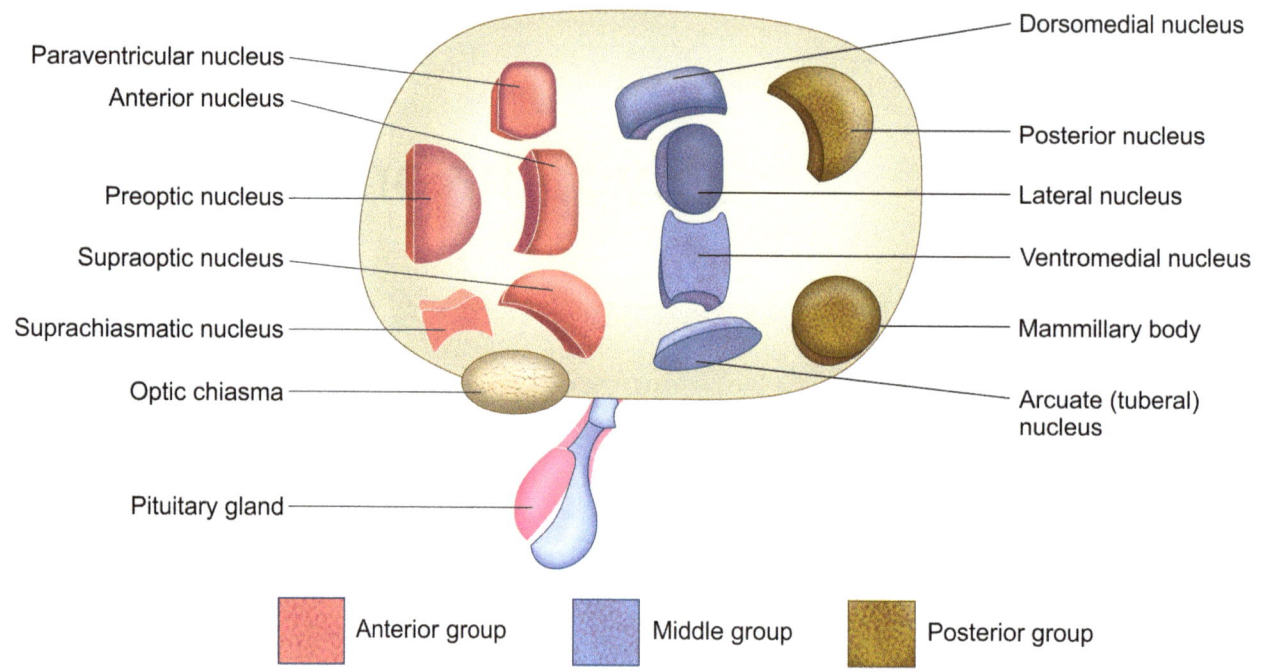

FIGURE 98.1: Nuclei of hypothalamus.

TABLE 98.2: Functions of hypothalamus.

Functions	Action/Center	Nuclei or parts involved
1. Control of anterior pituitary	By releasing hormones and inhibiting hormones	Discrete areas
2. Secretion of posterior pituitary hormones	Oxytocin Antidiuretic hormone (ADH)	Paraventricular nucleus Supraoptic nucleus
3. Control of adrenal cortex	By corticotropin-releasing hormone (CRH)	Paraventricular nucleus
4. Control of adrenal medulla	Catecholamines during emotion	Posterior nucleus Dorsomedial nucleus
5. Regulation of autonomic nervous system (ANS)	Sympathetic Parasympathetic	Posterior and lateral nuclei Anterior nucleus
6. Regulation of heart rate	Acceleration Inhibition	Posterior nucleus Lateral nucleus Preoptic nucleus Anterior nuclei
7. Regulation of blood pressure	Pressor effect Depressor effect	Posterior and lateral nuclei Preoptic area
8. Regulation of body temperature	Heat gain center Heat loss center	Posterior hypothalamus Anterior hypothalamus
9. Regulation of hunger and food intake	Feeding center Satiety center	Lateral nucleus Ventromedial nucleus
10. Regulation of water intake	Thirst center Water retention by ADH	Lateral nucleus Supraoptic nucleus
11. Regulation of sleep and wakefulness	Sleep Wakefulness	Anterior hypothalamus Mammillary body
12. Regulation of behavior and emotion	Reward center Punishment center	Ventromedial nucleus Posterior and lateral nuclei
13. Regulation of sexual function	Sexual cycle	Arcuate nucleus Posterior nucleus
14. Regulation of response to smell	Autonomic responses	Posterior hypothalamus
15. Role in circadian rhythm	Rhythmic changes	Suprachiasmatic nucleus

and paraventricular nuclei of hypothalamus. These two hormones are transported by means of **axonic** or **axoplasmic flow** through the fibers of **hypothalamo-hypophyseal tracts** to the posterior pituitary. Refer Chapter 50 for details.

2. CONTROL OF ANTERIOR PITUITARY

Hypothalamus controls the secretions of anterior pituitary gland by secreting releasing hormones and inhibitory hormones.

Hypothalamus secretes seven hormones:

i. Growth hormone-releasing hormone (GHRH).
ii. Growth hormone-releasing polypeptide (GHRP).
iii. Growth hormone inhibitory hormone (GHIH) or somatostatin.
iv. Thyrotropin-releasing hormone (TRH).
v. Corticotropin-releasing hormone (CRH).
vi. Gonadotropin-releasing hormone (GnRH).
vii. Prolactin inhibitory hormone (PIH).

All these hormones are transported from hypothalamus to the anterior pituitary by the **hypothalamo-hypophyseal portal blood vessels**. Details are given in Chapter 50.

3. REGULATION OF ADRENAL CORTEX

Hypothalamus controls adrenal cortex through anterior pituitary. Anterior pituitary regulates the adrenal cortex by secreting **adrenocorticotropic hormone (ACTH)**. ACTH secretion is in turn regulated by **corticotropin-releasing hormone (CRH)** which is secreted by the paraventricular nucleus of hypothalamus (Chapter 54).

4. REGULATION OF ADRENAL MEDULLA

Dorsomedial and posterior hypothalamic nuclei are excited by **emotional stimuli**. These hypothalamic nuclei, in turn, send impulses to adrenal medulla through sympathetic fibers and cause release of **catecholamines**, which are essential to cope up with emotional stress.

5. REGULATION OF AUTONOMIC NERVOUS SYSTEM

Hypothalamus controls the autonomic nervous system (ANS). The sympathetic division of ANS is regulated by posterior and lateral nuclei of hypothalamus. The parasympathetic division of ANS is controlled by anterior group of nuclei. Cerebral cortex influences ANS through hypothalamus.

6. REGULATION OF HEART RATE

Hypothalamus regulates heart rate through vasomotor center in the medulla oblongata. Stimulation of posterior and lateral nuclei of hypothalamus increases the heart rate. Stimulation of preoptic and anterior nuclei decreases the heart rate (Chapter 70).

7. REGULATION OF BLOOD PRESSURE

Hypothalamus regulates the blood pressure by acting on the vasomotor center. Stimulation of posterior and lateral nuclei increases arterial blood pressure and stimulation of preoptic area decreases the blood pressure (Chapter 71).

8. REGULATION OF BODY TEMPERATURE

Body temperature is regulated by hypothalamus which sets the normal range of body temperature. The **set point** under normal physiological conditions is 37°C.

Hypothalamus has two centers which regulate the body temperature:

i. **Heat loss center** that is present in preoptic nucleus of anterior hypothalamus.
ii. **Heat gain center** that is situated in posterior hypothalamic nucleus.

Regulation of body temperature is explained in Chapter 48.

9. REGULATION OF HUNGER AND FOOD INTAKE

Food intake is regulated by two centers present in hypothalamus:

i. Feeding center.
ii. Satiety center.

Feeding Center

Feeding center is in the lateral hypothalamic nucleus. Normally feeding center is always active. That means it has the tendency to induce food intake always.

In experimental conditions, the stimulation of this center in animals leads to uncontrolled hunger and increased food intake (**hyperphagia**) resulting in obesity. The destruction of feeding center leads to loss of appetite (**anorexia**) and the animal refuses to take food.

Satiety Center

Satiety center is in the ventromedial nucleus of the hypothalamus. Satiety center regulates food intake by temporary inhibition of feeding center after food intake.

Stimulation of this nucleus in animals causes total loss of appetite and cessation of food intake. Destruction of satiety center leads to hyperphagia and the animal becomes obese. This type of obesity is called **hypothalamic obesity**.

Mechanism of Regulation of Food Intake

Under normal physiological conditions, appetite and food intake are well balanced and continues in a cyclic manner. Feeding center and satiety center of hypothalamus are responsible for regulation of appetite and food intake.

Hypothalamic centers are regulated by the following mechanisms:

a. Glucostatic mechanism.
b. Lipostatic mechanism.
c. Peptide mechanism.
d. Hormonal mechanism.
e. Thermostatic mechanism.

Glucostatic Mechanism

Cells of the satiety center function as **glucostats** or **glucose receptors**. The glucostats are stimulated by increased

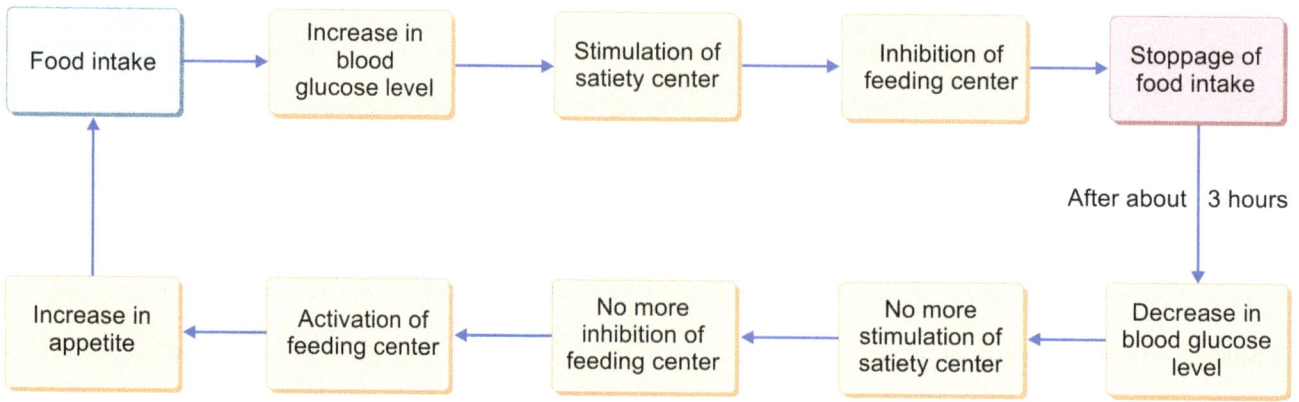

FIGURE 98.2: Glucostatic mechanism.

blood glucose level during food intake. This develops the feeling of 'fullness'. The satiety center in turn, inhibits the feeding center, resulting in stoppage of food intake.

After few hours of food intake, the blood glucose level decreases and satiety center, becomes inactive. So, the feeding center is no longer inhibited. Now it becomes active and increases the appetite and induces food intake. After taking food, once again blood glucose level increases and the cycle is repeated **(Fig. 98.2)**.

Lipostatic Mechanism

Leptin is a peptide secreted by **adipocytes** (cells of adipose tissue). It plays an important role in controlling the food intake and adipose tissue volume. Details of leptin are given in Chapter 57.

When the volume of adipose tissues increases, adipocytes secrete and release a large quantity of leptin into the blood. While circulating through brain, leptin acts on hypothalamus and inhibits the feeding center resulting in loss of appetite and stoppage of food intake.

Peptide Mechanism

Some peptides regulate the food intake either by stimulating or inhibiting the feeding center directly or indirectly.

Peptides which increase the food intake are:

i. Ghrelin.
ii. Neuropeptide Y.

Peptides which decrease food intake are:

i. Leptin.
ii. Peptide YY.

Hormonal Mechanism

Some of the endocrine hormones and GI hormones inhibit the food intake by acting through hypothalamus.

Hormones which inhibit food intake:

i. Somatostatin.
ii. Oxytocin.
iii. Glucagon.
iv. Pancreatic polypeptide.
v. Cholecystokinin.

Thermostatic Mechanism

Food intake is inversely proportional to body temperature. So, in **fever**, the food intake is decreased due to the influence of preoptic **thermoreceptors** on feeding center.

10. REGULATION OF WATER BALANCE

Hypothalamus regulates water content of the body by two mechanisms:

i. Thirst mechanism.
ii. ADH mechanism.

Thirst Mechanism

Thirst center is in the lateral nucleus of hypothalamus. There are some **osmoreceptors** in the areas adjacent to thirst center. When the ECF volume decreases, the osmolality of ECF is increased. If the osmolarity increases by 1 to 2%, the osmoreceptors are stimulated. Osmoreceptors in turn, activate the thirst center and thirst sensation is initiated. Now, the person feels thirsty and drinks water. Water intake increases ECF volume and decreases the osmolality **(Fig. 98.3)**.

ADH Mechanism

Simultaneously, when the volume of ECF decreases with increased osmolality, the supraoptic nucleus is stimulated and ADH is released. ADH causes retention of water by **facultative reabsorption** in the renal tubules. It increases the ECF volume and brings the osmolality back to the normal level.

On the contrary, when ECF volume is increased, the supraoptic nucleus is not stimulated and ADH is not secreted. In the absence of ADH, more amount of water is excreted through urine and the volume of ECF is brought back to normal.

11. REGULATION OF SLEEP AND WAKEFULNESS

Mammillary body in the posterior hypothalamus acts as the **wakefulness center**. Stimulation of mammillary body causes wakefulness and its lesion leads to sleep. Stimulation of anterior hypothalamus also leads to sleep.

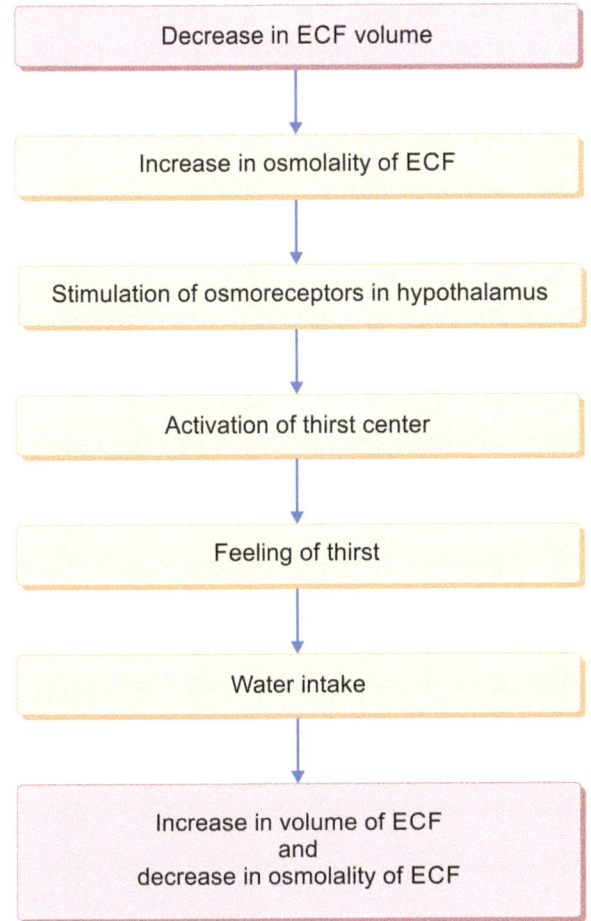

FIGURE 98.3: Thirst mechanism.

■ 12. ROLE IN BEHAVIOR AND EMOTIONAL CHANGES

Behavior of animals and human beings is mostly affected by two responding systems in hypothalamus and other structures of limbic system. These two systems act opposite to one another.

The responding systems are concerned with the affective nature of sensations, i.e. whether the sensations are pleasant or painful. These two qualities are called the **reward** (satisfaction) and **punishment** (aversion or avoidance). Hypothalamus has two centers for behavior and emotional changes:

i. Reward center.
ii. Punishment center.

Reward Center

It is situated in medial forebrain bundle and ventromedial nucleus of hypothalamus. Electrical stimulation of these areas in animals pleases or satisfies the animals.

Punishment Center

It is situated in posterior and lateral nuclei of hypothalamus. Electrical stimulation of these nuclei in animals leads to pain, fear, defense, escape reactions and other elements of punishment.

Role of Reward and Punishment Centers

Importance of reward and punishment centers lies in the **behavioral pattern** of the individuals. Almost all the activities of day to day life depend upon **reward and punishment**. While doing something, if the person is rewarded or feels satisfied, he or she continues to do so. If the person feels punished or unpleasant, he or she stops doing so. Thus, these two centers play an important role in the development of the behavioral pattern of a person.

Rage

Rage is the violent and aggressive emotional expression with extreme anger. It is common in animals when punishment centers in hypothalamus are stimulated. Reactions of rage are expressed by developing a defense posture which includes:

i. Extension of limbs with lifting of tail.
ii. Hissing and spitting.
iii. Piloerection.
iv. Wide opening of eyeballs with pupillary dilatation.
v. Severe savage attack even by mild provocation.

Sham Rage

Sham rage means **false rage**. It is an extreme emotional condition that resembles rage and occurs in some pathological conditions in humans. Sham rage is due to release of hypothalamus from the inhibitory influence of cortical control.

■ 13. REGULATION OF SEXUAL FUNCTION

Hypothalamus regulates sexual functions by secreting **gonadotropin-releasing hormone**. Arcuate and posterior hypothalamic nuclei are involved in the regulation of sexual functions.

■ 14. ROLE IN RESPONSE TO SMELL

Posterior hypothalamus along with other structures such as hippocampus and brainstem nuclei is responsible for the autonomic responses of body to olfactory stimuli. The responses include feeding activities and emotional responses like fear, excitement and pleasure.

■ 15. ROLE IN CIRCADIAN RHYTHM

Circadian rhythm is the regular recurrence of physiological processes or activities which occur in cycles of 24 hours. It is also called **diurnal rhythm**. The term circadian is a Latin word meaning 'around the day'.

Circadian rhythm occurs in response to recurring daylight and darkness. The cyclic changes taking place in various physiological processes are set by means of a hypothetical internal clock that is often called **biological clock**.

Suprachiasmatic nucleus of hypothalamus sets the biological clock by its connection with retina via retinohypothalamic fibers. Through the efferent fibers, it sends circadian signals to different parts and maintains the circadian rhythm of sleep, hormonal secretion, thirst, hunger, appetite, etc.

Whenever body is exposed to a new pattern of daylight/darkness rhythm, the biological clock is reset, provided the new pattern is regular. Accordingly, the circadian rhythm also changes.

APPLIED PHYSIOLOGY: DISORDERS OF HYPOTHALAMUS

Following disorders develop in hypothalamic lesion that occurs due to tumors, encephalitis or ischemia.

1. DIABETES INSIPIDUS

Diabetes insipidus is the condition characterized by excretion of large quantity of water through urine. Details are given in Chapter 50.

2. DYSTROPHIA ADIPOSOGENITALIS

It is characterized by obesity and sexual infantilism, associated with dwarfism (if the condition occurs during growing period). It is also called **Frohlich's syndrome**. Details are given in Chapter 50.

3. KALLMANN SYNDROME

Kallmann syndrome is a genetic disorder characterized by **hypogonadism**, associated with **anosmia** (loss of olfactory sensation) or **hyposmia** (decreased olfactory sensation). It is also called **hypogonadotropic hypogonadism**, since it occurs due to deficiency of gonadotropin-releasing hormone secreted by hypothalamus.

4. LAURENCE-MOON-BIEDL SYNDROME

This disorder of hypothalamus is characterized by **moon face** (facial contours become round by hiding the bony structures), obesity, **polydactylism** (having one or more extra fingers or toes), mental retardation and hypogenitalism.

5. NARCOLEPSY

Narcolepsy is a hypothalamic disorder with abnormal sleep pattern. There is sudden attack of uncontrollable desire for sleep and the person suddenly falls asleep. It occurs in the daytime.

6. CATAPLEXY

It is the sudden uncontrolled outbursts of emotion associated with narcolepsy. Due to emotional outburst like anger, fear or excitement, the person becomes completely exhausted with muscular weakness. The attack is brief and last for few seconds to a few minutes. The consciousness is not lost.

Cerebellum

CHAPTER OUTLINE

- PARTS
  - VERMIS
  - CEREBELLAR HEMISPHERES
- DIVISIONS
- VESTIBULOCEREBELLUM
  - COMPONENTS
  - FUNCTIONS
- SPINOCEREBELLUM
  - COMPONENTS
  - FUNCTIONS
- CORTICOCEREBELLUM
  - COMPONENTS
  - AFFERENT-EFFERENT CIRCUIT
  - FUNCTIONS
- APPLIED PHYSIOLOGY: CEREBELLAR LESIONS
  - DISTURBANCES IN TONE AND POSTURE
  - DISTURBANCES IN EQUILIBRIUM
  - DISTURBANCES IN MOVEMENTS

PARTS OF CEREBELLUM

Cerebellum consists of a narrow, worm-like central body called **vermis** and two lateral lobes, the right and left **cerebellar hemispheres (Fig. 99.1)**.

VERMIS

Part of vermis on the upper surface of cerebellum is known as **superior vermis** and the vermis on the under surface of cerebellum is called **inferior vermis**. Vermis of cerebellum is formed by nine parts which are listed in **Table 99.1**.

Nodulus has extension on either side called flocculus. Nodulus and flocculi are together called **flocculonodular lobe**. On either side of pyramid, there is another extension named **paraflocculus**.

CEREBELLAR HEMISPHERES

Cerebellar hemispheres are the extended portions on either side of the vermis. Each hemisphere has two portions:

1. Lobulus ansiformis or ansiform lobe.
2. Lobulus paramedianus or paramedian lobe.

DIVISIONS OF CEREBELLUM

Based on the functions, cerebellum is divided into three divisions:

1. Vestibulocerebellum.
2. Spinocerebellum.
3. Corticocerebellum.

TABLE 99.1: Parts of superior and inferior vermis.

Superior vermis	Inferior vermis
1. Lingula	6. Tuber
2. Central lobe	7. Pyramid
3. Culmen	8. Uvula
4. Lobulus simplex	9. Nodulus
5. Declive	

VESTIBULOCEREBELLUM (ARCHICEREBELLUM)

This part of cerebellum is connected with the **vestibular apparatus** and so it is known as vestibulocerebellum. Since, vestibulocerebellum is the **phylogenetically oldest** part of cerebellum, it is also called archicerebellum.

COMPONENTS OF VESTIBULOCEREBELLUM

Vestibulocerebellum includes the **flocculonodular lobe** that is formed by the **nodulus** of vermis and its lateral extensions called **flocculi (Fig. 99.1 and Table 99.2)**.

FUNCTIONS OF VESTIBULOCEREBELLUM

Vestibulocerebellum regulates muscle tone, posture and equilibrium by receiving information from vestibular apparatus regarding gravity and movements **(Table 99.3)**.

Mechanism of Action of Vestibulocerebellum

Normally, the vestibular nuclei of brainstem facilitate the movements of trunk, neck and limbs. And, medullary reticular formation inhibits the muscle tone.

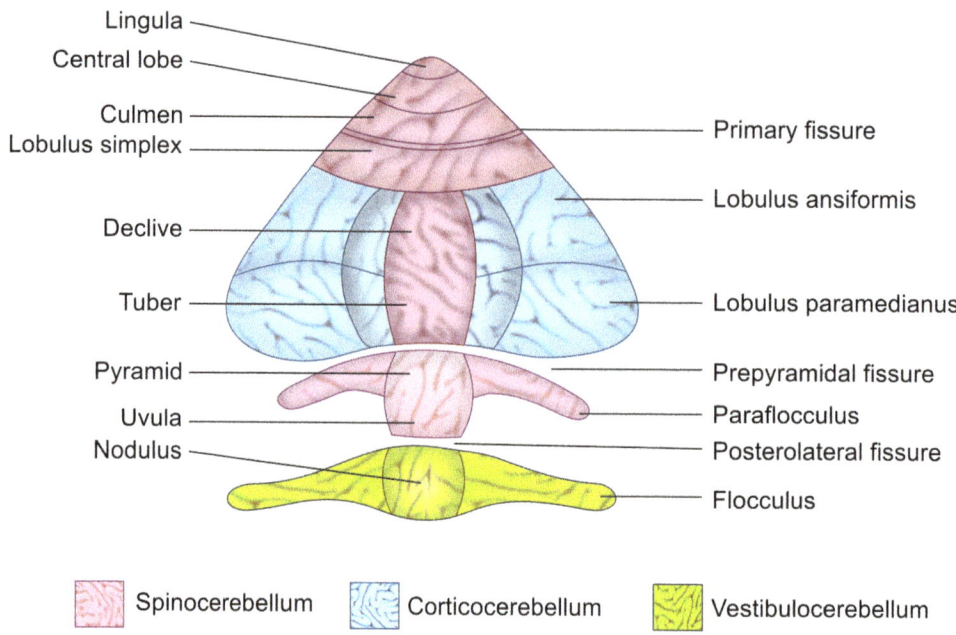

FIGURE 99.1: Parts and functional divisions of cerebellum.

After receiving information from vestibular apparatus, the vestibulocerebellum inhibits both vestibular nuclei and medullary reticular formation. As a result, the movements of neck, trunk and limbs are checked and the muscle tone increases. Because of these effects, any disturbance in posture and equilibrium is corrected.

Lesion of vestibulocerebellum results in hypotonia (reduction of muscle tone) and failure to maintain posture and equilibrium.

■ SPINOCEREBELLUM (PALEOCEREBELLUM)

Spinocerebellum or paleocerebellum is connected with **spinal cord**. It forms the **major receiving area** of cerebellum for sensory inputs. Spinocerebellum is also phylogenetically older part of cerebellum.

■ COMPONENTS OF SPINOCEREBELLUM

Spinocerebellum consists of medial portions of cerebellar hemisphere, paraflocculi and the parts of vermis, viz. lingula, central lobe, culmen, lobulus simplex, declive, tuber, pyramid and uvula **(Fig. 99.1 and Table 99.2)**.

■ FUNCTIONS OF SPINOCEREBELLUM

Spinocerebellum regulates **muscle tone, posture and equilibrium** by receiving sensory impulses from tactile receptors, proprioceptors, visual receptors and auditory receptors. It also receives the cortical impulses via pontine nuclei.

Spinocerebellum facilitates the discharge from **gamma motor neurons**. Increased discharge from gamma motor neurons increases the **muscle tone**. The lesion in spinocerebellum causes stoppage of discharge from the gamma motor neurons resulting in hypotonia and disturbances in posture.

Spinocerebellum also receives impulses from optic and auditory pathway and helps in adjustment of posture and equilibrium in response to visual and auditory impulses.

TABLE 99.2: Components of divisions of cerebellum.

Division	Components
Vestibulocerebellum	Flocculonodular lobe (nodulus and flocculi)
Spinocerebellum	Lingula Central lobe Culmen Lobulus simplex Declive Tuber Pyramid Uvula Paraflocculi Medial portions of cerebral hemispheres
Corticocerebellum	Lateral portions of cerebral hemispheres

■ CORTICOCEREBELLUM (NEOCEREBELLUM)

Corticocerebellum is largest part of cerebellum. Because of its connection with **cerebral cortex**, it is called corticocerebellum or **cerebrocerebellum**. It is phylogenetically newer part of cerebellum. So, it is also called **neocerebellum**. It is concerned with planning, programming and coordination.

■ COMPONENTS OF CORTICOCEREBELLUM

Corticocerebellum includes the lateral portions of cerebellar hemispheres **(Fig. 99.1 and Table 99.2)**.

■ AFFERENT-EFFERENT CIRCUIT (CEREBRO-CEREBELLO-CEREBRAL CONNECTIONS)

It is a neuronal pathway through which corticocerebellum controls the voluntary movements.

Fibers from motor areas 4 and 6 in frontal lobe of cerebral cortex enter the pontine nuclei. These fibers are called **corticopontine fibers (Fig. 99.2)**. From pontine

TABLE 99.3: Functions of cerebellum.

Functions		Division of cerebellum involved
1. Regulation of tone, posture and equilibrium	By receiving impulses from vestibular apparatus	Vestibulocerebellum
	By receiving impulses from proprioceptors in muscles, tendons and joints, tactile receptors, visual receptors and auditory receptors	Spinocerebellum
2. Regulation of coordinated movements	i. Damping action ii. Control of ballistic movements iii. Timing and programming the movements iv. Servomechanism v. Comparator function	Corticocerebellum (neocerebellum)

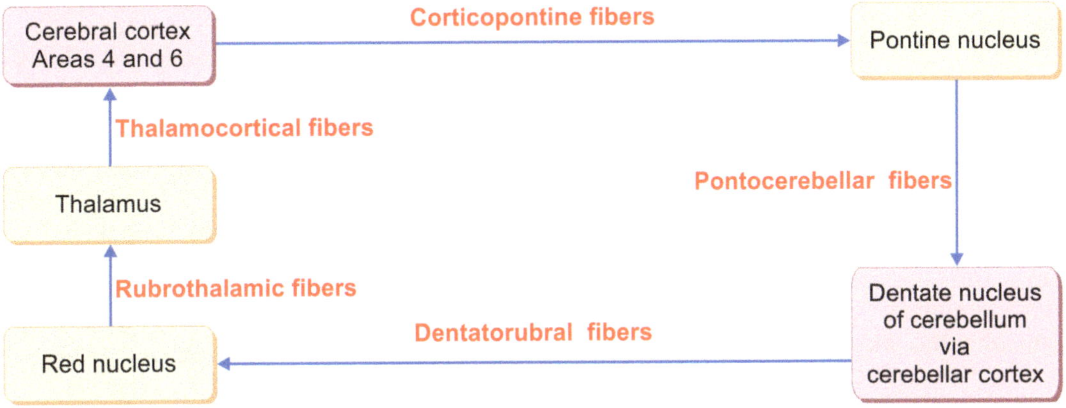

FIGURE 99.2: Schematic representation of cerebro-cerebello-cerebral circuit.

nuclei, the **pontocerebellar fibers** arise and pass through middle cerebellar peduncle of the opposite side and terminate in the cerebellar cortex. This pathway is called the **cerebropontocerebellar tract** or **corticopontocerebellar tract**.

Cerebellar cortex is, in turn, connected to the dentate nucleus. Fibers from the dentate nucleus pass via superior cerebellar peduncle and end in red nucleus of opposite side. These fibers are called **dentatorubral fibers**. From red nucleus, the **rubrothalamic fibers** go to thalamus. Thalamus is connected to areas 4 and 6 in motor cortex of cerebrum by **thalamocortical fibers**. This tract between dentate nucleus and cerebral cortex is called **dentatorubro-thalamocortical tract**.

■ FUNCTIONS OF CORTICOCEREBELLUM

Corticocerebellum is concerned with the integration and regulation of well **coordinated muscular activities**. It is because of its afferent-efferent connection with cerebral cortex through the cerebro-cerebello-cerebral circuit. Apart from its connections with cerebral cortex, cerebellum also receives feedback signals from the muscles through the nerve fibers of proprioceptors.

Mechanism of Action of Corticocerebellum

1. Damping action

Damping action refers to **prevention** of exaggerated muscular activity. This helps in making the voluntary movements **smooth and accurate**. All the voluntary muscular activities are initiated by motor areas of cerebral cortex. Simultaneously, corticocerebellum receives impulses from motor cortex as well as feedback signals from the muscles as soon as the muscular activity starts.

Corticocerebellum, in turn, sends information (impulses) to cerebral cortex to discharge only appropriate signals to the muscles and to cut off any extra impulses. Because of this damping action of corticocerebellum, the exaggeration of muscular activity is prevented and the movements become smooth and accurate. Literally, the word damping means any effect that decreases the amplitude of mechanical oscillation.

2. Control of ballistic movements

Ballistic movements are the **rapid alternate movements**, which take place in different parts of the body while doing any skilled or trained work like typing, cycling, dancing, etc. Corticocerebellum is responsible for **preplanning** the ballistic movements during learning process.

3. Timing and programming the movements

Corticocerebellum is responsible for timing and programming the movements particularly during **learning process**. While using a keyboard of a computer or while doing any other fast skilled work, a chain of movements occurs rapidly in a sequential manner. During the learning process of these skilled works, corticocerebellum plans the various sequential movements. It also plans schedule of time duration of each movement and the time interval between movements. All the information from corticocerebellum are communicated to **sensory motor area** of cerebral cortex and stored in the form of **memory**. So, after the learning process is over, these activities are executed easily and smoothly in sequential manner.

4. Servomechanism

Servomechanism is the **correction of any disturbance** or interference while performing skilled work. Once the skilled works are learnt, the sequential movements are executed without any interruption. Cerebellum lets the cerebral cortex to discharge the signals, which are already programmed and stored at sensory motor cortex, and, does not interfere much. However, if there is any disturbance or interference, the corticocerebellum immediately influences the cortex and corrects the movements.

5. Comparator function

Comparator function of the corticocerebellum is responsible for the integration and coordination of the various muscular activities.

On one side, cerebellum receives the information from **cerebral cortex** regarding the cortical impulses which are sent to the muscles. On the other side, it receives the **feedback information** (proprioceptive impulses) from the **muscles** regarding their actions under the instruction of cerebral cortex.

By receiving the messages from both ends, corticocerebellum compares the cortical commands for muscular activity and the **actual movements** carried out by the muscles. If any correction is to be done, then, corticocerebellum sends instructions (impulses) to the motor cortex.

Accordingly, the cerebral cortex corrects or modifies the signals to muscles, so that the movements become accurate, precise and smooth. This function of corticocerebellum is known as comparator function.

Simultaneously, it also receives the impulses from tactile receptors, eye and ear. Such additional information facilitates the comparator function of corticocerebellum.

■ APPLIED PHYSIOLOGY: CEREBELLAR LESIONS

Cerebellar lesions occur due to tumor, abscess, injury and excess alcohol intake. Cerebellar lesions lead to disturbances in posture, equilibrium and the movements. In unilateral lesion, symptoms appear on the affected side because cerebellum controls the same (**ipsilateral**) side of the body.

■ DISTURBANCES IN TONE AND POSTURE

Atonia or Hypotonia

Atonia is the loss of tone and hypotonia is reduction in tone of the muscle. Atonia or hypotonia occurs because of the loss of facilitatory impulses from cerebellum to gamma motor neurons in the spinal cord.

Attitude

Attitude of the body changes in unilateral lesion of the cerebellum.

Changes in the attitude are:

1. Rotation of head towards the opposite side (unaffected side).
2. Lowering of shoulder on the same side.
3. Abduction of leg on the affected side. The leg is rotated outward.
4. Weight of the body is thrown on the leg of unaffected side. So, the trunk is bent with concavity towards the affected side.

Deviation Movement

It is the lateral deviation of arms when both the arms are stretched and held in front of the body with closed eyes. In bilateral lesion, both the arms deviate and in unilateral lesion arm of the affected side deviates.

Effect on Deep Reflexes

Pendular movements occur while eliciting a tendon jerk particularly the knee jerk (Chapter 93).

■ DISTURBANCES IN EQUILIBRIUM

While Standing

While standing, the legs are spread to provide a broad base. And, the body sways side-to-side with the oscillations of the head.

While Moving: Gait

Gait means the **manner of walking**. In cerebellar lesion, a **staggering, reeling and drunken like gait** is observed.

■ DISTURBANCES IN MOVEMENTS

Disturbances in movements during cerebellar lesions are explained in **Table 99.4**.

TABLE 99.4: Disturbances in movements during cerebellar lesions.

Disturbance	Explanation
1. Ataxia	Lack of coordination of movements
2. Asynergia	Lack of coordination between different groups of muscles
3. Asthenia	Weakness, easy fatigability and slowness of muscles
4. Dysmetria	Inability to check the exact strength and duration of muscular contractions required for any voluntary act While reaching for an object, the arm may overshoot (hypermetria) or it may fall short (hypometria) of the object
5. Intention tremor	Tremor that occurs while attempting to do any voluntary act Refer Chapter 97 for details of tremor
6. Astasia	Unsteady voluntary movement
7. Nystagmus	To and fro movement of eyeball. Refer Chapter 104 for details of nystagmus
8. Rebound phenomenon	While attempting to do a movement against a resistance, and if the resistance is suddenly removed, the limb moves forcibly in the direction in which the attempt was made
9. Dysarthria	Disturbance in speech
10. Adiadochokinesis	Inability to do rapid alternate successive movements such as supination and pronation of arm

Chapter 100: Basal Ganglia

CHAPTER OUTLINE

- SITUATION
- COMPONENTS
  - CORPUS STRIATUM
  - SUBSTANTIA NIGRA
  - SUBTHALAMIC NUCLEUS OF LUYS
- FUNCTIONS
  - CONTROL OF MUSCLE TONE
  - CONTROL OF MOTOR ACTIVITY
  - CONTROL OF REFLEX MUSCULAR ACTIVITY
  - CONTROL OF AUTOMATIC ASSOCIATED MOVEMENTS
- ROLE IN AROUSAL MECHANISM
- APPLIED PHYSIOLOGY: DISORDERS
  - PARKINSON DISEASE
  - WILSON'S DISEASE
  - CHOREA
  - ATHETOSIS
  - CHOREOATHETOSIS
  - HUNTINGTON'S DISEASE
  - HEMIBALLISMUS
  - KERNICTERUS

SITUATION

Basal ganglia are the scattered masses of gray matter submerged in subcortical substance of cerebral hemisphere **(Fig. 100.1)**.

COMPONENTS OF BASAL GANGLIA

Basal ganglia include three primary components:

I. Corpus striatum.
II. Substantia nigra.
III. Subthalamic nucleus of Luys.

CORPUS STRIATUM

It is a mass of gray matter situated at the base of cerebral hemispheres in close relation to the thalamus **(Fig. 100.2)**.

Corpus striatum has two parts:

1. Caudate nucleus.
2. Lenticular nucleus which is divided into two portions:
   i. Putamen.
   ii. Globus pallidus.

SUBSTANTIA NIGRA

Substantia nigra is situated below red nucleus. It is made up of large pigmented and small non-pigmented cells. The pigment contains high quantity of iron.

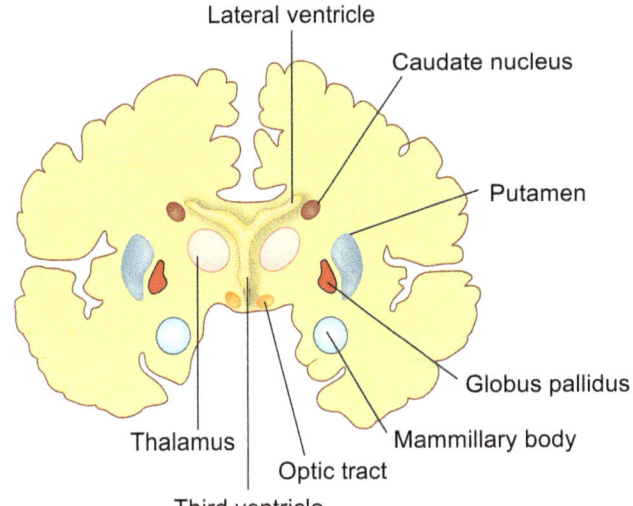

FIGURE 100.1: Basal ganglia.

SUBTHALAMIC NUCLEUS OF LUYS

This nucleus is situated lateral to red nucleus and dorsal to substantia nigra.

FUNCTIONS OF BASAL GANGLIA

As a part of **extrapyramidal system**, basal ganglia are concerned with regulation of muscle tone and integration

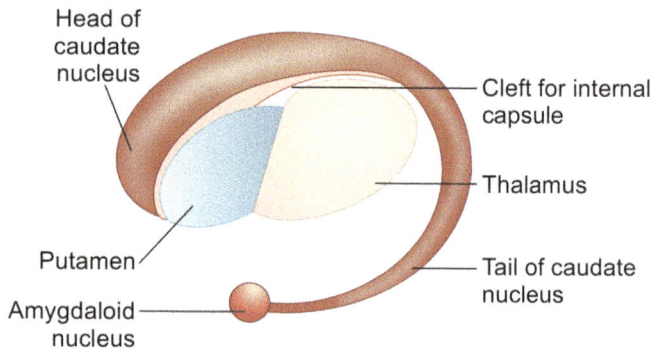

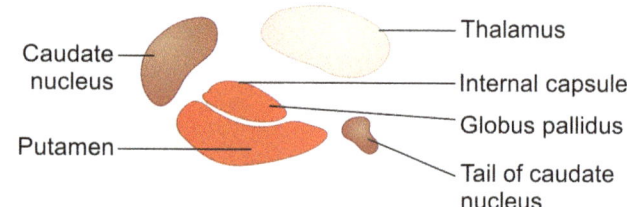

FIGURE 100.2: Corpus striatum.

and the regulation of motor activities. Various functions of basal ganglia are given below.

■ 1. CONTROL OF MUSCLE TONE

Basal ganglia control the muscle tone. In fact, the **gamma motor neurons** of spinal cord are responsible for the tone of the muscles. Basal ganglia decrease muscle tone by inhibiting the gamma motor neurons through descending inhibitory reticular system in brainstem.

■ 2. CONTROL OF MOTOR ACTIVITY

i. Regulation of Voluntary Movements

Voluntary motor activities are initiated by cerebral cortex. However, these movements are controlled by basal ganglia. During lesions of basal ganglia, the control mechanism is lost and so the movements become inaccurate and awkward.

Basal ganglia control the motor activities because of the nervous (neuronal) circuits between basal ganglia and other parts of brain which are involved in motor activity.

ii. Regulation of Conscious Movements

Basal ganglia regulate the conscious movements. This function of basal ganglia is also known as the **cognitive control** of activity. For example, when a stray dog barks at a man, immediately the person understands the situation, turns away and starts running.

iii. Regulation of Subconscious Movements

Basal ganglia regulate the subconscious movements which take place during trained motor activities, i.e. skilled activities such as writing the learnt alphabet, paper cutting, nail hammering, etc.

■ 3. CONTROL OF REFLEX MUSCULAR ACTIVITY

Some of the reflex muscular activities, particularly visual and labyrinthine reflexes, are important in the maintenance of posture. Basal ganglia are responsible for the coordination and integration of impulses for these reflex activities.

■ 4. CONTROL OF AUTOMATIC ASSOCIATED MOVEMENTS

Automatic associated movements are the movements in the body, which take place along with some motor activities. Examples are the swing of the arms while walking, appropriate facial expressions while talking or doing any work. Basal ganglia are responsible for the automatic associated movements.

■ 5. ROLE IN AROUSAL MECHANISM

Along with red nucleus, globus pallidus is involved in arousal mechanism because of their connections with reticular formation. Extensive lesion in globus pallidus causes drowsiness, leading to sleep.

■ APPLIED PHYSIOLOGY: DISORDERS OF BASAL GANGLIA

■ 1. PARKINSON DISEASE

Parkinson disease is a slow progressive degenerative disease of nervous system associated with destruction of dopamine producing cells in brain. It is named after the discoverer **James Parkinson**. It is also called **parkinsonism** or **paralysis agitans**.

Causes of Parkinson Disease

Parkinson disease occurs due to **lack of dopamine** caused by damage of basal ganglia. It is mostly due to the destruction of substantia nigra and the nigrostriatal pathway, which has **dopaminergic fibers**.

Causes for damage of basal ganglia:

  i. Viral infection of brain such as encephalitis.
 ii. Cerebral arteriosclerosis.
iii. Injury to basal ganglia.
 iv. Destruction or removal of dopamine from basal ganglia. It occurs mostly due to long-term treatment with drugs. Parkinsonism due to the drugs is known as **drug-induced parkinsonism**.
  v. Unknown causes: Parkinsonism can occur because of the destruction of basal ganglia due to some unknown causes. This type of parkinsonism is called **idiopathic parkinsonism**.

Signs and Symptoms of Parkinson Disease

Parkinson disease develops very slowly and the early signs and symptoms may be unnoticed for months or even for years. Often the symptoms start with a mild noticeable tremor in just one hand. When the tremor becomes remarkable, the disease causes slowing or freezing of movements followed by rigidity.

Common signs and symptoms of Parkinson disease are:

i. Tremor

Refer Chapter 97 for details of tremor. In Parkinson disease, static tremor or **resting tremor** occurs during rest. But it disappears while doing any work. It is also called **drum beating tremor**, as the movements are similar to beating a drum. The thumb moves rhythmically over the index and middle fingers. These movements are called **pill rolling movements**.

ii. Slowness of movements

Over the time, the movements start slowing down (**bradykinesia**) and it takes a long time even to perform a simple task. Gradually the patient becomes unable to initiate the voluntary activity (**akinesia**) or the voluntary movements are reduced (**hypokinesia**). It is because of hypertonicity of the muscles.

iii. Poverty of movements

Poverty of movements is the loss of all automatic associated movements. Because of absence of the automatic associated movements, the body becomes **statue like**. The face becomes **mask-like**, due to absence of appropriate expressions like blinking and smiling.

iv. Rigidity of limbs

Rigidity develops in limbs due to stiffness of muscles. **Muscular stiffness** occurs because of increased muscle tone which is due to the removal of inhibitory influence on gamma motor neurons. It affects both flexor and extensor muscles equally. So, the limbs become more **rigid like pillars**. The condition is called **lead pipe rigidity**. In later stages, the rigidity extends to neck and trunk.

v. Gait

Gait means **manner of walking**. The patient loses the normal gait. Gait in Parkinson disease is called **festinant gait**. The patient walks quickly in short steps by bending forward, as if he is going to catch up the center of gravity.

vi. Speech problems

Many patients develop speech problems. They may speak very softly or sometimes rapidly. The words are repeated many times. Finally, speech becomes slurred and they hesitate to speak.

vii. Emotional changes

Persons affected by Parkinson disease are often upset emotionally.

viii. Dementia

In later stages, some patients develop dementia (Chapter 107).

2. WILSON'S DISEASE

Wilson's disease is an inherited disorder characterized by **excess of copper** in the body tissues. It is also known as **progressive hepatolenticular degeneration**. This disease develops due to damage of the lenticular nucleus.

In Wilson disease, copper is deposited in the liver, brain, kidneys and eyes. Copper deposits cause damage of tissues. And the affected organs stop functioning. In addition to symptoms of Parkinson disease, liver failure and damage of central nervous system are the most predominant effects of this disorder. Wilson disease is fatal if not treated early.

3. CHOREA

It is an abnormal involuntary movement. Chorea means **rapid jerky movements**. It mostly involves the limbs. It is due to lesion in caudate nucleus and putamen.

4. ATHETOSIS

It is another type of abnormal involuntary movement, which includes **slow rhythmic** and **twisting movements**. It is because of the lesion in caudate nucleus and putamen.

5. CHOREOATHETOSIS

It is the condition characterized by aimless involuntary muscular movements. It is due to combined effects of chorea and athetosis.

6. HUNTINGTON'S DISEASE

Huntington's disease is an inherited progressive neural disorder due to the degeneration of neurons secreting GABA in corpus striatum and substantia nigra. It is characterized by **chorea, hypotonia** and **dementia**.

7. HEMIBALLISMUS

It is a disorder characterized by **violent involuntary abnormal movements** on one side of the body involving mostly the arm. While walking, the arm swings widely. Hemiballismus occurs due to degeneration of subthalamic nucleus of Luys.

8. KERNICTERUS

Kernicterus is a form of brain damage in infants caused by **severe jaundice**. Basal ganglia are the mainly affected parts of brain. Refer Chapter 19 for details.

Cerebral Cortex and Limbic System

CHAPTER OUTLINE

- **CEREBRUM**
- **MORPHOLOGY OF CEREBRAL CORTEX**
- **NEOCORTEX AND ALLOCORTEX**
- **LOBES OF CEREBRAL CORTEX**
- **CEREBRAL DOMINANCE**
- **BRODMANN AREAS**
- **FRONTAL LOBE**
  - PRECENTRAL CORTEX
  - PREFRONTAL CORTEX OR ORBITOFRONTAL CORTEX
  - APPLIED PHYSIOLOGY: FRONTAL LOBE SYNDROME
- **PARIETAL LOBE**
  - SOMESTHETIC AREA I
  - SOMESTHETIC AREA II
  - SOMESTHETIC ASSOCIATION AREA
- **APPLIED PHYSIOLOGY: EFFECTS OF LESION**
- **TEMPORAL LOBE**
  - PRIMARY AUDITORY AREA
  - SECONDARY AUDITORY AREA: AUDITOPSYCHIC AREA
  - AREA FOR EQUILIBRIUM
  - APPLIED PHYSIOLOGY: TEMPORAL LOBE SYNDROME
- **OCCIPITAL LOBE**
  - AREAS OF VISUAL CORTEX
  - APPLIED PHYSIOLOGY: EFFECTS OF LESION
- **LIMBIC SYSTEM**
  - COMPONENTS
  - FUNCTIONS

■ CEREBRUM

Cerebrum is the largest part of brain. Cerebrum is responsible for perception of all sensations and initiation of various movements of the body.

Cerebrum is formed by two structures:

1. Outer layer of **gray matter** called **cerebral cortex** which includes nerve cell bodies.
2. Inner layer of **white matter** which includes of nerve fibers.

■ MORPHOLOGY OF CEREBRAL CORTEX

Cerebral cortex is formed by two **hemispheres** which are separated anteriorly and posteriorly by a deep **vertical fissure** (deep furrow or groove). But the middle portions are connected by **corpus callosum**.

Each hemisphere, has three surfaces namely, lateral, medial and inferior surfaces. Surface of the cerebral cortex is characterized by complicated pattern of **sulci** (singular = sulcus) and **gyri** (singular = gyrus). Sulcus is a slight depression or groove and gyrus is a raised ridge.

Cerebral cortex is formed by outer **gray matter** which surrounds the inner **white matter**. It is formed by different types of nerve cells along with their processes and neuroglia which are arranged in **six layers**. It is not uniform throughout. It is thickest at the precentral gyrus, and thinnest at the frontal and occipital poles.

■ NEOCORTEX AND ALLOCORTEX

Part of the cerebral cortex that has **all six layers** of structures is called **neocortex**. It is also called **isocortex** or **neopallium**. It is the phylogenetically new structure of cerebral cortex. Neocortex forms the major portion of cerebral cortex.

Remaining part of the cerebral cortex is called **allocortex**. It has **less than six layers** of structures. This part of the cortex is called **allocortex**. It includes **archicortex** and **paleocortex** that form the part of limbic system.

■ LOBES OF CEREBRAL CORTEX

Neocortex of each cerebral hemisphere consists of four lobes (Figs. 101.1 to 101.3):

1. Frontal lobe.
2. Parietal lobe.
3. Occipital lobe.
4. Temporal lobe.

Chapter 101: Cerebral Cortex and Limbic System

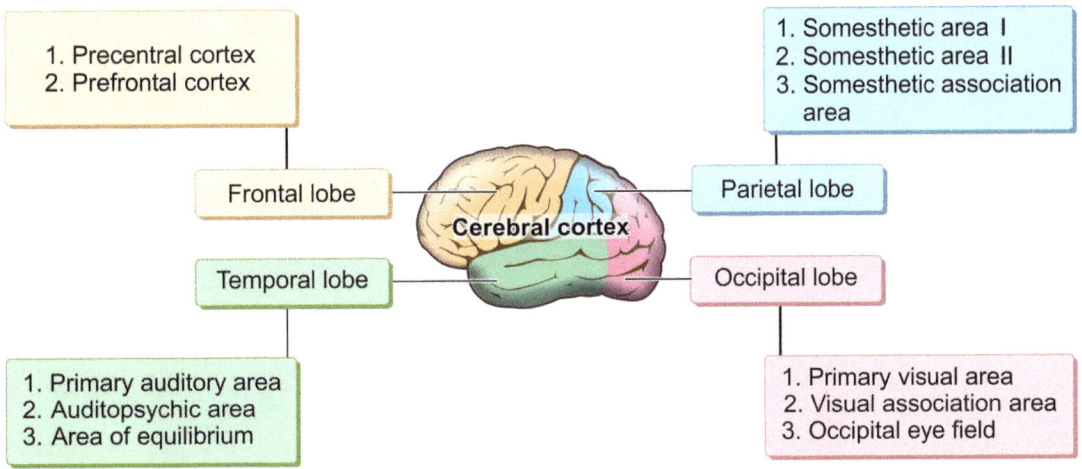

FIGURE 101.1: Parts of cerebral cortex.

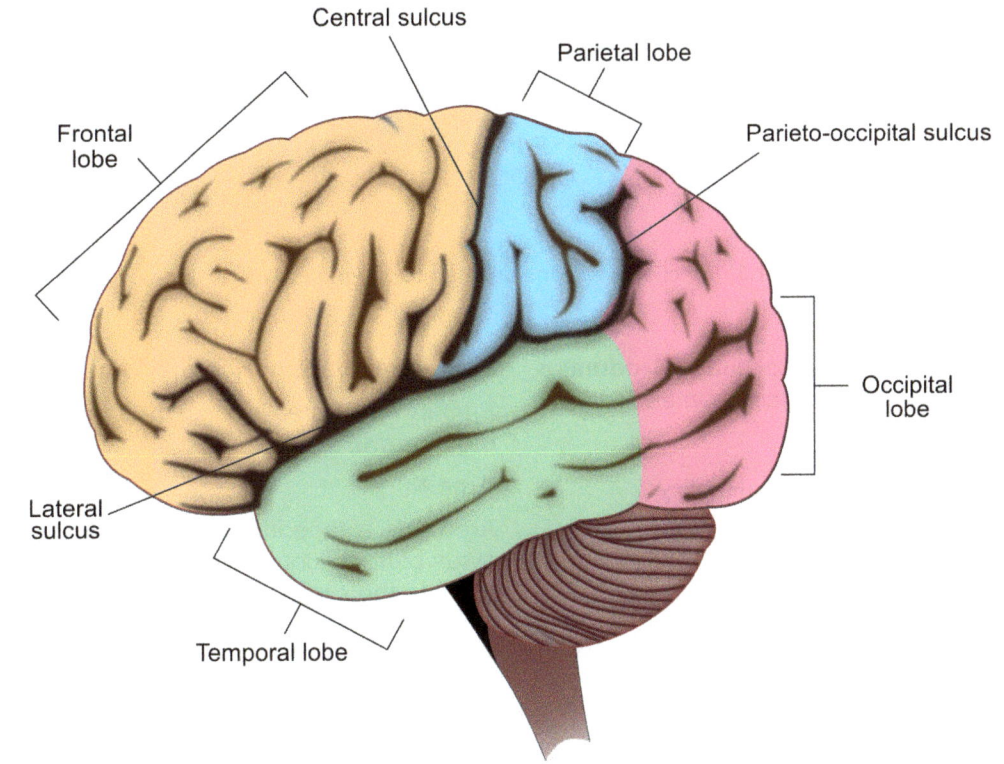

FIGURE 101.2: Lobes of cerebral cortex.

Lobes of each hemisphere are demarked by four main fissures and sulci:

1. **Central sulcus** or Rolandic fissure between frontal and parietal lobes.
2. **Parieto-occipital sulcus** between parietal and occipital lobe.
3. **Sylvian fissure** or **lateral sulcus** between parietal and temporal lobes.
4. **Callosomarginal fissure** between temporal lobe and limbic area.

CEREBRAL DOMINANCE

Cerebral dominance is defined as the dominance of one cerebral hemisphere over the other in the control of cerebral functions. The two cerebral hemispheres are not functionally equivalent.

Cerebral dominance is related to handedness, i.e. preference of the individual to use right or left hand. More than 90% of people are **right-handed**. In these individuals, the **left hemisphere** is **dominant** and it controls the analytical process and language-related functions such as speech, reading and writing. Hence, the left hemisphere of these persons is called **dominant hemisphere** or **categorical hemisphere**.

BRODMANN AREAS

Brodmann area is a region of cerebral cortex defined on the basis of organization of neurons. These areas were

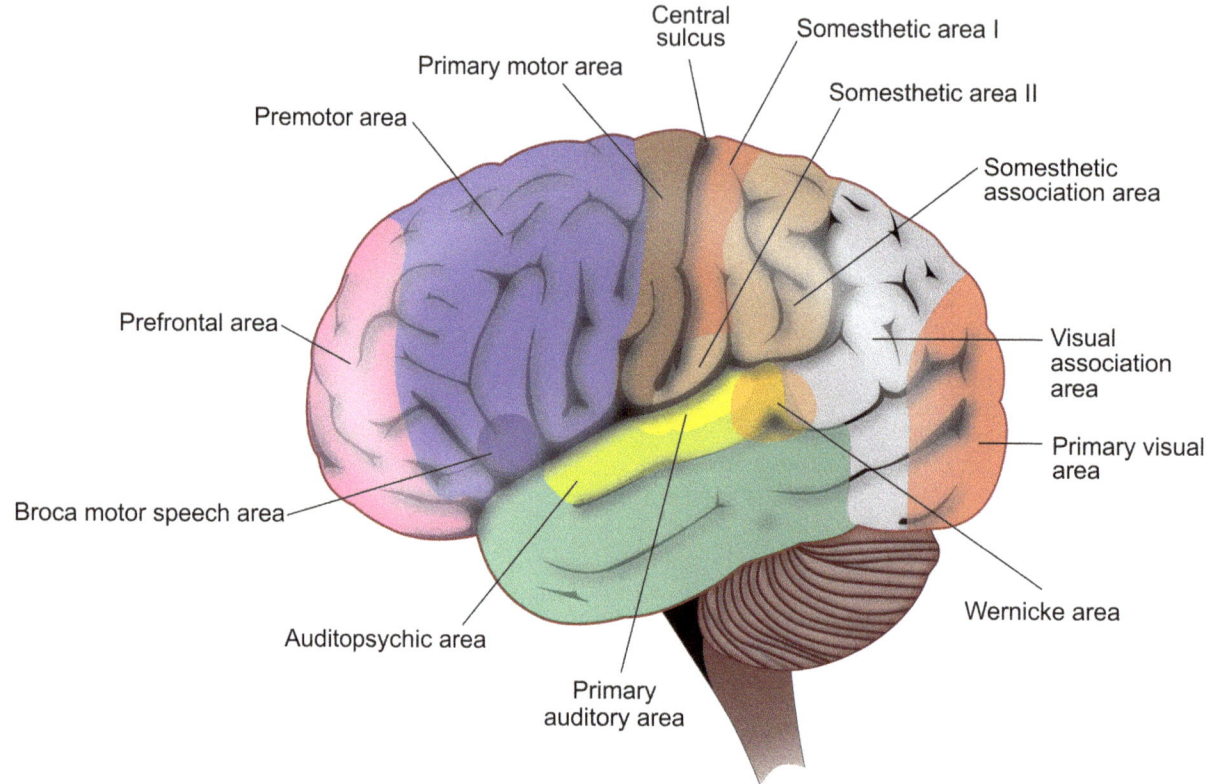

FIGURE 101.3: Functional regions on lateral surface of cerebral cortex.

originally defined and numbered by **Korbinian Brodmann**. Some of these areas were given specific names based on their functions.

■ FRONTAL LOBE OF CEREBRAL CORTEX

Frontal lobe forms one third of the cortical surface. It extends from frontal pole to the central sulcus and limited below by the lateral sulcus.

Frontal lobe of cerebral cortex is divided into two parts:

I. Precentral cortex situated posteriorly.
II. Prefrontal cortex situated anteriorly.

■ PRECENTRAL CORTEX

Posterior part of frontal lobe is called precentral cortex. It includes the lip of central sulcus, whole of precentral gyrus and posterior portions of superior, middle and inferior frontal gyri. It also extends to the medial surface.

This part is also called **excitomotor cortex** or area, since the stimulation of different points in this area causes activity of discrete skeletal muscle. Precentral cortex is further divided into three functional areas **(Fig. 101.3)**:

1. Primary motor area.
2. Premotor area.
3. Supplementary motor area.

1. *Primary Motor Area*

Primary motor area extends throughout the precentral gyrus and the adjoining lip of central sulcus. Areas 4 and 4S are present here **(Figs. 101.4 and 101.5)**.

Functions of primary motor area

Primary motor area is concerned with initiation of **voluntary movements** and speech.

Area 4

Area 4 is a tapering strip of area situated in precentral gyrus of frontal lobe **(Figs. 101.4 and 101.5)**.

It is the center for movement, as it sends all efferent (corticospinal) fibers of primary motor area. Through the fibers of corticospinal tracts, area 4 activates the **lower motor neurons** in the spinal cord. It activates both α-motor neurons and γ-motor neurons simultaneously by the process called **coactivation**.

Activation of α-motor neurons causes contraction of extrafusal fibers of the muscles. **Activation of γ-motor neurons** causes contraction of intrafusal fibers leading to increase in muscle tone.

Localization: Motor Homunculus

Muscles of various parts of the body are represented in area 4 in an inverted way from medial to lateral surface. Lower parts of body are represented in medial surface and upper parts of the body are represented in the lateral surface. Order of representation from medial to lateral surface is toes, ankle, knee, hip, trunk, shoulder, arm, elbow, wrist, hand fingers and face. However, parts of the face are not represented in inverted manner **(Fig. 101.6)**.

Area 4S

Area 4S is called **suppressor area**. It forms a narrow strip anterior to area 4. It scrutinizes and suppresses the extra

Chapter 101: Cerebral Cortex and Limbic System

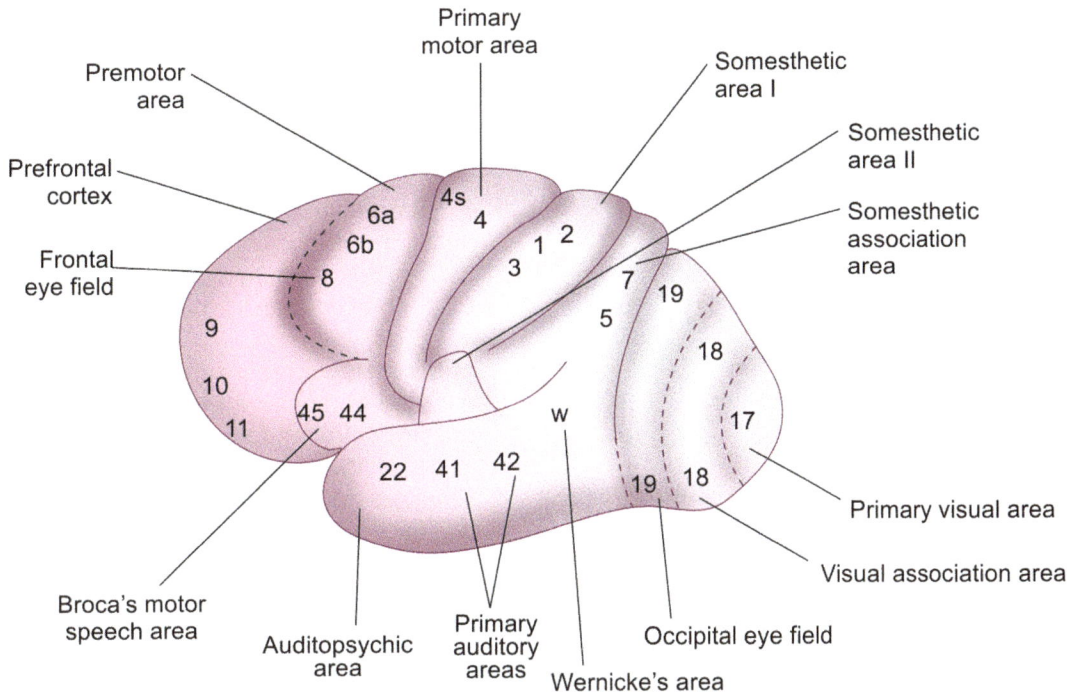

FIGURE 101.4: Lateral surface of cerebral cortex.

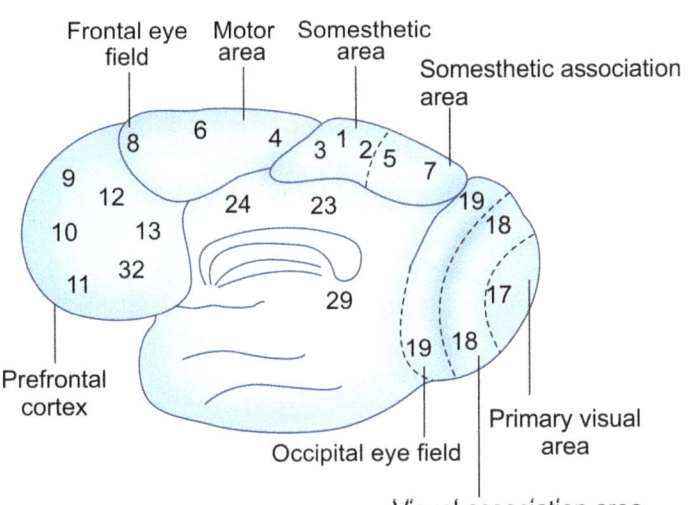

FIGURE 101.5: Medial surface of cerebral cortex.

impulses produced by area 4 and prevents **exaggeration of movements**.

2. Premotor Area

This has areas 6, 8, 44 and 45. Premotor area is anterior to primary motor area in the precentral cortex.

Functions of premotor area

Premotor area is concerned with control of **postural movements**.

Area 6

Area 6 is in the posterior portions of superior, middle and inferior frontal gyri. It is subdivided into 6a and 6b. It gives origin to some of the pyramidal tract fibers.

Area 6 has two functions:

i. It is concerned with **coordination of movements** initiated by area 4. It helps to make the skilled movements more accurate and smoother.
ii. It is **cortical center** for extrapyramidal system.

Area 8

Area 8 is called **frontal eye field**. It lies anterior to area 6 in the precentral cortex. It is concerned with movements of eyeball.

Frontal eye field is concerned with **conjugate movement** of eyeballs.

Areas 44 and 45: Broca's area

Broca's area is the **motor area for speech**. It includes areas 44 and 45. Broca's area is present in left hemisphere (dominant hemisphere) of right-handed persons and in the right hemisphere of left-handed persons. It is a special region of premotor cortex situated in inferior frontal gyrus.

Broca's area is responsible for movements of tongue, lips and larynx, which are involved in speech.

3. Supplementary Motor Area

It is situated in medial surface of frontal lobe rostral to primary motor area.

Functions of supplementary motor area

This area is concerned with coordination of **skilled movements**.

■ PREFRONTAL CORTEX OR ORBITOFRONTAL CORTEX

Prefrontal or orbitofrontal cortex is the anterior part of frontal lobe of cerebral cortex, in front of areas 8 and 44.

Section 10: Nervous System

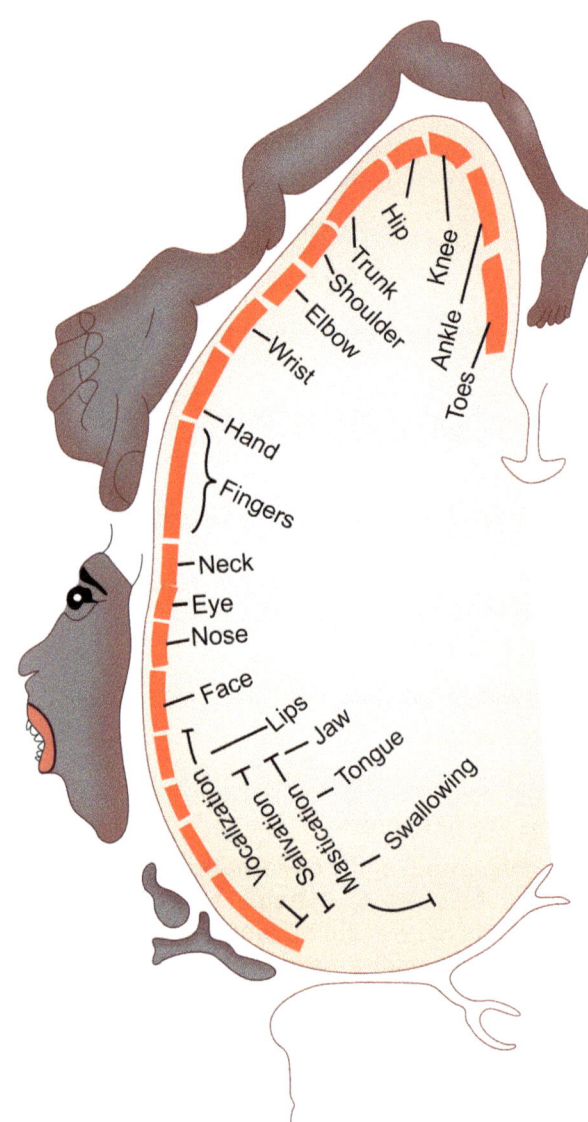

FIGURE 101.6: Topographical arrangement (homunculus) of motor areas in cerebral cortex.

It occupies the medial, lateral and inferior surfaces, and includes orbital gyri, medial frontal gyrus and the anterior portions of superior, middle and inferior frontal gyri.

Areas present in prefrontal cortex are 9, 10, 11, 12, 13, 14, 23, 24, 29 and 32. Areas 12, 13, 14, 23, 24, 29 and 32 are in medial surface. Areas 9, 10 and 11 are in lateral surface.

Area 13 is concerned with **emotional reactions**.

Functions of Prefrontal Cortex

1. It forms the center for the **higher functions** like emotion, learning, memory and social behavior. Short-term memories are registered here.
2. It is the center for **planned actions**.
3. It is the seat of intelligence. So, it is also called the **organ of mind**.
4. It is responsible for the **personality** of the individuals.
5. It is responsible for various **autonomic changes** during emotional conditions, because of its connections with hypothalamus and brainstem.

■ APPLIED PHYSIOLOGY: FRONTAL LOBE SYNDROME

Frontal lobe syndrome is a disorder caused by injury or ablation of prefrontal cortex.

Features of frontal lobe syndrome are:

1. Emotional instability: Lack of restraint leading to hostility, aggressiveness and restlessness.
2. Lack of concentration and lack of fixing attention.
3. Lack of initiation and difficulty in planning any course of action.
4. Impairment of recent memory occurs. However, the memory of remote events is not lost.
5. Loss of moral and social sense is common, and there is loss of love for family and friends.
6. There is failure to realize the seriousness of the condition. Patient has the sense of well-being and also has flight of ideas.
7. Functional abnormalities:
    i. Hyperphagia (increased food intake).
    ii. Loss of control over sphincter of the urinary bladder or rectum.
    iii. Disturbances in orientation.
    iv. Slight tremor.

■ PARIETAL LOBE

Parietal lobe extends from **central sulcus** and merges with occipital lobe behind and temporal lobe below. This lobe is separated from occipital lobe by **parieto-occipital sulcus** and from temporal lobe by **Sylvian sulcus**.

Parietal lobe is divided into three functional areas:

A. Somesthetic area I.
B. Somesthetic area II.
C. Somesthetic association area.

In addition to these three areas, a part of **sensory motor area** is also situated in parietal lobe (see below).

■ SOMESTHETIC AREA I

It is also called **somatosensory area I** or primary somesthetic or **primary sensory area**. It is present in the posterior lip of central sulcus, in the postcentral gyrus and in the paracentral lobule.

Areas

Somesthetic area I has three areas which are called **areas 3, 1 and 2**. Anterior part of this forms area 3 and posterior part forms areas 1 and 2.

Localization: Sensory Homunculus

Different sensory areas of the body are represented in somesthetic area I (**primary sensory area**) in an inverted manner as in the motor area. The toes are represented in lowest part of medial surface, legs at the upper border of hemispheres, then from above downwards knee, thigh, hip, trunk, upper limb, neck and face. The representation of face is not inverted. The representation of parts of face from above downwards are eyelids, nose, cheek, upper lip and lower lip **(Fig. 101.7)**.

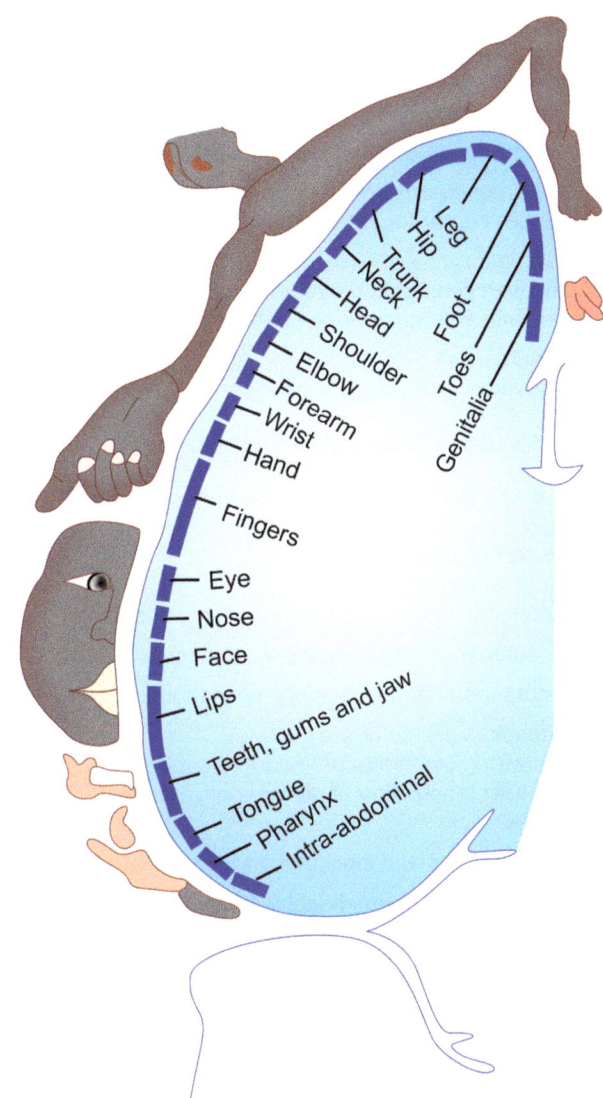

FIGURE 101.7: Topographical arrangement (homunculus) of sensory areas in cerebral cortex.

Functions of Somesthetic Area I

1. Somesthetic area I is responsible for **perception and integration** of cutaneous and kinesthetic sensations. It receives sensory impulses from cutaneous receptors (touch, pressure, pain, temperature) and proprioceptors of opposite side through thalamic radiation. Area 1 is concerned with sensory perception. The areas 2 and 3 are involved in the integration of these sensations.
2. This area sends **sensory feedback** to the premotor area. It is also concerned with the movements of head and eyeballs.
3. **Discriminative functions**: In addition to perception of cutaneous and kinesthetic sensation, this area is also responsible for recognizing the discriminative features of sensations (Chapter 97).

■ SOMESTHETIC AREA II

Somesthetic area II is situated in postcentral gyrus below the area of face of somesthetic area I. A part of this is buried in Sylvian sulcus. It is also known as **somatosensory area II**.

This area receives sensory impulses from somesthetic area I and from thalamus directly. This area is concerned with **perception of sensation**. Thus, the sensory parts of body have two representations, viz. in somesthetic area I and area II.

■ SOMESTHETIC ASSOCIATION AREA

This area is situated posterior to postcentral gyrus, above the auditory cortex and in front of visual cortex. It has two **areas, 5 and 7**. It is concerned with **synthesis of sensations** perceived by somesthetic area I.

Thus, the somesthetic association area forms the center for combined sensations like **stereognosis**. Lesion of this area causes astereognosis.

Sensory Motor Area

Sensory motor area is the area of cerebral cortex in which the precentral gyrus of frontal lobe (where motor areas are located) and postcentral gyrus of parietal lobe (where sensory areas are located) are knit together by association nerve fibers.

Function of this area is to store the **timing and programing** of various sequential movements of complicated skilled movements which are planned by **neocerebellum** (Chapter 99).

■ APPLIED PHYSIOLOGY: EFFECTS OF LESION

Lesion or ablation of parietal lobe (sensory cortex) results in the following disturbances:

1. Contralateral disturbance of cutaneous sensations.
2. Disturbances in kinesthetic sensations.
3. Loss of tactile localization and discrimination.

■ TEMPORAL LOBE

Temporal lobe of cerebral cortex includes three functional areas:

A. Primary auditory area.
B. Secondary auditory area.
C. Area for equilibrium.

■ PRIMARY AUDITORY AREA

Primary auditory area includes:

1. Area 41.
2. Area 42.
3. Wernicke's area.

Areas 41 and 42 are situated in anterior transverse gyrus and lateral surface of superior temporal gyrus. Wernicke's area is in upper part of superior temporal gyrus posterior to areas 41 and 42.

Functions of Primary Auditory Area

Primary auditory area is concerned with perception of auditory impulses, analysis of pitch and determination of intensity and source of sound.

Areas 41 and 42 are concerned only with the **perception** of auditory impulses (Table 101.1). **Wernicke's area** is responsible for the **interpretation of sound**. It

TABLE 101.1: Functions of cortical lobes.

Lobe			Functions
Frontal lobe	Precentral cortex	Primary motor area — Area 4	Initiates movements
		Primary motor area — Area 4S	Inhibits exaggeration of movements initiated by area 4
		Area 6	Coordinates movements initiated by area 4 Acts as higher center for extrapyramidal system
		Premotor area — Area 8	Frontal eye field Concerned with conjugate movements of eyeballs Concerned with voluntary movements of eyeballs
		Broca's area: Areas 44 and 45	Motor speech area: Initiates movements involved in speech
		Supplementary motor area —	Concerned with coordinated skilled movements
	Prefrontal cortex	Areas 9, 10, 11, 12, 13, 14, 23, 24, 29 and 32	Concerned with emotion, learning, memory and social behavior Act as the center for planned actions Form seat of intelligence Initiate autonomic changes during emotional conditions
Parietal lobe	Somesthetic area I	Area 1	Perceives cutaneous and kinesthetic sensations
		Areas 3 and 2	Integrate cutaneous and kinesthetic sensations
		Areas 3, 2 and 1	Send feedback to premotor area Concerned with movements of head and eyeballs Concerned with recognition of discriminative features of sensations
	Somesthetic area II	—	Perceives cutaneous and kinesthetic sensations
	Somesthetic association area	Areas 5 and 7	Synthesize sensations perceived by somesthetic area I Forms the center for combined sensations
Temporal lobe	Primary auditory area	Areas 41 and 42	Perceives auditory sensation
		Wernicke's area	Interprets auditory sensation (along with area 22)
	Secondary auditory area	Area 22	Interprets auditory sensation (along with Wernicke's area)
	Area for equilibrium	—	Concerned with maintenance of equilibrium of body
Occipital lobe	Primary visual area	Area 17	Perceives visual sensation
	Secondary visual area	Area 18	Interprets visual sensation
	Occipital eye field	Area 19	Concerned with reflex movement of eyeballs Concerned with associated movements of eyeballs while following a moving object

carries out this function with the help of auditopsychic area (area 22).

SECONDARY AUDITORY AREA: AUDITOPSYCHIC AREA

Secondary auditory area is also called auditopsychic area or auditory association area. It is the **area 22** and it occupies the superior temporal gyrus. This area is concerned with **interpretation of sound** along with Wernicke's area.

AREA FOR EQUILIBRIUM

This area is in the posterior part of superior temporal gyrus. It is concerned with the maintenance of equilibrium of the body. Stimulation of this area causes dizziness, swaying, falling and feeling of rotation.

APPLIED PHYSIOLOGY: TEMPORAL LOBE SYNDROME

Temporal lobe syndrome is otherwise known as **Kluver-Bucy syndrome**. It is the disorder caused by bilateral lesion or bilateral ablation of temporal lobe along with amygdaloid and uncus.

Manifestations of this syndrome are:

1. Aphasia: Disturbance in speech.
2. Auditory disturbances: Such as frequent attacks of tinnitus, auditory hallucinations with sounds like

buzzing, ringing or humming. **Tinnitus** means noise in the ear. **Hallucination** means feeling of a particular type of sensation without any stimulus.
3. Disturbances in smell and taste sensations.
4. Dreamy states: Patient is not aware of his or her own activities, and has the feeling of unreality.
5. Visual hallucinations associated with hemianopia.

OCCIPITAL LOBE: VISUAL CORTEX

Occipital lobe is also called the visual cortex.

AREAS OF VISUAL CORTEX

Occipital lobe consists of three functional areas:
1. Primary visual area: Area 17.
2. Visual association area: Area 18.
3. Occipital eye field: Area 19.

Functions

1. Primary visual area: Area 17 is concerned with **perception of visual impulses**.
2. Visual association area: Area 18 is concerned with **interpretation of visual impulses**.
3. Occipital eye field: Area 19 is concerned with **movement of eyes**.

APPLIED PHYSIOLOGY: EFFECTS OF LESION

Lesion in the upper or lower part of visual cortex results in hemianopia. Bilateral lesion leads to total blindness (Chapter 112).

LIMBIC SYSTEM OR LIMBIC LOBE

Limbic system or limbic lobe is a complex system of cortical and subcortical structures that form a ring around the hilus of cerebral hemisphere. Limbus means ring.

COMPONENTS OF LIMBIC SYSTEM

Structures of limbic system are classified into four groups:
1. Archicortical structures.
2. Paleocortical structures.
3. Juxtallocortical structures.
4. Subcortical structures.

1. Archicortical Structures

Archicortex forms **allocortex** along with **paleocortex**. Archicortex is the phylogenetically oldest structure. It is concerned with **memory.**

2. Paleocortical Structures

Paleocortex is in between archicortex and neocortex. It is concerned with **olfaction.**

3. Juxtallocortical Structures

Juxtallocortex or **mesocortex** is situated between paleocortex and neocortex.

4. Subcortical Structures

Structures situated below the level of cortex are called subcortical structures. Limbic system includes six subcortical structures **(Figs. 101.8 and 101.9).**

FUNCTIONS OF LIMBIC SYSTEM

1. Olfaction

Pyriform cortex and amygdaloid nucleus form the olfactory centers.

2. Regulation of Endocrine Glands

Hypothalamus plays an important role in regulation of endocrine secretion (Chapter 98).

3. Regulation of Autonomic Functions

Hypothalamus plays an important role in regulating the autonomic functions (Chapter 98) such as heart rate, blood pressure, water balance and body temperature.

4. Regulation of Food Intake

Along with amygdaloid complex, the feeding center and satiety center present in hypothalamus regulate food intake (Chapter 98).

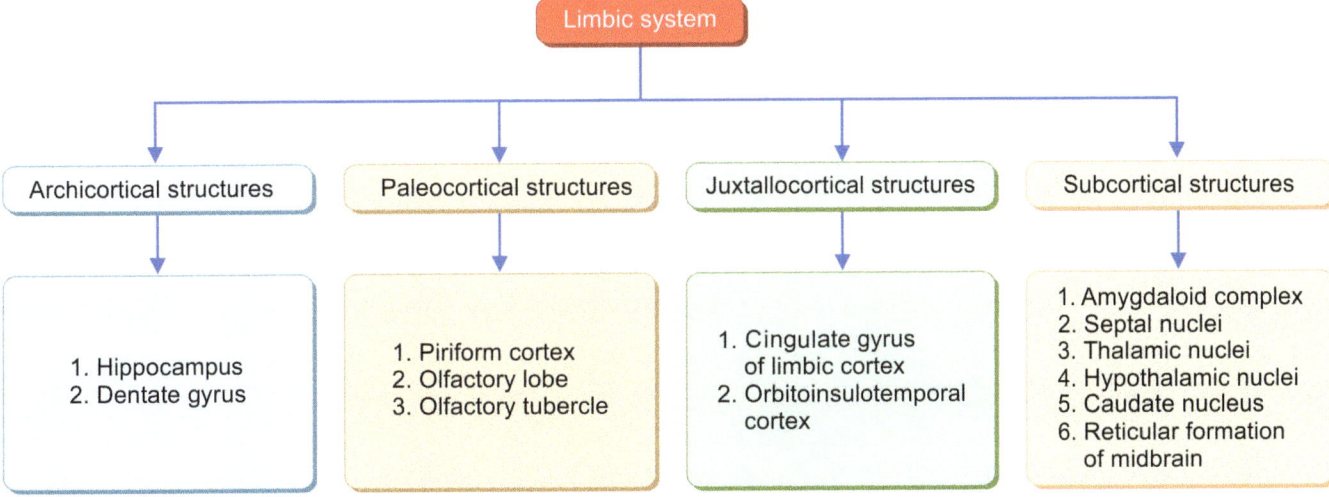

FIGURE 101.8: Components of limbic system.

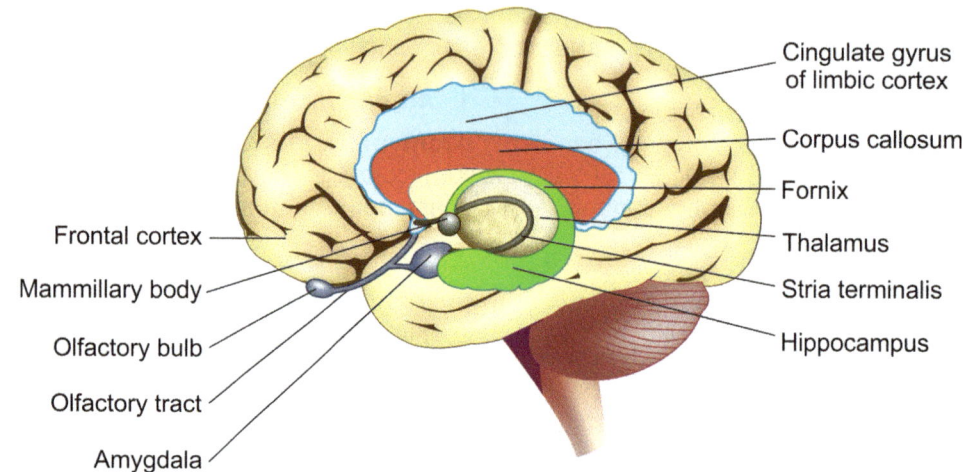

FIGURE 101.9: Limbic system.

5. Control of Circadian Rhythm

Hypothalamus is taking major role in the circadian fluctuations of various physiological activities.

6. Regulation of Sexual Functions

Hypothalamus is responsible for maintaining sexual functions.

7. Role in Emotional State

Emotional state of a person is maintained by hippocampus along with hypothalamus.

8. Role in Memory

Hippocampus plays an important role in memory (Chapter 107).

9. Role in Motivation

Reward and punishment centers present in hypothalamus and other structures of limbic system are responsible for motivation and the behavior pattern of human beings (Chapter 98).

Refer Chapter 98 for details of the hypothalamic functions.

Chapter 102: Reticular Formation

CHAPTER OUTLINE

- DEFINITION
- SITUATION
- DIVISIONS
- FUNCTIONS
- ASCENDING RETICULAR ACTIVATING SYSTEM (ARAS)
- DESCENDING RETICULAR SYSTEM

DEFINITION

Reticular formation is a diffused mass of neurons and nerve fibers forming an ill-defined **meshwork of reticulum** in the central portion of the brainstem.

SITUATION OF RETICULAR FORMATION

Reticular formation is situated in **brainstem**. It extends downwards into spinal cord and upwards up to thalamus and subthalamus.

DIVISIONS OF RETICULAR FORMATION

Reticular formation is divided into three divisions based on the location in brainstem:

1. Medullary reticular formation.
2. Pontine reticular formation.
3. Midbrain reticular formation.

Each division of reticular formation has its own collection of nuclei.

FUNCTIONS OF RETICULAR FORMATION

Based on functions, the reticular formation along with its connections is divided into two systems:

I. Ascending reticular activating system.
II. Descending reticular system.

ASCENDING RETICULAR ACTIVATING SYSTEM: ARAS

Ascending reticular activating system (ARAS) begins in lower part of brainstem, extends upwards through pons, midbrain, thalamus and finally projects throughout the cerebral cortex. It projects into cerebral cortex via subthalamus and thalamus.

ARAS receives fibers from the sensory pathways via long ascending spinal tracts **(Fig. 102.1)**.

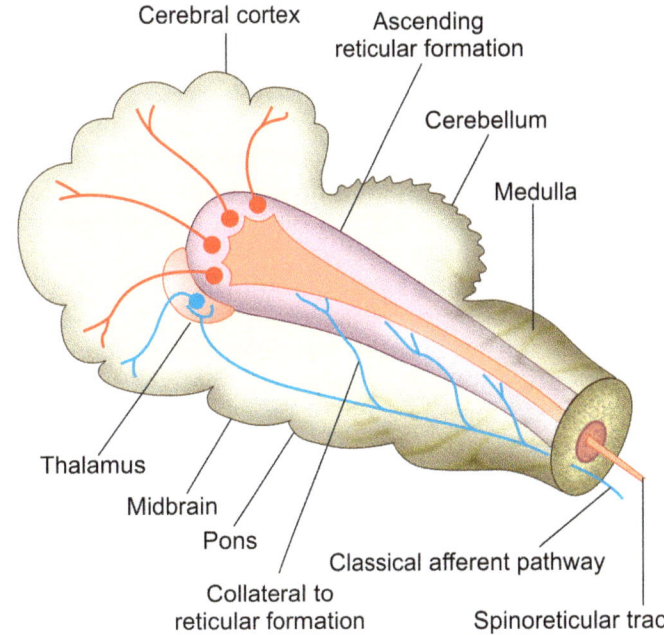

FIGURE 102.1: Ascending reticular formation.

Functions of ARAS

1. ARAS is concerned with arousal phenomenon, alertness, maintenance of attention and wakefulness. Hence the name ascending reticular activating system. Stimulation of midbrain reticular formation produces wakefulness by generalized activation of entire brain including cerebral cortex, thalamus, basal ganglia and brainstem.

Any type of sensory impulses such as impulses of proprioception, pain, auditory, visual, taste, and olfactory sensations cause sudden activation of the

ARAS producing arousal phenomenon in animals and human beings. Even the impulses of visceral sensations activate this system. Sympathetic stimulation and adrenaline cause arousal by affecting midbrain.
2. ARAS also causes emotional reactions.
3. ARAS plays an important role in regulating the learning processes and the development of conditioned reflexes.

Mechanism of Action of ARAS

Impulses of all the sensations reach the cerebral cortex through two channels:

1. Classical or specific sensory pathways.
2. Ascending reticular activating system or nonspecific sensory pathway.

Classical or specific sensory pathways

Classical sensory pathways are the pathways which transmit the sensory impulses from receptors to cerebral cortex via thalamus. Some of the pathways carry impulses of a particular sensation only. For example, the auditory stimulus transmitted by the auditory pathway reaches the auditory cortex via thalamus and causes perception of sound. Such classical sensory pathways are called **specific sensory pathways**.

Ascending reticular activating system or non-specific sensory pathway

All the sensory pathways send collaterals to diffused areas of ARAS. ARAS also receives afferents from spinal cord directly in the form of **spinoreticular tract**. ARAS in turn sends the impulses to almost all the areas of cerebral cortex and other parts of brain. Hence, this pathway is called the **nonspecific sensory pathway**.

The non-specific projection of ARAS into the cortex is responsible for the arousal, alertness and wakefulness. The sensory impulses transmitted directly to cortex via classical pathway causes perception of only the particular sensation. Whereas, the impulses transmitted to cortex via ARAS do not cause the perception of any particular sensation but cause the generalized activation of almost all the areas of cerebral cortex and other parts of brain. This leads to reactions of arousal, alertness and wakefulness.

ARAS in turn is controlled by the feedback signals from cerebral cortex. Also, an inhibitory system controls the activities of ARAS. The inhibitory system involves posterior hypothalamus, intralaminar and anterior thalamic nuclei and medullary area at the level of tractus solitarius.

Tumor or lesion in ARAS leads to sleeping sickness or coma. The impact of head injury on ARAS also causes coma.

■ DESCENDING RETICULAR SYSTEM

Descending reticular system includes reticular formation in brainstem, the reticulospinal tract and reticular formation in spiral cord.

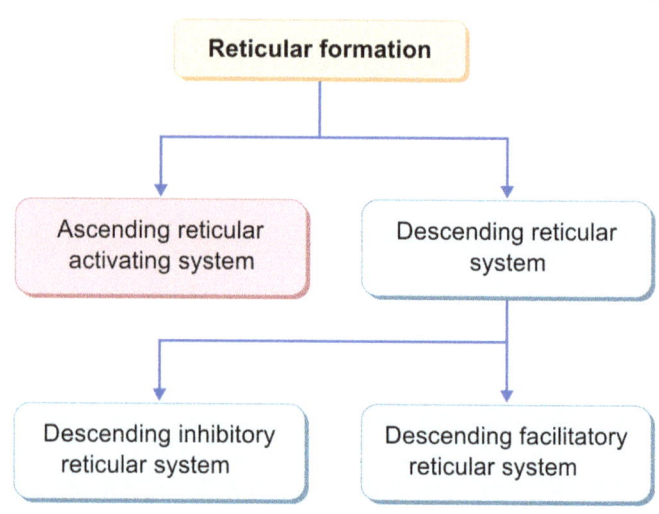

FIGURE 102.2: Functional divisions of reticular formation.

It modifies the activities of spinal motor neurons. Functionally, descending reticular system is divided into two subdivisions **(Fig. 102.2)**:

A. Descending facilitatory reticular system.
B. Descending inhibitory reticular system.

Descending Facilitatory Reticular System

Descending facilitatory reticular system is present in upper and lateral reticular formation.

Its functions are:

1. *Facilitation of somatomotor activities by:*
   i. Exciting the gamma motor neurons in spinal cord and increasing muscle tone.
   ii. Accelerating movements of the body.
   iii. Causing wakefulness and alertness.
2. *Facilitation of vegetative functions:* Descending facilitatory reticular system is the center for facilitation of the autonomic functions such as cardiac function, blood pressure, respiration, gastrointestinal function and body temperature.

Descending Inhibitory Reticular System

Descending inhibitory reticular system is located in a small area in lower and medial reticular formation.

Its functions are:

1. *Control of somatomotor activities by:*
   i. Inhibiting gamma motor neurons of spinal cord and decreasing muscle tone.
   ii. Inhibiting the α-motor neurons of spinal cord and producing smooth and accurate voluntary movements.
   iii. Controlling the reflex movements.
2. *Control of vegetative functions:* Descending inhibitory reticular system is the center for inhibition of several autonomic functions such as cardiac function, blood pressure, respiration, gastrointestinal function and body temperature.

Chapter 103: Proprioceptors, Posture and Equilibrium

CHAPTER OUTLINE

- PROPRIOCEPTORS
- MUSCLE SPINDLE
- GOLGI TENDON ORGAN
- PACINIAN CORPUSCLE
- FREE NERVE ENDING
- POSTURE
- BASIC PHENOMENA OF POSTURE
- MUSCLE TONE
- STRETCH REFLEX
- POSTURAL REFLEXES
- CLASSIFICATION OF POSTURAL REFLEXES
- STATIC REFLEXES
- STATOKINETIC REFLEXES

PROPRIOCEPTORS

Proprioceptors play a major role in the maintenance of posture and equilibrium. So, knowledge of proprioceptors is essential to understand maintenance of posture and equilibrium.

Proprioceptors are defined as the receptors, which give response to change in position of different parts of the body. These receptors are also called **kinesthetic receptors**.

Proprioceptors are situated in labyrinth, muscles, tendon of the muscles, joints, ligaments and fascia **(Table 103.1)**.

Different proprioceptors are:

1. Muscle spindle.
2. Golgi tendon organ.
3. Pacinian corpuscle.
4. Free nerve ending.
5. Proprioceptors in labyrinth.

Proprioceptors in labyrinth are described in Chapter 104.

MUSCLE SPINDLE

Muscle spindle is a spindle-shaped proprioceptor situated in the skeletal muscle. It is formed by modified skeletal muscle fibers called **intrafusal muscle fibers**.

Structure of Muscle Spindle

Muscle spindle has a central bulged portion and two tapering ends. Each muscle spindle is formed by 5 to 12 **intrafusal muscle fibers**. All these fibers are enclosed by a capsule, which is formed by connective tissue. Intrafusal fibers are attached to the capsule on either end. The capsule is attached to either side of extrafusal fibers or the tendon of the muscle. Thus, the intrafusal fibers are placed parallel to the extrafusal fibers.

Intrafusal fibers are thin and striated **(Fig. 103.1)**. Central portion of the intrafusal fibers does not contract because it has only few or no actin and myosin filaments. So, this portion acts only as a **receptor**. Only the end portion of the intrafusal fibers can contract. Discharge from the gamma motor neurons causes the contraction of intrafusal fibers.

Types of Intrafusal Fibers

Muscle spindle is formed by two types of intrafusal fibers.

1. Nuclear bag fiber

Central portion of this fiber is enlarged like a bag and contains many nuclei. Hence, it is called the nuclear bag fiber.

2. Nuclear chain fiber

In this fiber, the central portion is not bulged and the nuclei are arranged in the center in the form of a chain. Nuclear chain fiber is attached to the side of end portion of the nuclear bag fiber.

Nerve Supply to Muscle Spindle

Muscle spindle is innervated by both sensory and motor nerves. It is the **only receptor** in the body, which has both sensory and motor nerve supply.

TABLE 103.1: Proprioceptors.

Proprioceptor	Situation	Structure	Nerves	Function
Muscle spindle	Skeletal muscle	Fusiform with two tapering ends. Formed by intrafusal fibers	Sensory nerves: Aα and Aβ fibers. Motor nerves: Aγ fibers	1. Forms receptor for stretch reflex and thereby prevents muscle damage due to over stretching 2. Maintains muscle tone
Golgi tendon organ	Tendon of skeletal muscle	Formed by group of nerve endings encapsulated by collagen fibers	Sensory nerves: Iβ fibers	1. Prevents muscle damage by inhibiting forceful contraction 2. Forms the receptor for inverse stretch reflex and prevents muscle damage from overstretching 3. Forms the receptor for lengthening reaction
Pacinian corpuscle	Skin Fascia over muscles Tendons Tissues around joint Joint capsule	Concentric laminae encapsulated with connective tissue layers	Single unmyelinated C type sensory nerve fiber	Detects pressure and vibration sensations
Free nerve ending	Skin Muscle Tendon Fascia Joints	Uncapsulated ramified nerve fibers	Aδ fibers and C fibers	Detects pain, temperature and crude touch sensations
Crista ampullaris	Semicircular canals	Neuroepithelium consisting of hair cells supporting cells and epithelial cells	Fibers of vestibular division of vestibulocochlear (VIII cranial) nerve	Detects angular acceleration (rotatory movements) of the head
Macula	Otolith organ	Neuroepithelium consisting of hair cells supporting cells	Fibers of vestibular division of vestibulocochlear (VIII cranial) nerve	Detects angular acceleration (rotatory movements) of the head

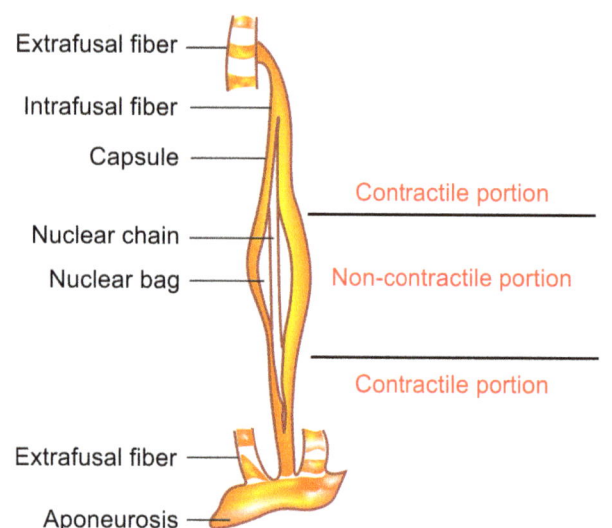

FIGURE 103.1: Muscle spindle.

Sensory nerve supply

Each muscle spindle receives two types of sensory nerve fibers:

1. *Primary sensory (afferent) nerve fiber:* It belongs to type **Iα (Aα) nerve fiber**. Each sensory (afferent) nerve fiber has two branches. One of the branches supplies the central portion of nuclear bag fiber **(Fig. 103.2)**. Another branch ends in the central portion of the nuclear chain fiber. The branches end in the form of rings around the central portion of the nuclear bag and nuclear chain fibers. Therefore, these nerve endings are called **annul spiral endings**.
2. *Secondary sensory (afferent) nerve fiber:* It is a type **IIβ (Aβ)** nerve fiber. It innervates only the nuclear chain fiber and ends near the end portion of nuclear chain fiber like the petals of the flower. So, the nerve ending is called the **flower spray ending**.

Motor nerve supply

Motor nerve fiber supplying the muscle spindle belongs to gamma motor neuron **(Aγ) type**.

1. *Motor (efferent) nerve supply to nuclear bag fiber:* Gamma motor nerve fiber supplying nuclear bag fiber ends as motor **end plate**. This nerve ending is called **plate ending**. Functionally, it is known as **dynamic gamma motor (efferent)** nerve fiber.
2. *Motor (efferent) nerve supply to nuclear chain fiber:* Gamma motor nerve fiber supplying the nuclear chain fiber divides into many branches, which form a network called **trail ending**. Functionally, it is known as **static gamma motor (efferent)** nerve fiber. Sometimes, it gives a branch to nuclear bag fiber also.

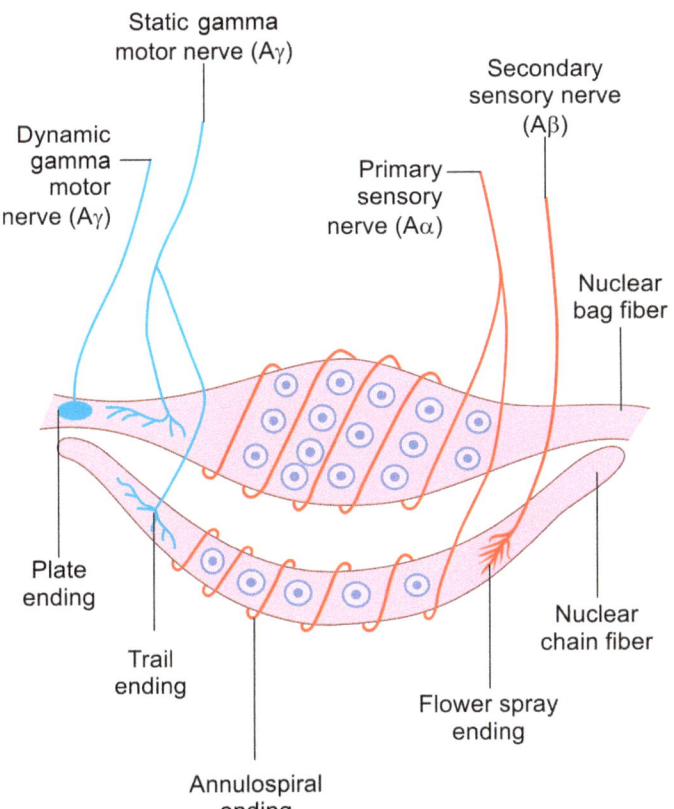

FIGURE 103.2: Nerve supply to muscle spindle. Red = Sensory nerve fibers. Blue = Motor nerve fibers. Letters in parenthesis = Type of nerve fibers.

Functions of Muscle Spindle

Muscle spindle gives response to change in the **length of the muscle**. It detects how much the muscle is being stretched and then sends the information to central nervous system via sensory nerve fibers. This information is processed in central nervous system to determine the position of different parts of the body.

By detecting the change in length of the muscle, the spindle plays an important role in **stretch reflex** and maintenance of **muscle tone** (see below).

■ GOLGI TENDON ORGAN

Golgi tendon organ is situated in the tendon of skeletal muscle near the attachment of extrafusal fibers. It is placed in series between the muscle fibers and the tendon. Golgi tendon organ is formed by a group of nerve endings covered by a connective tissue capsule (**Fig. 103.3**).

Nerve Supply to Golgi Tendon Organ

Sensory nerve fiber supplying Golgi tendon organ belongs to **Ib type**.

Functions of Golgi Tendon Organ

Golgi tendon organ gives response to the change in the **force** or **tension** developed in the skeletal muscle during contraction. Refer **Table 103.1** for other functions of Golgi tendon organ.

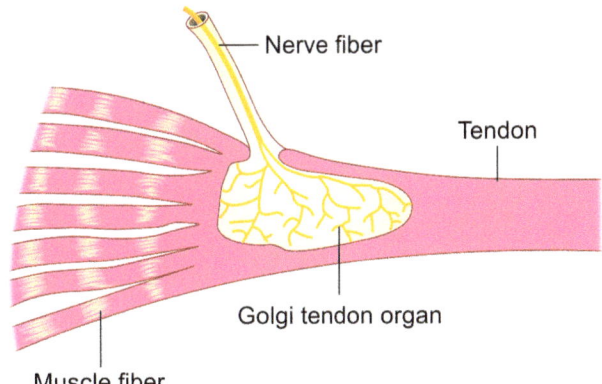

FIGURE 103.3: Golgi tendon apparatus.

■ PACINIAN CORPUSCLE

Pacinian corpuscle is a **mechanoreceptor** that senses pressure and vibration. It is situated in the deeper layers of skin. It is also situated in the tissues surrounding the joints such as fascia over the muscle, tendons and joint capsule. Pacinian corpuscles situated in these tissues send information about **joint position** to central nervous system.

■ FREE NERVE ENDING

Free nerve ending is the receptor for pain sensation situated in skin, muscles, tendon, fascia and joints. It is stimulated during some specific joint positions. In turn, it sends information about **joint position** to central nervous system.

■ POSTURE

Posture is defined as the position or attitude of the body while standing or sitting.

Maintenance of posture is carried out by subconscious **adjustment of tone** in different muscles in relation to every movement of the body. Significance of maintenance of posture is to make the movement smooth and accurate and to keep the body in equilibrium with line of gravity.

Postural movements are not active movements but **passive movements** associated with **redistribution of tone** in different groups of related muscles.

■ BASIC PHENOMENA OF POSTURE

Basic phenomena for maintenance of posture are the muscle tone and stretch reflex.

■ MUSCLE TONE

Definition

Muscle tone is defined as the state of continuous and passive partial contraction of the muscle with certain vigor and tension. It is also called **tonus**. It is also defined as resistance offered by the muscle to stretch.

Significance of Muscle Tone

Muscle tone plays an important role in maintenance of posture. Change in muscle tone enables movement of

530 Section 10: Nervous System

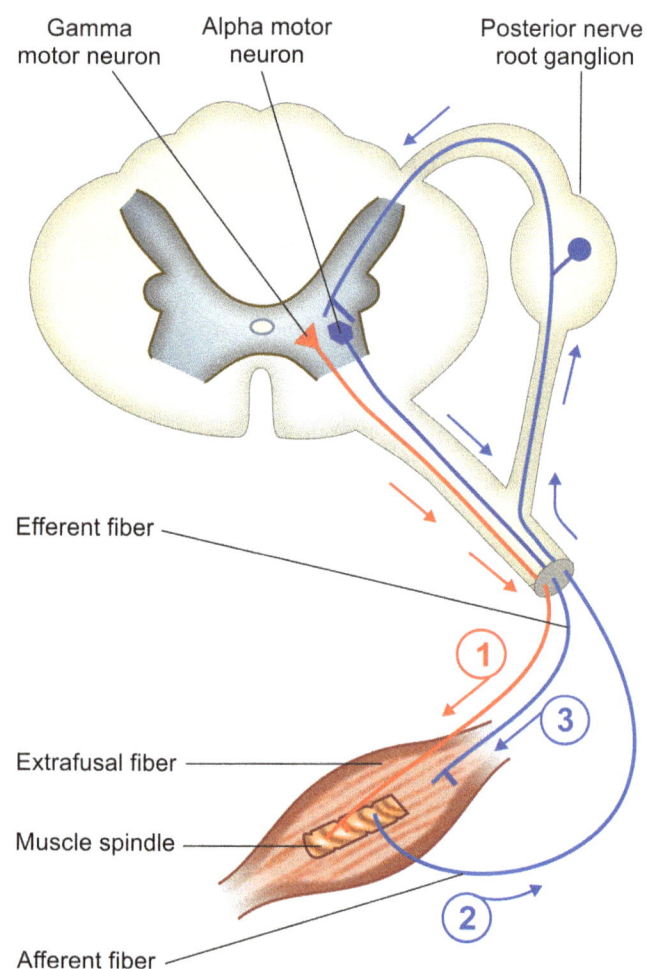

FIGURE 103.4: Development of muscle tone. 1. Impulses from γ-motor neuron stimulate muscle spindle. 2. Sensory (afferent) impulses from muscle spindle to α-motor neuron. 3. Motor (efferent) impulses from α-motor neuron produce partial contraction of extrafusal fibers and develop muscle tone.

different parts of the body. Muscle tone is present in all the skeletal muscles. However, it is more in the antigravity muscles such as extensors of lower limb, trunk muscles and neck muscles.

Development of Muscle Tone

Gamma motor neurons and muscle spindle are responsible for the development and maintenance of muscle tone **(Figs. 103.4 and 103.5)**.

Muscle tone is purely a reflex process. This reflex is a **spinal segmental reflex**. It is developed by continual synchronous discharge of motor impulses from the **gamma motor neurons** present in the anterior gray horn of the spinal cord.

Sequence of events

1. Impulses from the **gamma motor neurons** cause contraction of end portions of intrafusal fibers (stimulus). This stretches and activates the central portion of the intrafusal fibers.
2. Impulses from the central portion of intrafusal fibers pass through primary sensory nerve fibers (afferent fibers) and reach the anterior gray horn of spinal cord. These impulses stimulate the **alpha motor neurons** in anterior gray horn (center).
3. Alpha motor neurons in turn, send impulses to extrafusal fibers of the muscle through spinal nerve fibers (efferent fibers). These impulses produce **partial contraction** of the muscle fibers resulting in development of muscle tone (response).

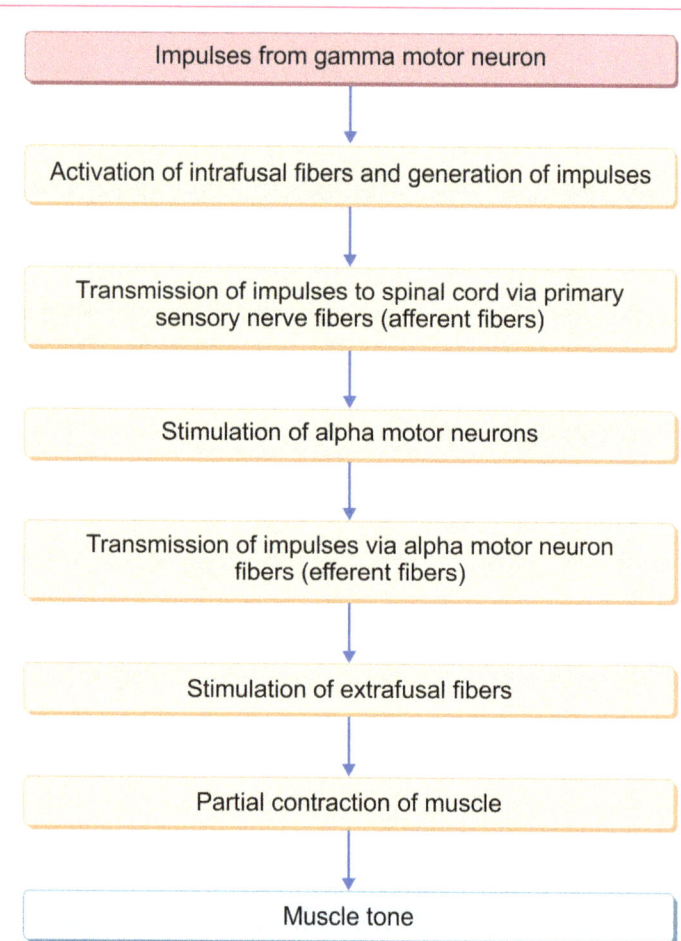

FIGURE 103.5: Schematic diagram showing development of muscle tone.

Regulation of Muscle Tone

Though muscle tone is developed by discharges from gamma motor neurons, it is maintained continuously and regulated by some **supraspinal centers** situated in different parts of brain. Some of these centers increase the muscle tone by sending facilitatory impulses while other centers decrease the muscle tone by inhibitory impulses.

■ STRETCH REFLEX

Stretch reflex is the reflex contraction of muscle when it is stretched. It is also called **myotatic reflex**. It is a **monosynaptic reflex** and the **quickest reflex**. Extensor muscles, particularly the antigravity muscles exhibit a severe and prolonged contraction during stretch reflex.

Stimulation of muscle spindle elicits the stretch reflex. Intrafusal muscle fibers are situated parallel to the extrafusal muscle fibers and are attached to the tendon

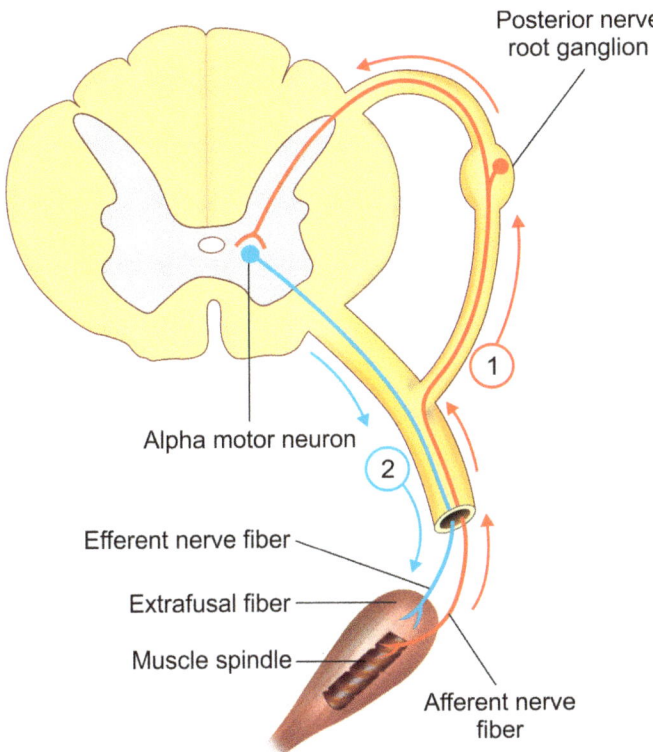

FIGURE 103.6: Stretch reflex. 1. Sensory (afferent) impulses from muscle spindle of stretched muscle. 2. Motor (efferent) impulses from α-motor neurons causing contraction of muscle.

of the muscle by means of capsule. So, stretching of the muscle causes stretching of the muscle spindle also. This stimulates the muscle spindle and it discharges the sensory impulses. These impulses are transmitted via the primary and secondary sensory (afferent) nerve fibers to the alpha motor neurons in spinal cord. Alpha motor neurons in turn send motor impulse to muscles through their fibers and cause contraction of extrafusal fibers **(Fig. 103.6)**.

Stretch reflex is the basic reflex involved in maintenance of posture. It is particularly responsible to maintain the body in an upright position.

■ POSTURAL REFLEXES

Postural reflexes are the reflexes which are responsible for the maintenance of posture. Sensory impulses for the maintenance of posture arise from proprioceptors, vestibular apparatus and retina of the eye and reach the centers in central nervous system.

Centers, which maintain the posture, are located at different levels of central nervous system particularly cerebral cortex, cerebellum, brainstem and spinal cord. These centers send motor impulses to the different groups of skeletal muscles so that appropriate movements occur to maintain the posture.

■ CLASSIFICATION OF POSTURAL REFLEXES

Postural reflexes are generally classified into two groups:

A. Static reflexes.
B. Statokinetic reflexes.

■ STATIC REFLEXES

Static reflexes are the postural reflexes that maintain posture at rest.

Static reflexes are of four types:

    I. General static reflexes or righting reflexes.
   II. Local static reflexes or supporting reflexes.
  III. Segmental static reflexes.
  IV. Statotonic or attitudinal reflexes.

I. *General Static Reflexes or Righting Reflexes*

General static or righting reflexes help to maintain an **upright position of the body** hence the name righting reflexes. Righting reflexes help to govern the orientation of the head in space, position of the head in relation to the body and appropriate adjustment of the limbs and eyes in relation to the position of the head, so that upright position of the body is maintained. Hence the name righting reflexes.

When a cat, held with its back downwards, is allowed to fall through the air, it lands upon its paws, with the head and body assuming the normal attitude in a flash. A fish resists any attempt to turn it from its normal position and if it is placed in water upon its back, it flips almost instantly into the normal swimming position. All these actions occur because of the righting reflexes.

Righting reflexes consist of a chain of reactions which occur one after another in an orderly sequence. Each reflex causes the development of the succeeding one.

Righting reflexes are divided into five types:

1. Labyrinthine righting reflexes acting upon the neck muscles.
2. Neck righting reflexes acting upon the body.
3. Body righting reflexes acting upon the head.
4. Body righting reflexes acting upon the body.
5. Optical righting reflexes.

First four reflexes are easily demonstrated on a **thalamic animal** or a **normal blindfolded animal**.

Sequential events of righting reflexes

1. When the animal is placed upon its back, the labyrinthine reflexes act on neck muscles and turn the head into its normal position in space, in relation to the body.
2. Proprioceptive reflexes from neck muscles then bring the body into its normal position in relation to position of head.
3. When resting upon a rigid support, these reflexes are reinforced by the body righting reflexes on head as well as on the body.
4. If the animal happens to be a labyrinthectomized one, then it makes an attempt to recover its upright position as a result of operation of the optical righting reaction. If the optical righting reflexes are abolished by covering the eyes, the righting ability is lost.
5. Optical righting reflexes are also demonstrated in 3 to 4 weeks old baby. When laid down on belly, i.e. prone position, the baby tries to raise the head to a vertical position.

TABLE 103.2: Static postural reflexes.

Types	Reflex	Center	Animal preparation to demonstrate
General static reflexes (righting reflexes)	1. Labyrinthine righting reflexes acting on the neck muscles 2. Neck righting reflexes acting on the body 3. Body righting reflexes acting on the head 4. Body righting reflexes acting on the body	Red nucleus situated in midbrain	Thalamic or normal blindfolded animal
	5. Optical righting reflexes	Occipital lobe	Labyrinthectomized animal
Local static reflexes	1. Positive supporting reflexes 2. Negative supporting reflexes	Spinal cord	Decorticate animal
Segmental static reflexes	1. Crossed extensor reflex	Spinal cord	Spinal animals
Statotonic or attitudinal reflexes	1. Tonic labyrinthine and neck reflexes acting on the limbs 2. Labyrinthine and neck reflexes acting on the eyes	Medulla oblongata	Decerebrate animal

Centers for righting reflexes

Centers for the first four righting reflexes are in the **red nucleus** situated in midbrain. The center for the optical righting reflexes is in the occipital lobe of **cerebral cortex** (Table 103.2).

II. Local Static Reflexes or Supporting Reflexes

Local static reflexes or supporting reflexes support the body in different positions against gravity and also protect the limbs against hyperextension or hyperflexion.

Supporting reflexes are classified into two types:

1. Positive supporting reflexes.
2. Negative supporting reflexes.

1. Positive supporting reflexes

Positive supporting reflexes are the reactions, which help to **fix the joints** and make the limbs **rigid like pillars**, so that limbs can support weight of the body **against gravity**.

Positive supporting reflexes are developed **while standing**. Body is supported against gravity while standing by the simultaneous reflex contractions of both extensor and flexor muscles and other opposing muscles. Impulses for these reflexes arise from proprioceptors present in the muscles, joints and tendons and the exteroceptors, particularly pressure receptors present in deeper layers of the skin of sole.

2. Negative supporting reflexes

Relaxation of the muscles and **unfixing of joints** enable the limbs to flex and move to a new position. It is called negative supporting reaction. It is brought about by raising the leg off the ground and plantar flexion of toes and ankle. When the leg is lifted off the ground, the exteroceptive impulses are stopped. When the toes and ankle joints are plantar flexed, the stretch stimulus for the plantar muscles is stopped. It causes **unlocking of the limbs** and facilitates new movement.

Centers for the supporting reflexes are located in the **spinal cord**.

III. Segmental Static Reflexes

Segmental static reflexes are essential for walking. During walking, in one leg, the flexors are active and the extensors are inhibited. On the opposite leg, the flexors are inhibited and extensors are active. Thus, the flexors and extensors of the same limb are not active simultaneously. It is known as **crossed extensor reflex**. It is due to the **reciprocal inhibition** and the neural mechanism responsible for this reflex is called **reciprocal innervation**.

Centers for these reflexes are situated in the **spinal cord**.

IV. Statotonic or Attitudinal Reflexes

Statotonic or attitudinal reflexes are developed according to the attitude of the body and are of two types:

1. Tonic labyrinthine and neck reflexes acting on limbs.
2. Labyrinthine and neck reflexes acting upon eyes.

1. Tonic labyrinthine and neck reflexes acting on limbs

These reflexes maintain the movements of limbs in accordance to position of head. These reflexes arise from labyrinth and neck muscles. When, head of an animal is dorsiflexed, all the four limbs are extended. And, when head is ventriflexed, all the four limbs are flexed.

2. Labyrinthine and neck reflexes acting upon eyes

These reflexes maintain the movements of eyes in accordance to position of head. These reflexes arise from labyrinth and neck muscles. Turning the head downward causes upward movement of the eyes. The eyes remain in this position as long as the position of the head is retained.

Centers for the statotonic reflexes are present in the **medulla oblongata**.

■ STATOKINETIC REFLEXES

Statokinetic reflexes are the postural reflexes that maintain posture during movement. These reflexes are concerned with both angular (rotatory), and linear (progressive) movements. **Vestibular apparatus** is responsible for these reflexes (Chapter 104).

Chapter 104: Vestibular Apparatus

CHAPTER OUTLINE

- **VESTIBULAR APPARATUS**
- **LABYRINTH**
- **FUNCTIONAL ANATOMY OF VESTIBULAR APPARATUS**
  - **SEMICIRCULAR CANALS**
  - **OTOLITH ORGAN OR VESTIBULE**
- **RECEPTOR ORGAN IN VESTIBULAR APPARATUS**
  - **CRISTA AMPULLARIS**
  - **MACULA**
- **NERVE SUPPLY TO VESTIBULAR APPARATUS**
- **FUNCTIONS OF VESTIBULAR APPARATUS**
  - **FUNCTIONS OF SEMICIRCULAR CANALS**
  - **FUNCTIONS OF OTOLITH ORGAN**
- **APPLIED PHYSIOLOGY**
  - **LABYRINTHECTOMY**
  - **MOTION SICKNESS**

■ VESTIBULAR APPARATUS

Vestibular apparatus is the part of **labyrinth** or **inner ear**. It plays an important role in maintaining posture and equilibrium through **statokinetic reflexes**. Other part of labyrinth is the cochlea, which is concerned with sensation of hearing.

■ LABYRINTH

Labyrinth (inner ear) consists of two structures, bony labyrinth and membranous labyrinth.

Bony labyrinth is a series of cavities or channels present in the petrous part of temporal bone. **Membranous labyrinth** is situated inside bony labyrinth (**Fig. 104.1**). The space between bony labyrinth and membranous labyrinth is filled with a fluid called **perilymph** which is similar to ECF in composition. Membranous labyrinth is filled with a fluid called **endolymph** which is similar to ICF in composition.

Membranous labyrinth consists of two portions:

1. **Cochlea** which is concerned with sensation of hearing (Chapter 116).
2. **Vestibular apparatus** which is concerned with posture and equilibrium.

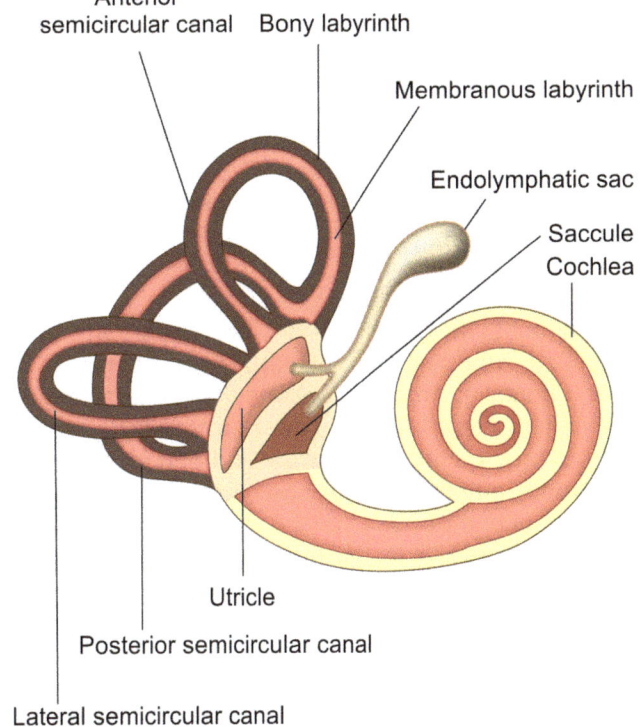

FIGURE 104.1: Labyrinth.

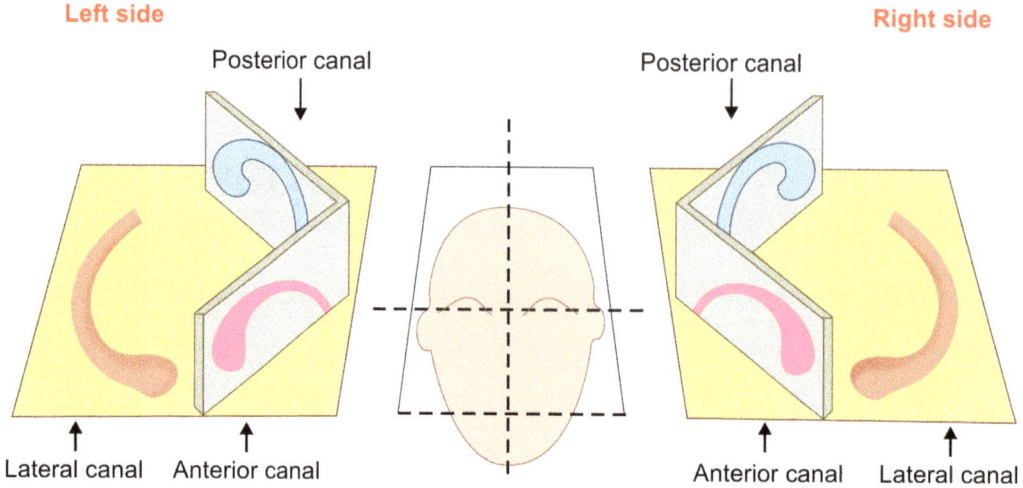

FIGURE 104.2: Position of semicircular canals.

FUNCTIONAL ANATOMY OF VESTIBULAR APPARATUS

Vestibular apparatus is formed by three semicircular canals and otolith organ or vestibule.

SEMICIRCULAR CANALS

Semicircular canals are:

1. Anterior or superior canal.
2. Posterior canal.
3. Lateral or horizontal or external canal.

Anterior and posterior canals are situated in **vertical plane** and the lateral canal is situated in **horizontal plane (Fig. 104.2)**.

When the head is tilted forward at an angle of 30°, lateral canals of both the sides are at horizontal plane parallel to earth with the convexities directed outward and a little backward. Anterior canals are at vertical plane and directed forward and outward at 45°. Posterior canals are also at vertical plane, but directed backward and outward at 45°.

Ampulla

Each semicircular canal has got two ends. One end is narrow and the other end is enlarged. The enlarged end is called ampulla. Ampulla contains the receptor organ of semicircular canals known as **crista ampullaris**. Ampulla of all the three canals and narrow end of horizontal canal open directly into the **utricle**. The narrow ends of anterior and posterior canals open into the utricle jointly, by forming the **common crus**. Thus, all the three semicircular canals open into the utricle by means of five openings. Utricle opens into **saccule**.

OTOLITH ORGAN OR VESTIBULE

Otolith organ or vestibule is formed by **utricle** and **saccule**. Often utricle and saccule are together called **otoliths**. Utricle communicates with saccule through **utriculosaccular duct**. Saccule communicates with cochlear duct through **ductus reuniens**. Another duct called **endolymphatic duct** arises from utriculosaccular duct. It ends in a bag-like structure called **endolymphatic sac**, which lies on the cranial surface of petrous bone.

RECEPTOR ORGAN IN VESTIBULAR APPARATUS

Receptor organ in semicircular canal is called **crista ampullaris** and that in otolith organ is called **macula**. These receptor organs contain the **proprioceptors**.

RECEPTOR ORGAN IN SEMICIRCULAR CANAL: CRISTA AMPULLARIS

Crista ampullaris is situated inside the ampulla of semicircular canals. It is formed by **receptor epithelium (neuroepithelium)** which consists of hair cells, supporting cells and secreting epithelial cells **(Fig. 104.3)**. The secreting epithelial cells secrete ground substance, **proteoglycan**. These cells are arranged in **planum semilunatum** (group of epithelial cells) around hair cells.

Hair Cells

Hair cells are the **receptor cells** of crista ampullaris. There are two types of hair cells, type I and type II hair

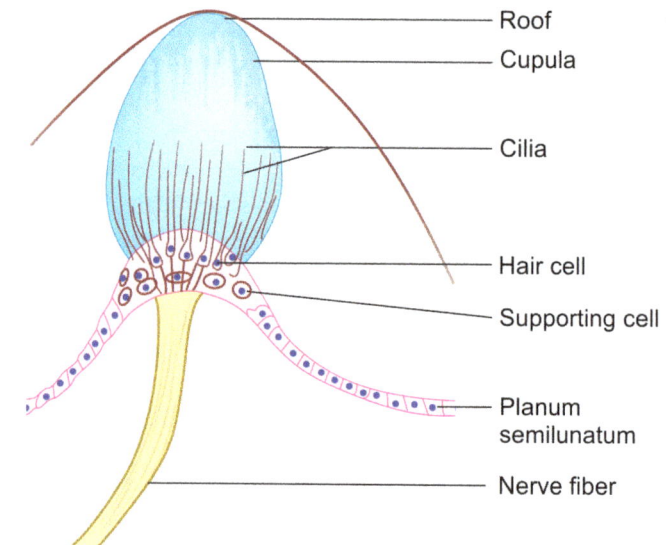

FIGURE 104.3: Crista ampullaris.

cells. Hair cells receive both afferent and efferent nerve terminals.

Type I hair cells

Type I hair cells are flask shaped. Afferent nerve terminates in the form of a **calyx** that surrounds the cell body. Efferent nerve terminal ends on the surface of the calyx.

Type II hair cells

These cells have a cylindrical or test tube shape. Both afferent and efferent nerve fibers terminate on the surface cell body without forming calyx.

Cilia of hair cells

Apex of each hair cell has a **cuticular plate**. From this plate, about 40 to 60 **cilia** arise which are called **stereocilia**. Each stereocilium is attached at its tip to the neighboring taller one by means of a fine process called tip link. Because of the tip links, all the stereocilia are held together. One of the cilia is very tall which is named as **kinocilium (Fig. 104.4)**.

Cupula

From crista ampullaris, a dome-shaped gelatinous structure extends up to the roof of the ampulla. It is known as cupula. The cupula encloses the cilia of hair cells. The cilia of hair cells are projected in the cupula.

■ RECEPTOR ORGAN IN OTOLITH ORGAN: MACULA

Receptor organ in otolith organ is called macula. Like crista ampullaris, the macula is also formed by **neuroepithelium** and supporting cells. Neuroepithelium of macula also has two types of hair cells, the type I and type II hair cells **(Fig. 104.5)**.

Otolith Membrane

Like crista ampullaris, macula is also covered by a gelatinous membrane called **otolith membrane**. It is a flat structure and not dome shaped like cupula. **Stereocilia and kinocilium** of each hair cell are embedded in otolith membrane. Otolith membrane contains some crystals, which are called ear dust, **otoconia** or **statoconia**. The otoconia are mainly constituted by calcium carbonate.

Situation of Macula

In utricle

In utricle the macula is situated in horizontal plane, so that the cilia from hair cells are in vertical direction.

In saccule

In saccule the macula is in vertical plane and the cilia are in horizontal direction.

■ NERVE SUPPLY TO VESTIBULAR APPARATUS

Impulses from the hair cells of crista ampullaris and maculae are transmitted to medulla oblongata and other parts of central nervous system through the fibers of **vestibular division** of **vestibulocochlear nerve** (VIII cranial nerve).

First order neurons of the sensory pathway are **bipolar** in nature. Dendrites of the bipolar cells have close contact with the basal part of hair cells. Axons of the first order neurons (bipolar cells) form the vestibular division of vestibulocochlear nerve.

Hair cells also have efferent nerve fiber which controls the hair cells.

■ FUNCTIONS OF VESTIBULAR APPARATUS

Receptors of semicircular canals give response to **rotatory movements** or **angular acceleration** of the head. And, the receptors of utricle and saccule give response to **linear acceleration** of head.

Thus, the vestibular apparatus is responsible for detecting the position of head during different movements. It also causes the reflex adjustments in the position of eyeball, head and body during postural changes.

■ FUNCTIONS OF SEMICIRCULAR CANALS

Semicircular canals are concerned with **angular (rotatory) acceleration**. Semicircular canals sense the **rotational movement**. Each semicircular canal is sensitive to rotation in a particular plane.

Superior Semicircular Canal

Superior semicircular canal gives response to rotation in **anteroposterior plane** (transverse axis), i.e. front to back movements like nodding the head while saying '**yes – yes**'.

Horizontal Semicircular Canal

This semicircular canal gives response to rotation in **horizontal plane** (vertical axis), i.e. side-to-side movements (left to right or right to left) like shaking the head while saying '**no – no**'.

Posterior Semicircular Canal

This semicircular canal gives response to rotation in the **vertical plane** (anteroposterior axis) by which head is rotated from **shoulder to shoulder**.

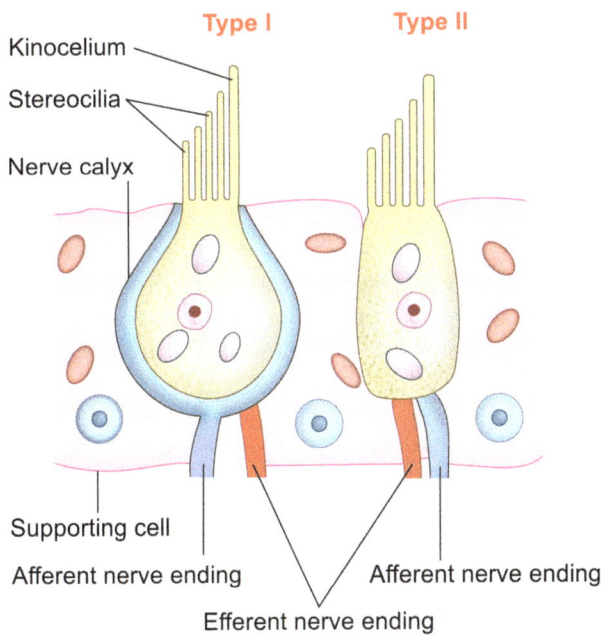

FIGURE 104.4: Hair cells of vestibular apparatus.

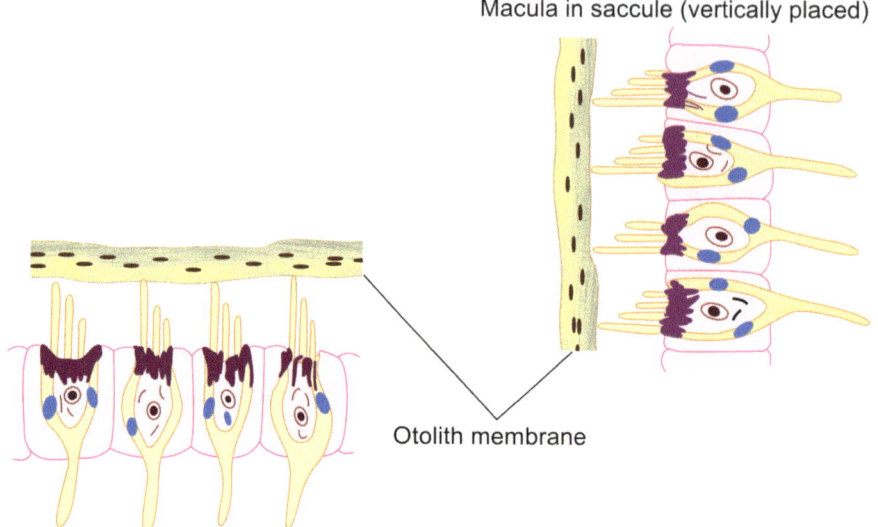

FIGURE 104.5: Macula in otolith organ.

Mechanism of Stimulation of Receptor Cells in Semicircular Canal

At the beginning of rotation, the receptor cells are stimulated by the movement of **endolymph** inside the semicircular canals. However, the receptors are stimulated only at the beginning and at the stoppage of rotatory movements. And during rotation at a constant speed, these receptors are not stimulated.

During rotation in clockwise direction

When a person rotates in **clockwise direction** in horizontal plane (vertical axis), **horizontal canal** moves in clockwise direction. But there is no corresponding movement of endolymph inside the canal at the beginning of rotation. Because of the inertia, endolymph remains static. This phenomenon causes relative displacement of endolymph in the direction opposite to that of the rotation of head. That is, the **fluid** is pushed in **anticlockwise direction**.

Thus, in the right horizontal semicircular canal, the **endolymph** flows towards the ampulla and, in the left canal, the fluid moves away from the ampulla (**Fig. 104.6**). The movement of endolymph in semicircular canal, in turn causes corresponding movement of gelatinous **cupula**. Thus, in the right horizontal canal, the cupula moves towards the ampulla. Whereas in the left canal the cupula moves away from ampulla. In any semicircular canal, when cupula moves towards the ampulla, the **stereocilia** of hair cells are pushed towards kinocilium leading to stimulation of **hair cells**. When the cupula moves away from ampulla, the stereocilia are pushed away from kinocilium and hair cells are not stimulated.

During rotation in anticlockwise direction

On the other hand, rotation in anticlockwise direction causes stimulation of hair cells in ampulla of horizontal canal in left ear only. Hair cells of horizontal canal in right ear are not stimulated. Stimulation of hair cells in left ear is followed by the process as in the case of clockwise rotation.

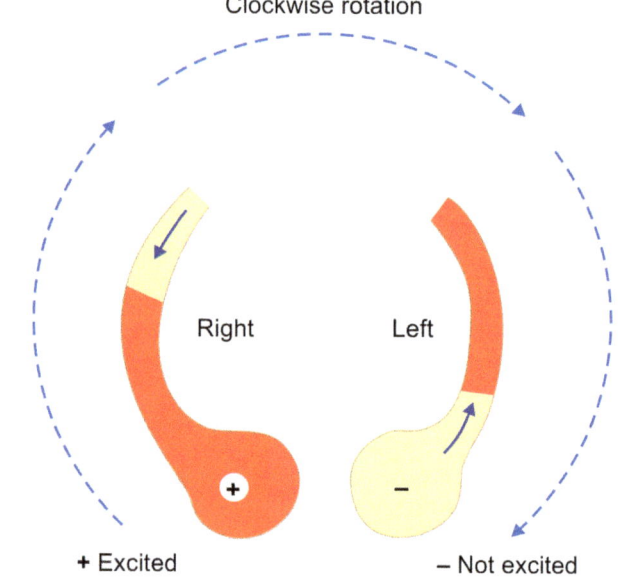

FIGURE 104.6: Movement of fluid and excitation of crista ampullaris in right horizontal semicircular canal during clockwise rotation.

Electrical Potential in Hair Cells: Mechanotransduction

Mechanotransduction is a type of sensory transduction (Chapter 91) in the receptor cells of vestibular apparatus by which the **mechanical energy** is converted into electrical energy (action potentials) in the vestibular nerve fiber.

Resting membrane potential in hair cells is about – 60 mV. Movement of stereocilia of hair cells towards kinocilium causes development of **mild depolarization** in hair cells up to – 50 mV which is called **receptor potential**.

Receptor potential in hair cells causes generation of action potential in nerve fibers distributed to hair cells.

Movement of stereocilia in the opposite direction (away from kinocilium) causes **hyperpolarization** of hair cells

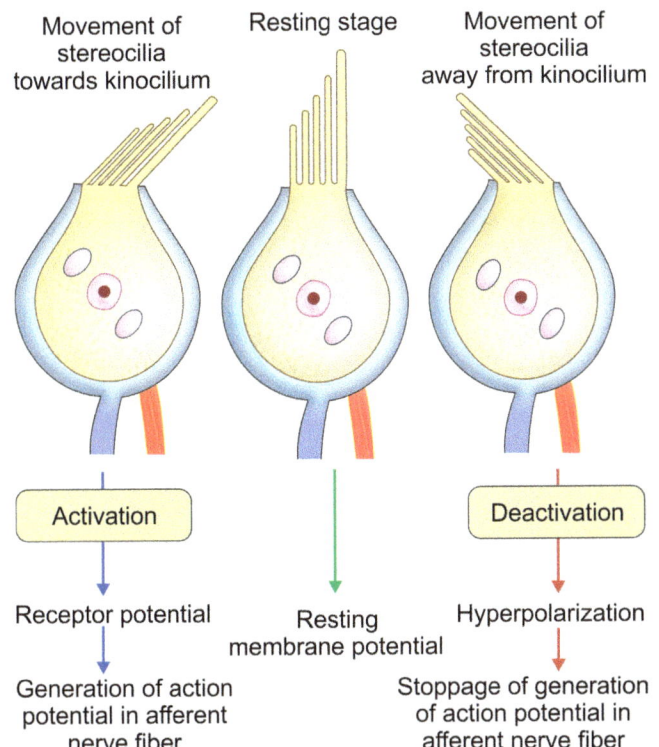

FIGURE 104.7: Mechanotransduction in hair cell of vestibular apparatus. During activation, receptor potential develops in hair cell. It causes development of action potential in afferent nerve fiber.

which stops generation of action potential in the nerve fibers **(Fig. 104.7)**.

Nystagmus

Nystagmus is the rapid involuntary **movements** of **eyeball**. It is common during rotation. It is due to the natural stimulatory effect of vestibular apparatus during rotational acceleration.

Movement of eyeball during nystagmus

Nystagmus has two components of movement, which occur alternately:

1. Slow component.
2. Quick component.

1. Slow component

At the beginning of rotation, since eyes are fixed at a particular object (point), eyeballs rotate slowly in the direction opposite to that of rotation of the head. It is called slow component of nystagmus. It is due to vestibulo-ocular reflex.

2. Quick component

When the slow movement of eyeballs is limited, the eyeballs move to a new fixation point in the direction of rotation of head. This movement to a new fixation point occurs with a jerk. So, it is called the quick component. Quick component of nystagmus is due to the activation of some centers in brainstem.

Vestibulo-ocular reflex and nystagmus

Nystagmus is a reflex phenomenon that occurs in order to maintain the visual fixation. Since the movements of eyeballs occur in response to the stimulation of vestibular apparatus this reflex is called the vestibulo-ocular reflex.

■ FUNCTIONS OF OTOLITH ORGAN

Otolith organ is concerned with linear acceleration and detects acceleration in both horizontal and vertical planes. Utricle responds during **horizontal acceleration** and saccule responds during **vertical acceleration**.

Function of Utricle

Position of hair cells of macula helps utricle to respond to horizontal acceleration. In the utricle, the macula is situated in horizontal plane with the cilia of hair cells in vertical plane **(Fig. 104.5)**. While moving horizontally, because of inertia the otoconia move in opposite direction and pull the cilia of hair cells resulting in stimulation of hair cells.

For example, when the body moves forward, the otoconia fall back in otolith membrane and pull the cilia of hair cells backward. Pulling of cilia causes stimulation of hair cells. Hair cells send information (impulses) to vestibular, cerebellar and reticular centers. These centers in turn send instructions to various muscles to maintain equilibrium of the body during the forward movement.

Function of Saccule

Macula of saccule is situated in vertical plane with the cilia of hair cells in horizontal plane. While moving vertically, as in the case of utricle, the otoconia of saccule move in opposite direction and pull the cilia resulting in stimulation of hair cells.

For example, while climbing up, the otoconia move down by pulling the cilia downwards. It stimulates the hair cells which in turn send information to the brain centers. And the action follows as in the case of movement in horizontal plane.

■ APPLIED PHYSIOLOGY

■ LABYRINTHECTOMY

Removal of labyrinthine apparatus on both sides leads to complete loss of equilibrium. The equilibrium could be maintained only by visual sensation. Postural reflexes are severely affected. There is loss of hearing sensation too.

Removal of labyrinthine apparatus on one side causes less effect on postural reflexes. However, severe autonomic symptoms such as nausea, vomiting and diarrhea occur.

■ MOTION SICKNESS

Motion sickness is defined as the syndrome of physiological response during movement (travel) to which the person is not adapted. It is characterized by nausea, vomiting, dizziness and other symptoms.

It can occur while traveling in any form of vehicle like automobile, ship, aircraft or spaceship. Motion sickness that occurs while traveling in a watercraft is called **seasickness**.

Cause

Motion sickness is due to excessive and repeated stimulation of vestibular apparatus.

Symptoms

1. Nausea and vomiting.
2. Sweating.
3. Diarrhea.
4. Excess salivation.
5. Discomfort.
6. Headache.
7. Disorientation.

Responses of motion sickness can be prevented by avoiding greasy and bulky food before travel and by taking **antiemetic drugs** (drugs preventing nausea and vomiting).

Chapter 105: Electroencephalogram (EEG) and Epilepsy

CHAPTER OUTLINE

- ELECTROENCEPHALOGRAM
  - DEFINITIONS
  - SIGNIFICANCE OF EEG
  - METHOD OF RECORDING EEG
  - WAVES OF EEG
- EEG DURING SLEEP
- EPILEPSY
  - DEFINITIONS
  - TYPES OF EPILEPSY

ELECTROENCEPHALOGRAM

DEFINITIONS

Electroencephalography is the study of electrical activities of brain. **Electroencephalogram (EEG)** is the graphical recording of electrical activities of brain. German psy-chiatrist **Hans Berger** was the first one to analyze the EEG waves, hence the EEG waves are called as **Berger waves**.

Electroencephalograph is the instrument used to record EEG.

SIGNIFICANCE OF EEG

Electroencephalogram is useful in the diagnosis of neurological and sleep disorders.

EEG pattern is altered in the following neurological disorders:

1. **Epilepsy**, which occurs due to excess discharge of impulses from cerebral cortex.
2. **Disorders of midbrain** which affect ascending reticular activating system.
3. **Subdural hematoma** during which there is collection of blood in subdural space over the cerebral cortex.

METHOD OF RECORDING EEG

For recording EEG the **scalp electrodes** from the instrument are placed over unopened skull or over the brain after opening the skull, or by piercing into the brain.

WAVES OF EEG

Electrical activity recorded by EEG may have synchronized or desynchronized waves. **Synchronized waves** are the regular and invariant waves, whereas **desynchronized waves** are irregular and variant.

Normally EEG has three frequency bands:

1. Alpha rhythm.
2. Beta rhythm.
3. Delta rhythm.

In children, in addition to these waves, theta rhythm appears.

1. Alpha Rhythm

Alpha waves are rhythmical waves, which appear at a frequency of 8 to 13 waves/second and with the amplitude of 50 μV. Alpha waves are **synchronized waves (Fig. 105.1)**.

Alpha waves are obtained in **inattentive brain** or **mind** as in drowsiness, light sleep or narcosis with closed eyes. These waves are abolished by any type of stimuli or mental effort and diminished when eyes are opened.

Alpha waves are most marked in parieto-occipital area.

Alpha block

Alpha block is the replacement of synchronized alpha waves in EEG by desynchronized and low voltage waves when the eyes are opened. Desynchronized waves do not have specific frequency. It occurs due to any form of sensory stimulation or mental concentration, such as solving arithmetic problems.

Desynchronization is the common term used for replacement of regular waves with irregular low voltage waves.

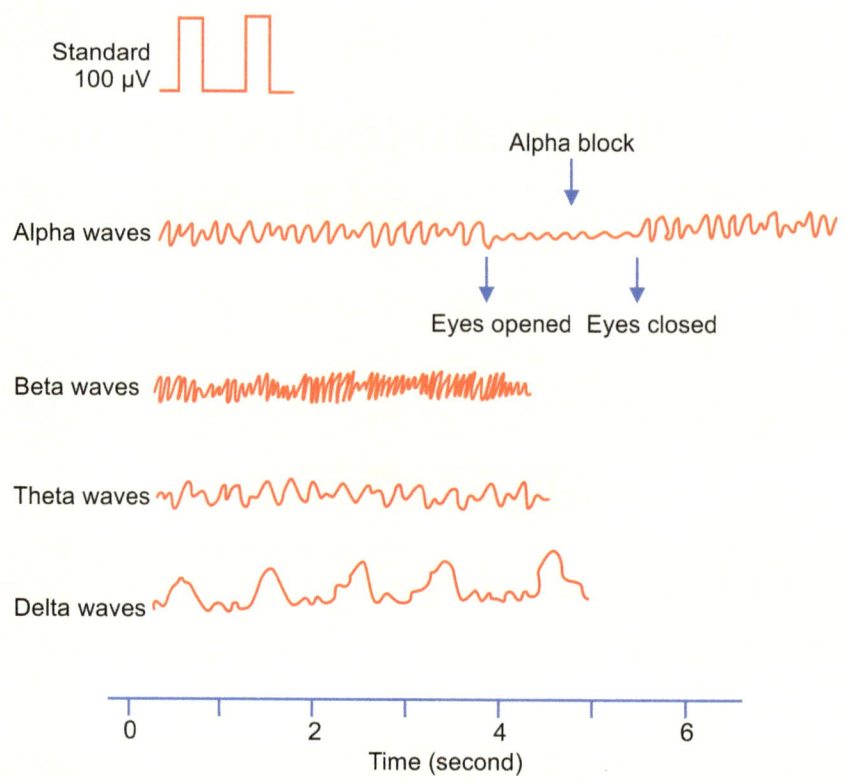

FIGURE 105.1: Waves of EEG.

TABLE 105.1: Properties of EEG waves.

Rhythm	Frequency (per second)	Amplitude (µV)
Alpha	8 to 13	50
Beta	15 to 80	5 to 10
Delta	1 to 4	20 to 200
Theta	4 to 7	10

2. Beta Rhythm

Beta waves are high frequency waves of 15 to 80 per second. But their amplitude is low, i.e. 5 to 10 µV **(Table 105.1)**. Beta waves are **desynchronized waves** and are recorded during mental activity or mental tension or arousal state. These waves are not affected by opening the eyes.

3. Delta Rhythm

Delta waves are low frequency and high amplitude waves. Frequency of these waves is 1 to 4 per second and the amplitude is 20 to 200 µV. Delta waves are common in early childhood during waking hours. In adults, these waves appear mostly during deep sleep.

Presence of delta waves in adults during conditions other than sleep indicates the pathological process in brain such as tumor, epilepsy, increased intracranial pressure and mental deficiency or depression. These waves are not affected by opening the eyes.

Theta Rhythm

Theta waves are obtained generally in children below 5 years of age. These waves are of low frequency and low voltage waves. Frequency of theta waves is 4 to 7 per second and the amplitude is about 10 µV.

EEG DURING SLEEP

Changes in the EEG pattern during sleep are described in Chapter 106.

EPILEPSY

DEFINITIONS

Epilepsy

Epilepsy is a brain disorder characterized by convulsive seizures or loss of consciousness or both.

Convulsion and Convulsive Seizure

Convulsion refers to uncontrolled involuntary muscular contractions. **Convulsive seizure** means sudden attack of uncontrolled involuntary muscular contractions. It occurs due to **paroxysmal** (sudden and usually recurring periodically) **uncontrolled discharge** of impulses from neurons of brain, particularly **cerebral cortex**.

Epileptic

Patient affected by epilepsy is called epileptic. The person with epilepsy remains normal in between seizures. Epileptic attack develops only when excitability of the neuron is increased, causing excessive neuronal discharge.

TYPES OF EPILEPSY

Epilepsy is divided into two categories:
1. Generalized epilepsy.
2. Localized epilepsy.

1. Generalized Epilepsy

Generalized epilepsy is the type of epilepsy that occurs due to excessive discharge of impulses from all parts of the brain. It is also called **general onset seizure** or **general onset epilepsy**.

Generalized epilepsy is subdivided into three types:

1. Grand mal.
2. Petit mal.
3. Psychomotor epilepsy.

Grand mal

Grand mal is characterized by sudden **loss of consciousness** followed by **convulsion**. Just before the onset of convulsions, the person feels the warning sensation in the form of some hallucination. It is called **epileptic aura**.

EEG shows fast waves with a frequency of 15 to 30 per second. Later slow and large waves appear. In between seizures, the EEG shows delta waves in all types of epileptics.

Cause for grand mal

Cause of grand mal epilepsy is the excess neural activity in all parts of the brain.

Petit mal

In this type of epilepsy, the person becomes **unconscious** suddenly without any warning. The unconsciousness lasts for a very short period of 3 to 30 seconds. Convulsions do not occur. However, the muscles of face show twitch-like contractions and there is blinking of eyes. Afterwards, the person recovers automatically and becomes normal. The frequency of attack may be once in many months or many attacks may appear in rapid series. It usually occurs in late childhood and disappears completely at the age of 30 or above.

EEG recording shows slow and large waves during the attack. Each wave is followed by a sharp spike. Delta waves appear in between the seizures.

Causes for petit mal

Causes of petit mal are head injury, stroke, brain tumor and brain infection.

Psychomotor epilepsy

It is characterized by **emotional outbursts** such as abnormal rage, sudden anxiety, fear or discomfort. There is amnesia or a confused mental state for some period. Some persons have the tendency to attack others bodily or rub their own face vigorously. In most cases, the persons are not aware of their activities.

The EEG recordings show low frequency rectangular waves, ranging between 2 and 4 per second.

Causes for psychomotor epilepsy

Causes of the psychomotor epilepsy are the abnormalities in temporal lobe and tumor in hypothalamus and other regions of limbic system such as amygdala and hippocampus.

2. Localized Epilepsy

Localized epilepsy is the epilepsy that occurs because of excess discharge of impulses from a **localized area of brain**. It is otherwise known as **local** or **focal epilepsy or local seizure** or **Jacksonian epilepsy**.

Abnormality starts from a particular area and spreads to adjacent areas, developing slow-spreading muscular contractions. Contractions usually start in the mouth region and spread down towards the legs.

Cause for localized epilepsy

Localized epilepsy is caused by brain tumor.

Chapter 106: Physiology of Sleep

CHAPTER OUTLINE

- SLEEP
- SLEEP REQUIREMENT
- PHYSIOLOGICAL CHANGES DURING SLEEP
- TYPES OF SLEEP
- STAGES OF SLEEP AND EEG PATTERN
- SLEEP CENTERS
- APPLIED PHYSIOLOGY

■ SLEEP

Sleep is the natural **state of rest** for mind and body with closed eyes characterized by partial or complete **loss of consciousness**. Loss of consciousness leads to decreased response to external stimuli and decreased body movements.

Depth of sleep is not constant throughout the sleeping period and it varies in different stages of sleep.

■ SLEEP REQUIREMENT

Sleep requirement is not constant.

Average sleep requirement per day at different age groups is:

Newborn infants	:	18 to 20 hours
Growing children	:	12 to 14 hours
Adults	:	7 to 9 hours
Old persons	:	5 to 7 hours

■ PHYSIOLOGICAL CHANGES DURING SLEEP

During sleep, most of the body functions are reduced to basal level. Important changes in the body during sleep are given below.

■ 1. PLASMA VOLUME

Plasma volume decreases by about 10% during sleep.

■ 2. CARDIOVASCULAR SYSTEM

Heart Rate

During sleep, the heart rate reduces. It varies between 45 and 60 beats per minute.

Blood Pressure

Systolic pressure falls to about 90 to 110 mm Hg. Lowest level is reached about 4th hour of sleep and remains at this level till a short time before waking up. Then, the pressure starts rising.

If sleep is disturbed by exciting dreams, the pressure is elevated above 130 mm Hg.

■ 3. RESPIRATORY SYSTEM

Rate and force of respiration are decreased. Respiration becomes irregular and **Cheyne-Stokes breathing** may develop.

■ 4. GASTROINTESTINAL TRACT

Salivary secretion decreases during sleep. Gastric secretion is not altered or may be increased slightly. Contraction of empty stomach is more vigorous.

■ 5. EXCRETORY SYSTEM

Formation of urine decreases and specific gravity of urine increases.

■ 6. SWEAT SECRETION

Sweat secretion increases during sleep.

■ 7. LACRIMAL SECRETION

Lacrimal secretion decreases during sleep.

■ 8. MUSCLE TONE

Tone in all the muscles of body except ocular muscles decreases very much during sleep. It is called **sleep paralysis**.

■ 9. REFLEXES

Certain reflexes particularly knee jerk, are abolished. **Babinski sign** becomes positive during deep sleep. Threshold for most of the reflexes increases. Pupils are constricted. Light reflex is retained. Eyeballs move up and down.

10. BRAIN

Brain is not inactive during sleep. There is a characteristic cycle of brain wave activity during sleep with irregular intervals of dreams. Electrical activity in the brain varies with stages of sleep (see below).

TYPES OF SLEEP

Sleep is of two types:
1. Non-rapid eye movement sleep, NREM sleep or non-REM sleep.
2. Rapid eye movement sleep or REM sleep.

1. NON-RAPID EYE MOVEMENT SLEEP (NREM SLEEP)

NREM sleep is the type of sleep without the movements of eyeballs. It is also called **slow wave sleep**. Dreams do not occur in this type of sleep and it occupies about 70 to 80% of total sleeping period. NREM sleep is followed by REM sleep.

2. RAPID EYE MOVEMENT SLEEP (REM SLEEP)

REM sleep is the type of sleep associated with rapid **conjugate movements** of the eyeballs which occurs frequently. Though the eyeballs move, the sleep is deep. So, it is also called **paradoxical sleep**. It occupies about 20 to 30% of sleeping period. Functionally, REM sleep is very important because it plays an important role in consolidation of memory. Dreams occur during this period.

Differences between the two types of sleep are given in **Table 106.1**.

STAGES OF SLEEP AND EEG PATTERN

Generally, everybody passes through **five stages of sleep**, i.e. four stages of NREM sleep followed by REM sleep. All these stages occur periodically in cycles. One complete sleep cycle takes about 90 to 110 minutes. Usually, adults have 5 or 6 **sleep cycles** every night.

Pattern of electroencephalogram (EEG) alters in each stage.

TABLE 106.1: REM sleep and NREM sleep.

Characteristics	REM sleep	NREM sleep
1. Rapid eye movement	Present	Absent
2. Dreams	Present	Absent
3. Muscle twitching	Present	Absent
4. Heart rate	Fluctuating	Stable
5. Blood pressure	Fluctuating	Stable
6. Respiration	Fluctuating	Stable
7. Body temperature	Fluctuating	Stable
8. Neurotransmitter	Noradrenaline	Serotonin

NREM SLEEP

Stage 1: Stage of Drowsiness

While feeling asleep and after going to bed, the person is in the **period of wakefulness**, i.e. while lying down, the eyes are closed and mind is relaxed. Then, the person proceeds to **drowsy state**. During drowsiness, the person can be awakened easily. Muscular activity slows down. Some persons may have feeling of falling followed by sudden muscular contractions. This period lasts for about 1 to 10 minutes.

EEG pattern in stage 1

During the stage of wakefulness, i.e. while lying down with closed eyes and relaxed mind, the **alpha waves** of EEG appear. Stage 1 of sleep is characterized by diminishing alpha waves and emerging **theta wave** activity in brain **(Fig. 106.1)**.

Stage 2: Stage of Light Sleep

When the person goes to **light sleep** from drowsiness, heart rate slows down and body temperature starts decreasing. Body prepares to go to deep sleep. This period lasts up to 20 minutes.

EEG pattern in stage 2

Theta wave continues in this stage also. In addition, theta waves are intermittently superimposed by **sleep spindles or spindle bursts** at a frequency of 14 per second. Sleep spindle is produced by electrical activity in thalamus and corticothalamic fibers.

During this stage of sleep, another type of wave called **K complex** also appears. It is a slow and large wave produced by the reaction to external stimuli while sleep.

Stage 3: Initial Stage of Deep Sleep

Stage 3 is the transitional period between light sleep and deep sleep. Hence, it is considered as **initial stage of deep sleep**.

EEG pattern in stage 3

During this stage, the spindle bursts and K complex disappear. Slow **delta waves** with high amplitude appear. Frequency decreases to 1 or 2 per second and amplitude increases to about 100 µV.

Stage 4: Stage of Deep Sleep

Earlier, stages 3 and 4 were separated. But nowadays these two stages are combined together. When the person enters **deep sleep**, it is difficult to wake up. If someone wakes him or her up, there may be a feeling of disorientation for few minutes. In spite of having potential sleep disturbances such as noise, some persons may sleep without any reaction.

These stages of sleep help rejuvenation of the body. There is release of many vital hormones which induce growth and development. Immune system is boosted. Muscles and tissues are repaired. Body builds up energy for next day.

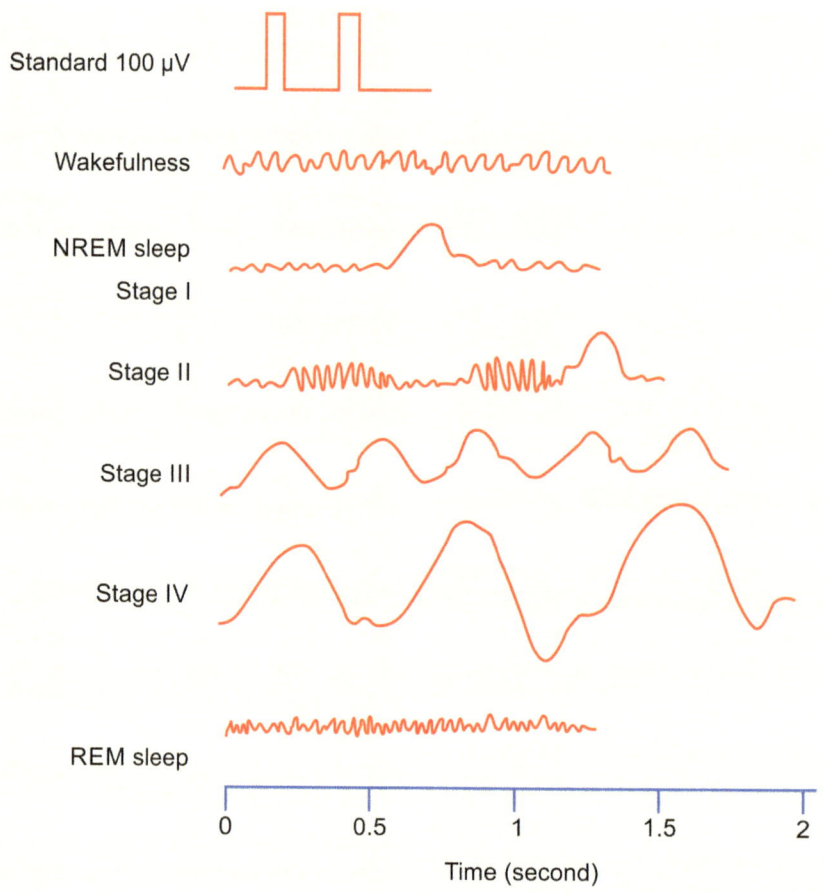

FIGURE 106.1: Electroencephalogram during wakefulness, different stages of NREM sleep and REM sleep.

During this stage, children may have bedwetting, nightmares and sleepwalking. Even some adults may experience, nightmares and sleepwalking.

In most of the people, stage 3 and stage 4 together last for about 40 to 60 minutes.

EEG pattern in stage 4

During this stage, **delta waves** become more prominent with low frequency and high amplitude.

■ REM SLEEP

Often, this is considered as **stage 5 of sleep**. During REM sleep, eyes move rapidly in all direction. Dreams occur. Muscles are relaxed or temporarily paralyzed. There is increase in heart rate and blood pressure. Respiration becomes rapid, shallow and irregular.

REM sleep during the first cycle of sleep lasts only for about 10 minutes. And the duration gradually increases in successive cycles and in final cycle it may last for about 1 hour.

EEG pattern in REM sleep

During REM sleep, electroencephalogram (EEG) shows irregular waves with high frequency and low amplitude. These waves are **desynchronized waves**.

■ SLEEP CENTERS

Sleep occurs due to the activity of some sleep inducing centers in brain. Complex pathways between the reticular formation of brainstem, diencephalon and cerebral cortex are involved in the onset and maintenance of sleep.

Brainstem has two centers which induce sleep which are:
1. Raphe nucleus.
2. Locus coeruleus

Inhibition of ascending reticular activating system also results in sleep.

Role of Raphe Nucleus

Raphe nucleus is situated in reticular formation of lower pons and medulla. Activation of this nucleus results in **NREM sleep**. It is due to release of **serotonin** by the nerve fibers arising from this nucleus. Serotonin induces NREM sleep.

Role of Locus Coeruleus

Locus coeruleus is situated in reticular formation of pons. Activation of this center produces **REM sleep**. **Noradrenaline** released by the nerve fibers arising from locus coeruleus induces REM sleep.

Inhibition of Ascending Reticular Activating System

Ascending reticular activating system (ARAS) is responsible for **wakefulness** because of its afferent and efferent connections with cerebral cortex. Inhibition of ARAS induces sleep. Lesion of ARAS leads to coma.

APPLIED PHYSIOLOGY: COMMON SLEEP DISORDERS

1. INSOMNIA

Insomnia is the **inability to sleep** or abnormal wakefulness. It occurs due to systemic illness or mental conditions such as psychiatric problems, alcoholic addiction and drug addiction.

2. HYPERSOMNIA

Hypersomnia is the **excess sleep** or excess need to sleep. It occurs because of lesion in floor of the third ventricle, brain tumors, encephalitis, chronic bronchitis and disease of muscles. Hypersomnia also occurs in endocrine disorders such as myxedema and diabetes insipidus.

3. NARCOLEPSY AND CATAPLEXY

Narcolepsy is the sudden attack of **uncontrollable sleep**. Cataplexy is sudden **outburst of emotion**. Both the diseases are due to hypothalamic disorders. Refer Chapter 98 for details.

4. SLEEP APNEA SYNDROME

Sleep apnea is the temporary stoppage of breathing repeatedly during sleep. Sleep apnea syndrome is the disorder that involves fluctuations in the rate and force of respiration during REM sleep with short apneic episode. Sleep apnea syndrome occurs in **obesity**, myxedema, enlargement of tonsil and lesion in brainstem.

Common features of this syndrome are **loud snoring**, restless movements, nocturnal insomnia, daytime sleepiness, morning headache and fatigue. In severe conditions, hypertension, right heart failure and stroke occur.

5. NIGHTMARE

Nightmare is a condition during sleep that is characterized by a sense of extreme **uneasiness** or discomfort or by frightful dreams. Discomfort is felt as of some heavy weight on the stomach or chest or as uncontrolled movement of the body. After a period of extreme anxiety, the subject wakes with a troubled state of mind.

Nightmare occurs due to improper food intake, digestive disorders or nervous disorders. It also occurs during drug withdrawal or alcohol withdrawal.

6. NIGHT TERROR

Night terror or **sleep terror** is a disorder similar to nightmare. It is common in children. The child awakes screaming in a state of fright and semiconsciousness. The child cannot recollect the attack in the morning.

7. SOMNAMBULISM

Somnambulism or **sleep walking** is getting up from bed and walking in the state of sleep. The episode lasts for few minutes to half an hour.

8. NOCTURNAL MICTURITION

Nocturnal micturition or enuresis is the involuntary voiding of urine at bed. It is also called **bedwetting**. It is common in children. Refer Chapter 46 for details.

9. MOVEMENT DISORDERS DURING SLEEP

Movement disorders occur immediately after falling asleep. **Sleep start** or **hypnic jerk** is the common movement disorder during sleep. It is characterized by **sudden jerks** of arms or legs. Sleep start is a physiological form of clonus.

Other movement disorders are teeth grinding (**bruxism**), banging the head and restless movement of arms or legs.

Chapter 107: Higher Intellectual Functions

CHAPTER OUTLINE

- **HIGHER INTELLECTUAL FUNCTIONS**
- **LEARNING**
  - DEFINITION
  - TYPES
- **MEMORY**
  - DEFINITION
  - TYPES
  - ANATOMICAL BASIS
  - PHYSIOLOGICAL BASIS
  - APPLIED PHYSIOLOGY
- **CONDITIONED REFLEXES**
  - DEFINITION
  - TYPES
- **SPEECH**
  - DEFINITION
  - MECHANISM
  - NERVOUS CONTROL
  - APPLIED PHYSIOLOGY

■ HIGHER INTELLECTUAL FUNCTIONS

Higher intellectual functions are very essential to make up the human mind. These functions are also called **higher brain functions** or **higher cortical functions**. Cerebral cortex is responsible for these functions. Important higher intellectual functions are learning, memory, conditioned reflexes and speech.

Conditioned reflex forms the basis of all higher intellectual functions.

■ LEARNING

■ DEFINITION

Learning is defined as the process by which **new information** is acquired.

■ TYPES OF LEARNING

Learning is of two types:

1. Non-associative learning.
2. Associative learning.

1. Non-associative Learning

It involves response of a person to only one type of stimulus. It is based on two factors.

i. Habituation

Habituation means getting used to something to which a person is constantly exposed. When a person is exposed to a stimulus repeatedly, he starts ignoring the stimulus slowly. During the first experience, the event (stimulus) is novel and evokes a response. However, it evokes less response when it is repeated. Finally, the person is habituated to the event and ignores it.

ii. Sensitization

Sensitization means a state in which the body becomes more sensitive to a stimulus. When a stimulus is applied repeatedly, habituation occurs. But if the same stimulus is combined with another type of stimulus, which may be pleasant or unpleasant, the person becomes more sensitive to the original stimulus.

For example, a woman gets habituated to different sounds around her and sleep is not disturbed by these sounds. However, she suddenly wakes up when her baby cries because she is sensitized to the crying sound of her baby.

2. Associative Learning

It involves learning about relations between two or more stimuli at a time. Classic example of associative learning is the conditioned reflex (see below).

■ MEMORY

■ DEFINITION

Memory is defined as the ability to recall the past experience. It is also defined as retention of learned materials.

TYPES OF MEMORY

Memory is classified by different methods, on the basis of various factors.

Short-term Memories and Long-term Memories

Short-term memory

Short-term memory is the recalling of events that happened very recently, i.e. within hours or days. It is also known as **recent memory**. For example, telephone number that is known today may be remembered till tomorrow. If it is not recalled repeatedly, it may be forgotten on 3rd day.

Long-term memory

It is otherwise called **remote memory**. It is the recalling of the events of weeks, months, years or sometimes lifetime. Examples are recalling 1st day of schooling, birthday celebration of previous year, picnic enjoyed last week, etc.

Explicit Memory and Implicit Memory

Explicit memory

Explicit memory is otherwise known as **declarative memory** or **recognition memory**. It is defined as the memory that involves **conscious recollection** of past experience. It consists of memories regarding the events which occurred in the external world around us. The information stored may be about a particular event that happened at a particular time and place. Examples are recollection of a birthday party celebrated three days ago; the events taken place while taking breakfast, etc.

Explicit memory involves hippocampus and medial part of temporal lobe.

Implicit memory

Implicit memory is otherwise known as **non-declarative memory** or **skilled memory**. It is defined as the memory in which past experience is utilized **without conscious awareness**. It helps to perform various skilled activities properly. For example, cycling, driving, playing tennis, dancing, typing, etc. are performed automatically without awareness.

Implicit memory involves the sensory and motor pathways.

ANATOMICAL BASIS OF MEMORY

Anatomical basis of memory is the **synapse** in brain. Memory encoding occurs at synaptic level. Synapse for memory coding is slightly different from other synapses. Two separate presynaptic terminals are present here. One of the terminals is **primary presynaptic terminal**, which ends on postsynaptic neuron as in conventional synapse. This terminal is called sensory terminal, because sensations are transmitted to the postsynaptic neuron through this terminal **(Fig. 107.1)**.

Another presynaptic terminal ends on the sensory terminal itself. This terminal is called **facilitator terminal**. When, sensory terminal is stimulated alone without facilitator terminal, the firing from sensory terminal leads to habituation, i.e. the firing decreases slowly. On the other

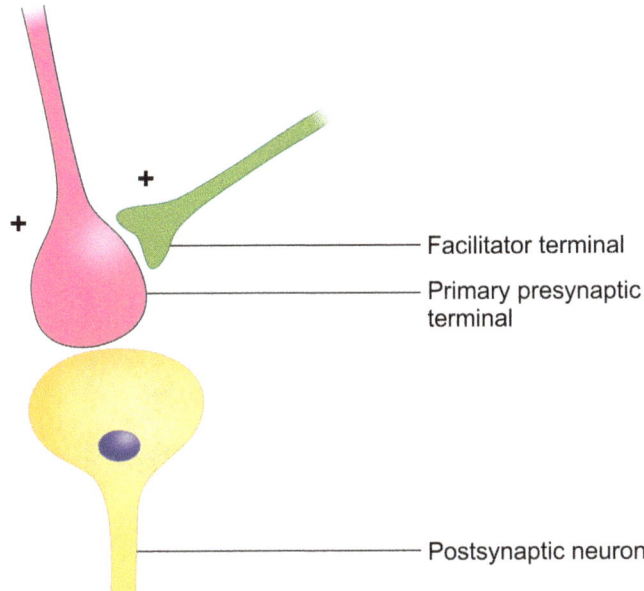

FIGURE 107.1: Synaptic terminal for memory encoding.

hand, if both the terminals are stimulated, facilitation occurs and the signals remain strong for long period, i.e. for few months to few years.

PHYSIOLOGICAL BASIS OF MEMORY

Memory is stored in brain by the alteration of synaptic transmission between the neurons involved in memory. Storage of memory may be facilitated or habituated.

Facilitation

It is the process by which the **memory storage** is enhanced. It involves increase in synaptic transmission and increased postsynaptic activity.

Habituation

It is the process by which the memory storage is attenuated (**attenuation** means decrease in strength, effect or value). It involves reduction in synaptic transmission and slow stoppage of postsynaptic activity.

Basis for Short-term Memory

Basic mechanism of memory is the development of new neuronal circuits by the formation of **new synapses** and facilitation of synaptic transmission. Number of presynaptic terminals and the size of the terminals are also increased.

Basis for Long-term Memory

When the neuronal circuit is reinforced by constant activity, the memory is consolidated and encoded into different areas of the brain. This encoding makes memory a permanent or long-term memory.

Sites of Encoding

Hippocampus and the Papez circuit (the closed circuit between hippocampus, thalamus, hypothalamus and corpus striatum) are the main sites for **memory encoding**.

Frontal and parietal areas are also involved in memory storage.

Consolidation of Memory

Consolidation is the process by which a short-term memory is crystallized into a long-term memory.

■ APPLIED PHYSIOLOGY: ABNORMALITIES OF MEMORY

1. Amnesia

Amnesia is the loss of memory. It is classified into two types:

i. *Anterograde amnesia:* Failure to establish new memories after the onset of amnesia. It occurs because of lesion in hippocampus.
ii. *Retrograde amnesia:* Failure to recall past remote long-term memory. It occurs in temporal lobe syndrome.

2. Dementia

Dementia is the progressive deterioration of intellect, emotional control, social behavior and motivation associated with loss of memory. It is an age-related disorder that occurs above the age of 65 years. When it occurs before the age of 65, it is called **presenile dementia.**

Causes of dementia

Dementia occurs because of many reasons. Most common cause of dementia is **Alzheimer disease**. Other common causes of dementia are hydrocephalus, Huntington chorea, Parkinson disease, viral encephalitis, HIV infection, hypothyroidism, hypoparathyroidism, Cushing's syndrome, alcoholic intoxication, poisoning by high dose of barbiturate, carbon monoxide, heavy metals, etc.

Features of dementia

Common features are loss of recent memory, lack of thinking and judgment and personality changes. As the disease progresses, psychiatric features begin to appear. Motor functions are also affected. Finally, the patient has to lead a vegetative life without any thinking power. The person is speechless and is unable to understand anything.

There is no effective treatment for this disorder. Physostigmine, which inhibits cholinesterase, causes moderate improvement.

3. Alzheimer Disease

Alzheimer disease is a progressive neurodegenerative disease. It is due to degeneration, loss of function and death of neurons in many parts of brain, particularly cerebral hemispheres, hippocampus and pons. There is reduction in the synthesis of most of the neurotransmitters, especially acetylcholine. Synthesis of acetylcholine decreases because of lack of enzyme choline acetyltransferase. Norepinephrine synthesis decreases because of degeneration of locus ceruleus. Dementia is the common feature of this disease.

■ CONDITIONED REFLEXES
■ DEFINITION

Conditioned reflex is the **acquired reflex** that requires learning, memory and recall of previous experience. It forms the basis of learning.

Unconditioned reflex is the **inborn reflex** which does not require previous experience.

■ TYPES OF CONDITIONED REFLEXES

Conditioned reflexes are of two types:

A. Classical conditioned reflexes.
B. Instrumental conditioned reflexes.

Classical Conditioned Reflexes

Classical conditioned reflexes are those reflexes, which are established by a **conditioned stimulus** followed by an **unconditioned stimulus**.

Method of study: Pavlov's bell-dog experiments

Classical conditioned reflexes are demonstrated by the classical **bell-dog experiments** (salivary secretion experiments) done by **Ivan Pavlov** and his associates.

In dogs, the duct of parotid gland or submandibular gland was taken outside through cheek or chin respectively and the salivary secretion was measured in drops by means of an electrical recorder.

Types of classical conditioned reflexes

Classical conditioned reflexes are classified into two groups:

I. Positive or excitatory conditioned reflexes.
II. Negative conditioned reflexes.

I. Positive conditioned reflexes

Positive conditioned reflexes are of three types:

1. *Primary conditioned reflex*

It is the reflex developed with **one unconditioned stimulus** and **one conditioned stimulus**. The dog is fed with **food** (unconditioned stimulus). Simultaneously a **flash of light** (conditioned stimulus) is also shown. Both the stimuli are repeated for some days. After the development of reflex, the flash of light (conditioned stimulus) alone causes salivary secretion without food (unconditioned stimulus).

2. *Secondary conditioned reflex*

It is the reflex developed with **one unconditioned stimulus** and **two conditioned stimuli**. After establishment of a conditioned reflex with one conditioned stimulus, another conditioned stimulus is applied along with the first one. For example, the animal is fed with food (unconditioned reflex) and simultaneously a flash of light (first conditioned stimulus), and a **bell sound** (second conditioned stimulus) are applied. After the development of the reflex, the second conditioned stimulus, the bell sound alone can cause salivary secretion.

3. *Tertiary conditioned reflex*

In this reflex, a third conditioned stimulus is added and the reflex is established. But, the reflex with more than three conditioned stimuli is not possible.

II. Negative conditioned reflexes

In negative conditioned reflexes, the established conditioned reflexes are inhibited by some factors. For example, some disturbing factors such as sudden entrance of a stranger or sudden noise can abolish the conditioned reflex and inhibit salivary secretion.

Instrumental or Operant Conditioned Reflexes

Instrumental or operant conditioned reflexes are the reflexes in which the behavior of the person is instrumental. This type of reflexes is developed by the conditioned stimulus followed by a **reward** or **punishment**.

For example, if the animal is rewarded by a banana by pressing a bar, the animal repeatedly presses the bar. If the animal is given a tasty food along with electric shock, the animal starts avoiding that food.

Instrumental conditioned reflexes play an important role during the learning processes of a child. These conditioned reflexes are also responsible for behavior pattern of an individual.

SPEECH

DEFINITION

Speech is defined as the expression of thoughts by production of articulate sound, bearing a definite meaning. When a sound is produced verbally, it is called the **speech**. If it is expressed by visual symbols, it is known as **writing**.

MECHANISM OF SPEECH

Speech depends upon the coordinated activities of **central speech apparatus** and **peripheral speech apparatus**. The central speech apparatus consists of higher centers, i.e. the cortical and subcortical centers. The peripheral speech apparatus includes larynx or sound box, pharynx, mouth, nasal cavities, tongue and lips.

NERVOUS CONTROL OF SPEECH

Speech is controlled by the following cortical areas.

A. Motor Areas

1. Broca's area

It is area 44. It is also called **speech center**. It is situated in lower part of lateral surface of prefrontal cortex. This area controls the movements of structures concerned with vocalization.

2. Upper frontal motor area

It is situated in the paracentral gyrus over the medial surface of the cerebral hemisphere. It controls the coordinated movements concerned with writing.

B. Sensory Areas

1. Auditopsychic area

Auditopsychic area is situated in the superior temporal gyrus. It is concerned with storage of memories of spoken words.

2. Visuopsychic area

It is present in angular gyrus of the parietal cortex. It is concerned with storage of memories of the visual symbols.

C. Wernicke's Area

This area is situated in the upper part of temporal lobe. It is responsible for understanding the auditory and visual information about any word.

APPLIED PHYSIOLOGY: DISORDERS OF SPEECH

1. Aphasia

Aphasia is the loss or **impairment of speech**. It is due to damage of speech centers which occurs during stroke, head injury, cerebral tumors, brain infections and degenerative disease such as Parkinson disease.

Head's classification of aphasia

Henry Head has classified aphasia into four types:

  i. *Verbal aphasia:* Disability in the formation of words.
  ii. *Syntactical aphasia:* Inability to arrange words in proper sequence.
  iii. *Semantic aphasia:* Inability to recognize the significance of words.
  iv. *Nominal aphasia:* Difficulty in naming the object due to failure in recognizing the meaning of words.

2. Dysarthria or Anarthria

Dysarthria or anarthria is the difficulty or **inability to speak** because of paralysis of muscles involved in articulation. The spoken and written words are understood. It is caused by damage of brain areas or the nerves that control muscles involved in speech. It occurs in conditions like stroke, brain injury and degenerative disease.

3. Dysphonia

Dysphonia is a voice disorder characterized by **hoarseness** and a sore or **dry throat**. Hoarseness means the difficulty in producing sound while trying to speak or a change in the pitch or loudness of voice. It occurs due to diseases of vocal cords or larynx.

4. Stammering

Stammering or shuttering is a speech disorder in which the normal flow of speech is disturbed by repetitions or stoppage of sound and words. It is associated with some unusual facial and body movements. Stammering is due to genetic factors, brain damage, neurological disorders or anxiety.

Chapter 108: Cerebrospinal Fluid

CHAPTER OUTLINE

- DEFINITION
- PROPERTIES AND COMPOSITION
- FORMATION
- CIRCULATION
- ABSORPTION
- PRESSURE EXERTED BY CSF
- FUNCTIONS
- COLLECTION
- BLOOD-BRAIN BARRIER
- BLOOD-CEREBROSPINAL FLUID BARRIER
- APPLIED PHYSIOLOGY: HYDROCEPHALUS

■ DEFINITION

Cerebrospinal fluid (CSF) is the clear, colorless and transparent fluid that circulates through **ventricles of brain**, **subarachnoid space** and **central canal** of spinal cord. It is a part of **ECF**.

■ PROPERTIES AND COMPOSITION OF CSF

Properties

Volume	: 150 mL
Rate of formation	: 0.3 mL per minute
Specific gravity	: 1.005
Reaction	: Alkaline.

Composition

Composition of CSF is given in **Figure 108.1**. CSF contains more amount of sodium than potassium since it is a part of ECF. CSF also contains some lymphocytes. CSF secreted by ventricle does not contain any cell. Lymphocytes are added when CSF flows in the spinal cord.

■ FORMATION OF CSF

CSF is formed by the **choroid plexuses** (tuft of capillaries) situated within the ventricles. It is formed by the process of **secretion** which involves active transport.

■ CIRCULATION OF CSF

Major quantity of CSF is formed in the **lateral ventricles** and passes through the **foramen of Monro** into the **third ventricle** (Figs. 108.2 and 108.3). From here, it passes to the **fourth ventricle** through **aqueductus Sylvius**. From fourth ventricle, CSF enters into the cisterna magna and cisterna lateralis through **foramen of Magendie** (central opening) and **foramen of Luschka** (lateral opening).

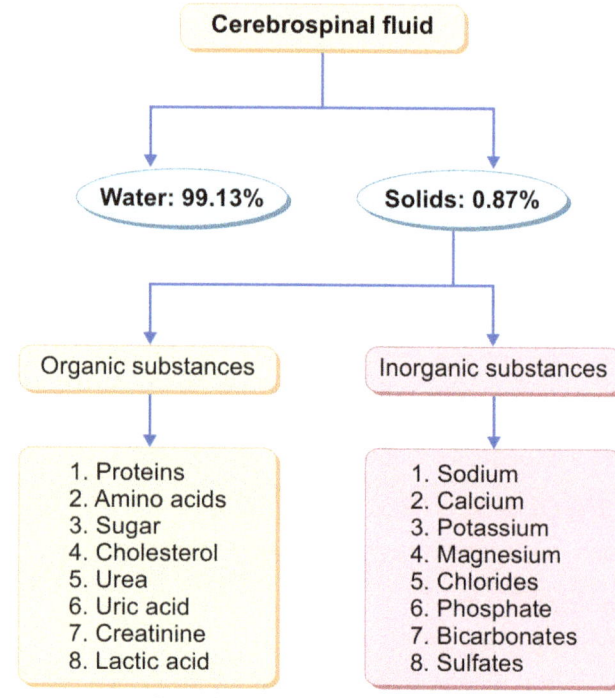

FIGURE 108.1: Composition of cerebrospinal fluid.

From **cisterna magna** and **cisterna lateralis**, CSF circulates through **subarachnoid space** over spinal cord and cerebral hemispheres. It also flows into **central canal** of spinal cord.

■ ABSORPTION OF CSF

CSF is mainly absorbed by the **arachnoid villi** into **dural sinuses** and **spinal veins**. Small amount is absorbed

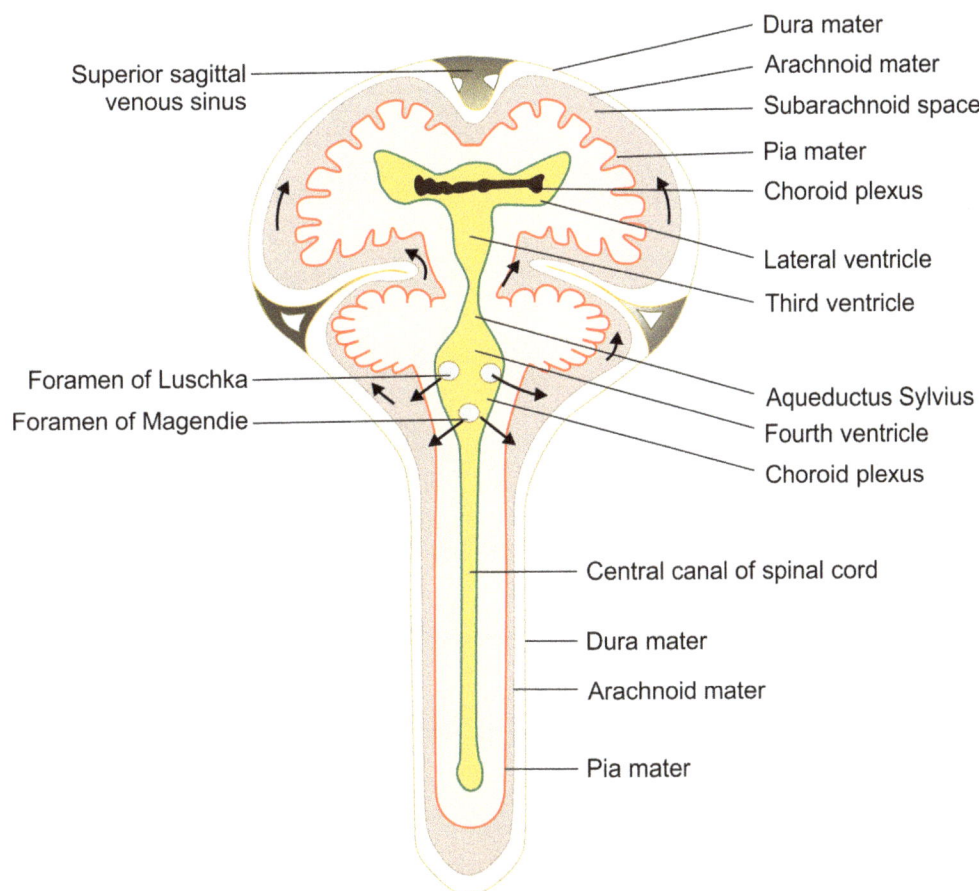

FIGURE 108.2: Circulation of cerebrospinal fluid.

into cervical lymphatics and perivascular spaces. The mechanism of absorption is by **filtration**.

Normally, about 500 mL of CSF is formed every day and an equal amount is absorbed.

■ PRESSURE EXERTED BY CSF

Pressure exerted by CSF varies in different position, viz.:
- Lateral recumbent position = 10 to 18 cm of H_2O
- Lying position = 13 cm of H_2O
- Sitting position = 30 cm of H_2O

Certain events like coughing, crying and compression of internal jugular vein increase the CSF pressure.

■ FUNCTIONS OF CSF

■ PROTECTIVE FUNCTION

CSF acts as **fluid buffer** and protects the brain from **shock**. Since, the specific gravity of brain and CSF is more or less same, brain floats in CSF. When head receives a blow, CSF acts like a cushion and prevents the movement of brain against the skull bone and thereby prevents the damage of brain.

But severe blow affecting brain results in contrecoup injury.

Contrecoup Injury

Contrecoup injury is the injury to brain, in which the damage is on the side opposite to the side on which head receives a severe blow.

When the head receives a severe blow, the brain moves forcefully and hits against the skull bone, leading to damage of brain tissues. Brain strikes against the skull bone at a point opposite to the point where the blow was applied. Hence the name contrecoup injury.

■ REGULATION OF CRANIAL CONTENT VOLUME

Regulation of cranial content volume is essential because, brain may be affected if the volume of cranial content increases. It happens in cerebral hemorrhage and brain tumors. Increase in cranial content volume is prevented by greater absorption of CSF to give space for the increasing cranial contents.

■ MEDIUM OF EXCHANGE

CSF is the medium through which many substances, particularly the nutritive substances and waste materials are exchanged between blood and brain tissues.

■ COLLECTION OF CSF

CSF is collected either by **cisternal puncture** or **lumbar puncture**. In cisternal puncture, the CSF is collected by passing a needle between the **occipital bone and atlas**, so that it enters the **cisterna magna**. In lumbar puncture, the **lumbar puncture needle** is introduced into the **subarachnoid space** in the lumbar region, between **third and fourth lumbar spines**.

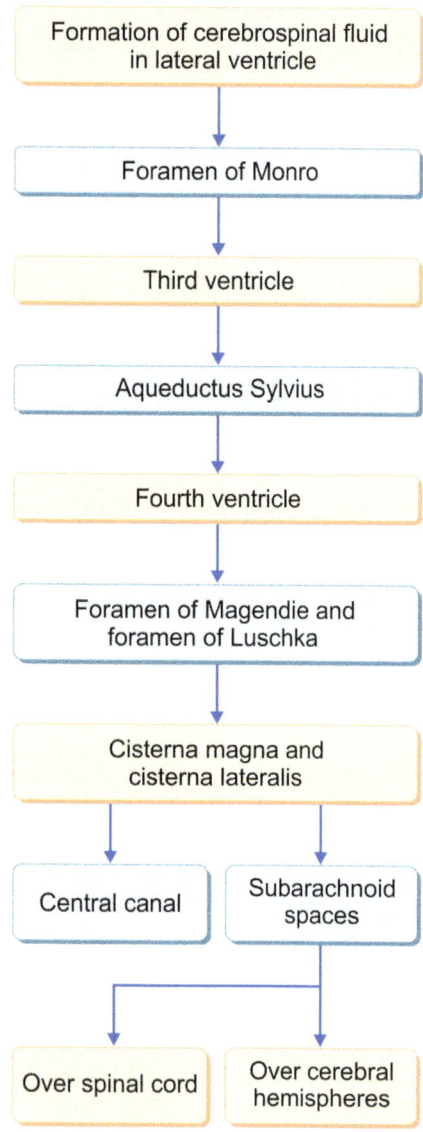

FIGURE 108.3: Schematic diagram of CSF circulation.

■ BLOOD-BRAIN BARRIER

Blood-brain barrier (BBB) is a **neuroprotective structure** that prevents the entry of many substances and pathogens from blood into the brain tissues. Barrier exists in the capillary membrane of all parts of the brain except in some areas of hypothalamus.

BBB is formed by **tight junctions** in the endothelial cells of the brain capillaries. The cytoplasmic foot processes of **astrocytes** (neuroglial cells) develop around the capillaries and reinforce the barrier.

■ FUNCTIONS OF BLOOD-BRAIN BARRIER

1. BBB acts as a mechanical barrier and prevents harmful chemical substances from entering brain.
2. BBB provides a healthy environment for brain tissues by preventing injurious materials and organisms.
3. BBB permits metabolic and essential materials into the brain tissues.

Substances which can pass through blood-brain barrier and the substances which cannot pass through blood-brain barrier are listed in **Box 108.1**.

BOX 108.1: Substances which can pass and substances which cannot pass through blood-brain barrier.

Substances which can pass through blood-brain barrier
1. Oxygen
2. Carbon dioxide
3. Water
4. Glucose
5. Amino acids
6. Electrolytes
7. Drugs such as L-dopa, 5-HT, sulfonamides, tetracycline and many lipid-soluble drugs
8. Lipid-soluble anesthetic gases such as ether and nitrous oxide
9. Other lipid-soluble substances
Substances which cannot pass through blood-brain barrier
1. Injurious chemical agents
2. Pathogens such as bacteria
3. Drugs such as penicillin and the catecholamines
4. Dopamine (so, parkinsonism is treated with L-dopa, instead of dopamine)
5. Bile pigments
However, since the barrier is not well developed in infants, the bile pigments enter the brain tissues. During jaundice due to erythroblastosis fetalis in infants, the bile pigments enter brain and causes damage of basal ganglia, leading to kernicterus (Chapter 19)

■ BLOOD-CEREBROSPINAL FLUID BARRIER

It is the barrier between the blood and cerebrospinal fluid that exists at the **choroid plexus**. The function of this barrier is similar to that of the BBB. It does not allow the movement of many substances from blood to cerebrospinal fluid. It allows the movement of only those substances, which are allowed by BBB.

■ APPLIED PHYSIOLOGY: HYDROCEPHALUS

Hydrocephalus is the **abnormal accumulation of CSF** in brain, associated with **enlargement of head**.

Types and Causes of Hydrocephalus

1. *Internal hydrocephalus or non-communicating hydrocephalus*

Internal hydrocephalus is the accumulation of CSF in **ventricles** of brain caused by **blockage of cerebral aqueduct**. It causes dilatation of ventricles resulting in enlargement of head and cortical atrophy.

2. *External hydrocephalus or communicating hydrocephalus*

External hydrocephalus is the accumulation of CSF in **subarachnoid space**. There is dilatation of ventricles and widening of subarachnoid space resulting in enlargement of head. It is due to **blockage of arachnoid villi**.

Features of Hydrocephalus

Hydrocephalus along with increased intracranial pressure causes headache and vomiting. In severe conditions, it leads to atrophy of brain, mental weakness and convulsions.

Chapter 109: Autonomic Nervous System

CHAPTER OUTLINE

- AUTONOMIC NERVOUS SYSTEM
- SYMPATHETIC DIVISION
- PARASYMPATHETIC DIVISION
- FUNCTIONS
- NEUROTRANSMITTERS
- SYMPATHOMIMETIC DRUGS
- SYMPATHETIC BLOCKERS
- PARASYMPATHOMIMETIC DRUGS
- PARASYMPATHETIC BLOCKERS
- GANGLIONIC BLOCKERS

■ AUTONOMIC NERVOUS SYSTEM

Autonomic nervous system (ANS) is a part of **peripheral nervous system** which is concerned with regulation of visceral or vegetative functions of the body. So, it is also called **vegetative** or **involuntary nervous system**.

■ DIVISIONS OF ANS

Autonomic nervous system is divided into two divisions:

1. Sympathetic division.
2. Parasympathetic division.

Differences between both the divisions of ANS are given in **Table 109.1**.

■ SYMPATHETIC DIVISION

It is otherwise called **thoracolumbar outflow** because, the preganglionic neurons are situated in lateral gray horns of 12 thoracic segments and first two lumbar segments of spinal cord. Fibers arising from here are called **preganglionic fibers**.

Preganglionic fibers leave the spinal cord through anterior nerve root and white rami communicants, and terminate in the postganglionic neurons, which are situated in the **sympathetic ganglia**.

Sympathetic division supplies smooth muscle fibers of all the visceral organs such as blood vessels, heart, lungs, glands, gastrointestinal organs, etc.

■ SYMPATHETIC GANGLIA

Ganglia of sympathetic division are classified into three groups:

I. Paravertebral or sympathetic chain ganglia.
II. Prevertebral or collateral ganglia.
III. Terminal or peripheral ganglia.

I. *Paravertebral or Sympathetic Chain Ganglia*

Paravertebral or sympathetic chain ganglia are present on either side of vertebral column. These ganglia are connected with each other by longitudinal fibers to form the sympathetic chains **(Fig. 109.1)**. Both the chains extend from skull to coccyx.

Ganglia of the sympathetic chain (trunk) on each side are divided into four groups.

1. Cervical ganglia   :   8 in number
2. Thoracic ganglia   :   12 in number
3. Lumbar ganglia   :   5 in number
4. Sacral ganglia   :   5 in number

II. *Prevertebral or Collateral Ganglia*

Prevertebral ganglia are situated in thorax, abdomen and pelvis in relation to aorta and its branches.

Prevertebral ganglia are:

1. Celiac ganglion.
2. Superior mesenteric ganglion.
3. Inferior mesenteric ganglion.

Prevertebral ganglia receive preganglionic fibers from T5 to L2 segments. The postganglionic fibers from these ganglia supply the visceral organs of thorax, abdomen and pelvis.

III. *Terminal or Peripheral Ganglia*

Terminal ganglia are situated within or close to structures innervated by them. Heart, bronchi, pancreas and urinary bladder are innervated by the terminal ganglia.

Sympathoadrenergic System

Sympathoadrenergic system is a functional and phylogenetic unit that includes sympathetic division and

TABLE 109.1: Actions of sympathetic and parasympathetic divisions of ANS.

Effector organ		Sympathetic division	Parasympathetic division
1. Eye	Ciliary muscle	Relaxation	Contraction
	Pupil	Dilatation	Constriction
2. Lacrimal glands		Decrease in secretion	Increase in secretion
3. Salivary glands		Secretion of thick saliva and Vasoconstriction	Secretion of watery saliva and Vasodilatation
4. Gastrointestinal tract	Motility	Inhibition	Acceleration
	Secretion	Decrease	Increase
	Sphincters	Constriction	Relaxation
	Smooth muscles	Relaxation	Contraction
5. Gallbladder		Relaxation	Contraction
6. Urinary bladder	Detrusor muscle	Relaxation	Contraction
	Internal sphincter	Constriction	Relaxation
7. Sweat glands		Increase in secretion	–
8. Heart: Rate and force		Increase	Decrease
9. Blood vessels		Constriction of all blood vessels, except those in heart and skeletal muscle	Dilatation
10. Bronchioles		Dilatation	Constriction

adrenal medulla. Adrenal medulla is a modified sympathetic ganglion.

■ PARASYMPATHETIC DIVISION

Parasympathetic division of ANS is otherwise called **craniosacral outflow** because the fibers of this division arise from brainstem and sacral segments of spinal cord. Cranial portion of parasympathetic division innervates the blood vessels of the head and neck, and many thoracoabdominal visceral organs.

Sacral portion of parasympathetic division innervates the smooth muscles forming the walls of viscera and the glands such as large intestine, liver, spleen, kidneys, bladder, genitalia, etc.

■ CRANIAL OUTFLOW OR CRANIAL PORTION OF PARASYMPATHETIC DIVISION

Cranial outflow or cranial portion of parasympathetic division arises from brainstem. It innervates the blood vessels of head and neck, and many thoracoabdominal visceral organs.

Cranial outflow includes the following cranial nerves:

1. Oculomotor nerve (III cranial nerve).
2. Facial nerve (VII cranial nerve).
3. Glossopharyngeal nerve (IX cranial nerve).
4. Vagus nerve (X cranial nerve).

Preganglionic fibers of these cranial nerves arise from neurons situated at two different levels:

1. Tectal or **midbrain outflow** (III cranial nerve).
2. Bulbar level or **bulbar outflow** (VII, IX and X cranial nerves).

Preganglionic fibers are longer and reach the postganglionic neurons, which are situated within the organs or close to the organs innervated by these nerves. Preganglionic fibers are myelinated, but the postganglionic fibers are nonmyelinated.

■ SACRAL OUTFLOW OR SACRAL PORTION OF PARASYMPATHETIC DIVISION

Sacral outflow or sacral portion of parasympathetic division arises from the sacral segments of spinal cord. It innervates smooth muscles forming the walls of viscera and the glands such as large intestine, liver, spleen, kidneys, bladder, genitalia, etc.

Preganglionic fibers arise from anterior gray horn cells of 2nd, 3rd and 4th sacral segments (from 1st also in some cases) of spinal cord and form the **pelvic nerve** (nervi erigens). Fibers end on postganglionic neurons, which are situated on or near the visceral organs. Fibers from postganglionic neurons supply descending colon, rectum, urinary bladder, internal sphincter, urethra and accessory sex organs.

Sacral parasympathetic fibers supply those visceral organs which are not supplied by **vagus**.

■ FUNCTIONS OF ANS

Autonomic nervous system is concerned with regulation of **vegetative functions**, which are beyond voluntary control. By controlling the various vegetative functions, ANS plays an important role in maintaining the constant internal environment (homeostasis).

Almost all the visceral organs are supplied by both sympathetic and parasympathetic divisions of ANS, and the two divisions produce antagonistic effects on each organ. When the fibers of one division supplying to an organ is sectioned or affected by lesion, the effects of fibers from other division on the organ become more prominent.

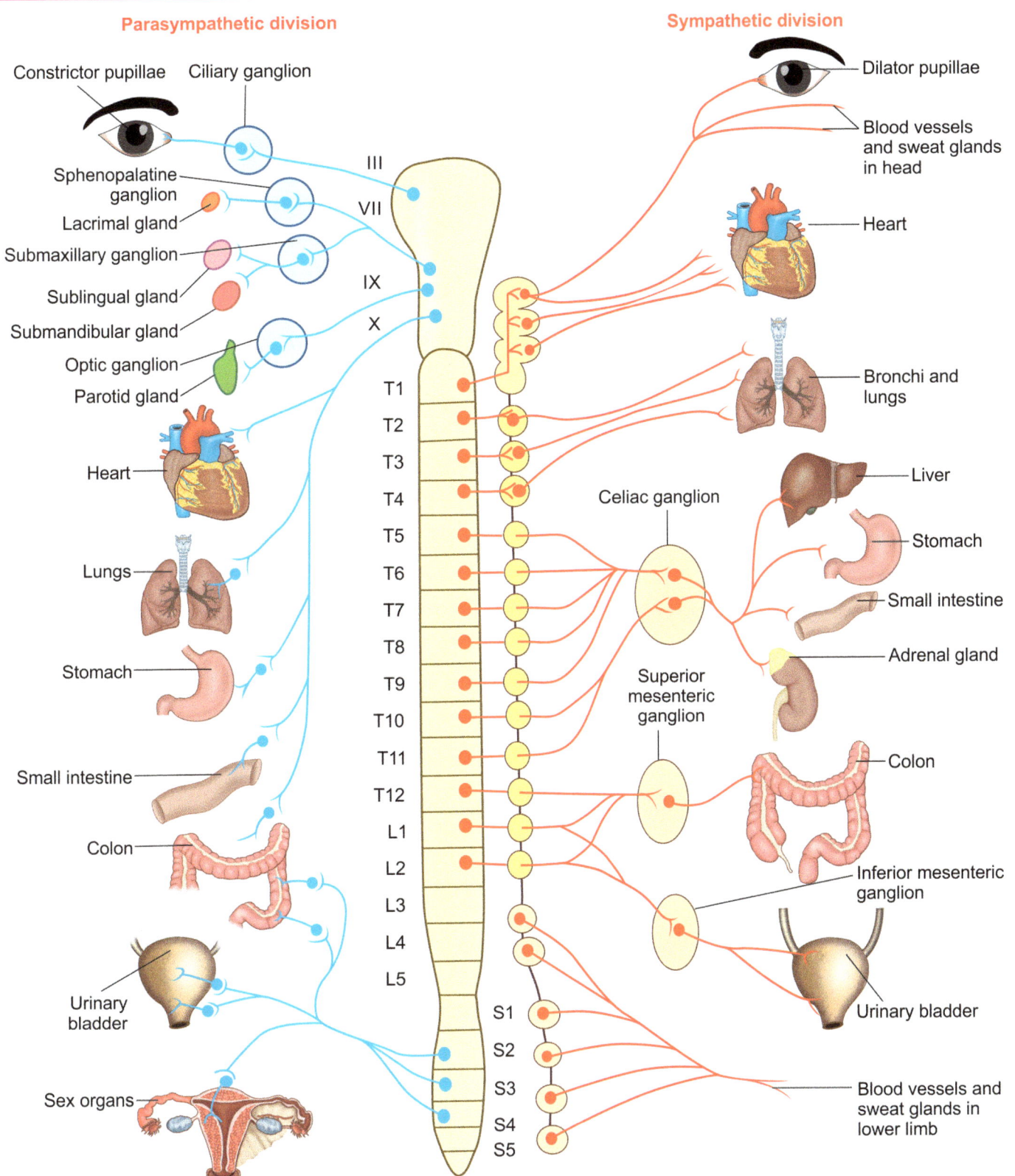

FIGURE 109.1: Autonomic nervous system.

Actions of the sympathetic and parasympathetic fibers on various structures are given in **Table 109.1**.

NEUROTRANSMITTERS OF ANS

Different nerve fibers of ANS execute the functions by releasing some neuro transmitter substances.

SYMPATHETIC FIBERS

1. Preganglionic fibers: Acetylcholine.
2. Postganglionic sympathetic noradrenergic fibers: Noradrenaline.
3. Postganglionic sympathetic cholinergic fibers: Acetylcholine.

Postganglionic sympathetic cholinergic nerve fibers supply sweat glands and blood vessels in heart and skeletal muscle.

PARASYMPATHETIC FIBERS

1. Preganglionic fibers : Acetylcholine.
2. Postganglionic fibers : Acetylcholine.

SYMPATHOMIMETIC DRUGS

Sympathomimetic drugs or **adrenaline-like** drugs are the drugs, which produce the effects of sympathetic stimulation. Adrenaline and noradrenaline produced in the body act only for a short duration of about 1 to 2 minutes. Whereas, sympathomimetic drugs injected intravenously act for a longer period of about 30 minutes to 2 hours.

Examples are phenylephrine, albuterol, ephedrine and amphetamine.

SYMPATHETIC BLOCKERS

Sympathetic blockers are the drugs that prevent actions of sympathetic neurotransmitter. Sympathetic blockers act on all levels.

Examples are **reserpine** and **quanethidine**.

PARASYMPATHOMIMETIC DRUGS

Parasympathomimetic drugs or acetylcholine (Ach) like drugs are drugs, which produce the effects of parasympathetic stimulation. ACh produced in the body acts only for a short period, whereas the injected ACh acts for a long time. Similarly, parasympathomimetic drugs also exhibit their actions for a longer time.

Parasympathomimetic drugs are as follows:

1. Drugs which Act on Muscarinic Receptors

Pilocarpine and **methacholine** produce their effects by acting on the **muscarinic receptors.**

2. Drugs which Prolong the Action of ACh

Action of ACh can be prolonged by preventing its destruction. Drugs like **neostigmine** and **physostigmine** inhibit the activity of acetylcholinesterase and so the ACh is not destroyed quickly.

PARASYMPATHETIC BLOCKERS

Parasympathetic blockers are drugs, which prevent the actions of parasympathetic neurotransmitter. Drugs **atropine**, **homatropine** and **scopolamine** inhibit the actions of ACh by blocking the muscarinic receptors.

GANGLIONIC BLOCKERS

Ganglionic blockers are the drugs that prevent the transmission of impulses from preganglionic neurons to postganglionic neurons. **Tetraethyl ammonium ion**, **hexamethonium ion** and **pentolinium** are some of the ganglionic blockers.

MODEL QUESTIONS IN NERVOUS SYSTEM

LONG QUESTIONS

1. What is neuron? Describe the structure of neuron and the properties of nerve fibers.
2. What are receptors? Classify them and explain their properties.
3. What is synapse? Explain the structure, functions and properties of synapse.
4. Define and classify reflex action. Explain reflex arc and the properties of reflexes.
5. Name the ascending tracts of the spinal cord and, explain spinothalamic tracts.
6. What are the tracts of spinal cord? Describe the spinocerebellar tracts.
7. Give an account of tracts in the posterior white funiculus of spinal cord.
8. Enumerate the descending tracts of spinal cord. Describe in detail the pyramidal tracts. Write a note on the effects of upper and lower motor neuron lesions.
9. What are the thalamic nuclei? Describe the functions and effects of lesions of thalamus.
10. Name the hypothalamic nuclei. Explain the functions and effects of lesions of hypothalamus.
11. What are the different divisions of cerebellum? Explain the functions of each division. Add a note on cerebellar lesions.
12. What are the components of basal ganglia? Give an account of functions and disorders of basal ganglia.
13. Name lobes of cerebral cortex? Describe the functions of each lobe. Add a note on frontal lobe syndrome.
14. Describe the receptor organ in vestibular apparatus and explain role of vestibular apparatus in maintenance of equilibrium.
15. Explain divisions and functions of autonomic nervous system. Add a note on neurotransmitters of autonomic nervous system.

SHORT QUESTIONS

1. Structure of neuron.
2. Classification of nerve fibers.
3. Properties of nerve fibers.
4. Saltatory conduction.
5. Wallerian degeneration.
6. Neuroglia.
7. Cutaneous receptors.
8. Generator (receptor) potential.
9. EPSP.
10. Synaptic transmission.
11. Reflex arc.
12. Properties of reflexes.
13. Superficial reflexes.
14. Deep reflexes.
15. Upper/Lower motor neuron lesion.
16. Pathway for fine touch sensations.
17. Pathway for pressure sensation.
18. Pathway for temperature sensations.
19. Pathway for conscious kinesthetic sensations.
20. Pathway for subconscious kinesthetic sensations.
21. Pathway for pain sensations.
22. Functions of thalamus.
23. Thalamic syndrome.
24. Regulation of food intake.
25. Disorders of hypothalamus.
26. Corticocerebellum (neocerebellum).
27. Spinocerebellum (paleocerebellum).
28. Vestibulocerebellum
29. Functions of basal ganglia.
30. Parkinsonism.
31. Frontal lobe of cerebral cortex.
32. Parietal lobe (or sensory areas) of cerebral cortex.
33. Functions of limbic system.
34. Muscle spindle.
35. Muscle tone.
36. Righting reflexes.
37. Semicircular canal.
38. Otolith organ.
39. Motion sickness.
40. EEG.
41. EEG pattern during sleep.
42. Learning.
43. Memory.
44. Conditioned reflexes.
45. Speech.
46. CSF.
47. Role of ANS in the regulation of cardiovascular functions.
48. Role of ANS in the regulation of gastrointestinal activity.
49. Functions of sympathetic division of ANS.
50. Functions of parasympathetic division of ANS.

VERY SHORT ANSWER QUESTIONS

1. Parts of brain.
2. Classification of neuron.
3. Myelin sheath.
4. Neurilemma and Schwann cells.
5. Myelinogenesis.
6. Nerve growth factor.
7. Action potential in nerve fiber.
8. Conduction through myelinated nerve fiber/saltatory conduction.
9. Degrees of injury to nerve fiber/Sunderland's classification.
10. Classify receptors on the basis of adaptation. Give examples.
11. Müller law.
12. Sensory transduction.
13. Classification of synapse.
14. Synaptic delay.
15. Functions of synapse.
16. IPSP.
17. Renshaw cell inhibition.

18. Bell-Magendie law.
19. Reflex arc.
20. Babinski reflex.
21. Segments of spinal cord and spinal nerves.
22. Types of neuron present in gray matter of spinal cord.
23. Classify tracts of fibers in spinal cord.
24. Name the ascending tracts situated in each white column of spinal cord.
25. Functions of ascending tracs situated in posterior white column of spinal cord.
26. Name the descending tracts of spinal cord and their situation.
27. Define Brown-Séquard syndrome.
28. Disk prolapse.
29. Types of somatic sensations.
30. Combined or synthetic sensations.
31. Paralysis.
32. Functions of red nucleus.
33. Thalamic phantom limb.
34. Nuclei of hypothalamus.
35. Rage and sham rage.
36. Laurence-Biedl-Moon syndrome.
37. Narcolepsy and cataplexy.
38. Timing and programming the skilled movements.
39. Servomechanism.
40. Automatic associated movements.
41. Components of basal ganglia.
42. Kernicterus.
43. Crista ampullaris/macula.
44. Nystagmus/vestibulo-ocular reflex.
45. Labyrinthectomy.
46. Alpha block.
47. Differences between REM sleep and non-REM sleep.
48. Definition of epilepsy, convulsion, convulsive seizures and epileptic seizure.
49. Short-term and long-term memories/explicit and implicit memories/sensory, primary and secondary memories.
50. Amnesia and dementia.
51. Alzheimer's disease.
52. Head's classification of aphasia.
53. Blood-CSF barrier.
54. Hydrocephalus.
55. Neurotransmitters of ANS.
56. Sympathomimetic drugs.
57. Sympathetic blockers.
58. Parasympathomimetic drugs.
59. Parasympathetic blockers.
60. Ganglionic blockers.

SECTION 11: SPECIAL SENSES

Chapter 110: Eye

CHAPTER OUTLINE

- SPECIAL SENSES
- FUNCTIONAL ANATOMY OF THE EYEBALL
  - MORPHOLOGY
  - ORBITAL CAVITY
  - EYELIDS
  - CONJUNCTIVA
  - LACRIMAL GLAND AND TEAR
- WALL OF THE EYEBALL
  - OUTER LAYER
  - MIDDLE LAYER
  - INNER LAYER
- FUNDUS OCULI
  - OPTIC DISK
  - MACULA LUTEA
- INTRAOCULAR FLUID
  - VITREOUS HUMOR
  - AQUEOUS HUMOR
- INTRAOCULAR PRESSURE
- LENS
  - STRUCTURE
  - CHANGES IN THE LENS DURING OLD AGE
- OCULAR MUSCLES
  - MUSCLES OF THE EYEBALL
  - INNERVATION OF OCULAR MUSCLES
- OCULAR MOVEMENTS
  - MOVEMENTS IN VERTICAL AXIS
  - MOVEMENTS IN TRANSVERSE AXIS
  - MOVEMENTS IN ANTEROPOSTERIOR AXIS
  - SIMULTANEOUS MOVEMENTS OF BOTH EYEBALLS
- APPLIED PHYSIOLOGY
  - GLAUCOMA
  - CATARACT

SPECIAL SENSES

Special senses or **special sensations** are the complex sensations which involve **specialized sense organs**. Special sensations are different from somatic sensations that arise from skin, muscles, tendons and joints (Chapter 95).

Special senses are:

1. Sensation of vision.
2. Sensation of hearing.
3. Sensation of taste.
4. Sensation of smell.

FUNCTIONAL ANATOMY OF EYEBALL

MORPHOLOGY

Human **eyeball** (**bulbus oculi**) is approximately globe shaped with a diameter of about 24 mm. It is slightly flattened from above downwards. Eyeball is made up of two segments, an anterior part and a posterior part.

Anterior part is small and forms one-sixth of the eyeball. Posterior part is larger and forms five-sixth of the eyeball. Radius of this part is about 8 mm. Posterior wall of this part is lined by the light-sensitive structure called **retina.**

Center of anterior curvature of the eyeball is called the **anterior pole**, and the center of posterior curvature is called the **posterior pole**. A line joining the two poles is called **optic axis**. And, another line joining a point in cornea little medial to anterior pole and the fovea centralis situated lateral to posterior pole is known as **visual axis**. Light rays pass through the visual axis of eyeball **(Fig. 110.1)**.

ORBITAL CAVITY

Except anterior 1/6, the eyeball is situated in the bony **orbital cavity** or eye socket. A thick layer of areolar tissue is interposed between the bone and the eye. It serves as a cushion to protect the eyeball from external force. Eyeballs are attached to **orbital cavity** by **ocular muscles**.

EYELIDS

Eyelids protect the eyeball from foreign particles coming in contact with its surface and cutoff the light during sleep.

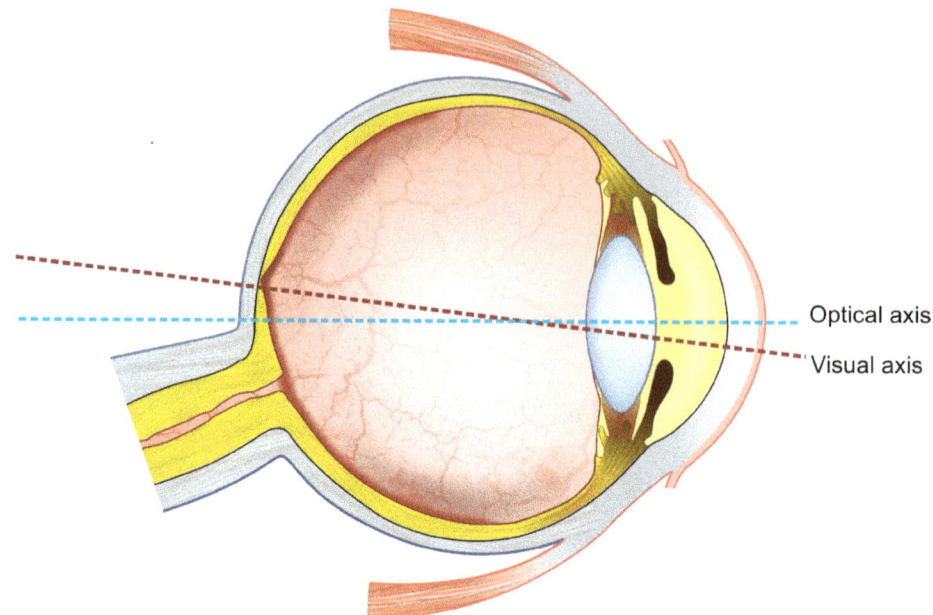

FIGURE 110.1: Optical and visual axis.

Eyelids are opened and closed voluntarily as well as reflexly.

Margins of eyelids have sensitive hairs called the **cilia**. Each cilium arises from a follicle, which is surrounded by a sensory nerve plexus. When the dust particle comes in contact with cilia, these sensory nerves are activated resulting in rapid blinking of eyelids. It prevents the dust particles from reaching the eyeball.

Opening between the two eyelids is called **palpebral fissure**. In adults, it is about 25 mm long. Its width is about 12 to 15 mm when opened.

CONJUNCTIVA

It is a thin **mucous membrane**, which covers the exposed part of the eye. After covering the anterior surface, the conjunctiva is reflected into the inner surfaces of the eyelids. The part of conjunctiva covering the eyeball is called the **bulbar portion**. The part covering the eyelid is called the **palpebral portion**.

LACRIMAL GLAND AND TEAR

Lacrimal gland is situated in the shelter of bone, forming the upper and outer border of wall of the eye socket. From the lacrimal gland, **tear** flows over the surface of conjunctiva and drains into nose via lacrimal ducts, lacrimal sac and nasolacrimal duct.

Tear

Tear is a hypertonic fluid. Due to its continuous washing and lubrication, the conjunctiva is kept moist and is protected from infection. Tear also contains the enzyme **lysozyme** that kills bacteria. Secretion of tears is controlled by the parasympathetic fibers of facial (VII cranial) nerve.

WALL OF THE EYEBALL

Wall of the eyeball is composed of three layers:

I. Outer layer, which includes cornea and sclera.
II. Middle layer, which includes choroid, ciliary body and iris.
III. Inner layer, the retina.

OUTER LAYER OR TUNICA EXTERNA OR TUNICA FIBROSA

Outer layer preserves the shape of eyeball. Anterior 1/6 of this layer is transparent and is known as **cornea**. It covers the **iris** and **pupil**. It is continuous with the sclera. **Sclera** forms posterior 5/6 of outer layer and it is tough, fibrous and opaque.

MIDDLE LAYER OR TUNICA MEDIA OR TUNICA VASCULOSA

This layer surrounds the eyeball completely except for a small opening in front known as the pupil.

Middle layer comprises three structures:

1. Choroid.
2. Ciliary body.
3. Iris.

1. Choroid

Choroid is the thin vascular layer of eyeball situated between sclera and retina. It forms posterior 5/6 of middle layer. Choroid is extended anteriorly up to the insertion of ciliary muscle (the level of **ora serrata**). Choroid is composed of a rich capillary plexus, numerous small arteries and veins.

2. Ciliary Body

Ciliary body is the thickened anterior part of middle layer of eye situated between choroid and iris. It is situated in front of ora serrata.

It is in the form of a ring. Its outer surface is separated from the sclera by perichoroidal space. Inner surface of the ciliary body faces the vitreous body and lens. The **suspensory ligaments** from the lens are attached to ciliary body. Anterior surface of ciliary body faces towards

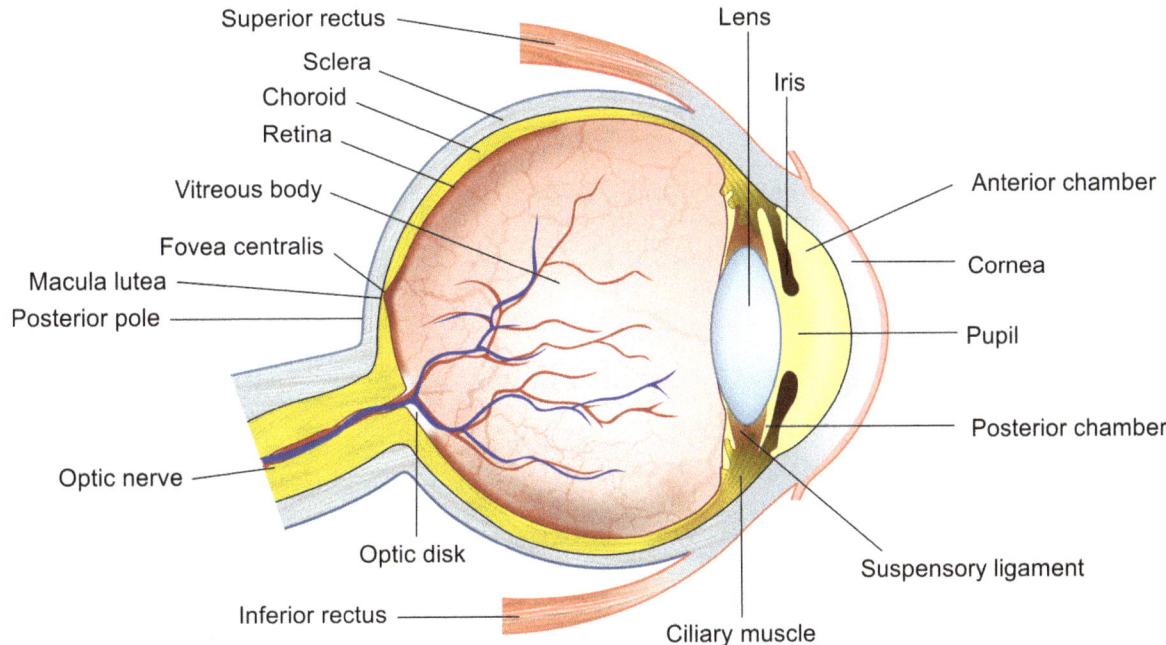

FIGURE 110.2: Structure of eyeball.

the center of cornea. From this surface, the iris arises (Fig. 110.2).

Ciliary body has three parts:
i. Orbiculus ciliaris.
ii. Ciliary body proper.
iii. Ciliary processes.

3. Iris

Iris is the thin-colored curtain-like structure of eyeball. It forms the anterior most part of middle layer (**Fig. 110.3**). It is like a thin **circular diaphragm**, placed in front of the lens. It has a circular opening in the center called **pupil**. Iris is a muscular structure and has two muscles:

Muscles of iris are:
i. **Constrictor papillae** or sphincter pupillae. Contraction of this muscle causes constriction of pupil.
ii. **Dilator papillae** or pupillary dilator muscle. Contraction of this muscle causes dilatation of pupil.

Activities of muscles of iris increase or decrease the diameter of the pupil and regulate the amount of light entering the eye. Thus, iris acts like the diaphragm of a camera.

Iris separates the space between cornea and lens into two chambers namely, the **anterior and posterior chambers**. Both the chambers communicate with each other through **pupil**. The lateral border of anterior chamber is angular in shape. It is called **iris angle** or angle of anterior chamber.

■ INNER LAYER OR TUNICA INTERNA OR TUNICA NERVOSA OR RETINA

Retina is the light-sensitive membrane that forms the innermost layer of eyeball. It extends from the margin of optic disk to just behind the ciliary body. Here, it ends abruptly as a dentated border known as **ora serrata**. Retina has the receptors of vision. Structurally, retina is made up of 10 layers:

Layers of retina from outside in:
1. Layer of pigment epithelium.
2. Layer of rods and cones.
3. External limiting membrane.
4. Outer nuclear layer.
5. Outer plexiform layer.
6. Inner nuclear layer.
7. Inner plexiform layer.
8. Ganglion cell layer.
9. Layer of nerve fibers.
10. Internal limiting membrane.

1. Layer of Pigment Epithelium

Pigment epithelial layer is the outermost layer situated adjacent to choroid. It is formed by a single layer of hexagonal epithelial cells which contain the pigment **melanin**.

2. Layer of Rods and Cones

This layer lies between pigment epithelial layer and external limiting membrane (**Fig. 110.4**). Rods and cones are the light sensitive portions of the **visual receptor cells**, the rod cells and the cone cells.

Receptor cells are arranged in a parallel fashion and are perpendicular to the inner surface of the eyeball.

3. External Limiting Membrane

It is a thin layer, formed by the chief supporting elements of retina called **Müller's fibers**.

4. Outer Nuclear Layer

Fibers and granules of rods and cones are present in this layer. The granules of rods and cones contain nucleus.

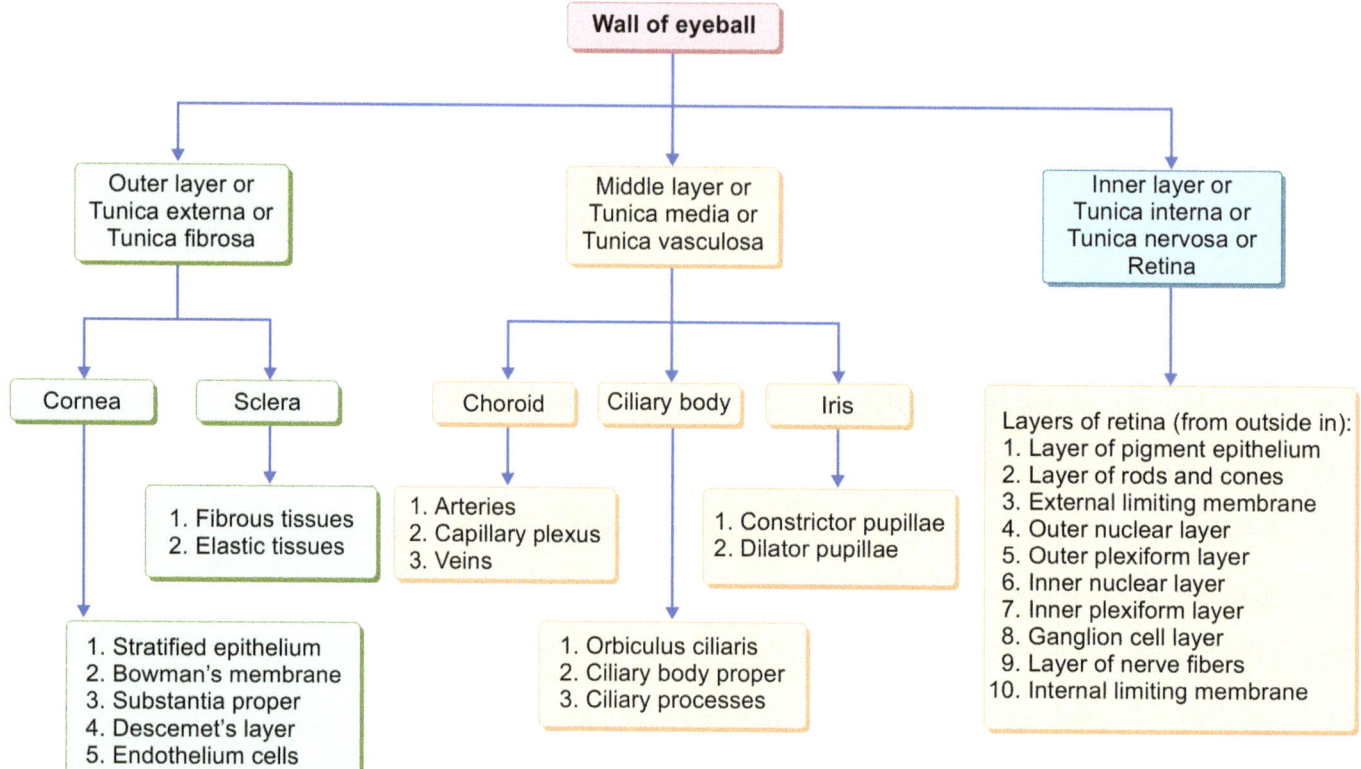

FIGURE 110.3: Wall of eyeball.

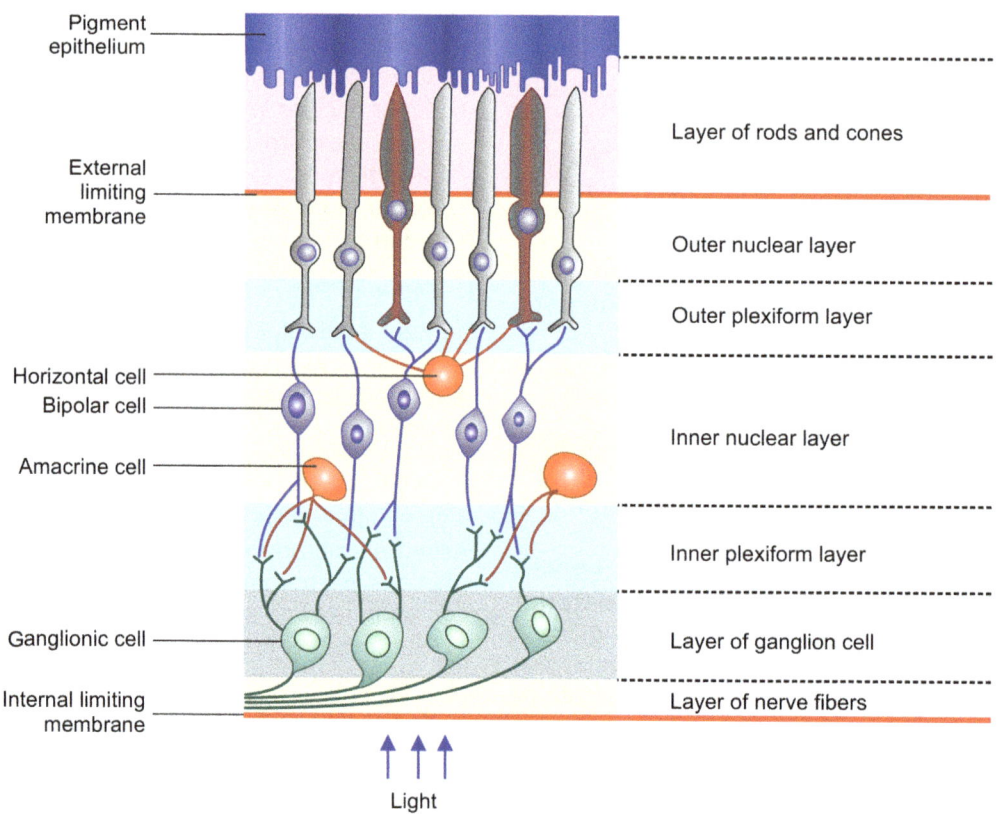

FIGURE 110.4: Layers of retina.

5. Outer Plexiform Layer

This layer contains reticular meshwork formed by the terminal fibers of rods and cones and the dendrites from bipolar cells, situated in the inner nuclear layer.

6. Inner Nuclear Layer

Inner nuclear layer contains small oval shaped flattened **bipolar cells**. Axons of the bipolar cells go inside and synapse with dendrites of ganglionic cells in the inner plexiform layer. Dendrites synapse with fibers of rods and cones in the outer plexiform layer.

Inner nuclear layer also contains nuclei of Müller's supporting fibers and some association neurons called **horizontal cells** and **amacrine cells**.

7. Inner Plexiform Layer

Inner plexiform layer of retina consists of synapses between dendrites of ganglionic cells and axons of bipolar cells.

8. Ganglion Cell Layer

Multipolar cells are present in this layer. Axons from ganglion cells are in the inner surface of the retina. These axons form the optic nerve. Dendrites of the ganglion cells synapse with axons of bipolar cells in the inner plexiform layer.

9. Layer of Nerve Fibers

This layer is formed by non-myelinated axons of **ganglionic cells**. After taking origin, the axons run horizontally to a short distance. Afterwards, the fibers converge towards the optic disk and form the **optic nerve**.

10. Internal Limiting Membrane

Internal limiting membrane forms the inner most layer of retina. It separates retina from the vitreous body. It is a hyaline membrane formed by the opposition of expanded ends of Müller fibers.

■ FUNDUS OCULI OR FUNDUS

Fundus oculi or **fundus** is the posterior part of interior of eyeball **(Fig. 110.5)**. It is examined by **ophthalmoscope**.

Fundus has two important structures:

1. Optic disk or optic papilla.
2. Macula lutea with fovea centralis.

■ OPTIC DISK: BLIND SPOT

Optic disk or **optic papilla** is a pale disk-like structure situated near the center of posterior wall of eyeball. It is formed by the convergence of axons from ganglion cells, while forming the optic nerve.

Optic disk contains all the layers of retina except rods and cones. Therefore, it is insensitive to light, i.e. the object is not seen if the image falls upon this area. Because of this, the optic disk is known as **blind spot**.

Blind Spot

Blind spot is a small portion of visual field of each eye that corresponds to the position of optic disk. Optic disk is

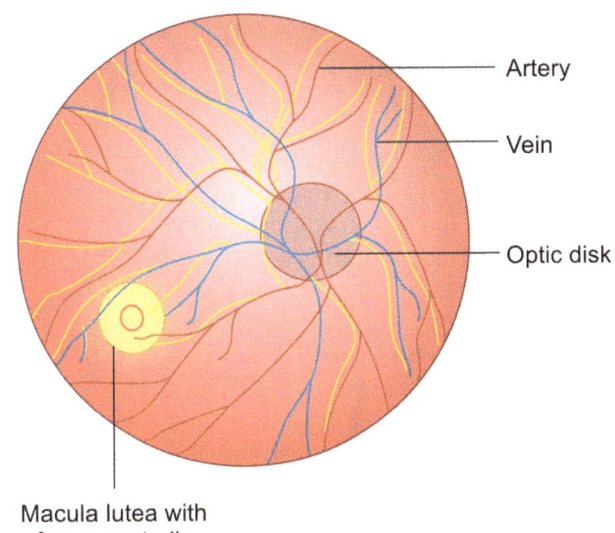

FIGURE 110.5: Fundus oculi.

insensitive to light because of absence of visual receptors. So, object is not seen if its image falls on optic disk. Therefore, a small blind spot is formed in visual field. Refer Chapter 111 for more details.

■ MACULA LUTEA

Macula lutea is a small yellowish area situated lateral to optic disk in retina. It is also called **yellow spot**. The yellow color of macula lutea is due to the presence of a **yellow pigment**. Macula lutea has fovea centralis in its center.

Fovea Centralis

Fovea centralis is a **minute depression** in the center of macula lutea. Fovea is the region of the most acute vision because it contains only cones. When one looks at an object, the eyeballs are directed towards the object, so that the image of that object falls on the fovea of each eye and the person can see the object very clearly. It is known as **foveal vision**.

Vision in other parts of retina is called peripheral or **extrafoveal vision**. It is less sensitive and enables the subject to gain only a dim and an ill-defined impression of surroundings.

■ INTRAOCULAR FLUID

Intraocular fluid (fluid in eyeball) is responsible for the maintenance of shape of the eyeball.

Intraocular fluid is of two types:

1. Vitreous humor.
2. Aqueous humor.

■ VITREOUS HUMOR OR VITREOUS BODY

Vitreous humor or vitreous body is a viscous fluid present behind the lens in the space between the lens and retina. It is a highly **viscous** and **gelatinous** substance. It is formed by a fine fibrillar network of **proteoglycan molecules**. Vitreous humor helps to maintain the shape of the eyeball.

AQUEOUS HUMOR

Aqueous humor is a **thin fluid** present in front of lens. It fills the space between the lens and cornea. This space is divided into anterior and posterior chambers by iris. Both the chambers communicate with each other through pupil.

Aqueous humor is formed by **ciliary processes**. It is derived from plasma within capillary network of ciliary process by diffusion, ultrafiltration and active transport through the epithelial cells lining the ciliary processes. After formation, aqueous humor reaches the posterior chamber by passing through the suspensory ligaments. From here, it reaches the anterior chamber via pupil.

From anterior chamber, the aqueous humor passes through the angle between cornea and iris, meshwork of **trabeculae** and **canal of Schlemm**, and reaches the venous system via anterior **ciliary vein**.

Functions of aqueous humor

Aqueous humor

i. Maintains shape of the eyeball.
ii. Maintains the intraocular pressure.
iii. Provides nutrients, oxygen and electrolytes to the avascular structures like lens and cornea.
iv. Removes metabolic end products from lens and cornea.

INTRAOCULAR PRESSURE

Intraocular pressure is the measure of **fluid pressure** in the eye exerted by **aqueous humor**. Normal intraocular pressure varies from 12 to 20 mm Hg. It is measured by tonometer. High intraocular pressure is associated with glaucoma (see below) and blindness.

LENS

Lens of the eyeball is **crystalline** in nature. It is situated behind the pupil. It is a biconvex, transparent and elastic structure. Lens is avascular and receives its nutrition mainly from the aqueous humor.

Lens refracts light rays and helps to focus the image of the objects on retina. The focal length of human lens is 44 mm and its refractory power is 23 D.

Lens is supported by the **suspensory ligaments** (zonular fibers) which are attached with **ciliary bodies**.

STRUCTURE OF LENS

Lens is formed from three components:

1. Capsule.
2. Anterior epithelium.
3. Lens substance.

1. Capsule

Capsule is a clear elastic membrane that covers the lens.

2. Anterior Epithelium

Anterior epithelium is a single layer of cuboidal epithelial cells, situated beneath the capsule. At the margins, epithelial cells are elongated. Epithelial cells give rise to lens fibers present in the lens substance.

3. Lens Substance

Lens is formed by long lens fibers derived from anterior epithelium. Lens fibers are **prismatic** in nature and are arranged in concentric layers.

CHANGES IN THE LENS DURING OLD AGE

In old age, the elastic property of lens is decreased due to the physical changes in lens and its capsule. It causes **presbyopia**.

In old age, lens also becomes opaque and this condition is called **cataract** (see below).

OCULAR MUSCLES

MUSCLES OF THE EYEBALL

Muscles of the eyeball are of two types:

I. Intrinsic muscles.
II. Extrinsic muscles.

I. Intrinsic Muscles

Intrinsic muscles are formed by smooth muscle fibers and are controlled by the autonomic nerves.

Intrinsic muscles of the eye are:

1. Constrictor pupillae.
2. Dilator pupillae.
3. Ciliary muscle.

II. Extrinsic Muscles

Extrinsic muscles are formed by skeletal muscle fibers and are controlled by the somatic nerves. The eyeball moves within the orbit by six extrinsic skeletal muscles (**Fig. 110.6**). One end of each muscle is attached to the eyeball and the other end to the wall of orbital cavity. There are four straight muscles (rectus) and two oblique muscles:

Extrinsic muscles of eye are:

1. Superior rectus.
2. Inferior rectus.
3. Medial or internal rectus.
4. Lateral or external rectus.
5. Superior oblique.
6. Inferior oblique.

INNERVATION OF OCULAR MUSCLES

Innervation of Intrinsic Muscles

Intrinsic muscles of eyeball are innervated by both sympathetic and parasympathetic divisions of autonomic nervous system.

Parasympathetic nerve fibers

Parasympathetic preganglionic fibers arise from **Edinger-Westphal nucleus** of III cranial nerve. After passing through III cranial nerve, these fibers synapse with postganglionic neurons in **ciliary ganglion**.

Postganglionic fibers arising from here pass through **short ciliary nerves** and innervate the **ciliary muscle** and **constrictor pupillae**.

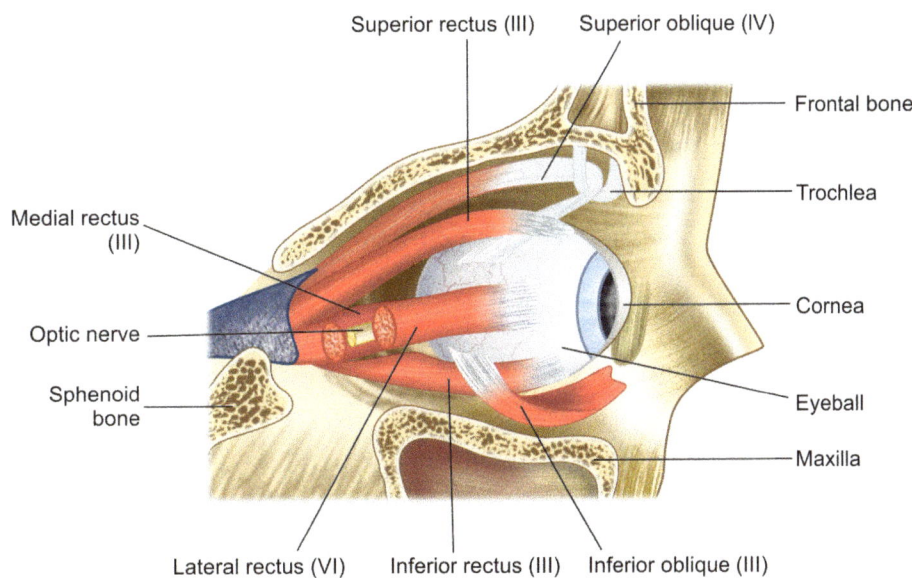

FIGURE 110.6: Extrinsic muscles of eyeball. Numbers in parenthesis indicate the cranial nerve supplying the muscle.

Stimulation of parasympathetic nerve fibers causes **contraction** of ciliary muscle and constrictor pupillae resulting in constriction of pupil.

Sympathetic nerve fibers

Sympathetic preganglionic nerve fibers arise from lateral horn of first thoracic segment of spinal cord, pass through **sympathetic chain** and synapse with neurons of **superior cervical sympathetic ganglion**.

Postganglionic fibers arising from this ganglion run along with carotid artery and its branches, to reach the intrinsic muscles of the eyeball.

Stimulation of sympathetic nerve fibers causes **relaxation** of ciliary muscle and **contraction** of dilator pupillae resulting in dilatation of pupil.

Innervation of Extrinsic Muscles

Extrinsic muscles of the eyeball are innervated by somatic motor nerve fibers. Somatic nerve fibers arise from the cranial nerve nuclei in brainstem and reach the ocular muscles via three cranial nerves:

1. Oculomotor nerve (third cranial nerve) which supplies:
   i. Superior rectus.
   ii. Inferior rectus.
   iii. Medial rectus (internal rectus).
   iv. Inferior oblique.
2. Trochlear nerve (fourth cranial nerve) which supplies the superior oblique.
3. Abducens nerve (sixth) which supplies the lateral rectus (external rectus).

■ OCULAR MOVEMENTS

Eyeball moves or rotates within the orbital socket in all the three primary axes, vertical, transverse and anteroposterior axis **(Fig. 110.7 and Table 110.1)**.

■ MOVEMENTS IN VERTICAL AXIS OR IN HORIZONTAL PLANE

1. Abduction or Lateral Movement or Outward Movement

Abduction of eyeball is due to the contraction of **lateral rectus** mainly. It is supported by the two **oblique muscles**.

2. Adduction or Medial Movement or Inward Movement

Adduction of the eyeball occurs because of the action of **medial or internal rectus,** along with action of superior **rectus** and **inferior rectus**.

■ MOVEMENTS IN TRANSVERSE AXIS OR IN SAGITTAL PLANE

1. Elevation or Upward Movement

Elevation of eyeball occurs because of the contraction of **superior rectus** and **inferior oblique muscles**.

2. Depression or Downward Movement

Depression of eyeball is brought out by **inferior rectus** and **superior oblique**.

■ MOVEMENTS IN ANTEROPOSTERIOR AXIS

Movements of eyeball in anteroposterior axis or in the frontal plane are called **torsion** or **wheel movements**. Torsion movements are two types, namely extorsion and intorsion.

1. Extorsion

During extorsion, the top of eyeball is rotated upward and outward direction away from nose. This movement is due to contraction of **inferior oblique and inferior rectus**.

2. Intorsion

During intorsion, the top of eyeball is rotated downward and inward direction towards nose. It is produced by the

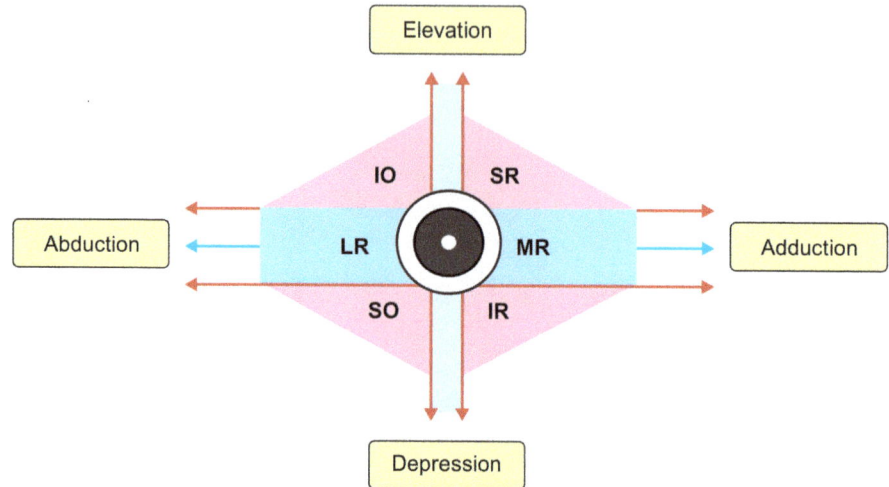

FIGURE 110.7: Diagram showing the movements of right eye. MR = Medial rectus. SO = Superior oblique. LR = Lateral rectus. IO = Inferior oblique. SR = Superior rectus. IR = Inferior rectus.

TABLE 110.1: Muscles taking part in ocular movements.

Movement	Primary muscle	Secondary muscle
1. Abduction	Lateral rectus	Superior oblique Inferior oblique
2. Adduction	Medial rectus	Superior rectus Inferior rectus
3. Elevation	Superior rectus	Inferior oblique
4. Depression	Inferior rectus	Superior oblique
5. Extorsion	Inferior oblique	Inferior rectus
6. Intorsion	Superior oblique	Superior rectus

contraction of **superior oblique** and **superior rectus muscles**.

SIMULTANEOUS MOVEMENTS OF BOTH EYEBALLS

Simultaneous movements of both eyeballs are of four types.

1. Conjugate Movement

Conjugate movement is the movement of both eyeballs in the **same direction**. Visual axes of both eyes remain parallel. It is due to contraction of **medial rectus** of one eye and **lateral rectus** of the other eye.

2. Disjugate Movement

Disjugate movement is the movement of both eyeballs in **opposite direction**. There are two types of disjugate movements, namely convergence and divergence.

i. *Convergence*: Convergence is the movement of both eyeballs towards nose. It is due to simultaneous contraction of medial rectus and simultaneous relaxation of lateral rectus of both eyes. Visual axes move close to each other. Convergence of eyeballs occurs during accommodation.

ii. *Divergence*: Divergence is the movement of both eyeballs towards temporal side. It is due to the simultaneous contraction of lateral rectus and simultaneous relaxation of medial rectus of both eyes. Visual axes of the eyes move away from each other.

3. Pursuit Movement

Pursuit movement is the movement of eyeballs along with object, when eyeballs follow a moving object.

4. Saccadic Movement

Saccadic movement is the quick jerky movement of both eyeballs when the fixation of eyes (gaze) is shifted from one object to another object. It is also called **optokinetic movement**.

APPLIED PHYSIOLOGY

GLAUCOMA

Glaucoma is an eye disease characterized by increase in intraocular pressure above 60 mm Hg resulting in damage of optic nerve and blindness. Intraocular pressure increases due to the blockage in the drainage of aqueous humor.

CATARACT

Cataract is the **opacity** or **cloudiness** in the natural lens of the eye. It is the major cause of blindness worldwide. When the lens becomes cloudy, light rays cannot pass through it easily, and vision is blurred. Cataract develops in old age after 55 to 60 years.

Lens is situated within the sealed capsule. Old cells die and accumulate within the capsule. Over years, the accumulation of cells is associated with accumulation of fluid and denaturation of the proteins in the lens fibers causing cloudiness of lens and blurred image.

Cataract is treated by surgery. The cloudy lens is removed from the eye through a surgical incision. Natural lens is replaced with a permanent, clear and plastic **intraocular lens implant** or IOL implant.

Chapter 111: Visual Process and Field of Vision

CHAPTER OUTLINE

- **VISUAL PROCESS**
  - IMAGE FORMING MECHANISM
  - NEURAL BASIS OF VISUAL PROCESS
  - STRUCTURE OF VISUAL RECEPTORS
  - FUNCTIONS OF VISUAL RECEPTORS
  - CHEMICAL BASIS OF VISUAL PROCESS
  - ELECTRICAL BASIS OF VISUAL PROCESS
  - ACUITY OF VISION
- **FIELD OF VISION**
  - DEFINITION
  - BINOCULAR AND MONOCULAR VISION
  - DIVISIONS OF VISUAL FIELD
  - CORRESPONDING RETINAL POINTS
  - BLIND SPOT
  - VISUAL FIELD AND RETINA
  - MAPPING OF VISUAL FIELD

VISUAL PROCESS

Visual process is the series of actions taking place during **visual perception**. When the image of an object is focused on **retina**, the energy in visual spectrum is converted into **electrical potentials** (impulses) by rods and cones of retina through some chemical reactions. Impulses from **rods and cones** reach the **cerebral cortex** through **optic nerve**. And, the sensation of vision is produced in cerebral cortex.

Thus, process of visual sensation can be explained on the basis of image formation, and neural, chemical and electrical phenomena.

IMAGE FORMING MECHANISM

While looking at an object, the light rays from the object are refracted and brought to a focus upon retina. The image falls on the retina in an inverted position and reversed side to side. In spite of this, the object is seen in an upright position. It is because of cerebral cortex.

Light rays are refracted by the lens and cornea. Refractory power is measured in diopter (D). A diopter is the reciprocal of focal length expressed in meters. Focal length of cornea is 24 mm and refractory power is 42 D. Focal length of lens is 44 mm and refractory power is 23 D.

NEURAL BASIS OF VISUAL PROCESS

Retina has the **visual receptors** which are also called **photoreceptors**. The photoreceptors are rods and cones. There are about 6 million cones and 12 million rods in the human eye. Distribution of the photoreceptors varies in different areas of retina. Fovea has only cones and no rods. While proceeding from fovea towards the periphery of retina, the rods increase and the cones decrease in number. At the periphery of the retina, only rods are present and cones are absent.

STRUCTURE OF VISUAL RECEPTORS

Structure of Rod Cell

Rod cells are cylindrical structures with a length of about 40 to 60 μ and a diameter of about 2 μ.

Each rod cell has four structures:

1. Outer segment.
2. Inner segment.
3. Cell body.
4. Synaptic terminal.

1. Outer segment

Outer segment of rod cell is long, slender and gives the rod like appearance. Outer segment of rod cell is formed by the modified cilia and it contains a pile of freely floating flat **membranous disks.** There are about 1,000 disks in each rod. Disks in rod cells are closed structures and contain the photosensitive pigment, the **rhodopsin.**

2. Inner segment

Inner segment is connected to outer segment by means of a modified **connecting cilium.** Inner segment contains many types of organelles with large number of mitochondria **(Fig. 111.1)**.

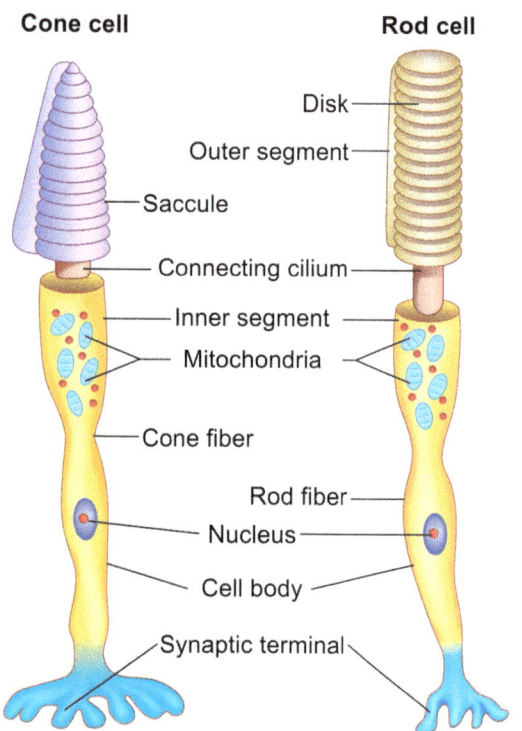

FIGURE 111.1: Structure of visual receptors.

3. Cell body

A rod fiber arises from inner segment of the rod cell and passes to outer nuclear layer through external limiting membrane. In outer nuclear layer, the enlarged portion of this fiber forms the cell body or rod granule that contains the nucleus.

4. Synaptic terminal

A thick fiber arising from cell body passes to outer plexiform layer and ends in a small and enlarged synaptic terminal or body. Synaptic terminal of the rod cell synapses with dendrites of **bipolar cells** and **horizontal cells**. Synaptic vesicles present in the synaptic terminal contain neurotransmitter, **glutamate.**

Structure of Cone Cell

Generally, the cone cell is flask shaped. It has a length of 35 to 40 μ and a diameter of about 5 μ.

Like rod cell, cone cell also has four parts:

1. Outer segment.
2. Inner segment.
3. Cell body.
4. Synaptic terminal.

1. Outer segment

Outer segment is small and conical without membranous disks. In cone, infoldings of cell membrane form **saccules**, which are the counterparts of rod disks.

Photopigment of cone is synthesized in the inner segment and incorporated into the folding of surface membrane forming **saccule.**

2. Inner segment

In cones also, the inner segment is connected to outer segment by a modified connecting cilium as in the case of rods. Though various types of organelles are present in this segment, the number of mitochondria is more.

3. Cell body

Cone fiber arising from inner segment is thick and it enters the inner nuclear layer through external limiting membrane. In the inner nuclear layer, cone fiber forms the cell body or cone granule that possesses nucleus.

4. Synaptic terminal

Fiber from cell body of cone leaves the inner nuclear layer and enters outer plexiform layer. Here, it ends in the form of an enlarged synaptic terminal or body. Synaptic vesicle present in the synaptic terminal of cone cell also possesses the neurotransmitter, **glutamate**.

■ FUNCTIONS OF VISUAL RECEPTORS

Functions of Rods

Rods are very sensitive to light and have a **low threshold**. So, the rods are responsible for **dim light vision** or **night vision** or **scotopic vision**. But rods are not responsible for acute vision or color vision. The vision by rod is black, white or in the combination of black and white namely, gray. Therefore, the colored objects appear faded or grayish in twilight.

Functions of Cones

Cones have **high threshold** for light stimulus. So, the cones are sensitive only to bright light. Therefore, the cone cells are responsible for **bright light vision** or **photopic vision** or **day light vision**. Cones are also responsible for **acuity of vision** and the **color vision**.

Differences between rods and cones are listed in **Table 111.1**.

■ CHEMICAL BASIS OF VISUAL PROCESS

Photosensitive pigments present in rods and cones form chemical basis of visual process. Chemical reactions of these pigments lead to the development of electrical activity in retina and generation of impulses (action potentials) in optic nerve. Photochemical changes in the visual receptors are called **Wald's visual cycle**.

Rhodopsin

Rhodopsin is the **photosensitive pigment** of rod cells. Rhodopsin is made up of a protein called **opsin** and a **chromophore**. Opsin present in rhodopsin is known as **scotopsin**. Chromophore is a chemical substance that develops color in the cell. The chromophore present in the rod cells is called **retinal**. The retinal is the aldehyde of vitamin A or **retinol**.

Photochemical Changes in Rhodopsin

During exposure to light, rhodopsin is bleached and it is split into **retinine** and the protein called **opsin** through

TABLE 111.1: Rods vs cones.

Features	Rods	Cones
1. Number in each eye	12 million	6 million
2. Length	40 to 60 μ	35 to 40 μ
3. Diameter	2 μ	5 μ
4. Shape	Cylindrical	Flask shaped
5. Outer segment	Long and slender	Small and conical
6. Sensitivity to light	More sensitive	Sensitive only to bright light
7. Threshold	Low	High
8. Type of vision responsible for	Dim light vision or night vision or scotopic vision	Bright light vision or day light vision or photopic vision
9. Acuity of vision	Not responsible	Responsible
10. Color vision	Not responsible	Responsible
11. Photosensitive pigment	Rhodopsin	Porphyropsin or iodopsin or cyanopsin

various intermediate photochemical reactions. The **metarhodopsin** produced during these reactions is the **activated rhodopsin**. It is responsible for development of receptor potential in rod cells.

Phototransduction: Visual Transduction

Phototransduction or visual transduction is the process in visual receptors by which **light energy** is converted into **electrical energy** (action potentials) in optic nerve fibers.

The resting membrane potential in other sensory receptor cells is usually between – 70 and – 90 mV. However, in the visual receptors in dark, the negativity is reduced and the resting membrane potential is about – 40 mV. When light falls on retina, the rhodopsin is converted into metarhodopsin. Metarhodopsin causes **mild hyperpolarization** which is called **receptor potential** in the rod cells.

Thus, the process of receptor potential in visual receptors is different from that of other sensory receptors. When other sensory receptors are excited, the electrical response is in the form of depolarization. But, in visual receptors, the response is in the form of **hyperpolarization**.

Significance of Hyperpolarization

Hyperpolarization in rod cells leads to the development of response in bipolar cells and ganglionic cells so that the action potentials are transmitted to cerebral cortex via optic pathway.

Photosensitive Pigment in Cone Cells

Photosensitive pigment in the cone cells are porphyropsin, iodopsin and cyanopsin. Only one of these pigments is present in each cone. Each type of cone pigment is sensitive to a particular color.

The processes involved in phototransduction in cone cells are similar to those in the rod cells.

Dark Adaptation

Dark adaptation is the process by which the person is able to see the objects in dim light. If a person enters a dim lighted room (darkroom) from a bright lighted area, he is blind for some time, i.e. he cannot see any object. After sometime his eyes get adapted and he starts seeing the objects slowly. Maximum duration for dark adaptation is about 20 minutes.

Causes for dark adaptation

1. *Resynthesis of rhodopsin:* Time required for dark adaptation is partly determined by the time to resynthesize rhodopsin. In bright light, much of the pigment is being bleached (broken down). But in dim light, it requires sometime for the regeneration of certain amount of rhodopsin, which is necessary for optimal rod function.
2. *Dilatation of pupil:* Dilatation of pupil during dark adaptation allows more and more light to enter the eye.

Light Adaptation

Light adaptation is the process in which eyes get adapted to bright light. When a person enters a bright lighted area from a dim lighted area, he feels discomfort due to the dazzling effect of bright light. After some time, when the eyes become adapted to light, he sees the objects around him without any discomfort. It is the mere disappearance of dark adaptation. The maximum period for light adaptation is about 5 minutes.

Causes for light adaptation

1. Reduced sensitivity of rods during light adaptation due to the breakdown of rhodopsin.
2. Constriction of pupil which reduces quantity of light rays entering the eye.

Night Blindness

Night blindness is defined as the loss of vision in dim light. It is otherwise called **nyctalopia** or defective dim light (scotopic) vision.

Causes of night blindness

Night blindness is due to **vitamin A deficiency.** Vitamin A is essential for function of visual receptors.

Deficiency of vitamin A occurs because of:
1. Diet containing less amount of vitamin A.
2. Decreased absorption of vitamin A from the intestine.

Initially, vitamin A deficiency causes **defective rod function**. Prolonged deficiency leads to **anatomical changes** in rods and cones, and finally the **degeneration** of other retinal layers occurs. So, retinal function can be restored, only if treatment is given with vitamin A before the visual receptors start degenerating.

■ ELECTRICAL BASIS OF VISUAL PROCESS

Definition

Electroretinogram (ERG) is the record of electrical activity in retina. When light rays stimulate the retina, potential changes occur, which can be recorded in the form of ERG. Recording ERG is a diagnostic procedure. It is useful in determining retinal disorders such as **cone dystrophy** (degeneration of cones) and **retinitis pigmentosa** (hyperactivity of the pigmented retinal epithelial cells, leading to damage of photoreceptors and blindness).

Waves of ERG

Electroretinogram has 4 waves namely 'A', 'B', 'C' and 'D' **(Fig. 111.2)**. 'A' is the only negative wave and other three are positive waves. 'A', 'B' and 'C' waves occur when light stimulus falls on retina. 'D' wave occurs when light stimulus is stopped. 'A' and 'B' waves arise from rods and cones. 'C' wave arises from pigment epithelial layer and 'D' wave arises from inner nuclear layer.

■ ACUITY OF VISION

Definition

Acuity of vision is the ability of the eye to determine the precise shape and details of the object. It is also called **visual acuity**. **Cones** of the retina are responsible for acuity of vision. Visual acuity is highly exhibited in **fovea centralis**, which contains only cones. It is greatly reduced during the refractive errors.

Test for Acuity of Vision

Acuity of vision is tested for distant vision as well as near vision. If there is any difficulty in seeing the distant object or the near object, the defect is known as **refractive errors**. The refractive errors are described separately in Chapter 115.

Distant vision

Snellen's chart is used to test the acuity of vision for **distant vision** in the diagnosis of refractive errors of the eye.

Near vision

Jaeger's chart is used to test the visual acuity for **near vision**.

■ FIELD OF VISION
■ DEFINITION

Part of the external world seen by one eye when it is fixed in one direction is called field of vision or **visual field** of that eye.

■ BINOCULAR AND MONOCULAR VISION

Binocular Vision

Binocular vision is the vision in which both the eyes are **used together**, so that a portion of external world is seen by the eyes together. In human and some animals, the eyeballs are placed in front of the head. So, the visual fields of both the eyes overlap. Because of this, a portion of the external world is seen by both the eyes.

Monocular Vision

It is the vision in which each eye is **used separately**. In some animals like dog, rabbit and horse, the eyeballs are present at the sides of head. So, the visual fields of both eyes overlap to a very small extent. Because of this, different portion of the external world is seen by each eye.

■ DIVISIONS OF VISUAL FIELD

Visual field of human eye has an angle of 160° in horizontal meridian and 135° in vertical meridian.

Visual field is divided into four parts:
1. Temporal field.
2. Nasal field.
3. Upper field.
4. Lower field.

Temporal and Nasal Fields

Visual field of each eye is divided into two unequal parts namely, outer or temporal field and the inner or nasal field by a vertical line passing through the fixation point **(Fig. 111.3)**.

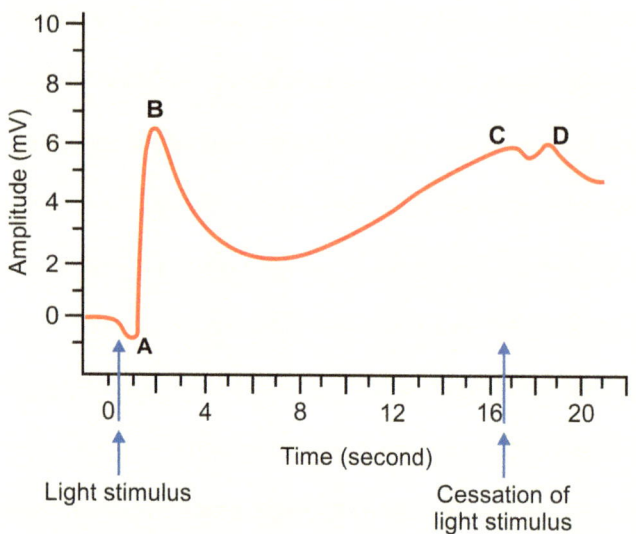

FIGURE 111.2: Electroretinogram.

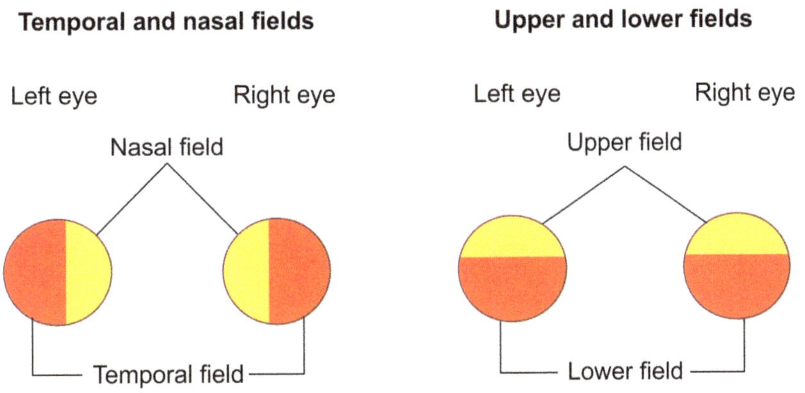

FIGURE 111.3: Divisions of visual field.

The **fixation point** is the meeting point of visual axis with the object.

Temporal part of visual field extends up to about 100°, but the nasal part extends only up to 60° because it is restricted by nose.

Upper and Lower Fields

Visual field of each eye is also divided into an upper field and a lower field by a horizontal line passing through the fixation point. The extent of the upper field is about 60° as it is restricted by upper eyelid and orbital margin. The extent of lower field is about 75°. It is restricted by cheek.

Thus, the visual field is restricted in all the sides except in the temporal part.

CORRESPONDING RETINAL POINTS

Corresponding retinal points are the area in retina of both eyes on which the light rays from the object falls. It occurs in the binocular vision. Two images developed on retina of both eyes are fused into a single sensation. So, we see the objects with single image.

Diplopia

Diplopia means **double vision**. Normal single sensation is because of the ocular muscles, which direct the axes of the eyes in such a way that the light rays from the object fall upon the corresponding points of both retinas. If the light rays do not fall on the corresponding retinal points, diplopia occurs.

BLIND SPOT

Blind spot is the small area of retina where visual receptors are absent. The **optic disk** in the retina does not have any visual receptors and, if the image of any object falls on the optic disk, the object cannot be seen. So, this part of the retina is blind, hence the name **blind spot**.

Normally, the darkness in the visual field due to the blind spot does not cause any inconvenience because the fixation of each eye is at different angles. Even when one eye is closed or blind, the person is not aware of blind spot. However, one can recognize blind spot by some experimental procedures.

VISUAL FIELD AND RETINA

Light rays from different halves of each visual field do not fall on the same halves of the retina. Light rays from temporal part of visual field of an eye fall on the nasal half of retina of that eye. Similarly, the light rays from nasal part of visual field fall on the temporal half of retina of the same side.

MAPPING OF VISUAL FIELD

Shape and extent of visual field is mapped out by means of an instrument called **perimeter**. The visual field is also determined by **Bjerrum screen** or by **confrontation test**.

Chapter 112: Visual Pathway

CHAPTER OUTLINE

- **VISUAL PATHWAY**
  - VISUAL RECEPTORS
  - FIRST ORDER NEURONS
  - SECOND ORDER NEURONS
  - THIRD ORDER NEURONS
- **COURSE OF VISUAL PATHWAY**
  - OPTIC NERVE
  - OPTIC CHIASMA
  - OPTIC TRACT
- **LATERAL GENICULATE BODY: SUBCORTICAL CENTER**
- **OPTIC RADIATION**
- **VISUAL CORTEX: CORTICAL CENTER**
- **APPLIED PHYSIOLOGY**
  - ANOPIA
  - HEMIANOPIA
  - EFFECTS OF LESION AT DIFFERENT LEVELS OF VISUAL PATHWAY

■ VISUAL PATHWAY

Visual pathway or **optic pathway** is the nervous pathway that carries the retinal impulses to cerebral cortex. In binocular vision, the light rays from temporal (outer) half of visual field (Chapter 111) fall upon the nasal part of corresponding retina. Light rays from nasal (inner) half of visual field fall upon the temporal part of retina.

■ VISUAL RECEPTORS

Rods and cones, which are present in the retina of eye, form the visual receptors. Fibers from the visual receptors synapse with dendrites of **bipolar cells** of inner nuclear layer of retina.

■ FIRST ORDER NEURONS

First order neurons are **bipolar cells** in the retina. Axons from the bipolar cells synapse with dendrites of ganglionic cells.

■ SECOND ORDER NEURONS

Second order neurons are the **ganglionic cells** in ganglionic cell layer of retina. Axons of the ganglionic cells form optic nerve. Optic nerve leaves the eye and terminates in lateral geniculate body.

■ THIRD ORDER NEURONS

Third order neurons are in the **lateral geniculate body**. Fibers arising from here reach the **visual cortex**.

■ COURSE OF VISUAL PATHWAY

Visual pathway consists of six components:

1. Optic nerve.
2. Optic chiasma.
3. Optic tract.
4. Lateral geniculate body.
5. Optic radiation.
6. Visual cortex.

■ 1. OPTIC NERVE

Optic nerve is formed by the **axons of ganglionic cells (Fig. 112.1)**. Optic nerve leaves the eye through **optic disk**. Fibers from temporal part of retina are in lateral part of the nerve and carry the impulses from nasal half of visual field of same eye. Fibers from nasal part of retina are in medial part of the nerve and carry the impulses from temporal half of visual field of same eye.

■ 2. OPTIC CHIASMA

Medial fibers of each optic nerve cross the midline and join the uncrossed lateral fibers of opposite side to form the optic tract **(Fig. 112.1)**. Area of crossing of the optic nerve fibers is called optic chiasma.

■ 3. OPTIC TRACT

Optic tract is formed by uncrossed fibers of optic nerve on the same side and crossed fibers of optic nerve from the opposite side. All the fibers of optic tract run backward and

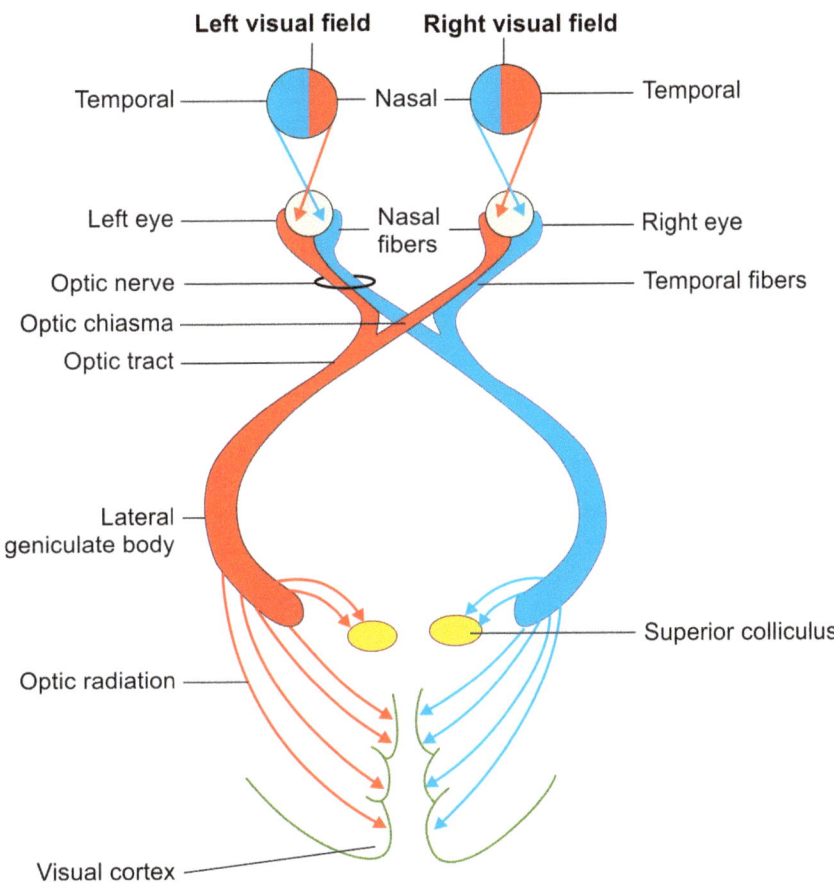

FIGURE 112.1: Visual pathway.

outward, and terminate in the lateral geniculate body in thalamus. Few fibers just pass through medial geniculate body and run towards superior colliculus in midbrain (see below).

Due to crossing of medial fibers in optic chiasma, the left optic tract carries impulses from temporal part of left retina and nasal part of right retina, i.e. it is responsible for vision in nasal half of left visual field and temporal half of right visual field. Right optic tract contains fibers from nasal half of left retina and temporal half of right retina. It is responsible for vision in temporal half of left visual field and nasal half of right visual field.

4. LATERAL GENICULATE BODY: SUBCORTICAL CENTER

Majority of the fibers of optic tract terminate in lateral geniculate body, which forms the **subcortical center** for visual sensation. From here, the **geniculocalcarine tract** or **optic radiation** arises. This tract is the last relay of visual pathway.

Some of the fibers from optic tract do not synapse in lateral geniculate body, but pass through it and terminate in one of the following centers:

i. **Superior colliculus** of midbrain which is concerned with **reflex movements of eyeballs** and head in response to optic stimulus.
ii. **Pretectal nucleus** of midbrain which is concerned with **light reflexes**.
iii. **Supraoptic nucleus** of hypothalamus which is concerned with the retinal **control of pituitary**.

5. OPTIC RADIATION

Fibers from lateral geniculate body pass through internal capsule and form optic radiation. Optic radiation ends in visual cortex **(Fig. 112.2)**.

6. VISUAL CORTEX: CORTICAL CENTER

Cortical center for vision is called visual cortex that is located on the medial surface of **occipital lobe**. It forms the walls and lips of calcarine fissure in medial surface of occipital lobe.

There is definite localization of retinal projections upon visual cortex. In fact, the point to point projection of retina upon visual cortex is well established. Peripheral retinal representation occupies the anterior part of visual cortex. Macular representation occupies the posterior part of visual cortex near the occipital pole.

Areas of Visual Cortex and Their Function

Three areas are present in visual cortex:

1. **Primary visual area (area 17)** which is concerned with perception of visual impulses.
2. **Visual association area (area 18)** which is concerned with interpretation of visual impulses.
3. **Occipital eye field (area 19)** which is concerned with movement of eyes.

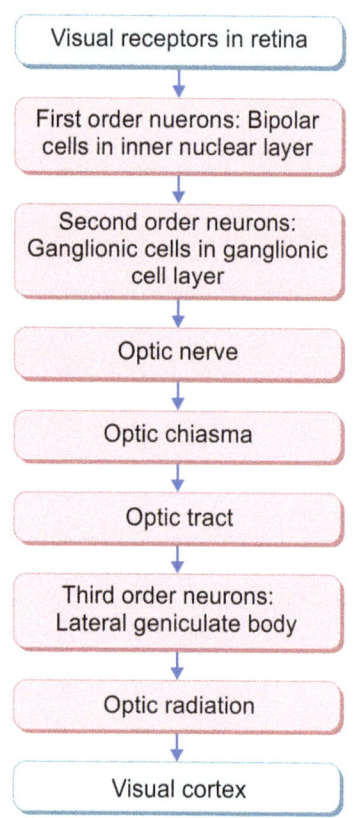

FIGURE 112.2: Schematic representation of visual pathway.

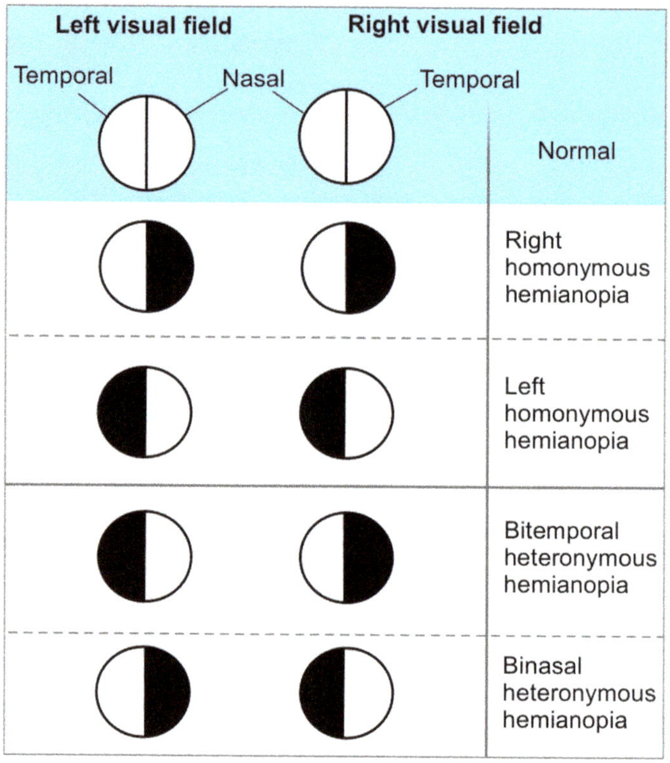

FIGURE 112.3: Types of hemianopia. Dark shade in circles indicates blindness.

APPLIED PHYSIOLOGY

Injury to any part of optic pathway causes visual defect and the nature of defect depends upon the location and extent of injury.

ANOPIA

Anopia or blindness is the loss of vision in one visual field.

HEMIANOPIA

Hemianopia is the loss of vision in one half of visual field (Figs. 112.3 to 112.5).

Hemianopia is classified into two types:
1. Homonymous hemianopia.
2. Heteronymous hemianopia.

1. Homonymous Hemianopia

Homonymous hemianopia means loss of vision in the **same halves** of both the visual fields. Loss of vision in right half of visual field of both eyes is known as **right homonymous hemianopia**. Similarly, **left homonymous hemianopia** means loss of vision in left half of visual field of both eyes.

2. Heteronymous Hemianopia

Heteronymous hemianopia means loss of vision in **opposite halves** of visual field. For example, **binasal heteronymous hemianopia** means loss of vision in right half of left visual field and left half of right visual field (nasal half of both visual fields).

Bitemporal heteronymous hemianopia is the loss of sight in left side of left visual field and right side of right visual field (temporal half of both visual fields).

EFFECTS OF LESION AT DIFFERENT LEVELS OF VISUAL PATHWAY

1. *Lesion of left optic nerve:* Total blindness (anopia) of left eye (Fig. 112.5: A).
2. *Lesion of right optic nerve:* Total blindness (anopia) of right eye (Fig. 112.5: B).
3. *Lesion of lateral fibers in left side of optic chiasma:* Left nasal hemianopia (Fig. 112.5: C).
4. *Lesion of lateral fibers in right side of optic chiasma:* Right nasal hemianopia (Fig. 112.5: D).
5. *Lesion of lateral fibers in both sides of optic chiasma:* Binasal hemianopia (Fig. 112.5: C + D).
6. *Lesion of medial fibers in optic chiasma:* Bitemporal hemianopia (Fig. 112.5: E).
7. *Lesion of left optic radiation:* Right homonymous hemianopia (Fig. 112.5: F).
8. *Lesion of right optic radiation:* Left homonymous hemianopia (Fig. 112.5: G).

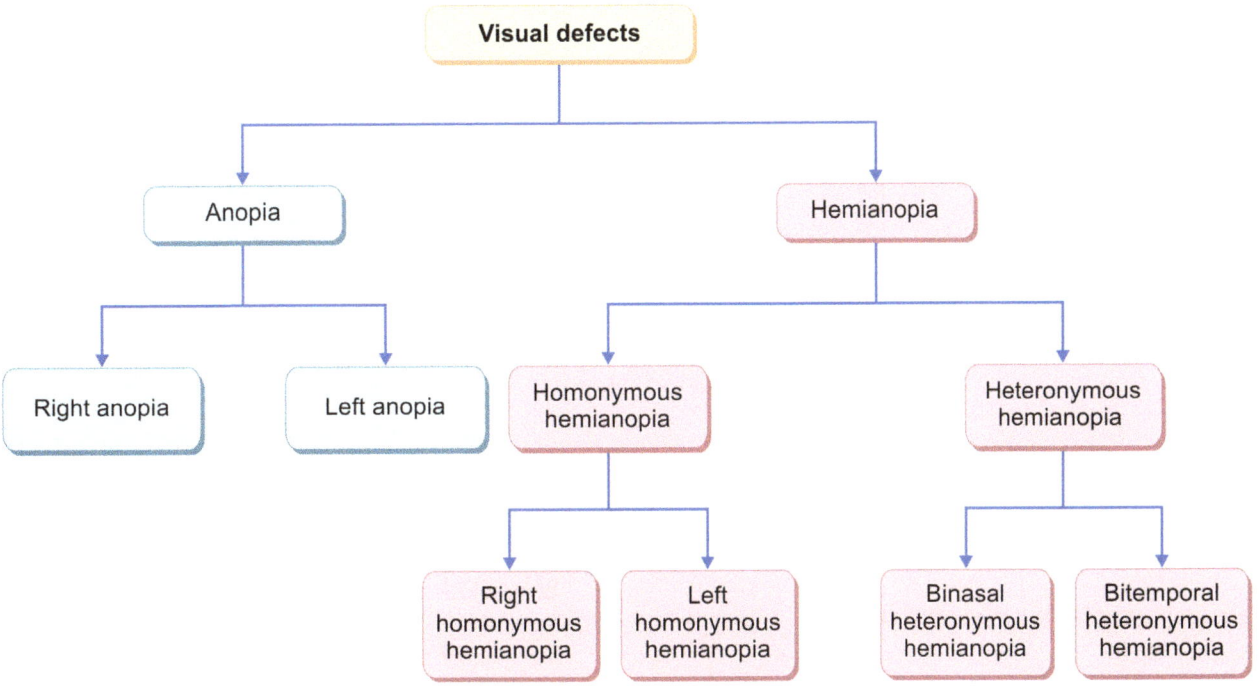

FIGURE 112.4: Visual defects.

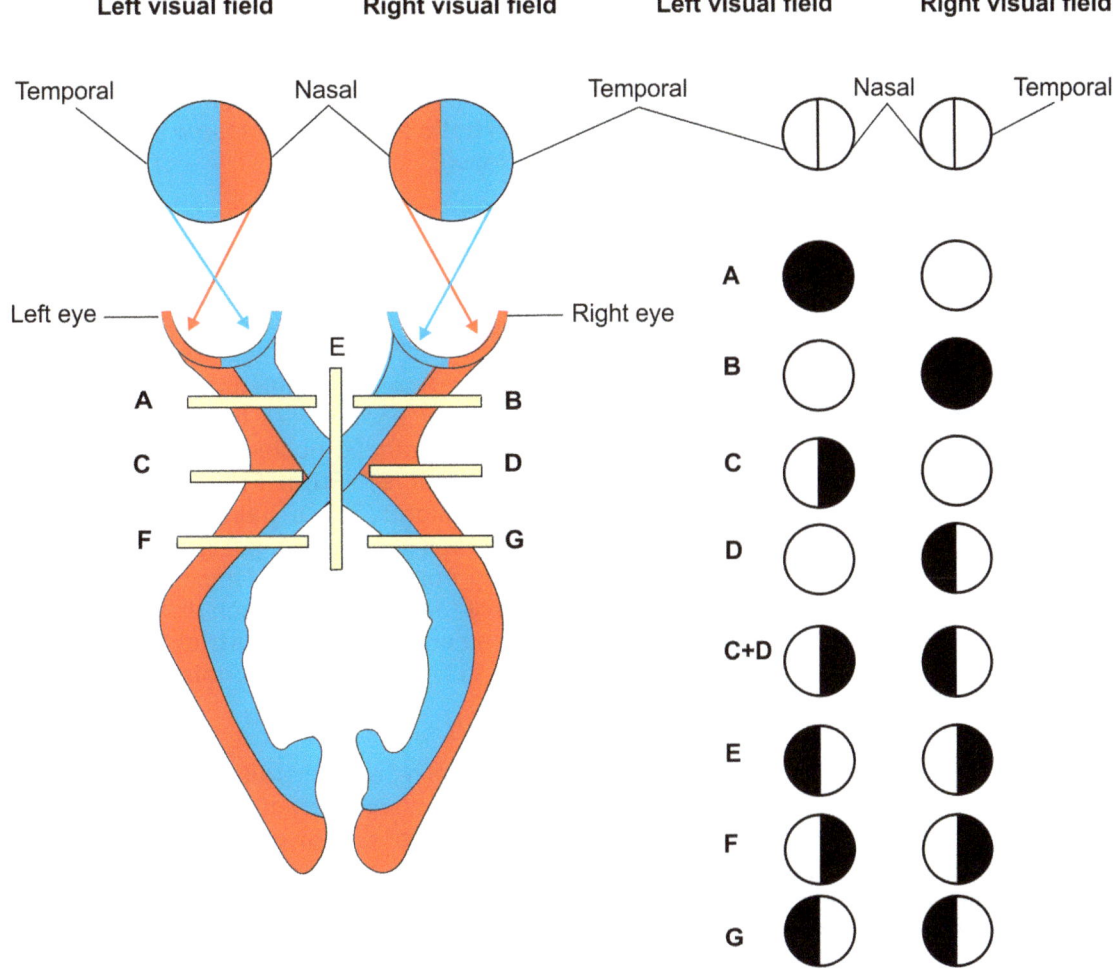

FIGURE 112.5: Effects of lesions of optic pathway. Dark shade in circles indicates blindness.

Chapter 113: Pupillary Reflexes

CHAPTER OUTLINE

- DEFINITION AND TYPES
- LIGHT REFLEX
  - PATHWAY FOR LIGHT REFLEX
- CILIOSPINAL REFLEX
- ACCOMMODATION
  - DEFINITION
  - MECHANISM OF ACCOMMODATION
- ACCOMMODATION REFLEX
- PATHWAY FOR ACCOMMODATION REFLEX
- APPLIED PHYSIOLOGY
  - PRESBYOPIA
  - ARGYLL ROBERTSON PUPIL
  - HORNER SYNDROME

DEFINITION AND TYPES

Pupillary reflexes are the **visceral reflexes**, which alter the **size of pupil**.

Pupillary reflexes are classified into three types:

1. Light reflex.
2. Ciliospinal reflex.
3. Accommodation reflex.

LIGHT REFLEX

It is the reflex in which the **pupil constricts** when light is flashed into the eyes. It is also called **pupillary light reflex**.

Light reflex is of two types:

1. **Direct light reflex** in which there is constriction of pupil in an eye when light is thrown into that eye. It is also called direct pupillary light reflex.
2. **Indirect light reflex** in which there is constriction of pupil in both eyes when light is thrown into one eye. It is otherwise called **consensual light reflex**.

PATHWAY FOR LIGHT REFLEX

Afferent Pathway

Pathway for light reflex is slightly deviated from visual pathway. When light falls on the eye, the visual receptors are stimulated. Afferent (sensory) impulses from the receptors pass through the optic nerve, optic chiasma and optic tract. At **midbrain**, some fibers get separated **from optic tract** and synapse with the neurons of pretectal nucleus.

Center

Pretectal nucleus of midbrain forms the center for light reflexes.

Efferent Pathway

Efferent (motor) impulses from pretectal nucleus are carried by short fibers to **Edinger-Westphal** nucleus (parasympathetic nucleus) of **oculomotor nerve** (third cranial nerve). From Edinger-Westphal nucleus, the preganglionic fibers pass through oculomotor nerve and reach the **ciliary ganglion**. Postganglionic fibers arising from the ciliary ganglion pass through the **short ciliary nerves** and reach the eyeball. These fibers cause contraction of **constrictor pupillae** muscle of iris **(Fig. 113.1)** resulting in **constriction of pupil**.

CILIOSPINAL REFLEX

Ciliospinal reflex is the **dilatation of pupil** in eyes caused by painful stimulation of **skin over neck**. It is due to the contraction of **dilator pupillae** muscle. Sensory impulses pass through cutaneous afferent nerve. Center is in first thoracic spinal segment. Efferent impulses pass through sympathetic fibers and reach dilator pupillae.

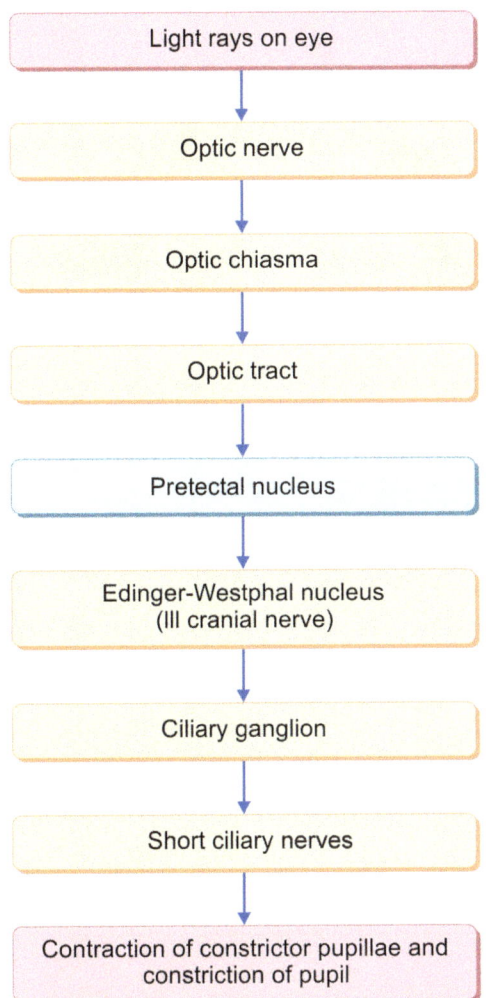

FIGURE 113.1: Pathway for light reflex.

ACCOMMODATION
DEFINITION

Accommodation is the adjustment of the eye to see either near or distant objects clearly. It is the process, by which light rays from near objects or distant objects are brought to a focus on the sensitive part of retina. It is achieved by various adjustments made in the eyeball.

MECHANISM OF ACCOMMODATION

During Distant Vision

Light rays from distant objects are approximately **parallel** and are less refracted while getting focused on retina. So, no adjustments are made in eye during distant vision.

During Near Vision

But, the light rays from near objects are **divergent**. So, to be focused on retina, these light rays must be **refracted (converged)** to a greater extent. Some adjustments are made in eyes in order to converge the light rays from the objects.

Adjustments in Eyeballs during Accommodation

Accommodation in near vision occurs by means of three adjustments made in the eyeballs:

1. Increase in anterior curvature of lens, so that the refractory power of lens is increased.
2. Convergence of both eyeballs which brings the retinal images on to the corresponding points.
3. Constriction of pupil that causes:
   i. Increase in the visual acuity.
   ii. Reduction in the quantity of light entering eye.
   iii. Increase in the depth of focus through more central part of lens as its convexity is increased.

Young-Helmholtz Theory

This theory describes how the curvature of lens increases and thereby, the refractive power of lens is enhanced. When the eyes are fixed on a distant object (distant vision), lens is flat due to the traction of **suspensory ligaments** which extend from the capsule of lens and are attached to the **ciliary processes**. The ciliary processes are attached to **choroid** through the ciliary muscle **(Fig. 113.2)**.

When the vision is shifted from the distant object to a near object (near vision), **ciliary muscle** contracts and draws the **choroid** forward. **Ciliary processes** are brought closer to lens. Because of this, the **suspensory ligaments** are slackened. Now, the tension on the lens is released. So, the **lens bulges** forward due to its elastic property. The anterior curvature (convexity) of lens increases greatly. A very little change occurs in posterior curvature.

In resting eye, the intraocular pressure sets up tension in choroids and pulls the ciliary processes backward and outward. Suspensory ligaments are tensed up and the lens becomes flat.

ACCOMMODATION REFLEX

Accommodation is a reflex action. When a person looks at a near object after seeing a far object, three adjustments are made in the eyeballs:

1. Increase in the anterior curvature of the lens due to contraction of the ciliary muscle.
2. Convergence of the eyeballs due to contraction of the medial recti.
3. Constriction of the pupil due to the contraction of constrictor pupillae of iris.

Thus, the accommodation reflex involves both skeletal muscle (medial recti) and smooth muscle (ciliary muscle and sphincter pupillae).

PATHWAY FOR ACCOMMODATION REFLEX

Afferent Pathway

Visual impulses from retina pass through the optic nerve, optic chiasma, optic tract, lateral geniculate body and optic radiation to visual cortex (area 17) of occipital lobe. From

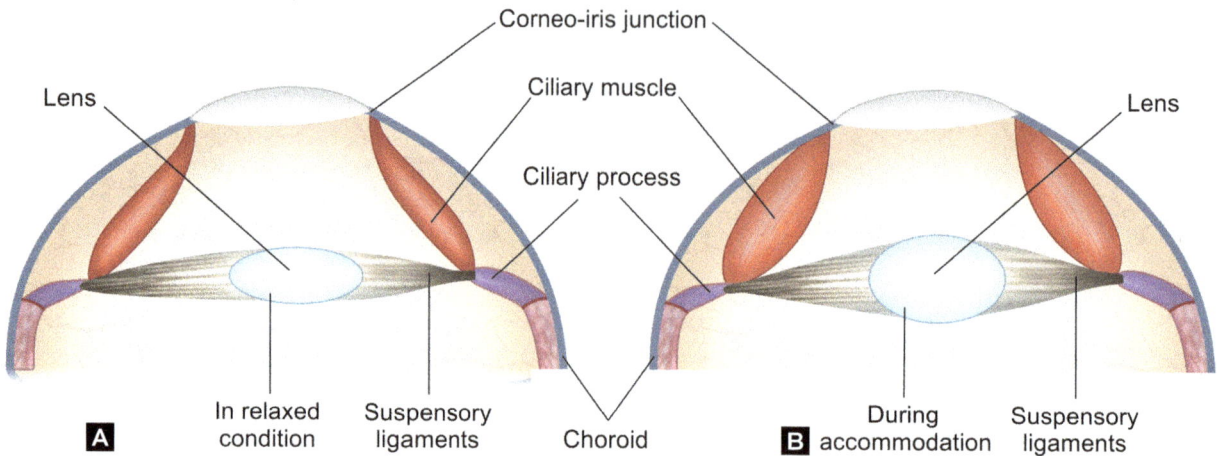

FIGURE 113.2: Accommodation. **A.** In relaxed condition; **B.** During accommodation.

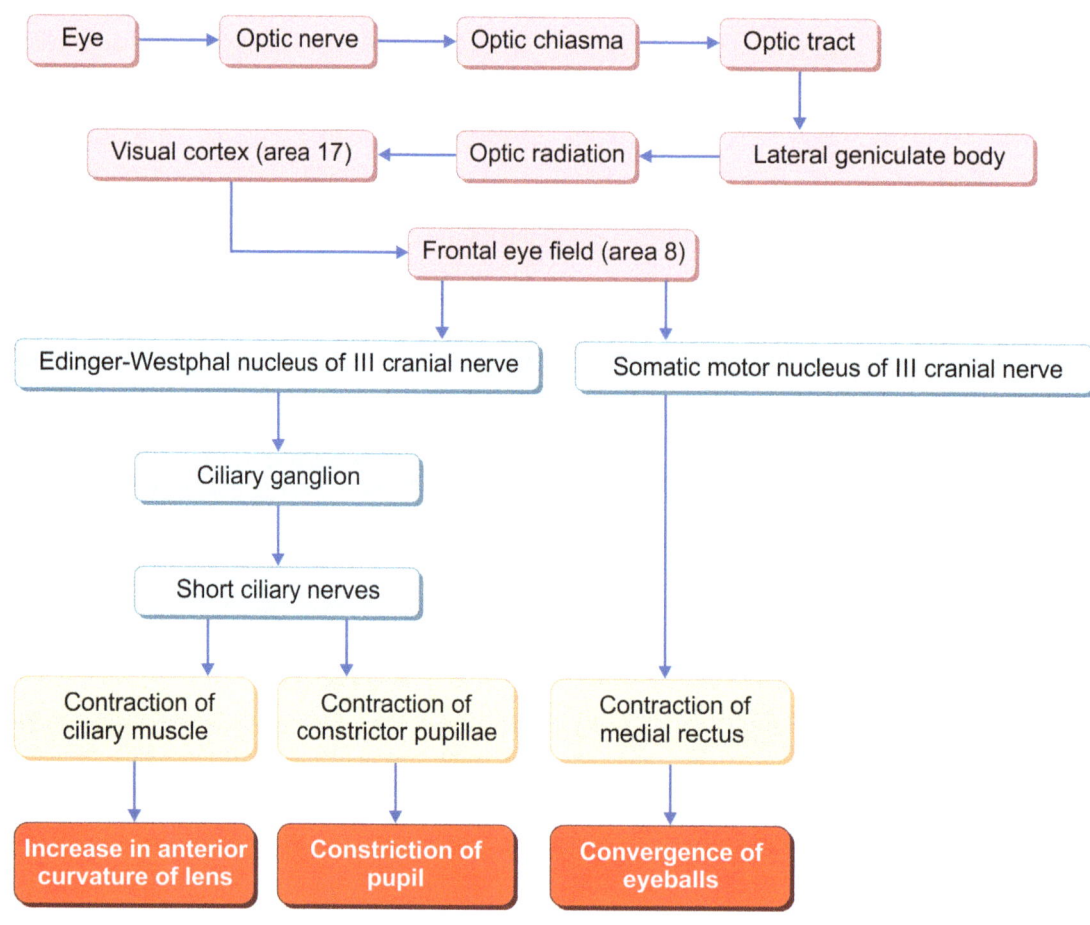

FIGURE 113.3: Pathway for accommodation reflex.

here, the **association fibers** carry the impulses to **frontal lobe** (Fig. 113.3).

Center

Center for accommodation lies in **frontal eye field** (area 8) that is situated in the frontal lobe of cerebral cortex.

Efferent Pathway

1. *Efferent fibers to ciliary muscle and sphincter pupillae*

From area 8, the **corticonuclear fibers** pass via internal capsule to the **Edinger-Westphal nucleus** of III cranial nerve. From here, the preganglionic fibers pass through the **III cranial nerve** to the **ciliary ganglion**. Postganglionic fibers from ciliary ganglion pass via the **short ciliary nerves** and supply the **ciliary muscle** and **the constrictor pupillae**.

2. Efferent fibers to medial rectus

Some of the fibers from **frontal eye field** terminate in the somatic **motor nucleus** of oculomotor nerve. Fibers from this nucleus supply the medial rectus.

APPLIED PHYSIOLOGY

1. PRESBYOPIA

Presbyopia is a condition characterized by progressive diminished ability of eyes to focus on near objects with age. It is due to gradual reduction in amplitude of accommodation because of failure to increase the anterior curvature of lens.

Since the amplitude of accommodation is decreased, near point is away from the eye. Details are given in Chapter 115.

2. ARGYLL ROBERTSON PUPIL

Argyll Robertson pupil is a clinical condition in which the **light reflex** is lost but the accommodation reflex is present. It is due to lesion in pretectal nucleus or rostral portion of Edinger-Westphal nucleus.

Argyll Robertson pupil is common in tertiary syphilis. It also occurs in diabetic and alcoholic neuropathy.

3. HORNER SYNDROME

Horner syndrome is an eye disorder caused by damage to **cervical sympathetic nerve**. It is also called Bernard-Horner syndrome, Claude **Bernard-Horner syndrome** or **oculosympathetic palsy.**

Symptoms of Horner syndrome appear on the affected side.

Symptoms are:

i. **Ptosis** (drooping of upper eyelid).
ii. Swelling of lower eyelid.
iii. **Miosis** or **myosis** (abnormal constriction of pupil).
iv. **Enophthalmos** (sinking of eyeball into its cavity).
v. Absence of sweating on affected side of the face.

Chapter 114: Color Vision

CHAPTER OUTLINE

- **VISIBLE SPECTRUM**
  - SPECTRAL COLORS
  - EXTRA SPECTRAL COLORS
  - PRIMARY COLORS
  - COMPLEMENTARY COLORS
- **CONES AND COLOR VISION: YOUNG-HELMHOLTZ TRICHROMATIC THEORY**
- **COLOR SENSITIVE AREAS IN RETINA**
- **APPLIED PHYSIOLOGY: COLOR BLINDNESS**
  - CLASSIFICATION OF COLOR BLINDNESS
  - TESTS FOR COLOR BLINDNESS

VISIBLE SPECTRUM

Human eye can recognize about 150 different colors in the **visible spectrum**. Discrimination and appreciation of colors depend upon the ability of cones in retina.

SPECTRAL COLORS

When sunlight or white light is passed through a glass **prism**, it is separated into a series of colored lights called the **visible spectrum**. And, the colors that form the spectrum are called the **spectral colors**. Spectral colors are violet, indigo, blue, green, yellow, orange and red, (**VIBGYOR** or **ROYGBIV**). In the spectrum, the colors occupy the position according to their wavelengths. Wavelength is the distance between two identical points in the wave of light energy. Accordingly, violet has got the minimum wavelength of about 3,000 Å and red has got the maximum wavelength of about 8,000 Å.

Light rays shorter than violet are called the **ultraviolet rays**. And, light rays longer than red are called **infrared rays**. But, these two extraordinary types of rays do not evoke the sensation of vision.

EXTRA SPECTRAL COLORS

Extra spectral colors are the colors other than those present in visible spectrum. These colors are formed by the combination of two or more spectral colors. For example, **purple** is the combination of violet and red. **Pink** is the combination of red and white.

PRIMARY COLORS

Primary colors are those, which when combined together produce the white. Primary colors are **red**, **green** and **blue**. These three colors in equal proportion give white.

COMPLEMENTARY COLORS

Complementary colors are the pair of two colors which produce white when mixed or combined in proper proportion. Examples of complementary colors are red and greenish blue; orange and cyan blue; yellow and indigo blue; violet and greenish yellow; and purple and green.

CONES AND COLOR VISION: YOUNG-HELMHOLTZ TRICHROMATIC THEORY

According to Young-Helmholtz theory, retina has three types of cones and each cone is supplied by a separate fiber of optic nerve. Each cone has its own photosensitive pigment and gives response to one of the primary colors namely, red, green and blue.

Different color sensations are produced by the stimulation of various combinations of the three types of cones. White is perceived by equal stimulation of all three types of cones.

COLOR SENSITIVE AREAS IN RETINA

Peripheral part of retina is devoid of cones, so it is insensitive to color and gives sensation of white, black and gray only. Central portion of retina, fovea centralis has

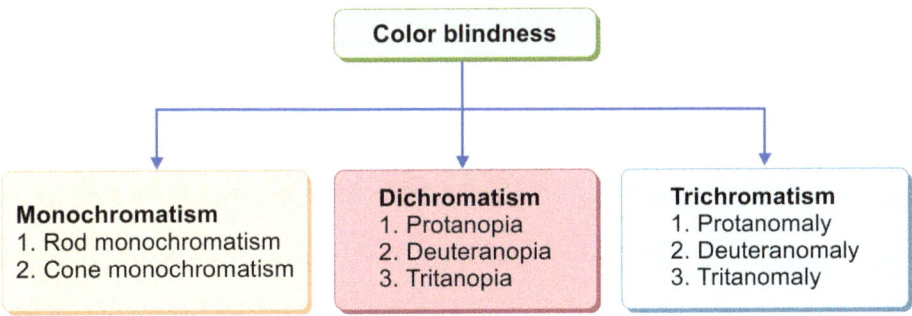

FIGURE 114.1: Color blindness.

more cones so, it is more sensitive to color. In extrafoveal regions, cones are mingled with rods.

Retinal area sensitive to blue is largest and to green is smallest. Red comes next to blue and then comes yellow. All the color areas of retina are mapped out by using **perimeter**.

APPLIED PHYSIOLOGY: COLOR BLINDNESS

Color blindness is the failure to appreciate one or more colors. It is common in 8% of males and only in 0.4% of females, as mostly the color blindness is an inherited **sex-linked recessive character**. In addition to hereditary conditions, color blindness occurs due to acquired conditions also, such as ocular diseases or injury, or disease of retina.

CLASSIFICATION OF COLOR BLINDNESS

Based on Young-Helmholtz trichromatic theory, color blindness is classified into three types:

1. Monochromatism.
2. Dichromatism.
3. Trichromatism.

1. Monochromatism

Monochromatism is the condition characterized by total inability to perceive color. It is also called **total color blindness** or **achromatopsia**. Monochromatism is very rare. Persons with monochromatism are called **monochromats**. The retina of monochromats is totally insensitive to color and they see the whole spectrum in only black, white and different shades of gray. So, their vision is similar to black and white photography.

2. Dichromatism

Dichromatism is the color blindness in which the subject can appreciate only two colors. Persons with this defect are called **dichromats**. They can match the entire spectrum of colors by only two primary colors because the receptors for third color are defective.

Dichromatism is classified into three groups.

i. Protanopia

Protanopia is the type of dichromatism caused by the defect in the receptor of **first primary color**, i.e. **red**. So, the red color cannot be appreciated. The persons having protanopia are called **protanopes**. They use blue and green to match the colors. Thus, they confuse red with green (Fig. 114.1).

ii. Deuteranopia

It is the dichromatism caused due to the defect in the receptor of the **second primary color**, i.e. **green**. **Deuteranopes** use blue and red colors and they cannot appreciate green color.

iii. Tritanopia

It is the dichromatism caused due to the defect in the receptor of **third primary color**, i.e. **blue**. **Tritanopes** use red and green colors and they cannot appreciate blue color.

3. Trichromatism

Trichromatism is the color blindness in which the intensity of one of the primary colors cannot be appreciated correctly though the affected persons are able to perceive all the three colors. Persons with this defect are called **trichromats**. Even the dark shades of one particular color look dull for them.

Trichromatism is classified into three types.

i. Protanomaly

Protanomaly is the type of trichromatism in which the perception for **red** is weak. So, to appreciate the red color, the person requires more intensity of red than a normal person.

ii. Deuteranomaly

Deuteranomaly is the trichromatism in which the perception for **green** is weak.

iii. Tritanomaly

Tritanomaly is the trichromatism with weak perception for **blue**.

TESTS FOR COLOR BLINDNESS

Color blindness is determined by using:

1. Ishihara's color charts.
2. Colored wool.
3. Edridge-Green lantern.

Chapter 115: Refractive Errors

CHAPTER OUTLINE

- REFRACTIVE ERRORS
- AMETROPIA
  - HYPERMETROPIA OR LONG SIGHTEDNESS
  - MYOPIA OR SHORT SIGHTEDNESS
- ANISOMETROPIA
- ASTIGMATISM
  - DEFINITION
  - CAUSE
  - TYPES
  - CORRECTION
- PRESBYOPIA
  - DEFINITION
  - CAUSES
  - CORRECTION

REFRACTIVE ERRORS

Refractive error is defined as inability of the eye to focus the image of objects accurately on retina.

AMETROPIA

Emmetropia is the vision with lens having normal refractive power. And eye with normal refractive power is called **emmetropic eye**.

Any deviation in refractive power from normal condition resulting in inadequate focusing on retina is called **ametropia** and the eye is called **ametropic eye**. The defect is due to the change in shape of the eyeball.

Ametropia is of two types:
1. Hypermetropia.
2. Myopia.

HYPERMETROPIA OR LONG SIGHTEDNESS

Hypermetropia is the eye defect characterized by the inability to focus on near object. It is otherwise known as **long sightedness** because the person can see the distant objects clearly, but not the near objects. It is also called **hyperopia**. In this defect, the distant vision is normal, but the near vision is affected (metras = measure).

Causes of Hypermetropia

Hypermetropia is due to **decreased anteroposterior diameter** of the eyeball. So, even though the refractive power of the lens is normal, the light rays are not converged enough to form a clear **image** on retina, i.e. the light rays are brought to a focus **behind retina**. It causes a blurred image of near objects. Hypermetropia occurs in childhood, if the eyeballs fail to develop to the correct size. It is common in old age also.

Correction of Hypermetropia

Hypermetropia is corrected by using **biconvex lens**. Light rays are converged by convex lens before entering the eye **(Fig. 115.1)**.

MYOPIA OR SHORT SIGHTEDNESS

Myopia is the defect characterized by inability of the eye to focus on distant object. It is otherwise called **short sightedness**, because the person can see near objects clearly, but not the distant objects.

Normally, in emmetropia, the far point is infinite. In myopia, the near vision is normal, but the far point is not infinite, i.e. it is at definite distance **(Fig. 115.1 and Table 115.1)**. In extreme conditions, it may be only a few centimeters away from the eye (myo = half closed; ops = eye).

Causes of Myopia

In myopia, refractive power of the lens is usually normal. But, **anteroposterior diameter** of the eyeball is abnormally **long**. Therefore, the **image** is brought to a focus a little **in front of retina**. In other words, refractory power of lens is too strong for the length of eyeball. The light rays, after coming to a focus, disperse again, so a blurred image is formed upon retina.

TABLE 115.1: Refractive errors.

Type of error	Cause	Correction
Hypermetropia	Decrease in anteroposterior diameter of the eyeball	Biconvex lens
Myopia	Increase in anteroposterior diameter of the eyeball	Biconcave lens
Anisometropia	Difference in refractive power of both eyes	Separate lens (biconcave or biconvex) for each eye as required
Astigmatism	Refractory power of lens is different in different meridians	
Regular astigmatism	Refractory power of lens is unequal in different meridians but uniform in one single meridian	Cylindrical lens
Irregular astigmatism	Refractory power of lens is unequal in different meridians as well as in different points in same meridian	
Presbyopia	Loss of elasticity in lens and weakness of ocular muscles due to old age	Biconvex lens

Correction of Myopia

In myopic eye, in order to form a clear image on the retina, light rays entering the eye must be divergent and not parallel. Thus, the myopic eye is corrected by using **biconcave lens**. Light rays are diverged by the concave lens before entering the eye **(Fig. 115.1)**.

ANISOMETROPIA

Anisometropia is the condition in which the two eyes have **unequal refractive power**. It is corrected by using different appropriate lens for each eye **(Table 115.1)**.

ASTIGMATISM

DEFINITION

Astigmatism is the condition in which the light rays are not brought to a sharp point upon retina. It is the common optical defect present in all eyes. When it is moderate, it is known as **physiological astigmatism**. When it is well marked, it is considered abnormal. For example, the stars appear as small dots of light to a person with normal eye. But in astigmatism, the stars appear as radiating short lines of light (a = not; stigma = point).

CAUSE OF ASTIGMATISM

Light rays pass through all meridians of a lens. In a normal eye, lens has approximately same curvature in all meridians. So, the light rays are refracted almost equally in all meridians and brought to a focus.

If the curvature is different in different meridians, vertical, horizontal and oblique, the refractive power is also different in different meridians. Meridian with greater curvature refracts the light rays more strongly than other meridians. So, these light rays are brought to a focus in front of the light rays, which pass through other meridians. Such irregularity of curvature of lens causes astigmatism.

TYPES OF ASTIGMATISM

Astigmatism is of two types:
1. Regular astigmatism.
2. Irregular astigmatism.

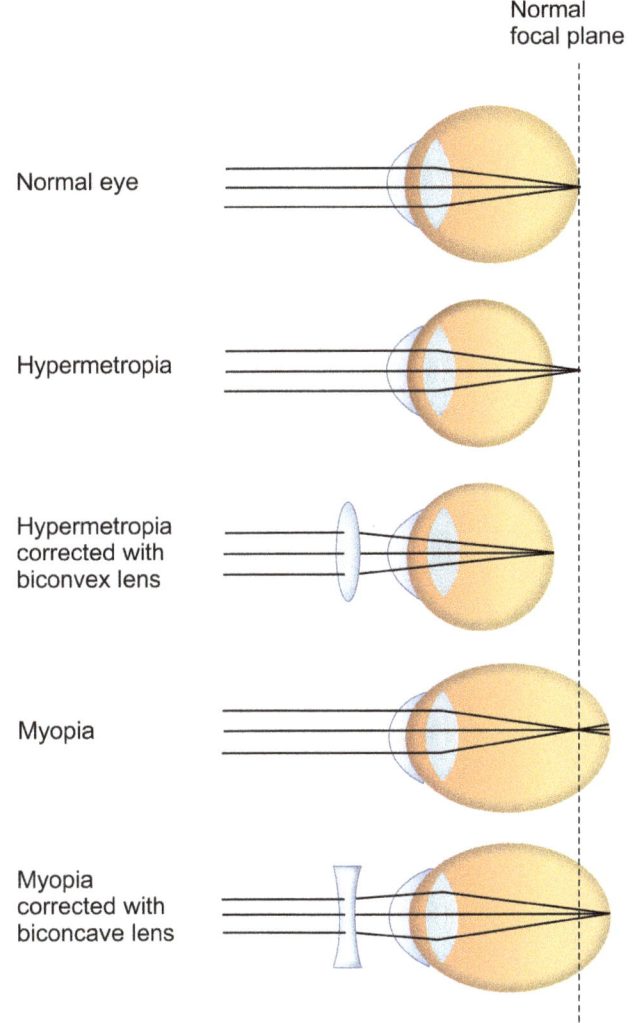

FIGURE 115.1: Refractive errors.

1. Regular Astigmatism

In this type of astigmatism, the refractive power is unequal in different meridians because of alteration of curvature in one meridian. But it is uniform in all points throughout the affected meridian.

2. Irregular Astigmatism

Here, the refractive power is unequal not only in different meridians but it is also unequal in different points of same meridian.

■ CORRECTION OF ASTIGMATISM

Astigmatism is corrected by using **cylindrical lens** having the convexity in the meridians corresponding to that of lens of eye having a lesser curvature, i.e. if the horizontal curvature of lens is less, the person should use cylindrical glass lens with the convexity in horizontal meridian.

■ PRESBYOPIA

■ DEFINITION

Presbyopia is the condition characterized by progressive decrease in the ability of eyes to focus on near objects with age. It is due to the gradual reduction in the **amplitude of accommodation**. Presbyopia starts developing after middle age and progresses as the age advances (presbyos = old; ops = eye).

In presbyopia, the distant vision is unaffected. Only the near vision is affected. The near point is away from eye. In presbyopia, the anterior curvature of lens does not increase during near vision. So, the light rays from near objects are not brought to a focus on retina.

■ CAUSES OF PRESBYOPIA

1. Decreased elasticity of lens is because of the physical changes in lens and its capsule during old age. So, the anterior curvature is not increased during near vision.
2. Decreased convergence of eyeballs due to the concomitant weakness of ocular muscles in old age.

■ CORRECTION OF PRESBYOPIA

Presbyopia is corrected by using **biconvex lens**.

Chapter 116: Ear

CHAPTER OUTLINE

- **EAR**
- **EXTERNAL EAR**
  - AURICLE OR PINNA
  - EXTERNAL AUDITORY MEATUS
- **MIDDLE EAR**
  - AUDITORY OSSICLES
  - AUDITORY MUSCLES
  - EUSTACHIAN TUBE
- **INTERNAL EAR**
  - COCHLEA
  - COMPARTMENTS OF COCHLEA
  - ORGAN OF CORTI
  - AUDITORY RECEPTORS

EAR

Ear consists of cochlea, the sense organ for hearing and vestibular apparatus, the sense organ for equilibrium. Ear consists of three parts namely, external ear, middle ear and internal ear **(Fig. 116.1)**.

EXTERNAL EAR

External ear is formed by two parts:

1. Auricle or pinna.
2. External auditory meatus.

AURICLE OR PINNA

Auricle or pinna of the external ear consists of **fibrocartilaginous plate** covered by connective tissue and skin. This plate is characteristically folded and ridged. Skin covering this plate contains many fine hairs and sebaceous glands. On the posterior surface of auricles, many sweat glands are present.

In many animals, auricle can be moved and turned to locate the source of sound or the auricle can be folded to avoid unwanted sound. But in man, extrinsic and intrinsic muscles of auricles are **rudimentary** and the movement is not possible. Depression of auricle, which forms the orifice of external auditory meatus, is called **concha.**

EXTERNAL AUDITORY MEATUS

External auditory meatus starts from the concha and extends inside as a slightly curved canal, with a length of about 55 mm.

External auditory meatus consists of two parts:

i. Outer cartilaginous part.
ii. Inner bony part.

i. Outer Cartilaginous Part

Outer cartilaginous part is the initial part of external auditory meatus made up of cartilage. It is covered by thick skin, which contains **stiff hairs**. These hairs prevent the entry of foreign particles.

Large **sebaceous glands** and **ceruminous glands** are also present in the skin covering this portion. Secretions of sebaceous glands, ceruminous glands and desquamated epithelial cells form the **earwax.**

ii. Inner Bony Part

Inner part of the external auditory meatus is also covered by skin, which adheres closely to periosteum. Only sebaceous glands are present here. Skin covering this portion is continuous with cuticular layer of tympanic membrane.

MIDDLE EAR

Middle ear or **tympanic cavity** is situated within the temporal bone. It is separated from external auditory meatus by a thin semitransparent membrane called **tympanic membrane (Fig. 116.2).**

Middle ear consists of three structures:

1. Auditory ossicles.
2. Auditory muscles.
3. Eustachian tube.

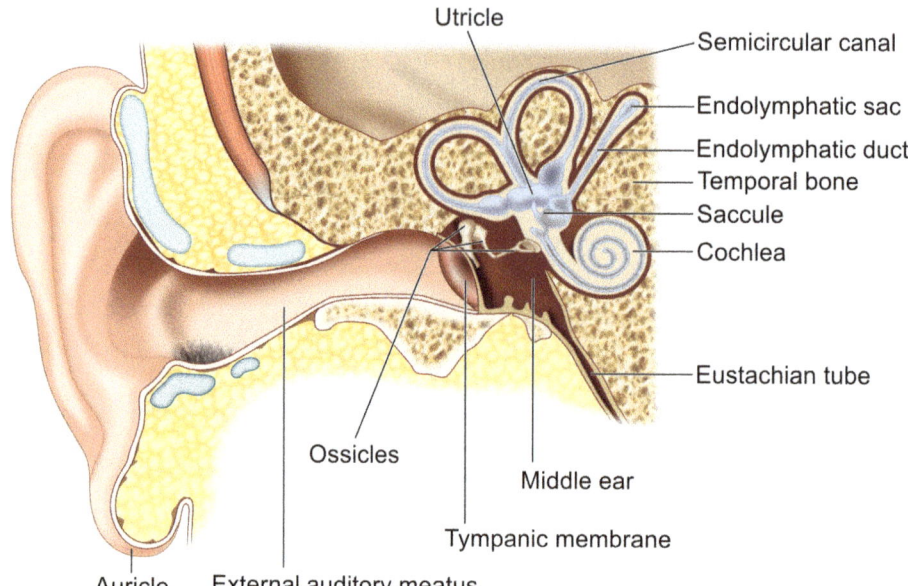

FIGURE 116.1: Diagram showing the structure of ear.

■ AUDITORY OSSICLES

Auditory ossicles are the three **miniature bones**, which are arranged in the form of a chain extending across middle ear from **tympanic membrane** to **oval window** (Fig. 116.2).

Auditory ossicles are:

1. Malleus.
2. Incus.
3. Stapes.

1. *Malleus*

Malleus is otherwise called **hammer**. It has a handle, head and neck. Handle is otherwise known as **manubrium**. It is attached to the tympanic membrane. Head or capitulum articulates with the body of next bone incus.

2. *Incus*

Incus is also known as **anvil**. It looks like a premolar tooth. Incus has a body, one long process and one short process. Anterior surface of the body articulates with head of malleus. The tip of the long process is like a knob, called **lenticular process** and it articulates with the next bone, stapes.

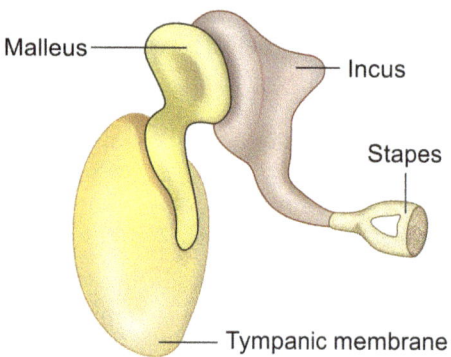

FIGURE 116.2: Tympanic membrane and auditory ossicles.

3. *Stapes*

Stapes is also called **stirrup**. It is the **smallest bone** present in the body. It has a head, neck, anterior crus, posterior crus and a footplate. Head articulates with incus. **Footplate** fits into the oval window.

■ AUDITORY MUSCLES

Two skeletal muscles are attached to the ossicles:

1. Tensor tympani.
2. Stapedius.

1. *Tensor Tympani*

Tensor tympani muscle arises from cartilaginous portion of eustachian tube. Its tendon is inserted on **manubrium of malleus** which is in turn attached to tympanic membrane. It is supplied by mandibular division of **trigeminal nerve.**

Tensor tympani muscle pulls and keeps the tympanic membrane stretched constantly.

2. *Stapedius*

Stapedius is the **smallest skeletal muscle** in human body with a length of just over 1 mm. It arises from interior pyramid of tympanic cavity. Its tendon is inserted into the posterior surface of neck of stapes. It is supplied by branch of **facial nerve.**

Stapedius prevents excess movements of stapes. When it contracts, it pulls the neck of stapes backwards and reduces the movement of footplate against the fluid in cochlea.

Tympanic Reflex

Tympanic reflex is an **attenuation reflex** characterized by involuntary contraction of tensor tympani and stapedius muscles, in response to a **loud noise**.

When both the muscles contract, manubrium of malleus moves inward and stapes is pulled outward. These two actions result in stiffness of auditory ossicles, so that the transmission of sound is decreased.

Significance of tympanic reflex

i. Tympanic reflex protects the tympanic membrane from being ruptured by loud sound.
ii. It also prevents fixation of footplate of stapes, against oval window, during exposure to loud sound.
iii. Tympanic reflex helps to protect the cochlea from damaging effects of loud sounds. Contraction of tensor tympani and stapedius during exposure to loud sound develops stiffness of the auditory ossicles so that, the transmission of sound into cochlea is decreased.

■ EUSTACHIAN TUBE

Eustachian tube or the auditory tube connects the middle ear with posterior part of nose and forms the passage of air between middle ear and atmosphere. So, the pressure on both sides of tympanic membrane is equalized.

■ INTERNAL EAR

Internal ear or **labyrinth** is a membranous structure, enclosed by a **bony labyrinth** in petrous part of temporal bone. It consists of the sense organs of hearing and equilibrium. Sense organ for hearing is the **cochlea**. And, the sense organ for equilibrium is the **vestibular apparatus**. Vestibular apparatus is already explained in Chapter 104.

■ COCHLEA

Cochlea is a coiled structure like a snail's shell (cochlea = snail's shell).

Cochlea consists of two structures:

1. Central conical axis formed by spongy bone called **modiolus**.
2. Bony spiral canal, which winds around the modiolus.

Bony spiral canal makes two and a half turns, starting from the base of the cochlea and ends at the top (apex) of cochlea. End of the canal is called **cupula**. Base of modiolus forms the bottom of internal auditory meatus, through which cochlear nerve fibers pass and enter the modiolus. Thus, a section through the axis of cochlea reveals the central **bony pillar,** modiolus and **periotic or osseous canal,** which coils around the modiolus.

From modiolus, a bony ridge called **osseous spiral lamina** projects into the canal, winding around modiolus like the thread of a screw. Spiral lamina follows the spiral turns of cochlea and ends at the cupula in a hook shaped process called **hamulus**.

■ COMPARTMENTS OF COCHLEA

Cochlea is divided into three compartments by two membranous partitions called **basilar membrane** and **vestibular membrane**.

Compartments of spiral canal of cochlea are:

1. Scala vestibuli.
2. Scala tympani.
3. Scala media.

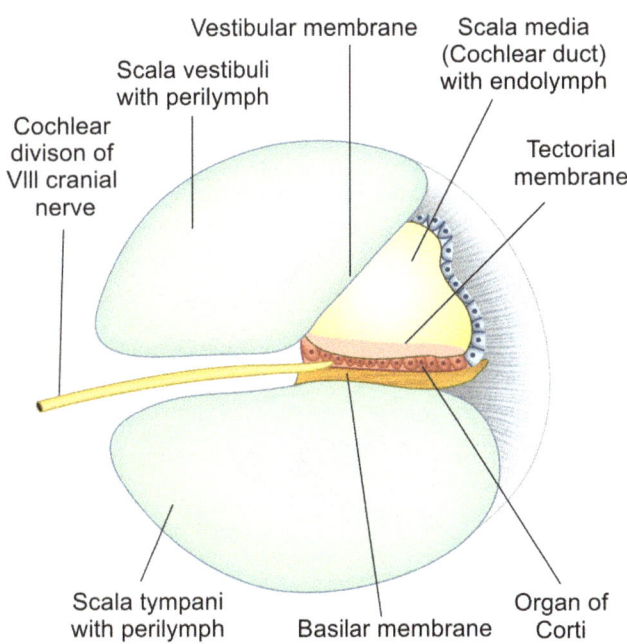

FIGURE 116.3: Cross-section of spiral canal of cochlea.

All the three compartments are filled with fluid. Scala vestibuli and scala tympani contain **perilymph**. The scala media is filled with **endolymph (Fig. 116.3)**.

1. Scala Vestibuli

Scala vestibuli lies above the scala media. It arises from **oval window** (fenestra vestibuli) which is closed by the **footplate of stapes**. It follows the osseous canal up to its apex. At the apex, it communicates with the scala tympani through a small canal called **helicotrema (Fig. 118.1)**.

2. Scala Tympani

It lies below the scala media. It is parallel to scala vestibuli and ends at the **round window**. The round window is closed by a strong thin membrane known as **secondary tympanic membrane**.

3. Scala Media

Scala media is otherwise called **cochlear duct**. It ends blindly at the apex and at the base of cochlea. The sensory part of cochlea called organ of Corti is situated on the upper surface of basilar membrane **(Fig. 116.3)**.

■ ORGAN OF CORTI

Organ of Corti is the receptor organ for hearing. It is the neuroepithelial structure situated in cochlea **(Fig. 116.4)**. It rests upon the lip of spiral lamina and the basilar membrane. It extends throughout the cochlear duct, except for a short distance on either end. The roof of the organ of Corti is formed by gelatinous tectorial membrane.

Structure

Organ of Corti is made up of the auditory receptors called the **hair cells** and various **supporting cells**. All the cells of organ of Corti are arranged in order from center towards periphery of the cochlea.

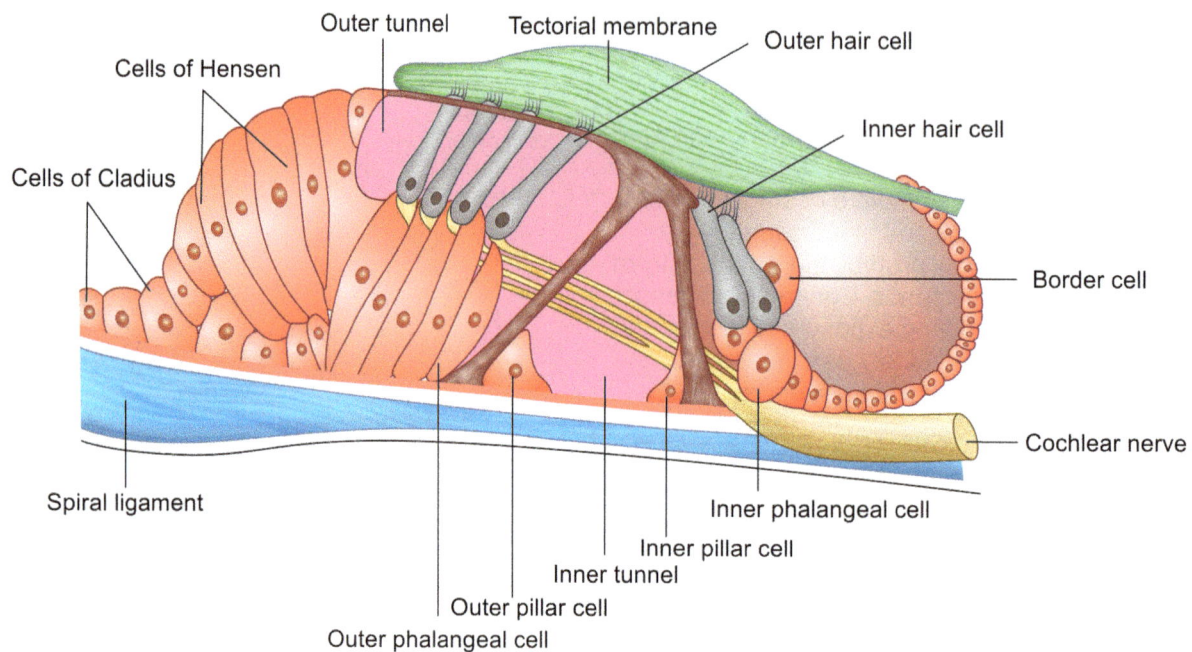

FIGURE 116.4: Organ of Corti.

Cells of organ of Corti:

1. Border cells.
2. Inner hair cells.
3. Inner phalangeal cells.
4. Inner pillar cells.
5. Outer pillar cells.
6. Outer phalangeal cells.
7. Outer hair cells.
8. Cells of Hensen.
9. Cells of Claudius.
10. Tectorial membrane and lamina reticularis.

■ AUDITORY RECEPTORS

Hair cells in organ of Corti are the receptors of the auditory sensation. The hair cells are of two types, outer hair cells and inner hair cells. Surface of the hair cell bears a **cuticular plate.** A number of short stiff hairs, called **stereocilia** arise from this cuticular plate.

Each hair cell has about 100 stereocilia. One of the stereocilia is larger and it is called **kinocilium.** Stereocilia are in contact with the **tectorial membrane.** Sensory nerve fibers are distributed around the hair cells.

Chapter 117: Auditory Pathway

CHAPTER OUTLINE

- **AUDITORY PATHWAY**
  - RECEPTORS
  - FIRST ORDER NEURONS
  - SECOND ORDER NEURONS
  - THIRD ORDER NEURONS
- **SUBCORTICAL AUDITORY CENTER**
- **CORTICAL AUDITORY CENTERS**
- **FUNCTIONS OF CORTICAL AUDITORY CENTERS**
- **APPLIED PHYSIOLOGY: EFFECT OF LESION**

AUDITORY PATHWAY

Fibers of auditory pathway pass through **cochlear division** of **vestibulocochlear nerve** (VIII cranial nerve). It is also known as **auditory nerve**.

RECEPTORS

Outer and inner **hair cells in organ of Corti** are the receptors of the auditory sensation (Chapter 116). Afferent nerve fibers which innervate the hair cells form the auditory nerve (see below).

FIRST ORDER NEURONS

First order neurons of the auditory pathway are the **bipolar cells** of **spiral ganglion** situated in the modiolus of cochlea (Fig. 117.1).

Dendrites of the bipolar cells are distributed around the **hair cells** of organ of Corti. Their axons leave ear as cochlear nerve fibers and enter medulla oblongata. Immediately after entering the medulla oblongata, the fibers divide into two groups which end on ventral and dorsal **cochlear nuclei** of the same side in medulla oblongata.

SECOND ORDER NEURONS

Neurons of dorsal and ventral cochlear nuclei in the medulla oblongata form the second order neurons of auditory pathway.

Axons of the second order neurons run in four different directions:

1. First group of fibers cross the midline and run to the opposite side to form **trapezoid body** and go to the superior **olivary nucleus**.
2. Second group of the fibers terminate at the superior olivary nucleus of same side via trapezoid body of the same side.
3. Third group of fibers run in the **lateral lemniscus** of the same side and terminate in the **nucleus of lateral lemniscus**.
4. Fourth group of fibers cross the midline as intermediate trapezoid fibers and join the nucleus of lateral lemniscus of opposite side.

THIRD ORDER NEURONS

Third order neurons are in the **superior olivary nucleus** and **nucleus of lateral lemniscus**. Fibers from here end in medial geniculate body.

SUBCORTICAL AUDITORY CENTER

Medial geniculate body forms the subcortical auditory center.

Fibers from medial geniculate body go to the temporal cortex, via internal capsule as **auditory radiation.** Some fibers from medial geniculate body go to **inferior colliculus** of tectum in midbrain. These fibers are involved in reflex movement of head, in response to auditory stimuli.

CORTICAL AUDITORY CENTERS

Cortical auditory centers are in the **temporal lobe** of cerebral cortex (Chapter 101).

Auditory areas are:

1. **Primary auditory area**, which includes area 41, area 42 and Wernicke's area.
2. **Secondary auditory area** or **auditopsychic area** or auditory association area, which includes area 22.

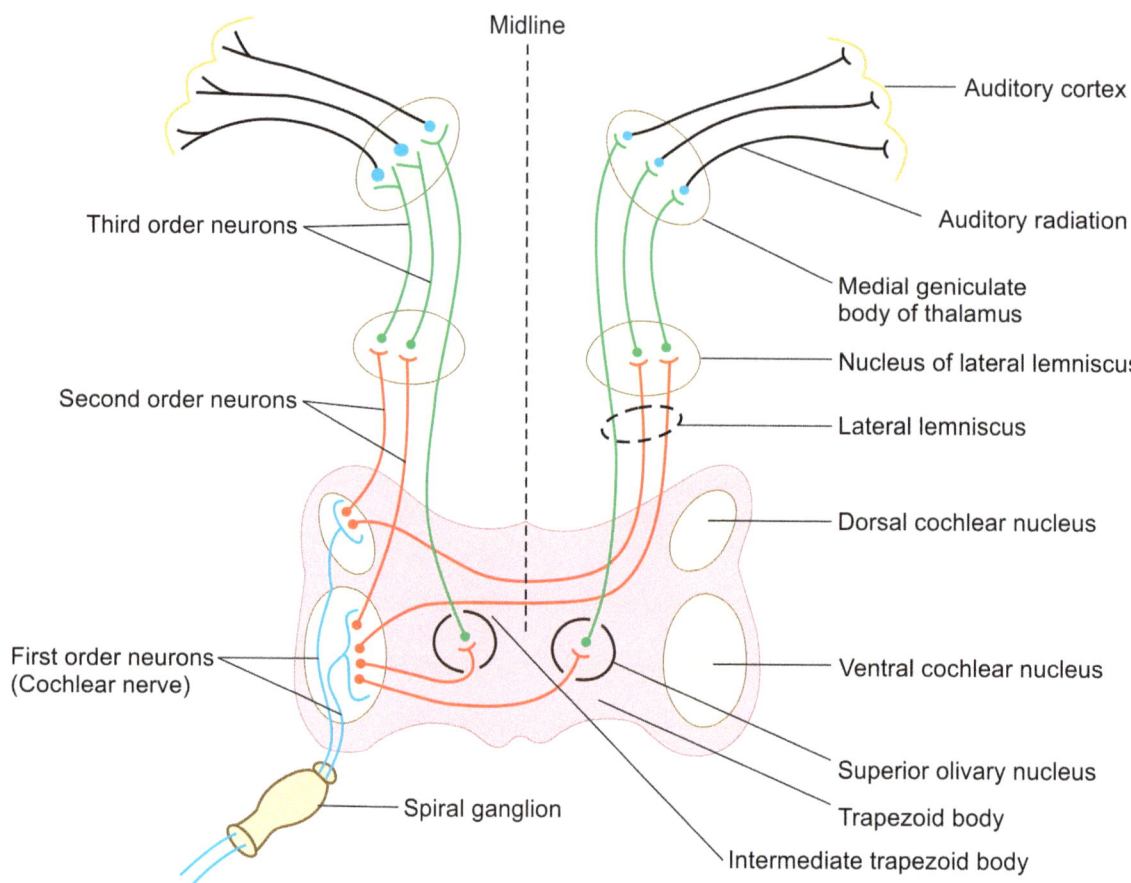

FIGURE 117.1: Auditory pathway. Blue = First order neuron. Red = Second order neuron. Green = Third order neuron. Black = Auditory radiation.

■ FUNCTIONS OF CORTICAL AUDITORY CENTERS

Cortical auditory centers are concerned with the perception of auditory impulses, analysis of pitch and intensity of sound and determination of source of sound.

Areas 41 and 42 are concerned with the perception of auditory impulses only. However, analysis and interpretation of sound are carried out by **Wernicke's area**, with the help of **area 22**.

■ APPLIED PHYSIOLOGY: EFFECT OF LESION

1. Lesion of cochlear nerve causes **deafness**.
2. Unilateral lesion of auditory pathway above the level of cochlear nuclei causes **diminished hearing**.
3. Degeneration of hair cells in organ of Corti leads to **gradual loss of hearing**. This is common in old age and the condition is called **presbycusis**.
4. Lesion in superior olivary nucleus results in **poor localization of sound**.

# Chapter 118: Mechanism of Hearing and Auditory Defects

CHAPTER OUTLINE

- PERCEPTION OF HEARING
- ROLE OF EXTERNAL EAR
- ROLE OF MIDDLE EAR
  - ROLE OF TYMPANIC MEMBRANE
  - ROLE OF AUDITORY OSSICLES
  - ROLE OF EUSTACHIAN TUBE
- ROLE OF INNER EAR
  - TRAVELING WAVE
  - EXCITATION OF HAIR CELLS
- ELECTRICAL EVENTS DURING PROCESS OF HEARING
  - SOUND TRANSDUCTION
  - RECEPTOR POTENTIAL
- PROPERTIES OF SOUND
- APPRECIATION OF PITCH OF THE SOUND: THEORIES OF HEARING
- APPRECIATION OF LOUDNESS OF SOUND
- LOCALIZATION OF SOUND
- AUDITORY DEFECTS
  - CONDUCTION DEAFNESS
  - NERVE DEAFNESS
- TESTS FOR HEARING
  - BEDSIDE TESTS
  - ROUTINE TESTS

PERCEPTION OF HEARING

Sound waves travel through external auditory meatus and produce vibrations in the tympanic membrane. Vibrations from tympanic membrane travel through malleus and incus and reach the stapes resulting in the movement of stapes. Movements of stapes produce vibrations in the fluids of cochlea and stimulate the hair cells in the organ of Corti. This, in turn, causes the generation of action potential (auditory impulses) in the auditory nerve fibers. When the auditory impulses reach the cerebral cortex, perception of hearing occurs.

ROLE OF EXTERNAL EAR

External ear directs the sound waves towards the tympanic membrane. The sound waves produce **pressure changes** over the surface of **tympanic membrane**.

ROLE OF MIDDLE EAR

ROLE OF TYMPANIC MEMBRANE

Due to the pressure changes produced by sound waves, the tympanic membrane vibrates, i.e. it moves in and out of middle ear. Thus, the tympanic membrane acts as a **resonator** that produces the vibration of sound.

ROLE OF AUDITORY OSSICLES

Vibrations set up in tympanic membrane are transmitted through the malleus and incus and reach the stapes, causing to and fro **movement of stapes** against oval window and against the perilymph present in scala vestibuli of cochlea.

Impedance Matching

Impedance matching is the process, by which the tympanic membrane and auditory ossicles convert the sound energy into the mechanical vibrations in the fluid of internal ear with **minimum loss of energy** by matching the impedance offered by the fluid.

Impedance means obstruction or opposition to the passage of sound waves. When sound waves reach the inner ear, the fluid (perilymph) in cochlea offers impedance, i.e. the fluid resists the transmission of sound due to its own inertia. Tympanic membrane and the auditory ossicles effectively reduce the sound impedance which is called the impedance matching.

Significance of impedance matching

Impedance matching is the most important function of middle ear. Because of impedance matching the sound waves (stimuli) are transmitted to cochlea with minimum loss of intensity. Without impedance matching conductive deafness occurs.

Types of Conduction

Conduction of sound from external ear to internal ear through middle ear occurs by three routes:

1. Ossicular conduction.
2. Air conduction.
3. Bone conduction.

1. Ossicular conduction

Ossicular conduction is the conduction of sound waves through middle ear by **auditory ossicles**. This is the normal way of conditions of the sound waves through middle ear.

2. Air conduction

Air conduction is the conduction of sound waves through air in middle ear. If the ossicular chain is broken, conduction occurs in an alternate route of air conduction. Air conduction is common in otosclerosis. **Otosclerosis** is the disease associated with fixation of stapes to oval window.

3. Bone conduction

It is the conduction of sound waves by **bones**. When middle ear is affected, bone conduction occurs. In this type of conduction, the sound waves are transmitted to cochlear fluid by the vibrations set up in the skull bones.

ROLE OF EUSTACHIAN TUBE

Eustachian tube is not concerned with hearing directly. However, it is responsible for **equalizing the pressure** on either side of tympanic membrane.

ROLE OF INNER EAR

TRAVELING WAVE

Movement of **footplate of stapes** against **oval window** causes movement of perilymph in scala vestibuli. This fluid does not move all the way from oval window toward round window through the helicotrema. It immediately hits the vestibular membrane near oval window and displaces the fluid in scala media **(Fig. 118.1)**. This causes bulging of basal portion of basilar membrane towards scala tympani.

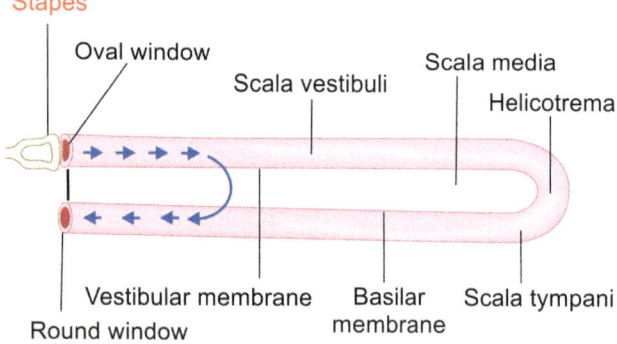

FIGURE 118.1: Diagrammatic representation of cochlea. Arrows show displacement of fluid.

Elastic tension developed in the bulged portion of basilar membrane initiates a wave called traveling wave. This wave travels along basilar membrane towards the helicotrema like arterial pulse wave.

Resonance Point

Resonance point is the part of **basilar membrane**, which is activated by traveling wave. In the beginning, each traveling wave is weak. While traveling through basilar membrane from base towards apex (helicotrema), the wave becomes stronger and stronger and at one point of basilar membrane, it becomes very strong and activates the basilar membrane. This part of basilar membrane which is activated by travelling wave is called resonance point. This resonance point of basilar membrane immediately vibrates back and forth. The traveling wave stops here and does not travel further.

EXCITATION OF HAIR CELLS

Stereocilia of hair cells in organ of Corti are embedded in tectorial membrane (Chapter 116). Hair cells are tightly fixed by cuticular lamina reticularis and the pillar cells of Corti **(Fig. 116.4)**.

When the traveling wave produces vibration of basilar membrane, all these structures move as a single unit. It causes movements of stereocilia leading to excitement of hair cells and generation of **receptor potential**.

ELECTRICAL EVENTS DURING PROCESS OF HEARING

SOUND TRANSDUCTION

Sound transduction or **auditory transduction** is a type of sensory transduction in the hair cell (receptor cells) in organ of Corti by which the **sound energy** is converted into **action potentials** in the auditory nerve fibers.

RECEPTOR POTENTIAL OR COCHLEAR MICROPHONIC POTENTIAL

Receptor potential or cochlear microphonic potential is the **mild depolarization** that is developed in the hair cells of cochlea when sound waves are transmitted to internal ear. The resting membrane potential in hair cells is about –60 mV. The sensory transduction mechanism in cochlear receptor cells is different from the mechanism in other sensory receptors.

Receptor potential in the hair cells causes generation of action potential in auditory nerve fibers.

PROPERTIES OF SOUND

Sound has two basic properties:

1. **Pitch** which depends upon the **frequency** of sound waves. Frequency of sound is expressed in **hertz**. The frequency of sound **audible to human ear** lies between 20 and 20,000 Hz or cycles/second. The range of greatest sensitivity lies between 2,000 and 3,000 Hz (cycles/second).
2. **Loudness** or **intensity** which depends upon the **amplitude** of sound waves. It is expressed in **decibel**

(dB). The threshold intensity of sound wave is not constant. It varies in accordance to the frequency of the sound.

APPRECIATION OF PITCH OF SOUND: THEORIES OF HEARING

Though many theories are postulated to explain the mechanism by which the pitch of the sound is appreciated only few theories are accepted so far. Accepted theories are given below.

1. Place Theory

According to this theory, the nerve fibers from different portions (places) of organ of Corti on basilar membrane give response to sounds of different frequency. Accordingly, the corresponding nerve fiber from organ of Corti gives information to the brain regarding the portion of organ of Corti that is stimulated.

2. Traveling Wave Theory

This theory explains how traveling wave is generated in the basilar membrane. The generation, movement and disappearance of traveling wave are already described earlier in this chapter.

APPRECIATION OF LOUDNESS OF SOUND

Appreciation of loudness of sound depends upon the activities of auditory nerve fibers.

When the loudness of sound increases, it produces longer vibrations which spread over longer area of basilar membrane. This activates large number of hair cells and recruits many auditory nerve fibers. So, the frequency of action potential is also increased.

LOCALIZATION OF SOUND

Sound localization is the ability to detect the source from where the sound is produced or the direction through which the sound wave is traveling. It is important for survival and it helps to protect us from moving objects such as vehicles. Cerebral cortex and medial geniculate body are responsible for localization of sound.

AUDITORY DEFECTS

Auditory defects may be either partial or complete.

Auditory defects are of two types:
1. Conduction deafness.
2. Nerve deafness.

1. CONDUCTION DEAFNESS

Conduction deafness occurs due to impairment in the transmission of sound waves in external ear or middle ear.

Causes of Conduction Deafness

i. Obstruction of external auditory meatus with dry wax or foreign bodies.
ii. Thickening of tympanic membrane due to infection.
iii. Perforation of tympanic membrane due to inequality of pressure on either side.
iv. **Otitis media** (inflammation of middle ear).
v. **Otosclerosis** (fixation of footplate of stapes against oval window).

2. NERVE DEAFNESS

Nerve deafness is caused by damage of any structure in cochlea such as hair cell, organ of Corti, basilar membrane or cochlear duct or the lesion in auditory pathway.

Causes of Nerve Deafness

i. Degeneration of hair cells.
ii. Damage of cochlea by prolonged exposure to loud noise.
iii. Tumor affecting VIII cranial nerve.

TEST FOR HEARING

Various tests are available to assess the sensation of hearing. However, some simple tests called **bedside tests** are usually carried before doing routine (conventional) hearing tests.

BEDSIDE TESTS

Bedside tests are simple tests which are useful to know whether the hearing is normal or less.

Bedside tests are:
1. Whispering test.
2. Tickling of watch test.

1. Whispering Test

The examiner stands about 60 cm away from the subject at his side and whispers some words. If the subject is not able to hear the whisper, then hearing deficit is suspected.

2. Tickling of Watch Test

Wrist watch with tickling sound is kept near the ear of the subject. The subject suffering from hearing defects cannot hear the tickling sound of watch.

ROUTINE TESTS

Routine tests for hearing are of three types:
1. Rinne test.
2. Weber test.
3. Audiometry.

First two tests are done by using a tuning fork with high frequency. A tuning fork with 512 cycles per second is used. By tuning fork tests, only the nature of auditory defect is determined. By audiometry, both nature and severity of auditory defects can be determined.

1. Rinne Test

Base of a vibrating tuning fork is placed on mastoid process, until the subject cannot feel the vibration and cannot hear the sound. When the subject does not hear the sound any more, the tuning fork is held in air in front of the ear of same side.

Normal person hears vibration in air even after the bone conduction ceases because, in normal conditions, air conduction via ossicles is better than bone conduction.

But in **conduction deafness**, the vibrations in air are not heard after cessation of bone conduction. Thus, in conduction deafness, the bone conduction is better than air conduction.

In **nerve deafness**, both air conduction and bone conduction are diminished or lost.

2. Weber Test

Base of a vibrating tuning fork is placed on the vertex of skull or the middle of forehead. Normal person hears the sound equally on both sides.

In unilateral **conduction deafness** (deafness in one ear), the sound is heard louder in diseased ear. In unaffected ear, there is a masking effect of environmental noise. So, the sound through bone conduction is not heard as clearly as on the affected side. In affected side, the sound is louder due to the absence of masking effect of environmental noise.

During unilateral **nerve deafness**, sound is heard louder in the normal ear.

3. Audiometry

Audiometry is the technique used to determine the nature and the severity of auditory defect. An electronic instrument called **audiometer** is used for this purpose. This instrument is capable of generating sound waves of different frequencies from lowest to highest. Intensity (loudness or volume) of sound also can be adjusted.

During the tests by audiometer, the subject's ability to hear the sounds with 8 to 10 different frequencies is observed and the hearing loss is determined for each frequency. By using these values, the audiogram is plotted.

Audiometer has an **electronic vibrator** also. It is used to test the bone conduction from mastoid process into the cochlea.

Chapter 119: Sensation of Taste

CHAPTER OUTLINE

- TASTE BUDS
- PATHWAY FOR TASTE SENSATION
- PRIMARY TASTE SENSATIONS
- SUBSTANCES PRODUCING DIFFERENT TASTE SENSATIONS
- TASTE TRANSDUCTION
- FLAVOR
- APPLIED PHYSIOLOGY: ABNORMALITIES OF TASTE SENSATION

TASTE BUDS

Taste buds are the sense organs for **taste** or **gustatory sensation**. Taste buds are ovoid bodies with a diameter of 50 to 70 μ.

SITUATION OF TASTE BUDS

Most of the taste buds are present on the **papillae of tongue**. Some taste buds are situated in the mucosa of epiglottis, palate, pharynx and proximal part of esophagus.

Types of papillae located on tongue:

1. Filiform papillae.
2. Fungiform papillae.
3. Circumvallate papillae.

1. Filiform Papillae

Filiform papillae are small and conical shaped papillae situated over the **dorsum of tongue**. These papillae contain only few taste buds.

2. Fungiform Papillae

Fungiform papillae are round in shape and are situated over the **anterior surface of tongue** near the tip. Numerous fungiform papillae are present. Number of taste buds in each papilla is moderate (up to 10).

3. Circumvallate Papillae

Circumvallate papillae are large structures arranged 'V' shape on the **posterior part of tongue** and are many in number. Each papilla contains many taste buds (up to 100).

STRUCTURE OF TASTE BUD

Taste bud is a bundle of taste receptor cells, with supporting cells embedded in the epithelial covering of the papillae

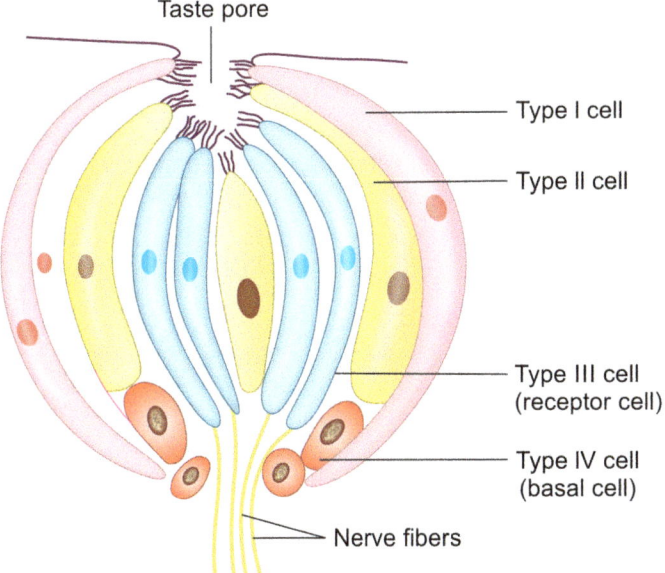

FIGURE 119.1: Taste bud.

(Fig. 119.1). Each taste bud contains about 40 cells, which are the modified epithelial cells. The cells of taste bud are divided into four groups:

Types of Cells in Taste Bud

1. Type I cells or sustentacular cells (supporting cells).
2. Type II cells (receptors cells).
3. Type III cells (receptor cells).
4. Type IV cells or basal cells (supporting cells).

Type I cells and type IV cells are **supporting cells**. Type II cells and type III cells are the **taste receptor cells**. Type I, II and III cells have projections called **microvilli**.

Microvilli project into an opening in the epithelium covering the tongue. The opening is called **taste pore**. All the cells of taste bud are surrounded by epithelial cells.

■ PATHWAY FOR TASTE SENSATION
■ RECEPTORS

Receptors for taste sensation are the **type II and III cells** of **taste buds**. Each taste bud is innervated by about 50 sensory nerve fibers and each nerve fiber supplies at least 5 taste buds.

■ FIRST ORDER NEURON

First order neurons of taste pathway are in the nuclei of three different cranial nerves, situated in medulla oblongata. Dendrites of the neurons are distributed to the taste buds. After arising from taste buds, the fibers reach the cranial nerve nuclei by running along the following nerves **(Fig. 119.2)**:

1. **Chorda tympani fibers** of facial nerve, which run from anterior two third of tongue.
2. **Glossopharyngeal nerve fibers**, which run from posterior one third of the tongue.
3. **Vagal fibers**, which run from taste buds in other regions.

Axons of the first order neurons run together in medulla oblongata and terminate in the nucleus of tractus solitarius.

■ SECOND ORDER NEURON

Second order neurons are in the **nucleus of tractus solitarius**. Axons of the second order neurons run through medial lemniscus and terminate in posteroventral nucleus of thalamus.

■ THIRD ORDER NEURON

Third order neurons are in the **posteroventral nucleus** of thalamus. Axons from the third order neurons project into cerebral cortex.

■ TASTE CENTER

Center for taste sensation is in the **opercular insular cortex** (lower part of postcentral gyrus) in parietal lobe of cerebral cortex.

■ PRIMARY TASTE SENSATIONS

Primary or fundamental taste sensations are divided into five types:

1. Sweet.
2. Salt.
3. Sour.
4. Bitter.
5. Umami.

Man can perceive more than 100 different tastes. Other taste sensations are just the combination of two or more primary sensations.

Combination of Taste Sensation with Other Sensations

Sometimes, taste sensation combines with other sensations to give rise to a different sensation. For example, combination of taste and smell, gives rise to **sensation of flavor**. Combination of taste with pain gives rise to **sensation of ginger**.

■ SUBSTANCES PRODUING DIFFERENT TASTE SENSATIONS
■ 1. SWEET TASTE

Sweet taste is produced mainly by organic substances like monosaccharides, polysaccharides, glycerol, alcohol, aldehydes, ketones and chloroform. Inorganic substances producing sweet taste sensations are lead and beryllium.

■ 2. SALT TASTE

Salt taste is produced by chlorides of sodium, potassium and ammonium, nitrates of sodium and potassium. Some sulfates, bromides and iodides also produce salt taste.

■ 3. SOUR TASTE

Sour taste is produced because of hydrogen ions in acids and acid salts.

■ 4. BITTER TASTE

Bitter taste is produced by **organic substances** like quinine, strychnine, morphine, glucosides, picric acid and bile salts, and inorganic substances like salts of calcium, magnesium and ammonium.

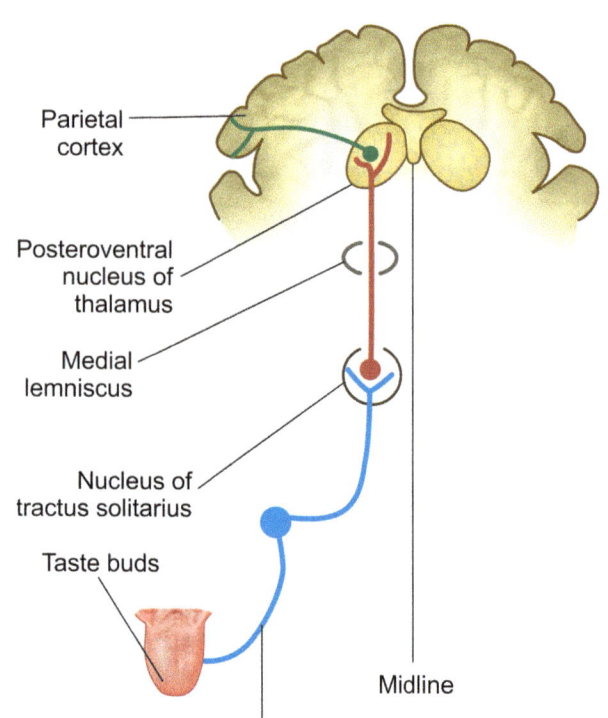

FIGURE 119.2: Pathway for taste sensation.

5. UMAMI

Umami is the recently recognized taste sensation. Umami is a Japanese word meaning '**delicious**'. Receptors of this taste sensation respond to monosodium glutamate which is a common ingredient in Asian food.

Threshold for Taste Sensations

Sweet taste sugar	: 1 in 200 dilution
Salt taste sodium chloride	: 1 in 400 dilution
Sour taste hydrochloric acid	: 1 in 15,000 dilution
Bitter taste quinine	: 1 in 20,00,000 dilution

Bitter taste has very low threshold and sweet taste has a high threshold. Threshold for umami is not known.

TASTE TRANSDUCTION

Taste transduction is the process in taste receptors by which **chemical energy** is converted into **electrical energy** (action potentials) in the taste nerve fibers. Taste receptors **chemoreceptors**, which are stimulated by substances dissolved in mouth by saliva. The dissolved substances act on microvilli of taste receptors exposed in the taste pore. It causes development of receptor potential in the receptor cells. This in turn, is responsible for the generation of action potential in the sensory neurons.

FLAVOR

Flavor of food is the combination of two chemical sensations, namely taste and smell sensations.

Taste of the food is detected by the receptors in taste buds and the information is sent to brain. Smell of the food is detected by olfactory receptors in nose and the information is sent to brain. Ultimately, both taste and smell sensations combine and allow us to detect the flavors of food.

Retronasal olfaction is linked with flavor of the food (Chapter 120).

APPLIED PHYSIOLOGY: ABNORMALITIES OF TASTE SENSATION

1. *Ageusia:* Loss of taste sensation.
2. *Hypogeusia:* Decrease in the taste sensation.
3. *Taste blindness:* Inability to recognize substances by taste due to genetic disorder.
4. *Dysgeusia:* Disturbance in the taste sensation like hallucinations of taste.

Chapter 120: Sensation of Smell

CHAPTER OUTLINE

- OLFACTORY RECEPTORS
- VOMERONASAL ORGAN
- OLFACTORY PATHWAY
- OLFACTORY TRANSDUCTION
- CLASSIFICATION OF ODOR
- THRESHOLD FOR OLFACTORY SENSATION
- ADAPTATION
- ORTHONASAL OLFACTION AND RETRONASAL OLFACTION
- APPLIED PHYSIOLOGY: ABNORMALITIES OF OLFACTORY SENSATION

■ OLFACTORY RECEPTORS

Olfactory receptors are situated in **olfactory mucous membrane** that lines nasal cavity. Olfactory mucous membrane consists of 10 to 20 million of **olfactory receptor cells** supported by the **sustentacular cells**. Mucosa also contains mucus secreting **Bowman glands** (Fig. 120.1).

Olfactory receptor cell is a **bipolar neuron**. Dendrite of this neuron is short. Expanded end of the dendrite is called **olfactory rod**. From the rod, about 10 to 12 cilia arise. **Cilia** are nonmyelinated with a length of 2 μ and a diameter of 0.1 μ. The cilia project to the surface of olfactory mucous membrane.

Mucus secreted by Bowman's glands continuously lines the olfactory mucosa. The mucus contains some proteins, which increase the actions of odoriferous substances on receptor cells.

■ VOMERONASAL ORGAN

Vomeronasal organ is an **accessory olfactory organ** found in many animals including mammals. It is enclosed in a cartilaginous capsule, which opens into the base of nasal cavity.

Olfactory receptors of this organ are sensitive to non-volatile substances such as scents and **pheromones**. Vomeronasal organ helps the animals to detect even the trace quantities of chemicals. Impulses from this organ are sent to amygdala and hypothalamus via accessory olfactory bulb.

■ VOMERONASAL ORGAN IN HUMAN BEINGS

In human beings, the vomeronasal organ was considered as vestigial or non-functional. Recently, it is claimed that vomeronasal organ is present in the form of **vomeronasal pits** on the anterior part of **nasal septum.** It is not known whether it is having olfactory function or not.

Receptors of vomeronasal pit detect human **pheromones** or **vomeropherins,** at a very low concentration in air. Refer Chapter 47 for details of pheromones. The subconscious detection of odorless chemical messengers in air is considered as the **sixth sense in human beings**.

■ OLFACTORY PATHWAY

Axons of the **bipolar olfactory receptors** pierce the **cribriform plate** of ethmoid bone and reach **the olfactory bulb**. Here, the axons synapse with dendrites of **mitral cells**. Different groups of these synapses form globular structures called **olfactory glomeruli**. Axons of mitral cells leave the olfactory bulb and form **olfactory tract**. Olfactory tract runs backwards and ends in **olfactory cortex**.

Olfactory cortex includes the structures, which form a part of limbic system. These structures are anterior olfactory nucleus, prepyriform cortex, olfactory tubercle and amygdala.

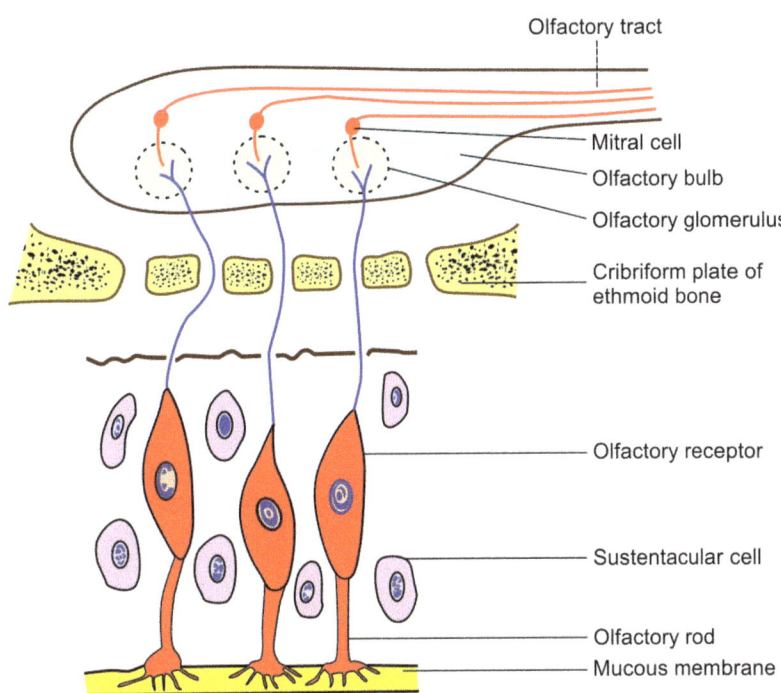

FIGURE 120.1: Olfactory mucous membrane and pathway for olfactory sensation.

OLFACTORY TRANSDUCTION

Olfactory transduction is the process in olfactory receptors by which **chemical energy** is converted into **electrical energy** (action potentials) in olfactory nerve fibers.

Odoriferous substance stimulates the olfactory receptors, only if it dissolves in mucus, covering the olfactory mucous membrane. Molecules of dissolved substance, bind with receptor proteins in the cilia and form substance-receptor complex. Substance-receptor complex activates adenyl cyclase that causes the formation of cyclic AMP. Cyclic AMP in turn, causes opening of sodium channels, leading to influx of sodium and generation of receptor potential.

Receptor potential causes generation of action potential in the axon of bipolar neuron.

CLASSIFICATION OF ODOR

Odor is classified into various types. Each type is produced by different substance.

SUBSTANCES PRODUCING DIFFERENT TYPES OF ODOR

1. *Aromatic or resinous odor:* Camphor, lavender, clove and bitter almonds.
2. *Ambrosial odor:* Musk.
3. *Burning odor:* Burning feathers, tobacco, roasted coffee and meat.
4. *Ethereal odor:* Fruits, ethers and beeswax.
5. *Fragrant or balsamic odor:* Flowers and perfumes.
6. *Garlic odor:* Garlic, onion and sulfur.
7. *Goat odor:* Caproic acid and sweet cheese.
8. *Nauseating odor:* Decayed vegetables and feces.
9. *Repulsive odor:* Bed bug.

THRESHOLD FOR OLFACTORY SENSATION

Ethyl ether	: 5.8 mg/L of air
Chloroform	: 3.3 mg/L of air
Peppermint oil	: 0.02 mg/L of air
Butyric acid	: 0.009 mg/L of air
Artificial musk	: 0.00004 mg/L of air
Methyl mercaptan	: 0.0000004 mg/L of air

Thus, the methyl mercaptan produces olfactory sensation even at a low concentration of 0.0000004 mg/L of air.

ADAPTATION

Olfactory receptors are phasic receptors and adapt very rapidly. Within one second, the adaptation occurs up to 50%.

ORTHONASAL OLFACTION AND RETRONASAL OLFACTION

Perception of smell occurs by two ways. One is via orthonasal olfaction and the other one is via retronasal olfaction.

Orthonasal Olfaction

Orthonasal olfaction is the **perception of smell** by means of **sniffing** into the **nose**. In this type of olfaction, the odor molecules pass through nostrils, reach the olfactory mucous membrane and stimulate the olfactory receptors.

Retronasal Olfaction

Retronasal olfaction is the **perception of odor** originating from **mouth** during **eating or drinking**. While chewing the food or while drinking, some of the odor molecules gently pass through the passage behind uvula, reach the nasal cavity and stimulate the olfactory receptors.

Retronasal olfaction is commonly linked with **flavor** of the food. Flavor is a combined sense which involves sensation of taste and sensation of smell.

■ APPLIED PHYSIOLOGY: ABNORMALITIES OF OLFACTORY SENSATION

1. *Anosmia:* Total loss of sensation of smell.
2. *Hyposmia:* Reduced ability to recognize and to detect any odor.
3. *Hyperosmia or olfactory hyperesthesia:* Increased or exaggerated olfactory sensation.

MODEL QUESTIONS IN SPECIAL SENSES

LONG QUESTIONS

1. Draw a diagram of visual pathway and explain it. Add note on hemianopia.
2. Explain the auditory pathway with suitable diagram. Add a note on auditory defects.
3. Explain the mechanism of hearing.

SHORT QUESTIONS

1. Retina.
2. Ocular muscles
3. Ocular movements.
4. Intraocular pressure.
5. Fundus oculi.
6. Lens of eye.
7. Visual receptors
8. Phototransduction.
9. Rhodopsin.
10. Dark adaptation.
11. Light adaptation.
12. Rhodopsin.
13. Effects of lesion in optic pathway.
14. Light reflex and its pathway.
15. Accommodation reflex and its pathway.
16. Color blindness.
17. Refractive errors.
18. Auditory ossicles and auditory muscles.
19. Cochlea/Organ of Corti.
20. Role of middle ear in hearing (functions of middle ear).
21. Traveling wave.
22. Auditory defects.
23. Taste buds.
24. Taste pathway.
25. Olfactory pathway.

VERY SHORT ANSWER QUESTIONS

1. Lacrimal gland and tear.
2. Ciliary body.
3. Iris.
4. Blind spot.
5. Vitreous humor/aqueous humor.
6. Cataract.
7. Photosensitive pigments in rod cells and cone cells.
8. Night blindness or nyctalopia.
9. ERG.
10. Acuity of vision and tests for acuity.
11. Divisions of visual field and mapping of visual field.
12. Corresponding retinal point and diplopia.
13. Subcortical and cortical centers for visual sensation.
14. Anopia and hemianopia.
15. Ciliospinal reflex.
16. Adjustments in eyeball during accommodation.
17. Young-Helmholtz theory.
18. Argyll Robertson pupil.
19. Horner syndrome.
20. Spectral colors, primary colors and complementary colors.
21. Monochromatism/dichromatism/trichromatism.
22. Myopia/hypermetropia/astigmatism.
23. Presbyopia.
24. Tympanic membrane.
25. Tympanic reflex.
26. Compartments and membranes of cochlea.
27. Subcortical and cortical centers for auditory sensation.
28. Effect of lesion of auditory pathway.
29. Types of conduction through middle ear.
30. Impedance matching.
31. Conduction deafness.
32. Nerve deafness.
33. Primary taste sensations.
34. Abnormalities of taste sensation.
35. Flavor.
36. Substances producing different odor.
37. Orthonasal and retronasal olfaction.
38. Abnormalities of olfactory sensation.

Index

Page numbers followed by *b* refer to box, *f* refer to figure, and *t* refer to table.

A

Abdominothoracic pump 352
Abduction 565
ABO
  agglutinogens, inheritance of 87
  blood groups 85, 86*t*
  group 86
    determination of 86
    inheritance of 87*t*
  incompatibility 88
  system 85
Abortion 281, 311, 321
Abrupt apnea, causes of 431
Absolute refractory period 114, 334, 452
Absorptive functions 162, 169, 171, 221
Accessory digestive organs 133, 134
Accessory olfactory organ 598
Accessory sex organs 285, 287, 296
  development of 290
Acclimatization 435
Accommodation 577, 578*f*
  amplitude of 584
  mechanism of 577
  reflex 577
    pathway for 578*f*
Acetoacetate 262
Acetone
  breath odor 265
  breathing 265
Acetylcholine 119, 122, 123, 130, 141, 231, 282, 358, 365, 450
  action of 123, 282
  destruction of 123, 124, 282
  receptor complex 123
  release of 123
  secretion of 282
  synthesis of 122
Acetylcholinesterase 123, 124
Acetyl-CoA synthetase 6
Achilles tendon reflex 471
Achlorhydria 151
Achromatopsia 581
Acid
  base balance 205
    maintenance of 182
    regulation of 35, 38, 398
  base disturbance 208*t*
  base status, distribution of 207
  citrate dextrose 82
  neutralization of 170
Acidic gastric juice 497
Acidophilic cells 233
Acidosis 32, 207, 265
Acinar cells 152
Acini 152
Acne, vulgaris 220
Acquired immune deficiency
  diseases 71
  syndrome 71, 72

Acromegalic face 239
Acromegalic gigantism 240
Acromegaly 239*f*
Acromicria, causes of 241
Actin filaments 14, 107
  part of 108*f*
Actin molecule 107
Action blood cells 269
Action potential curve 117
Activin 290
Actomyosin complex 119, 120
  formation of 120
Acute heart failure 389
  signs of 390
  symptoms of 390
Acute renal failure 211, 388
  causes of 211
  treatment for 211
Adaptation 452, 458, 599
Addison's anemia 57
Addison's disease 272, 273
  causes for primary 273
  types of 273
Addisonian crisis, causes of 273
Adduction 565
Adenine 9
Adenohypophysis 233
Adenosine
  diphosphate 18, 77, 120
  triphosphate 108, 120, 231
    resynthesis of 121
Adenyl cyclase, activated 231
Adherens junction 13, 14
Adhesiveness 74
Adipocytes 506
Adipose tissue 261
Adjacent muscle fibers 327
Adrenal cortex 189, 266, 297, 298, 313
  disorders of 271, 273*b*
  functional histology of 266
  hyperactivity of 271
  hyperplasia of 271
  hypoactivity of 272
  layer of 267*t*
  regulation of 505
Adrenal crisis 273
Adrenal gland 266, 266*f*
  functional anatomy of 266
  parts of 266
Adrenal insufficiency
  acute 273
  chronic 272
Adrenal medulla 274
  functional histology of 274
  regulation of 505
Adrenal sex hormones 270
Adrenaline 74, 130, 141, 274, 275, 556
  actions of 275
  apnea 276, 427
  mode of action of 275
  secreting cells 274

Adrenergic receptors 275, 275*t*
  types of 275
Adrenocorticotropic hormone 188, 234, 236, 270, 505
  secretion of 189, 269
Adrenogenital syndrome
  causes of 272
  symptoms of 272
Adult respiratory distress syndrome 401
Aerobic exercise 391, 392
Aerobic metabolism 392
Afferent arteriole 190
  constriction of 195
Afferent fibers 174
Afferent nerve 468
  fiber 450, 450*b*
Afferent neurons 448
Ageusia 597
Agglutination 70, 74, 86, 314
  absence of 314
Agglutinins 85, 87
Agglutinogens 85
Aggregation 74
Agranular cells 187
Agranulocytes 60
Air conduction 592
Airway resistance 404
Akinesia 515
Alanine 207
  transaminase 164
Albumin 37
Alcohol, excess intake of 175
Aldosterone 35, 206, 267
  antagonists 212
  escape 267
    mechanism of 267
    significance of 267
  influence of 206
  secretion, regulation of 268*f*
Alkaline 306
  phosphatase 164
Alkalinity 152
Alkalosis 207
Allergic reactions, delayed 67
Allocortex 516
Alpha-adrenergic receptors 275
Alpha-block 539
Alpha-granules 74
Alpha-motor neurons 494, 530
  activation of 518
Alpha-rhythm 539
Alpha-waves 543
Alveolar air 413
  composition of 413*t*
Alveolar cells 93, 397
Alveolar epithelial cells 401
Alveolar macrophages 63
Alveolar membrane 397
Alveolar sac 397
Alveolar ventilation 411
Alveoli 152
Alzheimer disease 548

Amacrine cells 563
Ameboid movement 62
Amelognosia 502
Amenorrhea 246, 308
Ametropia 582
Ametropic eye 582
Amino acid 19, 196
  glutamine 207
  number of 48*t*
  reabsorption of 198
  role of 262
  tyrosine 219, 274
Ammonia 207*f*
  mechanism 206, 207
Ammonium 81, 207
  acetoacetate 207
Amnesia 548
Ampulla of Vater 152, 156, 158
Amylolytic enzyme 140, 154, 167
Anacrotic limb 374
Anacrotic pulse 376
Anaerobic exercise 391, 392
Anaerobic metabolism 392
Anal canal 170
Anal sphincter
  external 134, 178
  internal 178
Analgesia system 498
Analgesic pathway 498, 498*f*
Anaphylaxis 389
Anarthria 549
Anastomosis 329
Androgen 270, 290
  binding protein 286
Androstenedione 290
Anemia 32, 43, 54-57
  aplastic 55-56, 57, 75
  classification of 55
  etiological classification of 56*t*
  extrinsic hemolytic 56
  hemolytic 55, 56, 58, 92
  hemorrhagic 55, 56
  intrinsic hemolytic 56
  mediterranean 57
  morphological classification of 55*t*
  severe 89
  signs of 57
  symptoms of 57
Anemic hypoxia
  causes of 428
  characteristic features of 428
Aneroid sphygmomanometer 369
Anesthetic agents 171
Angina pectoris 380
Angiotensin 188, 189, 196, 268
  actions of 188, 367
  converting enzyme 188, 367
    activity of 188
    secretion of 398
Angiotensinogen 188
Angular acceleration 535
Anisocytes 43

Anisometropia 583
Ankle jerk 471
Annul spiral endings 528
Anopia 574
Anorexia 151, 505
Anosmia 508, 600
Anovulatory cycle 309, 321
Anterior coronary veins 378
Anterior end knob 293
Anterior median fissure 473, 476
Anterior pituitary hormones 308
    regulation of secretion of 234
Anterior spinothalamic tract 476, 479f
    components of 480
Anterior vestibulospinal tract 484
Anteroposterior diameter 582
Antibiotics 171
Antibodies 56, 69, 70
    actions of 70
    direct actions of 69
    functions of 69
    mechanism of actions of 69
    molecule, structure of 69f
    structure of 69
    types of 69
Anticonvulsants 171
Antidepressants 171
Antidiuretic hormone 24, 35, 130, 188, 198, 200, 202, 228, 237
    action of 198
    activity of 198
    hypersecretion of 32
    mechanism of 506
    receptor antagonists, administration of 32
    role of 202
    secretion of 189
Antidromic vasodilator fibers 365
Antigen 67
    presentation of 67, 67f, 68, 94
    presenting cells 67, 67f, 68, 397
        role of 67, 68
Antigenic materials 67
Antihypertensive drugs 171
Antiparkinson drugs 171
Anti-insulin hormones 263
Antimicrobial peptides 397
Antiperistalsis, beginning of 175
Antiseptic action 162
Antrum 397
Aortic baroreceptors 359
Aortic nerve 359, 360
Aortic pressure
    changes 339
    significance of 339
Aortic regurgitation 376
Aortic valve 327
Aphasia 549
    Head's classification of 549
Apnea 173, 398, 427, 427
Apneic period 431
Apneusis 422, 427
Apneustic center 422
Apocrine glands 220, 220t
    control of 220
    secretory activity of 220
Apoferritin 41
Apoptosis 7, 11
    functional significance of 11
Apotransferrin 50
Appendicitis, major symptom of 171
Aquaporins 198, 237
Aqueductus Sylvius 550
Aqueous humor 564
    functions of 564
Arachidonic acid 282
Arachnoid mater 445

Arachnoid villi, blockage of 552
Archicerebellum 509
Arcuate artery 190
Arcuate fibers, internal 482
Argentaffin cells 167
Argyll Robertson pupil 579
Arrhythmia 344, 348
    ectopic 349
    homotopic 349
Arterial blood 208t, 211
    gases in 418t
    oxygen content in 354
    pressure 191, 246, 362, 363, 363t, 368
        maintaining 363
        mean 362
        measurement of 368
        regulation of 364
        variations of 363
Arterial hypoxia 428
Arterial pulse 374
    abnormal 376
    central 374
    formation of 374
    peripheral 374
    tracing 374
    transmission of 374
Arterial system 329
Arteriosclerosis 248, 364
Arteriovenous shunt 381
Artery
    branch of 182
    hepatic 158
Artificial immunization, passive 70
Artificial kidney 211
Artificial pacemaker 350
Artificial respiration 440, 441f
    methods of 440
    mouth-to-mouth method of 440, 441f
Ascending reticular
    activating system 525, 526, 544
    formation 525f
Ascorbic acid 196
Aspartate aminotransferase 164
Asphyxia 75, 430
    effects of 430
Aspiration, vacuum 321
Asplenia 95
Astereognosis 482, 502, 521
Asthenia 265
Astigmatism 583
    causes of 583
    correction of 584
    irregular 584
    physiological 583
    types of 583
Astrocytes 454
Ataxia 502
    posterior column 482
Atelectasis 432
Atherosclerosis 211, 245, 248, 364, 379
Athetoid hand 502
Athetosis 502, 515
Atmospheric air 416
Atmospheric pressure, normal 429
Atmospheric temperature 35
Atonia 512
Atonic bladder 217
ATP-driven proton pump 205, 206
Atretic follicles 296
Atrial diastole 336
Atrial fibrillation 349
Atrial flutter 349
Atrial natriuretic peptide 196, 267, 279
    effect of 280
    secretion of 267

Atrial repolarization 346
Atrial systole 336
Atrioventricular block 349
Atrioventricular ring 327
Atrioventricular valves 327
Atropine 142
Attenuation reflex 586
Attitudinal reflexes 532
Audiometer 594
Auditopsychic area 522, 549, 589
Auditory area, secondary 522, 589
Auditory defects 593
    mechanism of 591
Auditory meatus, external 585
Auditory muscles 586
Auditory nerve 589
Auditory ossicles 586, 586f, 592
    role of 591
Auditory pathway 589, 590f
Auditory radiation 589
Auditory receptors 588
Auditory transduction 592
Auerbach's plexus 134
    functions of 134
Auricle 585
Auscultatory areas 342f
Auscultatory method 369
Autoantibodies 72
Autoantigens 67, 72
Autocrine messengers 227
Autoimmune disease 38, 72, 125, 169, 247
Autoimmune disorder 125, 143
Autoimmunity 72
Automatic associated movements, control of 514
Automatic blood pressure instrument 369
Autonomic functions, regulation of 523
Autonomic nerve
    fibers 469
    role of 262
Autonomic nervous system 140, 214, 446, 553, 555f
    functions of 554
    neurotransmitters of 555
    regulation of 505
    sympathetic divisions of 140
Autophagosome 4, 6
Autophagy 5
Autophosphorylation 261
Autoregulation 191
Autorhythmicity 332
Autosomes 310
A-wave 376
Axillary pulse 375
Axillary temperature 222
Axoaxonic synapse 461
Axodendritic synapse 461
Axon, internal structure of 449
Axosomatic synapse 461
Ayerza's disease 43

B

Babinski reflex 470
Babinski sign 542
Bacillus cereus 58
Bacteria 98, 171
    destruction of 65
Bacterial infection 58
Bactericidal agents, secretion of 94
Bainbridge reflex 360, 360f
Ballistic movements, control of 511
Ballistocardiographic method 355
Ballistocardiography 355
Barometric pressure 434, 435t, 436, 437t

Baroreceptors 359, 424
    functions of 359, 365
    mechanism 365
    nerve supply to 359, 359f
    reflex 189
    role of 365
    situation of 359
Barrier methods 318
Bartholin's duct 138
Bartter's syndrome 204
Basal ganglia 277, 494, 513, 513f
    components of 513
    damage of 514
    disorders of 514
    functions of 513
Basal lamina 14, 122
    matrix of 123
Basal metabolic rate 245
    effect on 291
Basement membrane 193
Basilar membrane 587
    parts of 592
Basophilic cells 233
Basophilic erythroblast 45
Basophils 44, 45f, 61
    functions of 62
Bathmotropic action 328
B-cell
    activation of 68
    immunity 68
    receptor 68
Bedwetting 217, 545
Bell's palsy 142
Bell-dog experiments 548
Bell-Magendie law 465, 471
Benedict-Roth apparatus 354
Bernard-Horner syndrome 579
Beta-adrenergic receptors 275
Beta-globulin 50
Beta-granules 74
Beta-rhythm 540
Betz cells 482
Bezold-Jarisch reflex 361
Bicarbonate 159, 196, 207, 419
    concentration of 152
    ions, reabsorption of 205
    mechanism 206
    reabsorption of 198
Biceps jerk 471
Biconcave lens 583
Biconvex lens 582, 584
Bicuspid valve 325, 327
Bile
    acids
        primary 160
        secondary 160
    alteration of pH of 163
    canaliculus 157
    composition of 159, 159f
    concentration of 163
    ducts 157
    formation of 160f
    pigments
        circulation of 161, 161f
        excretion of 161
        formation of 161, 161f
    properties of 159
    salts 154, 160
        enterohepatic circulation of 160
        formation of 160
        functions of 160, 162
    secretion 159, 162
        regulation of 163
    storage of 159, 163
Biliary apparatus, extrahepatic 158
Biliary system 157, 158, 158f, 163
    functional anatomy of 157

Index

Bilirubin 41, 50, 161, 182
  direct 161
  encephalopathy 89
  normal plasma levels of 162
Biliverdin 50, 161
Binocular vision 570
Biot breathing, features of 431
Biphasic action potential 118
Bipolar cells 563, 568, 572
Bipolar limb leads 345
Bipolar neuron 448, 598
Bipolar olfactory receptors 598
Birth, respiration after 384
Bjerrum screen 571
Bladder, automatic 217
Bleeding
  disorders 83
  time 82
Blind spot 563, 571
Blindness 597
Blood 23, 27, 33
  brain barrier 13, 552, 552b
    functions of 552
  buffers 182
  calcium level 251, 254, 255, 256f
    maintenance of 251
    regulation of 182, 256, 256f
  cancer, types of 62
  cells 33
    destruction of 95
    formation of 94
    rupture of 58
  cerebrospinal fluid barrier 552
  cleansing function 193
  clot
    external 80
    composition of 33, 80
  clotting 74, 78, 80, 82
    intravascular 83
    stages of 79
  coagulation 25f, 38, 76, 78
    stages of 79f
  disorder 55
  effect on 291, 429
  elements of 60
  examination of 210
  flow 381, 382, 393
    lack of 11
    obstruction of 389
    regulation of 191
    velocity of 364
  functions of 35
  glucose level 263
    regulation of 263
    role of 262
  group 85, 86t, 89
    determination 41, 86f
    systems 85
  in ventricles, volume of 339
  indices 52, 54
    importance of 54
  loss 35
    anemia 55
    prevention of 75
  matching 87
  oxygen carrying capacity of 418
  phosphate level 252, 257f
  pressure 267, 276, 280, 312, 393, 542
    change in 365
    diastolic 362, 391
    regulation of 182, 364-366, 366f, 367, 367f, 368f, 505
    sudden fall in 211
    systolic 362
  properties of 33
  reservoir function 95

substitutes 91
sugar level
  maintenance of 263
  normal 263
  regulation of 263
testis barrier 286
transfusion 86, 91
  autologous 92
  hazards of 91
  heterologous 92
  indications of 91
typing
  principle of 86
  requisites for 86
vessels 143, 182, 188, 190, 246, 276, 325, 328, 384
  condition of wall of 375
  diameter of 364
  elasticity of 364
  hepatic 381
  walls, different 328t
viscosity of 38, 364
volume 34, 364, 388
  measurement of 30, 35
  normal 34
  regulation of 35
  variations of 34
B-lymphocytes 66, 70, 72
  specificity of 70
  storage of 67
  types of 67
Body 293
  built 363
  defense mechanism of 38, 95
  fluid 27, 392
    compartments of 27, 28f
    composition of 27
    concentration of 30
    distribution of 27
    volume, measurement of 28
  motor activities of 493
  parts of 222, 222t
  systems of 22
  temperature 222, 224
    normal 222
    regulation of 36, 140, 221, 224, 225f, 398, 505
    set point for 224
    variations of 222
  water, measurement of total 29
  weight 246
Bohr effect 419
Boiled starch 140
Bolus 139, 173
Bombay group 89
Bone 93, 251, 259, 592
  conduction 592
  diseases 254, 259
  effect on 298
  functions of 257
  growth, effect on 291
  marrow 93
  physiology of 251, 257
  remodeling, significance of 259
  smallest 586
  structure of 258
Bony labyrinth 533, 587
Bony spiral canal 587
Botulinum toxin 124
Bowman's capsule 183-185, 188, 190, 193, 194, 194f, 195, 202
  functional histology of 185
  visceral layer of 194
Bowman's glands 598
Brachial pulse 375
Brachioradialis jerk 471
Bradycardia 356, 361
Bradykinesia 515

Bradykinin 195
Bradypnea 427
Brain 143, 388, 445, 543
  attack 380
  damage 388
  inattentive 539
  lesions 225
  natriuretic peptide 196, 269, 280
  parts of 445, 446f
  synapse in 547
  ventricles of 550
Brainstem 484
  nuclei 494
Braxton Hicks contractions 313
Breast
  adenosis of 316
  cysts in 315
  disease
    benign, types of 315
  effect on 298
  fibroadenoma of 315
  hyperplasia of 315
  milk, advantages of 317
Breath holding time 421
Breathing 431
  capacity, maximum 410
  cessation of 175
  prolonged forced 43
  temporary arrest of 427
  work of 404, 404f
Broca's area 519, 549
Brodmann areas 517
Bronchial artery 398, 399
Bronchial asthma
  causes of 432
  features of 432
Bronchodilation 276
Bronchospasm 88
Brown adipose tissue 223
Brown fat tissue 223
Brown-Séquard syndrome 487
Brunner's glands 167
Brush bordered cells 153, 185
Bruxism 545
B-type natriuretic peptide 280
Buccal cavity 137
Buccal glands 138
Buccinator muscle 172
Bucket handle movement 401
Buffer action 37, 48
Bulbar outflow 554
Bulbourethral glands 288
Bulbs, capillary 96
Bulbus oculi 559
Bulk flow 16
Bulldog scalp 240
Bundle branches 333
Bungarotoxin 124
Burn shock 388
Burning sensation 392
Butter fat 147
Butyric acid 599

C

C cells 254
C wave 377
Caisson disease 437
Calcitonin 243, 254
  plasma level of 254
  role of 256, 257
  secretion, regulation of 254
Calcitriol 256, 279
Calcium 196, 255
  absorption of 255, 256
  calmodulin complex 129
  excretion of 255, 256
  ion

excess of 165
influx of 332
role of 119
transport of 18
level, normal value of 255
metabolism 254, 255f
phosphate crystals 254
pump 18
receptor 254
rigor 114
role of blood level of 252
types of 255
Callosomarginal fissure 517
Calyx 185, 535
Canal constitute internal anal sphincter 134
Canal of Schlemm 564
Canaliculi 145
Cancer development, risk of 315
Capillary blood
  flow, peculiarities of 382
  pressure 371, 372, 372f, 373
    regional variations of 372
Capillary membrane 196, 397
  permeability of 196
Capillary oncotic pressure 373
Capillary plexus 398
Capillary system, pattern of 381
Carbamino compounds 420
Carbamino proteins 420
Carbamylcholine 124
Carbhemoglobin 41, 420
Carbohydrate 3, 73
  digestion of 154
  functions of 3
  metabolism 235, 245, 260, 262, 269, 276
  molecules 3
Carbolic acid 58
Carbon dioxide 15, 354, 354f, 398, 415f, 417f, 420
  diffusing capacity for 415
  diffusion of 415, 416, 416f
  dissociation curve 420f
    normal 420
  excess of 130
  partial pressure of 207
  transport of 419, 420, 420f
Carbon monoxide 49, 432
  effects of 432
  poisoning 432
    chronic 43
    signs of 49
    symptoms of 49, 432
  sources of 49
Carbon monoxyhemoglobin 49
Carbon particles and silicon, removal of 94
Carbonic acid 147, 205, 398, 419
Carbonic anhydrase 147, 205, 419
  inhibitor 212
Carboxyhemoglobin 49
Carboxypeptidases 152, 154
  actions of 154
Carcinogens 5
Carcinoma 75
Cardiac bruit 343
Cardiac cycle 335, 336, 336f, 337t, 338, 339
  division of 335
  events of 335
  pressure changes during 338, 339, 339t
  ventricular events of 336
Cardiac diseases, shock due to 389
Cardiac failure
  congestive 212
  development of 440

Cardiac glands 145
Cardiac index, normal value of 351
Cardiac murmur 340, 343
Cardiac muscle 1, 103, 104, 114, 326, 331, 332, 334, 334f
    fiber 327f
    intercalated disk of 14
    properties of 331
    refractory period in 334
    structure of 326
Cardiac output 351, 354, 363, 393, 399
    distribution of 352
    measurement of 353, 354
    variations in 352
Cardiac sphincter 144
Cardioaccelerator
    center 357
    reflex 360, 360f
    tone 359
Cardiogenic shock, types of 389
Cardioinhibitory reflex 359, 360f
Cardioinhibitory tone 358
Cardiovascular accident 380
Cardiovascular system 1, 57, 126, 246, 312, 325, 388, 436, 542
    effects on 429
Carotid baroreceptors 359
Carotid pulse 375
Carotid sinus syncope 389
Carpopedal spasm 253, 253f
Carrier protein 17, 18f, 19f
Cartilage 1
Caruncula sublingualis 138
Caseinogens 153
Castle, intrinsic factor of 47, 167
Casts 210
Catacrotic limb 374
Catacrotic notch 374
Catalase 6, 50
Catamenia 305
Cataplexy 508, 545
Cataract 566
Catecholamines 274
    metabolism of 274, 275f
    plasma level of 274
    removal of 275
    stages of
        metabolism of 275
        synthesis of 274
    synthesis of 274, 275f
Catechol-O-methyltransferase 275
Cathelicidins 70, 397
Celiac disease 156, 169
Celiac ganglion 135
Celiac plexus 159
Celiac sprue 169
Cell 1
    body 568
    death 11
        unprogrammed 11
    junction 12, 13t
        different types of 12f
        proteins 12
    membrane 1, 2f, 15, 73
        carbohydrate of 3
        composition of 2
        functions of 3, 3b
        lipids of 2, 2f
        permeability of 230
        protein layers of 2
        selective permeability of 116
        simple diffusion through 16f
        structure of 2
    murder 11
    secretory function of 145t, 167t
    signaling 227
    structure of 1, 2f
    types of 167, 258, 595
Cellulose 140
Central nervous system 23, 215, 246, 269, 276, 445
    development of 246
    effects on 429
    manifestations of 265
    normal function of 246
    parts of 445f
Centrosome 4, 7
Cephalic phase 148, 154
Cephalin 154
Cerebellar
    ataxia 115
    hemispheres 509
    lesions 512t
Cerebellum 494, 509
    division of 509
    functions of 511t
    parts of 509, 510f
Cerebral
    aqueduct, blockage of 552
    blood flow
        normal 380
        regulation of 380
    blood vessels 380
    circulation 380
        importance of 380
    cortex 178, 359, 366, 476, 494, 512, 516, 520f, 521f, 532, 540, 567
        frontal lobe of 518
        functional gateway for 501
        lateral surface of 518f, 519f
        lobes of 516, 517f
        medial surface of 519f
        morphology of 516
        parts of 517f
        sensory area of 482
        temporal lobe of 589
    dominance 517
    palsy 115, 495
Cerebri, epiphysis of 278
Cerebro-cerebello-cerebral
    circuit 511f
    connections 510
Cerebropontocerebellar tract 511
Cerebrospinal fluid 445, 550
    absorption of 550
    circulation of 550, 551f
    collection of 551
    composition of 550, 550f
    formation of 550
    functions of 551
Cerebrum 516
Ceruminous glands 585
Cervical
    cap 319
    sympathetic
        ganglia 358
        nerve 579, 359
Cervix 296
    effect on 299
Chemical
    barriers 319
    energy 597, 599
    messengers 227, 228f
        classification of 227
    stimulus 110
    synapse 13, 462, 462f
        functional anatomy of 462
        structure of 462
    thermogenesis 224
Chemoattractants 62
Chemokines 70
Chemoreceptors 360, 424, 457, 458, 597
    central 425
    functions of 360, 366
    mechanism 366
    nerve supply to 359f, 360
    peripheral 425
    situation of 360
    types of 424
Chemoreflex, coronary 361
Chemotaxis 62
Chenodeoxycholic acid 160
Chest leads
    electrodes for 345f
    position of 345
    unipolar 345
Cheyne-Stokes breathing 428, 431, 542
    features of 431
Chicken chest 259
Chief cells 251
Chief sensory nucleus 480
Chloride 19, 197
Chloroform 599
Cholagogue 163
    action 161, 162
Cholecalciferol 252, 279
Cholecystectomy 163
Cholecystokinin 149, 150, 156, 169, 262
    action of 156
Cholelithiasis 165
Cholera 71
Choleretic action 161, 162
Cholestatic jaundice, causes of 164
Cholesterol 2, 73
    ester hydrolase 154
    excess of 165
Cholic acid 160
Choline 124
Cholinergic neurotransmitter 282
Cholinesterase inhibitors 124
Chondrocytes 235
Chorda tympani
    fibers 596
    syndrome 142
Chordae tendineae 327
Chorea 502, 515
Choreoathetosis 515
Choroid 560
    plexus 550, 552
Christmas disease 83
Chromaffin cells, types of 274
Chromatin 8
    network 45
Chromophil cells, classification of 233
Chromophobe
    cells 233
    tumor of 241
Chromophore 568
Chromosomal disorders 10, 10b, 115
Chromosome 8
    instability syndromes 10
Chronaxie
    determines, measurement of 111
    importance of 111
Chronic heart failure 389
    signs of 390
    symptoms of 390
Chronic renal failure
    causes of 211
    treatment for 211
Chvostek's sign 253
Chyme 156, 175
    formation of 146
Chymotrypsin
    actions of 153
    digests 153
Chymotrypsinogen 153
Cilia 560
Ciliary body 460, 560
Ciliary ganglion 579
Ciliary muscle 578, 579
Ciliospinal reflex 576
Circadian rhythm 278, 507
    control of 524
Circular diaphragm 561
Circulation, division of 329
Circulatory shock 265, 387
    types of 388, 388f
Circulatory system 23
Circumvallate papillae 595
Circus movement 349
Cisterna 5
    lateralis 550
    magna 550, 551
Cisternal puncture 551
Citrates
    mechanism of action of 82
    phosphate dextrose 82
    uses of 82
Clara cells 401
Clarke's nucleus 480
Classical conditioned reflexes, types of 548
Classical pills, mechanism of action of 321
Clathrin 20
Clear cells 243, 254
Clonus 471
Clostridium
    botulinum 124
    tetani 58
Clot
    lysis of 288, 306
    retraction 74, 80
Clotting
    mechanism, sequence of 78
    tests for 82
    time 82
Coal mines 49
Cochlea 533, 587, 592f
    compartments of 587
    spiral canal of 587f
Cochlear microphonic potential 592
Cochlear nerve 590
Cochlear nuclei 589
Coenzyme 154
Cohn's tubes 59
Cold
    blooded animals 224
    effects of 438
    rigor 114
    temperature 113
Collapse, stage of 430
Collateral arteries, coronary 379
Collateral ganglia 553
Collecting ducts 182, 185, 204
Colliculus
    inferior 589
    superior 573
Colloidal osmotic pressure 17, 194, 195
Colon
    descending 170
    hypertrophy of 171
Colony-forming
    blastocytes 44, 64
    cells, different units of 44
    unit 44, 46f
Colony-stimulating factor 64, 70
    secretion of 94

Color blindness 581*f*
 classification of 581
 tests for 581
 total 581
Color index 54
Color sensitive areas 580
Color vision 580
Colostrum 316
Columns of Bertin 181
Coma 32
 hyperosmolar 265
Common bile duct 152, 158
Computerized spirometer 407
Concha 585
Conditioned reflex 141, 149, 155, 469
 types of 548
Conduction deafness 593, 594
 causes of 593
Conduction, types of 592
Conductive system, parts of 333
Cone 580
 cells 569
 structure of 568
 dystrophy 570
 functions of 568
Configuration 50
Confrontation test 571
Congenital adrenal hyperplasia 273*f*
 causes of 273
 symptoms of 273
Conjugate movement 543, 566
Conjugated bilirubin
 excretion of 161
 fate of 161
Conjunctiva 560
Conn's syndrome 272
Connective tissue 1
Connexins 13
Conscious kinesthetic sensation 481*f*
Conscious movements, regulation of 514
Consciousness, loss of 541, 542
Consensual light reflex 576
Constipation, causes of 171
Constrictor papillae 561
Continuous murmur 343, 386
Contraceptive
 hormonal 321
 long-term 321
 methods 318, 320*t*
 pills 321
Contractile proteins 127
Contraction
 period 112
 point of 112
 time 112
 types of 111
Contrecoup injury 551
Conus medullaris 473
Convergence 465, 466*f*
Conveyor belts 7
Convoluted tubules 181
Convulsion 312, 540
 stage of 430
Cooley's anemia 57
Copper intrauterine contraceptive device 320
Core temperature 222
Corona radiata 302, 482
Coronary artery
 branch of 378
 disease 379
Coronary blood flow
 normal 378
 phasic changes in 379, 379*f*
 regulation of 379

Coronary blood vessels 378
Coronary circulation 378
Coronary perfusion pressure 379
Coronary sinus 378
Corpora cavernosa 288
Corpus albicans 305
Corpus hemorrhagicum 304
Corpus luteum 297, 298, 304, 304*f*, 305
 graviditatis 305
 development of 304
 fate of 305
 functions of 305
Corpus spongiosum 288
Corpus striatum 513, 514*f*
Corpuscular hemoglobin concentration, mean 54, 55
Cortex 97, 278, 295
Cortical auditory centers 589
 functions of 590
Cortical lobes, functions of 522*t*
Corticocerebellum
 components of 510
 functions of 511
 mechanism of action of 511
Corticomedullary junction 183
Corticonuclear fibers 578
Corticopontocerebellar tract 511
Corticospinal tract 483
Corticosteroids 266
Corticotrophs 234
Corticotropin-releasing hormone 188, 234, 505
 secretion of 189
Cortisol 163
 secretion, regulation of 271*f*
Cotransport 18
Cough reflex 397, 398
 causes of 398
 mechanism of 398
Cough syncope 389
Coumarin derivatives 81
Countercurrent exchanger 201, 202*f*
Countercurrent flow 200
Countercurrent multiplier 201, 201*f*
Countercurrent system, divisions of 201
Countertransport 18
Cracking voice 291
Cramps 115
Cranial content volume, regulation of 551
Cranial nerve nuclei 493
Cranial outflow 554
Craniosacral outflow 554
Creatine phosphate 121
Creatinin 182
Cretinism 249, 249*t*
 causes for 249
Cricopharyngeal muscle 173
Crista 6
 ampullaris 534, 534*f*
 excitation of 536*f*
Crohn's disease 169
Crossed extensor reflex 472, 472*f*, 532
Crude touch sensation, loss of 478
Cryptorchidism 290
Crypts of Lieberkühn 166
Crystalline 564
Crystals 210
C-type natriuretic peptide 269, 280
Cubic micron 54
Cuboidal epithelial cells 1
Cumulus oophorus 302
Cupula 535, 587
Cushing's disease 240, 271

Cushing's syndrome
 causes of 271
 signs of 271, 272*b*
 symptoms of 271, 272*b*
 tests for 271
Cusps 327
Cutaneous blood vessels, architecture of 382
Cutaneous circulation, functions of 383
Cutaneous receptors 456, 456*f*, 457*t*
Cuticular plate 535, 588
Cyanocobalamin 47
Cyanosis 32, 430-432
 causes for 431
 distribution of 432
Cyclic adenosine, monophosphate 231
Cystic fibrosis 156
Cystometrogram 215, 216, 216*f*
 segments of 216
Cytochrome, oxidase 50
Cytokines 70, 71*t*, 187
Cytoplasm 3, 73, 230
Cytoplasmic organelles 3*b*
 functions of 4*t*
Cytosine 9
Cytoskeleton 4, 7
Cytosol 3
Cytotoxic cells, activity of 68
Cytotoxic substances 62
Cytotoxic T cells
 mechanism of action of 68
 role of 68
Cytotoxic T lymphocytes 6

D

D antigen 87
D-amino acid oxidase 6
Dark adaptation, causes for 569
Dark band 106
Dead space 411
 measurement of 412, 412*f*
 normal value of 412
 physiological 412
 types of 411
Deafness 590
Decompression sickness
 prevention of 437
 symptoms of 437
Deep reflexes 469, 471*t*
Deep sea physiology 436
Deep sensations 490
Deep sleep
 initial stage of 543
 stages of 543
Defecation reflex 177, 177*f*
 pathway for 178
Defective rod function 570
Defensins 70, 397
Deglutition 172
 apnea 173, 398
 reflex 174, 398
 stages of 172, 173*f*
Dehydration 31, 54, 142, 195, 171, 241
 causes of 31
 classification of 31
 exhaustion 439
 mild 31
 severe 31
 shock 388
 signs of 31
 symptoms of 31
 treatment of 32
Dehydroepiandrosterone sulphate 312

Deiter nucleus 484
Delirium 32
Delta rhythm 540
Delta waves 543, 544
Dementia 515, 548
 causes of 548
 features of 548
Dendritic cells 67, 397
Dengue
 fever 54
 shock syndrome 54
Dense bodies 127
Dental caries 142
Dentatorubral fibers 511
Dentatorubro-thalamocortical tract 511
Deoxycholate 160
Deoxygenated blood 158, 398
Deoxyribonucleic acid 8, 154
 molecules of 8
 non-chromosomal 8
 structure of 9, 9*f*
Depolarization 117, 118
Depression 565
Dermatomal rule 498
Dermis 218
Desensitization 458
Desmosome 12-14
Desynchronization 539
Desynchronized waves 539, 540, 544
Detoxification 5
Detrusor muscle 213
 contraction of 216*f*
Deuteranomaly 581
Deuteranopia 581
Dextrinase converts dextrin 167
Diabetes insipidus 225, 241, 508
 causes of 241
Diabetes mellitus 72, 240, 264
 causes of 264
 classification of 264
 complications of 265
 diagnostic tests for 265
 non-insulin-dependent 264
 type I 264, 264*t*
 type II 264, 264*t*
Diabetic nephropathy 265
Diabetic neuropathy 265
Diabetic retinopathy 265
Dialysis 209, 211
Diapedesis 62
Diaphragm 319, 401
Diarrhea 151, 171
 causes of 171
 chronic 171
 features of 171
Dibenamine 142
Dichromatism 581
Diencephalon 445, 503
Dietary iron 50
Diffusion 15
DiGeorge's syndrome 71
Digestion 133
Digestive enzymes 139, 170, 317
Digestive function 139, 146, 162, 167, 168
Digestive glands, ducts of 126
Digestive juices 168
Digestive organs, primary 134
Digestive peristaltic contractions 174
Digestive process 133
Digestive system 22, 57, 126, 133, 313
 effects on 429
 functions of 133
Digests milk fats 140
Dihydrotestosterone 290

Dihydroxycholecalciferol
	action of 279
	formation of 279
	role of 256
Dihydroxyphenylalanine 219, 274, 275
Diiodo- tyrosine 244
Dilator papillae 561
Dilution method, uses of indicator 29
Dipalmitoylphosphatidylcholine 401
Diplegia 495
Diploid cells 8
Diplopia 571
Direct light reflex 576
Disjugate movement 566
Disk prolapse 487
Distal convoluted tubule 185, 204
Distant vision 570
	vision for 570
Disulfide
	bonds 69
	bridges 260
Diuresis 204, 212
Diuretics
	administration of 32
	agents 212
	types of 212
	uses of 212
Diurnal rhythm 507
Diurnal variation 278, 363
Divergence 465, 466f
Dopa decarboxylase 274
Dopamine 196, 274, 277
	beta-hydroxylase 274
	lack of 514
Doppler echocardiography 355
Dorsal funiculus 476
Dorsal respiratory group 421
Dorsal root 474
Dorsal spinocerebellar tract 479
Dorsal white column 476
Dorsalis pedis pulse 375
Double antigen-antibody reactions 314
Double lumen catheter 216
Double vision 571
Douglas bag 408, 413
Down syndrome 10, 115
Downhill movement 15
Downward movement 565
Drooling 142
Drowsiness 57
	stages of 543
Drowsy state 543
Drugs 182
	stimulating neuromuscular junction 124
Drum beating tremor 515
Ductless glands 228
Ducts of Bellini 182, 185
Ducts of Rivinus 138
Ductus arteriosus 384, 385
	closure of 386
Ductus reuniens 534
Ductus venosus, closure of 386
Duodenal ulcer 151
Duodenum 166
Dura mater 445
Dural sinuses 550
Dust particles, prevention of 397
Dwarfism 240, 249t
	types of 240b
Dye dilution technique 29
Dynamic gamma motor 528
Dynamic lung function tests 405
Dysarthria 549
Dysgeusia 597

Dysmenorrhea 308
Dysphonia 549
Dyspnea 57, 427, 428, 430, 431
	point 431
Dystrophia adiposogenitalis 241, 294, 508
	causes of 242
	symptoms of 242

E

Ear 585
	internal 587
	structure of 586f
Earwax 585
Eaton-Lambert myasthenic syndrome 125
Eccrine glands
	control of 220
	secretory activity of 220
Eccrine sweat glands 220t
Eclampsia 312
Ectopic foci 349
Ectoplasm 3
	microfilament of 7f
Edema 99
	extracellular 99, 100, 100b
	generalized 99
	local 99
	types of 99
Edinger-Westphal nucleus 564, 576, 578
Effector 23
	organ 468
Efferent arteriole 184, 190
	constriction of 195
Efferent fibers 174, 578, 579
Efferent nerve 468
	fiber 450, 450b
Efferent pathway 576
Effort syncope 389
Einthoven's triangle 344
Ejaculation 292
Ejaculatory duct 287
Ejection fraction 337, 351
Elastase 152, 154
Elastic resistance thorax 404
Electrical energy 569, 597, 599
Electrical stimulus 110
Electrical synapse 462, 462f
Electrocardiogram 344
Electrochemical gradient 196
Electrodes, position of 345f
Electroencephalogram 539, 539, 544f
Electrolyte
	balance
		effect on 298
		maintenance of 182
	imbalance 171
	loss 36
	reabsorption, inhibiting of 212
Electron
	dense layers 2
	transport system 6
Electronic vibrator 594
Electroretinogram 570, 570f
Elevated jugular venous pulse 377
Eliciting reflex, method of 470
Eliminates transfusion reactions 92
Elliptocytosis 43
Embolism 83
Embolus 83, 379
Embryo
	development of 311
	implantation of 311
Emergency contraceptive pills 321
Emmenia 305

Emmetropia 582
Emmetropic eye 582
Emotion 35, 223
	outburst of 545
Emphysema 43, 404, 433
Emulsion 161
End knob, posterior 293
End-diastolic volume 338, 339
Endemic colloid goiter 249
Endocardium 327
Endocrine
	disorders 208, 264
	function 152, 182, 311
	glands 228, 229f, 247
		major 229t
		regulation of 523
	hormones, role of 262
	messengers 227
	system 1, 23, 227, 313
Endocrinology 227
Endocytosis 19
Endogenous analgesia system 498
Endolymph 533, 536
Endolymphatic duct 534
Endolymphatic sac 534
Endometrium 296, 305, 306
Endomysium 105, 453
Endopeptidase 153
Endoplasm 3
Endoplasmic reticulum 3-5, 73
	integrated function of 5f
	types of 3
Endosmosis 17, 20, 31
Endosteum 258
Endothelial cells 21, 64, 398
Endothelial layer, capillary 185
Endothelin 130, 196, 368
Endothelium 414
	derived relaxing factor 130
Endplate potential
	development of 123
	properties of 124
End-systolic volume 337, 339
Energy
	minimum loss of 591
	production of 6
Enophthalmos 579
Enteric nervous system 134, 135
Enterochromaffin cells 145, 167
Enterocytes 166, 167
	secrete 167
Enteroendocrine cells 145
Enterogastric reflex 150
Enterohepatic circulation, significance of 159
Enterokinase 153, 167
Enteropeptidase 153
Enuresis 217
Enzymatic proteins 7
Enzyme 74
	cascade theory 78
	glutaminase 207
	hydrolytic 20
	iodinase 244
	lysozyme 560
	phenylalanine hydroxylase 274
	transport of 35
Eosinophils 44, 45f, 61
	functions of 62
Ephedrine 141
Epicardiac arteries 378
Epicardium 326
Epicritic sensations 489
Epidermis 218
Epididymis 287
Epilepsy 539, 540
	general onset 541

	generalized 541
	localized 541
	types of 540
Epileptic aura 541
Epimysium 105
Epiphyseal cartilage 258
Epiphyseal fusion 235
Epiphyseal plate 258
Epiphysis 258
	fusion of 298
Epithalial cells 13, 187, 210
	columnar 1
Epithelial tissue 1
Epithelium 414, 564
Equilibrium 527
	area for 522
Erb's sign 253
Erb-Westphal sign 253
Ergotamine 142
Erlanger-Gasser classification 450
Erythroblastosis fetalis 89, 92
	complications of 89
Erythroblasts, presence of 89
Erythrocyte 33, 40, 44, 46f, 63f
	development of 44
	maturation of 44, 47
	sedimentation rate 38, 52
		determination of 52
		normal values of 52, 53t
		variations of 53
Erythropoiesis 44, 46t, 47t
	factors necessary for 47
	process of 44
	site of 44
	stages of 45
Erythropoietin 47, 182, 279
	secreting 182
Esophageal balloon 402
Esophageal Doppler transducer technique 355
Esophageal sphincter, upper 173
Esophagus 126, 134
	peristaltic contractions of 174
Estrogen 163, 290, 297, 307, 311
	binding protein 286
	forms of 297
	functions of 297
	mode of action of 298
	secretion, regulation of 298, 299
Ethinyl estradiol 321
Ethyl ether 599
Ethylenediaminetetra acetic acid 52, 81
Eukaryotes 8
Eunuchism 242, 294
Eustachian tube 587
	role of 592
Excess secretory products, removal of 6
Excess sleep 545
Exchange transfusion
	indications of 92
	procedure for 92
Excitation-contraction coupling 119
Excitatory neurotransmitter 282, 467
Excitatory postsynaptic potential 462, 463
Excretion system 181
Excretory function 35, 140, 146, 162, 171, 182, 221, 311
Excretory products 161
Excretory system 22, 313, 542
Exercise
	mild 392
	severity of 392
	types of 391
Exocrine function 152

Index

Exocytosis 19, 20, 123
   mechanism of 20
   process of 21*f*
Exopeptidases 154
Exophthalmos, effect of 248
Exosmosis 17
Expired air 413, 413*t*
External ear 585
   role of 591
External sphincter, voluntary relaxation of 178
External urethral sphincter 213, 214
Exteroceptors 456, 457*f*
Extorsion 565
Extracellular fluid 1, 13, 16*f*, 18, 18*f*, 19*f*, 22, 27, 28*f*, 35, 123, 188*f*, 191, 212, 231, 267
   subunits of 27*t*
   volume 267
      measurement of 29
      regulation of 367
Extracellular materials, digestion of 5
Extrafoveal vision 563
Extraglomerular mesangial cells 187, 189
Extrahepatic jaundice, causes of 164
Extrapyramidal system 513
Extrapyramidal tracts 482, 484, 494
Extrasystole 349
Extrinsic muscles 564, 565*f*
   innervation of 565
Extrinsic pathway 80
Eye 559
   movement of 523
Eyeball 559
   conjugate movement of 519
   extrinsic muscles of 565*f*
   functional anatomy of 559
   movement of 537
   muscles of 564
   reflex movements of 573
   simultaneous movements of 566
   structure of 561*f*
   wall of 560, 562*f*
Eyelids 218, 559

F

F cells 263
Fabricius, bursa of 66
Facial nerve 136
   branch of 586
   chorda tympani branch of 140
Facial pulse 375
Facilitatory reticular system, descending 526
F-actin 107
Fallopian tubes 296
   effect on 298, 299
False labor contractions 313
Farrell and Ivy pouch, uses of 148
Fascia 105
Fasciculi 105
Fasciculus
   cuneatus 481
   dorsolateralis 480
   gracilis 481
Fast pain fibers 497
Fat 97
   absorption of 161
   deposition of 298
   emulsification of 160
   metabolism 235, 245, 262, 269, 276
   necrosis 316
   storage of 261
   surface tension of 161
Fatigue 465, 472
Fatty acids
   synthesis of 261
   transport of 261
Fatty liver 245
Faundice, extrahepatic 164
Feces, formation of 171
Feed-forward control system 25
Feminization 272
Femoral pulse 375
Fencing function 13
Fenestra 193
Ferrihemoglobin 49
Ferritin 41
Fertile period 318
Fertility control 318
Fertilization 287
   prevention of 319
Festinant gait 515
Fetal
   circulation 384, 385*f*
   hemoglobin 48
   lungs 384
      nonfunctioning of 384
Fetoplacental unit 312, 312*f*
Fetus, expulsion of 238
Fever, causes of 225
Fibers
   dopaminergic 514
   extrafusal 494
Fibrin monomer 80
Fibrinogen 37, 287
   conversion of 24, 89
Fibrinolysin 292, 306
Fibrinolysis 80
Fibrinolytic enzymes 80
Fibrin-stabilizing factor 74, 80
Fibrocartilaginous plate 585
Fick's principle 210, 353
   modification of 354
Fight reactions 276
Filaments 73
Filiform papillae 595
Filtration 16, 99
   fraction 194
   membrane 185, 193, 194*f*
   pores 184, 193
   process of 99
First heart sound 336, 340, 341
   reduplication of 341
Fissure 473
Flaccid paralysis 115
Flaccidity 115
Flavor 597
Flechsig's tract 479
Flexor reflexes 469
Flight reactions 276
Floating ribs 401
Flocculonodular lobe 509
Fluid
   buffer 551
   hypotonic 30, 31
   imbalance 31*b*
   loss 36
   movement of 28*f*, 536*f*
   pressure 564
Folic acid 47
   deficiency 47, 57
Follicle stimulating hormone 234, 236, 289, 298, 302, 307
Follicular cavity 243, 302
Follicular cells 243
Follicular sheath 302
Food
   flavor of 597
   intake, regulation of 505, 523
   particles, digestion of 133
   substances
      consumption of 133
      movement of 126
Foodstuffs, metabolism of 223
Footplate 586, 592
Foramen magnum 445, 473
Foramen of Luschka 550
Foramen of Magendie 550
Foramen of Monro 550
Foramen ovale, closure of 385
Forced expiratory volume 409, 409*f*
Forebrain 445
Fovea centralis 563, 570
Foveal vision 563
Fractional gastric analysis 151
Fractional test meal 151
Fragility 58, 59
   test 59
      results of 59*t*
   types of 59
Frank-Starling law 114, 353
Free bilirubin 161
Free fatty acids 219
Free nerve ending 457, 529
Fröhlich's syndrome 242, 294, 508
Frontal eye field 519, 578, 579
Frontal lobe 578
   syndrome 520
Frontal motor area, upper 549
Frostbite 438
Fruity breath odor 265
Functional residual capacity 406
   measurement of 408
Fundic glands 145
Fundus 144, 563
   oculi 563, 563*f*
Fungiform papillae 595
Funiculus, posterior 476

G

G cells 150
G proteins, role of 231
G-actin 107
Gait 515
Galactopoiesis 316
Gallbladder 163
   bile 160*f*, 160*t*
   disorders of 164
   epithelium, infection of 165
   functions of 163
Gallop rhythm 342
Gallstone
   features of 165
   formation
      causes for 165
      prevention of 161, 162
      presence of 165
Gamma globulins 38
Gamma glutamyl transferase 164
Gamma-aminobutyric acid, action of 463
Gamma-motor neurons 114, 484, 494, 514, 527, 530
   activation of 518
Ganglia, peripheral 553
Ganglion cell layer 563
Ganglionic blockers 556
Ganglionic cells 563, 572
   axons of 572
Gangrene 439
Gap junction 12, 13, 127
   functions of 13
   structure of 13
Garbage disposal system 6
Gases
   effects of 434
   exchange of 414
   transport of 418
Gastric
   acidity, measurement of 151
   amylase 146, 147, 150
   atrophy
      causes of 151
      features of 151
   content
      consistency of 175
      osmolar concentration of 175
      pH of 175
      volume of 175
   disorder 151
   function tests 150
   glands 145, 145*f*, 145*t*
      parietal cell of 148*f*
      structure of 145
   inhibitory peptide 149, 150, 262
   juice
      collection of 150
      composition of 146, 146*f*
      digestive enzymes of 147*t*
      enzymes of 147
      functions of 146
      hydrochloric acid of 147
      hyperacidity of 151
      properties of 146
      secretion of 25, 147
   lipase 146, 147, 149, 156
   phase, experimental evidences of 150
   pits 145
   secretion 144, 149
      actions of 150
      phases of 148
      regulation of 147, 149*f*
   ulcer 151
Gastrin 150, 156, 262
   actions of 150
   releasing peptide 150
Gastritis
   causes of 151
   features of 151
Gastrocnemius-sciatic preparation 111
Gastrocolic reflex 177, 178
Gastrointestinal disorder 175
Gastrointestinal hormones 283
   role of 262
Gastrointestinal mucosa 134
Gastrointestinal tract 66, 97, 126, 133, 133*f*, 134, 162, 171, 246, 252, 263, 542, 554
   hormones 150
   movements of 172
   wall of 134
Gate control
   significance of 499
   theory 499
Gate function 12
Gaucher's disease 75
Gelatinase 147
Gelatinous cupula, movement of 536
Gene 9
   expression 10
Genetic code
   transcription of 10
   translation of 11
Genetic disorders 9, 10
   causes of 9
Genetic mutation 10
Geniculate body
   lateral 572, 573
   medial 589
Geniculate ganglion 140

Geniculocalcarine tract 573
Genital ducts 126
Genital ridge 290
Genital tract, female 288
Genitalia, external 290
Germ cells 286, 296
Germ hill 302
Germinal center 97
Gestation period 313
Ghrelin 156
Giant cells 482
Giddiness 313
Gigantism
   causes of 239
   signs of 239
   symptoms of 239
Glands of Littre 213, 288
Glans penis 288
Glaucoma 566
Globin 41, 48
   formation of 50
   molecule 48
   polypeptide chains of 48t
Globulin 37
Glomerular blood flow, regulation of 189
Glomerular capillary 184, 190, 192
   membrane 193
   pressure 194, 195
Glomerular filtration 193, 194, 199
   rate 188, 189, 191, 194, 195, 210, 212
      measurement of 210
      regulation of 189
Glomerular interstitium, secrete matrix of 187
Glomerular mesangial cells 187, 189
   contraction of 196
Glomerulonephritis
   acute 211
   chronic 211
Glomerulotubular balance 197
Glomerulus 183, 184
Glossopharyngeal nerve 136, 140, 174
   fibers 596
Glottis, closure of 175
Glucagon 163, 262
   actions of 262
   regulation of secretion of 262
   role of 263
Glucocorticoids 256, 257, 268
   functions of 269
   mode of action of 270
   permissive action of 269
   regulation of secretion of 270
Gluconeogenesis 262
   inhibiting of 261
Glucose 196
   buffer system 263
   peripheral utilization of 260
   reabsorption of 198
   receptors 505
   renal threshold for 198
   storage of 261
   tolerance test 265
   transport of 19
   tubular maximum for 198
Glucostatic mechanism 505, 506f
Glucostats 505
Glucosuria 240, 265
Glutamate 568
Glutamic acid 207
Gluten-sensitive enteropathy 169
Glycerophosphate acetyltransferase 6
Glycine 50, 160, 207

Glycocalyx 3, 73
Glycocholic acid 160
Glycogen 74
   droplets 105
Glycogenesis 261
Glycogenolysis 262
   inhibiting of 261
Glycolipids 3, 73
Glycoproteins 3, 73, 80, 279
Goblet cells 167
Goiter
   hypothyroid 249
   idiopathic non-toxic 250
Goitrin 250
Goitrogens 250
Golgi apparatus 4, 5, 5f, 73, 105, 448
   functions of 5
Golgi neurons 448
Golgi tendon
   apparatus 529f
   organ 529
      functions of 529
Gonadotrophs 234
Gonadotropin releasing hormone 299, 234, 507
Gonads 143, 285
Goormaghtigh cells 187
Gower's tract 478
Graafian follicle 303, 303f, 310
Grand mal 541
Granular cells 188
Granules 73
Granulocyte 44, 46f, 60, 63f, 64
Granulosa cells 302
Granzymes 6
Graves' disease 72, 248
Gravitational force 436, 469
Growth
   factor, secretion of transforming 94
   hormone 234, 236, 256, 257, 290
      actions of 234
      inhibitory hormone 234-236
      receptor, genes of 240
      releasing hormone 234-236
      releasing polypeptide 234-236
   inducers 47
   plate 258
   stage of 289, 297
Guanine 9
Guanosine
   diphosphate 231
   triphosphate 231
Guerrilla face 239
Gustatory sensation 595
Guttural breathing 249
Gynecomastia 272

H

H antigen 89
Haemophilia, causes for 83
Hageman factor 79
Hair 57
   cells 535, 536, 536f, 537f, 588-592
      cilia of 535
      electrical potential in 536
      excitation of 592
   distribution, effect on 291
   follicles 218
Hairpin bend 185
Haldane effect, significance of 420
Halitosis 142
Hallucination 523

Hamburger phenomenon 419
Hamulus 587
Haploid cells 8
Hashimoto's thyroiditis 72, 248
Hassall corpuscles 278
Head
   enlargement of 552
   linear acceleration of 535
Hearing
   gradual loss of 590
   mechanism of 591
   perception of 591
   process of 592
   test for 593
   theories of 593
Heart 279, 325
   actions of 327, 328t
   attack 380
   block 349, 358
      complete 358
      partial 358
   conductive system of 333f, 334t
   disease, congenital 43
   failure 387, 389
      causes of 389
      congestive 389
      signs of 390
      symptoms of 390
      types of 389
   layers of wall of 326
   left side of 325
   motor nerve fibers to 357
   nerve supply to 358f
   rate 353, 356, 361f, 364, 392, 542
      normal 356
      regulation of 357, 505
   regulation of actions of 328
   right side of 325
   section of 326f
   septa of 326
   sound 340, 340t, 342
      abnormal 343
      appearance of 342
      different 340
      first 336, 340, 341
      fourth 336, 341
      production of 340
   valve 327, 327f, 343
      weakening of 343
Heartburn 151
Heat
   balance 223
   cramps 439
   effects of 438, 439
   exhaustion 439
   frustration 31
   gain 223
      center 224, 505
   initial 121
   loss 223
      center 224, 505
      prevention of 224, 438
      promotion of 224
   production 162, 438
      prevention of 224
      promotion of 224
Heatstroke 439
Heavy chain 69
Heavy menstrual bleeding 308
Helicobacter pylori 151
Helium
   dilution technique 408
   equilibration of 408
Helper T cells 67f
   activation of 67
   role of 67, 69

Hematemesis 151
Hematocrit 33
   value 33, 41
Hematopoietic function 182, 258
Hematopoietic growth factors 47, 64
Hematopoietic stem cells 44
Heme iron 50
Hemianopia
   bitemporal heteronymous 574
   heteronymous 574
   homonymous 574
   types of 574f
Hemiballismus 515
Hemidesmosome 12-14
Hemiplegia 495
Hemodialysis 211
Hemodilution 42
Hemoglobin 48, 219, 432
   abnormal 49
   adult 48
   content, normal 48
   derivative 49
      abnormal 49, 49t
   destruction of 50, 94
   dissociation curve 57
   formation 47
   functions of 48
   SS disease 56
   structure of 48
   synthesis 50
      substances necessary for 50
   types of normal 48, 49t
Hemoglobinopathies 49
Hemolysins 58
Hemolysis 35, 56, 58
Hemolytic disease 89
Hemolytic jaundice 58, 164
   causes of 164
Hemolytic transfusion reaction 88
Hemophilia 82, 83
   types of 83
Hemopoiesis 44
   stages of 46f
Hemopoietic function 146, 147, 162, 167, 169
Hemorrhage 35, 387
   accidental 387
   acute 56, 387
   capillary 387
   causes of 387
   chronic 56, 387
   effects of 387
   internal 387
   postpartum 387
   types of 387
Hemosiderin 50
Hemostasis 75, 76, 282
   stages of 76, 77f
Hemostatic agents 82
Hemothorax 404, 432
Henle's loop 201, 203, 204, 212
Heparin 81, 283, 398
   actions of 283
   mechanism of action of 81, 81f
   source of secretion of 283
   uses of 81
Hepatic cells 158
Hepatic circulation 381
Hepatic duct 157, 158
Hepatic jaundice, causes of 164
Hepatic lobule 158f
Hepatic plates 157
Hepatic portal vein 158
Hepatic sinusoids 158
Hepatic stage 44
Hepatic vein 158
Hepatitis 56, 70, 92, 164

Index 611

Hepatocellular jaundice, causes
   of 164
Hepatocytes 157, 159
Hering's nerve 359, 360
Hering-Breuer reflex 423, 424f
Hermaphroditism 285, 310
Heterophagy 5
Heterotopic arrhythmia 349
Hexamethonium ion 556
Hexapeptide 188
High atmospheric pressure 429
High barometric pressure 42
   effect of 436
High molecular weight kininogen 79
Hilum 181
Histamine 130, 283
   actions of 283
   source of secretion of 283
Histiocytes, fixed 93
Histocompatibility complex, major 67
Histone 8
Histotoxic hypoxia
   causes for 428
   characteristic features of 429
Hoarseness 549
Hodgkin's disease 75
Holger-Nielsen method 440, 441f
Hollow organs
   overdistension of 497
   spasm of 497
Homeostasis 22, 23
   role in 182
Homeostatic imbalance 25, 25b
Homeostatic system
   components of 23, 23f
   mechanism of action of 23
Hormonal action, mechanism of 230
Hormonal mechanism 150, 367, 506
Hormonal receptors, situation of
   229, 230f
Hormone 231, 317
   antidiabetogenic 263
   calorigenic 276
   classification of 228, 230t
   hypothalamic 308
      releasing 228
   inhibiting pancreatic secretion
      156
   life-protecting 269
   life-saving 267
   local 227, 229b, 281-283
   receptor 228
      complex 228, 231
   regulating tubular reabsorption
      197t
   replacement therapy 300
   role of 223, 256, 263, 315, 316,
      316f
   secretion of 305
   stimulating pancreatic secretion
      156
   transport of 35
Horner syndrome 579
Horse's gallop 342
Huge stature 239
Human chorionic gonadotropin 229,
   311, 314
   high level of 313
Human chorionic somatomammotropin, actions of 312
Human heart, different parts of 332t
Human immune deficiency virus 72,
   319
Human leukocyte antigen 67
Human sperm 293f
Humoral immunity, development
   of 68

Hunger contractions 174
Huntington's disease 515
Hyaline cartilage 258
Hyaluronidase 292, 310
Hydrocephalus
   causes of 552
   external 552
   features of 552
   internal 552
   types of 552
Hydrochloric acid 147, 151
   functions of 147
   secretion of 147, 148f, 151
Hydrocholeretic agents 163
Hydrogen 19f
   excretion of 207f
   ions
      concentration 268
      removal of 206
      secretion of 205, 206t
      transport of 18
   peroxide 6
   pump 18
Hydrolytic function 169
Hydrolyzes triglycerides 140
Hydrops fetalis 89
Hydrostatic pressure 194, 195
   capillary 372
Hydrothorax 404, 432
Hydroxycholecalciferol 279
Hydroxy-dehydroepiandrosterone
   sulfate 312
Hyperactive micturition reflex 217
Hyperaldosteronism 35, 271
   causes of 271
   primary 272
   types of 271
Hyperbaric oxygen 429, 430
Hyperbilirubinemia 162
Hypercalcemia 240, 254
Hypercapnia 294, 428, 430
   causes of 430
   effects of 430
Hyperemia, reactive 379
Hypergonadism
   causes of 294
   symptoms of 294
Hyperinsulinism
   causes of 265
   signs of 265
   symptoms of 265
Hypermetropia
   causes of 582
   correction of 582
Hyperosmia 600
Hyperparathyroidism, causes of 254
Hyperphagia 505
Hyperplasia 254, 271
Hyperpnea 427
   causes of 431
   stage of 430
Hyperpolarization 118, 463, 536,
      569
   mild 569
   significance of 569
Hyperproteinemia 39, 195
Hyperpyrexia 225
Hypersalivation 142
Hypersensitivity reactions, acute 62
Hypersomnia 545
Hypersplenism 56, 95
Hypertension 211, 265, 312, 369,
      370
   cardiovascular 370
   endocrine 370
   essential 370
   primary 370

   secondary 370, 370t
   systolic 370
   types of 370
Hyperthermia 225
Hyperthyroidism 35, 225, 247, 249
   causes for 248
   signs of 248
   symptoms of 248
   treatment for 250
Hypertonia, causes for 115
Hypertonic fluid 30
Hyperventilation 427, 443
   causes of 427
   effects of 428
Hypervolemia 35
Hypnic jerk 545
Hypocalcemia 253
Hypocalcemic tetany
   signs of 253
   symptoms of 253
Hypocapnia 294, 430
   effects of 430
Hypochlorhydria 313
Hypogastric ganglion 214
Hypogastric nerve 214
Hypoglycemia 236, 265
Hypogonadism 508
   causes of 294
   hypergonadotropic 294
   signs of 294
   symptoms of 294
Hypokalemia 171
Hypokinesia 515
Hypomenorrhea 308
Hypoparathyroidism, causes for 253
Hypophyseal stalk 233, 237
Hypophysis 2
Hypoproteinemia 39, 195
Hyposalivation
   permanent 142
   temporary 142
Hyposmia 600
Hyposplenia 95
Hypotension 361, 370
   secondary 370
   types of 370
Hypothalamic eunuchism 294
Hypothalamo-hypophyseal portal
   blood vessels 234, 505
Hypothalamo-hypophyseal tract
   237, 237f, 505
Hypothalamus 189, 359, 366, 503
   disorders of 508
   formation of 503
   functions of 503, 504t
   nuclei of 503, 503t, 504f
   role of 247, 270
   situation of 503
Hypothermia 225
Hypothyroidism 35, 248, 249
   treatment for 250
Hypotonia 115, 512
   causes for 115
Hypotonic saline solution 59
Hypoventilation 427, 428
   causes of 428
   effects of 428
Hypovolemia 35
Hypoxia 11, 47, 428, 434, 435
   causes of 428
   classification of 428
   effect of 429, 434
   hypokinetic 428
   immediate effects of 429
   stimulates kidney 42
   treatment for 429
   types of 429, 429t

Hypoxic hypoxia 428, 429
   causes for 428
   characteristic features of 428

I

Icterus 164
Idiopathic thrombocytopenic purpura
   83
Ileocecal junction 166
Ileocecal valve, pyloric sphincter
   of 166
Ileum 166
Immune deficiency diseases, con-
   genital 71
Immunity
   acquired 65
   cell-mediated 67, 68
   cellular 67
   development of 66f
   humoral 68
   innate 65
   non-specific 65
   specific 65
   types of 65
Immunization
   active 70
   passive 70
Immunoglobulin 38, 69, 140
Immunological test 314
Impulse transmission 461
Incus 586
Indicator dilution method 28, 355
Indirect light reflex 576
Infarction 84
Infatigability 452
Inferior vermis 509
   parts of 509t
Inflammation 433
Inflammatory bowel disease 169
Influenza 70
Ingestion 133
Inhibitory postsynaptic potential,
   development of 463
Inhibitory reticular system, descend-
   ing 526
Injury
   causes for 453
   degrees of 453
   fifth degree 453
   first degree 453
   fourth degree 453
Ink spot nucleus 45
Inner ear, role of 592
Inner matrix space 6
Inner medulla 181
Inner nuclear layer 563
Inner plexiform layer 563
Inorganic phosphate 120
Insomnia 545
Inspiration 402f
Inspiratory impulses, rhythmic dis-
   charge of 423
Inspiratory ramp 421, 423
   signals, significance of 423
Inspiratory reserve volume 405
Inspired air 413, 413t
Insulin 163, 260
   dependent diabetes mellitus 264
   receptor 261
   regulation of secretion of 262
   role of 263
Intercalated cells 185, 205
Intercalated disk 326
Intercalated duct 138
Intercellular communication 227
Intercellular junctions 12
Interconnecting gap junctions 127

Intercostal nerve 400
  fibers 423
Interdigestive phase 150
Interferons 70
Interleukins 70
  secretion of 94
Interlobular artery 190
Interlobular ducts 138
Interlobular veins 191
Intermediate filament 7, 7f, 14
Intermediate normoblast 45
Intermediate sulcus, posterior 473
Intermediolateral nucleus 475
Interoceptors 457, 458f
Interstitial cell stimulating hormone 234
Interstitial cells of Leydig 287
Interstitial connective tissues 182
Interstitial fluid 22, 99, 100, 200
  transport from 198
  volume, measurement of 30
Interventricular septum 326
Intestinal diseases 171
Intestinal gland 166, 166f, 167, 167t
Intestinal juice 176
Intestinal mucosa
  epithelial cells of 13
  secretes enterocrinin 169
Intestinal phase 150, 156
  initial stage of 150
  later stage of 150
Intestinal villi 166
Intestinal wall, structure of 125f
Intestine 134, 268
Intorsion 565
Intoxication, alcoholic 429
Intra-alveolar pressure
  measurement of 403
  normal values of 403, 403t
  significance of 403
Intra-atrial pressure, significance of 338
Intracellular chemical mediators 227
Intracellular edema 99, 100, 100b
Intracellular enzyme 231
Intracellular fluid 1, 16f, 18, 18f, 19f, 27, 28t
  volume, measurement of 30
Intrafusal fibers, types of 527
Intralaminar nuclei 500, 501f
Intralobular duct 152
Intraocular fluid 563
Intraocular lens implant 566
Intraocular pressure 564
Intrapleural fluid, functions of 396
Intrapleural pressure 401-402
  measurement of 402
  normal values of 402, 402t
  significance of 403
Intrapulmonary pressure 403
Intrarectal pressure 177
Intrathoracic pressure 402
Intrauterine contraceptive device 319, 320
  disadvantages of 320
  nonmedicated 319
Intraventricular pressure, significance of 338
Intrinsic muscles 564
  innervation of 564
Intrinsic prothrombin activator 74
Inulin, clearance 210
Inward movement 565
Iodide
  chloride pump 244
  oxidation of 244
  pump 244
  role of 247
  trapping 244
Iodine 244
  deficiency goiter 249
Iodotyrosine
  deiodinase 245
  residues 244
Ionized calcium 255
Iris, angle 561
Iron
  absorption of 50
  daily loss of 50
  deficiency anemia 43, 51, 57
  distribution of 50
  importance of 50
  lung chamber 441
  metabolism 48, 50
  storage of 50
  transport of 50
Ischemia 84, 497
Islets of Langerhans 260, 260f
Isoagglutinin 86
Isometric contraction 111, 119, 336
  period 336
  significance of 336
Isometric relaxation
  period 337
  significance of 337
Isotonic contraction 111, 119
Isotonic fluid 30
Isotonic simple muscle curve 112f
Isovolumetric contraction 336
Isthmus 296

J

J point 348
Jaeger's chart 570
Jaundice 88, 162, 164, 165
  cholestatic 164
  hemolytic 58, 164
  hepatic 164
  hepatocellular 164
  physiological 42
  severe 92
  types of 164, 164f, 165t
Jaw jerk 471
Jejunum 166
Joints, unfixing of 532
Jugular venous pulse tracing 376
Juxtacapillary receptors 424
Juxtacrine messengers 227
Juxtaglomerular apparatus 187, 187f, 189
  functions of 188
  structure of 187
Juxtaglomerular cells 187
Juxtallocortex 523
Juxtallocortical structures 523
Juxtamedullary nephrons 183, 183t, 185, 201

K

K complex 543
Kallikrein
  presence of 79
  syndrome 508
Kernicterus 89, 115, 515
Kidney 57, 143, 182, 279, 388
  blood vessels of 190
  different layers of 181
  effects on 429
  functional anatomy of 181
  longitudinal section of 182f
  regulate blood calcium 182
  transplantation 211
  tubular structures of 182
Kinesthetic receptors 527
Kinocilium 535, 588
Kluver-Bucy syndrome 522
Knee jerk 471
Korbinian brodmann 518
Korotkoff sounds, phases of 369t
Krause end bulb 457
Kulchitsky cells 145
Kupffer cells 63, 93, 157, 163
Kussmaul's breathing 265
Kussmaul's sign 377
Kyphosis 240, 259

L

Labial glands 138
Labor 281
Labyrinth 533, 533f, 587
Labyrinthectomy 537
Labyrinthine 532
Lacis cells 187
Lacrimal gland 554, 560
Lacrimal secretion 542
Lactase 167
Lactation, process of 316f
Lactic acid 130, 208
Lactoferrin of saliva 140
Lactogenesis 316
Lactotrophs 234
Lamina around central canal 476
Lamina propria 134
Landsteiner's law 85
Large intestinal juice 170f
  composition of 170
  parts of 170
Large intestine 134, 170
  disorders of 171
  functional anatomy of 170
  functions of 171
  movements of 177
  secretion of 170
Laryngeal stridor 253
Laurence-Moon-Biedl syndrome 508
Law of Laplace 216
Laxatives, action 161, 162
Lead pipe rigidity 515
Learning 546
  process 511
  types 546
Lecithin 154
Left optic
  nerve, lesion of 574
  radiation, lesion of 574
Leishman's stain 61
Lemniscus, lateral 589
Lens
  structure of 564
  substance 564
Lenticular process 586
Leptin 156, 283, 506
  actions of 283
  source of secretion of 283
Lesser petrosal nerve 140
Leukemia
  acute 75
  chronic 75
Leukocytes 33, 60, 397
  count
    normal 61
    variations in 61
Leukocytosis 61
Leukopenia 61, 62
Leukopoiesis 63, 63f, 64
Leukotrienes, actions of 282
Lewis blood group 89
Ligand gated sodium channels 16, 231
Light adaptation, causes for 569
Light band 106
Light chain 69
Light energy 569
Light rays, effects of 435
Light reflex 576
  pathway for 576, 577f
Light sleep, stages of 543
Limb
  ascending 185
  descending 185
  rigidity of 515
  unlocking of 532
Limbic system 516, 524f
  components of 523, 523f
  functions of 523
Lingual lipase 139, 140
Lingual mucus glands 138
Lingual serous glands 138
Lipid
  derivatives, role of 262
  digestion of 154
  layer, functions of 2
Lipolytic enzyme 140, 147, 154, 167
Lipoxins, actions of 282
Lips 137
Liquor folliculi 302
Lithium
  battery 350
  salts 81
Lithocholate 160
Liver 143, 157-159
  bile 160t
  cells 236
  cirrhosis of 165
  diseases 53
  disorders of 164
  dual functions of 157
  failure 56
  fats 245
  function tests 163
  functional anatomy of 157
  normal blood flow to 381
  posterior surface of 157f
  role of 263
Lobes 278
Locke's solution 38
Locus coeruleus, role of 544
Long bone, parts of 258f
Long refractory period, significance of 334
Loop diuretics 212
Loop of Henle 185, 201
  role of 201
Lordosis 259
Loud noise 586
Loud snoring 545
Lower esophageal sphincter
  constriction of 174
  relaxation of 174
  role of 174
Lower motor neuron 483, 494, 518
  lesion 472, 494t
  nuclei of 474
L-tubule 108
  cisterna of 109
  functions of 109
Lubrication function 162
Lumbar puncture, needle 551
Lumbar segments, upper 480
Lumbar spines 551
Lumbosacral vertebral defects 217
Lung 143, 182, 401, 414, 419
  capacity 406, 406f
  measurement of 406
  total 406, 408
  collapse of 432
  compliance, variations in 404f

covering of 395
elastic resistance of 404
function tests, types of 405
irritant receptors of 424
J receptors of 424
movements of 401
parenchyma 396
preventing collapsing tendency of 401
stretch receptors of 423
tissues, damage of 433
volumes 405, 406f
    measurment of 406
Lusitropic action 328
Lutein cells 304
Luteinizing hormone 234, 236, 289, 299, 302, 304, 307
Luteolysis 281
Luteum menstrualis 305
Lymph
  capillaries 96
  channels, system of 96
  composition of 98, 98f
  concentration of 98
  drainage 96f
  flow, rate of 98
  formation of 97
  glands 97
  node 93, 97
    cortex of 97
    distribution of 97
    functions of 97, 98
    structure of 97, 97f
    swelling of 97
  vessels 96
Lymphatic duct, right 96
Lymphatic system 23, 96
  drainage of 96
  organization of 96
Lymphatic vessels 97
Lymphocytes 45f, 61
  activity of 65
  development of 65
  functions of 63
  processing of 65
Lymphoid follicles
  primary 97
  secondary 97
Lymphoid stem cells 44
Lysocephalin 154
Lysolecithin 154
Lysosomal enzymes 5
  release of 259
Lysosomal function, mechanism of 5
Lysosomal proteins 7
Lysosome 4, 5
  functions of 5
  primary 6, 20
  secondary 6, 20
  specific functions of 6
  types of 5
Lysozyme 221

M

Macrocyte 43, 54
Macrocytic anemia 47
Macrocytic hypochromic anemia 55
Macrocytic normochromic anemia 55
Macrogenitosomia praecox 273f
Macromolecules, degradation of 6
Macrophages 20, 67, 68, 93, 94, 157, 397
  secrete colony-stimulating factor 94
Macula 535
  densa 187, 189

lutea 563
situation of 535
Magakaryocyte 63f
Major salivary glands 138f
  ducts of 138t
Malabsorption syndrome 169
Malaria 56
Male reproductive
  organs 285
  system 285, 286f
Male urethra 213
Malleus, manubrium of 586
Malpighian
  corpuscle 94, 183
  pyramids 181
Maltase 140
Mammary glands 126, 218, 238, 315
  development of 315
  effect on 299
  growth of 315
Mammillary body 506
Manubrium 400, 586
  sterni 400
Marey's law 360
Marey's reflex 359, 360f
Marginal nucleus 478
  neurons of 499
Marijuana 142
Mass peristalsis 177
Masseter muscle 172
Mast cells 81, 398
Mastication
  control of 172
  movements of 172
  muscles of 172
  significances of 172
Matrix junction 14
Maturation
  first phase of 289
  second phase of 289
  stage of 289, 297
Matured follicle, ovum of 310
Maximal stimulus 110
Maximum contraction, point of 112
Maximum relaxation, point of 112
Mean corpuscular volume 54, 55
Measles 70
Mechanical energy 458, 536
Mechanical stimuli 456
Mechanical trauma 59
Mechanically gated channels 16
Mechanism sneezing reflex 398
Mechanoreceptors 456, 529
Mechanotransduction 536
Medial fibers, lesion of 574
Medial lemniscus 482
Medial longitudinal fasciculus 484
Medial movement 565
Medial rectus 566f, 579
Median septum, posterior 473, 476
Median sulcus, posterior 473
Medical termination of pregnancy 321
Medulla 97, 278, 295
  oblongata 425, 482, 532
  reticular formation of 357
Medullary centers 421
  role of 423
Medullary gradient
  development of 200
  maintenance of 200, 201
Medullary hyperosmolarity 200
Medullary interstitial fluid, hyperosmolarity of 201
Medullary pyramids 181
Megacolon 171

Megakaryocyte 44, 46f, 75
Megaloblast 45
Megaloblastic anemia 43, 47, 54, 57
Meissner's corpuscle 457
Meissner's nerve plexus, functions of 135
Melanin, pigment 291
Melanocytes 218
Melatonin
  actions of 278
  secretion 278
Membrana granulosa 302
Membranous disks 567
Membranous labyrinth 533
Memory 523, 546
  abnormalities of 548
  anatomical basis of 547
  B cells, role of 69
  cells 67
  consolidation of 548
  declarative 547
  encoding, synaptic terminal for 547f
  explicit 547
  long-term 547
  non-declarative 547
  physiological basis of 547
  role in 524
  short-term 547
  skilled 547
  storage 547
  T cells, role of 68
  types of 547
Menarche 299, 301
Meninges 143
Meningocytes 93
Menopause 299-301
Menorrhagia 246, 248, 308, 387
Menses 305
Menstrual bleeding 305
Menstrual cramps 308
Menstrual cycle 223, 301, 307t
  duration of 301
  hormonal level during 309f
  ovarian changes during 301
  regulation of 308
  uterine changes during 305, 305f
  vagina during 308
Menstrual disorders 308
Menstrual phase 305
Menstrual symptoms 308
Menstruation 53, 305
  abnormal 308, 308t
Mental retardation 246
Mercury
  manometer 402
  toxicity of 369
Merkel disk 457
Mesangial cells, intraglomerular 187
Mesencephalon 446
Mesenchyme cells 37
Mesenteric circulation 381
Mesenteric ganglia 135
Mesoblastic stage 44
Mesocortex 523
Mesoepithelial cells 134
Meta-adrenaline 275
Metabolic acidosis 171, 207, 208
Metabolic activities 223
Metabolic alkalosis 207, 208
Metabolic disorders 277
Metabolic disturbances 207
Metabolic function 162, 257
Metabolism
  aerobic exercises 392
  anaerobic exercises 392
  effect on 298

Metabolites, removal of 113
Metanephrines 275
Metaphysis 258
Metarhodopsin 569
Metencephalon 446
Methacholine 556
Methemoglobin 49
Methyl mercaptan 599
Metrorrhagia 308
Microbodies 6
Microcytes 43, 54
Microcytic hypochromic anemia 55
Microfilaments 7
Microglia 93, 455
Microphone 342
Micropills 321
Microtubules 7, 7f, 73
  functions of 7
Microvessels 73
Microvilli 166
Micturition 213, 216
  abnormalities of 217
  higher centers for 217
  reflex 216, 217, 217f
  syncope 389
  urge for 216
  voluntary control of 216
Midbrain
  disorders of 539
  outflow 554
Middle ear 585
  role of 591
Middle tunica media 329
Midline nuclei 500, 501f
Migrating motor complex 177
Milk
  digestion of 153
  synthesis of 316
Milk ejection 316
  reflex 238, 238f, 316
Milk secretion
  initiation of 316
  maintenance of 316
Mineral metabolism 269
Mineralocorticoids 266
  functions of 267
  regulation of secretion of 268
Miniature bones 586
Miniature endplate potential, development of 123
Minimal stimulus 110
Minipills 321
Minor blood groups 90
Minor calyx 182, 185
Minor salivary glands 138
Minute volume, normal value of 351
Miosis 579
Mismatched blood transfusion, complications of 88f
Mitochondria 4, 6, 7, 50, 73, 105, 122, 448, 462
  functions of 6
  structure of 6f
Mitral cells 598
Mitral valve 327
  closure of 342
Mixed glands 138
Mixed nerve 473
Mixed venous blood 354
Mixing movements 176, 177
Modified cardiac muscle 332
Modulatory neuron 464
Molar glands 138
Mole 30
Molecules
  junctional adhesion 13
  movement of 196

Monoamine oxidase 275
Monochromatism 581
Monochromats 581
Monocular vision 570
Monocyte 44, 45f, 46f, 61, 62, 63f, 64, 94
    functions of 62
Monoiodotyrosine 244
Monophosphate 231
Monoplegia 495
Monosynaptic reflex 469, 530
Morning sickness 313
Morphology 60, 105, 559
Motion sickness 537
Motivation, role in 524
Motor activity
    control of 514
    integration of 501
Motor areas, topographical arrangement of 520f
Motor endplate 122
Motor homunculus 518
Motor impulses 448
Motor nerve
    fibers 529f
    supply 528
Motor neuron 493
    lesion of 494
    nuclei of 475
Motor nucleus 579
Motor pathways, classification of 494
Motor system, structure of 493
Motor unit 124
Mountain sickness, symptoms of 435
Mouth 134, 137
    functions of 137, 137t
Movement
    coordination of 519
    disorders 545
    exaggeration of 519
    poverty of 515
    slowness of 515
Mucin 140
    secretion of 163
Mucus
    cells 138
    functions of 147
    glands 138
    layer 134
    membrane 134, 560
    neck cells 145
Muffled sound 369
Müller maneuver 372t
    effects of 372
    uses of 372
Müller's experiment 372
Müller's fibers 561
Müller's law 458
Müllerian duct 290
Müllerian inhibiting substance 286
Müllerian regression factor 286, 290
Multilumen tube 156
Multiple sclerosis 487
Multipolar neurons 448
Multiunit muscle fibers 127
Multiunit smooth muscle 128t, 129
    fibers 127f
Mumps 70, 143
Murmur
    classification of 343
    diastolic 343
    systolic 343
Muscarine 141
Muscle 117, 172, 269
    abdominal 217
    after fatigue, recovery of 113

    cells 105
    classification of 103
    composition of 109
    contractile elements of 107
    contraction of 494, 531f
    cramps 439
    cross-section of 106f
    expiratory 400
    inspiratory 400
    intrafusal fibers of 494, 527
    involuntary 103, 126
    length of 529
    mass 105
    physiology 103
    proteins of 107
    relaxation of 120, 130
    tissue 1
    wastage 115
Muscle fiber 105, 326, 327
    number of 124
Muscle pump 352
    mechanism of 353f
Muscle spindle 527, 528f, 529f
    functions of 529
    structure of 527
Muscle tone 114, 115, 529, 542
    control of 514
    development of 530, 530f
    maintenance of 114
    regulation of 530
    significance of 529
Muscular activity 223
Muscular contraction 116, 119, 120
    energy for 120
    molecular basis of 119
Muscular disease 115
Muscular dystrophy 115
Muscular exercise 42
Muscular growth, effect on 291
Muscular layer 134
Muscular stiffness, types of 115
Muscularis mucosa 134
Musculoskeletal system 1
Myasthenia gravis 72, 115, 125, 279, 370
Myelencephalon 446
Myelin sheath
    chemistry of 449
    formation of 449
    functions of 449
Myelinated nerve fiber 449, 449f, 452, 452f
Myelinogenesis 449, 450
Myeloid stage 44
Myenteric nerve plexus 134
Myenteric plexus, dysfunction of 171
Myenteric reflex 150
Myocardial infarction 80, 265, 380
    stages of 80
Myocardial ischemia 379
Myocardium 326
Myocytes 105
Myofibril 105, 108, 127
    microscopic structure of 106
    portion of 106
Myofilaments 127
Myometrium 296
Myopathy 259
Myopia
    causes of 582
    correction of 583
Myosin
    filament 107, 108f
    head 107, 120f
    light chain kinase 129
    molecule 107, 107f
Myosis 579
Myotatic reflex 530

Myotonia, causes for 115
Myxedema
    causes for 248
    signs of 248
    symptoms of 248

N

Nails 57
Naphthalene balls 49
Narcolepsy 508, 545
Nasal septum, parts of 598
Nasogastric tubes 151
Natural killer cell 6, 68, 70, 397
    functions of 70
Nausea 57, 171, 175, 313
Near vision 570
Neck 293
    reflexes 532
Necrosis 11, 84
    causes for 11
Necrotic endometrium 306
Negative conditioned reflexes 549
Negative supporting reflexes 532
Neighboring cells 3
Neocerebellum 510
Neocortex 516
Neoplasm 142
Neostigmine 124
Nephrogenic diabetes insipidus 204, 241
Nephron
    classification of 183
    cortical 183
    parts of 186f, 203t
    structure of 184f
    superficial 183
    tubular portion of 185
    types of 183, 184f
Nerve 182, 215, 453
    branch of 182
    cell body 448, 454
    covering of 449
    cross-section of 449f
    functions of 215t
    growth factor 450
    impulse 451
    organization of 448
    plexus, intrinsic 135f
    root ganglion, posterior 476
Nerve deafness, causes of 593
Nerve fiber 122, 451t
    classification of 450
    degeneration of 452, 453f, 454
    forming analgesic pathway 499
    layer of 563
    properties of 451
    types of 451t, 529f
Nervous mechanism 150
Nervous regulation 169
Nervous system 23, 313, 445
    divisions of 445
    involuntary 553
    organization of 446f
    peripheral 446, 473, 553
Nervous tissue 1
Nervus intermedius of Wrisberg 140
Net filtration pressure 194
Neural messengers 227
Neurilemma 449
Neurocardiogenic syncope 389
Neurocrine 227
Neuroendocrine reflex 238
Neuroepithelium 534, 535
Neurofibrils 448
Neurogenic bladder, uninhibited 217
Neurogenic hypertension 370

Neuroglia 445, 447, 454
    functions of 455t
Neuroglial cells 455, 455f
    central 454
    classification of 454
    functions of 455
    peripheral 455
Neuroglycopenic symptoms 265
Neurohormone 237, 228
Neurohypophysis 233
Neurological disorders 217
Neuromodulators 466, 467
    chemistry of 467
    types of 467
Neuromuscular blockers 124
Neuromuscular junction 122, 124, 130, 230
    autoimmune disorder of 125
    disorders of 125
    inability of 125
    longitudinal section of 122f
    structure of 123
Neuromuscular system 57
Neuromuscular transmission 123, 123f
Neuron 1, 421, 447, 445, 474
    axon of 448
    classification of 447
    dendrite of 448
    dopaminergic 277
    expiratory 422
    first order 476, 496, 572, 589, 596
    inspiratory 421
    large alpha-motor 464
    organization of 474
    processes of 448
    second order 476, 478, 482, 497, 572, 589, 596
    situation 422
    structure of 448, 448f
    type of 422, 447f
    unipolar 447
Neuroplasm 448
Neuroprotective structure 552
Neurotransmitter 227, 450, 465, 466t, 497
    classification of 465
    release of 466
    substance 122, 196
    transport of 466
Neurotrophic factors 450
Neurotrophins
    functions of 450
    secretion of 450
    types of 450
Neutrophils 44, 45f, 61, 62
    functions of 62
Newton's third law of motion 355
Nicotinic receptors acetylcholine 123
Night blindness, causes of 569
Night terror 545
Nightmare 545
Nissl
    bodies 448
    granules 448
Nitric oxide 130
    endothelium-derived 196
Nitrobenzene 58
Nitrogen
    meter 412
    washout method 408, 412
Nitrogen narcosis 436
    mechanism of 437
    symptoms of 437
Nitrous oxide 49
Nocturnal micturition 217, 545
Non-antibody proteins 70

Index

Non-communicating hydrocephalus 552
Nonelastic viscous resistance 404
Nonheme iron 50
Non-hemolytic transfusion reaction 88
Non-myelinated nerve fiber 449, 449f, 452f
Nonoxynol-9 319
Non-pitting edema 100
Non-pregnant uterus 238
Non-rapid eye movement sleep 543
Non-self-antigens 67
Non-steroidal anti-inflammatory drugs 59, 151
Non-striated muscle 103
Non-toxic goiter 249, 249f
Noradrenaline 130, 196, 274, 275, 450
    actions of 275
    methylation of 274
    regulation of secretion of 277
    secreting 141
        cells 274
Normal electrocardiogram, waves of 346
Normocyte 54
Normocytic normochromic anemia 54, 55
Normotopic arrhythmia 348
Nuclear bag fiber 527
Nuclear chain fiber 527
Nuclear layer, outer 561
Nuclear membrane 8
Nuclease 152, 154
Nucleolus 8
Nucleoplasm 8
Nucleus 1, 4, 8, 105, 230, 232, 448, 474, 475
    cuneatus 482
    functions of 8, 8b
    gracilis 482
    lateral mass of 500, 501f
    locus ceruleus 499
    medial mass of 500, 501f
    posterior group of 500, 501f
    raphe 499
    structure of 8
Nutrition deficiency anemia 55-57
Nutritive function 35
Nutritive substances diffuse 99
Nystagmus 537

O

Obesity 545
Obligatory water reabsorption 198
Obstructive jaundice, causes of 164
Obstructive respiratory disease 410, 410t, 433
Obstructive shock, causes of 389
Occasional hematemesis 151
Occasional lipid droplets 105
Occasionally amenorrhea 246
Occipital bone and atlas 551
Occipital eye field 573
Occipital lobe 523, 573
Ocular movements 565
Ocular muscles 559, 564
    innervation of 564
Oculosympathetic palsy 579
Oddi, sphincter of 158
Odor
    classification of 599
    perception of 600
    types of 599
Olfaction 397, 523
Olfactory bulb 598
Olfactory cortex 598
Olfactory glomeruli 598
Olfactory hyperesthesia 600
Olfactory mucous membrane 598, 599f
Olfactory pathway 598
Olfactory receptors cells 598, 599
Olfactory rod 598
Olfactory sensation
    abnormalities of 600
    pathway for 599f
    threshold for 599
Olfactory tract 598
Olfactory transduction 599
Oligodendrocytes 455
Oligomenorrhea 246, 308
Oliguria 204
Olivary nucleus, superior 589
Olivospinal tract 486
Oncotic pressure 17, 37, 99
    in blood, maintenance of 38
Oocyte
    maturation inhibiting factor 302
    primary 296, 297, 310
    secondary 297, 310
Oogenesis, stages of 297
Oogonia 296
Opercular insular cortex 596
Ophthalmoscope 563
Opioids 498
Opportunistic infections 72
Opportunists 71
Opsin 568
Optic axis 559
Optic chiasma 572, 574
    left side of 574
    right side of 574
Optic disk 563, 571
Optic nerve 567, 572
Optic papilla 563
Optic pathway 572
    lesion of 575f
Optic radiation 573
Optic tract 572
Optical axis 560f
Optokinetic movement 566
Ora serrata 561
Oral anticoagulants 81
Oral cavity 137
Oral contraceptives 321
Oral rehydration
    solution 32
    therapy 32
Orbital cavity 559
Orbitofrontal cortex 519
Organ 1
    endocrine functions of 278
    of Corti 587, 588f, 591, 592
        cells of 588
    particularly lungs, functions of 156
Organic acids, accumulation of 208
Organic substances 28, 34b, 596
Orthochromatic erythroblast 45
Orthograde degeneration 453
Orthonasal olfaction 599, 600
Orthostatic hypotension 370, 389
Orthostatic syncope 370
Oscillatory method 369
Osmolality 30
Osmolarity 30
Osmole 30
Osmoreceptors 506
    role of 237
Osmosis 17, 17f
Osmotic diuresis 204, 212, 265
Osmotic fragility 59
Osmotic pressure 17, 43
Osseous
    spiral lamina 587
    tissue 257
Ossicular conduction 592
Osteoblastic activity 254, 259, 298
Osteoblasts 258
    fate of 258
    functions of 258, 259
Osteoclastic activity 252, 259
Osteoclasts 252, 258
Osteocytes, functions of 258
Osteogenic cells 235
Osteomalacia 259
Osteoporosis 259, 298
Osteoprogenitor cells 258
Otic ganglion 140
Otitis media 593
Otoconia 535
Otolith 534
    membrane 535
    organ 534, 535, 536f
        functions of 537
Otosclerosis 592, 593
Outer cortex 181
Oval window 586, 592
Ovarian follicles 302, 304f
    effect on 297
Ovarian hormones 297, 308
Ovary
    functions anatomy of 295
    functions of 297
    Graafian follicle of 310
Overhydration 32
Ovulation 303
    process of 304f
    stages of 303
    time, determination of 303, 304
Ovum 302
    development of 310
    fertilization of 306, 310
    implantation of 319, 320
    natured 297
Oxalate compounds 82
    mechanism of action of 82
    uses of 82
Oxygen 57, 99, 412
    consumption 354, 354f, 443
    content of 415t, 417f
    debt 443
    diffusing capacity for 415, 443
    diffusion of 415, 416, 416f
    entrance of 415
    lack of 130
    partial pressure of 425, 434, 435t
    poisoning 430
    pure 408
    species, reactive 94
    therapy, efficacy of 429
    toxicity 430
        causes of 430
        effects of 430
    transport of 418
Oxygenated blood 158, 398
Oxygenation 418
Oxygen-hemoglobin dissociation curve 418, 418f
Oxyntic cells 145
Oxyntic glands 145
Oxyphil cells 251
Oxytocin 130, 237

P

P cells 185
P wave 346
    amplitude of 346
    causes of 346
    duration of 346
    morphology of 346
Pacemaker 327
    abnormal 349
    cells 327, 332
    waves 129
Pacinian corpuscle 457, 459, 459f, 529
Packed cell volume 33, 41, 52, 53, 54f
    normal values of 53
Pain 478
    abdominal 171
    cardiac 380
    chest 88
    fibers, slow 497
    pathway, descending 498
    physiology of 496
    receptors 424
    suppression 499
Pain sensation 496, 497, 502
    benefits of 496
    center for 497
    components of 496
    pathway of 496, 497
Painful
    periods 308
    stimuli 361
Palatal glands 138
Palate 137
Pale muscles 112
Paleocerebellum 510
Paleocortex 523
Paleocortical structures 523
Palpatory method 368
Palpebral fissure 560
Pancreas 143, 152
    disorders of 156, 264
    dual functions of 152
    duct system in 152
    endocrine function of 260
    exocrine part of 152
Pancreatic amylase 154
Pancreatic duct 152
Pancreatic exocrine functions tests 156
Pancreatic juice 168, 176
    collection of 156
    composition of 152, 153f
    digestive
        enzymes of 155t
        functions of 152
    functions of 152
    neutralizing action of 154
    properties of 152
Pancreatic lipase 154
    lack of 156
Pancreatic polypeptide 156, 263
    actions of 263
    mode of action of 263
    regulation of secretion of 263
Pancreatic secretion 152, 156
    regulation of 154, 155f
Pancreatic somatostatin 263
Pancreatic tumor 151
Pancreatitis 156
Pancreozymin 149, 156
Paneth cells 167
Panhypopituitarism 241
Papilla 185
Papillary
    ducts 185
    muscles 327
Papillomas, intraductal 316
Para-aminohippuric acid 191, 210
Paracellular route 197

Paracortex 97
Paracrine messengers 227
Paradoxical sleep 543
Paraffin 219
Paraflocculus 509
Parafollicular cells 243, 254
Paralysis 115, 495
    agitans 514
    causes for 495
    types of 495, 495t
Paramyxovirus 143
Paraplegia 495
Parasites 171
Parasympathetic blockers 556
Parasympathetic depressants 142
Parasympathetic division
    cranial portion of 554
    sacral portion of 554
Parasympathetic fibers 140, 141, 556
    functions of 136, 141
Parasympathetic nerve 177f, 214
    fibers 136, 142, 178, 357, 564
        distribution of 357
    functions of 214, 357
    stimulation of 169
Parasympathetic preganglionic fibers 140
Parasympathetic stimulation 177
Parasympathetic tone 358
Parasympathetic vasodilator fibers 365
Parasympathomimetic drugs 141
Parathormone 163, 251
    actions of 251
    role of 256, 257
    secretion, regulation of 252
Parathyroid
    function tests 254
    poisoning 254
Parathyroid gland 251, 251f, 313
    disorders of 253
    functional histology of 251
    morphology of 251
    removal of 253
    surgical removal of 253
Parathyroidectomy 253
Paraventricular nucleus 237
Parietal cell 145, 147
Parietal lobe 520
Parietal pericardium 326
Parieto-occipital sulcus 517, 520
Parkinson disease 514
Parkinsonism 514
Parotid gland 138, 141f
Paroxysmal tachycardia 349
Partial pressure 417f
Parturition 25f, 281, 310, 313
    stages of 313
Passive movements 529
Passive transport, types of 16
Patellar tendon reflex 471
Patent ductus arteriosus 343, 376, 386
Pavlov bell-dog experiments 548
Pavlov pouch 148, 148f
    nerve supply of 148
    use of 148
Peak expiratory flow rate 410
Pectus carinatum 259
Pelvic bones, effect on 291
Pelvic colon 170
Pelvic nerve 136
    fibers of 178
Pelvis, organs of 286f, 295f
Pendular movement 176, 471
Penetrating granulosa cells 310
Penicillin 59

Penis 218, 288
Pentolinium 556
Pepsin 146, 147
    action of 147
Pepsinogen 147
    cells 145
    secretion of 147
Peptic activity, measurement of 151
Peptic ulcer, causes of 151
Peptide
    mechanism 506
    YY 150, 156
Pericardium 326
    inner visceral 326
Perilymph 533
Perimenopause 309
Perimetrium 296
Perimysium 105
Periodic breathing 427, 431, 432f
Periosteum 258
Peripheral membrane proteins 2
Peripheral resistance 353
Peristalsis 174
Peristaltic movements 176
Peristaltic rush 176
Peristaltic waves 174, 215
Peritoneal dialysis 211
Peritoneum 145
Peritonsillar abscess 142
Peritubular capillaries 190-192
Periventricular nucleus 499
Pernicious anemia 47, 54, 57, 75, 151
Peroxidase 50
Peroxisomes 4, 6, 7
    functions of 6
Persistent plasma hypotonicity 241
Perspiration 223
Pesticides 182
Petit mal 541
    causes for 541
Phagocytic function 94
Phagocytosis 19, 20, 62
    mechanism of 20
    process of 20f
Phagosomal contents 20
Phagosome 6, 20
Phantom limb, pain 460
Pharyngeal mucous membrane 137
Pharyngeal stage 173
Pharynx 134
    mechanical stimulation of 175
Phasic receptors 458
Phenylethanolamine-n-methyltrans-ferase 274, 275
Pheochrome cells 274
Pheochromocytoma 277
    causes of 277
    signs of 277
    symptoms of 277
Pheromones 220, 598
Phlebogram 377f
Phonocardiogram 342
Phosphate 196
    buffer system 207
    level
        normal value of 257
        regulation of 257
    mechanism 206
    metabolism 257
    role of blood level of 252
Phospholipase 154
Phospholipids 2
Phosphoryl choline 154
Phosphorylation 129
Photosensitive pigment 568, 569
Phototransduction 569

Phrenic nerve 400
    fibers 423
Physical stress 59
Physostigmine 124, 141
Pia mater 445
Picogram 54
Pigeon chest 259
Pigment epithelium, layer of 561
Pill
    method 321
    rolling movements 515
Pilocarpine 141, 556
Pineal gland 278
    functions of 278
    structure of 278
Pinna 585
Pinocytosis 19
    mechanism of 19
    process of 19f
Pitting edema 100
Pituicytes 237
Pituitary
    cachexia 241
    diabetes 239
    stalk 233
Pituitary gland 233
    disorders of 238, 239t
    divisions of 233
    parts of 234f
    role of 247
Place theory 593
Placenta 297, 311, 384, 395
    functions of 311
    premature detachment of 387
    secretes 298
Placental estrogen, actions of 311
Placental lactogen 312
Placental progesterone, actions of 311
Plague, atherosclerotic 379
Planum semilunatum 534
Plasma 34, 203, 204, 245
    clearance 210
    composition of 34f
    transfusion 91
Plasma cells 67
    proliferation of 69
    role of 69
Plasma protein 37, 100f, 194
    functions of 38
    level 39
    molecular weight of 37t
    normal values of 37
    origin of 37
    properties of 37
Plasma volume 542
    measurement of 29
    percentage of 211
Plasmapheresis 38
Plasmin 80
Plasminogen 80
Platelet 33, 45f, 73
    activating factor 74, 76, 77
    composition of 73
    cytoplasm of 74t
    development of 75
    disorders 75, 75b
    dysfunction of 75
    fate of 75
    functions of 74
    granules 74, 74t
    lifespan of 75
    morphology of 73
    plug, formation of 76
    properties of 74
    shape of 73
    structure of 73
    transfusion 91

    under electron microscope 73f
    variations of 74
Platelet-derived growth factor 74, 75, 94
    secretion of 94
Plethysmograph 406, 408
Pleural cavity 395
Pleural effusion 433
Plexiform layer, outer 563
Pluripotent hematopoietic stem cells 44
Pneumocytes 397
Pneumonia 433
Pneumotaxic center 422
Pneumothorax 404, 432
Podocytes 194
Poikilocytosis 43
Poikilothermic animals 224
Polar body, second 297
Polar cushion 188
Poliomyelitis 70
Polkissen cells 187
Polychromatic erythroblast 45
Polycystic kidney disease 211
Polycythemia 41, 42, 53, 54
    physiological 41, 42f
    primary 42
    secondary 42, 43
    vera 42
Polydipsia 241, 265
Polymenorrhea 246, 248, 308
Polymorphonuclear leukocytes 61
Polyphagia 265
Polypnea 427
Polysaccharide, conjugated 81
Polysome 11
Polysynaptic reflexes 469
Polyuria 204, 241, 265
Pontine centers 422
    role of 423
Popliteal pulse 375
Porphyrin 41, 48
Portal vein 384
Postcatacrotic wave 375
Postcoital pills 321
Posterior pituitary hormones 237
    secretion of 503
Posterolateral sulcus 473
Posteroventral nucleus 596
Postganglionic fibers 141, 214
Postganglionic sympathetic fibers 189
Posthepatic jaundice 164
    causes of 164
Postmenopausal syndrome 300
Postsynaptic inhibition 463
Postsynaptic membrane 122, 123, 462
Postsynaptic neuron 461
    dendrite of 461
Postural movements 519
Postural reflexes 531
    classification of 531
Postural syncope 389
Posture 35, 527, 529
    basic phenomena of 529
    maintenance of 529
Potassium 18
    channels 15, 463
    glycocholate 160
    ions 268
        efflux of 332
    retaining diuretics 212
    taurocholate 160
Power stroke 120
PP cells 263
P-R interval 348
    duration of 348

Index

Pre-Bötzinger complex 423
Precentral cortex 518
Precipitation 70
Pre-emulsified fats 140
Prefrontal cortex 519
    functions of 520
Preganglionic fibers 214, 553
Preganglionic parasympathetic nerve fibers 136
Pregnancy 42, 310
    hypertensive disorder of 312
    immunological test for 314*f*
    maintenance of 305
    pre-eclampsia of 312
    test 314
        strip 314
    toxemia of 312
Prehepatic jaundice 164
    causes of 164
Premenstrual syndrome 308
Premotor area, functions of 519
Preoptic nucleus 224
Prepubertal boys 294
Presbycusis 590
Presbyopia 579, 584
    causes of 584
    correction of 584
Presenile dementia 548
Pressure
    changes 591
    determining filtration 194
    diuresis 267, 367
    natriuresis 367
    receptors 478
    ventilator 442
Presynaptic inhibition 463, 464*f*
Presynaptic inhibitory neuron 464
Presynaptic membrane 122, 462
Presynaptic neuron 461
Pretectal nucleus 573, 576
Prevertebral ganglia 553
Primary auditory area 521, 589
    functions of 521
Primary colors 580
Primary motor area 518
    functions of 518
Primordial follicle 296, 302
Procarboxypeptidases 154
Procoagulants 82
Procollagenase, inactive 154
Proelastase, inactive 154
Proenzyme-enzyme conversion reactions 78
Proerythroblast 78
Profibrinolysin 292
Progestasert 320
Progesterone 298, 307, 311
    functions of 299
    mode of action of 299
    regulation of secretion of 299
Prognathism 239
Programmed cell death 11
Projection, law of 459, 460
Prokaryotes 8
Prolactin 234, 236
    inhibitory hormone 234
Proliferation, stage of 288, 297
Proline-rich proteins 140
Proprioceptors 458, 527, 528*t*
Propulsive movements 176, 177
Propylthiouracil 250
Prosencephalon 445
Prostacyclin 282, 368
    actions of 282
Prostaglandin 187, 195, 279, 281
    actions of 281
    administration of 322
    types of 281

Prostate gland 126, 287
Prostatic fluid 287
    functions of 287
Protanomaly 581
Protanopes 581
Protects mucous membrane 170
Protein 41, 73, 74, 97
    anabolism of 235, 298
    C, activated 81
    channels 15
    conservation 261
    deficiency anemia 57
    depletion 265
    digestion of 152, 153
    factories 7
    hormonal 7
    hormones 228
    integral 2
    kinase 232
    layers, functions of 3
    metabolism 234, 245, 261, 262, 269
    peripheral 2
    reserve 38
    role of 262
    sparing effect 261
    synthesis of 4, 235
    transmembrane 2
Proteoglycan 534
    meshwork 100
Proteolytic enzymes 94, 146, 152, 153, 167, 293, 310
Prothrombin activator, formation of 24, 79, 80
Prothrombin time 82
Protodiastole 337
Protopathic sensation 478, 489
Proximal convoluted tubule 185
Pseudohermaphroditism 273
Pseudohypoparathyroidism 253
Pseudomonas aeruginosa 58
Pseudopuberty 294
Psychomotor epilepsy, causes of 541
Psychotherapy 300
Pterygoid muscles 172
Ptosis 579
Ptyalism 142
Pudendal nerve 215, 217
    functions of 215
    inhibition of 178
Pulmonary artery 398
    pressure 399
Pulmonary blood
    flow 399
    pressure 399
    vessels 398
Pulmonary capillary 416*f*
    membrane 330
    pressure 399
Pulmonary circulation 330, 395, 398, 399
    regulation of 399
Pulmonary edema 433
Pulmonary function tests 405
Pulmonary hypertension 436
Pulmonary tuberculosis 52, 433
Pulmonary valve 327
Pulmonary veins 330
Pulmonary ventilation 411
    effect on 443
Pulse
    examination of 375
    points 375, 375*t*
    pressure 362
    rate 375*t*
    velocity of 374
Pulsus alternans 376

Pulsus deficit 376
Pulsus paradoxus 376
Pump handle movement 401
Pupil 561
    constricts 576
    dilatation of 569, 576
    size of 576
Pupillary light reflex 576
Pupillary reflexes 576
Purkinje fibers 333
Purpura 82, 83
    causes of 83
    types of 83
Purpuric spots 83
Pursuit movement 566
Pus 62
    cells 62, 210
Pyelonephritis 211
Pyknosis 45
Pyloric glands 145
Pyloric sphincter 144
Pylorus 144
Pyothorax 432
Pyramidal cells 482
Pyramidal decussation 483
Pyramidal lobules 286
Pyramidal tracts 482, 483, 483*f*, 494
Pyrexia 225
Pyrogens 225
Pyrrole rings 48

Q

QRS complex 346
    amplitude of 346
    causes of 346
    duration of 346
    morphology of 346
Q-T interval, duration of 348
Quadriplegia 495
Quadruple gallop 342
Quadruple heart sound 342
Quadruple rhythm 342

R

Rabbit antiserum 314
Radial periosteal reflex 471
Radial pulse 375
    examination of 375
    tracing 374*f*
Radiotherapy 142
Ramp fashion 423
Raphe nucleus, role of 544
Rapid alternate movements 511
Rapid eye movement sleep 543
Rapid filling 337
Rapid jerky movements 515
Ratchet theory 120
Reabsorption 99
    active 196
    mechanism of 196
    routes of 197, 197*f*
    site of 197
Rebound phenomenon 472
Receptive relaxation 174
Receptor cells, stimulation of 536
Receptor coated pit 20
Receptor epithelium 534
Receptor organ 535
Receptor potential, properties of 458
Receptor-mediated endocytosis 19, 20
    mechanism of 20, 20*f*
Reciprocal inhibition 472, 532
    significance of 472
Reciprocal innervation 472, 532
Recognition memory 547

Recording cystometrogram, method of 216
Recovery heat 121
Rectal temperature 222
Rectum 170
Rectus
    inferior 565, 566*f*
    lateral 566*f*
    muscles, superior 566, 566*f*
Red blood cell 30*f*, 31, 33, 40, 45*f*, 52, 60, 60*t*, 63*f*, 210, 314
    abnormal shape of 58
    count, normal 40
    dimensions of 40*f*
    fate of 41, 41*f*
    fragility of 58
    functions of 41
    immature 45
    lifespan of 41
    morphology of 40
    number of 41
    properties of 40
    shape of 43
    size of 43
    suspension stability of 38
Red cell transfusion 91
Red muscles 112
Red nucleus 532
Red pulp 94
Referred pain 497
    mechanism of 498
    sites of 497*f*
Reflex 470, 471, 542, 548
    acquired 469, 548
    action, stages of 149
    activity 468
        center for 501
    antigravity 569
    arc 468
        simple 468*f*
    autonomic 469
    classification of 468
    cutaneous 470*t*
    explicit 469
    failure, stages of 487
    general static 531, 532
    inborn 469, 548
    local static 532
    muscular activity, control of 514
    operant conditioned 549
    pathological 470
    positive supporting 532
    primary conditioned 548
    properties of 471
    protective 569
    quickest 530
    secondary conditioned 548
    significance of 468
    superficial 469
    supporting 532
Refractive errors 570, 582, 583*f*, 583*t*
Refractory period 114, 452
Regular astigmatism 583
Regulating vagal tone 361*f*
Regulatory T cells 68
Relative refractory period 334
Relaxin 312
Remote memory 547
Renal artery 190
Renal autoregulation 191
Renal blood flow 189, 190, 191*f*, 195, 210
    autoregulation of 192
    measurement of 191, 210
    regulation of 191
Renal blood vessels 190, 190*f*
Renal calculi 211

Renal capillaries 191f
Renal circulation 190-192
Renal clearance 210
Renal columns 181
Renal corpuscle 181, 183, 184f
   situation of 183
   structure of 183
Renal disease, end stage 211
Renal disorder 32, 56
Renal failure 142, 209, 211
Renal function tests 209
Renal glomerular capillaries 192
Renal hypertension 370
Renal ischemia 211
Renal pelvis 186
Renal physiology 181
Renal plasma flow 210, 211
   measurement of 210
Renal shutdown 88
Renal sinus 182
Renal stones 254
Renal system 126, 181
Renal threshold 197, 265
Renal tubular disorders 208
Renal tubule 183, 206t
   segments of 198
   transport from lumen of 198
Renal vein leaves 191
Renewal alveolar air 413
Renin 146, 147, 195, 279
   actions of 279
   secretion of 188
Renin-angiotensin
   mechanism 182, 367, 367f
   system 188, 188f
Renshaw cell inhibition 464, 464f
Replacement transfusion 92
Reproductive organs
   female 295, 295f
   primary 285
Reproductive system 57, 126, 285
   female 295, 296f
Resist pathogenic agents 65
Respiration 384
   chemical regulation of 426f
   diseases of 427
   disorders of 427
   effect on 299, 371, 429
   external 395
   internal 395
   mechanics of 400
   muscles of 400
   neonatal 384
   nervous regulation of 422f
   normal rate of 395
   normal rhythm of 423
   phases of 395
   regulation of 421
   types of 395
Respiratory acid 207
Respiratory acidosis 207
Respiratory alkalosis 207
Respiratory bronchioles 396
Respiratory centers 366, 421, 422t
   connections of 423
   integration of 423
Respiratory chain 6
Respiratory disorders 43, 432
Respiratory distress syndrome 388, 401
Respiratory disturbances 207
Respiratory exchange ratio 417
   normal values of 417
   values of 417t
Respiratory function 35, 311
Respiratory gases
   exchange of 414, 416
   transport of 48, 414

Respiratory membrane 397, 414, 415
   layers of 415, 415t
   structure of 414f
   thickness of 415
Respiratory minute volume 410
Respiratory movements 400
Respiratory muscles 404
   paralysis of 428
Respiratory organ 311
Respiratory patterns 427
Respiratory pressures 401, 402f
Respiratory protective reflexes 398
Respiratory pump 352, 403
Respiratory quotient 417, 443
Respiratory sinus arrhythmia 348, 359
Respiratory system 22, 57, 126, 313, 388, 436, 542
Respiratory tract 395, 396f
   functional anatomy of 395
   lower 396
   non-respiratory functions of 397
Respiratory unit 396, 396f
   structure of 396, 397f
Respirometer 406, 408
Resting heat 121
Resting membrane potential 116, 127
Resting tremor 514
Restlessness 57
Restrictive respiratory disease 410, 410t
Rete testis 287
Reticular cells 93
Reticular formation 525
   divisions of 525
   functional divisions of 526f
   functions of 525
   situation of 525
Reticular system, descending 526
Reticulocyte 45
Reticuloendothelial cells 93, 94
   classification of 93
Reticuloendothelial system 93, 94
Reticulospinal tract 484
Reticulum, meshwork of 525
Retina 559, 571, 580
   cones of 570
   layers of 561, 562f
Retinal points 571
Retinine 568
Retinitis pigmentosa 570
Retinol 568
Retrograde degeneration 454
Retronasal olfaction 597, 599, 600
Reverse chloride shift 419
Reverse peristaltic movement 281
Rheobasic strength 111
Rhesus antigen, inheritance of 87, 87f
Rhesus factor 87
Rhesus incompatibility 88f
Rhesus monkey 87
Rheumatic fever 53, 75
Rheumatoid arthritis 52, 53, 72, 95
Rhodopsin 567, 568
   activated 569
   resynthesis of 569
Rhombencephalon 446
Rhythm method 318
   advantages of 318
   disadvantages of 318
Rhythmicity 332
Rib cage, effect on 291
Ribonucleic acid 8, 10, 154
   structure of 10
   synthesis of 8

Ribosomal ribonucleic acid 7, 10
Ribosomes 4, 7, 105
   functions of 7
Rickets 259
   manifestations of 259
Right atrial reflex 360
Right atrium 360
Right optic
   nerve, lesion of 574
   radiation, lesion of 574
Righting reflexes
   center for 532
   sequential events of 531
Rigor mortis 114
   medicolegal importance of 114
Rinne test 593
Rod cell, structure of 567
Rods and cones 567
   layer of 561
Root, anterior 474
Rotational movement 535
Rotatory acceleration 535
Rotatory movements 535
Rough endoplasmic reticulum 3-5
   functions of 4
Rouleaux formation 40, 41f
R-R interval 348
   duration of 348
   significance of 348
Rubrospinal tract 486
Rubrothalamic fibers 511
Ruffini end organ 457
Ruptured blood vessel, repair of 75
Ryle tube 150

S

SA node 332
Saccadic movement 566
Saccule, functions of 537
Sacral outflow 554
Sacral parasympathetic nerves 497
Safe period 318
Saliva
   augmented secretion of 142
   composition of 138, 139, 139f
   digestive enzymes of 140t
   dripping of 140
   functions of 139
   lack of 143
   mucin of 139
   paralytic secretion of 142
   properties of 138
Salivary amylase 139, 140
Salivary glands 137, 138, 139f, 140, 142, 268, 554
   classification of 138
   duct system of 138
   structure of 138
Salivary secretion 137, 141, 142
   disorders of 142
   reflex regulation of 141
   regulation of 140
Salivatory nucleus
   inferior 140
   superior 140
Salt taste 596
Saltatory conduction 449, 452
   mechanism of 452
Sarcolemma 105
Sarcomere 107, 127
   components of 107
   electron microscopic study of 107
   extent of 107
   parts of 108f
Sarcoplasm 105
Sarcoplasmic reticulum 105, 108

Sarcotubular system 108, 108f, 127
   structures of 108
Scab 80
Scala media 587
Scala tympani 587
Scala vestibuli 587
Scalp electrodes 539
Scanty menstruation 308
Schwann cells 449
Scoliosis 259
Scopolamine 142
Scotopsin 568
Seasonal fertility 278
Sebaceous glands 218, 219, 585
   activation of 220
Sebum
   composition of 219
   functions of 219
Second degree injury 453
Second heart sound 337, 341, 343
   reduplication of 341
Secretary tubules 182
Secrete serotonin 76
Secrete somatomedin C 236
Secrete tetraiodothyronine 243
Secretin 150, 156, 262
Secretion of adrenaline, regulation of 277
Secretor antigens 89
Secretory function 6, 168, 171, 221
Secretory lysosomes 6
Secretory phase 306, 308
Secretory vesicles 6
Sedatives 171
Segmental artery 190
Segmental static reflexes 532
Seizures 32, 312
   convulsive 540
   general onset 541
Self-antigens 67, 72
Self-excitation 332
Semen 292
   clotting of 287, 288
   composition of 292, 293f
   properties of 292
Semicircular canal 534, 536
   functions of 535
   position of 534f
   posterior 535
   superior 535
Semilunar valves 327, 341
Seminal fluid 287
   functions of 287
Seminal vesicles 287
Seminiferous tubules 286
Semipermeable membrane 1, 17f
Senile decay 241
Senile red blood cell 58
   destruction of 94
Sensation
   abnormal 490b
   affective nature of 501
   classification of 490f
   discriminative nature of 501
   loss of 502
   perception of 521
   relay center for 500
   synthesis of 521
Sense organs, specialized 559
Sensitization 546
Sensory
   adaptation 458
   ataxia 482
   decussation 482
   feedback 521
   fibers 491
   function 221
   homunculus 520

impulses 448, 450
information, processing of 501
motor area 520, 521
transduction 458
Sensory areas 357, 549
  functions of 357
  primary 520
  topographical arrangement of 521f
Sensory nerve 468
  fibers 359, 529f
    destruction of 217
  supply 528
Sensory pathway 490, 491t
  classical 526
  disorders of 493t
  nonspecific 526
  specific 526
Septic shock 389
Septicemia 56
Sequential pills 321
Serosa 134
Serotonin 130
  actions of 282
  release of 544
  source of secretion of 282
Serous cells 138
Serous glands 138
Serous membrane 134
Sertoli cells 286
  in spermatogenesis, role of 289
Serum 34
  albumin 37
  oozing of 80
Servomechanism 512
Sex chromosomes 310
  and autosomes 8
Sex determination 310
  abnormalities of 310
Sex differentiation 290
Sex hormones, role of 47
Sex organs
  effect on 291
  primary 285
Sexual characters, effect on secondary 291, 298
Sexual function 246
  regulation of 507, 524
Sexual infantilism 242
Sexual life in females 299
Sexual sensations, center for 501
Sexually transmitted infections 319
Sham feeding 148
  procedure for 148
  uses of 148
Sheath of Schwann 449
Shivering 223, 224, 438
Shock 388, 389
  anaphylactic 389
  cardiac 88
  cardiogenic 389
  circulatory 265, 387
  electric 110
  hemorrhagic 388
  hypovolemic 388
  manifestations of 388
  neurogenic 388
Short ciliary nerves 579
Short sightedness 582
Short-loop feedback control 236
Shoulder, effect on 291
Shunt, physiological 378, 381, 399
Sialolithiasis 142
Sialorrhea 142
Sickle cell 43
  anemia 53, 56, 92
    severe 92
  disease 56

Sigmoid colon 170
Signaling cells 227
Silicon-coated container 82
Simmond's disease 241
  causes of 241
  symptoms of 241
Simple diffusion 15
Simple muscle
  curve 111
    periods of 112
  twitch 111
Simultaneously water diffuses 202
Single-unit smooth muscle 127, 127f, 128t
Sinoatrial block 349
Sinoatrial node 325, 333f
Sinus
  arrhythmia 348
  block 349
  bradycardia 349
  tachycardia 349
Sjögren's syndrome 142, 143
Skeletal muscle 1, 23, 103-105, 106t, 112, 114, 117f, 246, 276
  activities of 493
  circulation 382
  composition of 109f
  fibers of 103, 134, 451t
  mass 106f, 382, 393
  properties of 110
  smallest 586
  structure of 105, 106f
  triad of 108
Skin 23, 181, 218, 388, 456
  appendages of 218
  color of 218
  effect on 291
  functions of 221
  glands of 219
  layers of 218
  normal blood flow to 383
  pigmentation of 218
  structure of 218, 219f
Sleep
  and wakefulness, regulation of 506
  apnea syndrome 545
  centers 544
  disorders 545
  paralysis 542
  physiology of 542
  spindles 543
  stages of 543
  types of 543
  walking 545
Sliding theory explains 120
Sliva kills, lysozyme of 140
Slow wave rhythm 127
Small intestine 134, 166
  disorders of 169
  functional anatomy of 166
  functions of 168
  glands of 166
  movements of 176, 176f
  parts of 166
Smell
  perception of 600
  sensation of 598
Smooth endoplasmic reticulum 4, 5
  functions of 4
Smooth muscle 1, 103, 104, 115, 126, 128f, 130, 178, 276
  activities, control of 130
  cells 187
  contractile process in 129
  contraction of 130
    molecular basis of 129, 130f
  distribution of 126

functions of 126
relaxation of 130
structure of 126
tonic contraction of 129
Smooth muscle fibers 104t, 126, 127, 127f, 134
  contraction of 126
  relaxation of 126
  types of 127
Sneezing reflex 397, 398
  causes of 398
Snellen's chart 570
Sodium 159, 160
  chloride 195, 198, 202
    active reabsorption of 201
  citrate 52
  countertransport 19, 19f
  excretion 280
  ions 267
    rapid influx of 332
    slow influx of 332
  loss of 204
  primary active transport of 18
  reabsorption of 198
Sodium-dependent glucose transporter 198
Sodium-hydrogen
  antiport pump 205
  pump 206
Sodium-iodide symport pump 244
Sodium-potassium pump 18, 18f, 116
Somatic chromosomes 310
Somatic nerve supply 215
Somatic nervous system 446
Somatic reflexes 469
Somatic sensations 489
  types of 489
Somatomedin 235
  stimulate hypothalamus 236
Somatomotor activities
  control of 526
  facilitation of 526
Somatomotor system 489, 493
Somatosensory cortex 492f
Somatosensory system 489
Somatostatin 150, 156, 263
  actions of 263
  regulation of secretion of 263
Somatotrophs 234
Somatotropic hormone 234
Somesthetic association area 521
Somnambulism 545
Somnolence 246
Sound
  appreciation of pitch of 593
  energy 592
  localization of 593
  loudness of 593
  poor localization of 590
  properties of 592
  transduction 592
  waves, amplitude of 592
Sour taste 596
Space physiology 436
Spacecraft 436
Spacelab 436
Spastic paralysis 115
Spasticity 115
Spatial summation 465f, 471
Special sensations 489, 559
Spectral colors 580
Speech 549
  center 549
  impairment of 549
  mechanism of 549
  motor area for 519
  nervous control of 549

problems 515
role in 140
Sperm 292
  acrosome of 310
  count 292
  motility of 292
    maintenance of 287
  nutrition to 287
  pathway for 287f
  structure of 292
  survival time of 292
  tail of 293
Spermatids 289
Spermatocyte
  primary 289
  secondary 289
Spermatogenesis 288, 288f, 290
  hormones for 289t
  stages of 288
Spermatogenic cells 286
Spermatogonia 286, 289
Spermatozoa 288
Spermiation 289
Spermicidal action 319
Spermicidal gel 319
Spermicide 319
Spermiogenesis 289
Spherocytosis 43
Sphincter 144
  nerve supply to 214
  pupillae 578
Sphygmomanometer 368
Spinal cord 445, 473, 474, 475f, 476, 493, 532
  ascending tracts of 476, 476t, 477t
  central canal of 550
  column of 481f
  complete transection of 486
  covering of 473
  descending tracts of 482, 482t, 485t
  diseases of 487
  enlargement of 473
  extent of 473
  filum terminale of 473
  gray horns of 475t
  gray matter of 474
  hemisection of 487
  incomplete transection of 486
  internal structure of 474
  laminae of 475, 475t
  length of 473
  long tracts of 476
  sacral segments of 177f
  section of 474t
  segments of 473, 474f
  shape of 473
  short tracts of 476
  situation of 473
  tracts of 478f
  white matter of 476
Spinal disk 487
Spinal nerve 473, 474t
  roots 474
Spinal segmental reflex 530
Spinal tracts 476
Spinal veins 550
Spindle bursts 543
Spinocerebellar tracts 480f
Spinocerebellum 492f, 510
  components of 510
  functions of 510
Spino-olivary tract 480
Spinoreticular tract 480, 526
Spinotectal tract 480
Spinothalamic tract 479f
Spinovestibular tract 481

Spiral ganglion, bipolar cells of 589
Spirogram 406, 407f
Spirometer 406, 407f
　disadvantages of 408
Splanchnic circulation 381
Splanchnic nerve 146, 152
Splanchnic region 353
Spleen 93, 94
　functions of 94
　storage of blood in 381
Splenectomy 75
Splenic circulation 381
Splenic corpuscles 94
Splenic pulp destroy 95
Splenomegaly 95
Spontaneous pain 502
S-T segment 348
　duration of 348
Stagnant hypoxia 428
　causes of 428
　characteristic features of 428
Staircase phenomenon 334
Stapes, movement of 591
Staphylococcus aureus 58
Starling's law 130
Static exercise 391
Static gamma motor 528
Static lung function tests 405
Static postural reflexes 532t
Static reflexes 531
Statoconia 535
Statokinetic reflexes 532, 533
Statotonic reflexes 532
Steatorrhea 154, 156, 169
　causes of 156
Stellate ganglion 358
Stem cells 44, 45f, 63, 145
　factor 47
Stensen's duct 138
Stercobilinogen 162
Stereocilia 535, 536, 588, 592
Stereognosis 481f
Steroid 171
　hormone 228, 232
Sterols 219
Stethoscope 342, 368
Stiff hairs 585
Stimulus 110, 174, 451
　duration of 110
　external 129
　intensity of 110
　point of 111, 112
　qualities of 110
　strength of 112, 458
　types of 110
Stomach 126, 134, 144, 146
　emptying of 174, 175
　filling of 174
　functional anatomy of 144
　functions of 146
　glands of 145
　movements of 174
　parts of 144, 144f
　peristalsis of 174
　pyloric sphincter of 166
　wall, structure of 145
Storage function 146, 162, 221
Stratum
　corneum 218
　germinativum 218
　granulosum 218
　lucidum 218
　spinosum 218
Strength-duration curve 111, 111f
Streptokinase 80
Stretch receptors 215, 216, 360, 423
Stretch reflex 469, 529, 530, 531f

Stretched muscle, muscle spindle of 531f
Striated fibers 326
Striated muscle 103
Stroke 380, 495
　causes of 380
　symptoms of 380
　volume 351
Subarachnoid space 550, 551
Subclinical tetany 253
Subconscious kinesthetic sensation 478, 480f
Subconscious movements, regulation of 514
Subcortical auditory center 589
Subcutaneous tissue cells 93
Subdural hematoma 539
Subliminal stimuli, summation of 334
Sublingual glands 138, 140, 141f
Submandibular glands 138, 140
Submaxillary ganglion 140
Submaxillary glands 138, 141f
Submucus layer 134
Subneural clefts 123
Substance 283
　reabsorption of 198
　source of secretion of 283
Substantia
　gelatinosa of Rolando 478, 499
　nigra 513
Subthalamic nucleus of Luys 513
Succinylcholine 124
Succinyl-CoA 50
Succus entericus 168, 168f
　amylolytic enzymes of 167
　composition of 167
　digestive enzymes of 168t
　functions of 167
　properties of 167
　secretion of 169
Sucrase 167
Sulcus
　central 517, 520
　lateral 517
Sulfhemoglobin 49
Summation gallop 342
Sunstroke 439
Superior cervical ganglion 141
Superior vermis 509
　parts of 509t
Supinator jerk 471
Supplementary motor area 519
　functions of 519
Supporting cells 1, 286, 595
Suppressor area 518
Suppressor T cells 66
　role of 68
Supramaximal stimulus 110
Supraoptic nucleus 237, 573
Suprarenal glands 266
Supravaginal portion 296
Surface temperature 222
Surgical shock 388
Suspensory ligaments 560, 564
Sustentacular cells 598
Swallowing 172-174
　reflex 398
Sweat glands 218, 220, 268, 554
Sweat secretion 542
Sweet taste 596
Sylvian fissure 517
Sylvian sulcus 520
Sympathetic adrenergic nerve fibers 220
Sympathetic chain 565
　ganglia 553
Sympathetic depressants 142

Sympathetic fibers 141, 148, 555
　functions of 141
Sympathetic ganglia 553
Sympathetic nerve
　effects of 359
　fibers 135, 358, 565
　　distribution of 358
　　functions of 135
　functions of 214, 359
　mode of action of 359
　stimulation of 169
　supply 214
Sympathetic postganglionic fibers 359
Sympathetic stimulation 196
Sympathetic tone 359, 365
Sympathetic vasoconstrictor tone 365
Sympathetic vasodilator fibers 365
Sympathoadrenergic system 553
Sympathomimetic drugs 141, 556
Synapse
　classification of 461
　functions of 462
　inhibitory 463
　properties of 465
Synaptic cleft 122, 462
Synaptic inhibition, significance of 464
Synaptic vesicles 122, 462
Synchronized waves 539
Syncope, types of 389
Syncytium 326
　functional 127
Syndrome of inappropriate hypersecretion of antidiuretic hormone 204, 241
Synthetic estrogen 321
Synthetic function 162, 171
Synthetic progesterone 321
Synthetic sensations 490
Syphilis 487
Syringomyelia 487
Systemic arterial pressure 196
Systemic circulation 329
Systolic pressure, normal 362

T

T cell
　immunity 67
　receptor 67
　specificity of 68
T lymphocytes 64, 65
　processing of 279
　storage of 66
　types of 65
T wave 347
　amplitude of 347
　causes of 347
　duration of 347
　morphology of 347
Tabes dorsalis 487
Tachycardia 277, 356
Tachypnea 427
Tactile discrimination 481f
Tactile localization 481f
Tapping sound, appearance of 369
Target cells 227
Taste 595
　appreciation of 139
　center 596
　pore 596
　receptor cells 595
　sensation of 595
　transduction 597
Taste bud 595, 595f, 596
　structure of 595
　situation of 595

Taste sensation
　abnormalities of 597
　combination of 596
　pathway for 596, 596f
　primary 596
　threshold for 597
Taurine 160
Taurocholic acids 160
Tear 560
Tectorial membrane 588
Tectospinal tract 484
Telencephalon 445
Telereceptors 457
Temperature
　regulating capacity, loss of 438
　regulation, mechanism of 224
　sensations 478
Temporal lobe 521
　syndrome 522
Temporal muscle 172
Temporal pulse 375
Temporal summation 465f, 471
Temporary endocrine gland 305
Temporary hyposalivation 142
Tendon reflexes 469, 471t
Tensor tympani 586
Terapeutic plasma exchange 38
Terminal bronchiole 396
Terminal cisternae 108
Terminal ganglia 553
Terminal tubules 182
Termination of pregnancy 311
Teste
　descent of 290
　effects of 294
　extirpation of 294
　functional anatomy of 285
Testis
　coverings of 285
　endocrine functions of 290
　functions of 288
　gametogenic functions of 288
　lobules of 285
　parenchyma of 285
　structure of 286f
　undescended 291
Testosterone 290
　functions of 290, 291
　mode of action of 291
　secretion 290
　　regulation of 291, 292f
Tetanus 71, 113
Tetraethyl ammonium ion 556
Tetraiodothyronine 243
Tetraplegia 495
TH1 cells, role of 68
TH2 cells, role of 68
Thalamic hand 502
Thalamic lesion 501
Thalamic nuclei 500, 501f
Thalamic phantom limb 502
Thalamic reticular nucleus 500
Thalamic syndrome 502
Thalamocortical fibers 511
Thalamus 500
　functions of 500
　situation of 500
Thalassemia 49, 57
Thebesian veins 378
Theca folliculi, formation of 302
Theca interna 297
Thelarche 315
Therapeutic plasma exchange 38
Thermal indicator method 355
Thermal sensations 478
Thermal stimulus 110
Thermodilution technique 355

Index

Thermogenic effect 299
Thermoreceptors 506
Thermoregulatory disorders 225
Thermostatic mechanism 506
Theta rhythm 540
Theta wave 543
Thiocyanate 250
Thioureylenes 250
Third degree injury 453
Third heart sound 337, 341
Third order neuron 476, 497, 572, 589, 596
Thirst mechanism 507f
Thoracic cage 401
    movements of 400
Thoracic duct 96
Thoracic lid 400
Thoracic segment 474f, 475f
Thoracolumbar outflow 553
Thorax, abnormal 404
Thready pulse 376
Thrombasthenic purpura 83
Thrombin binding protein 81
Thrombin converts fibrinogen 80
Thrombocytes 33
    production of 182
Thrombocytopenic purpura 83
Thrombomodulin, production of 81
Thrombopoietin 75, 182, 279
Thrombosis 83
    causes of 83
    complications of 83
Thrombospondin 74
Thrombosthenin 80
Thromboxane 76, 282, 368
    actions of 282
Thrombus 83
Thymin 279
Thymine 9
Thymopoietin 279
Thymosin 279
Thymus 65, 278
    endocrine function of 279
    functions of 279
    secretes thymosin 65
    structure of 278
Thyroglobulin 243
    organification of 244
    synthesis 244
Thyroid 143
    adenoma 248
    disorders, treatment for 250
    follicles 243
    function tests 250
    peroxidase 244
    timulating hormone 23
Thyroid gland 243, 243f, 245, 254, 313
    diseases of 248
    disorders of 247
    functional histology of 243
    histology of 243f
    hormones of 243
    morphology of 243
    posterior surface of 251f
Thyroid hormones 232
    functions of 245
    mode of action of 247
    regulation of secretion of 247, 247f
    release of 245
    stages of synthesis of 244
    storage of 245
    synthesis of 244, 244f
    transport of 245
Thyroidectomy 253
Thyroid-stimulating hormone 24, 234, 236, 247, 248
    receptor antibodies 248

Thyrotoxicosis 247
Thyrotrophs 234
Thyrotropin releasing hormone 234, 247
Thyroxine 47, 243, 246
    binding
        globulin 245
        prealbumin 245
    hypersecretion of 245
    secretion of 24f
Tibialis pulse 375
Tight junction 12, 13, 552
    functions of 12
Tigroid appearance 448
Tigroid substances 448
Timed vital capacity 409
Tinnitus 523
Tissue 1
    fluid 99
        formation of 99, 100f
        functions of 99
    macrophage 63, 93
        system 93
    plasminogen activator 80
    resistance work 404
Tone
    adjustment of 529
    redistribution of 529
Tongue
    anterior part of 172
    anterior surface of 595
    dorsum of 595
    papillae of 595
    posterior part of 595
Tonic labyrinthine 532
Tonic receptors 458
Tonicity 30, 139
Tonsillitis 142
Tooth, decay of 142
Total body water 27
Total iron, regulation of 51
Total leukocyte count 61
Touch receptor 238, 458
Toxic goiter 249
Toxic substances 65
Toxins 98, 182
Toxoids 71
Trabeculae 564
Tracheobronchial tree 396, 396f
    components of 396
Tract of Burdach 481
Tract of Goll 481
Tract of Schultze 482
Tractus solitaries, nucleus of 596
Transcellular fluid 28f
Transcellular route 197
Transcytosis 19, 21
Transduction 458
Transferrin 50
Transfusion reactions 88
    severe 211
    signs of 88
    symptoms of 88
Transneuronal degeneration 454
Transplanted tissues 65
    rejection of 67
Transport mechanism 38
    across cell membrane, types of 21f
Transpulmonary pressure 403
Transverse colon 170
Transverse tubules 108
Trapezoid body 589
Traumatic shock 388
Traveling wave 592
    theory 593
Trehalose glucohydrolase 167
Tremor 514

Trephone substances, production of 38
Tributyrin 147
Triceps jerk 471
Trichromatism 581
Tricuspid valve 327
Trigeminal nerve 491, 492t
    division of 141, 586
    lingual branch of 140
    mandibular division of 172
    three divisions of 492f
Trigeminal pathway 492f
Triglycerides 219, 261
Trigone 213
Triiodothyronine 243
Triple heart sound 342
Tritanomaly 581
Tritanopia 581
Tropic hormones 234
Tropomyosin 108
    role of 119
Troponin 108
    role of 119
Trousseau's sign 253
True capillaries 381
Trypsin 153
    actions of 153
    autocatalytic action of 153
Trypsinogen 153
T-tubules 108
    functions of 108
Tubectomy 322
Tubercle bacilli 433
Tuberculosis 53, 70, 95, 211
Tubular cell 198
    transport from 198
Tubular epithelial cells 198
Tubular excretion 193
Tubular necrosis,. acute 211
Tubular portion 183
Tubular reabsorption 193, 196, 199
    regulation of 197
Tubular secretion 193, 198, 199
Tubulin 73
Tubuloglomerular feedback 191, 195, 195f
Tumor necrosis factors 70
    secretion of 94
Tunica adventitia, outer 329
Tunica albuginea 285, 296
Tunica externa 560
Tunica fibrosa 560
Tunica interna 561
    Inner 329
Tunica media 560
Tunica nervosa 561
Tunica vaginalis 285
Tunica vasculosa 285, 560
Turner's syndrome 10
Tympanic cavity 585
Tympanic membrane 585, 586, 586f
    role of 591
    surface of 591
Tympanic plexus 140
Tympanic reflex 586
    significance of 587
Typhoid 95
Tyrosine 244
    iodination of 244
    kinase 261

U

U wave 348
Ulcerative colitis 169
Ulnar pulse 375
Ultraviolet rays 580
    protection from 221

Umbilical cord 311
Umbilical vessels 384
Unconditioned reflex 141, 149, 154, 469
Unconjugated bilirubin 161
Unequal refractive power 583
Unipolar limb leads 345
Unstable resting membrane potential 332
Uphill transport 17
Upper motor neuron 483, 494
    lesion 472, 483
    effects of 494f
Upper respiratory tract 396
Upper right atrium 325
Urase 147
Urate oxidase 6
Urea 182, 202
    recirculation of 201, 202
Ureter 181
    blockage of 211
    pelvis of 185
Urethra 126, 181, 213, 214f, 215f, 217, 288
    external 288
    female 213
    functional anatomy of 213
    internal 288
Urethral constriction 211
Urethral sphincter 214, 215t
Uric acid 182, 196
Urinary bladder 126, 181, 186, 213, 214f, 215f, 554
    filling of 215
    functional anatomy of 213
    nerve supply to 214
Urinary function 213
Urinary output, normal 193
Urinary system 181f
Urinary tract, obstruction in 204
Urine 314
    acidification of 205, 206
    chemical analysis of 210
    composition of 209
    concentration of 200
    examination of 209, 210
    formation 193
        events of 194f
    osmolarity of 200
    passage of 185
    physical examination of 209
    properties of 209
Uriniferous tubules 182
    parts of 182
Urobilinogen 161
Uterine tissues, desquamated 306
Uterine vessels 384
Uterine wall, structure of 296
Uterus 126, 296
    contraction of 238
    divisions of 296
    effect on 297, 299
    section of 297f
Utilization time 111
Utricle 534
    functions of 537
Utriculosaccular duct 534

V

V wave 377
Vaccines 65, 70
Vacuoles 6
Vagal apnea 427
Vagal escape, causes for 358
Vagal fibers 596
Vagal tone 357
    regulation of 359

Vagal trunks 146
Vagina 296
   effect on 298
Vaginal portion 296
Vaginal sponge 319
Vagovagal reflex 150
Vague pain 259
Vagus nerve 136, 152, 174, 358
   effects of 358
   mode of action of 358
   stimulation of right 358
Valsalva experiment 371
Valsalva maneuver 371, 372*t*
   effects of 371
   uses of 371
Valvular diseases 343
Vanillylmandelic acid 275
Varicose vein 382
   causes for 382
Varicosities 130
Vas deferens 287
   ampulla of 287
Vas efferens 287
Vasa recta 201
   descending limb of 202
   role of 201
Vascular spasm 312
Vasectomy 322
Vasoactive intestinal
   peptide 149
   polypeptide 134, 150
Vasoconstriction 76
Vasoconstrictor area, functions of 357
Vasoconstrictor fibers 365
Vasodilatation 281
Vasodilator
   fibers 365
   local 368
Vasogenic shock 388
Vasomotor center 357, 365
   areas of 357
   mechanism of action of 365
Vasomotor system, components of 364
Vasomotor tone 365
Vasopressin 237
Vasopressor action 237
Vena cava
   inferior 191, 329
   superior 329
Venous blood
   gases in 418*t*
   oxygen content in 354
Venous blood pressure 371
   normal values of 371*b*
Venous drainage 378
Venous pressure 371
Venous pulse 374, 376
   abnormal 377
   examination of 376
Venous return 364, 393
Venous system 191, 329
Ventilation 411
   method 441
   volume, maximum 410

Ventilation-perfusion ratio 412
   significance of 413
   variations in 413
Ventral posterolateral nucleus 478, 482
Ventral respiratory group 422
Ventral root 474
Ventral spinocerebellar tract 478
Ventral white column 476
Ventricular diastole 335
Ventricular events 335
   subdivisions of 335*b*
Ventricular fibrillation 349
Ventricular muscle 331
Ventricular systole 335
Vermis 509
Vertebral canal 473
Vertical acceleration 537
Vertical plane 534
Vesicular follicle 302
Vestibular apparatus 532, 533, 535, 587
   functional anatomy of 534
   functions of 535
   hair cells of 535*f*, 537*f*
   receptor organ in 534
Vestibular membrane 587
Vestibular nucleus, lateral 484
Vestibulocerebellum 509
   components of 509
   functions of 509
   mechanism of action of 509
Vestibulocochlear nerve 589
   vestibular division of 535
Vestibulo-ocular reflex 537
Vestibulospinal tract, Lateral 484
Vibratory sensation 481*f*, 490
Villi, movements of 177
Viral infection, Acute 143
Viropause 293
Viruses 171
Visceral muscle 104
Visceral pain, causes of 497
Visceral reflexes 469, 576
Visceral smooth muscle fibers 127
Visceroreceptors 458
Viscosity 33
Viscus saliva 138
Vision
   acuity of 570
   field of 567, 570
Visual area, primary 573
Visual association area 573
Visual axis 560*f*
Visual cortex 523, 572, 573
   areas of 523, 573
Visual defects 575*f*
Visual field 571
   divisions of 570, 571*f*
   mapping of 571
Visual impulses
   interpretation of 523
   perception of 523
Visual pathway 572, 573*f*, 574*f*
   course of 572
   different levels of 574
Visual perception 567

Visual process 567
   electrical basis of 570
   neural basis of 567
Visual receptor 572
   cells 561
   functions of 568
   structure of 567, 568*f*
Visual transduction 569
Visuopsychic area 549
Vital capacity 406, 408
Vital organs 388
Vitamin 47
   A deficiency 569
   B12 47
      deficiency 57
   D activation of 252*f*, 279
   D3 279
   metabolism 245
Vitreous body 563
Vitreous humor 563
Vitronectin 74
Voice, effect on 291
Voltage-gated channels 15, 123
Volume ventilator 442
Voluntary apnea 427
Voluntary hyperventilation 427
Voluntary movements 483, 511
   regulation of 514
Voluntary muscle 103
Vomeronasal organ 598
Vomeronasal pit 598
Vomeronasal receptors 220, 221
Vomeropherins 220, 598
Vomiting 175, 313
   act of 175
   causes of 175
   mechanism of 175
   reflex 176
Vomitus 175
von Willebrand
   disease 83
   factor 74, 76, 83

W

Waddling gait 259
Wakefulness 544
   center 506
   period of 543
Wald's visual cycle 568
Wallerian degeneration 453
Waning, causes for 431
Warm temperature 113
Warm-blooded animals 224
Waste
   air 412
   blood 399
   disposal system 6
   ventilation 412
Watch test, tickling of 593
Water
   and electrolyte balance, regulation of 221
   balance 291
      maintenance of 24*f*, 31, 182, 398
      regulation of 35, 140, 506

   diuresis 204
   facultative reabsorption of 202, 237
   hammer pulse 376
   intoxication 32
      causes for 32
      treatment of 32
   loss mechanism 398
   metabolism 269
   pills 212
   reabsorption of 198
   soluble substances 15
Watery saliva 138
Waxing, causes for 431
Weber test 594
Wernicke's area 549, 590
Westergren method 52
Westergren stand 52
Westergren tube 52, 53*f*
Wharton's duct 138
Wheel movements 565
Wheezing 432
Whispering test 593
White blood cells 23, 33, 53, 60, 60*t*, 61*f*
   classification of 60
   functions of 62
   lifespan of 62, 62*t*
   properties of 62
White buffy coat 53
White column, anterior 476
White matter 445
   divisions of 476
White muscles 112
White pulp 94
Whole blood transfusion 91
Wilson's disease 515
Wintrobe method 52
Wintrobe stand 52
Wintrobe tube 52, 53*f*
Wirsung's duct 152
Wolffian duct 290
Womb 296
World Health Organization 32
Worn-out organelles
   cytoplasmic 5
   degradation of 6

X

X chromosomes 310
X wave 377
Xerostomia 142, 143
   causes of 142

Y

Y chromosomes 310
Y wave 377
Young-Helmholtz theory 577, 580

Z

Zollinger-Ellison syndrome 151
   causes of 151
Zona vasculosa 295
Zymogen granules 147, 152

EU GSPR Authorised Reprsentative
Logos Europe, 9 rue Nicolas Poussin
1700, La Rochelle, France
Phone: +33 (0) 6 67 93 73 78
E-mail: contact@logoseurope.eu